5
EDITION

SAUNDERS
Comprehensive Review
for the
NCLEX-PN®
EXAMINATION

LINDA ANNE SILVESTRI, PhD, RN

Instructor of Nursing

Salve Regina University
Newport, Rhode Island

President

Nursing Reviews, Inc.
Professional Nursing Seminars, Inc.
Charlestown, Rhode Island

Instructor

NCLEX-RN® and NCLEX-PN® Review Courses

ELSEVIER
SAUNDERS

3251 Riverport Lane
St. Louis, Missouri 63043

SAUNDERS COMPREHENSIVE REVIEW FOR THE NCLEX-PN® EXAMINATION   ISBN: 978-1-4557-0379-1

Notices

Knowledge and best practice in this field are constantly changing. As new research and experience broaden our understanding, changes in research methods, professional practices, or medical treatment may become necessary.

Practitioners and researchers must always rely on their own experience and knowledge in evaluating and using any information, methods, compounds, or experiments described herein. In using such information or methods they should be mindful of their own safety and the safety of others, including parties for whom they have a professional responsibility.

With respect to any drug or pharmaceutical products identified, readers are advised to check the most current information provided (i) on procedures featured or (ii) by the manufacturer of each product to be administered, to verify the recommended dose or formula, the method and duration of administration, and contraindications. It is the responsibility of practitioners, relying on their own experience and knowledge of their patients, to make diagnoses, to determine dosages and the best treatment for each individual patient, and to take all appropriate safety precautions.

To the fullest extent of the law, neither the Publisher nor the authors, contributors, or editors, assume any liability for any injury and/or damage to persons or property as a matter of products liability, negligence or otherwise, or from any use or operation of any methods, products, instructions, or ideas contained in the material herein.

NCLEX® and NCLEX-PN® are registered trademarks and service marks of the National Council of State Boards of Nursing, Inc.
Nursing Diagnoses—Definitions and Classification 2012–2014. Copyright © 2012, 1994–2012 by NANDA International. Used by arrangement with Blackwell Publishing Limited, a company of John Wiley & Sons, Inc. In order to make safe and effective judgments using NANDA-I diagnoses, it is essential that nurses refer to the definitions and defining characteristics of the diagnoses listed in this work.

Library of Congress Cataloging-in-Publication Data

Silvestri, Linda Anne.
    Saunders comprehensive review for the NCLEX-PN examination / Linda Anne Silvestri. – 5th ed.
       p. ; cm.
    Comprehensive review for the NCLEX-PN examination
    Includes bibliographical references and index.
    ISBN 978-1-4557-0379-1 (alk. paper)
    I. Title. II. Title: Comprehensive review for the NCLEX-PN examination.
    [DNLM: 1. Nursing, Practical–Examination Questions. 2. Nursing Care–Examination Questions. WY 18.2]
    610.73076–dc23   2012007881

Vice President: Loren Wilson
Executive Content Strategist: Kristin Geen
Content Development Specialist: Lauren Harms Milford
Publishing Services Manager: Jeff Patterson
Senior Project Manager: Clay S. Broeker
Multimedia Producer: Jason Gonulsen
Designer: Ashley Eberts

Printed in Canada

Last digit is the print number: 9 0 7 6 5 4 3 2

To my parents:
To my mother, Frances Mary,
and in loving memory of my father, Arnold Lawrence,
who taught me to always love, care, and be the best that I can be.

About the Author

Linda Anne Silvestri

As a child, I dreamed of becoming either a nurse or teacher. Initially I chose to become a nurse because I wanted to help others, especially those who were ill. Then I realized that both of my dreams could come true: I could be a nurse and a teacher. So I pursued my dreams.

I received my diploma in nursing from Cooley Dickinson Hospital School of Nursing in Northampton, Massachusetts. Afterward, I worked at Baystate Medical Center in Springfield, Massachusetts. At Baystate Medical Center, I cared for clients in acute medical-surgical units, the intensive care unit, the emergency department, pediatric units, and other acute care units. Later, I received an associate degree from Holyoke Community College in Holyoke, Massachusetts; my BSN from American International College in Springfield, Massachusetts; and my MSN from Anna Maria College in Paxton, Massachusetts, with a dual major in Nursing Management and Patient Education. I received my

PhD in Nursing from the University of Nevada—Las Vegas, and conducted research on self-efficacy and the predictors of NCLEX success. I am also a member of the Honor Society of Nursing, Sigma Theta Tau International, Phi Kappa Phi, the American Nurses Association, the National League for Nursing, the Western Institute of Nursing, the Eastern Nursing Research Society, and the Golden Key International Honour Society.

As a native of Springfield, Massachusetts, I began my teaching career as an instructor of medical-surgical nursing and leadership-management nursing at Baystate Medical Center School of Nursing in 1981. In 1989, I relocated to Rhode Island and began teaching medical-surgical nursing and psychiatric nursing to RN and LPN students at the Community College of Rhode Island. In 1994, I began teaching nursing at Salve Regina University in Newport, Rhode Island, and remain there as an adjunct faculty member.

My experiences as a student, nursing educator, and item writer for the NCLEX examinations aided me as I developed a comprehensive review course to prepare nursing students and graduates for the NCLEX examination. In 1991, I established Professional Nursing Seminars, Inc., and in 2000, I started Nursing Reviews, Inc. Both companies are dedicated to conducting review courses for the NCLEX-RN and the NCLEX-PN examinations and assisting nursing graduates to achieve their goals of becoming registered nurses or licensed practical/vocational nurses.

Today I conduct review courses for the NCLEX examinations throughout New England and am the author of numerous successful review products. I am so pleased that you have decided to join me in your journey to success in testing for nursing examinations and for the NCLEX-PN examination!

To All Future Licensed Practical/Vocational Nurses,

Congratulations to you!

You should be very proud and pleased with yourself on your most recent well-deserved accomplishment of completing your nursing program to become a licensed practical/vocational nurse. I know that you have worked very hard to become successful and that you have proven to yourself that indeed you can achieve your goals.

In my opinion, you are about to enter the most wonderful and rewarding profession that exists. Your willingness, desire, and ability to assist those who need nursing care will bring great satisfaction to your life. In the profession of nursing, your learning will be a lifelong process. This aspect of the profession makes it stimulating and dynamic. Your learning process will continue to expand and grow as the profession continues to evolve. Your next very important endeavor will be the learning process involved to achieve success in your examination to become a licensed practical/vocational nurse.

I am excited and pleased to be able to provide you with the *Saunders Pyramid to Success* products, which will help you prepare for your next important professional goal, becoming a licensed practical/vocational nurse. I want to thank all of my former nursing students whom I have assisted in their studies for the NCLEX exam for their willingness to offer ideas regarding their needs in preparing for licensure. Student ideas have certainly added a special uniqueness to all of the products available in the *Saunders Pyramid to Success*.

Saunders Pyramid to Success products provide you with everything that you need to ready yourself for the NCLEX exam. These products include material that is required for the NCLEX exam for all nursing students regardless of educational background, specific strengths, areas in need of improvement, or clinical experience during the nursing program.

So let's get started and begin our journey through the *Saunders Pyramid to Success*, and welcome to the wonderful profession of nursing!

Sincerely,

Linda Anne Silvestri

Linda Anne Silvestri

Contributors

James Guilbault Jr., BS, PharmD(c)
Massachusetts College of Pharmacy and Health Sciences
Boston, Massachusetts

Bryan F. King, LPN
Home Care Nurse
Family Care Visiting Nurse
Waterbury, Connecticut

Nicholas L. Silvestri, BA
Nursing Reviews, Inc.
Charlestown, Rhode Island

Laurent W. Valliere, BS, DD
Vice President
Professional Nursing Seminars, Inc.
Charlestown, Rhode Island

CONTENT AND ITEM EDITORS

Mary L. Dowell, PhD, RN, BC
Assistant Professor
San Antonio College
San Antonio, Texas

Marilyn L. Johnessee Greer, MS, RN
Associate Professor of Nursing
Rockford College
Rockford, Illinois

Jennifer Ponto, RN, BSN
Vocational Nursing Program
South Plains College
Levelland, Texas

Donna Russo, RN, MSN, CCRN, CNE
Nursing Instructor
ARIA Health School of Nursing
Philadelphia, Pennsylvania

Angela E. Silvestri, MSN, RN
NCLEX Instructor
Nursing Reviews, Inc.
Charlestown, Rhode Island

Bethany Hawes Sykes, EdD RN, CEN CCRN
Adjunct Faculty
Department of Nursing
Salve Regina University
Newport, Rhode Island

Linda Turchin, RN, MSN, CNE
Assistant Professor of Nursing
Fairmont State University
Fairmont, West Virginia

ANCILLARY EDITORS

Angela E. Silvestri, MSN, RN
NCLEX Instructor
Nursing Reviews, Inc.
Charlestown, Rhode Island

The author and publisher would also like to acknowledge the following individuals for contributions to the previous editions of this book:

Alicia M. Adams, MN, RN, CEN
Roosevelt, Utah

Katrina D. Allen, RN, MSN, CCRN
Chickasaw, Alabama

Sonya S. Beacham, MSN, RN
Wilmington, North Carolina

Carol Boswell, EdD, RN
Odessa, Texas

Sharen Brady, MSN, RN
Ogden, Utah

Joyce Campbell, RN, MSN, CCRN, FNP-C
Chattanooga, Tennessee

Brenda E. Caranicas, MS, RN
New Town, North Dakota

Brigitte L. Casteel, RN, BSN
Weber City, Virginia

Faith Chumchal Darilek, RN, MSN
Victoria, Texas

Jean DeCoffe, MSN, RN
Milton, Massachusetts

Stephanie A. Dupler
Lebanon, Pennslyvania

Mary Ann Hogan, MSN, RN, CS
Amherst, Massachusetts

Mary Joanne Hovey, MSN, RN
Wilmington, North Carolina

Lisa Ivers, BSN, RN
Hamilton, Ohio

Lula Johnson, MSN, RN
Detroit, Michigan

Misty D. Johnson, LPN
North Platte, Nebraska

Mary T. Kowalski, MSN, BA, RN
Ridgecrest, California

Nancy K. Maebius, PhD, RN
San Antonio, Texas

Barbara Magenheim, EdD, MSN, BSN, RN, CNE
Chandler, Arizona

Lois S. Marshall, PhD, RN
Miami, Florida

Beverly McNeese, RN
Baton Rouge, Louisiana

Jan H. Mearkle, MSN, RN, CSNP
Summit, Mississippi

Jo Ann Barnes Mullaney, PhD, RN, CS
Newport, Rhode Island

Victoria Oxendine, RN, MSN, FNPC
Wilmington, North Carolina

Joann E. Potts Peuterbaugh, MSN, RN
Alton, Illinois

Elizabeth Pratt, BSN, RNC
Magnolia, Arkansas

Bonnie L. Shipferling, PhD(c), MSN, BSBA, RN
Pasadena, Texas

Jennifer C. Spencer, RN, BSN
Wilmington, North Carolina

Louis M. Stackler, RN, BSN, MS
Tulsa, Oklahoma

Jacquelyn Stovall, RN, BSN
San Antonio, Texas

Ruth Chandley Threlkeld, MSN, BSN
Clark, Missouri

Julie Traynor, MS, RN
Devils Lake, North Dakota

Ann Leiphart Unholz, MS, RN
Highland Springs, Virginia

Paula A. Viau, PhD, RN
Kingston, Rhode Island

Margaret Wafstet, MN, RN
Missoula, Montana

Kim Webb, RN, MN
Tonkawa, Oklahoma

Mary Louise White, MSN, RN
University Center, Michigan

Patricia H. White, BSN, RNC
Wilmington, North Carolina

Reviewers

JuTun Andrews-King, RN, MSN
Professor of Nursing
Kankakee Community College
Kankakee, Illinois

Prince Appiah-Yeboah, MSN, BSN, RN
Nursing Instructor
Stone Academy
East Hartford, Connecticut

Jacqueline Brinkman Arnett, RN, BSN, CPN
Staff Development Coordinator
Life Care Centers of America
Mountain View Care Center
Tucson, Arizona

Nancy Bohnarczyk, RN, MA
Manager
Distinguished Lecturer Program
Visiting Nurse Service of New York
New York, New York

Kathleen Bredberg, MSN, RN
Director of Vocational Nursing Program
Grayson County College
Denison, Texas

Joanna E. Cain, BSN, RN
President and Founder
Auctorial Pursuits, Inc.
Austin, Texas

Annette Marie Coates, MSN, RN, CPNP-PC, PCNS-BC
Clinical Assistant Professor of Nursing
Purdue University—North Central
Westville, Indiana

Barbara W. Collier, RN, BSN
Nursing Instructor
Putnam Career and Technical Center
Eleanor, West Virginia

Brenda A. Davis, APRN, MSN, FNP
Professor
City Colleges of Chicago—Malcolm X College
Chicago, Illinois

Belinda Douglas, MSN, PMHNP-BC, GNP-BC
Four Rivers Regional Nursing Director
Ripley, Tennessee

Theressa J. Edwards, RN, BSN
Program Coordinator
Vocational Nursing
North Central Texas College
Gainesville, Texas

Shelley Fess, MS, RN, AOCN, CRNI
Assistant Professor
Monroe Community College
Rochester, New York

Sally J. Flesch, RN, BSN, MA, EdS, PhD
Professor of Nursing
Black Hawk College
Moline, Illinois

Sharon Forrest, RN, MSN
Nursing Education
Stone Academy
East Hartford, Connecticut

Jeanne Hately, MSN, RN, PLNC
Regional Nursing Director, Research and Development
Corinthian Colleges, Inc.
Santa Ana, California

Kimberly S. Howard, RN, BS
Practical Nursing Instructor
Cattaraugus-Allegany Board of Cooperative Educational
   Services
Olean, New York

Lauralee S. Krabill, RN, C, CNOR, MBA
Director
Sandusky Career Center School of Practical Nursing
Sandusky, Ohio

Cheryl A. Lehman, PhD, RN, CNS-BC, RN-BC, CRRN
Associate Professor, Clinical
University of Texas Health Science Center at San Antonio
Nurse Educator and Researcher
Audie L. Murphy Veterans Hospital
San Antonio, Texas

Sarah J. Murray, MSN-RN, ACNS-BC, CNRN
Kailua, Hawaii

William Murray, RN, BSN, MSN, ANCC
Army Nurse Corps
Honolulu, Hawaii

Deborah J. Perkins, RN, BSN
Vocational Nursing Faculty
Galveston College
Galveston, Texas

Wendy L. Radspinner, RN, MSN
Nurse Administrator/Division Director
Institute of Technology
Salem, Oregon

Suzette D. Reyes, BSN, MSN
Madigan Army Medical Center, Practical Nurse Course
    Deputy Director
AMEDD Center and School, Madigan
Army Medical Center
Tacoma, Washington

Elaine M. Rissel-Muscarella, RN, BSN
Erie-2 Chautaqua Cattaraugus Board of Cooperative
Educational Services
Jamestown, New York

Christina M. Rutledge, RN, MN, CNE
Junior Module Coordinator
Madigan Army Medical Center
Tacoma, Washington

Bruce Austin Scott, MSN, RN
Instructor
San Joaquin Delta College
Stockton, California

Janet Sherwin, RN, MSN, BLS
Associate Professor
Joliet Junior College
Joliet, Illinois

Miranda Stover, RN, BS, MSN
Assistant Professor
Iowa Lakes Community College
Emmetsburg, Iowa

Lori Stutte, RN, MSN, CEN
Assistant Professor
Cardinal Stritch University
Milwaukee, Wisconsin

Elizabeth Timmons, RN, BSN
Coordinator for Practical Nursing Program
Cass Career Center
Harrisonville, Missouri

Pamela J. Tipton, RN, BSN
Administrator
Practical Nursing Program
Pike-Lincoln Technical Center
Pike County Memorial Hospital
Eolia, Missouri

Laura Travis, MSN, RN
Health Careers Coordinator
Tennessee Technology Center at Dickson
Dickson, Tennessee

Olma Weaver, LVN, RN
Instructor
Coastal Bend College—Beeville Campus
Beeville, Texas

Preface

Welcome to the Saunders Pyramid to Success!

This book is one in a series of products designed to assist you in achieving your goal of becoming a licensed practical/vocational nurse. Reading it will provide you with an all-inclusive review of the nursing content areas that you'll need to know for the NCLEX-PN Examination. The content is completely updated to reflect the 2011 NCLEX-PN test plan, which is implemented by the National Council of State Boards of Nursing.

ORGANIZATION OF THIS BOOK

- 20 units
- 67 chapters: content review and 825 study questions
- Evolve site containing more than 3400 **additional** questions

NEW TO THIS EDITION

- Content reflects the latest NCLEX-PN test plan.
- Now in **full color** with over 80 new **illustrations**.
- All **questions** have been updated, and more than 300 new questions have been added, including **graphic option, audio, and video** questions

- **Priority Nursing Actions boxes** outline and explain clinical emergent situations requiring immediate action
- **Pyramid Alerts** call attention to important nursing concepts tested on the NCLEX-PN exam.
- **New Chapter 29, Health and Physical Assessment of the Adult Client,** highlights the key components of physical examination and health history often encountered on the NCLEX-PN exam.
- Chapter 16, **Basic Life Support,** has been heavily updated to reflect the new **CPR** guidelines from the American Heart Association.
- Chapter 12, **Nutritional Components of Care,** has been updated to reflect **MyPlate,** the new nutrition guidelines from the U.S. Department of Agriculture.

SPECIAL FEATURES OF THIS BOOK

Pyramid Terms

Each content area (chapter or unit) begins with **Pyramid Terms** and their definitions. They are also in **purple bold** throughout the chapter or unit.

Pyramid to Success

This introduction to a content area (chapter or unit), provides you with an overview, guidance, and direction regarding the focus of review in the particular content area and its relative importance to the 2011 NCLEX-PN test plan. It also provides you with Client Needs that are most pertinent to the content in that unit or chapter.

Pyramid Points

You will see these pyramids next to specific content throughout the book, pointing out content that is especially important in preparing for the NCLEX-PN examination.

End-of-Chapter Questions

At the end of each content chapter (Chapters 6 through 67), you will find a practice test, followed by an answer section. The questions may be multiple-choice or any of the alternate item format types. Each answer includes a rationale, test-taking strategy, level of cognitive ability, client need, integrated process, and nursing content area.

Using the Companion Evolve Site

The main Web site for Evolve is evolve.elsevier.com. There is a code located inside the front cover of your book that you'll need to use to access the companion Evolve site for this book. The site contains more than 4200 questions and has three main functions:

- **Pre-test and study calendar**: To assess your strengths and weaknesses, take the 75-question pre-test. Your results will generate a customized study calendar.
- **Study:** Select questions by content area, client need, integrated process, or alternate item format type. The answer, rationale, test-taking strategy, and reference(s) appear immediately after you answer each question.
- **Exam:** Select questions by content area, client need, integrated process, or alternate item format type. Then select the number of questions you'd like to take in an exam—10, 25, 50, or 100. The percentage of questions you answered correctly will be shown in a table, and you will then have the ability to go back and review the correct answers as well as the rationales, test-taking strategies, and reference(s).

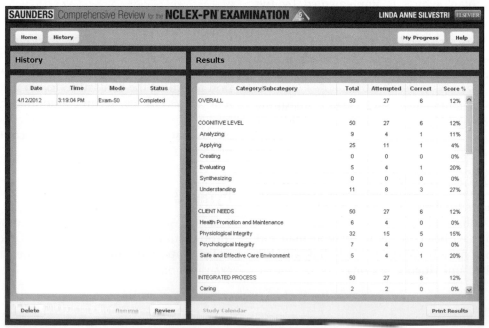

HOW TO USE THIS BOOK

Saunders Comprehensive Review for the NCLEX-PN® Examination is designed to help you with your successful journey to the peak of the *Saunders Pyramid to Success*: becoming a licensed practical/vocational nurse. As you begin your journey through this book, you will be introduced to all of the important points regarding the 2011 NCLEX-PN examination, the process of testing, and the unique and special tips on how to prepare yourself for this very important examination.

You should begin your process through the *Saunders Pyramid to Success* by reading all of Unit 1 and becoming familiar with the important points regarding the NCLEX-PN examination. Read the chapter from the nursing graduate who recently passed the examination and note what this graduate has to say about it. The test-taking strategy chapter will provide you with important strategies that will help you select the correct answer or narrow your choices when you must guess. Read this chapter and practice these strategies as you proceed through your journey with this book. Continue your journey by reading each of the chapters and content areas. Review the *Pyramid Terms* and the *Saunders Pyramid to Success* and identify the client needs specific to the test plan in that area. Read each of the content areas, focusing on the *Pyramid Points* and *Pyramid Alerts* that identify those areas most likely to be tested on the NCLEX-PN examination.

As you read each chapter, identify your strengths and those areas in need of further review. Highlight these areas and test your strengths and abilities by taking all of the practice tests provided at the end of the chapters. Be sure to read all of the rationales and the test-taking strategies. The rationale provides you with the significant information regarding both the correct and incorrect options. The test-taking strategy offers you the logical path to selecting the correct option. The strategy also identifies the content area that you need to review if you had difficulty with the question. Use the reference(s) listed so you can easily find the information that you need to review.

After you review all of the chapters in the book, turn to Unit 20, the Comprehensive Test. Take this test and then go over each question, answer, and rationale. Identify any areas requiring further review and then take the time to read through those areas again. After reviewing the book and taking the Comprehensive Test, proceed to the Evolve site and take the 75-question assessment pre-test. The results will provide you with feedback on your strengths and weaknesses and will generate a study calendar to guide you in your continued preparation for the NCLEX-PN.

After using this book to review specific content areas, continue on your journey through the *Saunders Pyramid to Success* with the companion book, *Saunders Q&A Review for the NCLEX-PN® Examination*, for additional practice questions. The companion book and its accompanying software offer you more than 3000 practice questions on specific areas outlined by the NCLEX-PN test plan. With practice questions uniquely focused on the client needs and the integrated processes, you can assess your level of competence.

Additional components of the *Saunders Pyramid to Success* are *Saunders Review Cards for the NCLEX-PN® Examination* and *Saunders Strategies for Success for the NCLEX-PN® Examination*. *Saunders Review Cards for the NCLEX-PN® Examination* provides you with more than 900 practice test questions, including multiple-choice questions and the new alternate item format questions such as fill-in-the-blank, multiple response, prioritizing (ordered response), and figure/illustration (hot spot) questions. The practice question is located on one side of the review card. The reverse side of the review card contains the correct answer, rationale, and question categories for the practice question on the front of the card. *Saunders Strategies for Test Success: Passing Nursing School and the NCLEX Exam* and its accompanying CD provide all of the test-taking strategies that will help you pass your nursing examinations and the NCLEX-PN. The chapters describe these test-taking strategies, include several sample questions that illustrate how to use the strategy, and provide an additional 500 practice questions, including multiple-choice and alternate item formats.

Good luck with your journey through the *Saunders Pyramid to Success*. I wish you continued success throughout your new career as a licensed practical/vocational nurse!

Acknowledgments

Sincere appreciation and warmest thanks are extended to the many individuals who in their own way have contributed to the publication of this book.

First, I want to thank all of my nursing students at the Community College of Rhode Island in Warwick who approached me in 1991 and persuaded me to help them prepare to take the NCLEX examination. Their enthusiasm and inspiration led to the commencement of my professional endeavors in conducting NCLEX review courses for nursing students. I also thank the numerous nursing students who have attended my review courses for their willingness to share their needs and ideas. Their input has certainly added a special uniqueness to this publication.

I wish to acknowledge all of the nursing faculty who taught in my NCLEX review courses. Their commitment, dedication, and expertise have certainly assisted nursing students in achieving success with the NCLEX examination. Additionally, a special acknowledgment goes to three very important people. A thank you to Laurent W. Valliere, or Larry, for his contribution to this publication, for teaching in my NCLEX review courses, and for his commitment and dedication in helping my nursing students prepare for the NCLEX examination from a non-academic point of view. I also thank Angela E. Silvestri for teaching in my review courses and for her tremendous assistance in preparing and editing the chapters and practice questions in this book. Her commitment and dedication has added to the excellent quality of this book. And I thank Dianne E. Fiorentino for researching and providing reference support for all of the practice questions in this book.

A special thank you and acknowledgment also goes to Nicholas L. Silvestri, who assisted me with many of the editing tasks needed to submit manuscript. I also thank James Guilbault Jr. for his assistance in researching medications for this book.

I sincerely acknowledge and thank some very special individuals from Elsevier. I thank Loren Wilson, Vice President, for her continuous and outstanding support as I prepared all of my NCLEX review products. I also thank Kristin Geen, Executive Content Strategist, for all of her assistance throughout the preparation of this edition and for her continuous enthusiasm, support, and expert professional guidance. And I thank Lauren Harms Milford, Content Development Specialist. Lauren, thank you so much for everything: your very creative ideas, your outstanding organizational skills, and your much-needed weekly priority lists. I also thank you for maintaining order for my several products and keeping track of all of the manuscript that I submitted. I could not have done this without you!

I want to acknowledge all of the staff in marketing. I also want to thank the very special people in the production department who were committed and dedicated to maintaining the excellent quality of this product. A special thank you goes to Jeff Patterson, Publishing Services Manager; Clay Broeker, Senior Project Manager; Jason Gonulsen, Multimedia Producer; and Ashley Eberts, Designer.

I would also like to acknowledge Patricia Mieg, former educational sales representative, who encouraged me to submit my ideas and initial work for the first edition of this book to the W.B. Saunders Company.

I want to acknowledge my parents, who opened my door of opportunity in education. I thank my mother, Frances Mary, for all of her love, support, and assistance as I continuously worked to achieve my professional goals. I thank my father, Arnold Lawrence, who always provided insightful words of encouragement. My memories of his love and support will always remain in my heart.

I also thank my sister, Dianne Elodia; my brother, Lawrence Peter; my nieces and nephews, Gina Marie, Angela, Katie, Karen, and Nicholas; and my husband, Larry, all of whom were continuously supportive, giving, and helpful during my research and preparation of this publication.

I want to acknowledge all of the contributors and reviewers of this publication for their thoughts and ideas. And a special thank you goes to Bryan F. King, LPN, a graduate from Stone Academy in Connecticut, for providing a chapter to this publication regarding his experiences with the NCLEX-PN examination.

I also need to thank Salve Regina University for the opportunity to educate nursing students in the baccalaureate nursing program and for its support during my research and writing of this publication. I would like to especially thank my colleagues Dr. Eileen Gray, Dr. Peggy Matteson, Dr. JoAnn Mullaney, Dr. Ellen McCarty, and Dr. Bethany Sykes for all of their support and encouragement.

I wish to acknowledge the Community College of Rhode Island, which provided me with the opportunity to educate nursing students in the Associate Degree of Nursing Program, and a special thank you goes to Patricia Miller, MSN, RN, and Michelina McClellan, MS, RN, from Baystate Medical Center, School of Nursing, in Springfield, Massachusetts, who were my first mentors in nursing education.

Lastly, a very special thank you to all of my nursing students—past, present, and future. Your love for and dedication to the profession of nursing and your commitment to provide health care will bring never-ending rewards!

Linda Anne Silvestri

Contents

NCLEX-PN® Exam Preparation

The NCLEX-PN® Examination

THE PYRAMID TO SUCCESS

Welcome to the Pyramid to Success

Saunders Comprehensive Review for the NCLEX-PN® Examination is specially designed to help you begin your successful journey to the peak of the pyramid, becoming a licensed practical/vocational nurse. As you begin your journey, you will be introduced to all the important points regarding the NCLEX-PN examination and the process of testing, and to the unique and special tips regarding how to prepare yourself for this important examination. You will read what a nursing graduate who recently passed the NCLEX-PN examination has to say about the test. Important test-taking strategies are detailed. These details will guide you in selecting the correct option or assist you in selecting an answer to a question at which you must guess.

Each of the content areas in this book begins with the Pyramid to Success. The Pyramid to Success addresses specific points related to the NCLEX-PN examination, including the Pyramid Terms and the Client Needs as identified in the test plan framework for the examination. Pyramid Terms are key words that are defined and are set in **bold purple** throughout each chapter to direct your attention to significant points for the examination. The Client Needs specific to the content of the chapter are identified.

Throughout each chapter, you will find Pyramid Point bullets that identify areas most likely to be tested on the NCLEX-PN examination. Read each chapter, and identify your strengths and areas that are in need of further review. Test your strengths and abilities by taking all the practice tests provided in this book and on the accompanying Evolve site. Be sure to read all the rationales and test-taking strategies. The rationale provides you with significant information regarding the correct and incorrect options. The test-taking strategy provides you with the logical path to selecting the correct option. The test-taking strategy also identifies the content area to review, if required. The reference source and page number are provided so that you can easily find the information that you need to review. Each question is coded with the Level of Cognitive Ability, the Client Needs category, the Integrated Process, and the nursing Content Area.

Following the completion of your comprehensive review in this book, continue on your journey through the Pyramid to Success with the companion book, *Saunders Q&A Review for the NCLEX-PN® Examination*, which provides you with more than 3200 practice questions based on the NCLEX-PN examination test plan framework, with a specific focus on Client Needs and Integrated Processes. Additional products in Saunders Pyramid to Success include *Saunders Strategies for Test Success: Passing Nursing School and the NCLEX® Exam*. This focuses on the test-taking strategies that will help you pass your nursing examinations while in nursing school and will prepare you for the NCLEX examination. The chapters describe various test-taking strategies and include sample questions that illustrate how to use the strategies; 1000 practice questions accompany this resource. Also included is a summary chart of the test-taking strategies, and information about cultural characteristics and practices, pharmacology strategies, medication and intravenous calculations, laboratory values, positioning guidelines, and therapeutic diets. Additional products include the *HESI/Saunders Online Review for the NCLEX-PN® Examination* and the *Saunders Q&A Review Cards for the NCLEX-PN® Examination*.

All the products in Saunders Pyramid to Success can be obtained online by visiting elsevierhealth.com or by calling 800-545-2522.

Let's begin our journey through the Pyramid to Success.

EXAMINATION PROCESS

An important step in the Pyramid to Success is to become as familiar as possible with the examination process. Candidates facing the challenge of this examination can experience significant anxiety. Knowing what the examination is all about and knowing what you will encounter during the process of testing will assist in alleviating fear and anxiety. The information contained in this chapter addresses the procedures related to the development of the NCLEX-PN examination test plan, the components of the test plan, and the answers to the questions most commonly asked by nursing students and graduates preparing to take the NCLEX-PN examination. The information contained in this chapter related to the test plan was obtained from the NCSBN Web site (http://www.ncsbn.org) and from the NCSBN test plan for the NCLEX-PN Examination (effective April 2014). You can obtain additional information regarding the test and its development by accessing the NCSBN Web site or by writing to the National Council of State Boards of Nursing, 111 East Wacker Drive, Suite 2900, Chicago, IL 60601. You are encouraged to access the NCSBN Web site because this site provides you with valuable information about the NCLEX and other resources available to an NCLEX candidate.

COMPUTER ADAPTIVE TESTING (CAT)

The acronym *CAT* stands for computer adaptive test, which means that the examination is created as the test-taker answers each question. All the test questions are categorized based on the test plan structure and the level of difficulty of the question. As you answer a question, the computer determines your competency based on the answer you selected. If you selected a correct answer to a question, the computer scans the question bank and selects a more difficult question. If you selected an incorrect answer, the computer scans the question bank and selects an easier question. This process continues until the test plan requirements are met and a reliable pass-or-fail decision is made.

When a test question is presented on the computer screen, you must answer it or the test will not move on. This means that you will not be able to skip questions, go back and review questions, or go back and change answers. In a CAT examination, once an answer is recorded, all subsequent questions administered depend, to an extent, on the answer selected for that question. Skipping and returning to earlier questions are not compatible with the logical methodology of a CAT. The inability to skip questions or go back to change previous answers will not be a disadvantage to you; you will not fall into that "trap" of changing a correct answer to an incorrect one with the CAT system.

If you are faced with a question that contains unfamiliar content, you may need to guess at the answer. There is no penalty for guessing on this examination. With most of the questions, the answer will be right there in front of you. If you need to guess, use your nursing knowledge and clinical experiences to their fullest extent and all the test-taking strategies that you have practiced in this review program.

You do not need any computer experience to take this examination. A keyboard tutorial is provided and administered to all test-takers at the start of the examination. The tutorial will instruct you on the use of the on-screen optional calculator, the use of the mouse, and how to record an answer. In addition to the traditional four-option, multiple-choice question, the tutorial provides instructions on how to respond to alternate item format questions. This tutorial is provided on the NCSBN Web site, and you are encouraged to view the tutorial when you are preparing for the NCLEX examination. Additionally, at the testing site, a proctor is present to assist in explaining the use of the computer to ensure your full understanding of how to proceed.

DEVELOPMENT OF THE TEST PLAN

The test plan for the NCLEX-PN examination is developed by the NCSBN. The NCLEX examination is a national examination; the NCSBN considers the legal scope of nursing practice as governed by state laws and regulations, including the nurse practice act, and uses these laws to define the areas on the examination that will assess the competence of the test-taker for licensure.

The NCSBN also conducts an important study every 3 years, known as a practice analysis study, to determine the framework for the test plan for the examination. The participants in this study include newly licensed practical or vocational nurses. From a list provided, the participants select the nursing activities that they perform, the frequency of performing these specific activities, the impact of the activities on maintaining client safety, and the setting where the activities were performed. A panel of content experts at the NCSBN analyzes the results of the study and makes decisions regarding the test plan framework. The results of this most recently conducted study provided the structure for the test plan implemented in April 2014.

TEST PLAN

The content of the NCLEX-PN examination reflects the activities identified in the practice analysis study conducted by the NCSBN. The questions are written to address Level of Cognitive Ability, Client Needs, and Integrated Processes as identified in the test plan developed by the NCSBN (Box 1-1).

Level of Cognitive Ability

Most questions on the NCLEX examination are written at the application level or higher levels of cognitive ability. Box 1-2 presents an example of a question that requires you to apply data.

Box 1-1 Examination Questions

Each examination question addresses the following:
- A Level of Cognitive Ability
- A Client Needs category
- An Integrated Process

Client Needs

In the test plan implemented in April 2014, the NCSBN has identified a test plan framework based on Client Needs. The NCSBN identifies four major categories of Client Needs. Some of these categories are divided further into subcategories. The Client Needs categories include Safe and Effective Care Environment, Health Promotion and Maintenance, Psychosocial Integrity, and Physiological Integrity (Table 1-1).

Safe and Effective Care Environment

The Safe and Effective Care Environment category includes two subcategories, Coordinated Care and Safety and Infection Control. According to the NCSBN, Coordinated Care addresses content that tests the nurse's knowledge, skills, and ability required to collaborate with health care members to facilitate effective client care. The NCSBN indicates that Safety and Infection Control addresses content that tests the nurse's knowledge, skills, and ability required

---

Box 1-2 Level of Cognitive Ability: Applying

The nurse notes blanching, coolness, and edema at the peripheral intravenous (IV) site. Based on these findings, the nurse should implement which most appropriate action?
1. Remove the IV
2. Apply a warm compress
3. Check for a blood return
4. Measure the area of infiltration

Answer: 1

This question requires that you focus on the data identified in the question and determine that the client is experiencing an infiltration. Next you need to consider the harmful effects of infiltration and determine the action to implement. Because infiltration can be damaging to the surrounding tissue, the most appropriate action is to remove the IV to prevent any further damage.

TABLE 1-1 Client Needs Categories and Percentage of Questions on the NCLEX-PN® Examination

Client Needs Category	Percentage of Questions
SAFE AND EFFECTIVE CARE ENVIRONMENT	
Coordinated Care	16-22
Safety and Infection Control	10-16
HEALTH PROMOTION AND MAINTENANCE	7-13
PSYCHOSOCIAL INTEGRITY	8-14
PHYSIOLOGICAL INTEGRITY	
Basic Care and Comfort	7-13
Pharmacological Therapies	11-17
Reduction of Risk Potential	10-16
Physiological Adaptation	7-13

Data from National Council of State Boards of Nursing. (2013). *2014 NCLEX-PN test plan.* Chicago.

---

to protect clients, families, significant others, visitors, and health care personnel from health and environmental hazards. Box 1-3 presents examples of questions that address these two subcategories.

Health Promotion and Maintenance

The Health Promotion and Maintenance category addresses the principles related to growth and development. According to the NCSBN, this Client Needs category also addresses content that tests the nurse's

---

Box 1-3 Safe and Effective Care Environment

Coordinated Care

The nurse has received the client assignment for the day. Which client should the nurse attend to first?
1. The client who has a nasogastric tube attached to intermittent suction
2. The client who needs to receive subcutaneous insulin before breakfast
3. The client who is 2 days postoperative and is complaining of incisional pain
4. The client who has a blood glucose level of 50 mg/dL and complains of blurred vision

Answer: 4

This question addresses the subcategory, Coordinated Care, in the Client Needs category, Safe and Effective Care Environment. It requires you to establish priorities by comparing the needs of each client and deciding which need is urgent. The client described in option 4 has a low blood glucose level and symptoms reflective of hypoglycemia. This client should be attended to first so that treatment can be implemented. Although the clients in options 1, 2, and 3 have needs that require attention, they are not the priority and can wait until the client in option 4 is stabilized.

Safety and Infection Control

The nurse prepares to care for a client on contact precautions who has a hospital-acquired infection caused by methicillin-resistant *Staphylococcus aureus* (MRSA). The client has an abdominal wound that requires irrigation and has a tracheostomy attached to a mechanical ventilator, which requires frequent suctioning. The nurse should assemble which necessary protective items before entering the client's room?
1. Gloves and a gown
2. Gloves, mask, and goggles
3. Gloves, mask, gown, and goggles
4. Gloves, gown, and shoe protectors

Answer: 3

This question addresses the subcategory, Safety and Infection Control, in the Client Needs category, Safe and Effective Care Environment. It addresses content related to protecting oneself from contracting an infection and requires that you consider the methods of possible transmission of infection, based on the client's condition. Because splashes of infective material can occur during the wound irrigation or suctioning of the tracheostomy, option 3 is correct.

knowledge, skills, and ability required to assist the client, family members, and significant others to prevent health problems; to recognize alterations in health; and to develop health practices that promote and support wellness. See Box 1-4 for an example of a question in this Client Needs category.

Psychosocial Integrity

The Psychosocial Integrity category addresses content that tests the nurse's knowledge, skills, and ability required to promote and support the ability of the client, client's family, and client's significant other to cope, adapt, and problem solve during stressful events. The NCSBN also indicates that this Client Needs category addresses the emotional, mental, and social well-being of the client, family, or significant other, and the knowledge, skills, and ability required to care for the client with an acute or chronic mental illness. See Box 1-5 for an example of a question in this Client Needs category.

Physiological Integrity

The Physiological Integrity category includes four subcategories, described by the NCSBN as follows.
- Basic Care and Comfort: Addresses content that tests the nurse's knowledge, skills, and ability required to provide comfort and assistance to the client in the performance of activities of daily living.
- Pharmacological Therapies: Addresses content that tests the nurse's knowledge, skills, and ability required to administer medications and parenteral therapies including dosage calculations and pharmacological pain management.
- Reduction of Risk Potential: Addresses content that tests the nurse's knowledge, skills, and ability

required to prevent complications or health problems related to the client's condition or any prescribed treatments or procedures.
- Physiological Adaptation: Addresses content that tests the nurse's knowledge, skills, and ability required to provide care to clients with acute, chronic, or life-threatening conditions.

See Box 1-6 for examples of questions in this Client Needs category.

Integrated Processes

The NCSBN identifies four processes that are fundamental to the practice of nursing. These processes are a component of the test plan and are incorporated throughout the major categories of Client Needs. The Integrated Process subcategories include:
- Caring
- Communication and Documentation
- Nursing Process (Clinical Problem-Solving Process)
  - Data Collection
  - Planning
  - Implementation
  - Evaluation
- Teaching and Learning

See Box 1-7 for an example of a question that incorporates the Integrated Process of caring.

TYPES OF QUESTIONS ON THE EXAMINATION

The types of questions that may be administered on the examination include:
- Multiple-choice
- Fill-in-the-blank

Box 1-4 Health Promotion and Maintenance

The nurse is choosing age-appropriate toys for a toddler. Which toy is the best choice for this age?
1. Puzzle
2. Toy soldiers
3. Large stacking blocks
4. A card game with large pictures

Answer: 3

This question addresses the Client Needs category, Health Promotion and Maintenance, and specifically relates to the principles of growth and development of a toddler. Toddlers like to master activities independently, such as stacking blocks. Because toddlers do not have the developmental ability to determine what could be harmful, toys that are safe need to be provided. A puzzle and toy soldiers provide objects that can be placed in the mouth and may be harmful for a toddler. A card game with large pictures may require cooperative play, which is more appropriate for a school-age child.

Box 1-5 Psychosocial Integrity

A client with coronary artery disease has selected guided imagery to help cope with psychological stress. Which client statement indicates an understanding of this stress reduction measure?
1. "This will help only if I play music at the same time."
2. "This will work for me only if I am alone in a quiet area."
3. "I need to do this only when I lie down in case I fall asleep."
4. "The best thing about this is that I can use it anywhere, anytime."

Answer: 4

This question addresses the Client Needs category, Psychosocial Integrity, and the content addresses coping mechanisms. Guided imagery involves the client's creation of an image in the mind, concentrating on the image, and gradually becoming less aware of the offending stimulus. It can be done anytime and anywhere; some clients may use other relaxation techniques or play music with it.

Box 1-6 Physiological Integrity

Basic Care and Comfort

A client with Parkinson's disease develops akinesia while ambulating, increasing the risk for falls. Which suggestion should the nurse provide to the client to alleviate this problem?

1. Use a wheelchair to move around.
2. Stand erect and use a cane to ambulate.
3. Keep the feet close together while ambulating and use a walker.
4. Consciously think about walking over imaginary lines on the floor.

Answer: 4

This question addresses the subcategory, Basic Care and Comfort, in the Client Needs category, Physiological Integrity, and addresses client mobility and promoting assistance in an activity of daily living to maintain safety. Clients with Parkinson's disease can develop bradykinesia (slow movement) or akinesia (freezing or no movement). Having these clients imagine lines on the floor to step over can keep them moving forward while remaining safe.

Pharmacological Therapies

The nurse should monitor a client receiving digoxin (Lanoxin) for which early manifestation of digoxin toxicity?

1. Anorexia
2. Facial pain
3. Photophobia
4. Yellow color perception

Answer: 1

This question addresses the subcategory, Pharmacological and Parenteral Therapies, in the Client Needs category, Physiological Integrity. Digoxin is a cardiac glycoside that is used to manage and treat heart failure and to control ventricular rates in clients with atrial fibrillation. The most common early manifestations of toxicity include gastrointestinal disturbances such as anorexia, nausea, and vomiting. Facial pain, personality changes, and ocular disturbances (photophobia, light flashes, halos around bright objects, yellow or green color perception) are also signs of toxicity, but are not early signs.

Reduction of Risk Potential

A magnetic resonance imaging (MRI) study is prescribed for a client with a suspected liver tumor. The nurse should implement which action to prepare the client for this test?

1. Keeps the client NPO for 6 hours before the test
2. Shaves the groin for insertion of a femoral catheter
3. Removes all metal-containing objects from the client
4. Instructs the client in breathing and inhalation techniques

Answer: 3

This question addresses the subcategory, Reduction of Risk Potential, in the Client Needs category, Physiological Integrity, and the nurse's responsibilities in preparing the client for the diagnostic test. In an MRI study, radiofrequency pulses in a magnetic field are converted into pictures. All metal objects, such as rings, bracelets, hairpins, and watches, should be removed. In addition, a history should be taken to ascertain whether the client has any internal metallic devices, such as orthopedic hardware, pacemakers, or shrapnel. NPO status is not necessary for an MRI study of the liver. The groin may be shaved for an angiogram, and inhalation techniques may be necessary for a ventilation/perfusion lung scan.

Physiological Adaptation

A client with renal insufficiency has a magnesium level of 3.6 mg/dL. Based on this laboratory result, the nurse should recognize which finding as significant?

1. Hyperpnea
2. Drowsiness
3. Hypertension
4. Physical hyperactivity

Answer: 2

This question addresses the subcategory, Physiological Adaptation, in the Client Needs category, Physiological Integrity. It addresses an alteration in body systems. The normal magnesium level is 1.6 to 2.6 mg/dL. A magnesium level of 3.6 mg/dL indicates hypermagnesemia. Neurological manifestations begin to occur when magnesium levels are elevated and are noted as neurological depression, such as drowsiness, sedation, lethargy, respiratory depression, muscle weakness, and areflexia. Bradycardia and hypotension also occur.

Box 1-7 Integrated Processes

A client is scheduled for angioplasty. The client says to the nurse, "I'm so afraid that it will hurt and will make me worse off than I am." Which response by the nurse is therapeutic?

1. "Can you tell me what you understand about the procedure?"
2. "Your fears are a sign that you really should have this procedure."
3. "Try not to worry. This is a well-known and easy procedure for the doctor."
4. "Those are very normal fears, but please be assured that everything will be okay."

Answer: 1

This question addresses the subcategory, Caring, in the category, Integrated Processes. Option 1 is a therapeutic communication technique that explores the client's feelings, determines the level of client understanding about the procedure, and displays caring. Option 2 demeans the client and does not encourage further sharing by the client. Option 3 diminishes the client's feelings by directing attention away from the client and to the health care provider's importance. Option 4 does not address the client's fears and puts the client's feelings on hold.

- Multiple-response
- Ordered response
- Figure
- Chart/exhibit
- Graphic option
- Audio
- Video

Some questions may require you to use the mouse and cursor on the computer. For example, you may be presented with a picture that displays the arterial vessels of an adult client. In this picture, you may be asked to "point and click" (using the mouse) on the area (hot spot) where the dorsalis pedis pulse could be felt. In all types of questions, the answer is scored as either right or wrong. Credit is not given for a partially correct answer. Additionally, all question types may include pictures, graphics, tables, charts, sound, or video. The NCSBN provides specific directions for you to follow with all question types to guide you in your process of testing. Be sure to read these directions as they appear on the computer screen. Examples of some of these types of questions are noted in this chapter. All question types are provided in this book and the accompanying Evolve site.

Multiple-Choice Questions

Most of the questions that you will be asked to answer will be in the multiple-choice format. These questions provide you with data about a client situation and four answers or options.

Fill-in-the-Blank Questions

Fill-in-the-blank questions may ask you to perform a medication calculation, determine an intravenous flow rate, or calculate an intake or output record on a client. You will need to type only a number (your answer) in the answer box. If the question requires rounding the answer, this needs to be performed at the end of the calculation. The rules for rounding an answer are provided in the tutorial provided by the NCSBN, and are also provided in the specific question. Additionally, you must type in a decimal point if necessary; however, it is not necessary to type a "0" before the decimal point. See Box 1-8 for an example.

Multiple-Response Questions

For a multiple-response question, you will be asked to select or check all the options, such as nursing interventions, that relate to the information in the question. No partial credit is given for correct selections. You need to do exactly as the question asks, which will be to select all the options that apply. See Box 1-9 for an example.

Box 1-8 Fill-in-the-Blank Question

A prescription reads: acetaminophen (Tylenol Extra Strength) liquid, 650 mg orally every 4 hours PRN for pain. The medication label reads: 500 mg/15 mL. The nurse prepares how many milliliters to administer one dose? **Fill in the blank.**

Answer: $\boxed{19.5}$ mL

Formula:

$$\frac{\text{Desired}}{\text{Available}} \times \text{Volume} = \text{mL}$$

$$\frac{650 \text{ mg}}{500 \text{ mg}} \times 15 \text{ mL} = 19.5 \text{ mL}$$

In this question, you need to use the formula for calculating a medication dose. When the dose is determined, you will need to type your numeric answer in the answer box. Always follow the specific directions noted on the computer screen when answering the question. Also, remember that there will be an on-screen calculator on the computer for your use.

Box 1-9 Multiple-Response Question

The emergency department nurse is caring for a child suspected of acute epiglottitis. Which interventions apply in the care of the child? **Select all that apply.**
- ☐ **1.** Obtain a throat culture.
- ☒ **2.** Ensure a patent airway.
- ☒ **3.** Prepare the child for a chest x-ray.
- ☐ **4.** Maintain the child in a supine position.
- ☒ **5.** Obtain a pediatric-size tracheostomy tray.
- ☒ **6.** Place the child on an oxygen saturation monitor.

In a multiple-response question, you will be asked to select or check all the options, such as interventions, that relate to the information in the question. To answer this question, recall that acute epiglottitis is a serious obstructive inflammatory process that requires immediate intervention. To reduce respiratory distress, the child should sit upright. Examination of the throat with a tongue depressor or attempting to obtain a throat culture is contraindicated because the examination can precipitate further obstruction. The child is placed on an oxygen saturation monitor to monitor oxygenation status. A lateral neck and chest x-ray is obtained to determine the degree of obstruction, if present. Tracheostomy and intubation may be necessary if respiratory distress is severe. Remember to follow the specific directions given on the computer screen.

Ordered Response

In this type of question, you will be asked to use the computer mouse to drag and drop your nursing actions in order of priority. Information will be presented in a question, and based on the data you need to determine what you will do first, second, third, and so forth. The unordered options will be located in boxes on the left side of the screen, and you need to move all options in order of priority to ordered response boxes on the right side of the screen. Specific directions for moving the options are provided with the question. See Box 1-10 for an example.

Figure Questions

A question with a picture or graphic will ask you to answer the question based on the picture or graphic. The question could contain a chart, a table, or a figure or illustration. You also may be asked to use the computer mouse to point and click on a specific area in the visual. A figure or illustration may appear in any type of question, including a multiple-choice question. See Box 1-11 for an example.

Chart/Exhibit Questions

In this type of question, you will be presented with a problem and a chart or exhibit. You will be provided with tabs or buttons that you need to click to obtain the information needed to answer the question. A prompt or message may appear that may indicate the need to click on a tab or button. See Box 1-12 for an example.

Graphic Option Questions

In this type of question, the option selections will be pictures rather than text. Each option will be preceded by a circle, and you will need to use the computer mouse to click in the circle that represents your answer choice. See Box 1-13 for an example.

Audio Questions

Audio questions will require listening to a sound to answer the question. These questions will prompt you to use the headset provided and click on the sound icon. You will be able to click on the volume button to adjust the volume to your comfort level, and you will be able to listen to the sound as many times as necessary. Content examples include, but are not limited to, various lung sounds, heart sounds, or bowel sounds. Examples of these question types are located on the accompanying Evolve site.

Video Questions

Video questions will require viewing an animation or video clip to answer the question. These questions will prompt you to click on the video icon. There may be sound associated with the animation and video, in which you will be prompted to use the headset. Content examples include, but are not limited to, data collection techniques, nursing procedures, or communication skills. Examples of these question types are located on the accompanying Evolve site.

REGISTERING TO TAKE THE EXAMINATION

It is important to obtain an NCLEX examination candidate bulletin from the NCSBN Web site at www.ncsbn. org because this bulletin provides all the information that you need to register for and schedule your

---

Box 1-10 Ordered Response Question

A nurse is preparing to suction a client who has a tracheostomy tube and gathers the supplies needed for the procedure. What is the order of priority of the actions that the nurse takes to perform this procedure? All options must be used.

Unordered Options	Ordered Response
Hyperoxygenate the client.	Place the client in a semi-Fowler's position.
Place the client in a semi-Fowler's position.	Turn on the suction device and set the regulator at 80 mm Hg.
Turn on the suction device and set the regulator at 80 mm Hg.	Apply gloves and attach the suction tubing to the suction catheter.
Apply gloves and attach the suction tubing to the suction catheter.	Hyperoxygenate the client.
Apply intermittent suction and slowly withdraw the catheter while rotating it back and forth.	Insert the catheter into the tracheostomy until resistance is met and then pull back 1 cm.
Insert the catheter into the tracheostomy until resistance is met and then pull back 1 cm.	Apply intermittent suction and slowly withdraw the catheter while rotating it back and forth.

   This question requires you to arrange in order of priority the nursing actions that should be taken to suction a client who has a tracheostomy tube. The nurse positions the client first, and then turns the suction device on and sets the regulator. The nurse then dons gloves and attaches the suction tubing to the suction catheter. The nurse hyperoxygenates the client before and after suctioning. The nurse then inserts the catheter into the tracheostomy until resistance is met and pulls back 1 cm, applies intermittent suction, and slowly withdraws the catheter while rotating it back and forth. Remember that the client and equipment are prepared before performing the procedure. Also, remember that on the NCLEX examination, you will use the computer mouse to place the unordered options in an ordered response.

examination. It also provides you with Web site and telephone information for NCLEX examination contacts. The initial step in the registration process is to submit an application to the state board of nursing in the state in which you intend to obtain licensure. You need to

obtain information from the board of nursing regarding the specific registration process because the process may vary from state to state. When you receive confirmation from the board of nursing that you have met all of the state requirements, you can register to take the NCLEX

Box 1-11 Figure Question

Rhythm strip. (From Ignatavicius, D., & Workman, M. [2013]. *Medical-surgical nursing: Patient-centered collaborative care* [7th ed.]. St. Louis: Saunders.)

A client who experienced a myocardial infarction is being monitored via cardiac telemetry. The nurse notes the sudden onset of this cardiac rhythm on the monitor and should plan to take which immediate action?
1. Take the client's blood pressure
2. Initiate cardiopulmonary resuscitation (CPR)
3. Place a nitroglycerin tablet under the client's tongue
4. Continue to monitor the client for 5 minutes and then contact the registered nurse (RN)

Answer: 2
This question requires you to identify the cardiac rhythm, and then determine the immediate nursing action. This cardiac rhythm identifies a coarse ventricular fibrillation (VF). The goals of treatment are to terminate VF promptly and convert it to an organized rhythm. The health care provider or an advanced cardiac life support (ACLS)–qualified nurse or other HCP must immediately defibrillate the client. If a defibrillator is not readily available, CPR is initiated until the defibrillator arrives. Options 1, 3, and 4 are incorrect actions and delay life-saving treatment.

Box 1-12 Chart/Exhibit Question

The nurse reviews the history and physical examination documented in the medical record of a client requesting a prescription for oral contraceptives. The nurse determines that oral contraceptives are contraindicated because of which documented item?

CLIENT'S CHART		
History and Physical	**Medications**	**Diagnostic Results**
Item 1: Has renal calculi Item 2: Had thrombophlebitis 1 year ago	Item 3: Multivitamin orally daily	Item 4: Electrocardiogram: normal

Answer: 2
This chart/exhibit question provides you with data from the client's medical record and asks you to identify the item that is a contraindication to the use of oral contraceptives. Oral contraceptives are contraindicated in women with a history of any of the following: thrombophlebitis and thromboembolic disorders, cardiovascular or cerebrovascular diseases (including stroke), any estrogen-dependent cancer or breast cancer, benign or malignant liver tumors, impaired liver function, hypertension, and diabetes mellitus with vascular involvement. Adverse effects of oral contraceptives include increased risk of superficial and deep vein thrombosis, pulmonary embolism, thrombotic stroke (or other types of strokes), myocardial infarction, and accelerations of pre-existing breast tumors.

Box 1-13 Graphic Option Question

The nurse should place the client in which position to administer a soapsuds enema?

1.

2.

3.

4.

Figures from Potter, P., & Perry, A. (2013). *Fundamentals of nursing* (8th ed.). St. Louis: Mosby.

Answer: 2
This question requires you to select the picture that represents your answer choice. To administer an enema, the nurse assists the client into the left side-lying (Sims) position with the right knee flexed. This position allows the enema solution to flow downward by gravity along the natural curve of the sigmoid colon and rectum, improving the retention of solution. Option 1 is a prone position. Option 3 is a dorsal recumbent position. Option 4 is a supine position.

examination with Pearson Vue. You may register for the examination through the Internet or by telephone. The NCLEX candidate Web site is http://www.pearsonvue. com/nclex.

Following the registration instructions and completing the registration forms precisely and accurately are important. Registration forms not properly completed or not accompanied by the proper fees in the required method of payment will be returned to you and will delay testing. You must pay a fee for taking the examination; you also may have to pay additional fees to the board of nursing in the state in which you are applying. You will then be made eligible by the licensure board and will receive an Authorization to Test (ATT) form via email. If you do not receive an ATT form within two weeks of registration, you should contact the candidate services at 1-866-496-2539 (U.S. candidates).

AUTHORIZATION TO TEST FORM AND SCHEDULING AN APPOINTMENT

You cannot make an appointment until the board of nursing declares eligibility and you receive an ATT form.

Note the validity dates on the ATT form, and schedule a date and time when you receive the ATT. The examination will take place at a Pearson Professional Center; U.S. candidates can make an appointment through the Internet (http://www.pearsonvue.com/nclex) or by telephone (1-866-496-2539). You can schedule an appointment at any Pearson Professional Center. You do not have to take the examination in the same state in which you are seeking licensure. A confirmation of your appointment with the appointment date and time and the directions to the testing center will be sent to you.

CHANGING YOUR APPOINTMENT

If for any reason you need to cancel or reschedule your appointment to test, you can make the change on the candidate Web site (http://www.pearsonvue.com/nclex) or by calling candidate services. The change needs to be made one full business day (24 hours) before your scheduled appointment. If you fail to arrive for the examination or fail to cancel your appointment to test without providing appropriate notice, you will forfeit your examination fee and your ATT form will be invalidated. This information will be reported to the board of nursing in the state in which you have applied for licensure, and you will be required to register and pay the testing fees again.

DAY OF THE EXAMINATION

It is important that you arrive at the testing center at least 30 minutes before the test is scheduled. If you arrive late for the scheduled testing appointment, you may be required to forfeit your examination appointment. If it is necessary to forfeit your appointment, you will need to re-register for the examination and pay an additional fee. The board of nursing will be notified that you did not take the test. A few days before your scheduled date of testing, take the time to drive to the testing center to determine its exact location, the length of time required to arrive to that destination, and any potential obstacles that might delay you, such as road construction, traffic, or parking sites.

You must have proper identification (ID) to be admitted to take the examination. Acceptable identification includes U.S. driver's license, passport, U.S. state ID, or U.S. military ID. All acceptable identification must be valid and not expired and contain a photograph and signature (in English). You do not need to bring the ATT form to the testing center on the day of the exam; however, the first and last names on your ID must match the names on the ATT form that was emailed to you. According to the NCSBN guidelines, any name discrepancies require legal documentation, such as a marriage license, divorce decree, or court action legal name change.

SPECIAL TESTING CIRCUMSTANCES

If you require special testing accommodations, you should contact the board of nursing before submitting a registration form. The board of nursing will provide the procedures for the request. The board of nursing must authorize special testing accommodations. Following board of nursing approval, the NCSBN reviews the requested accommodations and must approve the request. If the request is approved, the candidate will be notified and provided the procedure for registering for and scheduling the examination.

TESTING CENTER

The test center is designed to ensure complete security of the testing process. Strict candidate identification requirements have been established. You must bring the required form of identification. You will be asked to read the rules related to testing. A digital fingerprint and palm vein print will be taken, and this procedure is usually done twice. A digital signature and photograph will also be taken at the test center. These identity confirmations will accompany the NCLEX exam results. Additionally, if you leave the testing room for any reason, you may be required to perform these identity confirmation procedures again to be readmitted to the room.

Personal belongings are not allowed in the testing room. Secure storage, such as a locker and locker key, will be provided for you; however, storage space is limited. All electronic devices, including a cell phone, must be placed in a sealable bag provided by the proctor and kept in the locker. Any evidence of tampering of the bag could result in an incident and a result cancellation. In addition, the testing center will not assume responsibility for your personal belongings. The testing waiting areas are generally small; friends or family members who accompany you are not permitted to wait in the testing center while you are taking the examination.

Once you have completed the admission process, the proctor will escort you to the assigned computer. You will be seated at an individual work space area that includes computer equipment, appropriate lighting, and erasable note board or white board and a marker. No items, including unauthorized scratch paper, are allowed into the testing room. Eating, drinking, or the use of tobacco is not allowed in the testing room. You will be observed at all times by the test proctor while taking the examination. Additionally, video and audio recordings of all test sessions are made. Pearson Professional Centers has no control over the sounds made by typing on the computer by others. If these sounds are distracting, raise your hand to summon the proctor. Earplugs are available on request.

You must follow the directions given by the test center staff and must remain seated during the test except when authorized to leave. If you think that you have a problem with the computer, need an additional erasable or white board, need to take a break, or need the test proctor for any reason, you must raise your hand. You are also encouraged to access the candidate Web site (http://www.pearsonvue.com/nclex) to obtain additional information about the physical environment of the test center.

TESTING TIME

The maximum testing time is 5 hours; this period includes the tutorial, the sample items, all breaks, and the examination. All breaks are optional and count against testing time. If you take a break, you must leave the testing room and, when you return, you may be required to perform identity confirmation procedures to be readmitted.

LENGTH OF THE EXAMINATION

The minimum number of questions that you will need to answer is 85. Of these 85 questions, 25 will be pretest (unscored) questions. The maximum number of questions in the test is 205. Twenty-five of the total number of questions that you need to answer will be pretest (unscored) questions.

The pretest questions are questions that may be presented as scored questions on future examinations. These pretest questions are not identified as such. In other words, you do not know which questions are the pretest (unscored) questions.

PASS-OR-FAIL DECISIONS

All the examination questions are categorized by test plan area and level of difficulty. This is an important point to keep in mind when you consider how the computer makes a pass-or-fail decision because a pass-or-fail decision is not based on a percentage of correctly answered questions.

The NCSBN indicates that a pass or fail decision is governed by three different scenarios. The first scenario is the 95% Confidence Interval Rule, in which the computer stops administering test questions when it is 95% certain that the test-taker's ability is clearly above the passing standard or clearly below the passing standard. The second scenario is known as the Maximum-Length Exam, in which the final ability estimate of the test taker is considered. If the final ability estimate is above the passing standard, the test-taker passes; if it is below the passing standard, the test-taker fails.

The third scenario is the Run-Out-Of-Time-Rule (R.O.O.T). If the examination ends because the test-taker ran out of time, the computer may not have enough information with 95% certainty to make a clear pass-or-fail decision. If this is the case, the computer will review the test-taker's performance during testing. If the test-taker has not answered the minimum number of required questions, the test-taker fails. If the test-taker's ability estimate was consistently above the passing standard on the last 60 questions, the test-taker passes. If the test-taker's ability estimate falls to or below the passing standard, even once, the test-taker fails. Additional information about pass or fail decisions can be found in the 2014 NCLEX examination candidate bulletin located at www.ncsbn.org.

COMPLETING THE EXAMINATION

When the examination has ended, you will complete a brief computer-delivered questionnaire about your testing experience. After you complete this questionnaire, you need to raise your hand to summon the test proctor. The test proctor will collect and inventory all erasable or white boards and then permit you to leave.

PROCESSING RESULTS

Every computerized examination is scored twice, once by the computer at the testing center and again after the examination is transmitted to Pearson Professional Centers. No results are released at the test center. The board of nursing receives your result and you will be notified 2 days to 2 weeks after you take the examination. In some states, an unofficial result can be obtained via the Quick Results Service 2 business days after taking the examination. This can be done through the Internet or telephone, and there is a fee for this service. Information about obtaining your NCLEX result by this method can be obtained on the NCSBN Web site under candidate services.

CANDIDATE PERFORMANCE REPORT

A candidate performance report is provided to a test-taker who failed the examination. This report provides the test-taker with information about her or his strengths and weaknesses in relation to the test plan framework and provides a guide for studying and retaking the examination. If a retake is necessary, the candidate must wait 45 to 90 days between examination administration. Test-takers should refer to the state board of nursing in the state in which licensure is sought for procedures regarding when the examination can be taken again.

INTERSTATE ENDORSEMENT

Because the NCLEX-PN examination is a national examination, you can apply to take the examination in any state. When licensure is received, you can apply for interstate endorsement, which is obtaining another license in another state to practice nursing in that state. The procedures and requirements for interstate endorsement may vary from state to state, and these procedures can be obtained from the state board of nursing in the state in which endorsement is sought. You may also be allowed to practice nursing in another state if the state has enacted a Nurse Licensure Compact. The state boards of nursing can be accessed via the NCSBN Web site at http://www.ncsbn.org. States that participate in the Nurse Licensure Compact can also be located on this Web site.

NURSE LICENSURE COMPACT

It may be possible to hold one license from the state of residency and practice nursing in another state under the mutual recognition model of nursing licensure if the state has enacted a Nurse Licensure Compact. To obtain information about the Nurse Licensure Compact and the states that are part of this interstate compact, access the NCSBN Web site at http://www.ncsbn.org.

ADDITIONAL INFORMATION ABOUT THE EXAMINATION

Additional information regarding the NCLEX-PN examination can be obtained through the NCLEX examination candidate bulletin located on the NCSBN Web site and from the NCSBN, 111 East Wacker Drive, Suite 2900, Chicago, IL 60601. The telephone number for the NCLEX examinations department is 866-293-9600. The Web site is http://www.ncsbn.org.

Preparation for the NCLEX-PN® Examination: Transitional Issues for Foreign-Educated Nurses

You have taken an important first step—seeking the information that you need to know to become a licensed practical/vocational nurse in the United States. The challenge that is presented to you is one that requires great patience and endurance. The positive result of your endeavor will reward you professionally, however, and give you the personal satisfaction of knowing that you have become part of a family of skilled professionals.

NATIONAL COUNCIL OF STATE BOARDS OF NURSING

The National Council of State Boards of Nursing (NCSBN) is the agency that develops and administers the NCLEX-PN examination, the examination that you need to pass to become licensed as a nurse in the United States. Guidelines and procedures must be followed and documents must be sought and submitted to become eligible to take this examination. This chapter provides general information regarding the process you need to pursue to become a licensed practical/vocational nurse in the United States. An important first step in the process of obtaining information about becoming a nurse in the United States is to access the NCSBN Web site at http://www.ncsbn.org and obtain information provided for international nurses in the NCLEX Web site link. The NCSBN provides information about some of the documents you need to obtain as an international nurse seeking licensure as a nurse in the United States and about credentialing agencies. The NCSBN also provides a resource manual for international nurses that contains all of the necessary licensure information regarding the requirements for education, English proficiency, and immigration requirements such as visas and VisaScreens. You are encouraged to access the NCSBN Web site to obtain the most current information about seeking licensure as a nurse in the United States.

⚠ A first step is to access the NCSBN Web site at http://www.ncsbn.org and obtain information provided for international nurses on the NCLEX Web site.

STATE REQUIREMENTS FOR LICENSURE

An important factor to consider as you pursue this process is that some requirements may vary from state to state. You need to contact the board of nursing in the state in which you are planning to obtain licensure to determine the specific requirements and documents that you need to submit. Boards of nursing can decide either to use a credentialing agency to evaluate your documents or review your documents at the specific state board, known as in-house evaluation. When you contact the board of nursing in the state in which you intend to work as a nurse, inform them that you were educated outside of the United States and ask that they send you an application to apply for licensure by examination. Be sure to specify that you are applying for licensed practical/vocational nurse licensure. You should also ask about the specific documents needed to become eligible to take the NCLEX exam. You can obtain contact information for each state board of nursing through the NCSBN Web site at http://www.ncsbn.org. When you have accessed the NCSBN Web site, select the link titled "Boards of Nursing." Additionally, you can write to the NCSBN regarding the NCLEX exam. The address is 111 East Wacker Drive, Suite 2900, Chicago, IL 60601. The telephone number for the NCSBN is (866) 293-9600; the fax number is (312) 279-1036.

⚠ Contact the board of nursing in the state in which you are planning to obtain licensure to determine the specific requirements and documents that you need to submit. Documents that you need to submit vary state by state.

CREDENTIALING AGENCIES

The state board of nursing in the state in which you are seeking licensure may choose to use a credentialing agency to review your documents. It is necessary that you seek this information from the state board and use the credentialing agency that the state requires. The state board of nursing will provide you with the name and contact information of the credentialing agency. Seeking this information is important because you need to know where to send your required documents. Additionally, the NCSBN Web site (http://www.ncsbn.org) can provide information about credentialing agencies.

GENERAL LICENSURE REQUIREMENTS

Required documents may vary depending on the state requirements. These documents must be sent to either the state board of nursing or the credentialing agency specified by the state. Neither the credentialing agency nor the state board of nursing will accept these documents if they are sent directly from you. These documents must be official documents sent directly from the licensing authority or other agency in your home country to verify validity. Some of the general documents required are listed in Box 2-1; however, remember that the documents you need to submit vary state by state. Use the list provided in Box 2-1 as a checklist for yourself after you have found out about the documents you are required to submit.

Box 2-1 Some Documents Needed to Obtain Licensure

1. Proof of citizenship or lawful alien status
2. Work visa
3. VisaScreen certificate
4. Commission on Graduates of Foreign Nursing Schools (CGFNS) certificate
5. Criminal background check documents
6. Official transcripts of educational credentials sent directly to credentialing agency or board of nursing from home country school of nursing
7. Validation of a comparable nursing education as that provided in U.S. nursing programs. This may include theoretical instruction and clinical practice in a variety of nursing areas, including, but not limited to, medical nursing, surgical nursing, pediatric nursing, maternity and newborn nursing, community and public health nursing, and mental health nursing.
8. Validation of safe professional nursing practice in home country
9. Copy of nursing license or diploma or both
10. Proof of proficiency in the English language
11. Photograph(s)
12. Social security number
13. Application and fees

When all of your documents have been submitted, they will be reviewed. If you have met the eligibility requirements to take the NCLEX examination, you will be notified that you are eligible. Then you need to obtain an application to take the NCLEX exam from the state in which you intend to seek licensure and submit the required fees. Your application will be reviewed and processed, and you will be notified that you can make an appointment to take the NCLEX exam. Additional information about the application process for the NCLEX exam can be obtained at the NCSBN Web site at www.ncsbn.org. Box 2-2 provides a brief guide of the general steps to take in the licensure process.

⚠ Official documents must be sent directly from the licensing authority or other agency in your home country.

WORK VISA

A foreign-educated nurse who wants to work in the United States needs to obtain the proper work visa or visas. Obtaining the work visa is a U.S. federal government requirement. To obtain information about the work visa and the application process, contact the Department of Homeland Security (DHS), Office of U.S. Citizenship and Immigration Services (USCIS). The Web site is http://uscis.gov/graphics/howdoi/Health_Cert.htm.

VISASCREEN

U.S. immigration law requires certain health care professionals to complete a screening program successfully before receiving an occupational (work) visa (Section

Box 2-2 General Steps in the Licensure Process

1. Access the NCSBN Web site at http://www.ncsbn.org and read the literature provided for international nurses.
2. Contact the board of nursing in the state in which you are planning to obtain licensure to determine the specific requirements and documents that you need to submit.
3. Have the required documents sent from the appropriate agency in your home country.
4. When you are notified about eligibility to take the NCLEX exam, obtain the application form from the state in which you intend to obtain licensure, complete the form, and submit it with required fees.
5. Schedule an appointment to take the NCLEX exam when you receive your Authorization to Test (ATT) form.
6. Take the NCLEX exam.
7. Become a licensed practical/vocational nurse in the United States.

343 of the Illegal Immigration Reform and Immigration Responsibility Act of 1996). To become a nurse in the United States, you are required to obtain a VisaScreen certificate. You can ask about the VisaScreen certificate when you make your initial contact with the state board of nursing in which you are seeking licensure. The VisaScreen is a federal screening program, and the certificate needs to be obtained through an organization that offers this program.

⚠ Obtaining the work visa and the VisaScreen is a U.S. federal government requirement.

The Commission on Graduates of Foreign Nursing Schools (CGFNS) is an organization that offers this federal screening program. The VisaScreen components of this program include an educational analysis, license verification, assessment of proficiency in the English language, and an examination that tests nursing knowledge. When the applicant successfully achieves each component, the applicant is presented with a VisaScreen certificate. You can obtain information related to the VisaScreen through the CGFNS Web site at http://www.cgfns.org. The CGFNS Web site also provides you with specific information about the components of this program.

The Commission on Graduates of Foreign Nursing Schools (CGFNS) is also a credentialing agency and awards a CGFNS certificate to the applicant when all eligibility requirements are met. Some state boards of nursing use the CGFNS as a credentialing agency and require a CGFNS certificate, whereas others do not. Check with the state board of nursing regarding this certificate. The CGFNS certification program contains three parts, and you must complete all parts successfully to be awarded a CGFNS certificate. The three parts include a credentials review, a qualifying examination that tests nursing knowledge, and an English language proficiency examination. These components are similar to those needed to obtain the VisaScreen certificate. You can obtain information related to the CGFNS certificate through the CGFNS Web site at http://www.cgfns.org.

⚠ The NCLEX examination is administered in English only.

REGISTERING TO TAKE THE NCLEX® EXAM

When you have completed all state and federal requirements and received documentation that you are eligible to take the NCLEX examination, you can register for the exam. You need to obtain information from the state board of nursing in the state in which you are seeking licensure regarding the specific registration process because the process may vary from state to state. The

NCLEX candidate Web site is http://www.pearsonvue.com/nclex, and you are encouraged to access this site for additional information. Following the registration instructions and completing the registration forms precisely and accurately are important. You must pay a fee for taking the examination, and you may have to pay additional fees to the board of nursing in the state in which you are applying. When your eligibility is determined by the state licensure board, you will receive an Authorization to Test (ATT) form. You cannot make an appointment to test until the board of nursing declares eligibility and you receive an ATT form.

⚠ Registration forms for taking the NCLEX exam that are not properly completed or not accompanied by the proper fees in the required method of payment will be returned to you and will delay testing.

The examination takes place at a Pearson Professional Center, and you can make an appointment through the Internet or by telephone. You can schedule an appointment at any Pearson Professional Center. You do not have to take the exam in the state in which you are seeking licensure. NCLEX exam testing abroad is also available in some countries, and it is recommended that you visit the NCLEX Web site for current information about international testing sites. Chapter 1 contains additional information regarding the NCLEX exam and testing procedures. You can also obtain information about the registration process and testing procedures from the NCSBN Web site at http://www.ncsbn.org.

PREPARING TO TAKE THE NCLEX® EXAM

When you have successfully completed the requirements to become eligible to take the NCLEX exam, you have one more important goal to achieve: to pass the NCLEX exam.

⚠ Begin preparing for the NCLEX exam as soon as possible; start preparing even before you begin the licensure process.

I highly recommend adequate preparation for the NCLEX exam because the examination is difficult. An important step that you have taken in preparing is that you are using this book, *Saunders Comprehensive Review for the NCLEX-PN® Examination*. After you have reviewed the content and answered the practice questions, the next step in your journey to success is to use the companion book, *Saunders Q&A Review for the NCLEX-PN® Examination*; this book provides you with more than 3,200 practice questions based on the NCLEX-PN examination test plan framework, with a specific focus on Client Needs and Integrated Processes. Additional products in Saunders Pyramid to Success include *Saunders Strategies for Test Success: Passing Nursing School and the NCLEX® Exam*. This product focuses on the test-taking strategies that will prepare you for the NCLEX exam. The chapters describe all the test-taking strategies and include several sample questions that illustrate how to use the test-taking strategy. This book has 500 practice questions. All the practice questions reflect the framework and the content identified in the current NCLEX test plan and include multiple-choice and alternate item format questions. Several appendices are included that provide a review of test-taking strategies, cultural characteristics and practices, pharmacology strategies, medication and intravenous calculations, laboratory values, positioning guidelines, and therapeutic diets.

All the products in Saunders Pyramid to Success can be obtained online by visiting elsevierhealth.com or by calling 800-545-2522.

⚠ Stay positive and confident, and believe that you can achieve your goal.

Finally, never lose sight of your goal. Patience and dedication contribute significantly to your achieving the status of licensed practical/vocational nurse. Remember, success is climbing a mountain, facing the challenge of obstacles, and reaching the top of the mountain. I wish you the best success in your journey and beginning your career as a registered nurse in the United States.

Pathways to Success

Laurent W. Valliere, BS, DD

PYRAMID TO SUCCESS

Preparing to take the NCLEX-PN exam can produce a great deal of anxiety. You may be thinking that the NCLEX-PN is the most important exam that you will ever have to take, and that it reflects the culmination of everything for which you have worked so hard. The NCLEX-PN is an important exam, because receiving that nursing license means that you can begin your career as a licensed practical/vocational nurse. Your success on the NCLEX-PN involves expelling all thoughts from your mind that allow this exam to appear overwhelming and intimidating; such thoughts will take complete control over your destiny. A positive attitude, a structured plan for preparation, and maintaining control of your pathway to success will ensure your achievement of reaching the peak of the Pyramid to Success (Figure 3-1).

PATHWAYS TO SUCCESS (Box 3-1)

The Foundation

The foundation of Pathways to Success begins with a positive attitude, the belief that you will achieve success, and the development of control. It also includes the creation of a list of your personal short- and long-term goals and a plan for preparation. A positive attitude, belief in yourself, control, and a list of personal goals will lead you to becoming a licensed practical/vocational nurse. Without these components, your Pathway to Success leads to nowhere and has no end point. You will expend energy and valuable time in your journey, but you will lack control over where you are heading, and you will experience exhaustion without any accomplishment. Therefore, it is imperative that you take the time to develop that positive attitude and to establish your short- and long-term goals.

Where do you start? To begin this process, find a location that offers solitude. Sit or lie in a comfortable position, close your eyes, relax, inhale deeply, hold your breath to a count of 4, exhale slowly, and, again, relax. Repeat this breathing exercise several times until you begin to feel relaxed, free from anxiety, and in control of your destiny. Allow your mind to become void of

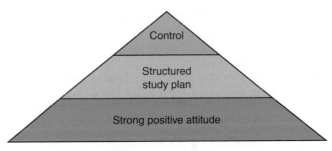

▲ **FIGURE 3-1** The Pyramid to Success.

all of the mind chatter; you are now in control, and your mind can see for miles. Your highway of life has a multitude of destinations to which you may travel. Next, reflect on all that you have accomplished and the path that brought you to where you are today. Journal your reflections as you plan the order of your journey to the Pyramid to Success.

The List

It is time to create "The List." "The List" is your set of short- and long-term goals. At this time, you may or may not have a scheduled date for taking the NCLEX-PN exam. Therefore, begin by developing the goals you wish to accomplish today, tomorrow, over the next month, and into the future. Allow yourself the opportunity to list all that is flowing from your mind. Write your goals in your personal journal. When "The List" is complete, put it away for 2 or 3 days. After that time, retrieve and review "The List," and begin the process of planning for preparing for the NCLEX-PN exam.

The Plan for Preparation

Now that you have "The List" in order, look at the goals that relate to studying for the licensing exam. The first task is to decide what study pattern works best for you. Think about what has worked most successfully for you in the past. There are questions that must be addressed to develop your plan for study. These questions are identified in Box 3-2.

Box 3-1 Pathways to Success

The Foundation
- Maintaining a positive attitude
- Thinking about realistic short- and long-term goals
- Preparing a plan for preparation
- Maintaining control

The List
- Journaling realistic short- and long-term goals

The Plan for Preparation
- Developing a study plan and schedule
- Deciding on the place to study
- Balancing personal and work obligations with the study schedule
- Sharing the study schedule and personal needs with others
- Implementing the study plan

Positive Pampering
- Planning time for exercise and fun activities
- Establishing healthy eating habits
- Including activities in the schedule that provide positive mental stimulation

Final Preparation
- Reviewing goals
- Identifying goals that have been achieved
- Remaining focused to complete the plan of study
- Writing down the date and time of the exam and posting it next to your name with the letters "LPN" or "LVN" after it, along with the word "YES!"
- Taking a test drive to the testing center
- Enjoying relaxing activities on the day before the exam

The Day of the Exam
- Grooming yourself for success
- Eating a healthy and nutritious breakfast
- Maintaining a confident and positive attitude
- Maintaining control
- Meeting the challenges of the day
- Reaching the peak of the Pyramid to Success

Box 3-2 Developing a Plan of Study

- Do I work better alone or in a group study environment?
- If I work best in a group, does the group consist of one, two, or more study partners?
- Who are these study partners?
- How long should my study sessions last?
- Does the time of day that I study make a difference for me?
- Do I retain more if I study in the morning?
- How does my work schedule affect my study pattern?
- How do I balance my family obligations with my need to study?
- Do I have a comfortable study area at home, or do I need to find another environment that is more conducive to my study needs?

you are determining a realistic amount of time for each session. Plan to schedule 2 hours of daily quality study time at the very least. If you can spend more than 2 hours studying, then by all means do so.

You may be asking yourself, "What do you mean by quality time?" Quality time means spending uninterrupted quiet time focusing on your study session. This may mean that you will have to isolate yourself for these study sessions. Think again about what has worked for you during nursing school when you studied for exams, and select a study place that has also worked for you in the past. If you have a special study room at home that you have always used, then plan your study sessions in that special room. If you have always studied at a library, then plan your study sessions for the library. If you plan to study at home, make the time spent studying uninterrupted and quiet. Sometimes it is difficult to balance your study time with your family obligations and possibly a work schedule, but if you can, plan your study time for when you know that you will be at home alone. Try to eliminate anything that may be distracting during your study time. For example, unplug your telephone or shut off your cell phone so that you will not be disturbed. If you have small children, plan your study time during their nap time or school hours.

Your plan must include the ways in which you will manage your study needs and the demands of your work, family, and friends. Take time to think about how you will balance your everyday commitments with your plan for study. Your family and friends are key players in your life, and they are going to become a part of your Pyramid to Success. After you have established your study needs, communicate your needs and the importance of your study plan for achieving your goal of becoming a licensed practical/vocational nurse to your family and friends.

A difficult part of the plan may be how you will deal with those family and friends who choose not to participate in your Plan for Success. What if an individual or

The plan must include a schedule. Use a calendar to plan and document the times and nursing content areas for your study sessions. Establish a realistic schedule that includes your daily, weekly, and future goals, and adhere to it. This consistency will provide advantages to you and those supporting you. A daily schedule allows you to plan your content areas for study more carefully. Stick to your plan of study. Adherence to the plan helps you develop a rhythm that can only enhance your retention and positive momentum. Those who are supporting you will share this rhythm, and they will be able to schedule their activities and life better because you are consistent with your study schedule. You are moving forward, and you are in control!

The length of the study session will depend on you and your ability to focus and concentrate. What you need to think about is quality rather than quantity when individuals choose to not be part of your plan? For example, what do you do if a friend asks you to go to a movie during your scheduled study time? Your friend may say, "Come on. Take some time off. You have plenty of time to study. Study later when we get back!" Then you are faced with a decision. You must weigh all of the factors carefully. You must keep your goals in mind and remember that your need for positive momentum is critical. Your decision may not be an easy one, but it must be one that will help you ensure that your goal of becoming a licensed practical/vocational nurse is achieved. Remember, positive momentum and meeting your goals are most important.

POSITIVE PAMPERING

What is positive pampering? This means that you must continue to care for yourself holistically. Positive momentum can be maintained only if you are properly balanced. Proper exercise, diet, and positive mental stimulation are critical to achieving your goal of becoming a licensed practical/vocational nurse. Just as you have developed a schedule for study, you should have a schedule that includes some fun and some form of physical activity. It is your choice—aerobics, running, walking, weight lifting, bowling, or whatever makes you feel good about yourself. Time spent away from the hard study schedule and devoted to some form of fun and physical exercise pays its rewards 100-fold. You will feel alive and more energetic with a schedule that includes these activities.

Establish healthy eating habits. Stay away from fatty foods, because they will slow you down. Eat lighter meals, and eat more frequently. Include complex carbohydrates in your diet for energy, and be careful to not include too much caffeine in your daily diet. Continue to feel good about yourself, because you are in control.

Take the time to pamper yourself with activities that make you feel even better about who you are. Make dinner reservations at your favorite restaurant with someone who is special and who is supporting your goal of becoming a licensed practical/vocational nurse. Take walks in a place that has a particular tranquillity that enables you to reflect on the positive momentum that you have achieved and maintained. Whatever it is and wherever it takes you, allow yourself the time to do some positive pampering.

FINAL PREPARATION

You have established the foundation of your Pyramid to Success. You have developed your list of goals and your study plan, and you have maintained your positive momentum. You are moving forward, and you are in control. When you receive your date and time for the NCLEX-PN exam, you may immediately think, "I'm not ready!" Stop thinking that way! Reflect on all that

you have achieved. Think about your goal achievement and the organization of the positive life momentum with which you have surrounded yourself. Think about all those individuals who love and support your effort to become a licensed practical/vocational nurse. Believe that the challenge that awaits you is one that you have successfully prepared for and that will lead you to your goal of becoming a licensed practical/vocational nurse!

Take a deep breath, and organize the remaining days so that they support your educational and personal needs. Support your positive momentum with a visual technique. Write your name in large letters, and write the letters "LPN" or "LVN" after it. Post one or more of these visual reinforcements in areas that you frequent. This form of visual motivational technique works for many individuals preparing for this exam.

Through all that you have accomplished to this point, it is imperative that you not fall into the trap of expecting too much of yourself. The idea of perfection must not drive you to a point that causes your positive momentum to hesitate. You must believe in who you are as you are, and you need to stay focused on your goal. Allow yourself the opportunity to continue to carry out your plan in a manner that is the most conducive to who you are. The date and time are in hand. Write down the date and time, and underneath write the word "YES!" Post this next to your note with your name plus "LPN" or "LVN."

You must ensure that you know how to get to the testing center. A test run is a must. Time the drive, and allow for road construction or whatever may occur to slow traffic down. On the test run, when you arrive at the testing facility, you may want to walk into it. Walk in and become familiar with the lobby and the surroundings. This may help to alleviate some of the peripheral nervousness associated with entering an unknown building. Remember, you must do whatever it takes to keep yourself in control. If familiarizing yourself with the facility will help you to maintain positive momentum, then by all means be sure to do so. Who is in control? You are!

It is time to check your study plan and make the necessary adjustments now that a firm date and time are set. Adjust your review so that it flows to your needs and so that your study plan ends 2 days before the exam. Remember that the mind is like a muscle. If it is overworked, it has no strength or stamina. Your strategy is to rest the body and mind on the day before the exam. Your need to stay in control and allow yourself the opportunity to be absolutely fresh and attentive on the day of the exam. This will help you to control the nervousness that is natural, achieve the clear thought processes required, and feel confident that you have done all that is necessary to prepare for and conquer this challenge. The day before the exam is to be one of pleasure. Treat yourself to what you enjoy the most.

Relax! You have prepared yourself well for the challenge of the next day. Allow yourself a good night's sleep, and wake up on the day of the exam knowing that you are absolutely ready to succeed. Look at your name with "LPN" or "LVN" after it next to the word "YES!"

THE DAY OF THE EXAM (Box 3-3)

Wake up believing in yourself and knowing that all you have accomplished is about to propel you to the professional level of becoming a licensed practical/vocational nurse. Allow yourself plenty of time, eat

---

Box 3-3 The Day of the Exam

Breathe—Inhale deeply, hold your breath to a count of 4, and exhale slowly.
Believe—Think positive thoughts about your achievements. Yes! This is your day!
Control—Yes! You are in command!
Visualize—See your name with the letters "LPN" or "LVN" after it!

---

a nutritious breakfast, and groom yourself for success. You are ready to meet the challenges of the day and overcome any obstacle that may face you. Today will soon be history, and tomorrow will bring you the envelope on which you read your name with the letters "LPN" or "LVN" after it.

Be proud and confident of your achievements. You have worked hard to achieve your goal of becoming a licensed practical/vocational nurse. If you believe in yourself and your goals, no one person or obstacle can move you off of the pathway that leads to success and to the peak of the Pyramid!

Congratulations! I wish you the very best in your career as a licensed practical/vocational nurse

The NCLEX-PN® Examination: From a Graduate's Perspective

Bryan F. King, LPN

Let me say, as a graduate, I was once in the position that you are now. I was full of worry and trepidation and anxious about taking the NCLEX. The best advice that I can give you is to RELAX! You have the knowledge you need to pass the NCLEX examination. The worst is almost over! You have sacrificed so much in the last several months. You *will* regain the time for the family life, socializing, religious practice, or whatever else you put aside in pursuit of becoming a nurse.

HOW TO PREPARE FOR THE NCLEX

When I was preparing for the NCLEX, I read the *Saunders Comprehensive Review for the NCLEX-PN®* book from cover to cover, reread it, and then answered the questions found in the practice tests. I then used the enclosed CD to review even further. By completing this self-study in my home office, away from any distractions, I found myself ready to face the very nerve-wracking experience of tackling the NCLEX head on. I also was very fortunate to have the luxury of my biggest supporter, my wife, who spent countless hours verbally testing me on the multitude of practice questions. Ask someone in your life, a friend or classmate or school instructor, if he or she will do the same for you.

There are lots of different types of study methods, so figure out what works for you. The methods I discuss above worked for me, so I used them consistently. Once you've figured out what works for you, stick with it, and then spend at least 2 to 5 days a week (Yes, I mean 8-hour days!) preparing for your exam.

APPLYING TO TAKE THE EXAM

As far as the application for the exam itself, I was very fortunate that my nursing school walked us through the entire process. We sat in a classroom and filled out the necessary paperwork, which was most helpful. (Remember, we are dealing with state bureaucracy and paperwork here, which can be very confusing to many!) If your nursing school doesn't offer this, see if you can get together with some other students to go through it together and make sure that you are filling it out correctly.

Then it was on to selecting the location and date to sit for the exam itself. In my case, I picked a primary and secondary choice for these items. I felt like I was back in the military as I played the "hurry up and wait" game. It was a big rush to apply but seemed like an eternity before I heard back from the state. Finally, I received notice of when and where I would sit for the exam. The most important advice I can give is to NOT study for the 2 days preceding your exam. You have worked so very hard, for so very long, that you need to have "me" time. Do something fun, clear your mind and, most of all, relax, relax, relax. Everything that you've learned up to that point is already stored in that brain of yours—you will be able to pull it back out on your big day.

TAKING THE EXAM

The night before your exam, I recommend that you get a good night's sleep, avoiding both alcohol and caffeine. Being well-rested was the key to my personal experience. I arrived at the testing center refreshed and focused, ready to face the challenge ahead. While I did have butterflies in my stomach, I knew that having a positive attitude was just as important as all those months of learning that I had just completed. Nonetheless, let me forewarn you that it is still a scary experience. When the computer shut down after only 88 questions, my self-doubt kicked in. I thought to myself that I had answered so many questions incorrectly, that I hadn't passed the exam. When I got home, my wife pointed out that I couldn't have possibly failed. With my mind still reeling she said, "Just do the math." I had completely forgotten how the exam is structured.

Let me explain how this test works, so you won't go through the same self-doubt that I experienced. At the time I sat for the NCLEX, you could get as few as 85 questions or as many as 205. The exam starts out on a basic level and if you answer the question correctly, the next question moves up a level. Conversely, if you answer incorrectly, it gives you a question at the basic level. Each time you answer correctly, successive questions become more difficult and if answered incorrectly, keeps you at the same level or drops down a level to allow you to redeem yourself. This exam gives you every chance available to pass! Don't become overly worried if your computer shuts down early.

RESULTS

I know it will be very difficult for you while you wait for your official results. You can now find out your results online within a day or two from the exam date but there is a fee associated with this service,. It will seem

like an eternity until you find out that you passed your nursing boards. Remember to keep a positive attitude before, during, and after this whole process. To lessen the stress while waiting for your results, treat yourself to a special occasion—dinner out with the family, a concert, a trip to a favorite place, or something else special to you.

BECOMING AN LPN

You have made a great decision in choosing to become a nurse. It is a richly rewarding profession. Your sense of satisfaction at the end of the day will be strong, knowing you made a difference in someone's life.

Congratulations, and I wish you the very best!

Test-Taking Strategies

I. PYRAMID TO SUCCESS (Box 5-1)

II. THE "WHAT IF…?" SYNDROME AND HOW TO AVOID READING INTO THE QUESTION (Box 5-2)

A. Pyramid points
1. Avoid asking yourself, "What if…?" because this will lead you right into the "forbidden" act of reading into the question.
2. Focus only on the information in the question, read every word, and make a decision regarding what the question is asking.
3. Look for the strategic words in the question, such as *side effect*, *adverse effect*, or *toxic effect*. Strategic words make a difference with regard to what the question is asking about.
4. For multiple-choice questions, multiple-response questions, or questions that require you to list options in order of priority, read every option presented before selecting your answers.
5. Always use the process of elimination when options are presented. After you have eliminated some options, reread the question before making your final choice or choices.

6. With questions that require you to fill in the blank, focus on the information in the question, and determine what the question is asking. If the question requires you to calculate a medication dose, an intravenous flow rate, or intake and output amounts, recheck your calculations, and always use the on-screen calculator to verify the answer.
7. Remember, avoid asking yourself the "forbidden" question "What if…?" when determining the answer to a question.

B. The Ingredients of a Question (Box 5-3)
1. The ingredients of a question include the event (which is a client or clinical situation), the event query, and the options or answers. A fill-in-the-blank

---

Box 5-1 Pyramid to Success

- Avoid asking yourself "What if…?," because this will lead you right into reading into the question.
- Focus only on the information in the question, read every word, and make a decision regarding what the question is asking.
- Look for the strategic words in the question. Strategic words make a difference with regard to what the question is asking about.
- Always use the process of elimination when options are presented. After you have eliminated some options, reread the question before making your final choice or choices.
- Determine if the question contains a positive or negative event query.
- Use all of your nursing knowledge, your clinical experiences, and your test-taking skills and strategies to answer the question.

Box 5-2 Practice Question: Avoiding the "What If…?" Syndrome and Reading into the Question

A nurse is changing the tapes on a tracheostomy tube. The client coughs, and the tube is dislodged. The initial nursing action is to:
1. Call the health care provider (HCP) to reinsert the tube.
2. Ventilate the client using a manual resuscitation bag.
3. Cover the tracheostomy site with a sterile dressing to prevent infection.
4. Call the respiratory therapy department to reinsert the tracheostomy tube.

Answer: 2
Test-Taking Strategy: Now, you may immediately think, "The tube is dislodged and I need the HCP." Read the question carefully, and note the strategic word "initial." Focus on the subject of the tube being dislodged. The question is asking you for a nursing action, so that is what you need to look for as you eliminate the incorrect options. Eliminate options 1 and 4, because they are comparable or alike and delay the initial intervention needed. Eliminate option 3, because this action will block the airway. If the tube is dislodged, the initial nursing action is to ventilate the client using a manual resuscitation bag. In addition, the use of the ABCs—airway, breathing, and circulation—will direct you to the correct option. Remember, avoid reading into the question!

question will not contain options, and some figure or illustration (hot spot) questions may or may not contain options.

2. The client or clinical event provides you with the content you need to think about when answering the question.
3. The event query asks something specific about the client or clinical event.
4. The options are all of the answers provided with the question.
5. With a multiple-choice question, there will be four options, and you must select one. Read every option carefully and think about the client or clinical event and the event query as you use the process of elimination.
6. With a multiple-response question, there most likely will be more than four options, and you must select all options that apply to the event in the question. Visualize the event, and use your nursing knowledge and clinical experiences to answer the question.
7. With a prioritizing (ordered-response) question, you will be required to list in order of priority (using the computer mouse and dragging and dropping the options) certain nursing interventions or other data. Visualize the event, and use your nursing knowledge and clinical experiences to answer the question.
8. A chart/exhibit question will most likely contain options. Read the question carefully and look at all of the information in the chart/exhibit before selecting an answer.

Box 5-3 Multiple-Choice Question: Event, Event Query, and Options

Event: After thoracic surgery, a client has two chest tubes inserted into the right pleural space that are attached to chest drainage systems.
Event Query: To promote optimal respiratory functioning, the nurse plans to implement which of the following?
Options:
1. Milk and strip the chest tubes once per shift.
2. Position the client on the back and the right side.
3. Encourage the client to cough and deep breathe every hour.
4. Maintain the client on bedrest until the chest tubes are removed.

Answer: 3
Test-Taking Strategy: Focus on the subject of promoting optimal respiratory functioning. Option 1 is eliminated first, because milking and stripping a chest tube is done only with a health care provider's prescription or when allowed by agency policy. Bedrest (option 4) does not promote respiratory function and is eliminated next. From the remaining options, recalling that positioning is done according to surgeon preference directs you to option 3.

III. THE STRATEGIC WORDS (Boxes 5-4 and 5-5)

A. Strategic words focus your attention on a critical point to consider when answering the question and will assist you with eliminating the incorrect options.
B. Some strategic words may indicate that all of the options are correct and that it will be necessary to prioritize to select the correct option.
C. As you read the question, look for the strategic words. Strategic words make a difference with regard to what the question is asking.

IV. THE SUBJECT OF THE QUESTION (Box 5-6)

A. The subject of the question is the specific topic that the question is asking about.
B. Identifying the subject of the question will assist with eliminating the incorrect options and direct you to the correct option.

V. POSITIVE AND NEGATIVE EVENT QUERIES (Boxes 5-7 and 5-8)

A. A positive event query uses strategic words that ask you to select an option that is correct. For example, the event query may read, "Which statement by a client *indicates an understanding* of the side effects of the prescribed medication?"

Box 5-4 Common Strategic Words

■ Early	■ Immediate
■ Late	■ Most likely
■ Best	■ Least likely
■ First	■ Most appropriate
■ Initial	■ Least appropriate

Box 5-5 Practice Question: Strategic Words

A client with a diagnosis of heart failure reports the occurrence of sudden shortness of breath and dyspnea. The nurse takes which immediate action?
1. Calls the health care provider
2. Administers oxygen
3. Elevates the head of the bed
4. Prepares to administer furosemide (Lasix)

Answer: 3
Test-Taking Strategy: Note the strategic word "immediate." Focusing on this strategic word and the client's symptoms (shortness of breath and dyspnea) will direct you to the correct option. Note that the question is asking for an immediate nursing action, so that is what you need to look for as you eliminate each incorrect option. Remember to look for strategic words!

B. A negative event query uses strategic words that ask you to select an option that is an incorrect item or statement. For example, the event query may read, "Which statement by a client *indicates a need for further teaching* about the side effects of the prescribed medication?"

Box 5-6 The Subject of the Question

The nurse is planning to teach a client in skeletal leg traction about measures to increase bed mobility. Which item would be most helpful for this client?
1. Television
2. Fracture bedpan
3. Overhead trapeze
4. Reading materials

Answer: 3

Test-Taking Strategy: Focus on the subject of increasing bed mobility. Also note the strategic words "most helpful." The use of an overhead trapeze is extremely helpful for assisting a client with moving about in bed and with getting on and off of the bedpan. Television and reading materials are helpful to reduce boredom and provide distraction. A fracture bedpan is useful for reducing discomfort with elimination. Remember to focus on the subject!

Box 5-7 Practice Question: Positive Event Query

The nurse has provided discharge instructions regarding nitroglycerin therapy to the client with angina. Which statement by the client indicates an understanding of the home use of the nitroglycerin?
1. "If I use the nitroglycerin and the pain does not subside in 15 minutes, I should go to the hospital."
2. "When I have pain, I should lie down and place a tablet under my tongue. If unrelieved in 5 minutes, I should call for an ambulance."
3. "When I have chest pain, I should put a tablet under my tongue. If I have a burning sensation, I should call my doctor immediately."
4. "When I experience chest pain, I can continue what I'm doing. If it doesn't go away in 10 minutes, I should use a nitroglycerin tablet."

Answer: 2

Test-Taking Strategy: This question identifies an example of a positive event query. Note the strategic words "indicates an understanding." The client taking sublingual nitroglycerin should recline after taking the medication, because lightheadedness and dizziness may occur as a result of postural hypotension. The client should call emergency medical services if relief is not obtained after 5 minutes. A burning sensation is a common side effect of nitroglycerin. Nitroglycerin should be taken with the onset of anginal pain. Remember, positive event queries ask you to select an option that is a correct item or statement!

VI. QUESTIONS THAT REQUIRE PRIORITIZING

A. Questions in the exam may require you to use the skill of prioritizing nursing actions.
B. Look for the strategic words in the question that indicate the need to prioritize (Box 5-9).
C. Remember, when a question requires prioritization, all options may be correct, and you need to determine the correct order of action
D. Strategies to use to prioritize include the ABCs—airway, breathing, and circulation; Maslow's Hierarchy of Needs theory; and the steps of the nursing process (clinical problem-solving process).
E. The ABCs (Box 5-10)
  1. Use the ABCs—airway, breathing, and circulation—when selecting an answer or determining the order of priority.
  2. Remember the order of priority: airway, breathing, and circulation.
  3. Airway is always the first priority!
F. Maslow's Hierarchy of Needs theory (Box 5-11 and Figure 5-1)

Box 5-8 Practice Question: Negative Event Query

A nurse has provided medication instructions to a client who will be taking warfarin sodium (Coumadin) indefinitely. Which statement by the client indicates a need for further teaching?
1. "I need to use a soft toothbrush."
2. "I need to use a straight razor for shaving."
3. "I need to avoid drinking alcohol while taking this medication."
4. "I need to carry identification about the medication being taken."

Answer: 2

Test-Taking Strategy: This question identifies an example of a negative event query. Note the strategic words "need for further teaching." These strategic words indicate that you need to select an option that identifies an incorrect client statement. Recalling that warfarin sodium is an anticoagulant and that the client is at risk for bleeding will direct you to the correct option. Remember that negative event queries ask you to select an option that is an incorrect item or statement!

Box 5-9 Common Strategic Words That Indicate the Need to Prioritize

- Best
- Essential
- First
- Highest priority
- Immediate
- Initial
- Most important
- Next
- Primary
- Vital

Box 5-10 Practice Question: Use of the ABCs

A client with a compound (open) fracture of the radius has a cast applied in the emergency department. The nurse provides home-care instructions and tells the client to seek medical attention if which of the following occurs?
1. Numbness and tingling are felt in the fingers.
2. The cast feels heavy and damp 24 hours after application.
3. The entire cast feels warm during the first 24 hours after application.
4. Bloody drainage is noted on the cast during the first 6 hours after application.

Answer: 1

Test-Taking Strategy: Use the ABCs—airway, breathing, and circulation—as a guide to direct you to the correct option. A limb encased in a cast is at risk for nerve damage and diminished circulation from increased pressure caused by edema. Signs of increased pressure and diminished circulation from the cast include numbness, tingling, and increased pain. Remember to use the ABCs—airway, breathing, and circulation—to prioritize.

Box 5-11 Practice Question: Maslow's Hierarchy of Needs Theory

A nurse is assigned to care for a client experiencing dystocia. When assisting with planning care, the nurse would consider the highest priority to be frequent:
1. Position changes and providing comfort measures
2. Explanations to family members about what is happening to the client
3. Monitoring for changes in the physical condition of the mother and fetus
4. Reinforcement of breathing techniques learned in childbirth preparatory classes

Answer: 3

Test-Taking Strategy: All of the options presented are correct and would be implemented during the care of this client. However, note the strategic words "highest priority," and use Maslow's Hierarchy of Needs theory to prioritize, remembering that physiological needs come first. Using this guideline will direct you to option 3. In addition, note that option 3 is the only option that addresses both the mother and the fetus.

Nursing Priorities From Maslow's Hierarchy

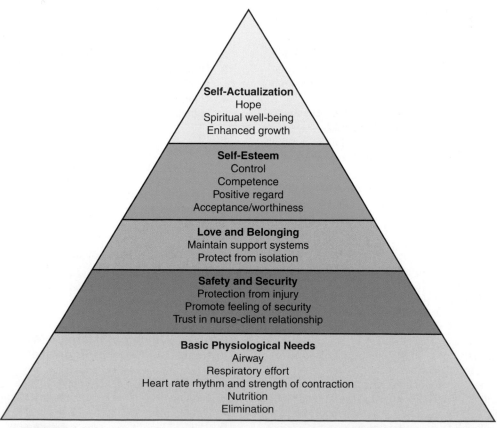

Self-Actualization
Hope
Spiritual well-being
Enhanced growth

Self-Esteem
Control
Competence
Positive regard
Acceptance/worthiness

Love and Belonging
Maintain support systems
Protect from isolation

Safety and Security
Protection from injury
Promote feeling of security
Trust in nurse-client relationship

Basic Physiological Needs
Airway
Respiratory effort
Heart rate rhythm and strength of contraction
Nutrition
Elimination

▲ **FIGURE 5-1** Using Maslow's Hierarchy of Needs theory to establish priorities. (From Harkreader, H., Hogan, M. A., & Thobaben, M. [2007]. *Fundamentals of nursing: Caring and clinical judgment* [3rd ed.]. Philadelphia: Saunders.)

1. According to Maslow's Hierarchy of Needs theory, physiological needs are the priority, followed by safety and security needs, love and belonging needs, self-esteem needs, and finally, self-actualization needs. Therefore, select the option or determine the order of priority by addressing physiological needs first.

2. When a physiological need is not addressed in the question or noted in one of the options, continue to use Maslow's Hierarchy of Needs theory as a guide, and look for the option that addresses safety.

G. Steps of the nursing process (clinical problem-solving process)

1. Use the steps of the nursing process (clinical problem-solving process) to prioritize.

2. The steps include data collection, planning, implementation, and evaluation and are followed in this order.

3. Data collection

   a. Data collection questions address the process of gathering subjective and objective data relative to the client, communicating and documenting information gained during data collection, and contributing to the formulation of nursing diagnoses.

   b. Remember that data collection is the first step of the nursing process (clinical problem-solving process).

   c. When you are asked a question regarding your initial or first nursing action, look for strategic words in the options that reflect the collection of data relative to the client (Box 5-12).

   d. If an option contains the concept of collection of client data, it is best to select that option (Box 5-13).

   e. If a data-collection action is not one of the options, follow the steps of the nursing process (clinical problem-solving process) as your guide to select your initial or first action.

   f. *Possible exception to the guideline:* If the question presents an emergency situation, read carefully. In an emergency situation, an intervention may be the priority.

4. Planning: Planning questions require providing input into plan development, assisting with the formulation of the goals of care, and assisting with the development of a plan of care (Box 5-14).

5. Implementation (Box 5-15)

   a. Implementation questions address the process of assisting with organizing and managing care, providing care to achieve established goals, and communicating and documenting nursing interventions thoroughly and accurately.

   b. Focus on a nursing action rather than on a medical action when you are answering a question, unless the question is asking you what prescribed medical action is anticipated.

Box 5-13 Practice Question: The Nursing Process/Data Collection

The nurse assists in developing a plan of care for an older client with diabetes mellitus. The nurse plans to first:

1. Structure menus for adherence to diet.
2. Teach with videotapes showing insulin administration to ensure competence.
3. Encourage dependence on others to prepare the client for the chronicity of the disease.
4. Determine the client's ability to read label markings on syringes and blood glucose monitoring equipment.

Answer: 4

Test-Taking Strategy: Note the strategic word "first." Use the steps of the nursing process to answer the question, remembering that data collection is the first step. The only option that addresses data collection is option 4. Options 1, 2, and 3 address the implementation step of the nursing process. Remember, data collection is the first step in the nursing process.

Box 5-14 Practice Question: The Nursing Process/Planning

A nurse reviews the plan of care for a client with a cataract and determines that which problem is the priority?

1. Concern about losing eyesight
2. Potential for injury related to decreased vision
3. Altered visual perception related to ocular lens opacity
4. Decreased ability to be active in the community

Answer: 3

Test-Taking Strategy: This question relates to the planning of nursing care and asks you to identify the priority problem. Use Maslow's Hierarchy of Needs theory to answer the question. Remembering that physiological needs are the priority will direct you to option 3. Potential for injury is a potential rather than an actual problem, and, according to Maslow's Hierarchy of Needs theory, safety is the second priority. Options 1 and 4 are psychosocial needs. Remember that planning is the second step of the nursing process!

Box 5-12 Data Collection: Strategic Words

- Check
- Collect
- Determine
- Find out
- Gather
- Identify
- Monitor
- Observe
- Obtain information
- Recognize

c. On the NCLEX-PN, the only client that you need to be concerned about is the client in the question that you are answering. Avoid the "What if...?" syndrome, and remember that the client in the question on the computer screen is your only assigned client.

d. Answer the question from a textbook and ideal perspective, and remember that the nurse has all the time and resources needed and readily available at the client's bedside; avoid the "What if...?" syndrome, and remember that you do not need to run to the treatment room to obtain sterile gauze, because it will be at the client's bedside.

6. Evaluation (Box 5-16)
   a. Evaluation questions focus on comparing the actual outcomes of care with the expected outcomes and on communicating and documenting findings.
   b. These questions focus on assisting with determining the client's response to care and on identifying factors that may interfere with achieving expected outcomes.
   c. With an evaluation question, watch for negative event queries, because they are frequently used with this type of question.

Box 5-15 Practice Question: The Nursing Process/Implementation

A nurse is checking the fundus of a postpartum woman and notes that the uterus is soft and spongy. Which nursing action is appropriate initially?
1. Notify the health care provider.
2. Encourage the mother to ambulate.
3. Massage the fundus gently until it is firm.
4. Document fundal position, consistency, and height.

Answer: 3
Test-Taking Strategy: Implementation questions address the process of organizing and managing care. Note the strategic word "initially." If the fundus is boggy (soft), it should be massaged gently until firm, and the nurse should observe for increased bleeding or clots. Remember that implementation is the third step of the nursing process!

Box 5-16 Practice Question: The Nursing Process/Evaluation

A client has just taken a dose of trimethobenzamide (Tigan). The nurse evaluates that the medication has been effective if the client states relief of:
1. Heartburn
2. Constipation
3. Abdominal pain
4. Nausea and vomiting

Answer: 4
Test-Taking Strategy: Note the strategic words "medication has been effective." These words indicate that this is an evaluation-type question. Recalling that this medication is an antiemetic will direct you to option 4. Remember that evaluation is the fourth step of the nursing process!

VII. CLIENT NEEDS

A. Safe and effective care environment
   1. These questions test the concepts that the nurse provides nursing care; collaborates with other health care team members to facilitate effective client care; and protects clients, significant others, and health care personnel from environmental hazards.
   2. Focus on safety with these types of questions, and remember the importance of handwashing, call bells, bed positioning, and the appropriate use of side rails.

B. Physiological integrity
   1. These questions test the concepts that the nurse provides comfort and assistance during the performance of activities of daily living; provides care related to the administration of medications; and monitors clients receiving parenteral therapies.
   2. These questions also address the nurse's ability to reduce the client's potential for developing complications or health problems related to treatments, procedures, or existing conditions and the nurse's role in providing care to clients with acute, chronic, or life-threatening physical health conditions.
   3. Focus on Maslow's Hierarchy of Needs theory for these types of questions, and remember that physiological needs are a priority and are addressed first.
   4. Use the ABCs—airway, breathing, and circulation—and the steps of the nursing process (clinical problem-solving process) when selecting an option that addresses physiological integrity.

C. Psychosocial integrity
   1. These questions test the concepts that the nurse provides nursing care that promotes and supports the emotional, mental, and social well-being of the client and significant others.
   2. Content addressed in these questions relates to supporting and promoting the client's or significant others' abilities to cope, adapt, or problem-solve in situations involving illnesses, disabilities, or stressful events such as abuse, neglect, or violence.

3. In this Client Needs category, you may be asked communication-type questions that relate to how you would respond to a client, a client's family members or significant others, or other health care team members.

4. Use therapeutic communication techniques to answer communication questions because of their effectiveness in the communication process.

5. Remember to select the option that focuses on the client's, the client's family members', or the client's significant others' thoughts, feelings, concerns, anxieties, and fears (Box 5-17).

D. Health promotion and maintenance

1. These questions test the concepts that the nurse provides and assists with directing nursing care to promote and maintain health.

2. Content addressed in these questions relates to assisting the client and significant others during the normal expected stages of growth and development from conception through advanced old age and to providing client care related to the prevention and early detection of health problems.

3. Use the Teaching and Learning Theory if the question addresses client teaching, remembering that client willingness, desire, and readiness to learn are the first priorities.

4. Watch for negative event queries, because they are frequently used in questions that address health promotion and maintenance and client education.

VIII. ELIMINATE COMPARABLE OR ALIKE OPTIONS (Box 5-18)

A. When reading the options, look for options that are comparable or alike; these options will include a similar concept or nursing action.

B. Comparable or alike options can be eliminated as possible answers.

IX. ELIMINATE OPTIONS THAT CONTAIN CLOSED-ENDED WORDS (Box 5-19)

A. Closed-ended words include all, always, every, must, none, never, and only.

B. Eliminate options with closed-ended words, because these words infer a fixed or extreme meaning. These types of options are usually incorrect.

C. Options that contain open-ended words such as may, usually, and generally should be considered as possible correct options.

Box 5-18 Practice Question: Eliminate Comparable or Alike Options

A nurse instructs an adolescent with iron-deficiency anemia about the administration of oral iron preparations. The nurse tells the adolescent that it is best to take the iron with:
1. Cola
2. Soda
3. Ginger ale
4. Tomato juice

Answer: 4
Test-Taking Strategy: Note that options 1, 2, and 3 are comparable or alike options in that they are carbonated beverages. Iron should be administered with vitamin-C–rich fluids, because vitamin C enhances the absorption of the iron preparation. Tomato juice contains a high content of ascorbic acid (vitamin C), whereas cola, soda, and ginger ale do not contain vitamin C. Remember to eliminate comparable or alike options!

Box 5-17 Practice Question: Communication

A client with a diagnosis of major depression says to the nurse, "I should have died. I've always been a failure." The nurse should make which therapeutic response to the client?
1. "I see a lot of positive things in you."
2. "You still have a great deal to live for."
3. "Feeling like a failure is part of your illness."
4. "You've been feeling like a failure for some time now?"

Answer: 4
Test-Taking Strategy: Remember the techniques that facilitate therapeutic communication to answer this question. Address the client's feelings and concerns. Option 4 is the only option that is stated in the form of a question and that is open-ended; this will encourage the verbalization of feelings. Remember to use therapeutic communication techniques and focus on the client.

Box 5-19 Practice Question: Eliminate Options That Contain Closed-Ended Words

A client will undergo a barium swallow, and the nurse provides preprocedure instructions to the client. The nurse instructs the client to:
1. Avoid eating or drinking after midnight before the test.
2. Take all routine medications on the morning of the test.
3. Have only a clear-liquid breakfast on the morning of the test.
4. Limit smoking to only two cigarettes on the morning of the test.

Answer: 1
Test-Taking Strategy: Note the closed-ended words *all* in option 2 and *only* in options 3 and 4. Remember to eliminate options that contain closed-ended words, because these options are usually incorrect. In addition, note that options 2, 3, and 4 are comparable or alike in that they all involve taking in something on the morning of the examination.

X. LOOK FOR THE UMBRELLA OPTION (Box 5-20)

A. When answering a question, look for the umbrella option.

B. The umbrella option is one that is a broad or universal statement and that usually contains the concepts of the other options within it.

C. The umbrella option will be the correct answer.

XI. USE THE GUIDELINES FOR DELEGATING AND ASSIGNMENT MAKING (Box 5-21)

A. You may be asked a question that will require you to decide how you will delegate a task or assign clients to other health care providers.

Box 5-20 Practice Question: Look for the Umbrella Option

A client who is admitted to the hospital is diagnosed with urethritis caused by chlamydial infection. The nurse implements which of the following precautions to prevent contraction of the infection during care?
1. Enteric precautions
2. Contact precautions
3. Standard precautions
4. Wearing gloves and a mask

Answer: 3

Test-Taking Strategy: Focus on the client's diagnosis and recall that this infection is sexually transmitted. Also, note that option 3 is the umbrella option. Remember, the umbrella option is a broad or universal option that includes the concepts of the other options in it!

Box 5-21 Practice Question: Use the Guidelines for Delegating and Assignment Making

A nurse is planning the client assignments for the day and most appropriately assigns which client to the nursing assistant?
1. A client on strict bedrest
2. A client with dyspnea who is receiving oxygen therapy
3. A client scheduled for transfer to the hospital for surgery
4. A client with a gastrostomy tube who requires tube feedings every 4 hours

Answer: 1

Test-Taking Strategy: Note that the question asks for the assignment to be delegated to the nursing assistant. When asked questions related to delegation, think about the role description of the employee and the needs of the client. A client scheduled for transfer to the hospital for surgery, a client with dyspnea who is receiving oxygen therapy, or a client with a gastrostomy tube who requires tube feedings every 4 hours has both physiological and psychosocial needs that require care by a licensed nurse. The nursing assistant has been trained to care for a client on bedrest. Remember to match the client's needs with the scope of practice of the health care provider!

B. Focus on the information in the question and the task or assignment that is to be delegated.

C. After you have determined what task or assignment is to be delegated, consider the client's needs, and match the client's needs with the scope of practice of the health care providers identified in the question.

D. The nurse practice act and any practice limitations define which aspects of care can be delegated and which must be performed by a nursing assistant, a licensed practical/vocational nurse, or a registered nurse.

E. Generally, noninvasive interventions such as skin care, range-of-motion exercises, ambulation, grooming, and hygiene measures can be assigned to a nursing assistant.

F. A licensed practical/vocational nurse can perform the tasks that a nursing assistant can in addition to certain invasive tasks such as dressings, suctioning, urinary catheterization, and administering oral, subcutaneous, intramuscular, and some intravenous piggyback (secondary) medications.

G. The registered nurse can perform the tasks that a licensed practical/vocational nurse can and is responsible for assessing, planning and supervising care, and initiating teaching.

XII. ANSWERING PHARMACOLOGY QUESTIONS (Box 5-22)

A. If you are familiar with the medication, use your nursing knowledge to answer the question.

B. Remember that the question will identify both the generic name and the trade name of the medication.

C. If the question identifies a medical diagnosis, then try to make a relationship between the medication and the diagnosis. For example, you can determine that cyclophosphamide (Neosar) is an antineoplastic

---

Box 5-22 Practice Question: Answering Pharmacology Questions

The nurse is preparing to administer atenolol (Tenormin) to a client. The nurse checks which of the following before administering the medication?
1. Temperature
2. Blood pressure
3. Potassium level
4. Blood glucose level

Answer: 2

Test-Taking Strategy: Focus on the name of the medication. Recall that most β-blocker medication names end with the letters -lol and that these medications are used to treat hypertension. This will direct you to option 2. Remember to focus on the medication name when answering pharmacology questions!

medication if the question refers to a client with breast cancer who is taking this medication.

D. Try to determine the classification of the medication being addressed to assist with answering the question. Identifying the classification will help with determining a medication's action and/or side effects; for example, diltiazem (*Cardizem*) is a cardiac medication.

E. Recognize the common side effects associated with each medication classification, and then relate the appropriate nursing interventions to each side effect. For example, if a side effect is hypertension, then the associated nursing intervention would be to monitor the blood pressure.

F. Learn the medications that belong to a classification by commonalities in their names; for example, medications that are xanthine bronchodilators end with the letters *-line* (e.g., theophyl*line*).

G. Look at the medication name, and use medical terminology to assist with determining the medication action; for example, *Lopressor* lowers (*Lo*) the blood pressure (*pressor*).

H. If the question requires a medication calculation, remember that an on-screen calculator is on the computer. Talk yourself through each step to be sure the answer makes sense, and recheck the calculation before answering the question, particularly if the answer seems like an unusual dosage.

I. Pyramid Points to remember
   1. Generally the client should not take an antacid with medication, because the antacid will affect the absorption of the medication.
   2. Enteric-coated and sustained-release tablets should not be crushed, and capsules should not be opened.
   3. The client should never adjust or change a medication dose or abruptly stop taking a medication.
   4. The nurse never adjusts or changes the client's medication dosage or discontinues a medication.
   5. The client needs to avoid taking any over-the-counter medications or herbal preparations unless they are approved for use by the health care provider.
   6. The client needs to avoid alcohol and smoking.
   7. Medications are never administered if the prescription is difficult to read or unclear or if it identifies a medication dose that is not a normal one.

Issues in Nursing

Cultural Diversity and Health Practices

PYRAMID TERMS

acculturation Process of learning norms, beliefs, and behavioral expectations of a group other than one's own group.

belief A theory accepted as true by a culture.

cultural assimilation Process in which individuals from a minority group are absorbed by the dominant culture and take on the characteristics of the dominant culture.

cultural competence Acquisition of knowledge, understanding, and appreciation of a culture that facilitates provision of culturally appropriate health care.

cultural diversity Differences among groups of people that result from ethnic, racial, and cultural variables.

cultural imposition Tendency to impose one's own beliefs, values, and patterns of behavior on individuals from another culture.

culture Dynamic network of knowledge, beliefs, patterns of behavior, ideas, attitudes, values, and norms that are unique to a particular group of people.

dominant culture Group whose values prevail within a society.

ethnic group People within a culture who share characteristics based on race, religion, color, national origin, or language.

ethnicity An individual's identification of self as part of an ethnic group.

ethnocentrism An assumption of cultural superiority and an inability to accept the ways of another culture.

minority group Ethnic, cultural, racial, or religious group that constitutes less than a numerical majority of the population.

race A grouping of people based on biological similarities. Members of a racial group have similar physical characteristics, such as blood group; facial features; and color of skin, hair, and eyes.

racism Discrimination directed toward individuals or groups who are perceived to be inferior.

stereotyping Expectation that all people within the same racial, ethnic, or cultural group act alike and share the same beliefs and attitudes.

subculture Social group within a culture that has distinctive characteristics, such as patterns of behavior or beliefs.

values Principles and standards that have meaning and worth to an individual, family, group, community, or culture.

PYRAMID TO SUCCESS

Nurses often care for clients who come from ethnic, cultural, or religious backgrounds that are different from their own. Awareness of and sensitivity to the unique health and illness beliefs and practices of people of different backgrounds are essential for the delivery of safe and effective care. Acknowledgment and acceptance of cultural differences with a nonjudgmental attitude are essential to providing culturally sensitive care. The NCLEX-PN exam test plan is unique and individualized to the client's culture and beliefs. The nurse needs to avoid stereotyping and needs to be aware that there are several subcultures within cultures and there are several dialects within languages. In nursing practice, the nurse needs to assess the client's perceived needs before planning and implementing nursing care. See Figure 6-1 for Giger and Davidhizar's Transcultural Assessment Model.

CLIENT NEEDS

Safe and Effective Care Environment

- Acting as a client advocate
- Ensuring ethical practices
- Ensuring legal rights and responsibilities
- Establishing priorities
- Maintaining confidentiality
- Providing continuity of care
- Respecting the client's control of personal environment and property
- Upholding client rights

Health Promotion and Maintenance

- Considering cultural issues related to family systems and family planning
- Respecting cultural preferences and lifestyle choices
- Promoting health and wellness
- Preventing disease
- Providing health screening
- Identifying changes related to the aging process

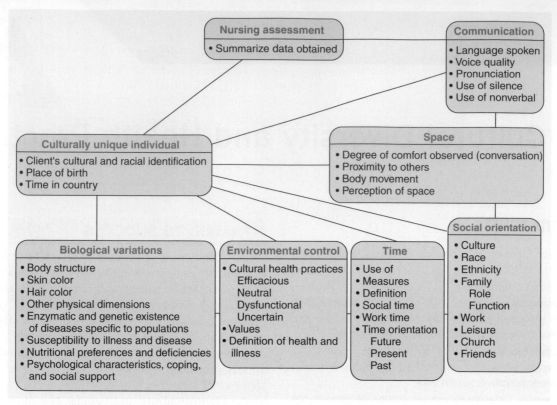

▲ **FIGURE 6-1** Giger and Davidhizar's Transcultural Assessment Model. (From Giger, J., & Davidhizar, R. [2008]. *Transcultural nursing: Assessment and intervention* [5th ed.]. St. Louis: Mosby.)

Psychosocial Integrity

- Providing a therapeutic environment
- Identifying clients who do not speak or understand English and determining how language needs will be met
- Assessing culture preferences and incorporating these preferences when planning and implementing care
- Respecting religious and spiritual influences on health (Box 6-1)
- Identifying support systems
- Identifying family dynamics as they relate to the client's culture
- Assessing the use of effective coping mechanisms
- Identifying end-of-life care issues

Physiological Integrity

- Identifying cultural differences for providing holistic client care
- Identifying cultural issues related to alternative and complementary therapies
- Identifying cultural issues related to receiving blood and blood products
- Implementing therapeutic procedures considering cultural preferences
- Providing nonpharmacological comfort interventions
- Providing nutrition and oral hydration (see Box 6-1)
- Providing palliative care

I. AFRICAN AMERICANS

A. Description: Citizens or residents of the United States who may have origins in any of the black populations in Africa.

B. Communication
   1. Members are competent in standard English.
   2. Head nodding does not always mean agreement.
   3. Prolonged eye contact may be interpreted as rudeness or aggressive behavior.
   4. Nonverbal communication may be important.
   5. Personal questions asked on initial contact with a person may be viewed as intrusive.

C. Time orientation and personal space preferences
   1. Time orientation varies according to age, socio-economics, and **subcultures** and may include past, present, or future orientation.
   2. Members may be late for an appointment because relationships and events that are occurring may be deemed more important than being on time.
   3. Members are comfortable with close personal space when interacting with family and friends.

D. Social roles
   1. Large extended family networks are important. Older adults are respected.
   2. Many households may be headed by a single-parent woman.
   3. Religious **beliefs** and church affiliation are sources of strength.

Box 6-1 Religions and Dietary Preferences

Seventh-Day Adventist (Church of God)
Alcohol and caffeinated beverages are usually prohibited.
Many are lacto ovo-vegetarians. Those who eat meat avoid
  pork.
Overeating is prohibited; 5 to 6 hours between meals without
  snacking is practiced.

Buddhism
Alcohol is usually prohibited.
Many are lacto-ovo-vegetarians.
Some eat fish, and some avoid only beef.

Roman Catholicism
They avoid meat on Ash Wednesday and Fridays during Lent.
They practice optional fasting during the Lenten season.
Children, pregnant women, and ill individuals are exempt
  from fasting.

Church of Jesus Christ of Latter-Day Saints (Mormon)
Alcohol, coffee, and tea are usually prohibited.
Consumption of meat is limited.
The first Sunday of the month is optional for fasting.

Hinduism
Many are vegetarians. Those who eat meat do not eat beef or
  pork.
Fasting rituals vary.
Children are not allowed to participate in fasting.

Islam
Pork, birds of prey, alcohol, and any meat product not ritually
  slaughtered are prohibited.

During the month of Ramadan, fasting occurs during the
  daytime.

Jehovah's Witness
Any foods to which blood has been added are prohibited.
They can eat animal flesh that has been drained.

Judaism
Orthodox believers need to adhere to dietary kosher laws:
- Meats allowed include animals that are vegetable eaters,
  cloven-hoofed animals, and animals that are ritually
  slaughtered.
- Fish that have scales and fins are allowed.
- Any combination of meat and milk is prohibited.
During Yom Kippur, 24-hour fasting is observed.
Pregnant women and seriously ill individuals are exempt from
  fasting.
During Passover, only unleavened bread is eaten.

Pentecostal (Assembly of God)
Alcohol is usually prohibited.
Members avoid consumption of anything to which blood has
  been added.
Some individuals avoid pork.

Eastern Orthodox
During Lent, all animal products, including dairy products, are
  forbidden.
Fasting occurs during Advent.
Exceptions from fasting include illness and pregnancy.

E. Health and illness
  1. Religious **beliefs** profoundly affect ideas about health and illness.
  2. Food preferences include such items as fried foods, chicken, pork, greens, and rice; some pregnant African-American women engage in pica.
F. Health risks
  1. Sickle cell anemia
  2. Hypertension
  3. Heart disease
  4. Cancer
  5. Lactose intolerance
  6. Diabetes mellitus
  7. Obesity
G. Interventions
  1. Assess each individual for cultural preferences because there are many individual and **subculture** variations.
  2. Build a relationship based on trust.
  3. Assess the meaning of the client's verbal and nonverbal behavior.
  4. Be flexible and avoid rigidity in scheduling care.
  5. Encourage family involvement.
  6. Alternative modes of healing include herbs, prayer, and laying on of hands practices.

⚠ Learn about the cultures of clients with whom you will be working; also, ask clients about their health care practices and preferences.

II. AMISH

A. Description: The Amish are known for simple living, plain dress, and reluctance to adopt modern conveniences and can be considered a distinct **ethnic group**; the various Amish church fellowships are Christian religious denominations that form a very traditional subgrouping of Mennonite churches. (See Box 6-2 for Amish communities.)
B. Cultural **beliefs** and preferences (Box 6-3)

⚠ Cultural beliefs and preferences vary depending on specific Amish community membership.

C. Interventions
  1. Assess each individual for cultural preferences because there may be individual and group variations.
  2. Speak to both the husband and the wife regarding health care decisions because they consider themselves partners in family life.

3. Health instructions must be given in simple, clear language.
4. Most Amish need to have church (bishop and community) permission to be hospitalized because the community will come together to help pay the costs.

Box 6-2 Amish Communities

Old Order Amish
Members live in rural communities in North America and are known for their plain dress and limited use of technology.

Amish Mennonites
This broad term is used for churches that split from the Old Order Amish. Some have a lifestyle similar to the Old Order Amish, whereas others do not.

Beachy Amish
Members have fewer limits on the use of technology and do not shun those who join Mennonite churches.

New Order Amish
This is the least restrictive Amish group. The use of electricity in the home is permitted, and shunning is not practiced.

5. Usually, Amish do not have health insurance because it is a "worldly product" and may show a lack of faith in God.
6. Barriers to modern health care include distance, lack of transportation, cost, and language (most do not understand scientific jargon).

⚠ Be alert to cues regarding eye contact, personal space, time concepts, and understanding of the recommended plan of care.

III. ASIAN AMERICANS

A. Description: Americans of Asian descent; can include **ethnic groups** such as Chinese Americans, Filipino Americans, Indian Americans, Vietnamese Americans, Korean Americans, Japanese Americans and others whose national origin is from the Asian continent.
B. Communication
   1. Languages include Chinese, Japanese, Korean, Filipino, Vietnamese, and English.
   2. Silence is valued.
   3. Eye contact may be considered inappropriate or disrespectful.

Box 6-3 Amish Cultural Beliefs and Preferences

Amish maintain a culture distinct and separate from the non-Amish.

They usually speak a German dialect called Pennsylvania Dutch.

German language is usually used during worship. English is usually learned in school.

Men follow the laws of the Hebrew Scriptures with regard to beards (mustaches are not grown because of the long-perceived association of mustaches with the military).

Men dress in plain, dark-colored suits; women wear plain dresses with long sleeves, as well as bonnets and aprons.

The wearing of jewelry, including wedding rings and wristwatches, is prohibited. Zippers, seen as labor-saving devices, are also forbidden.

During Rumspringa, a period that begins around the age of 16 years, youth decide whether to be baptized into the Amish church or leave the community. In some communities, Rumspringa is a time of relaxed standards.

Marriage outside the faith is usually not allowed.

Shunning is a practice in which a member is punished after violating religious rules and usually required to leave the community for a specified period of time.

Women are not allowed to hold positions of power in the congregational organization.

Family life has a patriarchal structure.

The husband is usually considered the authority figure in the family, but normal practice is to speak to both the husband and wife regarding health care decisions, because they consider themselves partners in family life. However, the nurse must consider client confidentiality and privacy before discussing such issues with both spouses.

Although the roles of women are considered equally important to those of men, they are very unequal in terms of authority.

Unmarried women remain under the authority of their fathers.

Wives are submissive to their husbands.

Amish generally remain separate from the rest of the world, physically and socially.

They reject materialism and worldliness.

Some Amish prefer not to be photographed.

They value living simply and may choose to avoid technology, such as electricity and cars.

Amish highly value responsibility, generosity, and helping others.

They often work as farmers, builders, quilters, and homemakers.

Some Amish use traditional health care and alternative health care measures and practices, such as healers, herbs, and massage.

They believe that health is a gift from God, but that clean living and a balanced diet help maintain it.

The Amish have fewer risk factors for disease than the general American population because of their practice of manual labor, consumption of fresh foods, and rare use of tobacco and alcohol; however, the risk of certain genetic disorders is increased because of intermarriage.

Sexual abuse of women is a problem in some communities.

Many choose not to have health insurance and maintain mutual aid funds for Amish members to help with medical costs.

4. Criticism or disagreement is not expressed verbally.
5. Head nodding does not always mean agreement.
6. The word "no" may be interpreted as disrespect for others.

C. Time orientation and personal space preferences
1. Time orientation reflects respect for the past, but includes emphasis on the present and future.
2. Formal personal space is preferred except with family and close friends.
3. Members usually do not touch others during conversation.
4. For some **cultures**, touching is unacceptable between members of the opposite gender.
5. The head is considered to be sacred in some **cultures**; touching someone on the head may be disrespectful.

D. Social roles
1. Members are devoted to tradition.
2. Large extended-family networks are common.
3. Loyalty to immediate and extended family and honor are valued.
4. Family unit is structured and hierarchical.
5. Men have the power and authority, and women are expected to be obedient.
6. Education is viewed as important.
7. Religions include Taoism, Buddhism, Confucianism, Shintoism, Hinduism, Islam, and Christianity.
8. Social organizations are strong within the community.

E. Health and illness
1. Health is a state of physical and spiritual harmony with nature and a balance between positive and negative energy forces (yin and yang).
2. A healthy body may be viewed as a gift from the ancestors.
3. Illness may be viewed as an imbalance between yin and yang.
4. Yin foods are cold and yang foods are hot; one eats cold foods when one has a hot illness, and one eats hot foods when one has a cold illness.
5. Illness may also be attributed to prolonged sitting or lying or to overexertion.
6. Food preferences include raw fish, rice, and vegetables.

F. Health risks
1. Hypertension
2. Heart disease
3. Cancer
4. Lactose intolerance
5. Thalassemia

G. Interventions
1. Assess each individual for cultural preferences because there are many individual and **subculture** variations.

2. Be aware of and respect physical boundaries; request permission to touch the client before doing so.
3. Limit eye contact.
4. Avoid gesturing with hands.
5. If possible, a female client prefers a female health care provider.
6. Clarify responses to questions and expectations of the health care provider.
7. Be flexible and avoid rigidity in scheduling care.
8. Encourage family involvement.
9. Alternative modes of healing include herbs, acupuncture, restoration of balance with foods, massage, and offering of prayers and incense.

⚠ If health care recommendations, interventions, or treatments do not fit within the client's cultural values, they will not be followed.

IV. HISPANIC AND LATINO AMERICANS

A. Description: Americans of origins in Latin countries; Mexican Americans, Cuban Americans, Colombian Americans, Dominican Americans, Puerto Rican Americans, Spanish Americans, and Salvadoran Americans are some Hispanic and Latino American subgroups.

B. Communication
1. Languages include primarily English and Spanish.
2. Members tend to be verbally expressive, yet confidentiality is important.
3. Avoiding eye contact with a person in authority may indicate respect and attentiveness.
4. Direct confrontation is usually disrespectful and the expression of negative feelings may be impolite.
5. Dramatic body language, such as gestures or facial expressions, may be used to express emotion or pain.

C. Time orientation and personal space preferences
1. Members are usually oriented more to the present.
2. Members may be late for an appointment because relationships and events that are occurring are valued more than being on time.
3. Members are comfortable in close proximity with family, friends, and acquaintances.
4. Members are very tactile and use embraces and handshakes.
5. Members value the physical presence of others.
6. Politeness and modesty are important.

D. Social roles
1. The nuclear family is the basic unit; also, large, extended-family networks are common.
2. The extended family is highly regarded.
3. Needs of the family take precedence over the needs of an individual family member.

4. Depending on age and **acculturation** factors, men are usually the decision makers and wage earners, and women are the caretakers and homemakers.

5. Religion usually is Catholicism, but may vary depending on origin.

6. Members usually have strong church affiliations.

7. Social organizations are strong within the community.

E. Health and illness

1. Health may be viewed as a reward from God or a result of good luck.

2. Some members believe that health results from a state of physical and emotional balance.

3. Illness may be viewed by some members to be a result of God's punishment for sins.

4. Some members may adhere to nontraditional health measures such as folk medicine.

F. Health risks

1. Hypertension
2. Heart disease
3. Diabetes mellitus
4. Obesity
5. Lactose intolerance
6. Parasites

G. Interventions

1. Assess each individual for cultural preferences because there are many individual and **subculture** variations.

2. Allow time for the client to discuss treatment options with family members.

3. Protect privacy.

4. Offer to call clergy because of the significance of religious preferences related to illnesses.

5. Ask permission before touching a child when planning to examine or care for him or her.

6. Be flexible regarding time of arrival for appointments and avoid rigidity in scheduling care.

7. Alternative modes of healing include herbs, consultation with lay healers, restoration of balance with hot or cold foods, prayer, and religious medals.

! Treat each client and individuals accompanying the client with respect and appreciate the differences and diversity of beliefs about health, illness, and treatment modalities.

V. NATIVE AMERICANS

A. Description: Term that the U.S. government uses to describe indigenous peoples from the regions of North America encompassed by the continental United States, including parts of Alaska and the island state of Hawaii; comprise a large number of distinct tribes, states, and **ethnic groups**, many of which survive as intact political communities.

B. Communication

1. There is much linguistic diversity, depending on origin.

2. Silence indicates respect for the speaker for some groups.

3. Some members may speak in a low tone of voice and expect others to be attentive.

4. Eye contact may be viewed as a sign of disrespect.

5. Body language is important.

C. Time orientation and personal space preferences

1. Members are oriented primarily to the present.

2. Personal space is important.

3. Members may lightly touch another person's hand during greetings.

4. Massage may be used for newborn to promote bonding between the infant and mother.

5. Some groups may prohibit touching of a dead body.

D. Social roles

1. Members are family oriented.

2. Basic family unit is the extended family, which often includes persons from several households.

3. In some groups, grandparents are viewed as family leaders.

4. Elders are honored.

5. Children are taught to respect traditions.

6. The father usually does all the work outside the home, and the mother assumes responsibility for domestic duties.

7. Sacred myths and legends provide spiritual guidance for some groups.

8. Most members adhere to some form of Christianity, and religion and healing practices are usually integrated.

9. Community social organizations are important.

E. Health and illness

1. Health is usually considered a state of harmony between the individual, family, and environment.

2. Some groups believe that illness is caused by supernatural forces and disequilibrium between the person and environment.

3. Traditional health and illness **beliefs** may continue to be observed by some groups, including natural and religious folk medicine tradition.

4. For some groups, food preferences include cornmeal, fish, game, fruits, and berries.

F. Health risks

1. Alcohol abuse
2. Obesity
3. Heart disease
4. Diabetes mellitus
5. Tuberculosis
6. Arthritis
7. Lactose intolerance
8. Gallbladder disease

G. Interventions
1. Assess each individual for cultural preferences because there may be individual variations.
2. Clarify communication.
3. Understand that the client may be attentive, even when eye contact is absent.
4. Be attentive to your own use of body language.
5. Obtain input from members of the extended family.
6. Encourage the client to personalize space in which health care is delivered; for example, encourage the client to bring personal items or objects to the hospital.
7. In the home, assess for the availability of running water, and modify infection control and hygiene practices as necessary.
8. Alternative modes of healing include herbs, restoration of balance between the person and the universe, and consultation with traditional healers.

⚠ If language barriers pose a problem, seek a qualified medical interpreter; avoid using ancillary staff or family members as interpreters.

VI. WHITE AMERICANS

A. Description: Term used to include U.S. citizens or residents having origins in any of the original people of Europe, the Middle East, or North Africa; the term is interchangeable with Caucasian American.
B. Communication
1. Languages include language of origin (e.g., Italian, Polish, French, Russian) and English.
2. Silence can be used to show respect or disrespect for another, depending on the situation.
3. Eye contact is usually viewed as indicating trustworthiness in most origins.
C. Time orientation and personal space preferences
1. Members are usually future oriented.
2. Time is valued; members tend to be on time and to be impatient with people who are not on time.
3. Some members may tend to avoid close physical contact.
4. Handshakes are usually used for formal greetings.
D. Social roles
1. The nuclear family is the basic unit; the extended family is also important.
2. The man is usually the dominant figure, but a variation of gender roles exists within families and relationships.
3. Religions are varied, depending on origin.
4. Community social organizations are important.
E. Health and illness
1. Health is usually viewed as an absence of disease or illness.

2. Many members usually have a tendency to be stoical when expressing physical concerns.
3. Members usually rely primarily on the modern Western health care delivery system.
4. Food preferences are based on origin; many members prefer items containing carbohydrates and red meat items.
F. Health risks
1. Cancer
2. Heart disease
3. Diabetes mellitus
4. Obesity
5. Hypertension
G. Interventions
1. Assess each individual for cultural preferences based on origin.
2. Build a relationship based on trust.
3. Assess the meaning of the client's verbal and nonverbal behavior.
4. Respect the client's personal space and time.
5. Be flexible and avoid rigidity in scheduling care.
6. Encourage family involvement.

VII. END-OF-LIFE CARE (Box 6-4)

A. Christian Science religion is unlikely to use medical means to prolong life.
B. People in the Jewish faith generally oppose prolonging life after irreversible brain damage.
C. Some Eastern Orthodox religions, Muslims, and Orthodox Jews may prohibit, oppose, or discourage autopsy.
D. Islam permits organ donation for the purpose of saving human life.
E. Amish permit organ donation with the exception of heart transplants (the heart is the soul of the body).
F. Buddhists in the United States encourage organ donation and consider it an act of mercy.
G. Some Mormon, Eastern Orthodox, Islamic, and Jewish (Conservative and Orthodox) faiths discourage, oppose, or prohibit cremation.
H. Hindus usually prefer cremation and cast the ashes in a holy river.
I. Hispanic and Latino groups
1. The family generally makes decisions and may request to withhold the diagnosis or prognosis from the client.
2. Extended-family members often are involved in end-of-life care (pregnant women may be prohibited from caring for dying clients or attending funerals).
3. Several family members may be at the dying client's bedside.
4. Vocal expression of grief and mourning are acceptable and expected.
5. Members usually refuse procedures that alter the body, such as organ donation or autopsy.
6. Dying at home may be considered bad luck.

J. African Americans
1. Members discuss issues with the spouse or older family member (elders are held in high respect).
2. Family is highly valued and is central to the care of terminally ill members.
3. Open displays of emotion are common and accepted.
4. Organ and blood donation are usually are not allowed.
5. Members prefer to die at home.

K. Asian Americans
1. Family members may make decisions about care and often do not tell the client the diagnosis or prognosis.
2. Dying at home may be considered bad luck.
3. Organ donation is usually not allowed.

L. Native Americans
1. Family meetings may be held to make decisions about end-of-life and the type of treatments that should be pursued.
2. Some groups avoid contact with the dying (may prefer to die in the hospital).

⚠ Provide individualized end-of-life care to clients and families.

VIII. COMPLEMENTARY AND ALTERNATIVE MEDICINE (CAM)

A. Description
1. Therapies are used in addition to conventional treatment to provide healing resources and focus on the mind-body connection.
2. High-risk therapies (therapies that are invasive) and low-risk therapies (those that are noninvasive) are included in CAM.

B. Whole medical systems
1. Traditional Chinese medicine (TCM): Focuses on restoring and maintaining a balanced flow of vital energy; interventions include acupressure, acupuncture, herbal therapies, diet, meditation, tai chi, and qi gong (exercise that focuses on breathing, visualization, and movement).
2. Ayurveda: Focuses on the balance of mind, body, and spirit; interventions include diet, medicinal

---

Box 6-4 Religion and End-of-Life Care

Christianity

Catholic and Orthodox
A priest anoints the sick.
Other sacraments before death include reconciliation and Holy Communion.

Protestant
No last rites are provided (anointing of the sick is accepted by some groups).
Prayers are given to offer comfort and support.

Church of Jesus Christ of Latter-Day Saints (Mormons)
A sacrament may be administered if the client requests.

Jehovah's Witness
Members do not believe in sacraments.
Members are excommunicated if they receive a blood transfusion.

Amish
Funerals are conducted in the home without a eulogy, flower decorations, or any other display. Caskets are plain and simple, without adornment.
At death, a woman is usually buried in her bridal dress.
One is believed to live on after death, either with eternal reward in heaven or punished in hell.

Islam
Second-degree male relatives such as cousins or uncles should be the contact person and determine whether the client or family should be given information about the client.
The client may choose to face Mecca (west or southwest in the United States).

The head should be elevated above the body.
Discussions about death usually are not welcomed.
Stopping medical treatment is against the will of Allah (Arabic word for God).
Grief may be expressed through slapping or hitting the body.
If possible, only a same-gender Muslim should handle the body after death. If this is not possible, non-Muslims should wear gloves so as not to touch the body.

Judaism
Prolongation of life is important (a client on life support must remain so until death).
A dying person should not be left alone (a rabbi's presence is desired).
Autopsy and cremation are usually not allowed.

Hinduism
Rituals include tying a thread around the neck or wrist of the dying person, sprinkling the person with special water, and placing a leaf of basil on their tongue.
After death, the sacred threads are not removed, and the body is not washed.

Buddhism
A shrine to Buddha may be placed in the client's room.
Time for meditation at the shrine is important and should be respected.
Clients may refuse medications that may alter their awareness (e.g., opioids).
After death, a monk may recite prayers for 1 hour (need not be done in the presence of the body).

herbs, detoxification, massage, breathing exercises, meditation, and yoga.
3. Homeopathy: Focuses on healing and interventions consisting of small doses of specially prepared plant and mineral extracts that assist in the innate healing process of the body.
4. Naturopathy: Focuses on enhancing the natural healing responses of the body; interventions include nutrition, herbology, hydrotherapy, acupuncture, physical therapies, and counseling.

C. Mind-body medicine
1. Mind-body medicine focuses on the interactions among the brain, mind, body, and behavior and on the powerful ways in which emotional, mental, social, spiritual, and behavioral factors can directly affect health.
2. Interventions include biofeedback, hypnosis, relaxation therapy, meditation, visual imagery, yoga, tai chi, qi gong, cognitive-behavioral therapies, group supports, autogenic training, and spirituality.

D. Biologically based practices (Box 6-5)
1. Biologically based therapies in CAM use substances found in nature, such as herbs, foods, and vitamins.
2. Therapies include botanicals, prebiotics and probiotics, whole-food diets, functional foods, animal-derived extracts, vitamins, minerals, fatty acids, amino acids, and proteins.

E. Manipulative and body-based practices
1. Interventions involve manipulation and movement of the body by a therapist.
2. Interventions include practices such as chiropractic and osteopathic manipulation, massage therapy, and reflexology.

F. Energy medicine
1. Energy therapies focus on energy originating within the body or on energy from other sources.

2. Interventions include sound energy therapy, light therapy, acupuncture, qi gong, reiki and johre, therapeutic touch, intercessory prayer, whole medical systems, and magnetic therapy.

IX. HERBAL THERAPIES (Box 6-6)

A. Herbal therapy is the use of herbs (plant or a plant part) for the therapeutic value on health.
B. Some herbs have been determined to be safe, but some herbs, even in small amounts, can be toxic.
C. If the client is taking prescription medications, the client should consult with the health care provider regarding the use of herbs because serious herb-medication interactions can occur.

Box 6-5 Biologically Based Practices

Aromatherapy
The use of topical or inhaled oils (plant extracts) that promote and maintain health

Herbal Therapies
The use of herbs derived mostly from plant sources that maintain and restore balance and health

Macrobiotic Diet
Diet high in whole-grain cereals, vegetables, beans, sea vegetables, and vegetarian soups
Elimination of meat, animal fat, eggs, poultry, dairy products, sugars, and artificially produced food from the diet

Orthomolecular Therapy
Focus on nutritional balance, including use of vitamins, essential amino acids, essential fats, and minerals

---

Box 6-6 Commonly Used Herbs and Health Products

Aloe: Anti-inflammatory and antimicrobial effect; accelerates wound healing
Angelica: Antispasmodic and vasodilator; balances the effects of estrogen
Bilberry: Improves microcirculation in the eyes
Black cohosh: Produces estrogen-like effects
Cat's claw: Antioxidant; stimulates the immune system, lowers blood pressure
Chamomile: Antispasmodic and anti-inflammatory; produces mild sedative effect
Dehydroepiandrosterone (DHEA): Converts to androgens and estrogen; slows the effects of aging; used for erectile dysfunction
Echinacea: Stimulates immune system
Evening primrose: Assists with metabolism of fatty acid
Feverfew: Anti-inflammatory; used for migraine headaches, arthritis, and fever
Garlic: Antioxidant; used to lower cholesterol levels
Ginger: Antiemetic; used for nausea and vomiting
Ginkgo biloba: Antioxidant; used to improve memory
Ginseng: Increases physical endurance and stamina; used for stress and fatigue
Glucosamine: Amino acid that assists in the synthesis of cartilage
Goldenseal: Anti-inflammatory and antimicrobial used to stimulate the immune system; has an anticoagulant effect and may increase blood pressure
Kava: Antianxiety and skeletal muscle relaxant; produces a sedative effect
Melatonin: A hormone that regulates sleep; used for insomnia
Milk thistle: Antioxidant; stimulates the production of new liver cells, reduces liver inflammation; used for liver and gallbladder disease
Peppermint oil: Antispasmodic; used for irritable bowel syndrome
St. John's wort: Antibacterial, antiviral, antidepressant
Saw palmetto: Antiestrogen activity; used for urinary tract infections and benign prostatic hypertrophy
Valerian: Used to treat nervous disorders such as anxiety, restlessness, and insomnia
Zinc: Antiviral; stimulates the immune system

D. Client teaching points
   1. Discuss herbal therapies with the health care provider before use.
   2. Contact the health care provider if any side effects of the herbal substance occur.
   3. Contact the health care provider before stopping the use of a prescription medication.
   4. Avoid using herbs to treat a serious medical condition such as heart disease.
   5. Avoid taking herbs if pregnant or attempting to get pregnant or if nursing.
   6. Do not give herbs to infants or young children.
   7. Purchase herbal supplements only from a reputable manufacturer. The label should contain the scientific name of the herb, name and address of the manufacturer, batch or lot number, date of manufacture, and expiration date.
   8. Adhere to the recommended dose. If herbal preparations are taken in high doses, they can be toxic.
   9. Moisture, sunlight, and heat may alter the components of herbal preparations.
   10. If surgery is planned, the herbal therapy may need to be discontinued 2 to 3 weeks before surgery.

⚠ Some herbs have been determined to be safe, but some herbs, even in small amounts, can be toxic. Inform the client to discuss herbal therapies with the health care provider before use.

X. LOW-RISK THERAPIES

A. Low-risk therapies are therapies that have no adverse effects and, when implementing care, can be used by the nurse who has training and experience in their use.
B. Common low-risk therapies
   1. Meditation
   2. Relaxation techniques
   3. Imagery
   4. Music therapy
   5. Massage
   6. Touch
   7. Laughter and humor
   8. Spiritual measures, such as prayer

MORE QUESTIONS ON EVOLVE!

Practice Questions

1. A client is diagnosed with cancer and is told that surgery followed by chemotherapy will be necessary. The client states to the nurse, "I have read a lot about complementary therapies. Do you think that I should try any?" The nurse responds by making which appropriate statement?
   1. "You need to ask your health care provider about it."
   2. "I would try anything that I could if I had cancer."
   3. "No, because it will interact with the chemotherapy."
   4. "There are many different forms of complementary therapies. Let's talk about these therapies."

2. A nurse is preparing to assist a Jewish client with eating lunch. A kosher meal is delivered to the client. Which nursing action is appropriate when assisting the client with the meal?
   1. Unwrapping the eating utensils for the client
   2. Replacing the plastic utensils with metal utensils
   3. Carefully transferring the food from paper plates to glass plates
   4. Asking the client to unwrap the utensils and allowing the client to prepare the meal for eating

3. A nurse is caring for a group of clients who are taking herbal medications at home. Which of the following clients should be instructed not to take herbal medications?
   1. A 60-year-old male client with rhinitis
   2. A 24-year-old male client with a lower back injury
   3. A 10-year-old female client with a urinary tract infection
   4. A 45-year-old female client with a history of migraine headaches

4. The client asks the student nurse about various herbal therapies available for the treatment of insomnia. The student could provide information about which of the following?
   1. Garlic
   2. Valerian
   3. Lavender
   4. Glucosamine

5. A nurse is assisting with collecting data from an African-American client admitted to the ambulatory care unit who is scheduled for a hernia repair. Which of the following information about the client is of least priority during the data collection?
   1. Respiratory
   2. Psychosocial
   3. Neurological
   4. Cardiovascular

6. A nurse is planning to reinforce nutrition instructions to an African-American client. When developing the plan, the nurse is aware that a common dietary practice of clients with African-American heritage is to eat:
   1. Raw fish
   2. Red meat
   3. Fried foods
   4. Rice as the basis for all meals

7. A nurse consults with a dietitian regarding the dietary preferences of an Asian-American client. Which of the following foods would the nurse likely include in the diet plan?
   1. Rice
   2. Fruits
   3. Red meat
   4. Fried foods

8. An antihypertensive medication has been prescribed for a client with hypertension. The client tells the nurse that she would like to take an herbal substance to help lower her blood pressure. The nurse should:
   1. Tell the client that herbal substances are not safe and should never be used.
   2. Advise the client to discuss the use of an herbal substance with the health care provider (HCP).
   3. Teach the client how to take her blood pressure so that it can be monitored closely.
   4. Tell the client that if she takes the herbal substance, she will need to have her blood pressure checked frequently.

9. A Hispanic-American mother brings her child to the clinic for an examination. Which of the following is most important when gathering data about the child?
   1. Avoiding eye contact
   2. Using body language only
   3. Avoiding speaking to the child
   4. Touching the child during the examination

10. A nursing student is asked to identify the practices and beliefs of the Amish society. **Select all that apply.**
    ❒ 1. Many choose not to have health insurance.
    ❒ 2. They believe that health is a gift from God.
    ❒ 3. The authority of women is equal to that of men.
    ❒ 4. They remain secluded and avoid helping others.
    ❒ 5. They use both traditional and alternative health care, such as healers, herbs, and massage.
    ❒ 6. Funerals are conducted in the home without a eulogy, flower decorations, or any other display. Caskets are plain and simple, without adornment.

ANSWERS

1. 4

Rationale: Complementary (alternative) therapies include a wide variety of treatment modalities that are used in addition to conventional treatment to treat a disease or illness. These therapies complement conventional treatment, but they should be approved by the person's health care provider to ensure that the treatment does not interact with prescribed therapy. Although the health care provider should approve the use of a complementary therapy and although some of these therapies can interact with the prescribed treatment plan, the statements in options 1 and 3 are inappropriate. Similarly, option 2 is an inappropriate response to the client. Option 4 addresses the client's question and encourages discussion.
Test-Taking Strategy: Use therapeutic communication techniques. Eliminate options 1, 2, and 3, because they are nontherapeutic. Option 4 is the only option that addresses the client's question and encourages discussion. Review therapeutic communication techniques if you had difficulty with this question.
Level of Cognitive Ability: Applying
Client Needs: Physiological Integrity
Integrated Process: Communication and Documentation
Content Area: Fundamental Skills: Cultural Diversity
References: Christensen, Kockrow, pp. 40–46, 416–418. 2011. *Foundations and adult health nursing.*
DeWit, pp. 1174–1176. 2009.

2. 4

Rationale: Kosher meals arrive on paper plates and with plastic utensils sealed. Health care providers should not unwrap the utensils or transfer the food to another serving dish. Although the nurse may want to be helpful by assisting the client with the meal, the only appropriate option for this client is option 4.

Test-Taking Strategy: Use the process of elimination and your knowledge regarding the rituals associated with kosher meals. Options 2 and 3 are comparable or alike and can be eliminated first. To choose from the remaining options, it is necessary to be familiar with kosher rituals. If you had difficulty with this question, review the dietary practices of the Jewish client.
Level of Cognitive Ability: Applying
Client Needs: Psychosocial Integrity
Integrated Process: Nursing Process/Implementation
Content Area: Fundamental Skills: Cultural Diversity
References: Jarvis, p. 178. 2012.
Nix, p. 256. 2009.
Schlenker, p. 5. 2011.

3. 3

Rationale: Children should not be given herbal therapies, especially in the home and without professional supervision. There are no general contraindications for the clients described in options 1, 2, and 4.
Test-Taking Strategy: Use the process of elimination and your knowledge regarding herbal therapies. Note the age in option 3 to direct you to this option. Options 1, 2, and 4 describe clients for which there are no contraindications and can thus be eliminated. If you had difficulty with this question, review the indications and contraindications for herbal therapies.
Level of Cognitive Ability: Analyzing
Client Needs: Safe and Effective Care Environment
Integrated Process: Nursing Process/Data Collection
Content Area: Fundamental Skills: Cultural Diversity
Reference: Christensen, Kockrow, p. 421. 2011. *Foundations and adult health nursing.*

4. 2

Rationale: Valerian has been used to treat insomnia, hyper-activity, and stress. It has also been used to treat nervous disorders such as anxiety and restlessness. Garlic is used as an antioxidant and to lower cholesterol levels. Glucosamine is an amino acid that assists with the synthesis of cartilage. Lavender is used as an antiseptic and fragrance for a mild sedative effect.

Test-Taking Strategy: Use the process of elimination and your knowledge regarding herbal therapies to assist with answering this question. Focus on the subject of a substance that may be used to treat insomnia, and remember that valerian has been used to treat insomnia. If you had difficulty with this question, review specific herbal therapies.

Level of Cognitive Ability: Understanding
Client Needs: Physiological Integrity
Integrated Process: Nursing Process/Implementation
Content Area: Fundamental Skills/Cultural Diversity
Reference: Christensen, Kockrow, p. 420. 2011. *Foundations and adult health nursing.*

5. 2

Rationale: The psychosocial data is the least priority during the initial admission data collection. In the African-American culture, it is considered intrusive to ask personal questions during the initial contact or meeting. Additionally, respiratory, neurological, and cardiovascular data include physiological assessments that would be the priority.

Test-Taking Strategy: Note the strategic words "least priority." Use Maslow's Hierarchy of Needs theory to answer the question. Options 1, 3, and 4 address physiological needs. Review the characteristics of the African-American culture if you had difficulty with this question.

Level of Cognitive Ability: Understanding
Client Needs: Physiological Integrity
Integrated Process: Nursing Process/Data Collection
Content Area: Fundamental Skills: Cultural Diversity
Reference: Christensen, Kockrow, p. 175. 2011. *Foundations and adult health nursing.*

6. 3

Rationale: African-American food preferences include chicken, pork, greens, rice, and fried foods. Asian Americans eat raw fish, rice, and soy sauce. Hispanic Americans prefer beans, fried foods, spicy foods, chili, and carbonated beverages. European Americans prefer carbohydrates and red meat.

Test-Taking Strategy: Use the process of elimination. Recalling that African Americans are at risk for hypertension and coronary artery disease will direct you to option 3. Review the food preferences of the African-American culture if you had difficulty with this question.

Level of Cognitive Ability: Understanding
Client Needs: Physiological Integrity
Integrated Process: Teaching and Learning
Content Area: Fundamental Skills: Cultural Diversity
References: Christensen, Kockrow, p. 177. 2011. *Foundations and adult health nursing.*
Nix, pp. 259–260. 2009.

7. 1

Rationale: Asian-American food preferences include raw fish, rice, and soy sauce. African-American food preferences include chicken, pork, greens, rice, and fried foods. Hispanic Americans prefer beans, fried foods, spicy foods, chili, and car-bonated beverages. European Americans prefer carbohydrates and red meat.

Test-Taking Strategy: Knowledge regarding the food practices and preferences related to various cultures is required to answer the question. Correlate rice with Asian Americans to answer questions similar to this one. Review the food preferences associated with the Asian-American culture if you had difficulty with this question.

Level of Cognitive Ability: Understanding
Client Needs: Physiological Integrity
Integrated Process: Nursing Process/Planning
Content Area: Fundamental Skills: Cultural Diversity
Reference: Nix, pp. 262–263. 2009.

8. 2

Rationale: Although herbal substances may have some bene-ficial effects, not all herbs are safe to use. Clients who are being treated with conventional medication therapy should be ad-vised to avoid herbal substances with similar pharmacological effects, because the combination may lead to an excessive reac-tion or unknown interaction effects. Therefore, the nurse would advise the client to discuss the use of the herbal sub-stance with the HCP.

Test-Taking Strategy: Use the process of elimination. Eliminate option 1 first because of the closed-ended word "never." Next, eliminate options 3 and 4, because they are comparable or alike. Review the limitations associated with the use of herbal substances if you had difficulty with this question.

Level of Cognitive Ability: Applying
Client Needs: Physiological Integrity
Integrated Process: Nursing Process/Implementation
Content Area: Fundamental Skills: Cultural Diversity
Reference: Christensen, Kockrow, pp. 85–86. 2011. *Founda-tions and adult health nursing.*

9. 4

Rationale: In the Hispanic-American culture, eye behavior is significant. It is believed that the "bad/evil eye" can be given to a child if a person looks at and admires a child without touching the child. Therefore, touching the child during the ex-amination is very important. Although avoiding eye contact in-dicates respect and attentiveness, this is not the most important intervention. Avoiding speaking to the child and using body language only are not therapeutic interventions.

Test-Taking Strategy: Use the process of elimination. Eliminate options 2 and 3 first, because they are comparable or alike. From the remaining options, select the intervention that is most ther-apeutic, which is touch. Review the characteristics of the His-panic-American culture if you had difficulty with this question.

Level of Cognitive Ability: Applying
Client Needs: Psychosocial Integrity
Integrated Process: Nursing Process/Data Collection
Content Area: Fundamental Skills: Cultural Diversity
Reference: Jarvis, p. 48. 2012.

❖ **10. 1, 2, 5, 6**

Rationale: The Amish society maintains a culture that is distinct and separate from the non-Amish society, and members generally remain separate from the rest of the world, both physically and socially. Family life has a patriarchal structure, and although the roles of women are considered equally important to those of men, they are very unequal in terms of authority. Amish society rejects materialism and worldliness. Members value living simply, and they may choose to avoid technology, such as electricity and cars. They highly value responsibility, generosity, and helping others, and they often work as farmers, builders, quilters, and homemakers. The Amish use traditional health care and alternative health care, such as healers, herbs, and massage. They believe that health is a gift from God, but that clean living and a balanced diet help maintain it. They may choose not to have health insurance and instead maintain mutual aid funds for those members who need help with medical costs. Funerals are conducted in the home without a eulogy, flower decorations, or any other display. Caskets are plain and simple, without adornment. At death, women are usually buried in their bridal dresses.

Test-Taking Strategy: Focus on the subject of the Amish society. Read each option, and think about the practices and beliefs of this society to answer the question. Review the characteristics of the Amish society if you had difficulty with this question.

Level of Cognitive Ability: Understanding

Client Needs: Psychosocial Integrity

Integrated Process: Teaching and Learning

Content Area: Fundamental Skills: Cultural Diversity

References: http://www.religioustolerance.org/amish.htm.

http://www.legalaffairs.org/issues/January-February-2005/feature_labi_janfeb05.msp

Ethical and Legal Issues

PYRAMID TERMS

advance directive Written document recognized by state law that provides directions concerning the provision of care when a client is unable to make his or her own treatment choices. The two basic types of advance directives include living wills and durable powers of attorney.

advocacy Acting on the behalf of the client and protecting the client's rights to make his or her own decisions.

confidentiality/information security In the health care system, refers to the protection of privacy of the client's personal health information.

consent Voluntary act whereby a person agrees to allow someone else to do something.

ethics The ideals of right and wrong; guiding principles that individuals may use to make decisions.

HIPAA (Health Insurance Portability and Accountability Act) Federal law that establishes standards for the privacy and security of health information and a standard for electronic data interchange of health information.

informed consent A client's understanding of the reason for the proposed intervention, with its benefits and risks, and agreement with the treatment by signing a consent form.

law A system composed of general rules governing conduct and the procedures for resolving disputes when rules are not followed.

malpractice Type of negligence. Failure to meet the standards of acceptable care, which results in harm to another person.

negligence Conduct that falls below a standard of care; failure to meet a client's needs either willfully or by omission or failure to act.

Patient's Bill of Rights The rights and responsibilities of clients receiving care.

values Beliefs and attitudes that may influence behavior and the process of decision making.

PYRAMID TO SUCCESS

Across all settings in the practice of nursing, nurses frequently are confronted with ethical and legal issues related to client care. The professional nurse has the responsibility to be aware of the ethical principles, laws, and guidelines related to providing safe and quality care to clients. In the Pyramid to Success, focus on ethical practices; the nurse practice act and client's rights, particularly confidentiality, information security, and informed consent; advocacy, documentation, and advance directives; and cultural, religious, and spiritual issues. Knowledgeable use of information technology, such as an electronic health record, is also an important role of the nurse.

CLIENT NEEDS

Safe and Effective Care Environment

- Acting as an advocate
- Advance directives documents
- Confidentiality and information security issues related to the client's health care
- Ensuring client rights
- Establishing priorities
- Ethical practice in health care
- Issues surrounding informed consent
- Legal responsibilities and information technology related to client care
- Quality improvement procedures
- Resource management
- Use of information technology

Health Promotion and Maintenance

- Developmental stages and transitions
- High-risk behaviors of the client
- Lifestyle choices of the client

Psychosocial Integrity

- Abuse and neglect issues
- Available support systems
- Chemical or other dependencies
- Coping mechanisms
- Cultural, spiritual, and religious issues
- End-of-life care and grief and loss

Physiological Integrity

- Alterations in body systems
- Palliative and comfort care for the client
- Unexpected responses to therapies

I. ETHICS

A. Description: The branch of philosophy concerned with the distinction between right and wrong based on a body of knowledge, not based only on opinions

B. Morality: Behavior in accordance with customs or tradition, usually reflecting personal or religious beliefs

C. Ethical principles: Codes that direct or govern nursing actions (Box 7-1)

D. **Values:** Beliefs and attitudes that may influence behavior and the process of decision making

E. **Values** clarification: Process of analyzing one's own **values** to understand oneself more completely regarding what is truly important

F. American Nurses Association Code of Ethics for Nurses. Web site: http://nursingworld.org/codeofethics.

G. Ethical dilemma
1. An ethical dilemma occurs when there is a conflict between two or more ethical principles.
2. No correct decision exists, and the nurse must make a choice between two alternatives that are equally unsatisfactory.
3. Such dilemmas may occur as a result of differences in cultural or religious beliefs.
4. Ethical reasoning is the process of thinking through what one should do in an orderly and systematic manner to provide justification for

actions based on principles. The nurse should gather all information to determine if an ethical dilemma exists, examine his or her own values, verbalize the problem, consider possible courses of action, negotiate the outcome, and evaluate the action taken.

H. Advocate
1. An advocate is a person who speaks up for or acts on the behalf of the client, protects the client's right to make his or her own decisions, and upholds the principle of fidelity.
2. An advocate represents the client's viewpoint to others.
3. An advocate avoids letting personal **values** influence **advocacy** for the client and supports the client's decision, even when it conflicts with the advocate's own preferences or choices.

I. **Ethics** committees
1. **Ethics** committees take a multidisciplinary approach to facilitate dialogue regarding ethical dilemmas.
2. These committees develop and establish policies and procedures to facilitate the prevention and resolution of dilemmas.

⚠ An important nursing responsibility is to act as a client advocate and protect the client's rights.

II. REGULATION OF NURSING PRACTICE

A. Nurse practice act
1. A nurse practice act is a series of statutes that have been enacted by each state legislature to regulate the practice of nursing in that state.
2. Nurse practice acts set educational requirements for the nurse, distinguish between nursing practice and medical practice, and define the scope of nursing practice.
3. Additional issues covered by nurse practice acts include licensure requirements for protection of the public, grounds for disciplinary action, rights of the nurse licensee if a disciplinary action is taken, and related topics.
4. All nurses are responsible for knowing the provisions of the act of the state or province in which they work.

B. Standards of care
1. Standards of care are guidelines that identify what the client can expect to receive in terms of nursing care.
2. The guidelines determine whether nurses have performed duties in an appropriate manner.
3. If a nurse does not perform duties within accepted standards of care, the nurse places himself or herself in jeopardy of legal action.
4. If a nurse is named as a defendant in a **malpractice** lawsuit and proceedings show that the nurse

Box 7-1 Ethical Principles

Autonomy	Respect for an individual's right to self-determination
Nonmaleficence	The obligation to do or cause no harm to another
Beneficence	The duty to do good to others and maintain a balance between benefits and harms. Paternalism is an undesirable outcome of beneficence, in which the health care provider decides what is best for the client and encourages the client to act against his or her own choices.
Justice	The equitable distribution of potential benefits and tasks determining the order in which clients should be provided care
Veracity	The obligation to tell the truth
Fidelity	The duty to do what one has promised

followed neither the accepted standards of care outlined by the state or province nurse practice act nor the policies of the employing institution, the nurse's legal liability is clear. He or she is liable.

C. Employee guidelines
1. Respondeat superior: The employer is held liable for any negligent acts of an employee if the alleged negligent act occurred during the employment relationship and was within the scope of the employee's responsibilities.
2. Contracts
   a. Nurses are responsible for carrying out the terms of a contractual agreement with the employing agency and the client.
   b. The nurse-employee relationship is governed by established employee handbooks and client care policies and procedures that create obligations, rights, and duties between those parties.
3. Institutional policies
   a. Written policies and procedures of the employing institution detail how nurses are to perform their duties.
   b. Policies and procedures are usually specific and describe the expected behavior on the part of the nurse.
   c. Although policies are not **laws**, courts generally rule against nurses who violate policies.
   d. If the nurse practices nursing according to client care policies and procedures established by the employer, functions within the job responsibility, and provides care consistently in a non-negligent manner, the nurse minimizes the potential for liability.

⚠ The nurse must follow the guidelines identified in the nurse practice act and agency policies and procedures when delivering client care.

D. Hospital staffing
1. Charges of abandonment may be made against nurses who "walk out" when staffing is inadequate.
2. Nurses in short staffing situations are obligated to make a report to the nursing administration.
E. Floating
1. Floating is an acceptable, legal practice used by health care facilities to alleviate understaffing and overstaffing.
2. Legally, a nurse cannot refuse to float unless a union contract guarantees that nurses can work only in a specified area or the nurse can prove lack of knowledge for the performance of assigned tasks.
3. Nurses in a floating situation must not assume responsibility beyond their level of experience or qualification.

4. Nurses who float should inform the supervisor of any lack of experience in caring for the type of clients on the new nursing unit.
5. The nurse should request and be given orientation to the new unit.
F. Disciplinary action
1. Boards of nursing may deny, revoke, or suspend any license to practice as a nurse, according to their statutory authority.
2. Some causes for disciplinary action are as follows:
   a. Unprofessional conduct
   b. Conduct that could affect the health and welfare of the public adversely
   c. Breach of client **confidentiality**
   d. Failure to use sufficient knowledge, skills, or nursing judgment
   e. Physically or verbally abusing a client
   f. Assuming duties without sufficient preparation
   g. Knowingly delegating to unlicensed personnel nursing care that places the client at risk for injury
   h. Failure to maintain an accurate record for each client
   i. Falsifying a client's record
   j. Leaving a nursing assignment without properly notifying appropriate personnel

III. LEGAL LIABILITY

A. Laws
1. Nurses are governed by civil and criminal **law** in roles as providers of services, employees of institutions, and private citizens.
2. A nurse has a personal and legal obligation to provide a standard of client care expected of a reasonably competent professional nurse.
3. Professional nurses are held responsible (liable) for harm resulting from their negligent acts or their failure to act.
B. Types of **laws** (Figure 7-1)
C. **Negligence** and **malpractice** (Box 7-2)
1. **Negligence** is conduct that falls below the standard of care.
2. **Negligence** can include acts of commission and acts of omission.
3. A nurse who does not meet appropriate standards of care may be held liable.
4. **Malpractice** is **negligence** on the part of a nurse.
5. **Malpractice** is determined if the nurse owed a duty to the client and did not carry out the duty and the client was injured because the nurse failed to perform the duty.
6. Proof of liability
   a. Duty: At the time of injury, a duty existed between the plaintiff and the defendant.
   b. Breach of duty: The defendant breached duty of care to the plaintiff.

c. Proximate cause: The breach of the duty was the legal cause of injury to the client.

d. Damage or injury: The plaintiff experienced injury or damages or both and can be compensated by **law**.

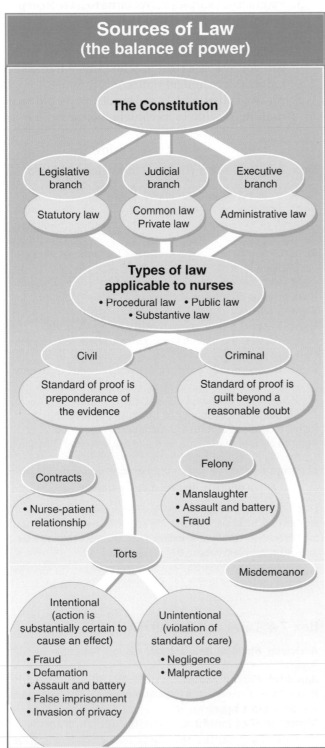

Sources of Law
(the balance of power)

The Constitution

Legislative branch

Judicial branch

Executive branch

Statutory law

Common law
Private law

Administrative law

Types of law
applicable to nurses
• Procedural law • Public law
• Substantive law

Civil

Criminal

Standard of proof is preponderance of the evidence

Standard of proof is guilt beyond a reasonable doubt

Felony

Contracts

• Manslaughter
• Assault and battery
• Fraud

• Nurse-patient relationship

Torts

Misdemeanor

Intentional (action is substantially certain to cause an effect)

Unintentional (violation of standard of care)

• Fraud
• Defamation
• Assault and battery
• False imprisonment
• Invasion of privacy

• Negligence
• Malpractice

▲ **FIGURE 7-1** Sources of law for nursing practice. (From Harkreader, H., & Hogan, M. A. [2007]. *Fundamentals of nursing: Caring and clinical judgment* [3rd ed.]. St. Louis: Saunders.)

⚠ The nurse must meet appropriate standards of care when delivering care to the client; otherwise the nurse would be held liable if the client is harmed.

D. Professional liability insurance

1. Nurses need their own liability insurance for protection against **malpractice** lawsuits.
2. Having their own insurance provides nurses protection as individuals. This allows a nurse to have an attorney present who has only the nurse's interests in mind.

E. Good Samaritan **laws**

1. State legislatures pass Good Samaritan **laws**, which may vary from state to state.
2. These **laws** encourage health care professionals to assist in emergency situations and limit liability and offer legal immunity for persons helping in an emergency, provided that they give reasonable care.
3. Immunity from suit applies only when all conditions of the state **law** are met, such as the health care provider receives no compensation for the care provided and the care given is not intentionally negligent.

F. Controlled substances

1. The nurse should adhere to facility policies and procedures concerning administration of controlled substances, which are governed by federal and state **laws**.
2. Controlled substances must be kept locked securely, and only authorized personnel should have access to them.

IV. COLLECTIVE BARGAINING

A. Collective bargaining is a formalized decision-making process between representatives of management and representatives of labor to negotiate wages and conditions of employment.

Box 7-2 Negligent Acts

Medication errors that result in injury to the client

Intravenous administration errors such as incorrect flow rates or failure to monitor a flow rate that results in injury to the client

Falls that occur as a result of failure to provide safety to the client

Failure to use sterile technique when indicated

Failure to check equipment for proper functioning

Burns sustained by the client as a result of failure to monitor bath temperature or equipment

Failure to monitor a client's condition

Failure to report changes in the client's condition to the health care provider (HCP)

Failure to provide a complete report to the oncoming nursing staff

Adapted from Potter, P., & Perry, A. (2009). *Fundamentals of nursing* (7th ed.). St. Louis: Mosby.

B. When collective bargaining breaks down because the parties cannot reach an agreement, the employees usually call a strike.

C. Striking presents a moral dilemma to many nurses because nursing practice is a service to people.

D. The United American Nurses (UAN) is an affiliate of the American Federation of Labor and Congress of Industrial Organizations (AFL-CIO) and the American Nurses Association. UAN staff nurses set the standard for RNs in organizing, collective bargaining, and contracts. Additional information can be obtained at http://www.uannurse.org.

V. LEGAL RISK AREAS

A. Assault
1. Assault occurs when a person puts another person in fear of a harmful or offensive contact.
2. The victim fears and believes that harm will result because of the threat.

B. Battery is an intentional touching of another's body without the other's **consent**.

C. Invasion of privacy includes violating **confidentiality**, intruding on private client or family matters, and sharing client information with unauthorized persons.

D. False imprisonment
1. False imprisonment occurs when a client is not allowed to leave a health care facility when there is no legal justification to detain the client.
2. False imprisonment occurs when restraining devices are used without an appropriate clinical need.
3. A client can sign an Against Medical Advice form when the client refuses care and is competent to make decisions.
4. The nurse should document circumstances in the medical record to avoid allegations by the client that cannot be defended.

E. Defamation is a false communication that causes damage to someone's reputation, either in writing (libel) or verbally (slander).

F. Fraud results from a deliberate deception intended to produce unlawful gains.

VI. CLIENT'S RIGHTS

A. Description
1. The client's rights document, also called the **Patient's Bill of Rights**, reflects acknowledgment of a client's right to participate in her or his health care with an emphasis on client autonomy.
2. The document provides a list of the rights of the client and responsibilities that the hospital cannot violate (Box 7-3).
3. The client's rights protect the client's ability to determine the level and type of care received. All health care agencies are required to have a Client's Bill of Rights posted in a visible area.

4. Several **laws** and standards pertain to client's rights (Box 7-4).

B. Rights for the mentally ill (Box 7-5)
1. The Mental Health Systems Act created rights for mentally ill people.
2. The Joint Commission has developed policy statements on the rights of mentally ill people.
3. Psychiatric facilities are required to have a client's bill of rights posted in a visible area.

C. Organ donation and transplantation
1. A client has the right to decide to become an organ donor and a right to refuse organ transplantation as a treatment option.
2. An individual who is at least 18 years old may indicate a wish to become a donor on his or

---

Box 7-3 Patient's Rights When Hospitalized

Right to considerate and respectful care

Right to be informed about diagnosis, possible treatments, likely outcome, and to discuss this information with the HCP

Right to know the names and roles of the persons who are involved in care

Right to consent or refuse a treatment

Right to have an advance directive

Right to privacy

Right to expect that medical records are confidential

Right to review the medical record and to have information explained

Right to expect that the hospital will provide necessary health services

Right to know if the hospital has relationships with outside parties that may influence treatment or care

Right to consent or refuse to take part in research

Right to be told of realistic care alternatives when hospital care is no longer appropriate

Right to know about hospital rules that affect treatment, and about charges and payment methods

From Christensen, B., & Kockrow, E. (2006). *Foundations of nursing* (5th ed.). St. Louis: Mosby; and modified from American Hospital Association. (1992). *A patient's bill of rights.* http://www.patienttalk.info/AHA-Patient_Bill_of_Rights.htm.

Box 7-4 Laws and Standards

American Hospital Association: Issued Patient's Bill of Rights

American Nurses Association: Developed the Code for Nurses, which defines the nurse's responsibility for upholding the client's rights

Mental Health Systems Act: Developed rights for mentally ill clients

The Joint Commission: Developed policy statements on the rights of mentally ill individuals her driver's license (state-specific) or in an **advance directive**.

3. The Uniform Anatomical Gift Act provides a list of individuals who can provide **informed consent** for the donation of a deceased individual's organs.

4. The United Network for Organ Sharing sets the criteria for organ donations.

5. Some organs, such as the heart, lungs, and liver, can be obtained only from a person who is on mechanical ventilation and has suffered brain death, whereas other organs or tissues can be removed several hours after death.

6. A donor must be free of infectious disease and cancer.

7. Requests to the deceased's family for organ donation usually are done by the HCP or nurse specially trained for making such requests.

8. Donation of organs does not delay funeral arrangements, no obvious evidence that the organs were removed from the body shows when the body is dressed, and the family incurs no cost for removal of the organs donated.

D. Religious beliefs: Refer to Chapter 6 for additional information regarding end-of-life-care.

Box 7-5 Rights for the Mentally Ill

Right to be treated with dignity and respect
Right to communicate with persons outside the hospital
Right to keep clothing and personal effects with them
Right to religious freedom
Right to be employed
Right to manage property
Right to execute wills
Right to enter into contractual agreements
Right to make purchases
Right to education
Right to habeas corpus (written request for release from the hospital)
Right to an independent psychiatric examination
Right to civil service status, including the right to vote
Right to retain licenses, privileges, or permits
Right to sue or be sued
Right to marry or divorce
Right to treatment in the least restrictive setting
Right not to be subject to unnecessary restraints
Right to privacy and confidentiality
Right to informed consent
Right to treatment and to refuse treatment
Right to refuse participation in experimental treatments or research

Adapted from Stuart, G., & Laraia, M. (2009). *Principles and practice of psychiatric nursing* (9th ed.). St. Louis: Mosby.

VII. INFORMED CONSENT

A. Description

1. **Informed consent** is the client's approval (or that of the client's legal representative) to have his or her body touched by a specific individual.

2. **Consents**, or releases, are legal documents that indicate the client's permission to perform surgery, perform a treatment or procedure, or give information to a third party.

3. There are different types of **consents** (Box 7-6).

4. **Informed consent** indicates the client's participation in the decision regarding health care.

5. The client must be informed, in understandable terms, of the risks and benefits of the surgery or treatment, what the consequences are for not having the surgery or procedure performed, treatment options, and the name of the health care provider performing the surgery or procedure.

6. A client's questions about the surgery or procedure must be answered before signing the **consent**.

Box 7-6 Types of Consents

Admission Agreement
Admission agreements are obtained at the time of admission and identify the health care agency's responsibility to the client.

Immunization Consent
An immunization consent may be required before the administration of certain immunizations. The consent indicates that the client was informed of the benefits and risks of the immunization.

Blood Transfusion Consent
A blood transfusion consent indicates that the client was informed of the benefits and risks of the transfusion. Some clients hold religious beliefs that would prohibit them from receiving a blood transfusion, even in a life-threatening situation.

Surgical Consent
Surgical consent is obtained for all surgical or invasive procedures or diagnostic tests that are invasive. The HCP, surgeon, or anesthesiologist who performs the operative or other procedure is responsible for explaining the procedure, its risks and benefits, and possible alternative options.

Research Consent
The research consent obtains permission from the client regarding participation in a research study. The consent informs the client about the possible risks, consequences, and benefits of the research.

Special Consents
Special consents are required for the use of restraints, photographing the client, disposal of body parts during surgery, donating organs after death, or performing an autopsy.

7. A **consent** must be signed freely by the client without threat or pressure and must be witnessed (witness must be an adult).

8. A client who has been medicated with sedating medications or any other medications that can affect the client's cognitive abilities should not be asked to sign a **consent form**.

9. Legally, the client must be mentally and emotionally competent to give **consent**.

10. If a client is declared mentally or emotionally incompetent, the next of kin, appointed guardian (appointed by the court), or durable power of attorney has legal authority to give **consent** (Box 7-7).

11. A competent client older than 18 years of age must sign the **consent**.

12. In most states, when a nurse is involved in the **informed consent** process, the nurse is witnessing only the signature of the client on the **informed consent** form.

13. An **informed consent** can be waived for urgent medical or surgical intervention as long as institutional policy so indicates.

14. A client has the right to refuse information and waive the **informed consent** and undergo treatment, but this decision must be documented in the medical record.

15. A client may withdraw **consent** at any time.

⚠️ An informed consent is a legal document, and the client must be informed, in understandable terms, of the risks and benefits of surgery, treatments, procedures, and plan of care. The client needs to be a participant in decisions regarding health care.

B. Minors
1. A minor is a client under legal age as defined by state statute (usually younger than 18 years).
2. A minor may not give legal **consent**, and **consent** must be obtained from a parent or the legal guardian.
3. Parental or guardian **consent** should be obtained before treatment is initiated for a minor except in the following cases: in an emergency; in

---

Box 7-7 Mentally or Emotionally Incompetent Clients

Declared incompetent
Unconscious
Under the influence of chemical agents such as alcohol or drugs
Chronic dementia or other mental deficiency that impairs thought processes and ability to make decisions

---

situations in which the **consent** of the minor is sufficient, including treatment related to substance abuse, treatment of a sexually transmitted infection, human immunodeficiency virus (HIV) testing and acquired immunodeficiency syndrome (AIDS) treatment, birth control services, pregnancy (excluding abortion), or psychiatric services; the minor is an emancipated minor; or a court order or other legal authorization has been obtained.

C. Emancipated minor
1. An emancipated minor has established independence from his or her parents through marriage, service in the armed forces, or by a court order.
2. An emancipated minor is considered legally capable of signing an **informed consent**.

VIII. HEALTH INSURANCE PORTABILITY AND ACCOUNTABILITY ACT

A. Description
1. The **Health Insurance Portability and Accountability Act (HIPAA)** describes how personal health information (PHI) may be used and how the client can obtain access to the information.
2. PHI includes individually identifiable information that relates to the client's past, present, or future health; treatment; and payment for health care services.
3. The act requires health care agencies to keep PHI private, provides information to the client about the legal responsibilities regarding privacy, and explains the client's rights with respect to PHI.
4. The client has various rights as a consumer of health care under **HIPAA**, and any client requests may need to be placed in writing. A fee may be attached to certain client requests.
5. The client may file a complaint if the client believes that privacy rights have been violated.

B. Client's rights include the right to do the following:
1. Inspect a copy of PHI.
2. Ask the health care agency to amend the PHI that is contained in a record if the PHI is inaccurate.
3. Request a list of disclosures made regarding the PHI as specified by **HIPAA**.
4. Request to restrict how the health care agency uses or discloses PHI regarding treatment, payment, or health care services, unless information is needed to provide emergency treatment.
5. Request that the health care agency communicates with the client in a certain way or at a certain location. The request must specify how or where the client wishes to be contacted.
6. Request a paper copy of the **HIPAA** notice.

C. Health care agency use and disclosure of PHI
1. The health care agency obtains PHI in the course of providing or administering health insurance benefits.
2. Use or disclosure of PHI may be done for the following:
   a. Health care payment purposes
   b. Health care operations purposes
   c. Treatment purposes
   d. Providing information about health care services
   e. Data aggregation purposes to make health care benefit decisions
   f. Administering health care benefits
3. There are additional uses or disclosures of PHI (Box 7-8)

IX. CONFIDENTIALITY AND INFORMATION SECURITY

A. Description
1. In the health care system, confidentiality refers to the protection of privacy of the client's PHI.
2. Clients have a right to privacy in the health care system.

3. A special relationship exists between the client and nurse, in which information discussed is not shared with a third party who is not directly involved in the client's care.
4. Violations of privacy occur in various ways (Box 7-9).

B. Nurse's responsibility
1. Nurses are bound to protect client **confidentiality** by most nurse practice acts, by ethical principles and standards, and by institutional and agency policies and procedures.
2. Disclosure of confidential information exposes the nurse to liability for invasion of the client's privacy.
3. The nurse needs to protect the client from indiscriminate disclosure of health care information that may cause harm (Box 7-10).

Box 7-8 Uses or Disclosures of Personal Health Information

Compliance with legal proceedings or for limited law enforcement purposes

To a family member or significant other in a medical emergency

To a personal representative appointed by the client or designated by law

For research purposes in limited circumstances

To a coroner, medical examiner, or funeral director about a deceased person

To an organ procurement organization in limited circumstances

To avert a serious threat to the client's health or safety or the health or safety of others

To a governmental agency authorized to oversee the health care system or government programs

To the Department of Health and Human Services for the investigation of compliance with the Health Insurance Portability and Accountability Act or to fulfill another lawful request

To federal officials for lawful intelligence or national security purposes

To protect health authorities for public health purposes

To appropriate military authorities if a client is a member of the armed forces

In accordance with a valid authorization signed by the client

Adapted from U.S. Department of Health and Human Services Office for Civil Rights. http://www.hhs.gov/ocr/privacy/hipaa/understanding/consumers/index.html.

Box 7-9 Violations and Invasion of Client Privacy

Taking photographs of the client

Release of medical information to an unauthorized person, such as a member of the press, family, friend, or neighbor of the client, without the client's permission

Use of the client's name or picture for the health care agency's sole advantage

Intrusion by the health care agency regarding the client's affairs

Publication of information about the client

Publication of embarrassing facts

Public disclosure of private information

Leaving the curtains or room door open while a treatment or procedure is being performed

Allowing individuals to observe a treatment or procedure without the client's consent

Leaving a confused or agitated client sitting in the nursing unit hallway

Interviewing a client in a room with only a curtain between clients or where conversation can be overheard

Accessing medical records when unauthorized to do so

Box 7-10 Maintenance of Confidentiality

Not discussing client issues with other clients or staff uninvolved in the client's care

Not sharing health care information with others without the client's consent (includes family members or friends of the client)

Keeping all information about a client private, and not revealing it to someone not directly involved in care

Discussing client information only in private and secluded areas

Protecting the medical record from all unauthorized readers

C. Medical records
1. Medical records are confidential.
2. The client has the right to read the medical record and have copies of the record.
3. Only staff members directly involved in care have legitimate access to a client's records. These may include HCPs and nurses caring for the client, technicians, therapists, social workers, unit secretaries, client advocates, administrators (e.g., for statistical analysis, staffing, quality care review). Others must ask permission from the client to review a record.
4. The medical record is sent to the records or the health information department after discharge of the client from the health care facility.

D. Information technology/computerized medical records
1. Health care employees should have access only to the client's records in the nursing unit or work area.
2. **Confidentiality/information security** can be protected by the use of special computer access codes to limit what employees have access to in computer systems.
3. The use of a password or identification code is needed to enter and sign off a computer system.
4. A password or identification code should never be shared with another person.
5. Personal passwords should be changed periodically to prevent unauthorized computer access.

E. When conducting research, any information provided by the client is not to be reported in any manner that identifies the client and is not to be made accessible to anyone outside the research team.

⚠ The nurse must always protect client confidentiality.

X. LEGAL SAFEGUARDS

A. Risk management
1. Risk management is a planned method to identify, analyze, and evaluate risks, followed by a plan for reducing the frequency of accidents and injuries.
2. Programs are based on a systematic reporting system for incidents or unusual occurrences.

B. Incident reports (Box 7-11)
1. The incident report is used as a means of identifying risk situations and improving client care.
2. Follow specific documentation guidelines.
3. Fill out the report completely, accurately, and factually.
4. The report form should not be copied or placed in the client's record.
5. Make no reference to the incident report form in the client's record.
6. The report is not a substitute for a complete entry in the client's record regarding the incident.

7. If a client injury or error in care occurred, assess the client frequently.

C. Safeguarding valuables
1. Client's valuables should be given to a family member or secured for safekeeping in a stored and locked designated location, such as the agency's safe. The location of the client's valuables should be documented per agency policy.
2. Many health care agencies require a client to sign a release to free the agency of the responsibility for lost valuables.
3. A client's wedding band can be taped in place unless a risk exists for swelling of the hands or fingers.
4. Religious items, such as medals or scapulars, may be pinned to the client's gown if allowed by agency policy.

D. HCP's prescriptions
1. A nurse is obligated to carry out a HCP's prescription (order) except when the nurse believes a prescription to be inappropriate or inaccurate.
2. A nurse carrying out an inaccurate prescription may be legally responsible for any harm suffered by the client.
3. The nurse should clarify with the HCP an unclear or inappropriate prescription.
4. If no resolution occurs regarding the prescription in question, the nurse should contact the nurse manager or supervisor.
5. The nurse should follow specific guidelines for telephone prescriptions (Box 7-12).
6. The nurse should ensure that all components of a medication prescription are documented (Box 7-13).

E. Documentation
1. Documentation is legally required by accrediting agencies, state licensing **laws**, and state nurse and medical practice acts.
2. The nurse should follow agency guidelines and procedures (Box 7-14).

F. Client and family teaching
1. Provide complete instructions in a language that the client or family can understand.

Box 7-11 Incidents That Need to Be Reported

Accidental omission of prescribed therapies
Circumstances that led to injury or a risk for client injury
Client falls
Medication administration errors
Needle-stick injuries
Procedure-related or equipment-related accidents
A visitor injury that occurred in the health care agency premises
A visitor who exhibits symptoms of a communicable disease

2. Document client and family teaching, what was taught, evaluation of understanding, and who was present during the teaching.
3. Inform the client of what could happen if information shared during teaching is not followed.

 The nurse should never carry out a prescription (order) if it is unclear or inappropriate. The HCP should be contacted immediately.

XI. ADVANCE DIRECTIVES

A. Patient Self-Determination Act
1. The Patient Self-Determination Act is a **law** that indicates clients must be provided with information about their rights to identify written directions about the care that they wish to receive in the event that they become incapacitated and are unable to make health care decisions.
2. On admission to a health care facility, the client is asked about the existence of an **advance directive**, and if one exists, it must be documented and included as part of the medical record; if the client signs an **advance directive** at the time of admission, it must be documented in the client's medical record.
3. The two basic types of **advance directives** include living wills and durable powers of attorney.
   a. Living will: lists the medical treatment that a client chooses to omit or refuse if the client becomes unable to make decisions and is terminally ill.
   b. Durable powers of attorney: appoints a person (health care proxy) chosen by the client to make health care decisions on the client's behalf when the client can no longer make decisions.

B. Do not resuscitate (DNR) orders
1. The DNR is an order written by a HCP when a client has indicated a desire to be allowed to die if he or she suffers cardiac or respiratory arrest.
2. The client or his or her legal representative must provide **informed consent** for the DNR status.
3. The DNR order must be defined clearly so that other treatment, not refused by the client, will be continued.
4. The DNR order must be reviewed regularly according to agency policy.
5. All health care personnel must know whether a client has a DNR order.
6. If a client does not have a DNR order, health care personnel need to make every effort to revive the client.
7. DNR protocols may vary state to state, and it is important for the nurse to know his or her state's protocols.

C. The nurse's role
1. Discussing **advance directives** with the client opens the communication channel to establish

---

Box 7-12 Telephone Prescriptions (Orders)

Date and time the entry.

Repeat the prescription to the HCP, and record the prescription.

Sign the prescription; begin with "t.o." (telephone order), write the HCP's name, and sign the prescription.

If another nurse witnessed the prescription, that nurse's signature follows.

The HCP needs to countersign the prescription within a timeframe according to agency policy.

Box 7-13 Components of a Medication Prescription (Order)

Date and time prescription was written
Medication name
Medication dosage
Route of administration
Frequency of administration
HCP's signature

Box 7-14 Documentation Guidelines: Narrative and Information Technology

Use a black-colored ink pen for narrative documentation.
Date and time entries.
Provide objective, factual, and complete documentation.
Document care, medications, treatments, and procedures as soon as possible after completion.
Document client responses to interventions.
Document consent for or refusal of treatments.
Document calls made to other health care providers.
Do not document for others or change documentation for other individuals.
Sign and title each entry.
Use quotes as appropriate for subjective data.
Use correct spelling, grammar, and punctuation.
Avoid unacceptable abbreviations.
Avoid judgmental or evaluative statements, such as "uncooperative client."
Do not leave blank spaces on documentation forms.
Follow agency policies when an error is made (draw one line through the error, initial, and date).
Follow agency guidelines regarding late entries.
Use only the user identification code, name, or password for computerized documentation.
Never lend access identification computer codes to another person. Change password at regular intervals.
Maintain privacy and confidentiality of documented information printed from the computer.

what is important to the client and what the client may view as promoting life versus prolonging dying.

2. The nurse needs to ensure that the client has been provided with information about the right to identify written directions about the care that the client wishes to receive.

3. On admission to a health care facility, the nurse determines whether an **advance directive** exists and ensures that it is part of the medical record.

4. The nurse ensures that the HCP is aware of the presence of an **advance directive**.

5. All health care workers need to follow the directions of an **advance directive** to be safe from liability.

6. Some agencies have specific policies that prohibit a nurse from signing as a witness to a legal document, such as a living will.

7. If allowed by the agency, when a nurse acts as a witness to a legal document, the nurse must document the event and the factual circumstances surrounding the signing in the medical record. Documentation as a witness should include who was present, any significant comments by the client, and the nurse's observations of the client's conduct during this process.

XII. REPORTING RESPONSIBILITIES

A. Nurses are required to report certain communicable diseases or criminal activities such as child or elder abuse or domestic violence; dog bite or other animal bite, gunshot, or stab wounds, assaults, and homicides; and suicides to the appropriate authorities.

B. Impaired nurse
1. If a nurse suspects that a co-worker is abusing chemicals and potentially jeopardizing a client's safety, the nurse must report the individual to the nursing administration in a confidential manner. (Client safety is always the first priority.)
2. Nursing administration notifies the board of nursing regarding the nurse's behavior.

C. Occupational Safety and Health Act (OSHA)
1. OSHA requires that an employer provide a safe workplace for employees according to regulations.
2. Employees can confidentially report working conditions that violate regulations.
3. An employee who reports unsafe working conditions cannot be retaliated against by the employer.

D. Sexual harassment
1. Sexual harassment is prohibited by state and federal **laws**.
2. Sexual harassment includes unwelcome conduct of a sexual nature.
3. Follow agency policies and procedures to handle reporting a concern or complaint.

MORE QUESTIONS ON EVOLVE!

Practice Questions

11. Which of the following is a recommended guideline for safe computerized charting?
1. Passwords to the computer system should only be changed if lost.
2. Computer terminals may be left unattended during client-care activities.
3. Report accidental deletions from the computerized file to the nursing manager or supervisor.
4. Copies of printouts from computerized files should be kept on a clipboard at the nurses' station for other nurses to access.

12. A licensed practical nurse (LPN) enters a client's room and finds the client sitting on the floor. The LPN calls the registered nurse who checks the client thoroughly and then assists the client back into bed. The LPN completes an incident report and the nursing supervisor and health care provider (HCP) are notified of the incident. Which of the following is the next nursing action regarding the incident?
1. Place the incident report in the client's chart.
2. Make a copy of the incident report for the HCP.
3. Document a complete entry in the client's record concerning the incident.
4. Document in the client's record that an incident report has been completed.

13. An unconscious client who is bleeding profusely is brought to the emergency department after a serious accident. Surgery is required immediately to save the client's life. With regard to informed consent for the surgical procedure, which of the following is the best action?
1. Call the nursing supervisor to initiate a court order for the surgical procedure.
2. Try calling the client's spouse to obtain telephone consent before the surgical procedure.
3. Ask the friend who accompanied the client to the emergency department to sign the consent form.
4. Transport the client to the operating department immediately, as required by the health care provider, without obtaining an informed consent.

14. A nurse arrives at work and is told to report (float) to the pediatric unit for the day because the unit is understaffed and needs additional nurses to care for the children. The nurse has never worked in the pediatric unit. Which of the following is the appropriate nursing action?
1. Call the hospital lawyer.
2. Call the nursing supervisor.

3. Refuse to float to the pediatric unit.
4. Report to the pediatric unit and identify tasks that can be safely performed.

15. A nurse enters a client's room and notes that the client's lawyer is present and that the client is preparing a living will. The living will requires that the client's signature be witnessed, and the client asks the nurse to witness the signature. Which of the following is the appropriate nursing action?
1. Decline to sign the will.
2. Sign the will as a witness to the signature only.
3. Call the hospital lawyer before signing the will.
4. Sign the will, clearly identifying credentials and employment agency.

16. A nurse enters a client's room and finds the client lying on the floor. The nurse calls the registered nurse, who checks the client and then calls the nursing supervisor and the health care provider to inform them of the occurrence. The nurse completes the incident report, understanding that it allows for the analysis of adverse client events through:
1. Providing clients with necessary stabilizing treatments
2. A method of promoting quality care and risk management
3. Determining the effectiveness of interventions in relation to outcomes
4. The appropriate method of reporting to local, state, and federal agencies

17. A nurse observes that a client received pain medication 1 hour ago from another nurse but the client still has severe pain. The nurse has previously observed this same occurrence. On the basis of the nurse practice act, the observing nurse plans to do which of the following?
1. Report the information to the police.
2. Call the impaired nurse organization.
3. Talk with the nurse who gave the medication.
4. Report the information to a nursing supervisor.

18. A client has died, and a nurse asks a family member about the funeral arrangements. The family member refuses to discuss the issue. The nurse's appropriate action is to:
1. Show acceptance of feelings.
2. Provide information needed for decision making.
3. Suggest a referral to a mental health professional.
4. Remain with the family member without discussing funeral arrangements.

19. A nurse lawyer provides an education session to the nursing staff regarding client rights. A nurse asks the lawyer to describe an example that may relate to invasion of client privacy. A nursing action that indicates a violation of this right is:
1. Threatening to place a client in restraints
2. Performing a surgical procedure without consent
3. Taking photographs of the client without consent
4. Telling the client that he or she cannot leave the hospital

20. An older woman is brought to the emergency department. When caring for the client, the nurse notes old and new ecchymotic areas on both of the client's arms and buttocks. The nurse asks the client how the bruises were sustained. The client, although reluctant, tells the nurse in confidence that her daughter frequently hits her if she gets in the way. Which of the following is the appropriate nursing response?
1. "I have a legal obligation to report this type of abuse."
2. "I promise I won't tell anyone, but let's see what we can do about this."
3. "Let's talk about ways that will prevent your daughter from hitting you."
4. "This should not be happening. If it happens again, you must call the emergency department."

ANSWERS

11. 3
Rationale: After any inadvertent deletions of permanent computerized records, the nurse should type an explanation into the computer file with the date, time, and his or her initials. The nurse should also contact the nursing manager or supervisor with a written explanation of the situation. Options 1, 2, and 4 represent unsafe charting actions. Only option 3 follows the guidelines for safe computer charting
Test-Taking Strategy: Use the process of elimination. Focusing on the subject of a safe guideline will direct you to option 3. Options 1, 2, and 4 represent unsafe charting actions. Review the guidelines for computerized documentation if you had difficulty with this question.
Level of Cognitive Ability: Understanding
Client Needs: Safe and Effective Care Environment

Integrated Process: Nursing Process/Implementation
Content Area: Leadership/Management: Ethical/Legal
Reference: Christensen, Kockrow, p. 155. 2011. *Foundations and adult health nursing.*

12. 3
Rationale: The incident report is confidential and privileged information, and it should not be copied, placed in the chart, or have any reference made to it in the client's record. The incident report is not a substitute for a complete entry in the client's record concerning the incident.
Test-Taking Strategy: Use the process of elimination. Eliminate options 1 and 4 first because they are comparable or alike. Recalling that incident reports should not be copied will direct you to option 3. Review the nursing responsibilities related to incident reports if you had difficulty with this question.

Level of Cognitive Ability: Applying
Client Needs: Safe and Effective Care Environment
Integrated Process: Communication and Documentation
Content Area: Leadership/Management: Ethical/Legal
Reference: Christensen, Kockrow, pp. 145, 148, 150. 2011. *Foundations and adult health nursing.*

13. 4
Rationale: Generally there are only two instances in which the informed consent of an adult client is not needed. One instance is when an emergency is present and delaying treatment for the purpose of obtaining informed consent would result in injury or death to the client. The second instance is when the client waives the right to give informed consent. Options 1, 2, and 3 are inappropriate.
Test-Taking Strategy: Use the process of elimination. Option 3 can easily be eliminated first. Note the strategic words "surgery is required immediately." Options 1 and 2 would delay treatment and should be eliminated. Review the issues surrounding informed consent if you had difficulty with this question.
Level of Cognitive Ability: Applying
Client Needs: Safe and Effective Care Environment
Integrated Process: Nursing Process/Implementation
Content Area: Leadership/Management: Ethical/Legal
Reference: Christensen, Kockrow, pp. 1260–1261. 2011. *Foundations and adult health nursing.*

14. 4
Rationale: Floating is an acceptable legal practice used by hospitals to solve their understaffing problems. Legally a nurse cannot refuse to float unless a union contract guarantees that the nurse can only work in a specified area or the nurse can prove a lack of knowledge for the performance of assigned tasks. When faced with this situation, the nurse should identify potential areas of harm to the client.
Test-Taking Strategy: Use the process of elimination. Options 1 and 3 can be eliminated first, because they are inappropriate. From the remaining options, eliminate option 2, because it is premature to call the nursing supervisor. Review the nursing responsibilities related to floating if you had difficulty with this question.
Level of Cognitive Ability: Applying
Client Needs: Safe and Effective Care Environment
Integrated Process: Nursing Process/Implementation
Content Area: Leadership/Management: Ethical/Legal
Reference: Linton, pp. 40–41. 2012.

15. 1
Rationale: Living wills are required to be in writing and signed by the client. The client's signature either must be witnessed by specified individuals or notarized. Many states prohibit any employee from being a witness, including a nurse in a facility in which the client is receiving care.
Test-Taking Strategy: Use the process of elimination. Options 2 and 4 are comparable or alike and should be eliminated first. From the remaining options, option 1 is the appropriate action. Review the legal implications associated with living wills if you had difficulty with this question.
Level of Cognitive Ability: Applying
Client Needs: Safe and Effective Care Environment
Integrated Process: Nursing Process/Implementation
Content Area: Leadership/Management: Ethical/Legal

Reference: Christensen, Kockrow, pp. 33, 236. 2011. *Foundations and adult health nursing.*

16. 2
Rationale: Proper documentation of unusual occurrences, incidents, accidents, and the nursing actions taken as a result of the occurrence are internal to the institution or agency. Documentation on the incident report allows the nurse and administration to review the quality of care and determine any potential risks present. Options 1, 3, and 4 are incorrect.
Test-Taking Strategy: Use the process of elimination. Eliminate options 1 and 3, because incident reports are not routinely filled out for interventions or treatment measures. Eliminate option 4, because incident reports are not used to report occurrences to other agencies; medical records are used for this purpose. Review the purpose of incident reports if you had difficulty with this question.
Level of Cognitive Ability: Understanding
Client Needs: Safe and Effective Care Environment
Integrated Process: Nursing Process/Implementation
Content Area: Leadership/Management: Ethical/Legal
Reference: Christensen, Kockrow, p. 150. 2011. *Foundations and adult health nursing.*

17. 4
Rationale: Nurse practice acts require reporting the suspicion of impaired nurses. The state board of nursing has jurisdiction over the practice of nursing and may develop plans for treatment and supervision. This suspicion needs to be reported to the nursing supervisor, who will then report to the board of nursing. Options 1 and 2 are inappropriate. Option 3 may cause a conflict.
Test-Taking Strategy: Use the principles related to following the channels of communication in a health care agency when answering this question. By reporting the information, the nurse alerts the institution to the potential problem and sets the stage for further investigation and appropriate action. Review the actions to take regarding reporting the suspicion of an impaired nurse if you had difficulty with this question.
Level of Cognitive Ability: Applying
Client Needs: Safe and Effective Care Environment
Integrated Process: Nursing Process/Planning
Content Area: Leadership/Management: Ethical/Legal
References: deWit, p. 1134. 2009.
Linton, p. 1341. 2012.

18. 4
Rationale: The family member is exhibiting the first stage of grief (denial), and the nurse should remain with the family member. Option 1 is an appropriate intervention for the acceptance or reorganization and restitution stage. Option 2 may be an appropriate intervention for the bargaining stage. Option 3 may be an appropriate intervention for depression.
Test-Taking Strategy: Use therapeutic communication techniques to direct you to option 4. Remember to address client and family feelings first. Review the grieving process and therapeutic communication techniques if you had difficulty with this question.
Level of Cognitive Ability: Applying
Client Needs: Psychosocial Integrity
Integrated Process: Caring
Content Area: Fundamental Skills: End-of-Life Care

References: Christensen, Kockrow, pp. 40–46. 2011. *Foundations and adult health nursing.*
Linton, pp. 377–378, 382. 2012.

19. 3

Rationale: Invasion of privacy takes place when an individual's private affairs are intruded on unreasonably. Threatening to place a client in restraints constitutes assault. Performing a surgical procedure without consent is an example of battery. Not allowing a client to leave the hospital constitutes false imprisonment.

Test-Taking Strategy: Use the process of elimination. Note the strategic words "invasion of client privacy." These words should direct you to option 3. Review the situations that constitute the invasion of client privacy if you had difficulty with this question.

Level of Cognitive Ability: Understanding
Client Needs: Safe and Effective Care Environment
Integrated Process: Nursing Process/Implementation
Content Area: Leadership/Management: Ethical/Legal
Reference: Linton, pp. 38–39. 2012.

20. 1

Rationale: Confidential issues are not to be discussed with nonmedical personnel or with the client's family or friends without the client's permission. Clients should be assured that information is kept confidential unless it places the nurse under a legal obligation. The nurse must report situations related to child, older adult abuse, and other types of abuse depending on state laws; gunshot wounds; stabbings; and certain infectious diseases.

Test-Taking Strategy: Use the process of elimination. Option 4 can be eliminated first, because this action does not protect the client from injury. Options 2 and 3 are comparable or alike and should be eliminated next. Review the nursing responsibilities related to reporting obligations if you had difficulty with this question.

Level of Cognitive Ability: Applying
Client Needs: Psychosocial Integrity
Integrated Process: Nursing Process/Implementation
Content Area: Leadership/Management: Ethical/Legal
Reference: deWit, p. 1089. 2009.

Leadership, Delegating, and Prioritizing Client Care

PYRAMID TERMS

accountability Moral concept that involves acceptance by a nurse of the consequences of a decision or action.

case management Health care delivery strategy that supports managed care. It is an interdisciplinary health care delivery approach that provides comprehensive client care using available resources to promote quality and cost-effective care.

critical pathway Clinical management care plan for providing client-centered care and for planning and monitoring the client's progress within an established time frame. Multidisciplinary collaboration and teamwork ensure shared decision making and quality client care.

delegation Process of transferring a selected nursing task in a situation to an individual who is competent to perform that specific task.

disaster Any human-made or natural event that causes destruction and devastation that cannot be alleviated without assistance; internal disasters are events that occur within a health care agency whereas external disasters are events that occur outside the health care agency.

emergency response plan A health care agency's preparedness and response plan in the event of a disaster.

evidence-based practice Approach to client care in which the nurse integrates the client's preferences, clinical expertise, and the best research evidence to deliver quality care.

leadership Interpersonal process that involves influencing others (followers) to achieve goals.

management Accomplishment of tasks or goals by oneself or by directing others.

prioritizing Deciding which needs or problems require immediate action and which ones could tolerate a delay in action until a later time because they are not urgent.

quality improvement Also known as performance improvement; focuses on processes or systems that significantly contribute to client safety and effective client care outcomes. Criteria are used to monitor outcomes of care and to determine the need for change to improve the quality of care.

triage Classifying procedure that ranks clients according to their need for medical care.

PYRAMID TO SUCCESS

A nurse is both a leader and a manager. As described in the NCLEX-PN exam test plan, a nurse needs to collaborate with other members of the multidisciplinary health care team to facilitate effective care. A primary Pyramid Point focuses on the skills required to prioritize client care activities. Pyramid Points also focus on concepts of management and supervision, leadership responsibilities, case management, quality improvement, the process of delegation, an emergency response plan, and triaging clients.

CLIENT NEEDS

Safe and Effective Care Environment

- Collaborating with members of the health care team
- Delegating client care activities and providing continuity of care
- Emergency response plan
- Establishing priorities related to client care activities
- Quality improvement
- Supervising the delivery of client care
- Triaging clients

Health Promotion and Maintenance

- Client's ability to perform self-care
- Disease prevention measures and health and wellness
- Health promotion programs
- Health screening
- Performing data collection techniques

Psychosocial Integrity

- Available support systems
- Cultural, spiritual, and religious issues
- Therapeutic interactions with others

Physiological Integrity

- Ensuring that palliative and comfort care is provided to the client
- Ensuring that emergencies are handled using a prioritization procedure
- Potential for alterations in body systems
- Unexpected responses to therapy

I. HEALTH CARE DELIVERY SYSTEMS

A. Managed care
1. Managed care is a broad term used to describe strategies used in the health care delivery system that reduce the costs of health care.
2. Client care is outcome driven and is managed by a case management process.
3. Managed care emphasizes the promotion of health, client education and responsible self-care, early identification of disease, and the use of health care resources.

B. Case management
1. Case management is a health care delivery strategy that supports managed care. It uses an interdisciplinary health care delivery approach that provides comprehensive client care throughout the client's illness using available resources to promote high-quality and cost-effective care.
2. Case management includes data collection and development of a plan of care, coordination of all services, referral, and follow-up.
3. Critical pathways are used, and variation analysis is conducted.

⚠ Case management involves collaboration with an interdisciplinary health care team.

C. Case manager
1. A case manager is a nurse who assumes responsibility for coordinating the client's care at admission and after discharge.
2. The case manager establishes a plan of care with the client, coordinates any consultations and referrals, and facilitates discharge.

D. Critical pathway
1. A critical pathway is a clinical management care plan for providing client-centered care and for planning and monitoring the client's progress within an established time frame; multidisciplinary collaboration and teamwork ensure shared decision making and quality client care.
2. All members of the health care team work with one plan to achieve the same client outcomes.
3. The goal of a critical pathway is to anticipate and recognize negative variance (i.e., problematic differences) early so that appropriate action can be taken and positive client outcomes can result.

4. Variation analysis
   a. Actual deviations or detours from a critical pathway are variances.
   b. Positive variance occurs when a client achieves maximum benefit and is discharged earlier than anticipated on the critical pathway.
   c. Negative variance occurs when untoward events prevent a timely discharge and the length of hospital stay is longer than planned for a client on a specific critical pathway.
   d. Variation analysis is a continuous process that the case manager and other caregivers conduct by comparing the specific client outcomes with the expected outcomes described on the critical pathway.
   e. Accurate monitoring of the critical pathway with variation analysis can estimate the financial impact of actual client outcomes on the health care facility, especially when the client is not achieving expected outcomes.
   f. If the variance is predictable, negotiation with health care insurers for cost coverage of an additional length of health care facility stay can maximize client care revenues.
   g. If the variance is not predicted and additional cost coverage is not negotiated with health care insurers, the hospital may not be reimbursed for a longer period of client care.

E. CareMaps
1. A CareMap is a model for a critical pathway.
2. The CareMap incorporates day-to-day expected client outcomes and outcomes anticipated at discharge or at the end of a treatment phase.
3. The CareMap outlines clinical assessments, treatments and procedures, dietary interventions, activity and exercise therapies, client education, and discharge planning.

F. Nursing care plan
1. A nursing care plan is a written guideline and communication tool that identifies the client's pertinent assessment data, problems and nursing diagnoses, goals, interventions, and expected outcomes.
2. The plan enhances continuity of care by identifying specific nursing actions necessary to achieve the goals of care.
3. The client and family are involved in developing the plan of care, and the plan identifies short- and long-term goals.
4. Client problems, goals, interventions, and expected outcomes are documented in the care plan, which provides a framework for evaluation of the client's response to nursing actions.

II. NURSING DELIVERY SYSTEMS

A. Functional nursing
1. Functional nursing involves a task approach to client care, with tasks being delegated to individual members of the team.

2. This type of system is task-oriented, and the team member focuses on the delegated task rather than the total client. This results in fragmentation of care and lack of accountability by the team member.

B. Team nursing
1. The team generally is led by a registered nurse (team leader) who is responsible for assessing, developing nursing diagnoses, planning, and evaluating each client's plan of care.
2. The team leader determines the work assignment. Each staff member works fully within the realm of his or her educational and clinical expertise and job description.
3. Each staff member is accountable for client care and outcomes of care delivered in accordance with the licensing and practice scope as determined by health care agency policy and state law.
4. Modular nursing is similar to team nursing, but takes into account the structure of the unit. The unit is divided into modules allowing nurses to care for a group of clients who are geographically close by.

C. Relationship-based practice (primary nursing)
1. Relationship-based practice (primary nursing) is concerned with keeping a nurse at the bedside, actively involved in client care, while planning goal-directed, individualized care.
2. One (primary) nurse is responsible for managing and coordinating the client's care while in the hospital and for discharge, and an associate nurse cares for the client when the primary nurse is off-duty.

D. Client-focused care
1. This is also known as the total care or case method. A nurse assumes total responsibility for planning and delivering care to a client.
2. The client may have different nurses assigned during a 24-hour period. However, the nurse provides all necessary care needed for the assigned time period.

III. PROFESSIONAL RESPONSIBILITIES

A. Accountability
1. The process in which individuals have an obligation (or duty) to act and are answerable for their actions
2. Involves assuming only the responsibilities that are within one's scope of practice and not assuming responsibility for activities in which competence has not been achieved
3. Involves admitting mistakes rather than blaming others and evaluating the outcomes of one's own actions
4. Includes a responsibility to the client to be competent, providing nursing care in accordance with standards of nursing practice, and adhering to the professional ethics codes

⚠ Accountability is accepting responsibility for one's actions. A nurse is always responsible for his or her actions when providing care to a client.

B. Leadership and management
1. Leadership is the interpersonal process that involves influencing others (followers) to achieve goals.
2. Management is the accomplishment of tasks or goals by oneself or by directing others.

C. Leader and manager approaches
1. Autocratic
   a. The leader or manager is focused and maintains strong control, makes decisions, and addresses all problems.
   b. The leader or manager dominates the group and commands rather than seeks suggestions or input.
2. Democratic
   a. This is also called participative.
   b. It is based on the belief that every group member should have input into the development of goals and problem solving.
   c. A democratic leader or manager acts primarily as a facilitator and resource person and is concerned for each member of the group.
   d. The democratic style is a more "talk with the members" style and much less authoritarian than the autocratic style.
3. Laissez-faire
   a. A laissez-faire leader or manager assumes a passive, nondirective, and inactive approach and relinquishes part or all of the responsibilities to the members of the group.
   b. Decision making is left to the group, with the laissez-faire leader or manager providing little, if any, guidance, support, or feedback.
4. Situational
   a. Situational style uses a combination of styles based on the current circumstances and events.
   b. Situational styles are assumed according to the needs of the group and the tasks to be achieved.
5. Bureaucratic
   a. The leader or manager believes that individuals are motivated by external forces.
   b. The leader/manager relies on organizational policies and procedures for decision making.

D. Effective leader and manager qualities (Box 8-1)
E. Problem-solving process and decision making
1. Problem solving involves obtaining information and using it to reach an acceptable solution to a problem.
2. Decision making involves identifying a problem and deciding which alternatives can best achieve objectives.

Box 8-1 Effective Leader and Manager Qualities

Effective communicator
Credible
Critical thinker
Initiator of action
Risk taker
Is persuasive and influences employees

TABLE 8-1 Similarities of the Problem-Solving Process and the Nursing Process

Problem-Solving Process	Nursing Process
Identifying a problem and collecting data about the problem	Data Collection
Deciding on a plan of action	Planning
Carrying out the plan	Implementation
Evaluating the plan	Evaluation

3. Steps of the problem-solving process are similar to the steps of the nursing process (Table 8-1).

IV. EMPOWERMENT

A. Empowerment is an interpersonal process of enabling others to do for themselves.

B. Empowerment occurs when individuals are able to influence what happens to them more effectively.

C. Empowerment involves open communication, mutual goal setting, and decision making.

D. Nurses can empower clients through teaching and advocacy.

V. FORMAL ORGANIZATIONS

A. An organization's mission statement communicates in broad terms its reason for existence; the geographic area that the organization serves; and attitudes, beliefs, and values from which the organization functions.

B. Goals and objectives are measurable activities specific to the development of designated services and programs of an organization.

C. The organizational chart depicts and communicates how activities are arranged, how authority relationships are defined, and how communication channels are established.

D. Policies, procedures, and protocols
    1. Policies are guidelines that define the organization's standpoint on courses of action.

2. Procedures are based on policy and define methods for tasks.
3. Protocols prescribe a specific course of action for a specific type of client or problem.

E. Centralization is the making of decisions by a few individuals at the top of the organization or by managers of a department or unit, and decisions are communicated thereafter to the employees.

F. Decentralization is the distribution of authority throughout the organization to allow for increased responsibility and delegation in decision making.

⚠ A nurse must follow policies, procedures, and protocols of the health care agency in which he or she is employed.

VI. EVIDENCE-BASED PRACTICE

A. Evidence-based practice is an approach to client care in which the nurse integrates the client's preferences, clinical expertise, and the best research evidence to deliver quality care.

B. Determining the client's personal, social, cultural, and religious preferences ensures individualization and is a component of implementing evidence-based practice.

C. A nurse needs to be an observer and identify and question situations that require change or result in a less than desirable outcome.

D. Use of information technology such as online resources, including research publications, provides current research findings related to areas of practice.

E. The nurse needs to follow evidence-based practice protocols developed by the institution and question the rationale for nursing approaches identified in the protocols as necessary.

⚠ Evidence-based practice requires that a nurse base nursing practice on evidence from clinical research studies. The nurse should also be alert to clinical issues that warrant investigation.

VII. QUALITY IMPROVEMENT

A. Also known as performance improvement, quality improvement focuses on processes or systems that significantly contribute to client safety and effective client care outcomes. Criteria are used to monitor outcomes of care and to determine the need for change to improve the quality of care.

B. Quality improvement processes or systems may be named quality assurance, continuous quality management, or continuous quality improvement.

C. When quality improvement is part of the philosophy of a health care agency, every staff member becomes involved in ways to improve client care and outcomes.

D. A retrospective ("looking back") audit is an evaluation method used to inspect the medical record after the client's discharge for documentation of compliance with the standards.

E. A concurrent ("at the same time") audit is an evaluation method used to inspect compliance of nurses with predetermined standards and criteria while the nurses are providing care during the client's stay.

F. Peer review is a process in which nurses employed in an organization evaluate the quality of nursing care delivered to the client.

G. The quality improvement process is similar to the nursing process and involves a multidisciplinary approach.

H. An outcome describes the most positive response to care; comparison of client responses to the expected outcomes indicates whether the interventions are effective, whether the client has progressed, how well standards are met, and whether changes are necessary.

I. A nurse is responsible for recognizing trends in nursing practice, identifying recurrent problems, and initiating opportunities to improve the quality of care.

 Quality improvement processes improve the quality of care delivery to clients and the safety of health care agencies.

 VIII. CONFLICT

A. Conflict arises from a perception of incompatibility or difference in beliefs, attitudes, values, goals, priorities, or decisions.

B. Types of conflict
1. Intrapersonal: Occurs within a person
2. Interpersonal: Occurs between and among clients, nurses, or other staff members
3. Organizational: Occurs when an employee confronts the policies and procedures of the organization

C. Modes of conflict resolution
1. Avoidance
   a. Avoiders are unassertive and uncooperative.
   b. Avoiders do not pursue their own needs, goals, or concerns, and they do not assist others to pursue theirs.
   c. Avoiders postpone dealing with the issue.
2. Accommodation
   a. Accommodators neglect their own needs, goals, or concerns (unassertive) while trying to satisfy those of others.
   b. Accommodators obey and serve others and often feel resentment and disappointment because they "get nothing in return."
3. Competition
   a. Competitors pursue their own needs and goals at the expense of others.

b. Competitors also may stand up for rights and defend important principles.
4. Compromise
   a. Compromisers are assertive and cooperative.
   b. Compromisers work creatively and openly to find the solution that most fully satisfies all important goals and concerns to be achieved.

IX. ROLES OF HEALTH CARE TEAM MEMBERS

A. Nurse roles are as follows:
1. Promote health and prevent disease
2. Provide comfort and care to clients
3. Make decisions
4. Act as client advocate
5. Manages client care
6. Communicate effectively
7. Educate clients, families, and communities and health care team members
8. Act as a resource person
9. Allocate resources in a cost-effective manner

B. Physician: A physician diagnoses and treats disease.

C. Physician assistant
1. A physician assistant acts to a limited extent in the role of the physician during the physician's absence
2. The physician assistant conducts physical examinations, performs diagnostic procedures, assists in the operating room and emergency department, and performs treatments.
3. Certified and licensed physician assistants in some states have prescriptive powers.

D. Physical therapist: A physical therapist assists in examining, testing, and treating physically disabled clients.

E. Occupational therapist: An occupational therapist develops adaptive devices that help chronically ill or handicapped clients perform activities of daily living.

F. Respiratory therapist: A respiratory therapist delivers treatments designed to improve the client's ventilation and oxygenation status.

G. Nutritionist: A nutritionist or dietitian assists in planning dietary measures to improve or maintain a client's nutritional status.

H. Continuing care nurse: This nurse coordinates discharge plans for the client.

I. Assistive personnel, including nursing assistants, unlicensed personnel, and client care technicians, help a nurse with specified tasks and functions.

J. Pharmacist: A pharmacist formulates and dispenses medications.

K. Social worker: A social worker counsels clients and families about home care services and assists the continuing care nurse with planning discharge.

L. Chaplain: A chaplain offers spiritual support and guidance to clients and families.

M. Administrative staff: Administrative or support staff members organize and schedule diagnostic tests and procedures and arrange for services needed by the client and family.

X. HEALTH CARE TEAM COLLABORATION

A. Client care planning can be accomplished through referrals to or consultations or collaborations with other health care specialists and through client care conferences, which involve members from all health care disciplines. This approach helps ensure continuity of care.

B. Reports
1. Reports should be factual, accurate, current, complete, and organized.
2. Reports should include essential background information, subjective data, objective data, any changes in the client's status, nursing diagnoses, treatments and procedures, medication administration, client teaching, discharge planning, family information, the client's response to treatments and procedures, and the client's priority needs.
3. Change of shift report
   a. The report facilitates continuity of care among nurses who are responsible for a client.
   b. The report may be written, oral, audiotaped, or provided during walking rounds at the client's bedside.
   c. The report describes the client's health status and informs the nurse on the next shift about the client's needs and priorities for care.
4. Telephone reports
   a. Purposes include informing a physician of a client's change in status, communicating information about a client's transfer to or from another unit or facility, and obtaining results of laboratory or diagnostic tests.
   b. The telephone report should be documented and should include when the call was made, who made the call, who was called, to whom information was given, what information was given, and what information was received.
5. Transfer reports
   a. Transferring nurse reports provide continuity of care and may be given by telephone or in person (Box 8-2).
   b. Receiving nurse should repeat transfer information to ensure client safety and ask questions to clarify information about the client's status.

XI. CONSULTATION WITH THE HEALTH CARE TEAM

A. Consultation is a process in which a specialist is sought to identify methods of care or treatment plans to meet the needs of a client.

> **Box 8-2 Transfer Reports**
>
> Client's name, age, physician, and diagnoses
> Current health status and plan of care
> Client's needs and priorities for care
> Any interventions that need to be performed after transfer, such as laboratory tests, medication administration, or dressing changes
> Need for any special equipment
> Additional considerations such as allergies, resuscitation status, precautionary considerations, or family issues

B. Consultation is needed when a nurse encounters a problem that cannot be solved using nursing knowledge, skills, and available resources.

C. Consultation also is needed when the exact problem remains unclear; a consultant can objectively and more clearly assess and identify the exact nature of the problem.

D. Rapid response teams are being developed within hospitals to provide nursing staff with internal consultative services provided by expert clinicians.

E. Rapid response teams are used to assist nursing staff with early detection and resolution of client problems.

XII. DISCHARGE PLANNING

A. Discharge planning begins when the client is admitted to the hospital or health care facility.

B. Discharge planning is a multidisciplinary process that ensures that the client has a plan for continuing care after leaving the health care facility and assists in the client's transition from one environment to another.

C. All caregivers need to be involved in discharge planning, and referrals to other health care professionals or agencies may be needed. A physician's prescription may be needed for the referral, and the referral needs to be approved by the client's health care insurer.

D. A nurse should anticipate the client's discharge needs and make the referral as soon as possible (involving the client and family in the referral process).

E. The nurse needs to assist in educating the client and family regarding care at home (Box 8-3).

XIII. DELEGATION AND ASSIGNMENTS

A. Delegation
1. Delegation is a process of transferring performance of a selected nursing task in a situation to an individual who is competent to perform that specific task.
2. Delegation involves achieving outcomes and sharing activities with other individuals who have the authority to accomplish the task.
3. The nurse practice act and any practice limitations define which aspects of care can be delegated.

4. Even though a task may be delegated to someone, the nurse who delegates maintains accountability for the task.

5. Only the task, not the ultimate accountability, may be delegated to another.

6. The five rights of delegation include the right task, right circumstances, right person, right direction/communication, and right supervision/evaluation.

⚠ Delegate only tasks for which you are responsible. A nurse who delegates is accountable for the task; the person who assumes responsibility for the task is also accountable.

B. Principles and guidelines of delegating (Box 8-4)
C. Assignments

1. Assignment is transferring performance of client care activities to specific staff members.

2. Guidelines for client care assignments
    a. Always ensure client safety.
    b. Be aware of individual variations in work abilities.
    c. Determine which tasks can be delegated and to whom.
    d. Match the task to the delegatee based on the nurse practice act and appropriate position descriptions.
    e. Provide directions that are clear, concise, accurate, and complete.
    f. Validate the delegatee's understanding of the directions.
    g. Communicate a feeling of confidence to the delegatee, and provide feedback promptly after the task is performed.
    h. Maintain continuity of care as much as possible when assigning client care.

XIV. TIME MANAGEMENT

A. Description
1. Time management is a technique designed to assist in completing tasks within a definite time period.

Box 8-3 Discharge Teaching

How to administer prescribed medications
Side effects of medications that need to be reported to the health care provider (HCP)
Prescribed dietary and activity measures
Complications of the medical condition that need to be reported to the HCP
How to perform prescribed treatments
How to use special equipment prescribed for the client
Schedule for home care services that are planned
How to access available community resources
When to obtain follow-up care

2. Learning how, when, and where to use one's time and establishing personal goals and time frames are part of time management.

3. Time management requires an ability to anticipate the day's activities, to combine activities when possible, and not to be interrupted by nonessential activities.

4. Time management involves efficiency in completing tasks as quickly as possible and effectiveness in deciding on the most important task to do (i.e., prioritizing) and doing it correctly.

B. Principles and guidelines
1. Identify tasks, obligations, and activities and write them down.

2. Organize the work day; identify which tasks must be completed in specified time frames.

3. Prioritize client needs according to importance.

4. Anticipate the needs of the day and provide time for unexpected and unplanned tasks that may arise.

5. Focus on beginning the daily tasks, working on the most important first while keeping goals in mind. Look at the final goal for the day, which helps in the breakdown of tasks into manageable parts.

6. Begin client rounds at the beginning of the shift, collecting data on each assigned client.

7. Delegate tasks when appropriate.

Box 8-4 Principles and Guidelines of Delegating

■ Delegate the right task to the right delegatee. Be familiar with the experience of the delegatees, their scopes of practice, their job descriptions, agency policy and procedures, and the state nurse practice act.

■ Provide clear directions about the task and ensure that the delegatee understands the expectations.

■ Determine the degree of supervision that may be required.

■ Provide the delegatee with the authority to complete the task. Provide a deadline for completion of the task.

■ Evaluate the outcome of care that has been delegated.

■ Provide feedback to the delegatee regarding his or her performance.

■ Generally, noninvasive interventions, such as skin care, range-of-motion exercises, ambulation, grooming, and hygiene measures, can be assigned to a nursing assistant.

■ Generally, a licensed practical nurse (LPN) or licensed vocational nurse (LVN) can perform not only the tasks that a nursing assistant can perform, but also certain invasive tasks, such as dressing changes, suctioning, urinary catheterization, and medication administration (oral, subcutaneous, intramuscular, and some piggyback [secondary] medications), according to the education and job description of the LPN or LVN.

■ A registered nurse (RN) can perform the tasks that an LPN or LVN can perform and is responsible for assessment and planning care, initiating teaching, and administering medications intravenously.

8. Keep a daily hour-by-hour log to assist in providing structure to the tasks that must be accomplished, and cross tasks off the list as they are accomplished.
9. Use health care agency resources wisely, anticipating resource needs, and gather the necessary supplies before beginning the task.
10. Organize paperwork and continuously document task completion and necessary client data throughout the day (i.e., documentation should be concurrent with completion of a task or observation of pertinent client data).
11. At the end of the day, evaluate the effectiveness of time management.

XV. PRIORITIZING CARE

A. Prioritizing is deciding which needs or problems require immediate action and which ones could tolerate a delay in response until a later time because they are not urgent.

B. Guidelines for prioritizing (Box 8-5)

C. Setting priorities for client teaching
1. Determine client's immediate learning needs.
2. Review the learning objectives established for the client.
3. Determine what the client perceives as important.
4. Assess the client's anxiety level and the time available to teach.

D. Prioritizing when caring for a group of clients (see Priority Nursing Actions)
1. Identify the problems of each client.
2. Review nursing diagnoses.

3. Determine which client problems are most urgent based on basic needs, the client's changing or unstable status, and complexity of the client's problems.
4. Anticipate the time that it may take to care for the priority needs of the clients.

▰▰▰▰ PRIORITY NURSING ACTIONS! ▰▰▰▰

Order of Priority in Assessing a Group of Clients

A nurse is assigned to the following clients. The order of priority in assessing the clients is as follows:
1. A client with heart failure who has a 4-lb weight gain since yesterday and is experiencing shortness of breath
2. A 24-hour postoperative client who had a wedge resection of the lung and has a closed chest tube drainage system
3. A client admitted to the hospital for observation who has absent bowel sounds
4. A client who is undergoing surgery for a hysterectomy on the following day

The nurse determines the order of priority by considering the needs of the client. The nurse also uses guidelines for prioritizing, such as the ABCs (airway, breathing, and circulation), Maslow's Hierarchy of Needs theory, and the steps of the nursing process. Clients 1 and 2 have conditions that relate to the respiratory system or cardiac system. These clients are the high priorities. Client 1 is the first priority because this client is experiencing shortness of breath (life-threatening). There is no indication that client 2 is experiencing any difficulty. Because client 4 is scheduled for surgery on the following day, this client would be the last priority (low priority), and the nurse would assess this client and prepare this client for surgery after other clients are assessed. Because absent bowel sounds could be an indication of a bowel obstruction (intermediate priority), this client would be the third priority.

Reference: Potter, P., & Perry, A. (2009). *Fundamentals of nursing* (7th ed., p. 307). St. Louis: Mosby.

Box 8-5 Guidelines for Prioritizing

- The nurse and the client mutually rank the client's needs in order of importance based on the client's preferences and expectations, safety, and physical and psychological needs. What the client sees as his or her priority needs may be different from what the nurse sees as the priority needs.
- Priorities are classified as high, intermediate, or low.
- Client needs that are life-threatening or that could result in harm to the client if they are left untreated are high priorities.
- Nonemergency and non–life-threatening client needs are intermediate priorities.
- Client needs that are not related directly to the client's illness or prognosis are low priorities.
- When providing care, the nurse needs to decide which needs or problems require immediate action and which ones could be delayed until a later time because they are not urgent.

- The nurse considers client problems that involve actual or life-threatening concerns before potential health-threatening concerns.
- When prioritizing care, the nurse must consider time constraints and available resources.
- Problems identified as important by the client must be given high priority.
- The nurse can use the ABCs—airway, breathing, and circulation—as a guide when determining priorities. Client needs related to maintaining a patent airway are always the priority.
- The nurse can use Maslow's Hierarchy of Needs theory as a guide to determine priorities and identify the levels of physiological needs, safety, love and belonging, self-esteem, and self-actualization. (Basic needs are met before moving to other needs in the hierarchy.)
- The nurse can use the steps of the nursing process as a guide to determine priorities, remembering that data collection is the first step of the nursing process.

5. Combine activities, if possible, to resolve more than one problem at a time.
6. Involve the client in his or her care as much as possible.

 Use the ABCs (airway, breathing, and circulation), Maslow's Hierarchy of Needs theory, and the steps of the nursing process (data collection is first) to prioritize.

XVI. DISASTERS AND EMERGENCY RESPONSE PLAN

A. Description
  1. A disaster is any human-made or natural event that causes destruction and devastation that cannot be alleviated without assistance (Box 8-6).
  2. Internal disasters are disasters that occur within a health care agency (e.g., health care agency fire, structural collapse, radiation spill), whereas external disasters are disasters that occur outside the health care agency (e.g., mass transit accident that could send hundreds of victims to emergency departments).
  3. An emergency response plan is a formal plan of action for coordinating the response of the health care agency staff in the event of a disaster in the health care agency or surrounding community.

B. American Red Cross (ARC)
  1. The ARC has been given authority by the federal government to provide disaster relief.
  2. All ARC disaster relief assistance is free, and local offices are located across the United States.
  3. The ARC participates with the government in developing and testing community disaster plans.
  4. The ARC identifies and trains personnel for emergency response.
  5. The ARC works with businesses and labor organizations to identify resources and individuals for disaster work.
  6. The ARC educates the public about ways to prepare for a disaster.
  7. The ARC operates shelters, provides assistance to meet immediate emergency needs, and provides disaster health services, including crisis counseling.
  8. The ARC handles inquiries from family members.
  9. The ARC coordinates relief activities with other agencies.
  10. Nurses are involved directly with the ARC and assume functions such as managers, supervisors, and educators of first aid; they also participate in emergency response plans and disaster relief programs and provide services, such as blood collection drives and immunization programs.

C. Phases of disaster management
  1. The Federal Emergency Management Agency (FEMA) identifies four disaster management phases: mitigation, preparedness, response, and recovery.
  2. Mitigation encompasses the following:
     a. Actions or measures that can prevent the occurrence of a disaster or reduce the damaging effects of a disaster
     b. Determination of the community hazards and community risks (actual and potential threats) before a disaster occurs
     c. Awareness of available community resources and community health personnel to facilitate mobilization of activities and minimize chaos and confusion if a disaster occurs
     d. Determination of the resources available for care to infants, older adults, disabled individuals, and individuals with chronic health problems
  3. Preparedness encompasses the following:
     a. Plans for rescue, evacuation, and caring for disaster victims
     b. Plans for training disaster personnel and gathering resources, equipment, and other materials needed for dealing with the disaster
     c. Identification of specific responsibilities for various emergency response personnel
     d. Establishment of a community emergency response plan and an effective public communication system
     e. Development of an emergency medical system and a plan for activation

---

Box 8-6 Types of Disasters

Human-Made Disasters
Dam failures resulting in flooding
Hazardous substance accidents such as pollution, chemical spills, or toxic gas leaks
Accidents involving release of radioactive material
Resource shortages such as food, water, and electricity
Structural collapse, fire, or explosions
Terrorist attacks such as bombing, riots, and bioterrorism
Mass transportation accidents

Natural Disasters
Blizzards
Communicable disease epidemics
Cyclones
Droughts
Earthquakes
Floods
Forest fires
Hailstorms
Hurricanes
Landslides
Mudslides
Tidal waves (tsunami)
Tornadoes
Volcanic eruptions

f. Verification of proper functioning of emergency equipment

g. Collection of anticipatory provisions and creation of a location for providing food, water, clothing, shelter, other supplies, and needed medicine

h. Inventory of supplies on a regular basis and replenishment of outdated supplies

i. Practice of community emergency response plans (mock disaster drills)

4. Response encompasses the following:

a. Putting disaster planning services into action and the actions taken to save lives and prevent further damage

b. Primary concerns include safety, physical health, and mental health of victims and members of the disaster response team

5. Recovery encompasses the following:

a. Actions taken to return to a normal situation after the disaster

b. Preventing debilitating effects and restoring personal, economic, and environmental health and stability to the community

D. Levels of disaster

1. FEMA identifies three levels of disaster with FEMA response (Box 8-7).

2. When a federal emergency has been declared, the federal response plan may take effect and activate emergency support functions.

3. The emergency support functions of the ARC include performing emergency first aid, sheltering, feeding, providing a disaster welfare information system, and coordinating bulk distribution of emergency relief supplies.

4. Disaster medical assistant teams (teams of specially trained personnel) can be activated and sent to a disaster site to provide triage and medical care to victims until they can be transported to a hospital.

E. Nurse's role in disaster planning

1. Personal and professional preparedness

a. Make personal and family preparations (Box 8-8).

b. Be aware of the disaster plan at the place of employment and in the community.

c. Maintain certification in disaster training and in cardiopulmonary resuscitation.

d. Participate in mock disaster drills, including a bomb threat drill.

e. Prepare professional emergency response items, such as a copy of nursing license, personal health care equipment such as a stethoscope, cash, warm clothing, record-keeping materials, and other nursing care supplies.

2. Disaster response

a. In the health care agency setting, if a disaster occurs, the agency disaster preparedness plan (emergency response plan) is activated immediately, and a nurse responds by following the directions identified in the plan.

b. In the community setting, if a nurse is the first responder to a disaster, the nurse cares for the victims by attending to the victims with life-threatening problems first. When rescue workers arrive at the scene, immediate plans for triage should begin. (See Priority Nursing Actions.)

Box 8-8 Emergency Plans and Supplies

Plan a meeting place for family members.
Identify where to go if an evacuation is necessary.
Determine when and how to turn off water, gas, and electricity at main switches.
Locate the safe spots in the home for each type of disaster.
Replace water supply every 3 months and food supply every 6 months.
Include the following supplies:

- A 3-day supply of water (1 gallon per person per day)
- A 3-day supply of nonperishable food
- Clothing and blankets
- First-aid kit
- Adequate supply of prescription medication
- Battery-operated radio
- Flashlight and batteries
- Credit card, cash, or traveler's checks
- Extra set of car keys and a full tank of gas in the car
- Sanitation supplies for washing, toileting, and disposing of trash
- Extra pair of eyeglasses
- Special items for infants, older adults, or disabled individuals
- Items needed for a pet such as food, water, and leash
- Important documents in a waterproof case

Box 8-7 Federal Emergency Management Agency (FEMA) Levels of Disaster

Level III Disaster
Minor disaster that involves a minimal level of damage, but could result in a presidential declaration of an emergency

Level II Disaster
Moderate disaster that is likely to result in a presidential declaration of an emergency, with moderate federal assistance

Level I Disaster
Massive disaster that involves significant damage and results in a presidential disaster declaration, with major federal involvement and full engagement of federal, regional, and national resources

▬▬ ▬PRIORITY NURSING ACTIONS! ▬▬

Triaging Clients at the Site of an Accident

A nurse is the first responder at the scene of a school bus accident. The nurse triages the victims from highest to lowest priority as follows:

1. Confused child with bright red blood pulsating from a leg wound
2. Child with a closed head wound and multiple compound fractures of the arms and legs
3. Child with a simple fracture of the arm
4. Sobbing child with several minor lacerations on the face, arms, and legs

Triage systems identify which victims are the priority and should be treated first. Rankings are based on immediacy of needs, including victims with immediate threat to life requiring immediate treatment (emergent), victims whose injuries are not life-threatening provided that they are treated within 1 to 2 hours (urgent), and victims with sustained local injuries who do not have immediate complications and can wait several hours for medical treatment (nonurgent). Victim 1 has a wound that is pulsating bright red blood; this indicates arterial puncture. The child is also confused, which indicates the presence of hypoxia and shock (emergent). Victim 2 has sustained multiple traumas, so this victim is also classified as emergent and would require immediate treatment; however, victim 1 is the higher priority because of the arterial puncture. Victim 3 sustained an injury that is not life threatening provided that the injury can be treated in 1 to 2 hours (urgent). Victim 4 sustained minor injuries that can wait several hours for treatment (nonurgent).

References: McKinney, E., James, S., Murray, S., & Ashwill, J. (2009). *Maternal-child nursing* (3rd ed., pp. 854, 849). St. Louis: Saunders; and Stanhope, M., & Lancaster, J. (2008). *Public health nursing: Population-centered health care in the community* (7th ed., p. 468). St. Louis: Mosby.

 In the event of a disaster, activate the emergency response plan immediately.

F. Triage
1. In a disaster or war, triage consists of brief assessment of victims that allows a nurse to classify victims according to the severity of the injury, urgency of treatment, and place for treatment.
2. In an emergency department, triage consists of brief assessment of clients that allows a nurse to classify clients according to their need for care and establishing priorities of care; the type of illness or injury, the severity of the problem, and the resources available govern the process.

 G. Emergency department triage system
1. A commonly used rating system in an emergency department is a three-tier system that uses the categories of emergent, urgent, and nonurgent; these

Box 8-9 Emergency Department Triage

Emergent (Red): Priority 1 (Highest)

This classification is assigned to clients who have life-threatening injuries and need immediate attention and continuous evaluation, but have a high probability for survival when stabilized.

Such clients include trauma victims, clients with chest pain, clients with severe respiratory distress or cardiac arrest, clients with limb amputation, clients with acute neurological deficits, and clients who have sustained chemical splashes to the eyes.

Urgent (Yellow): Priority 2

This classification is assigned to clients who require treatment and whose injuries have complications that are not life-threatening, provided that they are treated within 1 to 2 hours. These clients require continuous evaluation every 30 to 60 minutes thereafter.

Such clients include clients with a simple fracture, asthma without respiratory distress, fever, hypertension, abdominal pain, or a renal stone.

Nonurgent (Green): Priority 3

This classification is assigned to clients with local injuries who do not have immediate complications and who can wait several hours for medical treatment. These clients require evaluation every 1 to 2 hours thereafter.

Such clients include clients with conditions such as a minor laceration, sprain, or cold symptoms.

categories may be identified by color coding or numbers (Box 8-9).
2. A nurse needs to be familiar with the triage system of the health care agency.
3. When caring for a client who has died, the nurse needs to recognize the importance of family and religious rituals and provide support to loved ones.
4. Organ donation procedures of the health care agency need to be addressed if appropriate.

 Think survivability. If you are the first responder to a scene of a disaster, such as a train crash, the priority victim is the one whose life can be saved.

H. Client assessment in the emergency department
1. Primary assessment
   a. The purpose of primary assessment is to identify any client problem that poses an immediate or potential threat to life.
   b. A nurse gathers information primarily through objective data and, on finding any abnormalities, immediately initiates interventions.
   c. The nurse uses the ABCs—airway, breathing, and circulation—as a guide in assessing a client's needs and assesses a client who has sustained a traumatic injury for signs of a head injury or cervical spine injury.

2. Secondary assessment
   a. A nurse performs secondary assessment after the primary assessment and after treatment for any primary problems identified.
   b. Secondary assessment identifies any other life-threatening problems that a client might be experiencing.
   c. The nurse obtains subjective and objective data, including a history, general overview, vital sign measurements, neurological assessment, pain assessment, and complete or focused physical assessment.

MORE QUESTIONS ON EVOLVE!

Practice Questions

21. A nurse is recording an end-of-shift report for a client. What information needs to be included?
1. As-needed medications given that shift
2. Normal vital signs that have been normal since admission
3. All of the tests and treatments the client has had since admission
4. Total number of scheduled medications that the client received on that shift

22. A licensed practical nurse is planning the client assignments for the day. Which of the following is the most appropriate assignment for the nursing assistant?
1. A client who requires wound irrigation
2. A client who requires frequent ambulation
3. A client who is receiving continuous tube feedings
4. A client who requires frequent vital signs after a cardiac catheterization

23. A nurse employed in a long-term care facility is planning the client assignments for the shift. Which of the following clients would the nurse appropriately assign to the nursing assistant?
1. A client who requires a 24-hour urine collection
2. A client who requires twice-daily dressing changes
3. A diabetic client who requires daily insulin and the reinforcement of dietary measures
4. A client who is on a bowel management program and requires rectal suppositories and a daily enema

24. A nurse is assigned to care for four clients. When planning client rounds, which client would the nurse check first?
1. A client on a ventilator
2. A client in skeletal traction

3. A postoperative client preparing for discharge
4. A client admitted on the previous shift who has a diagnosis of gastroenteritis

25. A nurse employed in an emergency department is assigned to assist with the triage of clients arriving to the emergency department for treatment on the evening shift. The nurse would assign the highest priority to which of the following clients?
1. A client complaining of muscle aches, a headache, and malaise
2. A client who twisted her ankle when she fell while rollerblading
3. A client with a minor laceration on the index finger sustained while cutting an eggplant
4. A client with chest pain who states that he just ate pizza that was made with a very spicy sauce

26. A nurse is assigned to care for four clients. When planning client rounds, which client would the nurse collect data from first?
1. A client scheduled for a chest x-ray
2. A client requiring daily dressing changes
3. A postoperative client preparing for discharge
4. A client receiving oxygen via nasal cannula who had difficulty breathing during the previous shift

27. A licensed practical nurse is attending an agency orientation meeting about the nursing model of practice implemented in the facility. The nurse is told that the nursing model is a team nursing approach. The nurse understands that which of the following is a characteristic of this type of nursing model of practice?
1. A task approach method is used to provide care to clients.
2. Managed care concepts and tools are used when providing client care.
3. Nursing staff are led by a nurse when providing care to a group of clients.
4. A single registered nurse is responsible for providing nursing care to a group of clients.

28. A client experiences a cardiac arrest. The nurse leader quickly responds to the emergency and assigns clearly defined tasks to the work group. In this situation, the nurse is implementing which leadership style?
1. Autocratic
2. Situational
3. Democratic
4. Laissez-faire

29. A nurse has delegated several nursing tasks to staff members. The nurse's primary responsibility after the delegation of the tasks is to:

1. Document that the task was completed.
2. Assign the tasks that were not completed to the next nursing shift.
3. Allow each staff member to make judgments when performing the tasks.
4. Perform follow up with each staff member regarding the performance of the task and the outcomes related to the implementation of the task.

❖ **30.** The nurse on the day shift is assigned to care for the following six clients. List in order of priority how the nurse would plan to check the assigned clients.

(Number 1 is the client whom the nurse would check first, and number 6 is the last client.)
___ Client who requires before-breakfast insulin
___ Client who requires medications at 10:00 AM
___ Client who is scheduled for physical therapy in the afternoon
___ Client who has a tracheostomy and is on a mechanical ventilator
___ Client who is scheduled for a cardiac catheterization at 9:00 AM
___ Client who has been diagnosed with diabetes mellitus and who is scheduled for discharge to home

ANSWERS

21. 1
Rationale: End-of-shift report needs to be an efficient and accurate account of the client's condition during the last shift. It needs to include pertinent information about the client, such as tests and treatments; as-needed medications given or therapies performed during the past 24 hours, including the client's response to them; changes in the client's condition; scheduled tests and treatments; current problems; and any other special concerns. The total number of medications given or a list of all the tests and treatments that the client has had since admission are not necessary to include. Only significant vital signs need to be included.
Test-Taking Strategy: Remember that the purpose of end-of-shift reports is to communicate accurate and pertinent information about the client. The reporter does not have time to discuss extraneous or repetitive information, and the listener does not have time to listen to reports that include unneeded information. Review the information included in the end-of-shift report if you had difficulty with this question.
Level of Cognitive Ability: Applying
Client Needs: Safe and Effective Care Environment
Integrated Process: Communication and Documentation
Content Area: Leadership/Management: Delegating/Prioritizing
Reference: deWit, p. 30. 2009.

22. 2
Rationale: The nurse must determine the most appropriate assignment on the basis of the skills of the staff member and the needs of the client. In this case, the most appropriate assignment for a nursing assistant would be to care for the client who requires frequent ambulation. The nursing assistant is skilled in this task. The client who had a cardiac catheterization will require specific monitoring in addition to that of the vital signs. Wound irrigations and tube feedings are not performed by unlicensed personnel.
Test-Taking Strategy: Note the strategic words "most appropriate." Use the process of elimination, and recall the principles of delegation and the supervision of the work of others. Remember that work delegated to others must be done in a way that is consistent with the individual's level of expertise and that individual's licensure or lack of licensure. Review the principles of delegation if you had difficulty with this question.

Level of Cognitive Ability: Applying
Client Needs: Safe and Effective Care Environment
Integrated Process: Nursing Process/Planning
Content Area: Leadership/Management: Delegating/Prioritizing
Reference: Linton, p. 53. 2012.

23. 1
Rationale: The assignment of tasks needs to be implemented on the basis of the job description of the individual, the individual's level of clinical competence, and state law. Options 2, 3, and 4 involve care that requires the skill of a licensed nurse.
Test-Taking Strategy: Use the process of elimination and your knowledge regarding tasks that can be safely delegated to a nursing assistant. Eliminate options 2, 3, and 4, because these clients require care that needs to be provided by a licensed nurse. Review the principles related to assignments and delegation if you had difficulty with this question.
Level of Cognitive Ability: Applying
Client Needs: Safe and Effective Care Environment
Integrated Process: Nursing Process/Planning
Content Area: Leadership/Management: Delegating/Prioritizing
References: Christensen, Kockrow, p. 1260. 2011. *Foundations and adult health nursing.*
deWit, pp. 3–4. 2009.

24. 1
Rationale: The airway is always a high priority, and the nurse first checks the client on a ventilator. The clients described in options 2, 3, and 4 have needs that would be identified as intermediate priorities.
Test-Taking Strategy: Use Maslow's Hierarchy of Needs theory and the ABCs—airway, breathing, and circulation—to answer the question. Remember that the airway is always the first priority. Review the principles related to prioritizing if you had difficulty with this question.
Level of Cognitive Ability: Applying
Client Needs: Safe and Effective Care Environment
Integrated Process: Nursing Process/Planning
Content Area: Leadership/Management: Delegating/Prioritizing
References: Christensen, Kockrow, p. 1257. 2011. *Foundations and adult health nursing.*
deWit, pp. 28, 94–95. 2009.

25. 4

Rationale: In an emergency department, triage involves classifying clients according to their need for care, and it includes establishing priorities of care. The type of illness, the severity of the problem, and the resources available govern the process. Clients with trauma, chest pain, severe respiratory distress, cardiac arrest, limb amputation, or acute neurological deficits and those who sustained a chemical splash to the eyes are classified as emergent, and these clients are the number 1 priority. Clients with conditions such as simple fractures, asthma without respiratory distress, fever, hypertension, abdominal pain, or renal stones have urgent needs, and these clients are classified as the number 2 priority. Clients with conditions such as minor lacerations, sprains, or cold symptoms are classified as nonurgent, and they are the number 3 priority.

Test-Taking Strategy: Note the strategic words "highest priority." Use the ABCs—airway, breathing, and circulation—to direct you to option 4. A client who is experiencing chest pain is always classified as priority number 1 until a myocardial infarction has been ruled out. Review the triage classification system commonly used in the hospital emergency department if you had difficulty with this question.

Level of Cognitive Ability: Applying
Client Needs: Safe and Effective Care Environment
Integrated Process: Nursing Process/Implementation
Content Area: Leadership/Management: Delegating/Prioritizing
Reference: deWit, pp. 1074–1075. 2009.

26. 4

Rationale: The airway is always a high priority, and the nurse would attend to the client who has been experiencing an airway problem first. The clients described in options 1, 2, and 3 would have intermediate priority.

Test-Taking Strategy: Use the ABCs—airway, breathing, and circulation—to answer the question. Remember that the airway is always the first priority. Review the prioritizing principles if you had difficulty with this question.

Level of Cognitive Ability: Applying
Client Needs: Safe and Effective Care Environment
Integrated Process: Nursing Process/Planning
Content Area: Leadership/Management: Delegating/Prioritizing
Reference: deWit, pp. 94–95. 2009.

27. 3

Rationale: In team nursing, nursing personnel are led by a nurse when providing care to a group of clients. Option 1 identifies functional nursing. Option 2 identifies a component of case management. Option 4 identifies primary nursing.

Test-Taking Strategy: Note that the subject of the question relates to team nursing. Keep this subject in mind, and use the process of elimination. Option 3 is the only option that identifies the concept of a team approach. Review the various types of nursing delivery systems if you had difficulty with this question.

Level of Cognitive Ability: Understanding
Client Needs: Safe and Effective Care Environment
Integrated Process: Nursing Process/Implementation
Content Area: Leadership/Management: Delegating/Prioritizing
Reference: Linton, pp. 5, 51–52. 2012.

28. 1

Rationale: Autocratic leadership is an approach in which the leader retains all authority and is primarily concerned with task accomplishment. It is an effective leadership style to implement in an emergency or crisis situation. The leader assigns clearly defined tasks and establishes one-way communication with the work group, and he or she makes all decisions independently. Situational leadership is a comprehensive approach that incorporates the leader's style, the maturity of the work group, and the situation at hand. Democratic leadership is a people-centered approach that is primarily concerned with human relations and teamwork. This leadership style facilitates goal accomplishment and contributes to the growth and development of the staff. Laissez-faire leadership is a permissive style in which the leader gives up control and delegates all decision making to the work group.

Test-Taking Strategy: Use the process of elimination. Focusing on the data in the question and the nurse leader's actions will direct you to option 1. Review the various leadership styles if you had difficulty with this question.

Level of Cognitive Ability: Applying
Client Needs: Safe and Effective Care Environment
Integrated Process: Nursing Process/Implementation
Content Area: Leadership/Management: Delegating/Prioritizing
Reference: Linton, pp. 45–46. 2012.

29. 4

Rationale: The ultimate responsibility for a task lies with the person who delegated it. Therefore, it is the nurse's primary responsibility to follow up with each staff member regarding the performance of the task and the outcomes related to implementing the task. Not all staff members have the education, knowledge, and ability to make judgments about tasks being performed. The nurse documents that the task has been completed, but this would not be done until follow-up was implemented and outcomes were identified. It is not appropriate to assign the tasks that were not completed to the next nursing shift.

Test-Taking Strategy: Use the process of elimination, and note the strategic words "primary responsibility." Recalling that the ultimate responsibility for a task lies with the person who delegated it will direct you to option 4. Review the guidelines related to delegating if you had difficulty with this question.

Level of Cognitive Ability: Applying
Client Needs: Safe and Effective Care Environment
Integrated Process: Nursing Process/Implementation
Content Area: Leadership/Management: Delegating/Prioritizing
References: deWit, pp. 3–4. 2009.
Linton, p. 53. 2012.

30. 2, 4, 6, 1, 3, 5

Rationale: The airway is always a high priority, and the nurse first assesses the client who has a tracheostomy and is on a mechanical ventilator. The remaining order of priority is guided by time guidelines. Therefore, the nurse next administers before-breakfast insulin, assesses the client who is scheduled for a cardiac catheterization at 9:00 AM, and then administers medications scheduled for 10:00 AM. Finally, the nurse checks the client who is scheduled for discharge, and this is followed by checking the client who is scheduled for physical therapy in the afternoon.

Test-Taking Strategy: Use Maslow's Hierarchy of Needs theory and the ABCs—airway, breathing, and circulation. Focus only on the data identified in the question. Remember that the airway is always the first priority. Next, use time guidelines to plan the order of the remaining clients. Review the principles related to prioritizing if you had difficulty with this question.
Level of Cognitive Ability: Applying

Client Needs: Safe and Effective Care Environment
Integrated Process: Nursing Process/Planning
Content Area: Leadership/Management: Delegating/Prioritizing
References: Christensen, Kockrow, p. 1257. 2011. *Foundations and adult health nursing.*
deWit, pp. 94–95. 2009.

UNIT 3

Nursing Sciences

Fluids and Electrolytes

PYRAMID TERMS

calcium A mineral element needed for the process of bone formation, coagulation of blood, excitation of cardiac and skeletal muscle, maintenance of muscle tone, conduction of neuromuscular impulses, and synthesis and regulation of the endocrine and exocrine glands. The normal adult level is 8.6 to 10 mg/dL.

fluid volume deficit Dehydration in which the body's fluid intake is not sufficient to meet the body's fluid needs

fluid volume excess Fluid intake or fluid retention that exceeds the body's fluid needs; also called overhydration or fluid overload

homeostasis The tendency of biological systems to maintain relatively constant conditions in the internal environment while continuously interacting with and adjusting to changes originating within or outside of the system

hypercalcemia A serum calcium level that exceeds 10 mg/dL

hyperkalemia A serum potassium level that exceeds 5.1 mEq/L

hypermagnesemia A serum magnesium level that exceeds 2.6 mg/dL

hypernatremia A serum sodium level that exceeds 145 mEq/L

hyperphosphatemia A serum phosphorus level that exceeds 4.5 mg/dL

hypocalcemia A serum calcium level less than 8.6 mg/dL

hypokalemia A serum potassium level less than 3.5 mEq/L

hypomagnesemia A serum magnesium level less than 1.6 mg/dL

hyponatremia A serum sodium level less than 135 mEq/L

hypophosphatemia A serum phosphorus level less than 2.7 mg/dL

magnesium An element concentrated in the bone, cartilage, and within the cell itself that is required for the use of adenosine triphosphate as a source of energy. It is necessary for the action of numerous enzyme systems, such as carbohydrate metabolism, protein synthesis, nucleic acid synthesis, and the contraction of muscular tissue. It also regulates neuromuscular activity and the clotting mechanism. The normal adult level is 1.6 to 2.6 mg/dL.

potassium A principal electrolyte of intracellular fluid and the primary buffer within the cell itself; it is needed for nerve conduction, muscle function, acid–base balance, and osmotic pressure. In addition to calcium and magnesium, it controls the rate and force of contraction of the heart and, thus, cardiac output. The normal adult level is 3.5 to 5.1 mEq/L.

phosphorus An element needed for the generation of bony tissue; it functions in the metabolism of glucose and lipids, in the maintenance of acid-base balance, and in the storage and transfer of energy from one site in the body to another. Phosphorus levels are evaluated in relation to calcium levels because of their inverse relationship: when calcium levels are decreased, phosphorus levels are increased, and when phosphorus levels are decreased, calcium levels are increased. The normal adult level is 2.7 to 4.5 mg/dL.

sodium An abundant electrolyte that maintains osmotic pressure and acid–base balance and that transmits nerve impulses. The normal adult level is 135 to 145 mEq/L.

PYRAMID TO SUCCESS

Pyramid points focus primarily on the collection of data related to a fluid and electrolyte imbalance, interventions, and the evaluation of the expected outcomes. Fluid and electrolytes constitute a content area that is complex and sometimes difficult to understand. It is important to understand cell functions and properties and the concepts related to body fluids as outlined in this chapter. Review this content. Pyramid points also focus on the common fluid and electrolyte disturbances. Focus on the pyramid points related to the causes of imbalances or disturbances, data collection, and related treatments.

CLIENT NEEDS

Safe and Effective Care Environment

- Consulting with members of the health care team
- Establishing priorities for care
- Handling hazardous and infectious materials to prevent injury to health care personnel and others
- Maintaining medical and surgical asepsis and preventing infection in the client when samples for laboratory studies are obtained or when intravenous solutions are administered

- Maintaining standard, transmission-based, and other precautions to prevent the transmission of infection to self and others
- Preventing accidents and ensuring the safety of the client when an imbalance exists, particularly when changes in cardiovascular, respiratory, gastrointestinal, neuromuscular, renal, or central nervous systems occur or when the client is at risk for complications such as seizures, respiratory depression, or dysrhythmias

Health Promotion and Maintenance

- Implementing health screening and determining the potential risk for fluid and electrolyte imbalance
- Providing education related to medication and diet management
- Providing education related to the potential risk for fluid and electrolyte imbalance, measures to prevent an imbalance, signs and symptoms of an imbalance, and actions to take if signs and symptoms develop

Psychosocial Integrity

- Providing reassurance to the client who is experiencing a fluid or electrolyte imbalance
- Providing support and continuously informing the client of the purposes of prescribed interventions

Physiological Integrity

- Identifying clients who are at risk for fluid or electrolyte imbalance
- Monitoring laboratory values
- Monitoring for expected and unexpected responses to therapeutic interventions and documenting findings
- Assisting with managing emergencies related to fluid or electrolyte imbalance
- Monitoring for complications related to the imbalance

I. CELL PROPERTIES (Box 9-1)

II. CONCEPTS OF FLUID AND ELECTROLYTE BALANCE

A. Electrolytes
  1. Description: When a substance is dissolved in solution and some of its molecules split or dissociate into electrically charged atoms or ions (see Box 9-1)
  2. Measurement
    a. The metric system is used to measure volumes of fluids: liters (L) or milliliters (mL).
    b. The unit of measure that expresses the combining activity of an electrolyte is the milliequivalent (mEq).
B. Body fluid compartments (Box 9-2) (Figure 9-1)
  1. Fluid in each of the body compartments contains electrolytes.
  2. Each compartment has a particular composition of electrolytes that differs from that of other compartments.
  3. To function normally, body cells must have fluids and electrolytes in the right compartments and in the right amounts.
  4. Whenever an electrolyte moves out of a cell, another electrolyte moves in to take its place.
  5. The numbers of cations and anions must be the same for **homeostasis** to exist.
  6. Compartments are separated by semipermeable membranes.

Box 9-1 Cell Properties

Atom: The smallest part of an element that still has the properties of the element and that is composed of particles known as *protons* (positive charge), *neutrons* (neutral), and *electrons* (negative charge). Protons and neutrons are in the nucleus of the atom; therefore, the nucleus is positively charged. Electrons carry a negative charge and revolve around the nucleus. As long as the number of electrons is the same as the number of protons, there is no net charge on the atom—that is, it is neither positive nor negative. Atoms may gain, lose, or share electrons, and then they are no longer neutral.

Molecule: Two or more atoms that have combined to form a substance.

Ion: An atom that carries an electrical charge because it has either gained or lost electrons. Some ions carry a negative electrical charge, and some carry a positive charge.

Cation: An ion that carries a positive charge because it has given away or lost electrons. The result is fewer electrons than protons and a positive charge.

Anion: An ion that has gained electrons and therefore carries a negative charge. When an ion has gained or taken on electrons, it assumes a negative charge, and the result is a negatively charged ion.

Box 9-2 Body Fluid Compartments

Extracellular compartment: Refers to all fluid outside of the cells

Interstitial fluids: Fluid that is between the cells and the blood vessels

Intracellular compartment: Refers to all fluid inside the cells. Most body fluids are inside the cells.

Intravascular compartment: Fluid that is within blood vessels

C. Third-spacing
1. The accumulation and sequestration of trapped extracellular fluid in an actual or potential body space as a result of disease or injury
2. The trapped fluid represents a volume loss and is unavailable for normal physiological processes.
3. Fluid may be trapped in body spaces such as the pericardial, pleural, peritoneal, or joint cavities; the bowel; or the abdomen or within soft tissues after trauma or burns.
4. Assessing the intravascular fluid loss is difficult. It may not be reflected in weight changes or intake and output (I&O) records, and it may not become apparent until after organ malfunction occurs.

D. Edema
1. An excess accumulation of fluid in the interstitial spaces
2. Localized edema occurs as a result of traumatic injury from accidents or surgery, local inflammatory processes, or burns.
3. Generalized edema, also called *anasarca*, is an excessive accumulation of fluid in the interstitial space throughout the body as a result of a condition such as cardiac, renal, or liver failure.

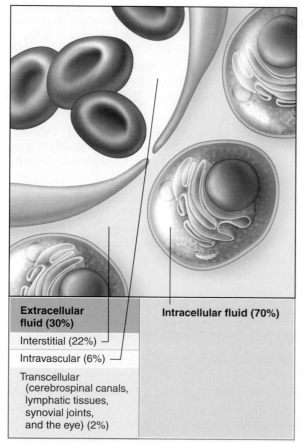

▲ **FIGURE 9-1** Distribution of fluid by compartments in the average adult. (From Harkreader, H., Hogan, M. A., & Thobaben, M. [2007]. *Fundamentals of nursing: Caring and clinical judgment* [3rd ed., p. 615]. St Louis: Saunders.)

E. Body fluid
1. Description
   a. Provides the transportation of nutrients to the cells and carries waste products from the cells
   b. Total body fluid (intracellular and extracellular) amounts to about 60% of body weight in the adult, 55% in the older adult, and 80% in the infant.
   c. Infants and older adults are at higher risk for fluid-related problems than younger adults; children have a greater proportion of body water than adults; and the older adult has the least proportion of body water.
   d. A loss of 10% of body fluid in the adult is serious and a 20% loss can be fatal.
2. Constituents of body fluids
   a. Body fluids consist of water and dissolved substances.
   b. The largest single fluid constituent of the body is water.

⚠ Infants and older adults need to be monitored closely for fluid imbalances.

F. Body fluid transport
1. Diffusion
   a. Diffusion is the process whereby a solute (substance that is dissolved) may spread through a solution or solvent (solution in which the solute is dissolved).
   b. Diffusion of a solute spreads the molecules from an area of higher concentration to an area of lower concentration.
   c. Diffusion occurs within fluid compartments and from one compartment to another if the barrier between the compartments is permeable to the diffusing substances.
2. Osmosis
   a. Osmosis is the movement of solvent molecules across a membrane in response to a concentration gradient, usually from a solution of lower to one of higher solute concentration.
   b. When a more concentrated solution is on one side of a selectively permeable membrane and a less concentrated solution is on the other side, a pull called *osmotic pressure* draws the water through the membrane to the more concentrated side, or the side with more solute.
3. Filtration
   a. Filtration is the movement of solutes and solvents by hydrostatic pressure.
   b. The movement is from an area of greater pressure to an area of lesser pressure.
4. Hydrostatic pressure
   a. The force exerted by the weight of a solution
   b. When a difference exists in the hydrostatic pressure on two sides of a membrane, water

and diffusible solutes move out of the solution that has the higher hydrostatic pressure by the process of filtration.

5. Osmolality
   a. Refers to the number of osmotically active particles per kilogram of water; it is the concentration of a solution.
   b. In the body, osmotic pressure is measured in milliosmols (mOsm).
   c. The normal osmolality of plasma is 270 to 300 (mOsm/kg) water.

G. Movement of body fluid
   1. Description
      a. Cell membranes separate the interstitial fluid from the intravascular fluid.
      b. Cell membranes are selectively permeable; that is, the cell membrane and the capillary wall allow water and some solutes free passage through them.
      c. Several forces affect the movement of water and solutes through the walls of cells and capillaries.
      d. The greater the number of particles in the concentrated solution, the more pull there will be to move the water through the membrane.
      e. If the body loses more electrolytes than fluids, as can happen with diarrhea, then the extracellular fluid will contain fewer electrolytes or less solute than the intracellular fluid.
      f. Fluids and electrolytes must be kept in balance for health; when they remain out of balance, death can occur.
   2. Isotonic solutions (Table 9-1)
      a. When the solutions on both sides of a selectively permeable membrane have established equilibrium or are equal in concentration, they are isotonic.
      b. Isotonic solutions are isotonic to human cells, and thus very little osmosis occurs. Isotonic solutions have the same osmolality as body fluids.

3. Hypotonic solutions (see Table 9-1)
   a. When a solution contains a lower concentration of salt or solute than another more concentrated solution, it is considered hypotonic.
   b. A hypotonic solution has less salt or more water than an isotonic solution. These solutions have lower osmolality than body fluids.
   c. Hypotonic solutions are hypotonic to the cells; therefore, osmosis would continue in an attempt to bring about balance or equality.
4. Hypertonic solutions: A solution that has a higher concentration of solutes than another less concentrated solution is hypertonic. These solutions have a higher osmolality than body fluids. (see Table 9-1)

H. Body fluid excretion (Table 9-2)
   1. Description
      a. Fluids leave the body by several routes, including the skin, lungs, gastrointestinal (GI) tract, and kidneys.
      b. The kidneys excrete the largest quantity of fluid.
      c. As long as all organs are functioning normally, the body can maintain balance in its fluid content.
   2. Skin
      a. Water is lost through the skin by diffusion in the range of 600 to 800 mL/day and includes loss through perspiration.
      b. The amount of water lost by perspiration will vary according to the temperature of the environment and the body, but the average amount of loss is 100 mL/day.
      c. Water lost through the skin by diffusion is called *insensible loss* (the individual is unaware of losing that water).
   3. Lungs
      a. Water is lost from the lungs through expired air that is saturated with water vapor.
      b. The amount of water lost from the lungs will vary with the rate and the depth of respiration.
      c. The average amount of water lost from the lungs ranges from 400 to 600 mL/day.
      d. Water lost from the lungs is called *insensible loss.*

TABLE 9-1 Tonicity of Intravenous Fluids

Solution	Tonicity
0.45% saline (½ normal saline [NS])	Hypotonic
0.9% saline (NS)	Isotonic
5% dextrose in water (D_5W)	Isotonic
5% dextrose in 0.225% saline ($D_5/\frac{1}{4}$ NS)	Isotonic
Lactated Ringer's solution	Isotonic
5% dextrose in lactated Ringer's solution	Hypertonic
5% dextrose in 0.45% saline ($D_5/\frac{1}{2}$ NS)	Hypertonic
5% dextrose in 0.9% saline ($D_5/$NS)	Hypertonic
10% dextrose in water ($D_{10}W$)	Hypertonic

TABLE 9-2 Daily Body Fluid Excretion or Loss

Where Fluid Is Lost or Excreted	Amount Lost or Excreted (mL)
Skin	600-800
Lungs	400-600
Feces	100
Kidneys	1500

4. GI tract
   a. Large quantities of water are secreted into the GI tract, but almost all of this fluid is reabsorbed.
   b. A very large volume of electrolyte-containing liquids moves into the GI tract and then returns again into the extracellular fluid.
   c. The average amount of water lost in the feces is about 100 mL/day.
   d. Severe diarrhea will result in the loss of large quantities of fluids and electrolytes.
5. Kidneys
   a. Kidneys play a major role in regulating the fluid and electrolyte balance and excrete the largest quantity of fluid.
   b. Normal kidneys can adjust the amount of water and electrolytes leaving the body.
   c. The quantity of fluid excreted by the kidneys is determined by the amount of water ingested and the amount of waste and solutes excreted.
   d. The usual urine output is approximately 1500 mL/day; however, this will vary greatly, depending on fluid intake, the amount of perspiration, and other factors.

⚠ The client with diarrhea is at high risk for a fluid and electrolyte imbalance.

I. Body fluid replacement
   1. Water enters the body through three sources: orally ingested liquids, water in foods, and water formed by the oxidation of foods.
   2. Amounts
      a. The average total amount of water taken into the body by all three sources is 2500 mL/day.
      b. About 10 mL of water is released by the metabolism of each 100 calories of fat, carbohydrates, or proteins.
   3. Electrolytes
      a. Electrolytes are present in both foods and liquids.
      b. With a normal diet, an excess of essential electrolytes is taken in, and the unused electrolytes are excreted.
   J. Maintaining fluid and electrolyte balance
   1. Description
      a. **Homeostasis** is a term that indicates the relative stability of the internal environment.
      b. Concentration and composition of body fluids must be nearly constant.
      c. When one of the substances in a client is deficient—either fluid or electrolytes—the substance must be replaced normally by the intake of food and water or by therapy such as intravenous (IV) solutions and medications.
      d. When the client has an excess of fluid or electrolytes, therapy is directed toward assisting the body with eliminating the excess.

2. The kidneys play a major role in controlling the balance of fluid and electrolytes.
3. The adrenal glands, through the secretion of aldosterone, also aid with controlling the extracellular fluid volume by regulating the amount of **sodium** reabsorbed by the kidneys.
4. Antidiuretic hormone from the pituitary gland regulates the osmotic pressure of extracellular fluid by regulating the amount of water reabsorbed by the kidney.

III. FLUID VOLUME DEFICIT

A. Description
   1. Dehydration occurs when the body's fluid intake is not sufficient to meet the body's fluid needs.
   2. The goal of treatment is to restore fluid volume, replace electrolytes as needed, and eliminate the cause of the **fluid volume deficit**.
B. Causes
   1. Vomiting and/or diarrhea
   2. Continuous GI irrigation
   3. GI suctioning
   4. Ileostomy or colostomy drainage
   5. Draining wounds, burns, or fistulas
   6. Increased urine output from the use of diuretics
C. Data collection
   1. Thirst
   2. Poor skin turgor and dry mucous membranes
   3. Increased heart rate, thready pulse, and postural hypotension
   4. Rapid weight loss
   5. Flat neck or hand veins
   6. Dizziness or weakness
   7. Decrease in urine volume and dark, concentrated urine
   8. Increased specific gravity of the urine
   9. Confusion
   10. Increased hematocrit level
D. Interventions
   1. The cause of the **fluid volume deficit** is treated (for example antidiarrheal, antiemetic, antimicrobial medications may be prescribed), and fluids are replaced through administration of intravenous solutions (lactated Ringer's solution, 0.9% normal saline) as prescribed and oral rehydration.
   2. Monitor vital signs.
   3. Check mucous membranes and skin turgor.
   4. Monitor weight daily.
   5. Monitor I&O.
   6. Test urine for specific gravity.
   7. Monitor hematocrit and electrolyte levels; prepare to correct electrolyte imbalance if needed.

IV. FLUID VOLUME EXCESS

A. Description

1. Fluid intake or retention exceeds the body's fluid needs.
2. Also called *overhydration* or *fluid overload*
3. The goals of treatment are to restore fluid balance; correct electrolyte imbalances, if present; and eliminate or control the underlying cause of the overload (impaired cardiac or renal function can lead to **fluid volume excess**).

 B. Data collection

1. Cough and dyspnea
2. Lung crackles
3. Increased respirations and heart rate
4. Increased blood pressure and bounding pulse
5. Pitting edema
6. Weight gain
7. Neck and hand vein distention
8. Decreased hematocrit level
9. Confusion
10. Increased blood urea nitrogen (BUN) level

 C. Interventions

1. Monitor vital signs.
2. Position the client in semi-Fowler's position.
3. Check for edema.
4. Monitor I&O.
5. Monitor daily weight.
6. Administer diuretics as prescribed.
7. Monitor hematocrit and electrolyte levels.
8. Restrict fluids as prescribed.
9. Provide a low-**sodium** diet as prescribed.

⚠ A client with renal failure is at high risk for fluid volume excess.

 V. HYPOKALEMIA (Table 9-3)

A. Description (Box 9-3)

1. Hypokalemia is a serum **potassium** level lower than 3.5 mEq/L.
2. **Potassium** deficit is potentially life threatening because every body system is affected.

 B. Interventions

1. Monitor vital signs.
2. Monitor neuromuscular activity.
3. Monitor I&O.
4. Check renal function before administering **potassium**.
5. Administer **potassium** supplements as prescribed (orally or monitor by IV).
6. Oral **potassium** chloride has an unpleasant taste and should be taken with juice or other desired liquid.
7. Oral **potassium** preparations can cause GI irritation and should not be taken on an empty stomach.

8. If the client complains of abdominal pain, distention, nausea, vomiting, diarrhea, or GI bleeding, the oral **potassium** may need to be discontinued.
9. When **potassium** is added to an IV solution, shake the bag and invert it to ensure that the **potassium** is evenly distributed.

TABLE 9-3 Potassium Imbalances

Hypokalemia	Hyperkalemia
CAUSES	
Use of non–potassium-sparing diuretics	Renal failure
Diarrhea	Intestinal obstruction
Vomiting	Cell damage
Inadequate intake of potassium	Excessive oral or parenteral administration of potassium; potassium-sparing diuretics
Excessive gastric suction	Acidosis
Excessive fistula drainage	Addison's disease
Cushing's syndrome	Excessive use of potassium-based salt substitutes
Chronic use of corticosteroids or laxatives	Transfusion of stored blood (the breakdown of older red blood cells releases potassium)
Renal disease	
Parenteral nutrition	
Uncontrolled diabetes	
Alkalosis	
SIGNS AND SYMPTOMS	
Leg and abdominal cramps	Muscle weakness
Lethargy and weakness	Paresthesias
Shallow respirations and thready pulse	Hypotension
Confusion	Diarrhea
Decreased or absent reflexes	Hyperactive bowel sounds
Hypoactive bowel sounds and ileus	Wide, flat P waves; widened QRS complex; prolonged PR interval; depressed ST segment; and narrow, peaked T waves
Postural hypotension	
Peaked P waves; flat T waves; depressed ST segment and U waves	

Box 9-3 Potassium

Normal Value
3.5 to 5.1 mEq/L

Common Food Sources
Avocados
Bananas
Cantaloupes
Carrots
Fish
Mushrooms
Oranges
Potatoes
Pork, beef, and veal
Raisins
Spinach
Strawberries
Tomatoes

10. An IV bolus injection of concentrated **potassium** is never administered; it is always diluted.
11. A client receiving more than 10 mEq/hr should be placed on a cardiac monitor. The infusion is controlled by an infusion device.
12. Monitor for cardiac changes during the administration of **potassium**.
13. Monitor electrolyte values.
14. Monitor the IV site; if phlebitis or infiltration occurs, the IV should be stopped immediately and restarted at another site.
15. Instruct the client not to use salt substitutes containing **potassium** unless prescribed by the health care provider.

⚠️ Potassium is never administered by IV push, intramuscular, or subcutaneous routes. IV potassium is always diluted and administered using an infusion device.

 VI. HYPERKALEMIA (see Table 9-3)

A. Description: **Hyperkalemia** is a serum **potassium** level that exceeds 5.1 mEq/L (see Box 9-3).
B. Interventions
  1. Monitor vital signs.
  2. Monitor for cardiac changes.
  3. Decrease **potassium** intake.
  4. Administer **potassium**-excreting diuretics as prescribed if renal function is not impaired.
  5. Monitor I&O.
  6. Monitor laboratory values.
  7. Emergency treatment includes the rapid IV administration of dextrose with regular insulin to move excess **potassium** into the cells.
  8. Administer **sodium** polystyrene sulfonate (Kayexalate) orally or by enema as prescribed, which releases **sodium** ions in exchange for primarily **potassium** ions and absorbs the **potassium** into the GI tract for excretion.
  9. Monitor for **calcium** and **magnesium** loss when using Kayexalate.
  10. Monitor renal function.
  11. Prepare for dialysis if **potassium** levels are critically high.
  12. When blood transfusions are prescribed for a client with a **potassium** imbalance, the client should receive fresh blood, if possible. Transfusions of stored blood may elevate the **potassium** level, because the breakdown of older blood cells releases **potassium**.
  13. Instruct the client to avoid foods high in **potassium**.
  14. Instruct the client to avoid the use of salt substitutes or other **potassium**-containing substances.

⚠️ Monitor the serum potassium level closely when a client is receiving a potassium-sparing diuretic!

 VII. HYPONATREMIA (Table 9-4)

A. Description
  1. Hyponatremia is a serum **sodium** level less than 135 mEq/L (Box 9-4).
  2. **Sodium** imbalances are usually associated with fluid imbalances.
B. Interventions
  1. Monitor vital signs.
  2. Monitor I&O.
  3. Monitor weight.
  4. Assess skin turgor and mucous membranes.
  5. Restrict water intake and avoid tap-water enemas.
  6. Use normal saline solution rather than sterile water for irrigation.
  7. Administer **sodium** replacement as prescribed and monitor electrolyte values.
  8. Encourage foods that contain **sodium** (see Box 9-4).
  9. If the client is taking lithium, monitor the lithium level, because **hyponatremia** can cause diminished lithium excretion that can result in toxicity.

⚠️ Hyponatremia precipitates lithium toxicity in a client taking lithium (Lithobid).

TABLE 9-4 Sodium Imbalances

Hyponatremia	Hypernatremia
CAUSES	
Inadequate sodium intake (nothing by mouth)	Decreased water intake
Gastrointestinal suction	Fever
Excessive intake of water	Excessive perspiration
Irrigation of gastrointestinal tubes with plain water	Dehydration
Potent diuretics	Hyperventilation
Increased perspiration	Watery diarrhea
Draining skin lesions	Enteral nutrition and parenteral nutrition deplete the cells of water
Burns	Diabetes insipidus
Nausea and vomiting	Cushing's syndrome
Diabetic ketoacidosis	Impaired renal function
Syndrome of inappropriate antidiuretic hormone secretion	Use of corticosteroids
Retention of fluid, such as with kidney or heart failure	Excessive administration of sodium bicarbonate
SIGNS AND SYMPTOMS	
Rapid, thready pulse	Dry mucous membranes
Postural blood pressure changes	Loss of skin turgor
Weakness	Thirst
Abdominal cramping	Flushed skin
Poor skin turgor	Elevated temperature
Muscle twitching and seizures	Oliguria
Apprehension	Muscle twitching
	Fatigue
	Confusion
	Seizures

VIII. HYPERNATREMIA (see Table 9-4)

A. Description: **Hypernatremia** is a serum **sodium** level that exceeds 145 mEq/L (see Box 9-4).

B. Interventions
1. Monitor vital signs.
2. Monitor I&O.
3. Monitor electrolyte levels.
4. Prepare to administer intravenous infusions if hypernatremia is caused by fluid loss.
5. Restrict dietary **sodium as prescribed** (see Box 9-4).
6. Increase water intake orally; provide water between meals or tube feedings and encourage the client to drink 8 to 10 glasses of water daily if hypernatremia is caused by fluid loss.

IX. HYPOCALCEMIA (Table 9-5)

A. Description: **Hypocalcemia** is a serum **calcium** level less than 8.6 mg/dL (Box 9-5).

B. Interventions
1. Monitor vital signs.
2. Monitor for the presence of Chvostek's and Trousseau's signs (Figure 9-2).
3. Provide a quiet environment and avoid overstimulation.
4. Initiate seizure precautions.
5. Administer **calcium** orally or monitor IV **calcium** administration as prescribed.
6. Administer vitamin D as prescribed to aid in the absorption of **calcium** from the intestinal tract.
7. Keep 10% **calcium** gluconate available for acute **calcium** deficit.
8. Monitor **calcium** levels closely after thyroid surgery.
9. Instruct the client who is taking **calcium**-excreting medications to have serum **calcium** levels checked periodically.

TABLE 9-5 Calcium Imbalances

Hypocalcemia	Hypercalcemia
CAUSES	
Inadequate dietary intake of calcium	Excessive intake of calcium supplements, milk, and antacid products that contain calcium
Inhibited absorption of calcium from the intestinal tract	
Inadequate vitamin D consumption	Excessive intake of vitamin D
Diarrhea	Increased bone resorption or destruction from conditions such as bone tumors, fractures, osteoporosis, and immobility
Long-term immobilization and bone demineralization	
Excessive gastrointestinal losses from diarrhea or wound draining	Decreased excretion of calcium
End-stage renal disease	Renal disease
Calcium-excreting medications such as diuretics, caffeine, anticonvulsants, heparin, laxatives, and nicotine	Use of thiazide diuretics
	Hyperparathyroidism
	Use of lithium
	Use of glucocorticoids
Decreased secretion of parathyroid hormone	Adrenal insufficiency
Acute pancreatitis	
Crohn's disease	
Excessive administration of blood	
SIGNS AND SYMPTOMS	
Tachycardia	Increased heart rate and blood pressure
Hypotension	
Paresthesias	Bounding pulse
Twitching	Bradycardia (late stage)
Cramps	Shortened QT interval and widened T wave
Tetany	
Positive Chvostek's or Trousseau's sign	Muscle weakness (hypotonicity)
	Diminished deep tendon reflexes
Diarrhea	Nausea and vomiting
Hyperactive bowel sounds	Constipation
Prolongation of QT interval	Abdominal distention
	Confusion, lethargy, and coma

Box 9-4 Sodium

Normal Value
135 to 145 mEq/L

Common Food Sources
Bacon
Butter
Canned foods
Cheese, such as American or cottage cheese
Hot dogs
Ketchup
Lunch meats
Milk
Mustard
Processed foods
Snack foods
Soy sauce
Table salt
White and whole-wheat bread

Box 9-5 Calcium

Normal Value
8.6 to 10 mg/dL

Common Food Sources
Cheese
Collard greens
Milk and soy milk
Rhubarb
Sardines
Spinach
Tofu
Yogurt

10. Teach the client about the proper use of antacids or laxatives.
11. Instruct the client to consume foods high in **calcium** (see Box 9-5).

X. HYPERCALCEMIA (see Table 9-5)

A. Description: **Hypercalcemia** is a serum **calcium** level that exceeds 10 mg/dL (see Box 9-5).
B. Interventions
   1. Monitor vital signs.
   2. Monitor for dysrhythmias.
   3. Restrict **calcium** intake.
   4. Increase mobility.
   5. Assist with passive range-of-motion exercises when ambulation is not possible.
   6. Move clients carefully.
   7. Monitor for the development of pathological fractures.
   8. Monitor for severe flank or abdominal pain and strain urine to check for urinary stones.
   9. Monitor level of consciousness.
   10. Monitor for confusion and neurological changes.
   11. Avoid large doses of vitamin D supplements.
   12. Avoid the use of thiazide diuretics.
   13. Prepare for the administration of phosphate as prescribed.
   14. Prepare for the administration of calcitonin (Calcimar) as prescribed to increase the incorporation of **calcium** into the bones.
   15. Prepare the client with severe **hypercalcemia** unresponsive to medications for dialysis.

XI. HYPOMAGNESEMIA (Table 9-6)

A. Description: **Hypomagnesemia** is a serum **magnesium** level less than 1.6 mg/dL (Box 9-6).

B. Interventions
   1. Monitor vital signs.
   2. Monitor for dysrhythmias.
   3. Monitor for neuromuscular changes.
   4. Monitor I&O.
   5. Initiate seizure precautions.
   6. Administer **magnesium** supplements and monitor laboratory values.
   7. Monitor serum **magnesium** levels every 12 to 24 hours when client is receiving **magnesium** by IV.
   8. Monitor for reduced deep tendon reflexes that suggest **hypermagnesemia** during the administration of **magnesium**.
   9. Instruct the client to eat food that is high in **magnesium** (see Box 9-6).

XII. HYPERMAGNESEMIA (see Table 9-6)

A. Description: **Hypermagnesemia** is a serum **magnesium** level that exceeds 2.6 mg/dL (see Box 9-6).
B. Interventions
   1. Monitor vital signs.
   2. Monitor for respiratory depression.
   3. Monitor for hypotension, bradycardia, and dysrhythmias.
   4. Monitor neurological and muscular activity.
   5. Monitor level of consciousness.
   6. Remove the source of the excess **magnesium**.
   7. Monitor laboratory values.
   8. Increase renal excretion by increasing oral fluids or administering loop diuretics as prescribed.
   9. Instruct the client to avoid the use of laxatives and antacids that contain **magnesium**.

⚠ Calcium gluconate is the antidote for magnesium overdose!

▲ **FIGURE 9-2** Tests for hypocalcemia. **A,** Chvostek's sign is a contraction of facial muscles in response to a light tap over the facial nerve in front of the ear. **B,** Trousseau's sign is a carpal spasm induced by inflating a blood pressure cuff (**C**) above the systolic pressure for a few minutes. (From Lewis, S., Heitkemper, M., & Dirksen, S. [2011]. *Medical-surgical nursing: Patient-centered collaborative care* [8th ed.]. St Louis: Mosby.)

XIII. HYPOPHOSPHATEMIA (Table 9-7)

A. Description: Hypophosphatemia is a serum **phosphorus** level less than 2.7 mg/dL (Box 9-7).

B. Interventions
1. Monitor vital signs.
2. Monitor respiratory status.
3. Move the client carefully.
4. Administer phosphate as prescribed.
5. Check the renal system before administering phosphate.
6. Monitor **calcium, phosphorus, sodium,** and chloride levels.
7. Administer vitamin D.
8. Monitor for decreased neuromuscular activity.
9. Monitor for **calcium** excess and kidney stones.
10. Monitor for hematological changes.
11. Decrease intake of **calcium**-rich foods and increase intake of meats and whole grains that contain **phosphorus** (see Box 9-7).
12. Instruct the client regarding the use of antacids.

 A decrease in the serum phosphorus level is accompanied by an increase in the serum calcium level, and an increase in the serum phosphorus level is accompanied by a decrease in the serum calcium level.

TABLE 9-6 Magnesium Imbalances

Hypomagnesemia	Hypermagnesemia
CAUSES	
Malnutrition	Overuse of antacids or laxatives that contain magnesium
Diarrhea	
Celiac disease	Renal insufficiency and renal failure
Crohn's disease	Treatment of preeclampsia with magnesium
Alcoholism	
Prolonged gastric suctioning	
Ileostomy, colostomy, or intestinal fistulas	
Acute pancreatitis	
Diabetic ketoacidosis	
Eclampsia	
Chemotherapy	
Sepsis	
SIGNS AND SYMPTOMS	
Twitching	Hypotension
Paresthesias	Bradycardia
Hyperactive reflexes	Weak pulse
Irritability	Sweating and flushing
Confusion	Respiratory depression
Positive Chvostek's or Trousseau's sign	Loss of deep tendon reflexes
Shallow respirations	Prolonged PR interval and widened QRS complexes
Tetany	
Seizures	
Tachycardia	
Tall T waves and depressed ST segment	

TABLE 9-7 Phosphorus Imbalances

Hypophosphatemia	Hyperphosphatemia
CAUSES	
Decreased nutritional intake of phosphorus and malnutrition	Excessive dietary intake of phosphorus
Use of magnesium-based or aluminum-hydroxide–based antacids	Overuse of phosphate-containing laxatives or enemas
Renal failure	Vitamin D intoxication
Hyperparathyroidism	Hypoparathyroidism
Malignancy	Renal insufficiency
Hypercalcemia	Chemotherapy
Alcohol withdrawal	
Diabetic ketoacidosis	
Respiratory alkalosis	
SIGNS AND SYMPTOMS	
Confusion	Neuromuscular irritability
Seizures	Muscle weakness
Weakness	Hyperactive reflexes
Decreased deep tendon reflexes	Tetany
Shallow respirations	Positive Chvostek's or Trousseau's sign
Increased bleeding tendency	
Immunosuppression	
Bone pain	

Box 9-6 Magnesium

Normal Value
1.6 to 2.6 mg/dL

Common Food Sources
Avocados
Canned white tuna fish
Cauliflower
Oatmeal
Green leafy vegetables, such as spinach and broccoli
Yogurt
Milk
Peanut butter
Peas
Pork, beef, and chicken
Potatoes
Raisins

Box 9-7 Phosphorus

Normal Value
2.7 to 4.5 mg/dL

Common Food Sources
Fish
Organ meats
Nuts
Pork, beef, and chicken
Whole-grain breads and cereals

XIV. HYPERPHOSPHATEMIA (see Table 9-7)

A. Description: **Hyperphosphatemia** is a serum **phosphorus** level that exceeds 4.5 mg/dL (see Box 9-7).

B. Interventions

1. Increase the fecal excretion of **phosphorus** by binding **phosphorus** from food in the GI tract with the use of aluminum hydroxide gel.
2. Monitor laboratory values.
3. Prepare for dialysis if prescribed.
4. Monitor for signs of **hypocalcemia**.
5. Administer **calcium** as prescribed if **hypocalcemia** exists.
6. Monitor for neuromuscular irritability.
7. Monitor for hyperreflexia, tetany, and seizures.
8. Monitor for Trousseau's and Chvostek's signs.
9. Instruct the client to avoid phosphate-containing medications, including laxatives and enemas.
10. Instruct the client to decrease intake of foods high in **phosphorus**.
11. Instruct the client regarding how to take phosphate-binding medications, emphasizing that these should be taken with meals or immediately after meals.

MORE QUESTIONS ON EVOLVE!

Practice Questions

31. A nurse is caring for a client with cirrhosis. The nurse notes that the client is dyspneic and crackles are heard on auscultation of the lungs. What additional signs would the nurse expect to note in this client if a fluid volume excess is present?
1. Rapid weight loss
2. Flat hand and neck veins
3. A weak and thready pulse
4. An increase in blood pressure

32. The nurse is reviewing the health records of assigned clients. The nurse plans care knowing that which client is at risk for a potassium deficit?
1. The client with Addison's disease
2. The client with metabolic acidosis
3. The client with intestinal obstruction
4. The client receiving nasogastric suction

33. A nurse reviews a client's electrolyte results and notes a potassium level of 5.5 mEq/L. The nurse understands that a potassium value at this level would be noted with which condition?
1. Diarrhea
2. Traumatic burn
3. Cushing's syndrome
4. Overuse of laxatives

34. A nurse reviews a client's electrolyte results and notes that the potassium level is 5.4 mEq/L. Which of the following would the nurse note on the cardiac monitor as a result of this laboratory value?
1. ST elevation
2. Peaked P wave
3. Prominent U wave
4. Narrow, peaked T waves

35. A nurse is reading the health care provider's (HCP's) progress notes in the client's record and sees that the HCP has documented "insensible fluid loss of approximately 800 mL daily." The nurse understands that this type of fluid loss can occur through:
1. The skin
2. Urinary output
3. Wound drainage
4. The gastrointestinal tract

36. A nurse is reviewing the health records of assigned clients. The nurse plans care knowing that which client is at the lowest risk for the development of third-spacing?
1. The client with sepsis
2. The client with cirrhosis
3. The client with renal failure
4. The client with diabetes mellitus

37. A nurse is reviewing the health records of assigned clients. The nurse plans care knowing that which client is at risk for fluid volume deficit?
1. The client with cirrhosis
2. The client with a colostomy
3. The client with decreased kidney function
4. The client with congestive heart failure (CHF)

38. A nurse is caring for a client who has been taking diuretics on a long-term basis. A fluid volume deficit is suspected. Which finding would be noted in the client with this condition?
1. Gurgling respirations
2. Increased blood pressure
3. Decreased hematocrit level
4. Increased specific gravity of the urine

39. A nurse reviews electrolyte values and notes a sodium level of 130 mEq/L. The nurse understands that this sodium level would be noted in a client with which condition?
1. The client with watery diarrhea
2. The client with diabetes insipidus
3. The client with an inadequate daily water intake
4. The client with the syndrome of inappropriate secretion of antidiuretic hormone (SIADH)

40. A nurse is caring for a client with leukemia and notes that the client has poor skin turgor and flat neck and hand veins. The nurse suspects hyponatremia. What additional signs would the nurse expect to note in this client if hyponatremia is present?
    1. Intense thirst
    2. Slow bounding pulse
    3. Dry mucous membranes
    4. Postural blood pressure changes

41. A nurse is caring for a client with a diagnosis of hyperparathyroidism. Laboratory studies are performed, and the serum calcium level is 12.0 mg/dL. On the basis of this laboratory value, the nurse takes which action?
    1. Documents the value in the client's record
    2. Informs the registered nurse of the laboratory value
    3. Places the laboratory result form in the client's record
    4. Reassures the client that the laboratory result is normal

42. A nurse reviews the client's serum calcium level and notes that the level is 8.0 mg/dL. The nurse understands that which condition would cause this serum calcium level?
    1. Prolonged bedrest
    2. Adrenal insufficiency
    3. Hyperparathyroidism
    4. Excessive ingestion of vitamin D

43. A nurse is caring for a client with a suspected diagnosis of hypercalcemia. Which of the following signs would be an indication of this diagnosis?
    1. Twitching
    2. Positive Trousseau's sign
    3. Hyperactive bowel sounds
    4. Generalized muscle weakness

44. A nurse is instructing a client on how to decrease the intake of calcium in the diet. The nurse tells the client that which food item contains the least amount of calcium?
    1. Milk
    2. Butter
    3. Spinach
    4. Collard greens

45. A nurse is caring for a client with hyperparathyroidism and notes that the client's serum calcium level is 13 mg/dL. Which medication should the nurse prepare to administer as prescribed to the client?
    1. Calcium chloride
    2. Calcium gluconate
    3. Calcitonin (Miacalcin)
    4. Large doses of vitamin D

ANSWERS

31. 4

Rationale: Findings associated with fluid volume excess include cough, dyspnea, crackles, tachypnea, tachycardia, an elevated blood pressure, a bounding pulse, an elevated central venous pressure, weight gain, edema, neck and hand vein distention, an altered level of consciousness, and a decreased hematocrit level.

Test-Taking Strategy: Use the process of elimination. Note that options 1, 2, and 3 are comparable or alike. Each of these signs relates to a decrease in fluid volume. Option 4 reflects an increase. If you had difficulty with this question, review the signs noted in clients with fluid volume excess.

Level of Cognitive Ability: Understanding
Client Needs: Physiological Integrity
Integrated Process: Nursing Process/Data Collection
Content Area: Fundamental Skills: Fluids & Electrolytes/Acid-Base
Reference: Linton, p. 208. 2012.

32. 4

Rationale: Potassium-rich gastrointestinal (GI) fluids are lost through GI suction, which places the client at risk for hypokalemia. The client with intestinal obstruction, Addison's disease, and metabolic acidosis is at risk for hyperkalemia.

Test-Taking Strategy: Read the question carefully, and note that it asks for the client who is at risk for hypokalemia. Read each option, and think about the electrolyte loss that can occur with each condition. Option 4 clearly identifies a loss of body fluid. If you had difficulty with this question, review the causes of hypokalemia.

Level of Cognitive Ability: Analyzing
Client Needs: Physiological Integrity
Integrated Process: Nursing Process/Planning
Content Area: Fundamental Skills: Fluids & Electrolytes/Acid-Base
Reference: Linton, p. 209. 2012.

33. 2

Rationale: A serum potassium level that exceeds 5.1 mEq/L is indicative of hyperkalemia. Clients who experience the cellular shifting of potassium, as in the early stages of massive cell destruction (i.e., with trauma, burns, sepsis, or metabolic or respiratory acidosis), are at risk for hyperkalemia. The client with Cushing's syndrome or diarrhea and the client who has been overusing laxatives are at risk for hypokalemia.

Test-Taking Strategy: Use the process of elimination, and eliminate options 1 and 4 first, because they are comparable or alike and reflect a gastrointestinal loss. From the remaining options, recalling that cell destruction causes potassium shifts will direct you to the correct option. Remember that Cushing's syndrome presents a risk for hypokalemia and that Addison's disease presents a risk for hyperkalemia. Review the causes of hyperkalemia if you had difficulty with this question.

Level of Cognitive Ability: Analyzing
Client Needs: Physiological Integrity
Integrated Process: Nursing Process/Data Collection
Content Area: Fundamental Skills: Fluids & Electrolytes/ Acid-Base
Reference: deWit, pp. 46, 48–49. 2009.

34. 4

Rationale: A serum potassium level of 5.4 mEq/L is indicative of hyperkalemia. Cardiac changes include a wide, flat P wave; a prolonged PR interval; a widened QRS complex; narrow, peaked T waves; and a depressed ST segment.
Test-Taking Strategy: From the information in the question, you need to determine that this condition is a hyperkalemic one. From this point, it is necessary to know the cardiac changes that are expected when hyperkalemia exists. Review these cardiac changes if you had difficulty with this question.
Level of Cognitive Ability: Analyzing
Client Needs: Physiological Integrity
Integrated Process: Nursing Process/Data Collection
Content Area: Fundamental Skills: Fluids & Electrolytes/ Acid-Base
References: Christensen, Kockrow, pp. 668–669. 2011. *Foundations and adult health nursing.*
Ignatavicius, Workman, pp. 190–191. 2010.

35. 1

Rationale: Sensible losses are those that the person is aware of, such as those that occur through wound drainage, GI tract losses, and urination. Insensible losses may occur without the person's awareness. Insensible losses occur daily through the skin and the lungs.
Test-Taking Strategy: Note that the subject of the question is insensible fluid loss. Use the process of elimination, and note that options 2, 3, and 4 are comparable or alike. These types of losses can be measured for accurate output. Fluid loss through the skin cannot be accurately measured, only approximated. If you had difficulty with this question, review the differences between sensible and insensible fluid loss.
Level of Cognitive Ability: Understanding
Client Needs: Physiological Integrity
Integrated Process: Nursing Process/Data Collection
Content Area: Fundamental Skills: Fluids & Electrolytes/ Acid-Base
Reference: Alexander, Corrigan, Gorski, Hankins, Perucca, pp. 184, 449–450. 2010.

36. 4

Rationale: Fluid that shifts into the interstitial spaces and remains there is referred to as *third-space fluid.* Common sites for third-spacing include the abdomen, pleural cavity, peritoneal cavity, and pericardial sac. Third-space fluid is physiologically useless because it does not circulate to provide nutrients for the cells. Risk factors include liver or kidney disease, major trauma, burns, sepsis, wound healing, major surgery, malignancy, malabsorption syndrome, malnutrition, alcoholism, and older age.
Test-Taking Strategy: Note the strategic words "lowest risk." These words indicate a negative event query and ask you to select the client who is at least risk for third-spacing. Eliminate options 2 and 3 first, because it is likely that fluid balance

disturbances will occur with these conditions. From the remaining options, sepsis is the option that is the most acute and therefore the most similar to options 2 and 3. Review the risk factors associated with third-spacing if you had difficulty with this question.
Level of Cognitive Ability: Analyzing
Client Needs: Physiological Integrity
Integrated Process: Nursing Process/Planning
Content Area: Fundamental Skills: Fluids & Electrolytes/ Acid-Base
Reference: deWit, pp. 43–44. 2009.

37. 2

Rationale: Causes of a fluid volume deficit include vomiting, diarrhea, conditions that cause increased respirations or increased urinary output, insufficient intravenous fluid replacement, draining fistulas, ileostomy, and colostomy. A client with cirrhosis, CHF, or decreased kidney function is at risk for fluid volume excess.
Test-Taking Strategy: Read the question carefully, and note that it asks for the client who is at risk for a deficit. Read each option, and think about the fluid imbalance that can occur in each client. The clients presented in options 1, 3, and 4 retain fluid. The only condition that can cause a fluid volume deficit is the condition noted in option 2. If you had difficulty with this question, review the causes of fluid volume deficit.
Level of Cognitive Ability: Analyzing
Client Needs: Physiological Integrity
Integrated Process: Nursing Process/Planning
Content Area: Fundamental Skills: Fluids & Electrolytes/ Acid-Base
References: deWit, p. 678. 2009.
Linton, p. 206. 2012.

38. 4

Rationale: Findings in a client with a fluid volume deficit include increased respirations and heart rate, decreased central venous pressure, weight loss, poor skin turgor, dry mucous membranes, decreased urine volume, increased specific gravity of the urine, dark-colored and odorous urine, an increased hematocrit level, and an altered level of consciousness. The signs in options 1, 2, and 3 are seen in a client with fluid volume excess.
Test-Taking Strategy: Use the process of elimination. Eliminate options 1 and 2 first. Gurgling respirations and increased blood pressure are noted in clients with fluid volume excess. Remember that the specific gravity of urine is increased in a client with a fluid volume deficit. If you had difficulty with this question, review the findings noted in a client with a fluid volume deficit.
Level of Cognitive Ability: Understanding
Client Needs: Physiological Integrity
Integrated Process: Nursing Process/Data Collection
Content Area: Fundamental Skills: Fluids & Electrolytes/ Acid-Base
Reference: Linton, p. 205. 2012.

39. 4

Rationale: Hyponatremia is a serum sodium level less than 135 mEq/L. Hyponatremia can result secondary to SIADH. The client with an inadequate daily water intake, watery diarrhea, or diabetes insipidus is at risk for hypernatremia.

Test-Taking Strategy: Knowledge regarding the normal sodium level and the causes of hyponatremia is required to answer the question. Remember that hyponatremia can result secondary to SIADH. Review the causes of hyponatremia if you had difficulty with this question.

Level of Cognitive Ability: Analyzing
Client Needs: Physiological Integrity
Integrated Process: Nursing Process/Data Collection
Content Area: Fundamental Skills: Fluids & Electrolytes/Acid-Base
Reference: deWit, pp. 891–892. 2009.

40. 4

Rationale: Postural blood pressure changes occur in the client with hyponatremia. Dry mucous membranes and intense thirst are seen in clients with hypernatremia. A slow, bounding pulse is not indicative of hyponatremia. In a client with hyponatremia, a rapid thready pulse is noted.

Test-Taking Strategy: Use the process of elimination, and note the information provided in the question. Eliminate options 1 and 3 first, because they are comparable or alike (a client with dry mucous membranes is likely to have intense thirst). From the remaining options, it is necessary to recall the signs of hyponatremia. Review the signs associated with hyponatremia if you had difficulty with this question.

Level of Cognitive Ability: Analyzing
Client Needs: Physiological Integrity
Integrated Process: Nursing Process/Data Collection
Content Area: Fundamental Skills: Fluids & Electrolytes/Acid-Base
Reference: deWit, p. 46. 2009.

41. 2

Rationale: The normal serum calcium level ranges from 8.6 to 10.0 mg/dL. The client is experiencing hypercalcemia, and the nurse would inform the registered nurse of the laboratory value. Because the client is experiencing hypercalcemia, options 1, 3, and 4 are incorrect.

Test-Taking Strategy: Focus on the laboratory value in the question to determine that the client is experiencing hypercalcemia. Note that options 1, 3, and 4 are comparable or alike and indicate that no action would be taken to report the value. Review the normal calcium level if you had difficulty with this question.

Level of Cognitive Ability: Applying
Client Needs: Physiological Integrity
Integrated Process: Nursing Process/Implementation
Content Area: Fundamental Skills: Fluids & Electrolytes/Acid-Base
Reference: deWit, pp. 47–49. 2009.

42. 1

Rationale: The normal serum calcium level is 8.6 to 10.0 mg/dL. A client with a serum calcium level of 8.0 mg/dL is experiencing hypocalcemia. The excessive ingestion of vitamin D, adrenal insufficiency, and hyperparathyroidism are causative factors associated with hypercalcemia. Although immobilization can initially cause hypercalcemia, the long-term effect of prolonged bedrest is hypocalcemia.

Test-Taking Strategy: Knowledge regarding the normal serum calcium level will assist you with determining that the client is experiencing hypocalcemia. This should help you to eliminate option 4. Recalling the causative factors associated with hypocalcemia is necessary to select the correct option from those remaining. Remember that the long-term effect of prolonged bedrest is hypocalcemia. If you had difficulty with the question, review the causative factors associated with hypocalcemia.

Level of Cognitive Ability: Understanding
Client Needs: Physiological Integrity
Integrated Process: Nursing Process/Data Collection
Content Area: Fundamental Skills: Fluids & Electrolytes/Acid-Base
References: Christensen, Kockrow, pp. 376, 670. 2011. *Foundations of nursing.*
deWit, pp. 47, 49. 2009.

43. 4

Rationale: Generalized muscle weakness is seen in clients with hypercalcemia. Options 1, 2, and 3 identify signs of hypocalcemia.

Test-Taking Strategy: Use the process of elimination. Note that options 1, 2, and 3 are comparable or alike, because they all reflect a hyperactivity of body systems. The option that is different is option 4. Review the signs of hypercalcemia if you had difficulty with this question.

Level of Cognitive Ability: Analyzing
Client Needs: Physiological Integrity
Integrated Process: Nursing Process/Data Collection
Content Area: Fundamental Skills: Fluids & Electrolytes/Acid-Base
Reference: Christensen, Kockrow, p. 670. 2011. *Foundations of nursing.*

44. 2

Rationale: Butter comes from milk fat and does not contain significant amounts of calcium. Milk, spinach, and collard greens are calcium-containing foods and should be avoided by the client on a calcium-restricted diet.

Test-Taking Strategy: Note the strategic words "least amount." These words indicate a negative event query and ask you to select the item that is lowest in calcium. Option 1 can be easily eliminated first. Eliminate options 3 and 4 next, because they are comparable or alike. Review the foods that are high and low in calcium if you had difficulty with this question.

Level of Cognitive Ability: Applying
Client Needs: Physiological Integrity
Integrated Process: Teaching and Learning
Content Area: Fundamental Skills: Fluids & Electrolytes/Acid-Base
Reference: Peckenpaugh, p. 111. 2010.

45. 3

Rationale: The normal serum calcium level is 8.6 to 10.0 mg/dL. This client is experiencing hypercalcemia. Calcium gluconate and calcium chloride are medications used for the treatment of tetany, which occurs as a result of acute hypocalcemia. In hypercalcemia, large doses of vitamin D need to be avoided. Calcitonin, a thyroid hormone, decreases the plasma calcium level by inhibiting bone resorption and lowering the serum calcium concentration.

Test-Taking Strategy: Recalling the normal serum calcium level will assist you with determining that the client is experiencing hypercalcemia. With this knowledge, you can easily eliminate options 1 and 2, because you would not administer medication that adds calcium to the body. Remembering that excessive vitamin D is a causative factor of hypercalcemia will assist you with eliminating option 4.

If you had difficulty with this question, review the treatment of hypercalcemia.

Level of Cognitive Ability: Analyzing
Client Needs: Physiological Integrity
Integrated Process: Nursing Process/Planning
Content Area: Pharmacology
References: Hodgson, Kizior, pp. 163–164. 2011. Christensen, Kockrow, pp. 670–671. 2011. *Foundations of nursing.*

Acid-Base Balance

PYRAMID TERMS

Allen's test A test to assess for collateral circulation to the hand by evaluating the patency of the radial and ulnar arteries

metabolic acidosis A total concentration of buffer base that is lower than normal with a relative increase in the hydrogen ion concentration. This results from loss of buffer bases or retention of too much acid without sufficient bases and occurs in conditions such as renal failure and diabetic ketoacidosis, from the production of lactic acid, and from the ingestion of toxins such as acetylsalicyclic acid (aspirin).

metabolic alkalosis A deficit or loss of hydrogen ions or acids or an excess of base (bicarbonate) that results from an accumulation of base or a loss of acid without a comparable loss of base in the body fluids. This occurs in conditions resulting in hypovolemia, the loss of gastric fluid, excessive bicarbonate intake, massive transfusion of whole blood, and hyperaldosteronism.

respiratory acidosis A total concentration of buffer base that is lower than normal with a relative increase in hydrogen ion concentration; thus a greater number of hydrogen ions is circulating in the blood than the buffer system can absorb. This is caused by primary defects in the function of the lungs or by changes in normal respiratory patterns as a result of secondary problems. Any condition that causes an obstruction of the airway or depresses respiratory status can cause respiratory acidosis.

respiratory alkalosis A deficit of carbonic acid or a decrease in hydrogen ion concentration that results from an accumulation of base or a loss of acid without a comparable loss of base in the body fluids. This occurs in conditions that cause overstimulation of the respiratory status.

PYRAMID TO SUCCESS

Acid-base imbalance is a content area that is sometimes viewed as difficult to understand. You must understand the description of each imbalance and then review the causes of each disorder, correlating the pathophysiology with each cause. From this point, note the signs and symptoms related to each disorder and the treatment associated with the clinical manifestations. The maintenance of a patent airway is a priority. The nurse also needs to monitor the vital signs, cardiovascular status, neurological status, intake and output, laboratory values, and arterial blood gas values. Remember that safety and seizure precautions may need to be initiated.

CLIENT NEEDS

Safe and Effective Care Environment

- Establishing priorities
- Maintaining medical and surgical asepsis
- Maintaining standard, transmission-based, and other precautions
- Obtaining informed consent for invasive procedures
- Preventing accidents
- Providing safety for the client during the implementation of various treatments for the acid-base imbalance

Health Promotion and Maintenance

- Identifying clients at risk for an acid-base imbalance
- Performing data-collection techniques
- Preventing disease
- Promoting health and wellness
- Teaching the client and family about the prevention, early detection, and treatment measures of health disorders

Psychosocial Integrity

- Identifying support systems
- Monitoring for sensory and perceptual alterations
- Providing emotional support to the client and family

Physiological Integrity

- Administering and monitoring medications, intravenous fluids, and other therapeutic interventions
- Assisting with diagnostic tests
- Monitoring for alterations in body systems
- Monitoring for changes in status and complications
- Monitoring for the expected effects of pharmacological and parenteral therapies

- Monitoring laboratory values
- Reducing the likelihood that an acid-base imbalance will occur
- Providing for basic care and comfort

I. HYDROGEN IONS, ACIDS, AND BASES

A. Hydrogen (H^+) ions
1. Vital to life, because H^+ ions determine the pH of the body, which must be maintained in a narrow range
2. Expressed as pH; the pH scale is determined by the number of H^+ ions and goes from 1 to 14; 7 is considered neutral.
3. The number of H^+ ions in the body fluid determines whether it is acid (acidic), alkaline (alkalosis), or neutral.
4. The pH of body fluid is between 7.35 and 7.45.

B. Acids
1. Produced as end products of metabolism
2. Contain H^+ ions
3. Are H^+ ion donors. They give up H^+ ions to neutralize or decrease the strength of an acid or to form a weaker base.

C. Bases
1. Contain no H^+ ions
2. Are H^+ ion acceptors. They accept H^+ ions from acids to neutralize or decrease the strength of a base or to form a weaker acid.
3. Normal serum levels of bicarbonate (HCO_3^-) are 22 to 27 mEq/L.

II. REGULATORY SYSTEMS FOR HYDROGEN CONCENTRATION IN THE BLOOD

A. Buffers
1. The fastest-acting regulatory system
2. Provide immediate protection against changes in H^+ ion concentration in the extracellular fluid (i.e., absorb or release H^+ ions as needed)
3. Serve as a transport mechanism that carries excess H^+ ions to the lungs
4. Once the primary buffer systems react, they are consumed, and this leaves the body less able to withstand further stress until they are replaced.

B. Primary buffer systems in extracellular fluid
1. Hemoglobin system
   a. Red blood cells contain hemoglobin.
   b. System maintains the acid-base balance by a process called *chloride shift.*
   c. Chloride shifts in and out of the red blood cells in response to the levels of oxygen (O_2) in the blood.
   d. For each chloride ion that leaves a red blood cell, a bicarbonate ion enters.
   e. For each chloride ion that enters a red blood cell, a bicarbonate ion leaves.

2. Plasma proteins system
   a. Functions in conjunction with the liver to vary the amount of H^+ ions in the chemical structure of plasma proteins
   b. Plasma proteins have the ability to attract or release H^+ ions as the body needs them.
3. Carbonic acid–bicarbonate (HCO_3^-) system
   a. Primary buffer system in the body
   b. Maintains a pH of 7.4, with a ratio of 20 parts HCO_3^- to 1 part carbonic acid (H_2CO_3) (20:1)
   c. This ratio (20:1) determines the concentration of H^+ ions in body fluid.
   d. The carbonic acid concentration is controlled by the excretion of carbon dioxide (CO_2) by the lungs. The rate and depth of respirations change in response to CO_2 levels.
   e. The kidneys control the bicarbonate (HCO_3^-) concentration and selectively retain or excrete HCO_3^- in response to bodily needs.
4. Phosphate buffer system
   a. Present in the cells and body fluids and is especially active in the kidneys
   b. Acts like HCO_3^- and neutralizes excess hydrogen (H^+) ions

C. Lungs
1. The body's second defense. They interact with the buffer system to maintain the acid-base balance.
2. In acidosis, the pH decreases and the respiratory rate and depth increase in an attempt to exhale acids. The carbonic acid created by the neutralizing action of HCO_3^- can be carried to the lungs, where it is reduced to CO_2 and water and is exhaled. Thus, H^+ ions are inactivated and exhaled.
3. In alkalosis, the pH increases and the respiratory rate and depth decrease. CO_2 is retained, and carbonic acid increases to neutralize and decrease the strength of excess HCO_3.
4. The action of the lungs is reversible for controlling an excess or deficit.
5. The lungs can hold H^+ ions until the deficit is corrected or can inactivate H^+ ions, changing the ions to water molecules to be exhaled along with CO_2, thus correcting the excess.
6. The lungs can inactivate only H^+ ions carried by carbonic acid. Excess H^+ ions created by other problems must be excreted by the kidneys.

⚠ Monitor the client's respiratory status closely. In acidosis, the respiratory rate and depth increase in an attempt to exhale acids. In alkalosis, the respiratory rate and depth decrease. CO_2 is retained to neutralize and decrease the strength of excess bicarbonate.

D. Kidneys
1. The ultimate correction of acid-base disturbances is dependent on the kidneys, although the renal excretion of acids and alkali (bases) occurs more slowly.
2. Compensation requires a few hours to several days; however, it is a more thorough and selective process than that of other regulators, such as the buffer systems and the lungs.
3. In acidosis, the pH decreases and excess H^+ ions are secreted into the tubules and combine with buffers for excretion in the urine.
4. In alkalosis, the pH increases and excess HCO_3^- ions move into the tubules, combine with sodium, and are excreted in the urine.
5. Selective regulation of HCO_3^- in the kidneys
   a. The kidneys restore HCO_3^- by excreting H^+ ions and retaining HCO_3^- ions.
   b. Excess H^+ ions are excreted in the urine in the form of phosphoric acid.
   c. The alteration of certain amino acids in the renal tubules results in the diffusion of ammonia into the kidneys. The ammonia combines with excess H^+ ions and is excreted into the urine.

E. Potassium (Figure 10-1)
1. Plays an exchange role in maintaining the acid-base balance
2. The body changes the potassium (K) level by drawing H^+ ions into the cell or by pushing them out of the cell.
3. In acidosis, the body protects itself from the acidic state by moving H^+ ions into the cell. Therefore, K moves out to make room for H^+ ions; the K serum level increases.
4. In alkalosis, the cells release H^+ ions into the blood in an attempt to increase the acidity of the blood; this forces the serum potassium into the cell and the serum potassium level decreases.

⚠ When the client experiences an acid-base imbalance, monitor the potassium level closely because the potassium moves in or out of the cells in an attempt to maintain acid-base balance.

III. RESPIRATORY ACIDOSIS

A. Description: The total concentration of buffer base is lower than normal, with a relative increase in H^+ ion concentration; thus, a greater number of H^+ ions are circulating in the blood than can be absorbed by the buffer system
B. Causes (Box 10-1)
1. Caused by primary defects in the function of the lungs or by changes in normal respiratory patterns
2. Any condition that causes an obstruction of the airway or that depresses respiratory status can cause **respiratory acidosis**.
C. Data collection
1. In an attempt to compensate, the respiratory rate and depth increase.
2. The pH is less than 7.35, and the partial pressure of CO_2 (P_{CO_2}) is greater than 45 mm Hg.
3. Headache
4. Restlessness

  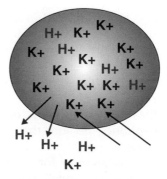

Under normal conditions, the intracellular potassium content is much greater than that of the extracellular fluid. The concentration of hydrogen ions is low in both compartments.

In acidosis, the extracellular hydrogen ion content increases, and the hydrogen ions move into the intracellular fluid. To keep the intracellular fluid electrically neutral, an equal number of potassium ions leave the cell, creating a relative hyperkalemia.

In alkalosis, more hydrogen ions are present in the intracellular fluid than in the extracellular fluid. Hydrogen ions move from the intracellular fluid into the extracellular fluid. To keep the intracellular fluid electrically neutral, potassium ions move from the extracellular fluid into the intracellular fluid, creating a relative hypokalemia.

▲ **FIGURE 10-1** Movement of potassium in response to changes in the extracellular fluid hydrogen ion concentration. (From Ignatavicius, D., & Workman, M. [2010]. *Medical-surgical nursing: Patient-centered collaborative care* [6th ed.]. St. Louis: Saunders. © M. Linda Workman. All rights reserved.)

Box 10-1 Causes of Respiratory Acidosis

- Asthma
- Atelectasis
- Brain trauma
- Bronchiectasis
- Bronchitis
- Central nervous system depression
- Emphysema
- Hypoventilation
- Medications
- Pneumonia
- Pulmonary edema
- Respiratory failure or depression

Box 10-2 Causes of Respiratory Alkalosis

- Anxiety
- Fever
- Hyperventilation
- Hypoxia
- Hysteria
- Overventilation by mechanical ventilators
- Pain

⚠ If the client has a condition that causes overstimulation of the respiratory system, monitor the client for respiratory alkalosis.

5. Mental status changes, such as drowsiness and confusion
6. Visual disturbances
7. Diaphoresis
8. Cyanosis as the hypoxia becomes more acute
9. Hyperkalemia
10. Rapid, irregular pulse
11. Dysrhythmias leading to ventricular fibrillation

D. Interventions
1. Maintain a patent airway
2. Monitor for signs of respiratory distress
3. Administer O_2 as prescribed
4. Place the client in semi-Fowler's position unless contraindicated.
5. Encourage and assist the client to turn, cough, and deep breathe.
6. Prepare to administer respiratory treatments as prescribed.
7. Encourage hydration to thin secretions unless excess fluid intake is contraindicated.
8. Suction the client's airway if necessary and if not contraindicated.
9. Monitor electrolyte values, especially the potassium level.
10. Avoid the use of tranquilizers, opioids, and sedatives/hypnotics, because they further depress respirations.
11. Administer antibiotics for infection or other medications (e.g., bronchodilators, opioid antagonists) as prescribed.
12. Prepare for endotracheal intubation and mechanical ventilation if CO_2 levels rise above 50 mm Hg and if signs of acute respiratory distress are present.

IV. RESPIRATORY ALKALOSIS

A. Description: A deficit of carbonic acid and a decrease in H^+ ion concentration that results from the accumulation of base or the loss of acid without a comparable loss of base in the body fluids
B. Causes: Conditions that cause overstimulation of the respiratory status (Box 10-2)

C. Data collection
1. Initially hyperventilation and respiratory stimulation cause abnormal rapid and deep respirations (tachypnea). In an attempt to compensate, the kidneys excrete excess circulating bicarbonate into the urine.
2. The pH is greater than 7.45, and the P_{CO_2} is less than 35 mm Hg.
3. Headache
4. Lightheadedness, vertigo
5. Mental status changes
6. Paresthesias, such as tingling of the fingers and toes
7. Hypokalemia, hypocalcemia
8. Tetany, convulsions

D. Interventions
1. Maintain a patent airway and monitor for respiratory distress.
2. Provide emotional support and reassurance to the client.
3. Encourage appropriate breathing patterns.
4. Assist with breathing techniques and breathing aids as prescribed.
   a. Voluntary holding of breath or slowed breathing
   b. Rebreathing exhaled CO_2 by methods such as using a paper bag or a rebreathing mask as prescribed.
5. Provide cautious care with ventilator clients so that they are not forced to take breaths too deeply or rapidly.
6. Monitor electrolyte values, particularly potassium and calcium levels.
7. Administer medications (antianxiety or antipyretic) as prescribed.
8. Prepare to assist with administering calcium gluconate for tetany as prescribed.

V. METABOLIC ACIDOSIS

A. Description: A total concentration of buffer base that is lower than normal, with a relative increase in the H^+ ion concentration resulting from loss of too much base and/or retention of too much acid

Box 10-3 Causes of Metabolic Acidosis

- Diabetes mellitus or diabetic ketoacidosis
- Excessive ingestion of acetylsalicylic acid (aspirin)
- Gastrointestinal fistulas
- High-fat diet
- Insufficient metabolism of carbohydrates
- Lactic acidosis
- Malnutrition
- Renal insufficiency or renal failure
- Severe diarrhea
- Starvation

B. Causes (Box 10-3)

1. Diabetes mellitus or diabetic ketoacidosis: An insufficient supply of insulin causes increased fat metabolism, leading to an excess accumulation of ketones or other acids; HCO_3^- then ends up being depleted.
2. Renal insufficiency or renal failure results in the following:
   a. Increased waste products of protein metabolism are retained.
   b. Acids increase, and HCO_3^- is unable to maintain the acid-base balance.
3. Insufficient metabolism of carbohydrates: When an insufficient supply of O_2 is available for the proper burning of carbohydrates, the lactic acid concentration increases, and lactic acidosis results.
4. Excessive ingestion of acetylsalicylic acid (aspirin) causes an increase in the H^+ ion concentration.
5. Severe diarrhea: Intestinal and pancreatic secretions are normally alkaline; therefore, excessive loss of base leads to acidosis.
6. Malnutrition/starvation: Improper metabolism of nutrients causes fat catabolism leading to an excess buildup of ketones and acids.
7. High-fat diet: A high intake of fat causes the waste products of fat metabolism to be accumulated much too rapidly, which leads to a buildup of ketones and acids.

⚠ An insufficient supply of insulin in a client with diabetes mellitus can result in metabolic acidosis known as *diabetic ketoacidosis*.

C. Data collection

1. To compensate for the acidosis, hyperpnea with Kussmaul's respirations (deep and fast) occurs as the lungs attempt to exhale the excess CO_2.
2. The pH is less than 7.35, and the HCO_3^- ion level is less than 22 mEq/L.
3. Headache
4. Nausea, vomiting, diarrhea
5. Fruity-smelling breath as a result of improper fat metabolism
6. Central nervous system (CNS) depression: mental dullness, drowsiness, stupor, coma

7. Hypotension
8. Hyperkalemia

D. Interventions

1. Based on the cause of the acidosis
2. Maintain a patent airway and monitor for signs of respiratory distress.
3. Assess the level of consciousness for CNS depression.
4. Monitor intake and output and assist with fluid and electrolyte replacement as prescribed.
5. Initiate safety and seizure precautions.
6. Monitor the serum K level closely; as **metabolic acidosis** resolves, K moves back into the cell, and the serum K level decreases.
7. Give medications as prescribed, depending on cause (e.g., antidiarrheals if diarrhea is the cause).

⚠ Monitor the client experiencing severe diarrhea for manifestations of metabolic acidosis.

E. Interventions for diabetes mellitus and diabetic ketoacidosis

1. Give insulin as prescribed to hasten the movement of serum glucose into the cell, thereby decreasing the concurrent ketosis.
2. When glucose is being properly metabolized, the body stops converting fats to glucose.
3. Monitor for circulatory collapse caused by polyuria, which can result from the hyperglycemic state. Osmotic diuresis may lead to extracellular volume deficit.

F. Interventions for renal failure

1. Dialysis may be used to remove protein and waste products, thereby decreasing the acidosis.
2. A diet low in protein and high in calories decreases the amount of protein waste products, which in turn lessens the acidosis.

VI. METABOLIC ALKALOSIS

A. Description: A deficit of carbonic acid and a decrease in hydrogen ion concentration that results from the accumulation of base or from a loss of acid without a comparable loss of base in the body fluids

B. Causes (Box 10-4)

C. Data collection

1. To compensate, respiratory rate and depth decrease to conserve CO_2.
2. Nausea, vomiting
3. Dizziness
4. Numbness and tingling in the extremities
5. Twitching in the extremities
6. Hypokalemia, hypocalcemia
7. Dysrhythmia: tachycardia

⚠ Monitor the client experiencing excessive vomiting or the client with gastrointestinal suctioning for manifestations of metabolic alkalosis.

Box 10-4 Causes of Metabolic Alkalosis

- Diuretics
- Excessive vomiting or gastrointestinal suctioning
- Excessive intake of antacids
- Hyperaldosteronism
- Ingestion or parenteral injection of excess sodium bicarbonate
- Massive transfusion of whole blood

Box 10-5 Normal Blood Gas Values

- pH: 7.35 to 7.45
- P_{CO_2}: 35 to 45 mm Hg
- HCO_3^-: 22 to 27 mEq/L
- PO_2: 80 to 100 mm Hg

Box 10-6 Performing Allen's Test

Direct pressure is applied over the client's ulnar and radial arteries simultaneously.

While pressure is applied, the client is asked to open and close the hand repeatedly; the hand should blanch.

Pressure is released from the ulnar artery while still compressing the radial artery, and the color of the extremity distal to the pressure point is assessed.

If pinkness fails to return within 6 seconds, the collateral flow by the ulnar artery is insufficient to provide adequate blood flow to the hand should the radial artery become occluded as a result of the puncture. In this situation the radial artery should not be used for obtaining a blood specimen.

D. Interventions

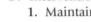

1. Maintain a patent airway and monitor for signs of respiratory distress.
2. Monitor potassium and calcium serum blood levels
3. Institute safety precautions
4. Prepare to administer medications as prescribed to promote the excretion of HCO_3^- by the kidneys.
5. Prepare to replace potassium chloride as prescribed.
6. Prepare to treat the underlying cause of the alkalosis.

VII. ARTERIAL BLOOD GASES (Box 10-5)

A. Description: Levels reflect the ability of the lungs to exchange O_2 and CO_2, the effectiveness of the kidneys for balancing the retention and elimination of HCO_3^-, and the effectiveness of the heart as a pump.

B. Obtaining an arterial blood gas specimen
1. Obtain vital signs
2. **Allen's test** is performed to determine the presence of collateral circulation (Box 10-6).
3. Identify factors that may affect the accuracy of the results, such as changes in the O_2 settings on respiratory assistive devices, suctioning within the past 20 minutes, and client activities.
4. Assist with the specimen draw by preparing a heparinized syringe.
5. Provide emotional support to the client.
6. Apply pressure immediately to the puncture site for 5 minutes or for 10 minutes if the client is taking anticoagulants.
7. Record the client's temperature and the type of supplemental O_2 that the client is receiving on the laboratory form.
8. Appropriately label the specimen, and transport it on ice to the laboratory.

C. Respiratory acid-base imbalances (Table 10-1)
1. Remember that the respiratory function indicator is the P_{CO_2}.
2. In a respiratory imbalance, you will find an opposite relationship between the pH and the P_{CO_2}. In other words, the pH will be elevated when the P_{CO_2} is decreased (alkalosis), or the pH will be decreased in the presence of an elevated P_{CO_2} (acidosis).
3. Remember that the pH is decreased in an acidotic condition and elevated in an alkalotic condition.

4. Look at the pH and the P_{CO_2} to determine if the condition is a respiratory problem.
5. **Respiratory acidosis**
   a. The pH is decreased
   b. The P_{CO_2} is elevated
6. Respiratory alkalosis
   a. The pH is elevated
   b. The P_{CO_2} is decreased

D. Metabolic acid-base imbalances (see Table 10-1)
1. Remember that the metabolic function indicator is the HCO_3^-.
2. In a metabolic imbalance, you will find a corresponding relationship between the pH and the HCO_3^-. In other words, the pH will be elevated and the HCO_3^- will be elevated (alkalosis), or the pH will be decreased and the HCO_3^- will be decreased (acidosis).
3. Remember that the pH is decreased in an acidotic condition and elevated in an alkalotic condition.
4. Look at the pH and the HCO_3^- concentration to determine if the condition is a metabolic problem.
5. **Metabolic acidosis**
   a. The pH is decreased.
   b. The HCO_3^- is decreased.
6. **Metabolic alkalosis**
   a. The pH is elevated.
   b. The HCO_3^- is elevated.

E. Steps for analyzing arterial blood gas results (Box 10-7).

TABLE 10-1 Acid-Base Imbalances: Significant Laboratory Value Changes that Normally Occur

Imbalance	pH	HCO_3^-	Pao_2	$Paco_2$	K^+
Respiratory acidosis	Decreased	Increased	Decreased	Increased	Increased
Respiratory alkalosis	Increased	Decreased	Normal	Decreased	Decreased
Metabolic acidosis	Decreased	Decreased	Normal	Normal or decreased	Increased
Metabolic alkalosis	Increased	Increased	Normal	Normal or increased	Decreased

HCO_3^-, Bicarbonate; K^+, potassium; Pao_2, partial pressure of oxygen in arterial blood; $Paco_2$, partial pressure of carbon dioxide in arterial blood.

Box 10-7 Analyzing Arterial Blood Gas Results

If you can remember the following pyramid points and steps, you will be able to analyze any blood gas report.

Pyramid Points

In acidosis, the pH is down.
In alkalosis, the pH is up.
The respiratory function indicator is the partial pressure of carbon dioxide (Pco_2) value.
The metabolic function indicator is the bicarbonate (HCO_3^-) level.

Pyramid Steps

Look at the blood gas report.

Pyramid Step 1

Look at the pH. Is it up or down? If it is up, it reflects alkalosis. If it is down, it reflects acidosis.

Pyramid Step 2

Look at the Pco_2 level. Is it up or down? If it reflects an opposite relationship to the pH, then you know that the condition is a respiratory imbalance. If it does not reflect an opposite relationship to the pH, then move on to pyramid step 3.

Pyramid Step 3

Look at the HCO_3^- level. Does the HCO_3^- level reflect a corresponding relationship to the pH? If it does, then the condition is a metabolic imbalance.

MORE QUESTIONS ON EVOLVE!

Practice Questions

46. A client has the following laboratory values: a pH of 7.55, an HCO_3^- level of 22 mm Hg, and a Pco_2 of 30 mm Hg. What should the nurse do?
    1. Perform Allen's test.
    2. Prepare the client for dialysis.
    3. Administer insulin as prescribed.
    4. Encourage the client to slow down breathing.

47. The nurse is told that the blood gas results indicate a pH of 7.50 and a Pco_2 of 32 mm Hg. The nurse determines that these results indicate:
    1. Metabolic acidosis
    2. Metabolic alkalosis
    3. Respiratory acidosis
    4. Respiratory alkalosis

48. A client is scheduled for blood to be drawn from the radial artery for an arterial blood gas (ABG) determination. A nurse assists with performing Allen's test before drawing the blood to determine the adequacy of the:
    1. Ulnar circulation
    2. Carotid circulation
    3. Femoral circulation
    4. Brachial circulation

49. A nurse is caring for a client with a nasogastric tube that is attached to low suction. The nurse monitors the client closely for which acid-base disorder that is most likely to occur in this situation?
    1. Metabolic acidosis
    2. Metabolic alkalosis
    3. Respiratory acidosis
    4. Respiratory alkalosis

50. A nurse is caring for a client with severe diarrhea. The nurse monitors the client closely, understanding that this client is at risk for developing which acid-base disorder?
    1. Metabolic acidosis
    2. Metabolic alkalosis
    3. Respiratory acidosis
    4. Respiratory alkalosis

51. A nurse is caring for a client with diabetic ketoacidosis and documents that the client is experiencing Kussmaul's respirations. Based on this documentation, which of the following did the nurse most likely observe?
    1. Respirations that cease for several seconds
    2. Respirations that are regular but abnormally slow
    3. Respirations that are labored and increased in depth and rate
    4. Respirations that are abnormally deep, regular, and increased in rate

52. A nurse is caring for a client with a diagnosis of chronic obstructive pulmonary disease (COPD). The nurse monitors the client for which acid-base imbalance that most likely occurs in clients with this condition?
    1. Metabolic acidosis
    2. Metabolic alkalosis
    3. Respiratory acidosis
    4. Respiratory alkalosis

53. The registered nurse reviews the results of the arterial blood gases with the licensed practical nurse (LPN) and tells the LPN that the client is experiencing respiratory acidosis. The LPN would expect to note which of the following on the laboratory result form?
    1. pH 7.50, Pco_2 52 mm Hg
    2. pH 7.35, Pco_2 40 mm Hg
    3. pH 7.25, Pco_2 50 mm Hg
    4. pH 7.50, Pco_2 30 mm Hg

54. A nurse is caring for a client with respiratory insufficiency. The arterial blood gas results indicate a pH of 7.50 and a Pco_2 of 30 mm Hg, and the nurse is told that the client is experiencing respiratory alkalosis. Which of the following additional laboratory values would the nurse expect to note?
    1. A sodium level of 145 mEq/L
    2. A potassium level of 3.2 mEq/L
    3. A magnesium level of 2.4 mg/dL
    4. A phosphorus level of 4.0 mg/dL

55. A client is scheduled for an arterial blood gas specimen to be drawn, and the nurse assists with performing Allen's test on the client. Number the steps for performing Allen's test in order of priority. (Number 1 is the first step, and number 6 is the last step.)
    ___ Document the findings.
    ___ Explain the procedure to the client.
    ___ Release pressure from the ulnar artery.
    ___ Apply pressure over the ulnar and radial arteries.
    ___ Ask the client to open and close the hand repeatedly.
    ___ Assess the color of the extremity distal to the pressure point.

ANSWERS

46. 4

Rationale: The client is in respiratory alkalosis based on the laboratory results of a high pH and a low Pco_2 level. Interventions for respiratory alkalosis are the voluntary holding of breath or slowed breathing and the rebreathing of exhaled CO_2 by methods such as using a paper bag or a rebreathing mask as prescribed. Option 1 would be incorrect, because the blood specimen has already been drawn, and the laboratory results have been completed. Options 2 and 3 are interventions for metabolic acidosis.
Test-Taking Strategy: First determine the laboratory results. Because the pH is high and the Pco_2 level is low, a respiratory problem is occurring. Using the process of elimination, you can determine that only one intervention deals with respirations. Review the interventions for respiratory alkalosis if you had difficulty with this question.
Level of Cognitive Ability: Analyzing
Client Needs: Physiological Integrity
Integrated Process: Nursing Process/Implementation
Content Area: Fundamental Skills: Fluids & Electrolytes/Acid-Base
Reference: deWit, pp. 52, 54. 2009.

47. 4

Rationale: The normal pH is 7.35 to 7.45. In a respiratory condition, an opposite relationship will be seen between the pH and the Pco_2, as is seen in option 4. In an alkalotic condition, the pH is increased. Options 1 and 3 indicate acidosis, and option 2 indicates a metabolic condition.
Test-Taking Strategy: Remember that with a respiratory condition, you will find an opposite relationship between the pH and the Pco_2 level. Therefore, options 1 and 2 can be eliminated. Remembering that the pH is increased in an alkalotic condition

helps you to eliminate option 3. Review the steps related to reading blood gas values if you had difficulty with this question.
Level of Cognitive Ability: Analyzing
Client Needs: Physiological Integrity
Integrated Process: Nursing Process/Data Collection
Content Area: Fundamental Skills: Fluids & Electrolytes/Acid-Base
Reference: deWit, p. 52. 2009.

48. 1

Rationale: Before performing a radial puncture to obtain an arterial specimen for ABGs, Allen's test should be performed to determine adequate ulnar circulation. Failure to assess collateral circulation could result in severe ischemic injury to the hand if damage to the radial artery occurs with arterial puncture. Options 2, 3, and 4 are not associated with this test.
Test-Taking Strategy: Use the process of elimination. Note the relationship between the words "radial artery" in the question and option 1. Review Allen's test if you had difficulty with this question.
Level of Cognitive Ability: Evaluating
Client Needs: Physiological Integrity
Integrated Process: Nursing Process/Evaluation
Content Area: Fundamental Skills: Fluids & Electrolytes/Acid-Base
Reference: Pagana, Pagana, p. 118. 2009.

49. 2

Rationale: The loss of gastric fluid via nasogastric suction or vomiting causes metabolic alkalosis as a result of the loss of hydrochloric acid; this results in an alkalotic condition. Options 3 and 4 deal with respiratory problems. Option 1 relates to acidosis.

Test-Taking Strategy: Remember that hydrochloric acid is lost when the client is receiving nasogastric suctioning. This will direct you to the options that identify an alkalotic condition. Because the question addresses a situation other than a respiratory one, the acid-base disorder would be a metabolic condition. Review the causes of metabolic alkalosis if you had difficulty with this question.
Level of Cognitive Ability: Analyzing
Client Needs: Physiological Integrity
Integrated Process: Nursing Process/Data Collection
Content Area: Fundamental Skills: Fluids & Electrolytes/Acid-Base
Reference: deWit, p. 54. 2009.

50. 1

Rationale: Intestinal secretions high in bicarbonate may be lost through enteric drainage tubes, an ileostomy, or diarrhea. The decreased bicarbonate level creates the actual base deficit of metabolic acidosis. Options 2, 3, and 4 are unlikely to occur in a client with severe diarrhea.
Test-Taking Strategy: Note that the condition described in the question is a gastrointestinal disorder; this will direct you to thinking about a metabolic disorder. Remembering that intestinal fluids are primarily alkaline will assist you with selecting the correct option. When excess bicarbonate is lost, acidosis will result. Review the causes of metabolic acidosis if you had difficulty with this question.
Level of Cognitive Ability: Analyzing
Client Needs: Physiological Integrity
Integrated Process: Nursing Process/Data Collection
Content Area: Fundamental Skills: Fluids & Electrolytes/Acid-Base
Reference: deWit, pp. 53–54. 2009.

51. 4

Rationale: Kussmaul's respirations are abnormally deep, regular, and increased in rate. In apnea, respirations cease for several seconds. In bradypnea, respirations are regular but abnormally slow. In hyperpnea, respirations are labored and increased in depth and rate.
Test-Taking Strategy: Knowledge regarding the descriptions of alterations in breathing patterns is required to answer this question. Remember that Kussmaul's respirations occur in clients with diabetic ketoacidosis. Review the data collection findings in diabetic ketoacidosis if you had difficulty with this question.
Level of Cognitive Ability: Understanding
Client Needs: Physiological Integrity
Integrated Process: Nursing Process/Data Collection
Content Area: Fundamental Skills: Fluids & Electrolytes/Acid-Base
Reference: Christensen, Kockrow, p. 525. 2011. *Adult health nursing.*

52. 3

Rationale: Respiratory acidosis most often occurs as a result of primary defects in the function of the lungs or changes in normal respiratory patterns from secondary problems. Chronic respiratory acidosis is most commonly caused by COPD. Acute respiratory acidosis also occurs in clients with COPD when superimposed respiratory infection or concurrent respiratory disease increases the work of breathing. Options 1, 2, and 4 are not likely to occur unless other conditions complicate the COPD.
Test-Taking Strategy: Use the process of elimination. Remembering that primary defects in the function of the lungs result in respiratory acidosis will direct you to the correct option. Review the causes of respiratory acidosis if you had difficulty with this question.
Level of Cognitive Ability: Analyzing
Client Needs: Physiological Integrity
Integrated Process: Nursing Process/Data Collection
Content Area: Fundamental Skills: Fluids & Electrolytes/Acid-Base
Reference: deWit, pp. 52–53. 2009.

53. 3

Rationale: The normal pH is 7.35 to 7.45, and the normal P_{CO_2} value is 35 to 45 mm Hg. In respiratory acidosis, the pH is down and the P_{CO_2} is up. Option 3 is the only option that reflects an acidotic condition. Options 1 and 4 reflect an elevated pH, which indicates an alkalotic condition. Option 2 reflects a normal blood gas result.
Test-Taking Strategy: Remember that with a respiratory imbalance, you will find an opposite relationship between the pH and the P_{CO_2} value. In addition, remember that the pH is down in an acidotic condition. Review the interpretation of arterial blood gas results if you had difficulty with this question.
Level of Cognitive Ability: Analyzing
Client Needs: Physiological Integrity
Integrated Process: Nursing Process/Data Collection
Content Area: Fundamental Skills: Fluids & Electrolytes/Acid-Base
Reference: deWit, p. 52. 2009.

54. 2

Rationale: Clinical manifestations of respiratory alkalosis include tachypnea, mental status changes, dizziness, pallor around the mouth, spasms of the muscles of the hands, and hypokalemia. Options 1, 3, and 4 identify normal laboratory results.
Test-Taking Strategy: Recalling the clinical manifestations of respiratory alkalosis and the normal laboratory values will assist you with answering this question. By the process of elimination, you can then determine that the only abnormal laboratory value is the potassium level. Review the clinical manifestations of respiratory alkalosis if you had difficulty with this question.
Level of Cognitive Ability: Analyzing
Client Needs: Physiological Integrity
Integrated Process: Nursing Process/Data Collection
Content Area: Fundamental Skills: Fluids & Electrolytes/Acid-Base
Reference: deWit, p. 54. 2009.

55. 6, 1, 4, 2, 3, 5

Rationale: Allen's test is performed before obtaining an arterial blood specimen from the radial artery to determine the presence of adequate collateral circulation and the adequacy of the ulnar artery. Failure to determine the presence of adequate collateral circulation could result in severe ischemic injury to the hand if damage to the radial artery occurs with arterial puncture. The nurse would first explain the procedure to the client. To perform the test, the nurse applies direct pressure over the client's ulnar and radial arteries simultaneously. While pressure is applied, the nurse asks the client to open and close the hand repeatedly; the hand should blanch. The nurse then releases pressure from the ulnar artery while compressing the radial artery and assesses the color of the extremity distal to the pressure point. If pinkness fails to return within 6 seconds, the ulnar artery is insufficient, which indicates that the radial artery should not be used for obtaining a blood specimen. Finally, the nurse documents the findings.

Test-Taking Strategy: Recalling that Allen's test needs to be explained to the client will assist you with determining the first action. Next, think about the purpose and reason for performing this test, and visualize the procedure. This will help you to determine the steps for performing the test. Review Allen's test if you had difficulty with this question.
Level of Cognitive Ability: Applying
Client Needs: Physiological Integrity
Integrated Process: Nursing Process/Data Collection
Content Area: Fundamental Skills: Fluids & Electrolytes/Acid-Base
Reference: Linton, pp. 549, 552. 2012.

Laboratory Values

PYRAMID TERMS

blood The liquid pumped by the heart through the arteries, veins, and capillaries. It is composed of a clear yellow fluid (plasma) and cell types with different functions (Figure 11-1).

blood cell Any of the formed elements of the blood, including red cells (erythrocytes), white cells (leukocytes), and platelets (thrombocytes).

plasma The watery, straw-colored fluid part of the lymph and blood in which the formed elements (blood cells) are suspended. Plasma is made up of water, electrolytes, protein, glucose, fats, bilirubin, and gases, and is essential for carrying the cellular elements of the blood through the circulation.

serum The clear and thin fluid part of the blood that remains after coagulation. Serum contains no blood cells, platelets, or fibrinogen.

venipuncture Puncture into a vein to obtain a blood specimen for testing. The antecubital veins are the veins of choice because of ease of access.

PYRAMID TO SUCCESS

This chapter identifies the normal adult values for the most common laboratory tests. (See Box 11-1 for common laboratory abbreviations.) If you are familiar with the normal values, you will be able to determine if an abnormality exists when a laboratory value is presented in a question. It is unlikely that a question on the NCLEX-PN will simply ask you what a normal value may be. The questions on the NCLEX-PN related to laboratory values will require you to identify whether the laboratory value is normal or abnormal, and then you will be required to think about the effects of the laboratory value in terms of the client. Pyramid points focus on knowledge of the normal values for the most common laboratory tests, the therapeutic serum levels of commonly prescribed medications, and interventions based on the findings. When a question is presented on the NCLEX-PN regarding a specific laboratory value, note the disorder presented in the question and the associated body organ that is affected as a result of the disorder. This process will assist you in determining the correct

answer. For example, if the question is asking you about the immune status of a client who is receiving chemotherapy, the assessment of the laboratory values will focus on the white blood cell (WBC) count and on the neutrophils, because this client may be at risk for infection. For the client who is receiving chemotherapy and who has a low WBC count, the plan of care focuses on the immune system and the protection of the client from infection. Implementation focuses on preventive interventions related to infection, perhaps even protective isolation measures. Evaluation may focus on the maintenance of a normal temperature in the client.

CLIENT NEEDS

Safe and Effective Care Environment

- Applying principles of infection control
- Ensuring medical and surgical asepsis when obtaining a specimen
- Implementing procedures for handling hazardous and infectious materials
- Maintaining confidentiality
- Maintaining standard, transmission-based, and other precautions
- Obtaining informed consent for specific procedures
- Verifying the identity of the client

Health Promotion and Maintenance

- Discussing the importance of follow-up laboratory studies
- Identifying community resources available for the follow-up
- Implementing posttest procedures
- Monitoring for signs and symptoms that indicate the need to notify the health care provider
- Preparing the client for the laboratory test

Psychosocial Integrity

- Communicating the purpose of the laboratory test to the client

▲ **FIGURE 11-1** Approximate values for the components of blood in a normal adult. (Adapted from Thibodeau, G. A., & Patton, K. T. [2010]. *The human body in health and disease* [5th ed.]. St. Louis: Mosby.)

Box 11-1 Pyramid Abbreviations

Abbreviation	Description
g/dL	Grams per deciliter
mcg/dL	Micrograms per deciliter
mg/dL	Milligrams per deciliter
mEq/L	Milliequivalents per liter
units/L	Units per liter
mm/hr	Millimeters per hour
IU/L	International units per liter
mcg/mL	Micrograms per milliliter
ng/mL	Nanograms per milliliter
microunits/mL	Microunits per milliliter
mL/kg	Milliliters per kilogram
mm³	Millimeters cubed
µL	Microliters
pg/mL	Picogram per milliliter

- Communicating with the client regarding the laboratory results
- Describing specific interventions or home-care measures required based on the results
- Providing emotional support during testing

Physiological Integrity

- Determining the need to implement specific actions based on the laboratory results
- Identifying normal values for the most common laboratory tests
- Identifying therapeutic serum medication levels of commonly prescribed medications
- Monitoring for clinical manifestations associated with an abnormal laboratory value
- Monitoring for potential complications related to a test
- Providing comfort measures
- Reporting significant laboratory values

⚠ Drawing blood specimens from an extremity in which an intravenous solution is infusing can produce an inaccurate result. Prolonged use of a tourniquet and clenching and unclenching the hand before venous sampling can increase the blood level of potassium, producing an inaccurate result.

TABLE 11-1 Normal Adult Electrolyte Values

Electrolyte	Value
Sodium	135-145 mEq/L
Potassium	3.5-5.1 mEq/L
Chloride	98-107 mEq/L
Bicarbonate (venous)	22-29 mEq/L

I. ELECTROLYTES (Table 11-1)

A. **Serum** sodium
1. Description
   a. A major cation of extracellular fluid
   b. Maintains osmotic pressures and acid-base balance and assists with the transmission of nerve impulses
   c. Absorbed from the small intestine and excreted in the urine in amounts that depend on dietary intake
   d. Minimum daily requirement of sodium is approximately 15 mEq
2. Nursing consideration: Drawing **blood** samples in the extremity in which an intravenous (IV) solution of sodium chloride is infusing increases the level, producing an inaccurate result

B. **Serum** potassium (K)
1. Description
   a. A major intracellular cation; regulates cellular water balance, electrical conduction in muscle cells, and acid-base balance
   b. The body obtains K through dietary ingestion, and the kidneys either preserve or excrete K, depending on cellular need
   c. K levels are used to evaluate cardiac function, renal function, gastrointestinal function, and the need for IV replacement therapy
2. Nursing considerations
   a. Use of a tourniquet and clenching and unclenching the hand before venous sampling can increase the value
   b. **Blood** is not drawn from an extremity site with an IV infusion containing potassium
   c. If the client is receiving K supplementation, note this on the laboratory form
   d. Clients with elevated WBC and platelet counts may have falsely elevated K levels

C. **Serum** chloride
1. Description
   a. A hydrochloric acid salt that is the most abundant body anion in the extracellular fluid
   b. Functions to counterbalance cations, such as sodium, and acts as a buffer during oxygen and carbon dioxide exchange in red **blood cells** (RBCs)
   c. Aids in digestion and maintaining osmotic pressure and water balance
2. Nursing considerations
   a. Draw **blood** from an extremity that does not have normal saline infusing into it
   b. Do not allow the client to clench and unclench the hand before a **blood** draw
   c. Any condition accompanied by prolonged vomiting, diarrhea, or both will alter levels

D. **Serum** bicarbonate
1. Description: Part of the bicarbonate-carbonic acid buffering system; mainly responsible for regulating the pH of body fluids
2. Nursing considerations
   a. Ingestion of acidic or alkaline solutions may cause increased or decreased results, respectively
   b. Prolonged tourniquet application before the **blood** draw increases the **serum** bicarbonate level

II. COAGULATION STUDIES

A. Activated partial thromboplastin time (aPTT)
1. Description
   a. Evaluates how well the coagulation sequence is functioning by measuring the amount of time it takes in seconds for recalcified citrated plasma to clot after partial thromboplastin is added to it
   b. Screens for deficiencies and inhibitors of all factors except VII and XIII
   c. Most commonly used to monitor heparin therapy and to screen for coagulation disorders
2. Value: 20 to 36 seconds, depending on the type of activator used
3. Nursing considerations
   a. If the client is receiving intermittent heparin therapy, draw the **blood** sample 1 hour before the next scheduled dose
   b. Do not draw samples from an arm into which heparin is infusing
   c. Transport the specimen to the laboratory immediately
   d. Provide pressure to the venipuncture site for 3 to 5 minutes
   e. The aPTT should be between 1.5 and 2.5 times normal when the client is receiving heparin therapy.

⚠ If the aPTT value is prolonged (longer than 90 seconds), in a client receiving IV heparin therapy, initiate bleeding precautions.

B. Prothrombin time (PT) and international normalized ratio (INR)
1. Description

a. Prothrombin is a vitamin K–dependent glyco-protein produced by the liver that is necessary for firm fibrin clot formation

b. Each laboratory establishes a normal or control PT value based on the method used to perform the test

c. The PT measures the amount of time it takes for clot formation and is used to monitor response to warfarin sodium (Coumadin) therapy or screen for dysfunction of the extrinsic clotting system that results from liver disease, vitamin K deficiency, or disseminated intravascular coagulation

d. A PT value within 2 seconds (plus or minus) of the control value is considered normal

e. The INR is frequently used to measure the effects of oral anticoagulants

f. The INR standardized the PT ratio and is calculated in the laboratory setting by raising the observed PT ratio to the power of the international sensitivity index specific to the thromboplastin reagent used

2. Values

a. PT: 9.6 to 11.8 seconds (adult male); 9.5 to 11.3 seconds (adult female)

b. INR: 2 to 3 for standard warfarin sodium (Coumadin) therapy

c. INR: 3 to 4.5 for high-dose warfarin sodium (Coumadin) therapy

3. Nursing considerations

a. A baseline PT should be determined before anticoagulation therapy is started; note the time of collection on the laboratory form

b. Apply direct pressure to the **venipuncture** site for 3 to 5 minutes if a coagulation defect is present

c. Concurrent warfarin sodium (Coumadin) therapy with heparin therapy can lengthen the PT for up to 5 hours after dosing

d. Diets high in green leafy vegetables can increase the absorption of vitamin K, which shortens the PT

e. Oral anticoagulation therapy usually maintains the PT at 1.5 to 2 times the laboratory control value

f. A PT longer than 30 seconds places the client at risk for bleeding

⚠ If the PT value is longer than 30 seconds in a client receiving warfarin therapy, initiate bleeding precautions.

C. Clotting time

1. Description: The time required for the interaction of all factors involved in the clotting process

2. Value: 8 to 15 minutes

3. Nursing considerations

a. The client should not receive heparin therapy for 3 hours before specimen collection because the heparin therapy will affect the results

b. The test result is prolonged by any anticoagulant therapy, test-tube agitation, or exposure of the specimen to high temperatures

D. Platelet count

1. Description

a. Platelets function in hemostatic plug formation, clot retraction, and coagulation factor activation

b. Platelets are produced by the bone marrow to function in hemostasis

2. Value: 150,000 to 400,000 cells/mm^3

3. Nursing considerations

a. Monitor the **venipuncture** site for bleeding in clients with known thrombocytopenia

b. High altitudes, chronic cold weather, and exercise increase platelet counts

c. Bleeding precautions should be instituted in clients with low platelet counts

⚠ Monitor the platelet count closely in clients receiving chemotherapy because of the risk for thrombocytopenia.

E. D-dimer test

1. A blood test that measures clot formation and lysis that results from the degradation of fibrin.

2. Helps to diagnose the presence of thrombus in conditions such as deep vein thrombosis, pulmonary embolism, or stroke; it is also used to diagnose disseminated intravascular coagulation (DIC) and monitor the effectiveness of treatment

III. ERYTHROCYTE STUDIES

A. Erythrocyte sedimentation rate

1. Description

a. The rate at which erythrocytes settle out of anticoagulated **blood** in 1 hour

b. A nonspecific test used to detect illnesses associated with acute and chronic infection, inflammation, advanced neoplasm, and tissue necrosis or infarction

2. Value: 0 to 30 mm/hour, depending on the age of the client

3. Nursing consideration: Fasting is not necessary, but a fatty meal may cause **plasma** alterations

B. Hemoglobin and hematocrit (Table 11-2)

1. Description

a. Hemoglobin is the main component of erythrocytes and serves as the vehicle for the transportation of oxygen and carbon dioxide

b. Hemoglobin determinations are important for identifying anemia

TABLE 11-2 Normal Adult Hemoglobin, Hematocrit, Iron, and Red Blood Cell Levels

Blood Component	Normal Value
HEMOGLOBIN	
Male adult	14-16.5 g/dL
Female adult	12-15 g/dL
HEMATOCRIT	
Male adult	42%-52%
Female adult	35%-47%
IRON	
Male adult	65-175 mcg/dL
Female adult	50-170 mcg/dL
RED BLOOD CELLS	
Male adult	4.5-6.2 million cells/μL
Female adult	4.0-5.5 million cells/μL

TABLE 11-3 Normal Adult Serum Enzyme and Cardiac Marker Values

Serum Enzyme	Normal Value
Creatine kinase (CK)	26 174 units/L
CK ISOENZYMES	
CK-MB	0%-5% of total
CK-MM	95%-100% of total
CK-BB	0%
Lactate dehydrogenase	140-280 units/L
LACTATE DEHYDROGENASE ISOENZYMES	
LDH_1	14%-26%
LDH_2	29%-39%
LDH_3	20%-26%
LDH_4	8%-16%
LDH_5	6%-16%
TROPONINS	
Troponin I	<0.6 ng/mL >1.5 ng/mL indicates myocardial infarction
Troponin T	>0.1-0.2 ng/mL indicates myocardial infarction
Myoglobin	<90 mcg/L; an elevation could indicate myocardial infarction
Natriuretic peptides	ANP: 22 to 27 pg/mL BNP: Less than 100 pg/mL CNP: Not yet determined

c. Hematocrit represents RBC mass and is an important measurement in the identification of anemia or polycythemia

2. Nursing consideration: Fasting is not required

C. Serum iron (Table 11-2)
   1. Description
      a. Iron is found predominantly in hemoglobin
      b. Iron acts as a carrier of oxygen from the lungs to the tissues and indirectly aids in the return of carbon dioxide to the lungs
      c. Helps with diagnosing anemias and hemolytic disorders
   2. Nursing consideration: Level of iron will be increased if the client has ingested iron before the test

D. RBC count (Table 11-2)
   1. Description
      a. RBCs function in hemoglobin transport, which results in the delivery of oxygen to the body tissues
      b. RBCs are formed by red bone marrow, have a life span of 120 days, and are removed from the **blood** by the liver, spleen, and bone marrow
      c. Helps with diagnosing anemias and **blood** dyscrasias
      d. Evaluates the body's ability to produce RBCs in sufficient numbers
   2. Nursing consideration: Fasting is not required

IV. SERUM ENZYMES/CARDIAC MARKERS (Table 11-3)

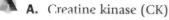

A. Creatine kinase (CK)
   1. Description
      a. An enzyme found in muscle and brain tissue; it reflects tissue breakdown resulting from cell trauma

b. The CK level begins to rise within 6 hours of muscle damage, peaks at 18 hours, and returns to normal in 2 to 3 days.
      c. The test is performed to detect myocardial or skeletal muscle damage or central nervous system damage; the normal CK value is 26 to 174 units/L
      d. Isoenzymes include CK-MB (cardiac), CK-BB (brain), and CK-MM (muscle)
      e. CK-MB is found mainly in cardiac muscle, CK-BB is found mainly in brain tissue, and CK-MM is found mainly in skeletal muscle
   2. Nursing considerations
      a. If the test is performed to evaluate skeletal muscle, instruct the client to avoid strenuous physical activity for 24 hours before the test
      b. Instruct the client to avoid the ingestion of alcohol for 24 hours before the test
      c. Invasive procedures and intramuscular injections may falsely elevate CK levels

B. Lactate dehydrogenase (LDH)
   1. Description
      a. The LDH isoenzymes affected by acute myocardial infarction are LDH_1 and LDH_2
      b. The LDH level begins to increase approximately 24 hours after myocardial infarction and peaks in 48 to 72 hours. It returns to normal thereafter, usually within 7 to 14 days.

c. The presence of an LDH flip (when LDH$_1$ is higher than LDH$_2$) is helpful for diagnosing a myocardial infarction.

2. Nursing considerations
   a. LDH isoenzyme levels should be interpreted in view of the clinical findings.
   b. Testing should be repeated on 3 consecutive days.

C. Troponins
1. Description
   a. Troponins are regulatory proteins found in striated muscle (skeletal and myocardial).
   b. Increased amounts of troponins are released into the bloodstream when an infarction causes damage to the myocardium.
   c. Levels elevate as early as 3 hours after myocardial injury. Troponin I levels may remain elevated for 7 to 10 days and troponin T levels may remain elevated for up to 10 to 14 days.
   d. Serial measurements are important to compare with a baseline test.
2. Nursing considerations:
   a. Testing is repeated after 12 hours and followed by daily testing for 3 to 5 days
   b. Rotate **venipuncture** sites

D. Myoglobin
1. Description
   a. An oxygen-binding protein found in striated (cardiac and skeletal) muscle that releases oxygen at very low tensions
   b. Any injury to skeletal muscle will cause a release of myoglobin into the **blood**
2. Nursing considerations
   a. The level can rise as early as 2 hours after a myocardial infarction, with a rapid decline in the level seen after 7 hours.
   b. Because the myoglobin level is not cardiac specific and rises and falls so rapidly, its use for diagnosing myocardial infarction may be limited.

E. Natriuretic peptides
1. Natriuretic peptides are neuroendocrine peptides that are used to identify clients with congestive heart failure (CHF).
2. There are three major peptides: atrial natriuretic peptides (ANP) synthesized in atrial cardiac muscle, brain natriuretic peptides (BNP) synthesized in cardiac ventricular muscle, and C-type natriuretic peptides (CNP) synthesized by endothelial cells.
3. BNP is the primary marker for identifying CHF as the cause of dyspnea.

⚠ The higher the BNP level, the more severe the CHF. If the BNP is elevated, the dyspnea is a result of CHF. If it is normal, the dyspnea is a result of a pulmonary problem.

V. SERUM GASTROINTESTINAL STUDIES

A. Albumin
1. Description
   a. A main **plasma** protein of **blood**
   b. Maintains oncotic pressure and transports bilirubin, fatty acids, medications, hormones, and other substances that are insoluble in water
   c. Increased in conditions such as dehydration, diarrhea, and metastatic carcinoma; decreased in conditions such as acute infection, ascites, and alcoholism
   d. The presence of detectable albumin or protein in the urine is indicative of abnormal renal function.
2. Value: 3.4 to 5 g/dL
3. Nursing considerations: Fasting is not required.

B. Alkaline phosphatase
1. Description
   a. An enzyme normally found in bone, liver, intestine, and placenta
   b. The blood level rises during periods of bone growth, liver disease, and bile duct obstruction.
2. Value: 4.5 to 13 King-Armstrong units/dL
3. Nursing considerations
   a. The client may need to fast 12 hours before the test.
   b. Hepatotoxic medications administered within 12 hours before specimen collection can cause falsely elevated values.
   c. Transport the specimen to the laboratory immediately.

C. Ammonia
1. Description
   a. Ammonia is a by-product of protein catabolism. Most of it is created by bacteria acting on proteins present in the gut.
   b. It is metabolized by the liver and excreted by the kidneys as urea.
   c. Elevated levels resulting from hepatic dysfunction may lead to encephalopathy.
   d. Venous ammonia levels are not a reliable indicator of hepatic coma.
2. Value: 10 to 80 mcg/dL
3. Nursing considerations
   a. Instruct the client to fast, except for water, and refrain from smoking for 8 to 10 hours before the test. Smoking increases ammonia levels.
   b. Place the specimen in ice and transport it to the laboratory immediately.

D. Alanine aminotransferase (ALT)
1. Description: Used to identify hepatocellular disease of the liver and to monitor improvement or worsening of the disease
2. Value: 4 to 6 international units/L
3. Nursing considerations

a. Previous intramuscular injections may cause elevated levels.

b. No fasting is required.

E. Aspartate aminotransferase (AST)

1. Description: used to evaluate a client with suspected hepatocellular disease (may also be used along with other cardiac markers to evaluate coronary artery occlusive disease)

2. Value: 0 to 35 units/L

3. Nursing considerations

a. Previous intramuscular injections may cause elevated levels.

b. No fasting is required.

F. Amylase

1. Description

a. This enzyme, produced by the pancreas and salivary glands, aids in the digestion of complex carbohydrates and is excreted by the kidneys.

b. In acute pancreatitis, the amylase level is greatly increased. The level starts rising 3 to 6 hours after the onset of pain, peaks at about 24 hours, and returns to normal 2 to 3 days after the onset of pain.

2. Value: 25 to 151 units/L

3. Nursing considerations

a. On the laboratory form, list medications that the client has taken during the 24 hours before the test.

b. Note that many medications may cause false-positive or -negative results.

c. Results are invalidated if the specimen was obtained less than 72 hours after cholecystography with radiopaque dyes.

G. Lipase

1. Description

a. This pancreatic enzyme converts fats and triglycerides into fatty acids and glycerol.

b. Elevated lipase levels occur in pancreatic disorders. Elevations may not occur until 24 to 36 hours after the onset of illness and may remain elevated for up to 14 days.

2. Value: 10 to 140 units/L

3. Nursing considerations: Endoscopic retrograde cholangiopancreatography may increase lipase activity.

H. Bilirubin

1. Description

a. Produced by the liver, spleen, and bone marrow; also a by-product of hemoglobin breakdown

b. Total bilirubin can be broken down into direct bilirubin, which is primarily excreted via the intestinal tract, and indirect bilirubin, which circulates primarily in the bloodstream

c. Total bilirubin levels increase with any type of jaundice, whereas direct and indirect levels rise depending on the cause of the jaundice.

2. Values

a. Bilirubin, direct: 0 to 0.3 mg/dL

b. Bilirubin, indirect: 0.1 to 1 mg/dL

c. Bilirubin, total: Less than 1.5 mg/dL

3. Nursing considerations

a. Instruct the client to eat a diet low in yellow foods, avoiding foods such as carrots, yams, yellow beans, and pumpkin for 3 to 4 days before the **blood** is drawn.

b. Instruct the client to fast for 4 hours before the **blood** is drawn.

c. Note that results will be elevated with the ingestion of alcohol or the administration of morphine sulfate, theophylline, ascorbic acid (vitamin C), or acetylsalicylic acid (aspirin).

d. Results are invalidated if the client has undergone a radioactive scan within 24 hours before the test.

I. Lipids

1. Description

a. **Blood** lipids consist primarily of cholesterol, triglycerides, and phospholipids.

b. Lipid assessment includes total cholesterol, high-density lipoprotein (HDL), low-density lipoprotein (LDL), and triglycerides.

c. Cholesterol is present in all body tissues and is a major component of LDLs, brain and nerve cells, cell membranes, and some gallbladder stones.

d. Triglycerides constitute a major part of very low-density lipoproteins (VLDLs) and a small part of LDLs.

e. Triglycerides are synthesized in the liver from fatty acids, protein, and glucose and they are obtained from the diet.

f. Increased cholesterol, LDL, and triglyceride levels place the client at risk for coronary artery disease.

g. HDLs help protect against the risk of coronary artery disease.

2. Values

a. Cholesterol: 140 to 199 mg/dL

b. LDLs: Less than 130 mg/dL

c. HDLs: 30 to 70 mg/dL

d. Triglycerides: Less than 200 mg/dL

3. Nursing considerations

a. Oral contraceptives may increase the lipid level.

b. Instruct the client to abstain from foods and fluid, except for water, for 12 to 14 hours before the test and from alcohol for 24 hours before the test.

c. Instruct the client that the evening meal before the test should be free from high-cholesterol foods.

J. Protein

1. Description

a. Reflects the total amount of albumin and globulins in the **serum**.
b. Regulates osmotic pressure and is necessary for the formation of many hormones, enzymes and antibodies. It is a major source of building material for blood, skin, hair, nails, and internal organs.
c. Increased in conditions such as Addison's disease, autoimmune collagen disorders, chronic infection, and Crohn's disease
d. Decreased in conditions such as burns, cirrhosis, edema, and severe hepatic disease
2. Value: 6 to 8 g/dL
3. Nursing considerations
a. Do not draw in an extremity with an IV infusion.
b. Instruct the client to avoid a high-fat diet for 8 hours before the test.

K. Uric acid
1. Description
a. Formed as the purines adenine and guanine are metabolized continuously during the formation and degradation of DNA and RNA and from the metabolism of dietary purines
b. Elevated amounts of uric acid deposit in joints and soft tissue and cause gout
c. Conditions of increased cell turnover, as well as slowed renal excretion of uric acid, may cause uricemia.
d. Elevated amounts of urinary uric acid form precipitates of urate stones in the kidneys.
2. Values
a. Male: 4.5 to 8 mg/dL
b. Female: 2.5 to 6.2 mg/dL
3. Nursing considerations
a. Instruct the client to fast for 8 hours before the test as prescribed.
b. Theophylline, caffeine, and vitamin C may cause falsely elevated results.

⚠ Clients with liver disease often have prolonged clotting times; therefore provide prolonged pressure at the venipuncture site and monitor the site closely for bleeding.

VI. GLUCOSE STUDIES

A. Fasting **blood** glucose
1. Description
a. Glucose is a monosaccharide found in fruits and formed from the digestion of carbohydrates and the conversion of glycogen by the liver.
b. Glucose is the body's main source of cellular energy, and it is essential for brain and erythrocyte function.

c. Fasting **blood** glucose levels are used to help diagnose diabetes mellitus and hypoglycemia (Table 11-4).
2. Nursing considerations
a. Instruct the client to fast for 8 to 12 hours before the test.
b. Instruct a client with diabetes mellitus to withhold morning insulin or oral hypoglycemic medication until after the **blood** is drawn.

B. Glucose tolerance test (see Table 11-4)
1. Description
a. Aids in the diagnosis of diabetes mellitus
b. If the glucose levels peak at higher than normal at 1 to 2 hours after the injection or ingestion of glucose and are slower than normal to return to fasting levels, then diabetes mellitus is confirmed.
2. Nursing considerations
a. Instruct the client to eat a high-carbohydrate (200- to 300-g) diet for 3 days before the test.
b. Instruct the client to avoid alcohol, coffee, and smoking for 36 hours before the test.
c. Instruct the client to fast for 10 to 16 hours before the test.
d. Instruct the client to avoid strenuous exercise for 8 hours before and after the test.
e. Instruct the client with diabetes mellitus to withhold morning insulin or oral hypoglycemic medication.
f. Instruct the client that the test will take 3 to 5 hours and that it requires the IV or oral administration of glucose and multiple **blood** samples.

C. Glycosylated hemoglobin
1. Description
a. Glycosylated hemoglobin is **blood** glucose that is bound to hemoglobin.
b. Hemoglobin A (HbA_{1c}) is a reflection of how well **blood** glucose levels have been controlled for up to the past 3 to 4 months.

TABLE 11-4 Normal Adult Glucose Values

Point of Measurement	Normal Value
Glucose, fasting	70-110 mg/dL
Glucose monitoring (capillary blood)	60-110 mg/dL
Glucose tolerance test, oral	
Baseline fasting	70-110 mg/dL
30-minute fasting	110-170 mg/dL
60-minute fasting	120-170 mg/dL
90-minute fasting	100-140 mg/dL
120-minute fasting	70-120 mg/dL
Glucose, 2-hour postprandial	<140 mg/dL

c. Hyperglycemia in clients with diabetes is usually a cause of an increase in the HbA_{1c} level.
2. Values
   a. Values are expressed as a percentage of the total hemoglobin.
   b. Good control of diabetes: 7% or less
   c. Fair control of diabetes: 7% to 8%
   d. Poor control of diabetes: 8% or more
3. Nursing considerations: Fasting is not required before the test.

D. Glycosylated **serum** albumin (fructosamine)
1. Description
   a. Reflects the average **serum** glucose levels over a period of 2 to 3 weeks
   b. More sensitive to recent changes than the HbA_{1c} test
2. Values: Normal ranges vary according to method of testing used; nondiabetic client, 1.5 to 2.7 mmol/L; diabetic client, 2.0 to 5.0 mmol/L
3. Nursing considerations: The client needs to fast for 12 hours before the test.

E. Diabetes mellitus autoantibody panel
1. Description: Used to evaluate insulin resistance and to identify type 1 diabetes and clients with a suspected allergy to insulin
2. Value: Less than 1:4 titer with no antibody detected
3. Nursing considerations
   a. Radioactive scans within 7 days before the test may interfere with test results
   b. No fasting is required

VII. RENAL FUNCTION STUDIES

A. Serum creatinine
1. Description
   a. Very specific indicator of renal function
   b. Increased levels indicate a slowing of the glomerular filtration rate.
2. Value: 0.6 to 1.3 mg/dL
3. Nursing considerations: Instruct the client to avoid excessive exercise for 8 hours before the test and excessive red meat intake for 24 hours before the test.

B. Blood urea nitrogen
1. Description
   a. Urea nitrogen is the nitrogen portion of urea, a substance formed in the liver through an enzymatic protein breakdown process.
   b. Urea is normally freely filtered through the renal glomeruli, with a small amount reabsorbed in the tubules and the remainder excreted into the urine.
   c. Elevated levels indicate a slowing of the glomerular filtration rate.

2. Value: 8 to 25 mg/dL
3. Nursing considerations: Creatinine and urea nitrogen levels should be analyzed when renal function is evaluated.

VIII. ELEMENTS

A. Calcium
1. Description
   a. A cation that is absorbed into the bloodstream from dietary sources and functions in bone formation, nerve impulse transmission, and the contraction of myocardial and skeletal muscles
   b. Aids in **blood** clotting by converting prothrombin to thrombin
2. Value: 8.6 to 10 mg/dL
3. Nursing considerations
   a. Instruct the client to eat a diet with normal calcium levels (800 mg/day) for 3 days before the test.
   b. Instruct the client that fasting may be required for 8 hours before the test.

B. Magnesium
1. Description
   a. Used as an index to determine metabolic activity and renal function
   b. Magnesium is needed for the **blood**-clotting process, regulates neuromuscular activity, acts as a cofactor that modifies the activity of many enzymes, and has an effect on the metabolism of calcium
2. Value: 1.6 to 2.6 mg/dL
3. Nursing considerations
   a. Prolonged use of magnesium products will cause increased levels of magnesium.
   b. Long-term parenteral nutrition therapy or excessive loss of body fluids may decrease serum levels.

C. Phosphorus
1. Description
   a. Important in bone formation, energy storage and release, urinary acid–base buffering, and carbohydrate metabolism
   b. Absorbed from food and excreted by the kidneys
   c. High concentrations of phosphorus are stored in bone and skeletal muscle
2. Value: 2.7 to 4.5 mg/dL
3. Nursing considerations: Instruct the client to fast before the test.

IX. THYROID STUDIES

A. Description
1. Performed if a thyroid disorder is suspected
2. Helps to differentiate primary thyroid disease from secondary causes and abnormalities in thyroxine-binding globulin levels

B. Values
1. Thyroid-stimulating hormone (thyrotropin): 0.2 to 5.4 microunits/mL
2. Thyroxine (T4): 5 to 12 mcg/dL
3. Thyroxine, free (FT4): 0.8 to 2.4 ng/dL
4. Triiodothyronine (T3): 80 to 230 ng/dL

C. Nursing considerations: Test results may be invalid if the client has undergone a radionuclide scan within 7 days before the test.

X. WHITE BLOOD CELL COUNT

A. Description
1. WBCs function in the body's immune defense system.
2. The WBC count assesses leukocyte distribution.

B. Value: 4500 to 11,000 cells/mm^3 (Table 11-5)

C. Nursing considerations
1. A "shift to the left" means that there is an increased number of immature neutrophils in the peripheral **blood**.
2. A low total WBC count with a left shift indicates a recovery from bone marrow depression or an infection of such intensity that the demand for neutrophils in the tissue is greater than the capacity of the bone marrow to release them into the circulation.
3. A high total WBC count with a left shift indicates an increased release of neutrophils by the bone marrow in response to an overwhelming infection or inflammation.
4. A "shift to the right" means that cells have more than the usual number of nuclear segments. This is found with liver disease, Down syndrome, and megaloblastic and pernicious anemia.

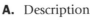 Monitor the WBC count closely in clients receiving chemotherapy because of the risk for neutropenia.

XI. HEPATITIS TESTS

A. Description
1. Tests include radioimmunoassay, enzyme-linked immunosorbent assay (ELISA), and microparticle enzyme immunoassay.

TABLE 11-5 Normal Adult White Blood Cell Differential Count

Cell Type	Percentage and Count
Neutrophils	56%; 1800-7800 cells/mm^3
Bands	3%; 0-700 cells/mm^3
Eosinophils	2.7%; 0-450 cells/mm^3
Basophils	0.3%; 0-200 cells/mm^3
Lymphocytes	34%; 1000-4800 cells/mm^3
Monocytes	4%; 0-800 cells/mm^3

2. Serologic tests for specific hepatitis virus markers assist with defining the specific type of hepatitis.

B. Values
1. The presence of immunoglobulin M (IgM) antibody to hepatitis A virus (IgM anti-HAV) and total antibody to hepatitis A virus (total anti-HAV) identify the disease.
2. Detection of hepatitis B core antigen (HBcAg), envelope antigen (HbeAg), and surface antigen (HbsAg) or their corresponding antibodies constitutes hepatitis B assessment.
3. Hepatitis C is confirmed by the presence of antibodies to hepatitis C.
4. Serologic hepatitis D virus (HDV) determination is made by the detection of the hepatitis D antigen (HDAg) early in the course of the infection and anti-HDV antibody in later disease stages.
5. Specific serologic tests for hepatitis E virus include the detection of IgM and immunoglobulin G antibodies to hepatitis E.
6. Hepatitis G virus (HGV) has been found in some **blood** donors (donated **blood**), IV drug users, hemodialysis clients, and clients with hemophilia; however HGV does not appear to cause significant liver disease.

C. Nursing considerations: If the radioimmunoassay technique is being used, the injection of radionuclides within 1 week before the **blood** test may falsely elevate results.

XII. HUMAN IMMUNODEFICIENCY VIRUS (HIV) AND ACQUIRED IMMUNODEFICIENCY SYNDROME (AIDS) TESTING

A. Description
1. Detects HIV, which is the cause of AIDS
2. Common tests used to determine the presence of antibodies to HIV include ELISA, Western blot (WB), and immunofluorescence assay (IFA).
3. A single reactive ELISA test by itself cannot be used to diagnose HIV and should be repeated in duplicate with the same blood sample. If the result is repeatedly reactive, follow-up tests using WB or IFA should be performed.
4. A positive WB or IFA is considered confirmatory for HIV.
5. A positive ELISA that fails to be confirmed by WB or IFA should not be considered negative, and repeat testing should take place in 3 to 6 months.

B. CD4 T-cell counts
1. Monitors the progression of HIV
2. As the disease progresses, there is usually a decrease in the CD4$^+$ T-cell count and a resultant decrease in immunity.
3. The normal CD4$^+$ T-cell count is between 500 and 1600 cells/mm^3.

4. Generally the immune system remains healthy with CD4$^+$ T-cell counts greater than 500 cells/mm^3.
5. Immune system problems occur when the CD4$^+$ T cell count is between 200 and 499 cells/mm^3.
6. Severe immune system problems occur when the CD4$^+$ T-cell count is less than 200 cells/mm^3.

C. CD4$^+$ to CD8$^+$ ratio
1. Monitors the progression of the disease
2. The normal ratio is approximately 2:1.

D. Viral culture involves placing the infected client's **blood cells** in a culture medium and measuring the amount of reverse transcriptase activity over a specified period of time.

E. Viral load testing measures the presence of HIV viral genetic material (RNA) or other viral protein in the client's **blood**.

F. The p24 antigen assay quantifies the amount of HIV viral core protein in the client's **serum**.

G. Oral testing for HIV
1. Uses a device that is placed against the gum and cheek for 2 minutes
2. Fluid (not saliva) is drawn into an absorbable pad. This fluid contains antibodies in an HIV-positive individual.
3. The pad is placed in a solution, and a specified observable change is noted if the test is positive.
4. If the result is positive, a **blood** test is needed to confirm the results.

H. Home test kits for HIV
1. In one at-home test kit, a drop of **blood** is placed on a test card with a special code number. The card is mailed to the laboratory for testing for HIV antibodies.
2. The individual receives the results by calling a special telephone number and entering the special code number. Test results are then given.

I. Nursing considerations
1. Maintain issues of confidentiality surrounding HIV and AIDS testing
2. Follow prescribed state regulations and protocols related to reporting positive test results.

XIII. URINE TESTS (Table 11-6)

XIV. THERAPEUTIC SERUM MEDICATION LEVELS (Table 11-7)

A. If the result is below the therapeutic level, the client may not be compliant with the medicine regimen or the dose may need to be increased. Notify the registered nurse (RN) or health care provider (HCP).

B. If the result is within the range, the medication can be administered as prescribed.

C. If the result is above the therapeutic level (toxic), the dose is too high. The client may not understand the medicine regimen and may be taking too much or may have organ dysfunction, leading to poor metabolism/elimination of the medication. Hold the dose and notify the RN or HCP.

TABLE 11-6 Normal Adult Values Urine Tests

Name of Test	Value
Color	Pale yellow
Odor	Specific aromatic odor similar to ammonia
Turbidity	Clear
pH	4.5-7.8
Specific gravity	1.016-1.022
Glucose	<0.5 g/day
Ketones	None
Protein	0.8 mg/dL
Bilirubin	None
Casts	None to few
Crystals	None
Bacteria	<1000 colonies/mL
Red blood cells	0-2
White blood cells	0-5
Chloride	110-250 mEq/24 hours
Magnesium	7.3-12.2 mg/dL per day
Potassium	25-125 mEq/24 hours
Sodium	40-220 mEq/24 hours
Uric acid	250-750 mg/24 hours

TABLE 11-7 Therapeutic Serum Medication Levels

Medication	Therapeutic Range
Acetaminophen (Tylenol)	10-20 mcg/mL
Carbamazepine (Tegretol)	5-12 mcg/mL
Digoxin (Lanoxin)	0.5-2 ng/mL
Gentamicin	5-10 mcg/mL
Lithium (Lithobid)	0.5-1.3 mEq/L
Magnesium sulfate	4-7 mg/dL
Phenytoin (Dilantin)	10-20 mcg/mL
Salicylates	100-250 mcg/mL
Theophylline	10-20 mcg/mL
Tobramycin (Nebcin)	5-10 mcg/mL
Valproic acid (Depakene)	50-100 mcg/mL

MORE QUESTIONS ON EVOLVE!

Practice Questions

56. A nurse is told that the laboratory result for the serum digoxin level is 2.4 ng/mL. The nurse plans to do which of the following?
1. Hold the medication.
2. Check the client's last respiratory rate.
3. Record the normal value on the client's flow sheet.
4. Administer the next dose of the medication as scheduled.

57. A client with atrial fibrillation who is receiving maintenance therapy with warfarin sodium (Coumadin) has a prothrombin time (PT) of 30 seconds. The nurse anticipates that which of the following will be prescribed?
1. Adding a dose of heparin
2. Holding the next dose of warfarin sodium
3. Increasing the next dose of warfarin sodium
4. Administering the next dose of warfarin sodium

58. An adult client who had preadmission testing before surgery has blood drawn for the determination of serum electrolyte levels. The nurse identifies which of the following as an abnormal value?
1. Sodium, 148 mEq/L
2. Chloride, 101 mEq/L
3. Potassium, 3.8 mEq/L
4. Bicarbonate, 26 mEq/L

59. An adult client with a critically high potassium level has received sodium polystyrene sulfonate (Kayexalate). The nurse determines that the medication has brought the potassium level back into normal range when the serum potassium level is:
1. 3.3 mEq/L
2. 4.9 mEq/L
3. 5.8 mEq/L
4. 6.2 mEq/L

60. The adult client with a history of cardiac disease is due for a morning dose of furosemide (Lasix). The nurse reviews the client's record and reports which of the following serum potassium levels before administering the dose of furosemide?
1. 3.2 mEq/L
2. 3.8 mEq/L
3. 4.2 mEq/L
4. 4.8 mEq/L

61. A client with diabetes mellitus has a blood sample drawn for the determination of a fasting blood glucose level. The nurse identifies which of the following results as a critical value?
1. 150 mg/dL
2. 200 mg/dL
3. 220 mg/dL
4. 340 mg/dL

62. An adult client with a history of gastrointestinal bleeding has a platelet count of 300,000 cells/mL. Which of the following actions by the nurse is most appropriate after reading this report?
1. Report the abnormally low count.
2. Report the abnormally high count.
3. Place the client on bleeding precautions.
4. Place the normal report in the client's medical record.

63. A nurse is reviewing the laboratory results of an adult client with Addison's disease. The nurse determines that the magnesium level is normal if it is which of the following?
1. 2 mg/dL
2. 3 mg/dL
3. 4 mg/dL
4. 5 mg/dL

64. An adult male client has had laboratory work done as part of a routine physical examination. The nurse reviews the client's record and determines that the client may have a mild degree of renal insufficiency if which of the following serum creatinine levels is found?
1. 0.6 mg/dL
2. 1.1 mg/dL
3. 1.9 mg/dL
4. 3.5 mg/dL

65. A client with a seizure disorder is taking phenytoin (Dilantin). A sample for a serum phenytoin level is drawn, and the nurse determines that the medication therapy is within therapeutic range if the laboratory result is:
1. 3 mcg/mL
2. 8 mcg/mL
3. 16 mcg/mL
4. 24 mcg/mL

66. An adult client with hepatic cirrhosis has been consuming a diet with optimal amounts of protein. The nurse evaluates the client's status as most satisfactory if the total protein level is which of the following values?
1. 0.4 g/dL
2. 3.7 g/dL
3. 6.4 g/dL
4. 9.0 g/dL

67. An adult client was diagnosed with acute pancreatitis 9 days ago. The nurse interprets that the client is recovering from this episode if the serum lipase level drops to which of the following values, which is just beneath the upper limit of normal?
1. 20 units/L
2. 80 units/L
3. 135 units/L
4. 250 units/L

68. A client arrives in the emergency department complaining of chest pain that began 4 hours ago. A troponin T blood specimen is obtained, and the results indicate a level of 0.6 ng/mL. The nurse interprets that this result indicates:
1. A normal level
2. A low value that indicates possible gastritis
3. A level that indicates a myocardial infarction
4. A level that indicates the presence of possible angina

69. An adult female client has a hemoglobin level of 10.8 g/dL. The nurse interprets that this result is most likely the result of which of the following factors in the client's history?
1. Heart failure
2. Dehydration
3. Iron deficiency anemia
4. Chronic obstructive pulmonary disease (COPD)

70. An adult male client admitted with dehydration has received fluid volume replacement. The nurse determines that the client has had adequate fluid resuscitation if the client's repeat hematocrit level has decreased to which of the following values in the normal range?
1. 34%
2. 39%
3. 48%
4. 56%

ANSWERS

56. 1
Rationale: The normal therapeutic range for digoxin is 0.5 to 2 ng/mL. A value of 2.4 ng/mL exceeds the therapeutic range and could be toxic to the client. The nursing action is to hold further doses of digoxin. Option 3 is incorrect, because the value is not normal. Option 4 would cause the client to become more toxic. The next dose should not be administered automatically. Checking the client's respiratory rate is not applicable at this time.
Test-Taking Strategy: Recall that the normal therapeutic range for digoxin is 0.5 to 2 ng/mL. Noting that the value is high will direct you to option 1. Review the therapeutic level of digoxin if you had difficulty with this question.
Level of Cognitive Ability: Applying
Client Needs: Physiological Integrity
Integrated Process: Nursing Process/Implementation
Content Area: Fundamental Skills: Laboratory Values
References: Christensen, Kockrow, p. 318. 2011. *Adult health nursing.*
Pagana, Pagana, p. 354. 2009.

57. 2
Rationale: The normal PT is 9.6 to 11.8 seconds for the adult male and 9.5 to 11.3 seconds for the adult female. Because the value stated is extremely high (and perhaps near the critical range), the nurse should anticipate that the client would not receive further doses at this time. If the level were too high, then the antidote (vitamin K) may be prescribed. Options 1, 3, and 4 would make the client more toxic and prone to bleeding.
Test-Taking Strategy: Note that the PT is 30 seconds. Noting that the PT value is high will direct you to option 2. Review this laboratory value if you had difficulty with this question.
Level of Cognitive Ability: Analyzing
Client Needs: Physiological Integrity
Integrated Process: Nursing Process/Planning
Content Area: Fundamental Skills: Laboratory Values
Reference: Pagana, Pagana, pp. 776–779. 2009.

58. 1
Rationale: The normal serum electrolyte ranges for adults are as follows: sodium, 135 to 145 mEq/L; potassium, 3.5 to 5.1 mEq/L; chloride, 98 to 107 mEq/L; and bicarbonate (venous), 22 to 29 mEq/L. The only abnormal value identified is the serum sodium level.
Test-Taking Strategy: Focus on the subject of an abnormal value. Recalling the normal serum electrolyte values will direct you to option 1. Review the normal electrolyte values if you had difficulty with this question.
Level of Cognitive Ability: Understanding
Client Needs: Physiological Integrity
Integrated Process: Nursing Process/Data Collection
Content Area: Fundamental Skills: Laboratory Values
Reference: deWit, p. 45. 2009.

59. 2
Rationale: The normal serum potassium level in the adult is 3.5 to 5.1 mEq/L. Option 2 is the only option that reflects a normal potassium value.
Test-Taking Strategy: Note the strategic words "critically high." You would expect that this medication is administered to lower the potassium level. Recalling the normal serum potassium level will direct you to option 2. Review this normal level if you had difficulty with this question.
Level of Cognitive Ability: Understanding
Client Needs: Physiological Integrity
Integrated Process: Nursing Process/Evaluation
Content Area: Fundamental Skills: Laboratory Values
Reference: deWit, p. 45. 2009.

60. 1
Rationale: The normal adult serum potassium level is 3.5 to 5.1 mEq/L. Option 1 is the only value that falls below the therapeutic range. Administering furosemide (Lasix) to a client with a low potassium level and a cardiac history could precipitate ventricular dysrhythmias in the client.

Test-Taking Strategy: Use the process of elimination. Recalling the normal serum potassium level will assist you with identifying the value that is not within normal range. This will direct you to option 1. Review the normal adult serum potassium level if you had difficulty with this question.
Level of Cognitive Ability: Understanding
Client Needs: Physiological Integrity
Integrated Process: Nursing Process/Implementation
Content Area: Fundamental Skills: Laboratory Values
References: deWit, p. 45. 2009.
Pagana, Pagana, p. 745. 2009.

61. 4
Rationale: The normal fasting blood glucose level is 70 to 110 mg/dL in the adult client. A critical level is considered to be one that exceeds 250 to 300 mg/dL, depending on the health care provider's preference. This makes option 4 the correct choice.
Test-Taking Strategy: Use the process of elimination and your knowledge of the normal fasting blood glucose level to answer the question. Noting the strategic words "critical value" will direct you to option 4, the highest value. Review this laboratory test if you had difficulty with this question.
Level of Cognitive Ability: Understanding
Client Needs: Physiological Integrity
Integrated Process: Nursing Process/Data Collection
Content Area: Fundamental Skills: Laboratory Values
References: Christensen, Kockrow, p. 512. 2011. *Adult health nursing.*
Pagana, Pagana, p. 477. 2009.

62. 4
Rationale: A normal platelet count ranges from 150,000 to 400,000 cells/mm3. The nurse should place the report that contains the normal laboratory value into the client's medical record.
Test-Taking Strategy: Use the process of elimination. Remember that options that are comparable or alike are not likely to be correct. With this in mind, eliminate options 1 and 3 first. From the remaining options, recalling the normal range for this laboratory test will direct you to option 4. Review the normal platelet count if you had difficulty with this question.
Level of Cognitive Ability: Applying
Client Needs: Physiological Integrity
Integrated Process: Nursing Process/Implementation
Content Area: Fundamental Skills: Laboratory Values
Reference: Pagana, Pagana, p. 731. 2009.

63. 1
Rationale: The normal magnesium level in an adult client is 1.6 to 2.6 mg/dL. Options 2, 3, and 4 indicate elevated values.
Test-Taking Strategy: Knowledge regarding the normal magnesium level in an adult client is required to answer this question. Remember that the normal magnesium level in an adult client is 1.6 to 2.6 mg/dL. Review this laboratory test if you had difficulty with this question.
Level of Cognitive Ability: Understanding
Client Needs: Physiological Integrity
Integrated Process: Nursing Process/Data Collection
Content Area: Fundamental Skills: Laboratory Values
Reference: Pagana, Pagana, p. 630. 2009.

64. 3
Rationale: The normal serum creatinine level is 0.6 to 1.3 mg/dL. The client with a mild degree of renal insufficiency would have a slightly elevated level, which would be the value of 1.9 mg/dL. Creatinine levels of 3.5 mg/dL may be associated with acute or chronic renal failure.
Test-Taking Strategy: Note the strategic word "mild." This tells you that the correct option will be an abnormal value but perhaps not the most abnormal of all of the options. Use your knowledge of the normal serum creatinine level to direct you to option 3. Review the normal value of this laboratory test if you had difficulty with this question.
Level of Cognitive Ability: Understanding
Client Needs: Physiological Integrity
Integrated Process: Nursing Process/Data Collection
Content Area: Fundamental Skills: Laboratory Values
Reference: deWit, p. 820. 2009.

65. 3
Rationale: The therapeutic range for serum phenytoin (Dilantin) level is 10 to 20 mcg/mL. If the level is below the therapeutic range, as in options 1 and 2, then the client may continue to experience seizure activity. If the level is too high, as in option 4, the client could experience phenytoin toxicity.
Test-Taking Strategy: Focus on the subject of effective medication therapy. Remember that the therapeutic range for serum phenytoin (Dilantin) level is 10 to 20 mcg/mL. Review this normal range if you had difficulty with this question.
Level of Cognitive Ability: Understanding
Client Needs: Physiological Integrity
Integrated Process: Nursing Process/Evaluation
Content Area: Fundamental Skills: Laboratory Values
Reference: Pagana, Pagana, p. 355. 2009.

66. 3
Rationale: The normal range for the protein level in the adult client is 6 to 8 g/dL, which makes option 3 the correct choice. Options 1 and 2 indicate low levels. Option 4 indicates an elevated level.
Test-Taking Strategy: Note the strategic words "most satisfactory." Recalling the normal protein level will direct you to option 3. Review this normal level if you had difficulty with this question.
Level of Cognitive Ability: Understanding
Client Needs: Physiological Integrity
Integrated Process: Nursing Process/Evaluation
Content Area: Fundamental Skills: Laboratory Values
Reference: Pagana, Pagana, p. 769. 2009.

67. 3
Rationale: The normal serum lipase level is 10 to 140 units/L. Option 3 is the only choice that contains a value just beneath the upper limit of normal. The client who is recovering from acute pancreatitis usually has elevated lipase levels for approximately 10 days after the onset of symptoms. This makes lipase a valuable test for monitoring the client's pancreatic function.
Test-Taking Strategy: Note the strategic words "just beneath the upper limit of normal." Recalling the normal lipase level will direct you to option 3. Review this normal level if you had difficulty with this question

Level of Cognitive Ability: Understanding
Client Needs: Physiological Integrity
Integrated Process: Nursing Process/Evaluation
Content Area: Fundamental Skills: Laboratory Values
Reference: Pagana, Pagana, p. 596. 2009.

68. 3

Rationale: Troponins are regulatory proteins that are found in striated muscle. The troponins function together in the contractile apparatus for striated muscle in the skeletal muscle and the myocardium. Increased amounts of troponins are released into the bloodstream when an infarction causes damage to the myocardium. A troponin T level greater than 0.1 to 0.2 ng/mL is consistent with a myocardial infarction. A normal troponin I level is less than 0.6 ng/mL, whereas a level greater than 1.5 ng/mL is consistent with a myocardial infarction. A troponin T level of 0.6 is not normal, so option 1 is incorrect. Troponin T does not test for angina or gastritis; thus options 2 and 4 are incorrect.
Test-Taking Strategy: Note that the subject of the question relates to the troponin T level. Recalling that a level greater than 0.1 to 0.2 ng/mL is consistent with a myocardial infarction will direct you to option 3. Review this diagnostic test if you had difficulty with this question.
Level of Cognitive Ability: Analyzing
Client Needs: Physiological Integrity
Integrated Process: Nursing Process/Evaluation
Content Area: Fundamental Skills: Laboratory Values
References: Christensen, Kockrow, p. 311. 2011. *Adult health nursing.*
Pagana, Pagana, p. 943. 2009.

69. 3

Rationale: The normal hemoglobin level for an adult female client is 12 to 15 g/dL. A low hemoglobin level usually indicates anemia. Iron deficiency anemia can result in lower hemoglobin levels. Options 1, 2, and 4 may increase hemoglobin. Heart failure and COPD may increase the hemoglobin level as a result of the body's need for more oxygen-carrying capacity. Dehydration may increase the hemoglobin level by hemoconcentration.
Test-Taking Strategy: Use the process of elimination. Evaluate each condition presented in the options with regard to whether it is likely to raise or lower the hemoglobin level. This will direct you to option 3. Review the normal hemoglobin level and the causes of a low level if you had difficulty with this question.
Level of Cognitive Ability: Analyzing
Client Needs: Physiological Integrity
Integrated Process: Nursing Process/Data Collection
Content Area: Fundamental Skills: Laboratory Values
References: Christensen, Kockrow, pp. 275–276. 2011. *Adult health nursing.*
deWit, p. 362. 2009.

70. 3

Rationale: The normal hematocrit level for an adult male is 42% to 52%. Thus, option 3 is the only correct choice. The client who is dehydrated has an elevated level as a result of hemoconcentration. The client's level may be expected to drift back down to within the normal range after the fluid volume has been adequately restored. Option 4 is too high, and options 1 and 2 are low.
Test-Taking Strategy: Use the process of elimination, and note the strategic words "normal range." Recalling the normal hematocrit level for an adult male will direct you to option 3. Review this normal value if you had difficulty with this question.
Level of Cognitive Ability: Evaluating
Client Needs: Physiological Integrity
Integrated Process: Nursing Process/Evaluation
Content Area: Fundamental Skills: Laboratory Values
References: Christensen, Kockrow, p. 263. 2011. *Adult health nursing.*
Pagana, Pagana, p. 506. 2009.

Nutritional Components of Care

PYRAMID TERMS

absorption Passage of digested nutrients through the wall of the stomach or small intestine into the blood or lymph system.

enteral nutrition Administration of nutrition with liquefied foods into the gastrointestinal tract via a tube.

fat emulsion (lipids) A white, opaque solution administered intravenously during parenteral nutrition therapy to prevent fatty acid deficiency.

malnutrition Deficiency of the nutrients required for the development and maintenance of the human body.

metabolism Ongoing chemical process within the body that converts digested nutrients into energy for the functioning of body cells.

nutrients Carbohydrates, fats or lipids, proteins, vitamins, minerals, and water that must be supplied in adequate amounts to provide energy, growth, development, and maintenance of the human body.

parenteral nutrition (PN) Administration of a nutritionally complete formula through a central or peripheral intravenous (IV) catheter. In the clinical setting, the term *PN* may be used interchangeably with the term *total parenteral nutrition (TPN)* or *hyperalimentation*.

peripheral parenteral nutrition (PPN) Parenteral nutrition administered through a peripheral vein in an extremity. PN solutions administered peripherally are not as calorically dense as those administered through a central vein.

PYRAMID TO SUCCESS

Nutrition is a basic need that must be met for all clients. Nurses must have the knowledge required to educate and care for healthy clients and for clients with nutritional needs or disorders that require alterations in dietary measures. The NCLEX-PN examination addresses the dietary measures required for basic needs and for particular body-system alterations. When presented with a question related to nutrition, consider the client's diagnosis and the particular requirement or restriction necessary for the treatment of the disorder. Pyramid points focus on the common types of therapeutic diets, nutrients contained in food items, enteral feedings, and parenteral nutrition (PN).

CLIENT NEEDS

Safe and Effective Care Environment

- Consulting with members of the health care team, such as a dietitian regarding dietary needs
- Discussing home safety for storing and cooking foods
- Handling hazardous and infectious materials
- Maintaining standard, transmission-based, and asepsis to prevent infection
- Obtaining informed consent for invasive procedures, such as central line placement

Health Promotion and Maintenance

- Performing data collection techniques
- Reinforcing dietary teaching about diet and foods to avoid or increase
- Reinforcing client and family education regarding the administration of enteral nutrition or PN at home

Psychosocial Integrity

- Considering cultural and religious preferences related to nutritional patterns and lifestyle choices
- Discussing role changes related to the need for enteral nutrition or PN at home
- Identifying coping mechanisms
- Identifying support systems in the home to assist with administration of enteral nutrition or PN

Physiological Integrity

- Assessing elimination patterns
- Checking for adverse, expected, and side effects of PN and enteral therapy for nutrition
- Monitoring for alterations in body systems
- Monitoring enteral feedings and the client's ability to tolerate feedings
- Monitoring for expected effects of nutritional therapy
- Monitoring fluid and electrolyte balance
- Monitoring laboratory values
- Monitoring nutritional intake and oral hydration

- Monitoring for potential complications/adverse effects of nutritional therapy
- Providing assistive devices for eating

I. NUTRIENTS

A. Carbohydrates
1. Carbohydrates are the preferred source of energy and provide 4 cal/g
2. Carbohydrates promote normal fat **metabolism,** spare protein, and enhance lower gastrointestinal (GI) function
3. Major food sources of carbohydrates include milk, grains, fruits, and vegetables
4. Inadequate carbohydrate intake affects **metabolism**

B. Fats (Box 12-1)
1. Fats provide a concentrated source and a stored form of energy and 9 cal/g
2. Fats protect internal organs and maintain body temperature
3. Fats enhance the **absorption** of the fat-soluble vitamins
4. Inadequate fat intake leads to clinical manifestations of sensitivity to cold, skin lesions, increased risk of infection, and amenorrhea in women
5. Diets high in fat can lead to obesity and increase the risk of cardiovascular disease and some cancers

C. Proteins
1. Amino acids, which make up proteins, are critical to all aspects of the growth and development of body tissues and provide 4 cal/g
2. Proteins build and repair body tissues, regulate fluid balance, maintain acid-base balance, produce antibodies, provide energy, and produce enzymes and hormones
3. Essential amino acids (EAAs) are required in the diet because the body cannot manufacture them
4. High-quality proteins or complete proteins such as eggs, dairy products, meat, fish, and poultry contain adequate amounts of EAAs
5. Foods that do not contain EAAs in sufficient amounts are lower-quality or incomplete proteins.
6. Inadequate protein intake can cause protein energy **malnutrition** and severe wasting of fat and muscle tissue

D. Vitamins (Box 12-2)
1. Vitamins facilitate **metabolism** of proteins, fats, and carbohydrates and act as catalysts for metabolic functions.
2. Vitamins promote life and growth processes, and maintain and regulate body functions
3. Fat-soluble vitamins A, D, E, and K can be stored in the body, so an excess can cause toxicity
4. The B vitamins and vitamin C are water soluble, are not stored in the body, and can be excreted in the urine
5. Vitamin K acts as a catalyst for facilitating blood-clotting factors, especially prothrombin
6. Vitamin C functions in the production of collagen, a vital component in wound healing
7. Vitamin A maintains eyesight and epithelial linings
8. Folic acid helps prevent neural-tube birth defects

Box 12-1 Food Sources of Fat

Cholesterol
Animal products
Egg yolks
Liver and organ meats
Shellfish

Monounsaturated Fats
Duck and goose
Eggs
Olive and peanut oils

Polyunsaturated Fats
Safflower oil
Corn oil
Sunflower oil

Saturated Fats
Beef
Butter
Luncheon meats
Hard yellow cheeses

Box 12-2 Food Sources of Vitamins

Water Soluble
- Folic acid: Green, leafy vegetables; liver, beef, and fish; legumes; grapefruit and oranges
- Niacin: Meats, poultry, fish, beans, peanuts, grains
- Vitamin B_1 (thiamine): Pork, nuts, whole-grain cereals, legumes
- Vitamin B_2 (riboflavin): Milk, lean meats, fish, grains
- Vitamin B_6 (pyridoxine): Yeast, corn, meat, poultry, fish
- Vitamin B_{12} (cobalamin): Meat, liver (only found in animal products)
- Vitamin C (ascorbic acid): Citrus fruits, tomatoes, broccoli, cabbage

Fat Soluble
- Vitamin A: Liver, egg yolk, whole milk, green or orange vegetables, fruits
- Vitamin D: Fortified milk, fish oils, cereals
- Vitamin E: Vegetable oils; green, leafy vegetables; cereals; apricots; apples; peaches
- Vitamin K: Green, leafy vegetables; cauliflower; cabbage

E. Minerals (Box 12-3)

1. Minerals are components of hormones, cells, tissues, and bones
2. Minerals act as catalysts for chemical reactions and enhancers of cell function
3. Almost all foods contain some form of minerals
4. A deficiency of minerals can occur in chronically ill or hospitalized clients

⚠ Always check the client's ability to eat and swallow and promote independence in eating as much as is possible.

Box 12-3 Food Sources of Minerals

Calcium
- Broccoli
- Carrots
- Cheese
- Collard greens
- Green beans
- Milk
- Rhubarb
- Spinach
- Tofu
- Yogurt

Chloride
- Salt

Magnesium
- Avocados
- Canned white tuna
- Cauliflower
- Cooked rolled oats
- Green, leafy vegetables
- Milk
- Peanut butter
- Peas
- Pork, beef, chicken
- Potatoes
- Raisins
- Yogurt

Phosphorus
- Fish
- Nuts
- Organ meats
- Pork, beef, chicken
- Whole-grain breads and cereals

Potassium
- Avocados
- Bananas
- Cantaloupe
- Carrots
- Fish

- Mushrooms
- Oranges
- Pork, beef, veal
- Potatoes
- Raisins
- Spinach
- Strawberries
- Tomatoes

Sodium
- American cheese
- Bacon
- Butter
- Canned food
- Cottage cheese
- Cured pork
- Hot dogs
- Ketchup
- Lunch meat
- Milk
- Mustard
- Processed food
- Snack food
- Soy sauce
- Table salt
- White and whole-wheat bread

Iron
- Breads and cereals
- Dark green vegetables
- Dried fruits
- Egg yolk
- Legumes
- Liver
- Meats

Zinc
- Eggs
- Green, leafy vegetables
- Meats
- Protein-rich foods

II. MYPLATE (Figure 12-1)

A. Provides a balanced diet that includes grains, vegetables, fruits, dairy products, and protein foods

B. Guidelines

1. Avoid eating oversized portions of foods
2. Fill half of the plate with fruits and vegetables
3. Vary the type of vegetables and fruits eaten
4. Select at least half of the grains as whole grains
5. Ensure that foods from the dairy group are high in calcium
6. Drink milk that is fat-free or low fat (1%)
7. Eat protein foods that are lean
8. Select fresh foods over frozen or canned foods
9. Drink water rather than liquids that contain sugar

C. Web site: http://www.choosemyplate.gov

III. THERAPEUTIC DIETS

A. Clear liquid diet

1. Indications
   a. Serves the primary function of providing fluids and electrolytes to prevent dehydration
   b. Initial feeding after complete bowel rest
   c. Used initially to feed a malnourished person or a person who has not had any oral intake for some time
   d. Bowel preparation for surgery or tests
   e. Postsurgical diet
   f. Initial diet in gastroenteritis and pancreatitis
2. Nursing considerations
   a. Sources of fuel and many nutrients needed by the client are deficient in a clear liquid diet
   b. The body digests and absorbs clear liquids easily

▲ **FIGURE 12-1** MyPlate. (From U.S. Department of Agriculture. http://www.choosemyplate.gov.)

c. Contributes to little or no residue in the GI tract

d. Can be unappetizing and boring

e. As a transition diet, clear liquids are intended for short-term use only

f. Consists of foods that are relatively transparent to light and clear and are liquid at body or room temperature

g. Sources include such items as water, bouillon, clear broth, carbonated beverages, gelatin, hard candy, lemonade, popsicles, and regular or decaffeinated coffee or tea

h. The nurse should limit the amount of caffeine consumed by the client, because caffeine can cause an upset stomach and sleeplessness

i. Client may have salt or sugar

j. Dairy products and fruit juices with pulp are not clear liquids

⚠ Monitor the client's hydration status by checking intake and output, weight, monitoring for edema, and monitoring for signs of dehydration.

B. Full liquid diet

1. Indication: May be used as a transition diet after clear liquids after surgery or for clients who have difficulty chewing, swallowing, or tolerating solid foods

2. Nursing considerations

a. A full liquid diet is nutritionally deficient in energy (calories) and many **nutrients**

b. The diet includes both clear and opaque liquid foods and those that are liquid at body temperature

c. Sources include all clear liquids and such items as plain ice cream, sherbet, breakfast drinks, milk, pudding, custard, soups that are strained, and strained vegetable juices

⚠ Provide nutritional supplements such as those high in protein, as prescribed for the client on a liquid diet.

C. Mechanically altered diet

1. Indications

a. Provides foods that have been mechanically altered in texture to require minimal chewing

b. Used for clients who have difficulty chewing but who tolerate more variety in texture than a liquid diet offers

c. Used for clients who have dental problems, have undergone surgery of the head or neck, or have dysphagia (requires swallowing evaluation and may require thickened liquids)

2. Nursing considerations

a. Degree of texture modification depends on individual need, including puréed, mashed, ground, or chopped

b. Foods to be avoided in mechanically altered diets include nuts; dried fruit; raw fruits and vegetables; fried foods; chocolate candy; tough, smoked, or salted meats; and foods with coarse textures

D. Soft diet

1. Indications

a. Used for clients with difficulty chewing or swallowing

b. Used for clients with ulcerations of the mouth or gums, broken jaws, or dysphagia and for those who have experienced oral surgery, plastic surgery of the head or neck, or stroke

2. Nursing considerations

a. Clients with mouth sores should be served foods at cooler temperatures.

b. Clients who have difficulty chewing and swallowing because of the reduced flow of saliva can increase salivary flow by sucking on sour candy.

c. Encourage the client to eat a variety of foods.

d. Provide plenty of fluids with meals to make the chewing and swallowing of foods easier.

e. Drinking fluids through a straw may be easier than drinking from a cup or glass.

f. All foods and seasonings are permitted; however liquid, chopped, or puréed foods or regular foods with a soft consistency are tolerated best.

g. Avoid foods that contain nuts or seeds, which can easily become trapped in the mouth and cause discomfort.

h. Raw fruits and vegetables, fried foods, and whole grains are avoided.

⚠ Consider the client's disease or illness and how it may affect his or her nutritional status.

E. Low-residue, low-fiber diet

1. Indications

a. Supplies foods that are least likely to form an obstruction when the intestinal tract is narrowed by inflammation or scarring or when GI motility is slowed

b. Used for inflammatory bowel disease, partial obstructions of the intestinal tract, gastroenteritis, diarrhea, or other GI disorders

2. Nursing considerations

a. Foods high in carbohydrates are usually low in residue. They include white bread, cereals, and pasta.

b. Foods to be avoided are raw fruits (except bananas), nuts and seeds, plant fiber, some vegetables and some whole grains.

c. Dairy products are limited to two servings a day.

F. High-residue, high-fiber diet
1. Indications
   a. Used for clients with constipation; irritable bowel syndrome, when the primary symptom is alternating constipation and diarrhea; and asymptomatic diverticular disease
   b. Helps regulate blood glucose in clients with diabetes mellitus
   c. Helps control blood cholesterol in clients with heart disease
2. Nursing considerations
   a. Provides 20 to 25 g of dietary fiber daily
   b. Adds volume and weight to the stool and speeds the movement of undigested materials through the intestine
   c. Consists of fruits, vegetables, and whole-grain products
   d. Increase fiber gradually and provide adequate fluids to reduce possible undesirable side effects such as abdominal cramps, bloating, diarrhea, and dehydration
   e. Gas-forming foods should be limited (Box 12-4)

G. Cardiac diet (see Box 12-1 and Box 12-5)
1. Indications
   a. Indicated for atherosclerosis, diabetes mellitus, hyperlipidemia, hypertension, myocardial infarction, nephrotic syndrome, and renal failure
   b. Reduces the risk of heart disease

Box 12-4 Gas-Forming Foods

■ Apples	■ Figs
■ Artichokes	■ Honey
■ Barley	■ Melons
■ Beans	■ Milk
■ Bran	■ Molasses
■ Broccoli	■ Nuts
■ Brussels sprouts	■ Onions
■ Cabbage	■ Radishes
■ Celery	■ Soybeans
■ Cherries	■ Wheat
■ Coconuts	■ Yeast
■ Eggplant	

Box 12-5 Sodium-Free Spices and Flavorings

■ Allspice	■ Ginger
■ Almond extract	■ Lemon extract
■ Bay leaves	■ Maple extract
■ Caraway seeds	■ Marjoram
■ Cinnamon	■ Mustard powder
■ Curry powder	■ Nutmeg
■ Garlic and garlic powder	

---

2. Nursing considerations: Limit the total amount of fats (polyunsaturated fats, monounsaturated fats, saturated fats, and trans fats), cholesterol, and sodium.

H. Fat-restricted diet
1. Indications
   a. Used to reduce symptoms of abdominal pain, steatorrhea, flatulence, and diarrhea associated with high intakes of dietary fat, and to decrease nutrient losses caused by the ingestion of dietary fat in individuals with malabsorptive disorders
   b. Used for clients with malabsorption disorders, pancreatitis, gallbladder disease, and gastroesophageal reflux
2. Nursing considerations
   a. Restricts the total amount of fat, including saturated fats, trans fats, polyunsaturated fats, and monounsaturated fats
   b. Clients with malabsorption may also have difficulty tolerating fiber and lactose.
   c. Vitamin and mineral deficiencies may occur in clients with diarrhea or steatorrhea.
   d. A fecal-fat test indicates fat malabsorption with the excretion of more than 6 to 8 g fat (or more than 10% of the fat consumed) per day during the 3 days of specimen collection.

I. High-calorie, high-protein diet
1. Indications: Severe stress, burns, cancer, human immunodeficiency virus infection, acquired immunodeficiency syndrome, chronic obstructive pulmonary disease, respiratory failure, or any other type of debilitating disease
2. Nursing considerations
   a. Encourage nutrient-dense, high-calorie, high-protein foods such as whole milk and milk products, peanut butter, nuts, seeds, beef, chicken, fish, pork, and eggs.
   b. Some high-calorie foods include sugar, cream, gravy, oil, butter, mayonnaise, dried fruit, avocados, and honey.
   c. Encourage snacks between meals, such as milkshakes, instant breakfasts, and nutritional supplements.

▲ Calorie counts assist in determining the client's total nutritional intake and can identify a deficit or excess intake.

J. Carbohydrate-consistent diet
1. Indications: Diabetes mellitus, hypoglycemia, hyperglycemia, and obesity
2. Nursing considerations
   a. The Exchange System for Meal Planning, developed by the American Dietetic Association and the American Diabetes Association, is a food guide that may be recommended

b. The Exchange System groups foods according to the amounts of carbohydrates, fats, and proteins that they contain.

c. Major food groups include the carbohydrate group, the meat and meat substitute group, and the fat group.

d. The MyPlate diet may also be recommended.

K. Sodium-restricted diet

1. Indications: Hypertension, heart failure, renal disease, cardiac disease, and liver disease

2. Nursing considerations (see Box 12-5)

a. Individualized; can include 4 g of sodium daily (no-added-salt diet), 2 to 3 g of sodium daily (moderate restriction), 1 g of sodium daily (strict restriction), or 500 mg of sodium daily (severe and seldom prescribed)

b. Encourage the intake of fresh rather than processed foods, which contain higher amounts of sodium.

c. Canned, frozen, instant, smoked, pickled, and boxed items usually contain higher amounts of sodium. Lunch meats, soy sauce, salad dressings, fast foods, soups, and snacks such as potato chips and pretzels also contain large amounts of sodium.

d. Certain medications contain significant amounts of sodium.

e. Salt substitutes may be used to improve palatability. Most salt substitutes contain large amounts of potassium and should not be used by clients with renal disease.

L. Protein-restricted diet

1. Indications: Acute renal failure, chronic renal disease, cirrhosis of the liver, and hepatic coma

2. Nursing considerations

a. Provides enough protein to maintain nutritional status but not an amount that will allow the buildup of waste products from protein **metabolism** (40 to 60 g of protein daily)

b. The smaller the amount of protein allowed, the more important it becomes that all protein included in the diet be of high biological value (contain all essential amino acids in recommended proportions).

c. An adequate total energy intake from foods is critical for clients on protein-restricted diets. (Protein will be used for energy rather than for protein synthesis.)

d. Special low-protein products, such as pastas, bread, cookies, wafers, and gelatin made with wheat starch, can improve energy intake and add variety to the diet.

e. Carbohydrates in powdered or liquid form can also provide additional energy.

f. Vegetables and fruits contain some protein. For very low-protein diets, these foods must be calculated into the diet.

g. Foods from the milk, meat, bread, and starch groups are limited.

M. Renal diet (see Box 12-3)

1. Indications: Acute and chronic renal failure, and those clients requiring hemodialysis or peritoneal dialysis

2. Nursing considerations

a. Controlled amounts of protein, sodium, phosphorus, calcium, potassium, and fluids may be prescribed; may also require modifications of the amounts of fiber, cholesterol, and fat based on individual requirements

b. Most clients who are receiving dialysis need to restrict fluids (Box 12-6).

⚠ Initial data collection includes identifying food and medication interactions.

N. Potassium-modified diet (see Box 12-3)

1. Indications

a. A low-potassium diet is indicated for hyperkalemia, which may be the result of impaired renal function, hypoaldosteronism, Addison's disease, angiotensin-converting enzyme inhibitor medications, immunosuppressive medications, potassium-sparing diuretics, and chronic hyperkalemia

b. A high-potassium diet is indicated for hypokalemia, which may be the result of renal tubular acidosis, GI losses (diarrhea, vomiting), intracellular shifts, potassium-wasting diuretics, antibiotics, mineralocorticoid or glucocorticoid excess caused by primary or secondary aldosteronism, Cushing's syndrome, or exogenous steroid use.

2. Nursing considerations

a. Foods that are low in potassium include applesauce, green beans, cabbage, lettuce, peppers, grapes, blueberries, cooked summer squash, cooked turnip greens, fresh pineapple, and raspberries

b. Refer to Box 12-3 for foods that are high in potassium

O. High-calcium diet

1. Indications: Calcium is needed during bone growth and in adulthood to prevent osteoporosis and facilitate vascular contraction and vasodilation, muscle contraction, and nerve transmission

---

Box 12-6 Measures to Relieve Thirst

Chew gum or suck hard candy.
Freeze fluids so that they take longer to consume.
Add lemon juice to water to make it more refreshing.
Gargle with refrigerated mouthwash.

2. Nursing considerations
   a. Primary dietary sources of calcium are dairy products (see Box 12-3)
   b. Clients with lactose intolerance need to incorporate sources of calcium other than dairy products into their dietary patterns regularly
P. Low-purine diet
   1. Indications: Gout, kidney stones, and elevated uric acid levels
   2. Nursing considerations
      a. Purine is a precursor of uric acid, which forms stones and crystals
      b. Foods to restrict include anchovies, herring, mackerel, sardines, scallops, glandular meats, gravies, meat extracts, wild game, goose, and sweetbreads
Q. High-iron diet
   1. Indication: Anemia
   2. Nursing considerations
      a. The high-iron diet replaces an iron deficit caused by inadequate intake or loss
      b. The diet includes organ meats; meat; egg yolks; whole-wheat products; dark green, leafy vegetables; dried fruit; and legumes (see Box 12-3)
R. Miscellaneous diets: See Chapter 9 (Boxes 9-3, 9-4, 9-5, 9-6, and 9-7) for foods high in potassium, sodium, calcium, magnesium, and phosphorus

IV. VEGETARIAN DIETS

A. Types (Box 12-7)
B. Nursing considerations
   1. Ensure that the client eats a sufficient amount of varied foods to meet normal nutrient and energy needs.
   2. Reinforce to clients about consuming complementary proteins over the course of each day to ensure that all EAAs are provided.

3. Potential deficiencies in vegetarian diets include protein, vitamin B_{12}, zinc, iron, calcium, omega-3 fatty acids, and vitamin D (if limited exposure to sunlight).
4. To enhance the **absorption** of iron, vegetarians should include a good source of iron and vitamin C with each meal.
5. Foods commonly eaten include tofu, tempeh, soy milk and soy products, meat analogues, legumes, nuts, seeds, sprouts, and a variety of fruits and vegetables.
6. Soy protein is considered equivalent in quality to animal proteins.

⚠ Body mass index (BMI) can be calculated by dividing the client's weight in kilograms by height in meters squared. For example, a client who weighs 75 kg (165 pounds) and is 1.8 m^2 (5 feet 9 inches tall) has a BMI of 23.15 (75 divided by 1.8 m^2 [3.24] = 23.15).

V. ENTERAL NUTRITION

A. Description: Provides liquefied foods to the GI tract via a tube
B. Indications
   1. When the GI tract is functional but oral intake is not meeting estimated nutrient needs
   2. Used for clients with swallowing problems, burns, major trauma, liver or other organ failure, or severe **malnutrition**
C. Nursing considerations
   1. Clients with lactose intolerance (diarrhea, bloating, cramping) need to be placed on lactose-free formulas
   2. See Chapter 19 for information about the administration of GI tube feedings
D. Complications of **enteral nutrition** (Box 12-8)

Box 12-7 Types of Semi-Vegetarian and Vegetarian Diets

Pescatarian
Abstains from eating all meat and animal flesh with the exception of fish.

Flexitarian/Semi-Vegetarian
Consumes mostly a vegetarian diet, but occasionally eats meat.

Vegetarian (Lacto/Ovo-Vegetarian)
Does not consume beef, pork, poultry, fish, shellfish or animal flesh of any kind, but does eat eggs and dairy products.
■ A lacto-vegetarian does not eat eggs, but does eat dairy products.
■ An ovo-vegetarian does not eat meat or dairy products, but does eat eggs.

Vegan
Does not consume meat of any kind and also does not eat eggs, dairy products, or processed foods containing these or other animal-derived ingredients such as gelatin.

Raw Vegan/Raw Food Diet
Consumes unprocessed vegan foods that have not been heated above 115° F (46° C).

Macrobiotic
Consumes unprocessed vegan foods, such as whole grains and fruits and vegetables, and occasionally consumes fish; also consumes Asian vegetables, such as daikon, and sea vegetables, such as seaweed.

VI. PARENTERAL NUTRITION (PN)

A. Description
1. Supplies necessary **nutrients** via the veins.
2. Supplies carbohydrates in the form of dextrose; fats in a special emulsified form; proteins in the form of amino acids; vitamins; minerals; electrolytes; and water
3. Prevents subcutaneous fat and muscle protein from being catabolized by the body for energy

B. Indications
1. Clients with severely dysfunctional or nonfunctional GI tracts who are unable to process **nutrients** may benefit from **PN.**
2. Clients who can take some oral nutrition (but not enough to meet their nutrient requirements) may benefit from **PN.**
3. Clients with multiple GI surgeries, GI trauma, severe intolerance to enteral feedings, or intestinal obstructions or those who need to rest the bowel for healing may benefit from **PN.**
4. Clients with acquired immunodeficiency syndrome, cancer, burn injuries, or **malnutrition** or those who have received chemotherapy may benefit from **PN.**
5. **PN** is the least desirable form of nutrition. It is used when there is no other alternative.

C. Administration of **PN**
1. Central vein
   a. **PN** is administered through a central vein when the client requires larger concentrations of carbohydrates (>10% glucose concentration).
   b. The subclavian or internal jugular vein is used when **PN** is a short-term intervention (less than 4 weeks).
   c. When **PN** is anticipated for an extended period (longer than 4 weeks), a more permanent catheter (e.g., a peripherally inserted central catheter [PICC] line), a tunneled catheter, or an implanted vascular access device is used.
2. Peripheral vein
   a. **PN** can be administered through a peripheral vein, typically in the arm, via a PICC line.
   b. **PN** administered through a peripheral vein delivers isotonic or mildly hypertonic solutions.

⚠ The delivery of hypertonic solutions into peripheral veins can cause sclerosis, phlebitis, or swelling. Monitor closely for these complications.

D. Fat emulsion (lipids)
1. **Lipids** provide nonprotein calories and prevent or correct fatty-acid deficiency.
2. Lipid solutions are isotonic and therefore can be administered through a peripheral or central vein.
3. Most **fat emulsions** are prepared from soybean or safflower oil with egg yolk to provide emulsification. The primary components are linoleic, oleic, palmitic, linolenic, and stearic acids.
4. **Lipids** contain egg yolk phospholipids and should not be given to clients with egg allergies.
5. Glucose-intolerant clients or those with diabetes mellitus may benefit from receiving a larger percentage of their **PN** from **lipids**. This can help control blood glucose levels and lower insulin requirements as a result of decreased infused dextrose.
6. The bottle is examined for the separation of the emulsion into layers, fat globules, and the accumulation of froth. If observed, do not use the solution and return it to the pharmacy.
7. Additives should not be put into the **fat emulsion** solution.
8. The solution is infused initially at 1 mL/minute. Monitor the vital signs every 10 minutes, and observe for adverse reactions for the first 30 minutes. If signs of an adverse reaction occur, stop the infusion and notify the registered nurse (Box 12-9).
9. If no adverse reaction occurs, the flow rate is adjusted to the prescribed rate.
10. Serum **lipids** are checked 4 hours after discontinuing the infusion.

Box 12-8 Complications of Enteral Feeding

- Aspiration
- Diarrhea
- Displacement of tube
- Nasal and mouth mucosal damage
- Obstruction of tube
- Refeeding syndrome

Box 12-9 Signs of an Adverse Reaction to Lipids

- Chest and back pain
- Chills
- Cyanosis
- Diaphoresis
- Dyspnea
- Fever
- Flushing
- Headache
- Nausea and vomiting
- Pressure over the eyes
- Rash
- Thrombophlebitis
- Vertigo

⚠ Fat emulsions (lipids) contain egg yolk phospholipids and should not be given to clients with egg allergies.

E. Additional additives to **PN** solutions
1. Vitamins are usually added to meet needs and prevent deficiencies.
2. Minerals and trace elements may be added to promote normal metabolism.
3. Electrolytes may be added to correct losses related to organ dysfunction and disease processes.
4. Water amounts in **PN** are determined by electrolyte balance and fluid requirements.
5. Insulin may be added to control blood glucose level because of the high concentration of glucose in the **PN** solution.
6. Heparin may be added to reduce the build-up of fibrinous clot at the tip of centrally inserted catheters.

VII. COMPLICATIONS OF PARENTERAL NUTRITION (Table 12-1)

VIII. NURSING CONSIDERATIONS

A. Always check the **PN** solution with the health care provider's (HCP's) prescription to ensure that the prescribed components are contained in the solution.

B. To prevent infection and solution incompatibility, intravenous medications and blood are not given through the **PN** line.
C. Monitor electrolytes, albumin, and liver and renal function studies.
D. In severely dehydrated clients, the albumin level may drop initially as the treatment restores hydration.
E. With severely malnourished clients, monitor for "refeeding syndrome" (i.e., a rapid drop in the potassium, magnesium, and phosphate serum levels).
F. Abnormal liver function values may indicate intolerance to or an excess of **fat emulsion** or problems with the **metabolism** of glucose and protein.
G. Abnormal renal function tests may indicate an excess of amino acids.
H. **PN** solutions should be refrigerated and administered within 24 hours from the time that they were prepared (remove from the refrigerator 0.5 to 1 hour before use).
I. **PN** solutions that are cloudy or darkened should not be used and should be returned to the pharmacy.
J. Additions to **PN** solutions should be made in the pharmacy and not in the nursing unit.

TABLE 12-1 Complications of Parenteral Nutrition

Complication	Possible Cause	Signs/Symptoms	Intervention	Prevention
Air embolism	• Catheter system is opened or IV tubing is disconnected • Air entry occurs on IV tubing changes	• Apprehension • Chest pain • Dyspnea • Hypotension • Loud churning sound heard over the pericardium on auscultation • Rapid and weak pulse • Respiratory distress	• Clamp the catheter • Place the client in a left-side-lying position with the head lower than the feet • Notify the HCP • Administer oxygen	• Make sure all catheter connections are secure • Clamp the catheter when not in use • Instruct the client in Valsalva's maneuver for tubing and cap changes • For tubing and cap changes, place the client in Trendelenburg's position (if not contraindicated) with the head turned in the opposite direction of the insertion site
Hyperglycemia	• Client is receiving solution too quickly • Not enough insulin • Infection	• Coma (when severe) • Confusion • Diaphoresis • Elevated blood glucose level (>200 mg/dL) • Excessive thirst • Fatigue • Kussmaul's respirations • Restlessness • Weakness	• Notify the HCP • May need to slow the infusion rate • Administer regular insulin as prescribed • Monitor blood glucose levels	• Assess the client for a history of glucose intolerance • Assess the client's medication history • Begin infusion at a slow rate as prescribed • Monitor blood glucose levels • Use strict aseptic technique

K. Discontinuing **PN** therapy

1. The flow rate is gradually decreased for 1 to 2 hours while increasing oral intake. (This assists with the prevention of hypoglycemia.)
2. After catheter removal, change the dressing daily until the wound heals.
3. Encourage oral nourishment.

4. Record oral intake, body weight, and laboratory results of serum electrolyte and glucose levels.

IX. HOME CARE INSTRUCTIONS (Box 12-10)

TABLE 12-1 Complications of Parenteral Nutrition—cont'd

Complication	Possible Cause	Signs/Symptoms	Intervention	Prevention
Hypervolemia	• Excessive fluid administration or administration of fluid too rapidly • Renal dysfunction • Heart failure • Hepatic failure	• Bounding pulse • Crackles on lung auscultation • Headache • Increased blood pressure • Jugular vein distention • Weight gain greater than desired	• Slow or stop the IV infusion • Restrict fluids • Diuretics • Use dialysis (in extreme cases)	• Assess the client's history for risk for hypervolemia • Administer solution via an electronic infusion device • Monitor intake and output • Monitor weight daily
Hypoglycemia	• PN abruptly discontinued • Too much insulin is being administered	• Anxiety • Diaphoresis • Hunger • Low blood glucose level (<70 mg/dL) • Shakiness • Weakness	• Administer IV dextrose • Monitor blood glucose levels	• Gradually decrease PN solution when discontinuing it • Infuse 10% dextrose at the same rate as the PN to prevent hypoglycemia when the PN solution is discontinued • Monitor glucose levels when insulin is being given
Infection	• Poor aseptic technique • Catheter contamination • Contamination of solution	• Chills • Fever • Elevated white blood cell count • Erythema or drainage at the insertion site	• Notify the HCP • Assist the HCP with removal of catheter • Send the catheter tip to the laboratory for culture • Prepare to obtain blood cultures • Prepare for antibiotic administration	• Use strict aseptic technique • Monitor temperature • Assess the IV site for signs of infection • Change site dressing, solution, and tubing as specified by agency policy • Do not disconnect tubing unnecessarily
Pneumothorax	• Inexact catheter placement	• Absence of breath sounds on affected side • Chest or shoulder pain • Sudden shortness of breath • Tachycardia • Cyanosis	• Small pneumothorax may resolve • Larger pneumothorax may require chest tube	• Monitor for signs of pneumothorax • Obtain a chest x-ray after the insertion of the catheter to ensure proper placement • PN is not initiated until correct catheter placement is verified and the absence of pneumothorax is confirmed

HCP, Health care provider, *IV*, intravenous; *PN*, parenteral nutrition.
Adapted from Ignatavicius, D., & Workman, M. (2010). *Medical-surgical nursing: Patient-centered collaborative care* (6th ed.). St. Louis: Saunders.

Box 12-10 Home-Care Instructions

Reinforce to the client and caregiver how to administer and maintain parenteral nutrition fluids.

Reinforce to the client and the caregiver how to change a sterile dressing.

Obtain a daily weight at the same time of day in the same clothes.

Stress that weight gain of more than 3 lb/week may indicate excessive fluid intake and should be reported.

Monitor the blood glucose level, and report abnormalities immediately.

Check for signs and symptoms of infection, thrombosis, air embolism, and catheter displacement.

Reinforce to the client and caregiver about the importance of reporting signs and symptoms of complications.

With regard to symptoms of thrombosis, the client should report edema of the arm or at the catheter insertion site, neck pain, and jugular vein distention.

The leakage of fluid from the insertion site or pain or discomfort as the fluids are infused may indicate the displacement of the catheter. This must be reported immediately.

Reinforce to the client and caregiver about the importance of follow-up care.

MORE QUESTIONS ON EVOLVE!

Practice Questions

71. A client is having problems with blood clotting. Which food item would the nurse encourage the client to eat?
1. Legumes
2. Citrus fruits
3. Vegetable oils
4. Green, leafy vegetables

72. A client has acute diverticulitis. Which principle should the nurse keep in mind while planning care for this client?
1. Avoid high-fiber foods.
2. Use a fluid-restricted diet.
3. Increase seed and nut intake.
4. Increase raw fruits and vegetables.

73. A client is a lacto vegetarian. Which food item would the nurse remove from the tray?
1. Eggs
2. Milk
3. Cheese
4. Broccoli

74. A low-sodium diet has been prescribed for a client with hypertension. Which of the following foods, if selected from the menu by the client, would indicate an understanding of this diet?
1. Baked turkey
2. Tomato soup

3. Boiled shrimp
4. Chicken gumbo

75. A nurse is providing dietary instructions to a client with gout. The nurse tells the client to avoid which food item?
1. Scallops
2. Chocolate
3. Corn bread
4. Macaroni products

76. A clear liquid diet has been prescribed for a client with gastroenteritis. Which item would be the most appropriate to offer to the client?
1. Soft custard
2. Orange juice
3. Fat-free broth
4. Strained soup

77. A client with heart disease is instructed regarding a low-fat diet. The nurse determines that the client understands the diet if the client states that a food item to avoid is:
1. Apples
2. Cheese
3. Oranges
4. Skim milk

78. A nurse instructs a client to increase the amount of riboflavin in the diet. The nurse tells the client to select which food item that is high in riboflavin?
1. Milk
2. Tomatoes
3. Citrus fruits
4. Green, leafy vegetables

79. A client with a burn injury is transferred to the nursing unit, and a regular diet has been prescribed. The nurse encourages the client to eat which dietary items to promote wound healing?
1. Veal, potatoes, gelatin, and orange juice
2. Chicken breast, broccoli, strawberries, and milk
3. Peanut butter and jelly sandwich, cantaloupe, and tea
4. Spaghetti with tomato sauce, garlic bread, and ginger ale

80. A nurse has completed diet teaching for a client who has been prescribed a low-sodium diet to treat hypertension. The nurse determines that further teaching is necessary when the client makes which of these statements?
1. "This diet will help lower my blood pressure."
2. "Fresh foods such as fruits and vegetables are high in sodium."
3. "This diet is not a replacement for my antihypertensive medications."
4. "The reason I need to lower my salt intake is to reduce fluid retention."

ANSWERS

71. 4

Rationale: Green, leafy vegetables are high in vitamin K, which acts as a catalyst for facilitating blood-clotting factors. Legumes are high in folic acid and thiamine. Citrus fruits are high in vitamin C, which helps with wound healing. Vegetable oil is high in vitamin E, which acts as an antioxidant.

Test-Taking Strategy: First, focus on the client's problem, and recall that vitamin K is involved in the clotting process. Next, determine the food sources that are high in vitamin K. Review the functions of vitamin K and the foods that are high in vitamin K if you had difficulty with this question.

Level of Cognitive Ability: Applying
Client Needs: Physiological Integrity
Integrated Process: Teaching and Learning
Content Area: Fundamental Skills: Nutrition
References: deWit, p. 747. 2009.
Schlenker, Roth, pp. 108, 110. 2011.

72. 1

Rationale: Diet therapy for acute diverticulitis involves allowing the bowel to rest by avoiding high-fiber foods. Fluids are encouraged rather than restricted. Seeds and nuts are to be avoided so that they do not become trapped in the diverticula and cause irritation. Raw fruits and vegetables are high in fiber.

Test-Taking Strategy: Use the process of elimination, and focus on the client's diagnosis of acute diverticulitis. Recalling foods that are allowed and not allowed when a client has diverticulitis and that high-fiber foods are avoided during the acute phase will direct you to option 1. Review diet therapy for acute diverticulitis if you had difficulty with this question.

Level of Cognitive Ability: Understanding
Client Needs: Physiological Integrity
Integrated Process: Nursing Process/Planning
Content Area: Fundamental Skills: Nutrition
References: deWit, pp. 714–715. 2009.
Schlenker, Roth, p. 463. 2011.

73. 1

Rationale: Eggs are not consumed by lacto vegetarians. Other dairy and plant products are eaten by lacto vegetarians.

Test-Taking Strategy: Note the words "remove from the tray." This indicates that the food item in question is not appropriate for a lacto vegetarian. Of the options listed, eggs are the food items that are not consumed by lacto vegetarians; however, they are eaten by lacto-ovo vegetarians. Review vegetarian diets if you had difficulty with this question.

Level of Cognitive Ability: Applying
Client Needs: Physiological Integrity
Integrated Process: Nursing Process/Implementation
Content Area: Fundamental Skills: Nutrition
References: Nix, pp. 51–52. 2009.
Peckenpaugh, p. 11. 2010.

74. 1

Rationale: Regular soup (1 cup) contains 900 mg of sodium. Fresh shellfish (1 oz) contains 50 mg of sodium. Poultry (1 oz) contains 25 mg of sodium.

Test-Taking Strategy: Use the process of elimination. Eliminate options 2 and 4 first, because they are comparable or alike. Also, recall that canned foods are high in sodium. From the remaining options, select option 1, remembering that shellfish is also high in sodium, even if it is boiled. Review the foods that are high in sodium if you had difficulty with this question.

Level of Cognitive Ability: Evaluating
Client Needs: Physiological Integrity
Integrated Process: Nursing Process/Evaluation
Content Area: Fundamental Skills: Nutrition
References: deWit, pp. 48, 440–441. 2009.
Schlenker, Roth, pp. 144–145. 2011.

75. 1

Rationale: Scallops should be omitted from the diet of a client who has gout because of the high purine content. The food items identified in options 2, 3, and 4 have negligible purine content and may be consumed by the client with gout.

Test-Taking Strategy: Use the process of elimination and note the strategic word "avoid." Focus on the client's diagnosis of gout. Recalling the food items that are high in purine will direct you to option 1. Review the foods that are high in purine if you had difficulty with this question.

Level of Cognitive Ability: Applying
Client Needs: Physiological Integrity
Integrated Process: Teaching and Learning
Content Area: Fundamental Skills: Nutrition
Reference: Linton, pp. 952–953. 2012.

76. 3

Rationale: A clear liquid diet consists of foods that are relatively transparent. The food items in options 1, 2, and 4 would be included in a full liquid diet.

Test-Taking Strategy: Remember that a clear liquid diet consists of foods that are relatively transparent. By the process of elimination, you should easily select option 3, because this is the only food item that is transparent. Review the food items that are allowed on clear liquid and full liquid diets if you had difficulty with this question.

Level of Cognitive Ability: Applying
Client Needs: Physiological Integrity
Integrated Process: Nursing Process/Implementation
Content Area: Fundamental Skills: Nutrition
References: Nix, p. 330. 2009.
Schlenker, Roth, p. 376. 2011.

77. 2

Rationale: Fruits, vegetables, and skim milk contain minimal amounts of fat. Cheese is high in fat.

Test-Taking Strategy: Use the process of elimination and your knowledge regarding the fat content of fruit to eliminate options 1 and 3. Recalling that cheese is high in fat will direct you to option 2. Review the foods that are high in fat if you had difficulty with this question.

Level of Cognitive Ability: Evaluating
Client Needs: Physiological Integrity
Integrated Process: Nursing Process/Evaluation
Content Area: Fundamental Skills: Nutrition
References: deWit, p. 491. 2009.
Nix, p. 38. 2009.

78. 1

Rationale: Food sources of riboflavin include milk, lean meats, fish, and grains. Tomatoes and citrus fruits are high in vitamin C. Green leafy vegetables are high in folic acid.

Test-Taking Strategy: Knowledge regarding food items that are high in riboflavin is required to answer this question. Remember that milk is a food source of riboflavin. Review the foods that contain riboflavin if you had difficulty with this question.

Level of Cognitive Ability: Applying
Client Needs: Physiological Integrity
Integrated Process: Teaching and Learning
Content Area: Fundamental Skills: Nutrition
Reference: Schlenker, Roth, p. 116. 2011.

79. 2

Rationale: Protein and vitamin C are necessary for wound healing. Poultry and milk are good sources of protein. Broccoli and strawberries are good sources of vitamin C. Peanut butter is a source of niacin. Gelatin and jelly have no nutrient value. Spaghetti is a complex carbohydrate.

Test-Taking Strategy: Focus on the subject of promoting wound healing, and recall that protein and vitamin C are necessary for wound healing. Eliminate options 1 and 3 first, because gelatin and jelly have no nutrient value related to healing. From the remaining options, select option 2 over option 4 because of the greater nutrient value of the foods listed in option 2. Review the foods that are high in protein and vitamin C if you had difficulty with this question.

Level of Cognitive Ability: Applying
Client Needs: Physiological Integrity
Integrated Process: Nursing Process/Implementation
Content Area: Fundamental Skills: Nutrition
References: deWit, p. 100. 2009.
Nix, pp. 436–437. 2009.

80. 2

Rationale: A low-sodium diet is used as an adjunct to antihypertensive medications for the treatment of hypertension. Sodium retains fluid, which leads to hypertension secondary to increased fluid volume. Fresh foods such as fruits and vegetables are low in sodium.

Test-Taking Strategy: Use the process of elimination, and note the strategic words "further teaching is necessary." These words indicate a negative event query and ask you to select an option that is an incorrect statement. Eliminate options 1, 3, and 4, because these are accurate statements related to hypertension. In addition, remember that fresh foods are low in sodium. Review the purpose of a low-sodium diet if you had difficulty with this question.

Level of Cognitive Ability: Evaluating
Client Needs: Physiological Integrity
Integrated Process: Teaching and Learning
Content Area: Fundamental Skills: Nutrition
References: Linton, p. 686. 2012.
Peckenpaugh, pp. 113, 282. 2010.

Intravenous Therapy and Blood Administration

PYRAMID TERMS

ABO A type of antigen system. The ABO type of the donor should be compatible with the recipient's.

air embolism Caused by a bolus of air that enters the vein through an inadequately primed intravenous line from a loose connection, during a tubing change or the removal of the intravenous catheter.

compatibility Matching of blood from two persons by two different types of antigen systems, ABO and Rh, present on the membrane surface of the red blood cells, to prevent a transfusion reaction (Table 13-1).

crossmatching The testing of the donor's blood and the recipient's blood for compatibility.

fluid (circulatory) overload A complication that results from the infusion of blood at a rate that is too rapid for the body size, cardiac status, or clinical condition of the recipient.

infiltration Seepage of intravenous fluid out of the vein and into the surrounding interstitial spaces.

phlebitis An inflammation of the vein that can occur from either mechanical or chemical (medication) trauma or from a local infection.

Rh factor Rh stands for Rhesus factor. The presence or absence of Rh antigens on the surface of the red blood cells (RBCs) determines the classification as Rh positive or Rh negative. A person who has the factor is Rh positive; a person who lacks the factor is Rh negative.

transfusion reaction A hemolytic transfusion reaction caused by blood type or Rh factor incompatibility. An allergic transfusion reaction is most often seen among clients with a history of allergy. A febrile transfusion reaction most commonly occurs among clients with antibodies directed against the transfused white blood cells. A bacterial transfusion reaction occurs after the transfusion of contaminated blood products

PYRAMID TO SUCCESS

The nurse is responsible for monitoring clients who are receiving parenteral therapies. The pyramid points focus on safety related to monitoring an infusion rate and monitoring for complications related to the intravenous (IV) line. Focus on the signs and symptoms of infiltration, phlebitis, circulatory overload, and air embolism and the treatment measures associated with each. The pyramid points also focus on safety related to monitoring a client who is receiving a blood transfusion and monitoring for complications related to the transfusion. Focus on the signs and symptoms of a transfusion reaction and the immediate interventions that should be employed if a transfusion reaction occurs. The documentation of the expected and unexpected effects of the therapy is also a pyramid point.

CLIENT NEEDS

Safe and Effective Care Environment

- Establishing priorities
- Handling hazardous or infectious materials
- Implementing standard, transmission-based, and surgical asepsis during handling of equipment and supplies
- Monitoring the client during the IV infusion
- Obtaining informed consent for therapy
- Preventing errors in the monitoring of IV lines and electronic IV infusion devices
- Providing continuity of care

Health Promotion and Maintenance

- Considering lifestyle choices related to the transfusion
- Implementing techniques for the collection of physical data
- Reinforcing teaching about the signs of a transfusion reaction
- Considering lifestyle choices related to home care of an intravenous (IV) line
- Reinforcing teaching to the client and family about at home care of the IV line

Psychosocial Integrity

- Considering religious, spiritual, and cultural matters related to blood administration
- Communicating regarding the procedure for IV infusion and blood administration

TABLE 13-1 Compatibility Chart for Red Blood Cell Transfusions

	Recipient			
Donor	A	B	AB	O
A	X		X	
B		X	X	
AB			X	
O	X	X	X	X

From Ignatavicius, D., & Workman, M. (2010). *Medical-surgical nursing: Patient-centered collaborative care* (6th ed.). St. Louis: Saunders.

■ Identifying coping mechanisms of the client and support systems in the home for caring for an IV line

Physiological Integrity

■ Ensuring the safe administration of the IV infusion and blood transfusion
■ Monitoring for complications of IV therapy and blood administration
■ Monitoring for expected effects of IV therapy and blood administration
■ Monitoring IV infusion sites and rates
■ Monitoring laboratory values related to IV therapy and blood administration
■ Documenting the client's response to treatment

I. INTRAVENOUS THERAPY (see Chapter 9 and Table 9-1)

A. Used to sustain clients who are unable to take substances orally
B. Replaces water, electrolytes, and nutrients more rapidly than oral administration
C. Provides immediate access to the vascular system for the rapid delivery of specific solutions without the time required for gastrointestinal tract absorption
D. Provides a vascular route for the administration of medication or blood components

II. INTRAVENOUS DEVICES

A. IV cannulas
  1. Steel needles or butterfly sets
    a. Wing-tipped needle with a metal cannula and plastic wings; the needle is 0.5 to 1.5 inches in length with needle gauge sizes from 16 to 26
    b. **Infiltration** is more common with these devices as a result of their stiffness.
    c. May commonly be used with children and older clients, whose veins are likely to be small or fragile. An armboard may be needed for a short infusion.

  2. Plastic cannulas
    a. Used primarily for short-term therapy, especially if rapid infusion is necessary; more comfortable for the client
    b. Can cause a catheter embolism if the tip of the cannula breaks
B. IV gauges
  1. The gauge refers to the diameter of the lumen of the needle or cannula.
  2. The smaller the gauge number, the larger the outside diameter of the cannula.
  3. The gauge size used depends on the solution to be administered and the diameter of the available vein.
  4. For rapid emergency fluid administration, blood products, or anesthetics, a large needle (e.g., 14-, 16-, 18-, or 19-gauge) is used.
  5. For standard IV fluid infusion, a 20- or 22-gauge needle is used.
  6. If the client has very small veins, a 24- to 25-gauge needle is used.
C. IV containers
  1. May be glass or plastic
  2. Squeeze the plastic bag to ensure that it is intact. Check the glass bottle for any punctures or cracks.
  3. The expiration date of IV fluid and all supplies should be checked.

⚠ Do not write on a plastic IV bag with a marking pen because the ink may be absorbed through the plastic into the solution. Use a label and a ballpoint pen for marking the bag, placing the label onto the bag.

D. IV tubing (Figure 13-1)
  1. Contains a spike end for the bag or bottle, a drip chamber, a roller clamp, a Y site, and an adapter end for attachment to the cannula or needle that is inserted into the client's vein
  2. Shorter secondary tubing is used for piggyback solutions, connecting them to the injection sites nearest to the drip chamber (Figure 13-2).
  3. Special tubing is used for medication that absorbs into plastic. (Check specific medication administration guidelines.)
  4. Vented and nonvented tubing are available.
    a. A vent allows air to enter the IV container as the fluid leaves.
    b. A vented adapter can be used to add a vent to a nonvented IV tubing system.
    c. Use nonvented tubing for flexible containers.
    d. Use vented tubing for glass or rigid plastic containers to allow air to enter and displace the fluid as it leaves. Fluid will not flow from a rigid IV container unless it is vented.

▲ **FIGURE 13-1** Intravenous tubing. (From Kee, J., & Marshall, S. [2009]. *Clinical calculations: With applications to general and specialty areas* [6th ed.]. Philadelphia: Saunders.)

 Extension tubing can be added to an IV tubing set to provide extra length to the tubing. Add extension tubing to the IV tubing set for children, clients who are restless, or clients who have special mobility needs.

E. Drip chambers (Figure 13-3)
   1. Microdrip chamber
      a. Normally has a short, vertical, metal piece where the drop forms
      b. Delivers about 60 gtt/mL
      c. Read the tubing package to determine how many drops per milliliter are delivered (drop factor).
      d. Used if fluid will be infused at a slow rate (less than 50 mL/hour), if the solution contains medication that needs to be titrated, and in the pediatric, older adult, and fluid-restricted client
   2. Macrodrip chamber
      a. Used if the solution is thick or needs to infuse rapidly
      b. Drop factor varies from 10 to 20 gtt/mL depending on the manufacturer
      c. Read the tubing package to determine how many drops per milliliter are delivered (drop factor).

F. Filters: May be used in IV lines to trap small particles and provide protection by preventing particles from entering the client's veins

G. Needleless systems: Include recessed needles, plastic cannulas, or one-way valves that decrease exposure to contaminated needles

H. Intermittent infusion sets: Used when intravascular accessibility is desired for the intermittent administration of medications or solutions
   1. Require periodic flushing as well as before and after medication administration.
   2. Normal saline is typically used to flush intermittent infusion sets. Hospital policy should be reviewed regarding amount of flush solution to instill.

I. Electronic infusion devices: Control the amount of fluid or medication infusing (for example, patient-controlled analgesia [PCA]).

 Check electronic IV infusion devices frequently. Although these devices are electronic, this does not ensure that they are infusing solutions and medications accurately.

III. LATEX ALLERGY

A. Ask the client about an allergy to latex.

B. IV supplies that may contain latex include IV catheters, IV tubing, IV ports (particularly IV rubber

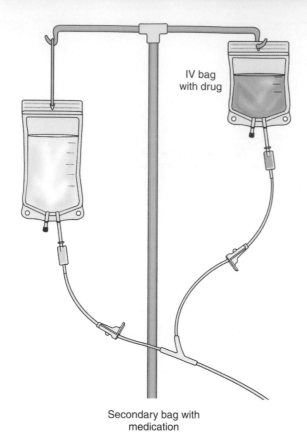

▲ FIGURE 13-2 Secondary bag with medication. (From Kee, J., & Marshall, S. [2009]. *Clinical calculations: With applications to general and specialty areas* [6th ed.]. Philadelphia: Saunders.)

Secondary bag with
medication

Macrodrip
10–20 gtt/ml

Microdrip
60 gtt/ml

▲ FIGURE 13-3 Macrodrip and microdrip sets. (From Kee, J., & Marshall, S. [2009]. *Clinical calculations: With applications to general and specialty areas* [6th ed.]. Philadelphia: Saunders.)

injection ports), rubber stoppers on multidose vials, and adhesive tape. Manufacturers typically label packaging when the item is latex-free.
C. Latex-safe IV supplies need to be used for clients with latex allergy.
D. Refer to Chapter 61 for additional information about latex allergy.

Box 13-1 Peripheral Intravenous Sites to Avoid

- Edematous extremity
- The lower extremities
- An arm that is weak, traumatized, or paralyzed
- The arm on the same side as a mastectomy
- An arm that has an arteriovenous fistula or a shunt for dialysis
- A skin area that is infected

IV. PERIPHERAL IV SITES

A. The most frequently used sites are the veins of the forearm, because the bones of the forearm act as a natural support and splint.
B. Veins in the lower extremities are not suitable because of the risk of thrombus formation and possible pooling in areas of decreased venous return (Box 13-1).
C. Veins in the scalp and feet may be suitable sites for infants.
D. Bending the elbow on the arm with an IV may easily obstruct the flow of the solution, thereby causing **infiltration**.
E. Avoid checking the blood pressure on the arm receiving the IV infusion.
F. Do not place restraints over the venipuncture site.
G. An armboard may be prescribed when the venipuncture site is located in an area of flexion.

V. ADMINISTERING IV SOLUTIONS

A. The IV solution should be checked against the health care provider's (HCP's) prescriptions for the type, amount, percentage of solution, and rate of flow.
B. Wash hands thoroughly and use sterile technique when working with an IV.
C. When preparing a new solution for administration, clamp the tubing, attach the spike end of the tubing to the IV bag, and then prime the tubing to remove air from the tubing and IV system.
D. Change the IV tubing according to agency policy.
E. Do not let an IV bag or bottle hang for more than 24 hours.
F. Do not allow the IV tubing to touch the floor.
G. Change the IV dressing as specified by agency policy or when the dressing is wet or contaminated.
H. Label the tubing, dressing, and solution bags clearly, including the date and time when changed.

VI. PRECAUTIONS

A. On insertion, can cause initial pain and discomfort for the client
B. An IV puncture provides a route of entry for microorganisms into the body.

C. Fluid (circulatory) overload or electrolyte imbalances can occur from an excessive or too-rapid infusion of fluids. An IV infusion should be checked at least once per hour in an adult client.

D. Incompatibilities between certain solutions can occur.

⚠️ A client with congestive heart failure usually is not given a solution containing saline because this type of fluid promotes the retention of water and would therefore exacerbate heart failure by increasing the fluid overload.

⚠️ A client with diabetes mellitus usually does not receive dextrose (glucose) solutions because the solution can increase the blood glucose level.

VII. COMPLICATIONS (Table 13-2)

A. Infection
   1. Description
      a. The entry of microorganisms into the body through the venipuncture site
      b. Venipuncture interrupts the integrity of the skin, which is the first line of defense against infection.
      c. The longer the therapy continues, the greater the risk of infection.
      d. Infection can occur locally at the IV insertion site or systemically from the entry of microorganisms into the body.
   2. At-risk clients
      a. Clients who are immunocompromised as a result of diseases such as cancer or acquired immunodeficiency syndrome
      b. Clients receiving treatments such as chemotherapy who have an altered or lowered white blood cell count
      c. Older clients, because aging alters the effectiveness of the immune system
      d. Clients with diabetes mellitus
   3. Prevention and interventions
      a. Maintain strict asepsis when caring for the IV site.
      b. Monitor the vital signs, particularly the temperature.
      c. Monitor for local inflammation at the IV site.
      d. Check fluid containers for cracks, leaks, cloudiness, or other evidence of contamination.
      e. Change the tubing and site dressing according to agency policy.
      f. Antimicrobial solution is used to clean the IV site.
      g. Ensure that the IV solution is not hanging for more than 24 hours.
      h. Monitor for systemic infection. This includes malaise, headache, chills, fever, nausea, vomiting, backache, and tachycardia.

TABLE 13-2 Signs of Complications of Intravenous Therapy

Complication	Signs
Infection	Elevated temperature, chills, and fever Redness, warmth, edema, and pain at the insertion site Elevated white blood cell count
Infiltration	Edema, pain, and coolness at site May or may not have a blood return
Phlebitis	Heat, redness, and tenderness at site Not swollen or hard Sluggish IV infusion
Thrombophlebitis	Hard, cord-like vein Heat, redness, and tenderness at site Sluggish IV infusion
Catheter embolism	Decrease in BP Pain along vein Weak, rapid pulse Cyanosis of nail beds Loss of consciousness
Fluid (circulatory) overload	Increased BP Rapid breathing Dyspnea Moist cough and crackles
Air embolism	Tachycardia Chest pain and dyspnea Cyanosis Hypotension Decreased level of consciousness
Electrolyte overload	Clinical manifestations will be specific to the elevated electrolyte

BP, Blood pressure; *IV*, intravenous.

      i. If infection occurs, the IV is discontinued and the HCP is notified. Blood cultures may be prescribed.
      j. Refer to the Priority Nursing Actions box for instructions on removing an IV.

B. Infiltration
   1. Description
      a. A form of tissue damage; may also be called *extravasation*
      b. Seepage of the IV fluid out of the vein and into the surrounding tissues
      c. Occurs when an IV device has become dislodged or perforates the wall of the vein
   2. Prevention and interventions
      a. IV sites over an area of flexion are avoided.
      b. Anchor the cannula and loop of tubing securely with tape
      c. Use an armboard or splint as prescribed if the client is restless or active.
      d. Monitor the IV site for pain, edema, or coolness, and compare it with the opposite extremity.
      e. Monitor the IV rate for a decrease or cessation of flow.

b. Anchor the cannula and loop of tubing securely with tape.

c. Use an armboard or splint as prescribed if the client is restless or active.

d. If **phlebitis** occurs, the IV device is removed immediately.

e. The HCP is notified if **phlebitis** is suspected, and warm, moist compresses are applied if prescribed.

D. Catheter embolism

1. Description: An obstruction that results from the breakage of the catheter tip during IV insertion or removal

2. Prevention and interventions

   a. Inspect the catheter before insertion.

   b. Remove the IV catheter carefully, and inspect the catheter when removed.

   c. If the catheter tip has broken off, the HCP is notified. A tourniquet is placed high on the limb of the IV site as prescribed, an x-ray study is obtained, and the client may require surgery to remove the catheter pieces.

E. Fluid (circulatory) overload

1. Description: Results from the administration of fluids too rapidly or in a client who is at risk for **fluid overload**

2. Prevention and interventions

   a. Identify clients who are at risk for **fluid overload**.

   b. Calculate and monitor the drip rate frequently.

   c. Use an electronic IV infusion device and frequently check settings for clients who are at risk for **fluid overload**.

   d. If **fluid overload** occurs, the HCP is notified.

⚠ Clients with respiratory, cardiac, renal, or liver disease, older clients, and very young persons are at risk for circulatory overload and cannot tolerate an excessive fluid volume.

F. Air embolism

1. Description: A bolus of air enters the vein through an inadequately primed IV line, from a loose connection, or during a tubing change or the removal of the IV.

2. Prevention and interventions

   a. Prime the tubing with fluid before use, and monitor for any air bubbles in the tubing.

   b. Secure all connections.

   c. Replace IV fluid before the bag or bottle is empty.

   d. If an **air embolism** is suspected, the tubing is clamped, the client is turned on his or her left side with the head of the bed lowered (Trendelenburg position) to trap the air in the right atrium, and the HCP is notified.

▰▰▰ PRIORITY NURSING ACTIONS! ▰▰▰

Steps for Removing a Peripheral Intravenous (IV) Line

1. Check the HCP's prescription and explain the procedure to the client. Ask the client to hold the extremity still during cannula/needle removal.

2. Turn the IV tubing clamp off and remove the dressing and tape covering the site while stabilizing the catheter.

3. Apply light pressure with sterile gauze or other material as specified by agency procedure over the site and withdraw the catheter using a slow steady movement keeping the hub parallel to the skin.

4. Apply pressure for 2 to 3 minutes using dry sterile gauze (apply pressure for a longer period of time if the client has a bleeding disorder or is taking anticoagulant medication).

5. Inspect the site for redness, drainage, or swelling and check the catheter for intactness.

6. Document the procedure and the client's response.

The nurse checks for a HCP's prescription to remove the IV line and then explains the procedure to the client. The nurse asks the client to hold the extremity still during removal. The IV tubing clamp is placed in the off position and the dressing and tape is removed. The nurse is careful to stabilize the catheter so that it is not pulled, resulting in vein trauma. Light pressure is applied over the site to stabilize the catheter and it is removed using a slow steady movement keeping the hub parallel to the skin. Pressure is applied until hemostasis occurs. The site is inspected for redness, drainage, or swelling and the catheter is checked for intactness to ensure that any part of it has not broken off. Finally the nurse documents the procedure and the client's response.

Reference: Elkin, M., Perry, A., & Potter, P. (2007). *Nursing interventions & clinical skills* (4th ed., pp. 620–621). St. Louis: Mosby.

---

f. If **infiltration** has occurred, the IV device is removed immediately.

g. If **infiltration** has occurred, the extremity is elevated, and compresses (warm or cool, depending on the IV solution that was infusing and the HCP's prescription) are applied over the affected area.

h. Do not rub an infiltrated area because this can cause the development of a hematoma.

C. Phlebitis and thrombophlebitis

1. Description

   a. An inflammation of the vein that can occur from mechanical or chemical (medication) trauma or local infection

   b. **Phlebitis** can cause the development of a clot (thrombophlebitis).

2. Prevention and interventions

   a. An IV cannula smaller than the vein is used. Very small veins are avoided when administering irritating solutions. Veins over an area of flexion are avoided.

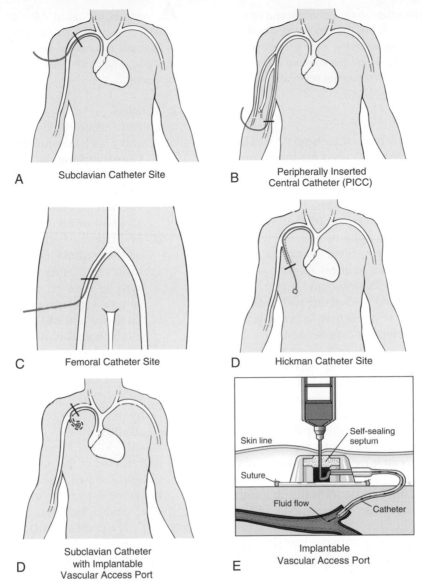

A Subclavian Catheter Site	B Peripherally Inserted Central Catheter (PICC)
C Femoral Catheter Site	D Hickman Catheter Site
D Subclavian Catheter with Implantable Vascular Access Port	E Implantable Vascular Access Port

▲ **FIGURE 13-4** Central venous access sites and access port. (From Kee, J., & Marshall, S. [2009]. *Clinical calculations: With applications to general and specialty areas* [6th ed.]. Philadelphia: Saunders.)

G. Electrolyte overload

1. Description: An electrolyte imbalance caused by too-rapid or excessive infusion or use of an inappropriate IV solution
2. Prevention and interventions
   a. Review laboratory value reports.
   b. Verify the correct solution and additives.
   c. Calculate and monitor the flow rate.
   d. Use an electronic infusion device and frequently check the settings.
   e. Place a sticker on the bag or bottle if a medication has been added to an IV solution.

⚠ Lactated Ringer's solution contains potassium and should not be administered to clients with renal failure.

⚠ Always document the occurrence of a complication, data collection findings, actions taken, and the client's response.

VIII. CENTRAL VENOUS CATHETERS (Figure 13-4)

A. Description

1. Used to deliver hyperosmolar solutions, measure central venous pressure, and infuse parenteral nutrition and multiple IV infusions or medications
2. Catheter position is determined by x-ray study after insertion.
3. May have a single, double, or triple lumen
4. May be inserted peripherally and threaded through the basilic or cephalic vein into the superior vena cava, inserted centrally through the internal jugular or subclavian veins, or surgically tunneled through subcutaneous tissue into the cephalic vein
5. With multilumen catheters, more than one medication can be administered at the same time without incompatibility problems, and there is only one insertion site for care.

⚠ For central line insertion, tubing change, and line removal, place the client in the Trendelenburg's position if not contraindicated or in the supine position, and instruct the client to perform the Valsalva maneuver to increase pressure in the central veins when the IV system is open.

B. Tunneled central venous catheters
  1. A more permanent type of catheter (e.g., Hickman, Broviac, Groshong) used for long-term IV therapy
  2. May be single or multilumen
  3. Inserted in the operating room. The catheter is threaded into the lower part of the vena cava at the entrance of the right atrium.
  4. The catheter will be fitted with an intermittent infusion device to allow access as needed and to keep the system closed and intact.
  5. Patency is maintained by flushing with a diluted heparin solution or a normal saline solution, depending on the type of catheter and according to agency policy.

C. Vascular access ports (implantable ports)
  1. Surgically implanted under the skin (e.g., Port-a-Cath, Mediport, Infusaport); used for the long-term administration of repeated IV therapy
  2. For access, the port requires palpation and injection through the skin into the self-sealing port with a noncoring needle, such as a Huber-point needle.
  3. Patency is maintained by periodic flushing with a diluted heparin solution as prescribed and per agency policy.

D. Peripherally inserted central catheter line (PICC)
  1. Used for long-term IV therapy, frequently in the home
  2. The basilic vein is usually used, but the median cubital and cephalic veins in the antecubital area can also be used.
  3. Threaded so that the catheter tip may terminate in the subclavian vein or the superior vena cava
  4. A small amount of bleeding may occur at the time of insertion and continue for 24 hours, but bleeding thereafter is not expected.
  5. **Phlebitis** is a common complication.
  6. Insertion is below the heart level; therefore **air embolism** is not common.

IX. BLOOD ADMINISTRATION

A. Types of blood components
  1. Red blood cells (RBCs)
    a. Used to replace erythrocytes; infusion time for 1 unit is usually between 2 and 4 hours
    b. Evaluation of an effective response is based on the resolution of the symptoms of anemia and an increase of the erythrocyte count

⚠ Washed red blood cells (depleted of plasma, platelets, and leukocytes) may be prescribed for a client with a history of allergic transfusion reactions or those who underwent hematopoietic stem cell transplant.

  2. Platelets
    a. Platelets are used to treat thrombocytopenia and platelet dysfunctions.
    b. **Crossmatching** is not required but is usually done (platelet concentrates contain few RBCs).
    c. Platelets are administered rapidly usually over 15 to 30 minutes.
    d. Evaluation of an effective response is based on the improvement of the platelet count.
  3. Fresh-frozen plasma
    a. May be used to provide clotting factors or volume expansion; contains no platelets
    b. **Rh factor** and **ABO compatibility** are required for the transfusion of plasma products
    c. Fresh frozen plasma is infused after thawing and administered rapidly, usually over 15 to 30 minutes.
    d. Evaluation of an effective response is assessed by monitoring coagulation studies.

B. Compatibility
  1. Client (the recipient) blood samples are drawn and labeled at the bedside at the time the blood sample is drawn. The client is asked to state his or her name, which is compared with the identification band or bracelet.
  2. The recipient's **ABO** and **Rh factor** are identified.
  3. An antibody screen is done to determine the presence of antibodies other than anti-A and anti-B.
  4. **Crossmatching** is done, in which donor RBCs are combined with the recipient's serum and Coombs' serum. The **crossmatch** is compatible if no RBC agglutination occurs.
  5. The universal RBC donor is O negative. The universal recipient is AB positive.

⚠ The donor's blood and the recipient's blood must be tested for compatibility. If the blood is not compatible, a life-threatening transfusion reaction can occur.

C. Precautions and nursing responsibilities (Box 13-2)

⚠ Stay with the client for the first 15 minutes of the infusion of the blood and monitor the client for signs and symptoms of a transfusion reaction. The first 15 minutes of the transfusion are the most critical, and the nurse must stay with the client.

Box 13-2 Precautions and Nursing Responsibilities

General Precautions

- A large volume of refrigerated blood infused rapidly through a central venous catheter into the ventricle of the heart can cause cardiac dysrhythmias.
- No solution other than normal saline should be added to blood components.
- Medications are never added to blood components or piggybacked into a blood transfusion.
- To avoid the risk of septicemia, infusions (1 unit) should not exceed the prescribed time for administration (2 to 4 hours for PRBCs); follow evidence-based practice guidelines and agency procedure.
- The blood administration set should be changed with each unit of blood, or according to agency policy, to reduce the risk of septicemia.
- Always check the blood bag for the date of expiration; components expire at midnight on the day marked on the bag unless otherwise specified.
- Inspect the blood bag for leaks, abnormal color, clots, and bubbles.
- Blood must be administered as soon as possible (within 20 to 30 minutes) from its being received from the blood bank, because this is the maximum allowable time out of monitored storage.
- Never refrigerate blood in refrigerators other than those used in blood banks; if the blood is not administered within 20 to 30 minutes, return it to the blood bank.
- The recommended rate of infusion varies with the blood component being transfused and depends on the client's condition; generally, blood is infused as quickly as the client's condition allows; caution should be taken to avoid circulatory overload.
- The nurse should measure vital signs and check the lung sounds before the transfusion and again after the first 15 minutes and every hour until 1 hour after the transfusion is completed.

Blood Bank Precautions

- Blood will be released from the blood bank only to personnel specified by agency policy.
- The name and identification number of the intended recipient must be provided to the blood bank, and a documented permanent record of this information must be maintained.
- Blood should be transported from the blood bank to only one client at a time to prevent blood delivery to the wrong client.

Client Identity and Compatibility

- Check the physician's prescription for the administration of the blood product.
- The most critical phase of the transfusion is confirming product compatibility and verifying client identity.
- Two licensed nurses need to check the physician's prescription, the client's identity, and the client's identification band or bracelet and number, verifying that the name and number are identical to those on the blood component tag.
- At the bedside, the nurse asks the client to state his or her name, and the nurse compares the name with the name on the identification band or bracelet.
- The nurse checks the blood bag tag, label, and blood requisition form to ensure that ABO and Rh types are compatible.
- If the nurse notes any inconsistencies when verifying client identity and compatibility, the nurse notifies the blood bank immediately.

Client Assessment

- Assess for any cultural or religious beliefs regarding blood transfusions (e.g., a Jehovah's Witness cannot receive blood or blood products; this group believes that blood transfusions have eternal consequences).
- Ensure that an informed consent has been obtained.
- Explain the procedure to the client and determine whether the client has ever received a blood transfusion or experienced any previous reactions to blood transfusions.
- Check the client's vital signs and assess renal, circulatory, and respiratory status and the client's ability to tolerate intravenously administered fluids.
- If the client's temperature is elevated, notify the physician before beginning the transfusion; a fever may be a cause for delaying the transfusion in addition to masking a possible symptom of an acute transfusion reaction.

Administration of the Transfusion

- Maintain standard and transmission-based precautions and surgical asepsis as necessary.
- Assist the registered nurse in administering the blood.
- Always check the bag for the volume of the blood component.
- Blood products should be infused through administration sets designed specifically for blood; use a Y-tubing or straight tubing blood administration set that contains a filter designed to trap fibrin clots and other debris that accumulate during blood storage
- Premedicate the client with acetaminophen (Tylenol) or diphenhydramine (Benadryl), as prescribed, if the client has a history of adverse reactions; if prescribed, oral medications should be administered 30 minutes before the transfusion is started, and intravenously administered medications may be given immediately before the transfusion is started.
- Instruct the client to report anything unusual immediately.
- Determine the rate of infusion by the physician's prescription or, if not specified, by agency policy.
- Begin the transfusion slowly under close supervision; if no reaction is noted within the first 15 minutes, the flow can be increased to the prescribed rate.
- During the transfusion, monitor the client for signs and symptoms of a transfusion reaction; the first 15 minutes of the transfusion are the most critical, and the nurse must stay with the client.
- If a major ABO incompatibility exists or a severe allergic reaction occurs, the reaction is usually evident within the first 50 mL of the transfusion.

Continued

Box 13-2 Precautions and Nursing Responsibilities—cont'd

Administration of the Transfusion, cont'd

- Document the client's tolerance to the administration of the blood product.
- Monitor appropriate laboratory values and document effectiveness of treatment related to the specific type of blood product.

Reactions to the Transfusion

- If a transfusion reaction occurs, stop the transfusion, change the IV tubing down to the IV site, keep the IV

line open with normal saline, notify the physician and blood bank, and return the blood bag and tubing to the blood bank. (Refer to Priority Nursing Actions)

- Do not leave the client alone, and monitor the client for any life-threatening symptoms.
- Obtain appropriate laboratory samples according to agency policies, such as blood and urine samples (free hemoglobin indicates that red blood cells were hemolyzed).

■■■ PRIORITY NURSING ACTIONS! ■■■

Steps to Take in the Care of a Client Experiencing a Transfusion Reaction

1. Stop the transfusion.
2. Change the intravenous (IV) tubing down to the IV site and keep the IV line open with normal saline.
3. Notify the physician and blood bank.
4. Stay with the client, observing signs and symptoms and monitoring vital signs as often as every 5 minutes.
5. Assist to administer emergency medications as prescribed.
6. Obtain a urine specimen for laboratory studies (and perform any other laboratory studies as prescribed).
7. Return blood bag, tubing, attached labels, and transfusion record to the blood bank. and return the blood bag and tubing to the blood bank.
8. Document the occurrence, actions taken, and the client's response.

If the client exhibits signs of a transfusion reaction, the nurse immediately stops the transfusion and changes the IV tubing down to the IV site to prevent the entrance of additional blood solution into the client. Normal saline solution is hung and infused to keep the IV line open in the event that emergency medications need to be administered. The registered nurse and physician are notified. The nurse also notifies the blood bank of the occurrence. The nurse stays with the client and monitors the client closely while other personnel obtain needed supplies to treat the client. As prescribed by the physician, the nurse assists to administer emergency medications. The nurse then obtains a urine specimen for laboratory studies and performs any other laboratory studies as prescribed to check for free hemoglobin indicating that red blood cells were hemolyzed. The blood bag, tubing, attached labels, and transfusion record are returned to the blood bank so that the blood bank can check the items to determine the reason that the reaction occurred. Finally the nurse documents the occurrence, the actions taken, and the client's response.

Reference: Potter, P., & Perry, A. (2009). *Fundamentals of nursing* (7th ed.). St. Louis: Mosby.

D. Transfusion reactions
1. Immediate transfusion reaction
   a. Chills and diaphoresis
   b. Muscle aches, back pain, or chest pain
   c. Rashes, hives, itching, and swelling
   d. Rapid, thready pulse
   e. Dyspnea, cough, or wheezing
   f. Pallor and cyanosis
   g. Apprehension
   h. Tingling and numbness
   i. Headache
   j. Nausea, vomiting, abdominal cramping, and diarrhea
2. Delayed transfusion reaction
   a. Reactions can occur days to years after a transfusion
   b. Signs include fever, mild jaundice, and a decreased hematocrit level.
3. Refer to Priority Nursing Actions for caring for a client experiencing a transfusion reaction.

MORE QUESTIONS ON EVOLVE!

Practice Questions

81. A nurse is assisting with caring for a client who will receive a unit of blood. Just before the infusion, it is most important for the nurse to check the client's:
1. Vital signs
2. Skin color
3. Oxygen saturation
4. Latest hematocrit level

82. A client who is receiving a blood transfusion rings the call bell for the nurse. When entering the room, the nurse notes that the client is flushed, dyspneic, and complaining of generalized itching. The nurse interprets that the client is experiencing:
1. Bacteremia
2. Fluid overload
3. Hypovolemic shock
4. A transfusion reaction

83. A client who was receiving a blood transfusion has experienced a transfusion reaction. The nurse sends the blood bag that was used for the client to which of the following areas?
    1. The pharmacy
    2. The laboratory
    3. The blood bank
    4. The risk-management department

84. A nurse takes a client's temperature before giving a blood transfusion. The temperature is 100° F orally. The nurse reports the finding to the registered nurse and anticipates that which of the following actions will take place?
    1. The transfusion will begin as prescribed.
    2. The blood will be held, and the health care provider will be notified.
    3. The transfusion will begin after the administration of an antihistamine.
    4. The transfusion will begin after the administration of 600 mg of acetaminophen (Tylenol).

85. A nurse is assisting with caring for a client who has received a transfusion of platelets. The nurse determines that the client is benefiting most from this therapy if the client exhibits which of the following?
    1. An increased hematocrit level
    2. An increased hemoglobin level
    3. A decline of the temperature to normal
    4. A decrease in oozing from puncture sites and gums

86. A client has a prescription to receive 1000 mL of 5% dextrose in 0.45% sodium chloride. After gathering the appropriate equipment, the nurse takes which action first before spiking the IV bag with the tubing?
    1. Uncaps the distal end of the tubing
    2. Uncaps the spike portion of the tubing
    3. Opens the roller clamp on the IV tubing
    4. Closes the roller clamp on the IV tubing

87. A nurse is doing a routine assessment of a client's peripheral IV site. The nurse notes that the site is cool, pale, and swollen and that the IV has stopped running. The nurse determines that which of the following has probably occurred?
    1. Phlebitis
    2. Infection
    3. Infiltration
    4. Thrombosis

88. A nurse is assigned to care for a client with a peripheral IV infusion. The nurse is providing hygiene care to the client and would avoid which of the following while changing the client's hospital gown?

1. Using a hospital gown with snaps at the sleeves
2. Disconnecting the IV tubing from the catheter in the vein
3. Checking the IV flow rate immediately after changing the hospital gown
4. Putting the bag and tubing through the sleeve, followed by the client's arm

89. A nurse is making a worksheet and listing the tasks that need to be performed for assigned adult clients during the shift. The nurse writes on the plan to check the IV of an assigned client who is receiving fluid replacement therapy at least every:
    1. 1 hour
    2. 2 hours
    3. 3 hours
    4. 4 hours

90. A nurse is checking the insertion site of a peripheral IV catheter. The nurse notes the site to be reddened, warm, painful, and slightly edematous in the area of the vein proximal to the IV catheter. The nurse interprets that this is likely the result of:
    1. Phlebitis of the vein
    2. Infiltration of the IV line
    3. Hypersensitivity to the IV solution
    4. An allergic reaction to the IV catheter material

91. A nurse has been instructed to discontinue an IV line. The nurse removes the catheter by withdrawing the catheter while applying pressure to the site with a(n):
    1. Band-Aid
    2. Alcohol swab
    3. Betadine swab
    4. Sterile 2 × 2 gauze

92. A nurse is preparing an IV solution and tubing for a client who requires IV fluids. While preparing to prime the tubing, the tubing drops and hits the top of the medication cart. The nurse should plan to do which of the following?
    1. Change the IV tubing.
    2. Wipe the tubing with Betadine.
    3. Scrub the tubing with an alcohol swab.
    4. Scrub the tubing before attaching it to the IV bag.

93. A client is going to be transfused with a unit of packed red blood cells. The nurse understands that it is necessary to remain with the client for what time period after the transfusion is started?
    1. 5 minutes
    2. 15 minutes
    3. 30 minutes
    4. 45 minutes

94. A nurse is assisting with caring for a client who is receiving a unit of packed red blood cells. The nurse tells the client that it is most important to report which of the following signs immediately?
1. Sore throat or earache
2. Chills, itching, or rash
3. Unusual sleepiness or fatigue
4. Mild discomfort at the catheter site

95. Which of these clients are most likely to develop fluid (circulatory) overload? **Select all that apply.**
❏ 1. A premature infant
❏ 2. A 101-year-old man
❏ 3. A client on renal dialysis
❏ 4. A client with diabetes mellitus
❏ 5. A 29-year-old woman with pneumonia
❏ 6. A client with congestive heart failure

ANSWERS

81. 1
Rationale: A change in the vital signs may indicate that a transfusion reaction is occurring. The nurse assesses the client's vital signs before the procedure to obtain a baseline, every 15 minutes for the first half hour after beginning the transfusion, and every half hour thereafter. Options 2, 3, and 4 may be checked but are not the most important.
Test-Taking Strategy: Note the strategic words "just before" and "most important." This tells you that more than one option may be partially or totally correct. Recalling the signs of a blood transfusion reaction will direct you to option 1. In addition, option 1 is the umbrella choice. Review the blood infusion procedure if you had difficulty with this question.
Level of Cognitive Ability: Applying
Client Needs: Physiological Integrity
Integrated Process: Nursing Process/Data Collection
Content Area: Fundamental Skills: Medications/Blood & IV Therapy
Reference: Christensen, Kockrow, p. 547. 2011. *Foundations and adult health nursing.*

82. 4
Rationale: The signs and symptoms exhibited by the client are consistent with a transfusion reaction. With bacteremia, the client would have a fever, which is not part of the clinical picture presented. With fluid (circulatory) overload, the client would have crackles in addition to dyspnea. There is no correlation between the signs mentioned in the question and hypovolemic shock. The signs identified in the question are indicative of an allergic reaction, which is one type of blood transfusion reaction.
Test-Taking Strategy: Use the process of elimination, and focus on the data in the question. Recalling the signs of a transfusion reaction will direct you to option 4. Review the complications of blood administration and the signs of a transfusion reaction if you had difficulty with this question.
Level of Cognitive Ability: Analyzing
Client Needs: Physiological Integrity
Integrated Process: Nursing Process/Data Collection
Content Area: Fundamental Skills: Medications/Blood & IV Therapy
Reference: Christensen, Kockrow, p. 548. 2011. *Foundations and adult health nursing.*

83. 3
Rationale: The nurse prepares to return the blood transfusion bag containing any remaining blood to the blood bank. This allows the blood bank to complete any follow-up testing procedures that are needed after a transfusion reaction has been documented. Options 1, 2, and 4 are incorrect.

Test-Taking Strategy: Use the process of elimination. Recalling that blood is obtained from the blood bank will help you to eliminate each of the incorrect options. Review the procedures to follow when a blood transfusion reaction occurs if you had difficulty with this question.
Level of Cognitive Ability: Applying
Client Needs: Physiological Integrity
Integrated Process: Nursing Process/Implementation
Content Area: Fundamental Skills: Medications/Blood & IV Therapy
Reference: Christensen, Kockrow, p. 547. 2011. *Foundations and adult health nursing.*

84. 2
Rationale: If the client has a temperature of 100° F or more, the unit of blood should be held until the health care provider is notified and has the opportunity to give further prescriptions. The other options are incorrect actions.
Test-Taking Strategy: Use the process of elimination. Eliminate options 1, 3, and 4, because they are comparable or alike. Remember that if the temperature is elevated, the physician needs to be notified before a blood transfusion is initiated. Review the procedures related to the administration of a blood transfusion if you had difficulty with this question.
Level of Cognitive Ability: Applying
Client Needs: Physiological Integrity
Integrated Process: Nursing Process/Implementation
Content Area: Fundamental Skills: Medications/Blood & IV Therapy
References: Christensen, Kockrow, p. 548. 2011. *Foundations and adult health nursing.*
deWit, pp. 395–396. 2009.

85. 4
Rationale: Platelets are necessary for proper blood clotting. The client with insufficient platelets may exhibit frank bleeding or the oozing of blood from puncture sites, wounds, and mucous membranes. The client's temperature would decline to normal after the infusion of granulocytes if those transfused cells were then instrumental in fighting infection in the body. Increased hemoglobin and hematocrit levels would be seen when the client has received a transfusion of red blood cells.
Test-Taking Strategy: Use the process of elimination. Recalling that bleeding is a concern when the platelets are low will easily direct you to option 4. Review the action of platelets if you had difficulty with this question.
Level of Cognitive Ability: Evaluating
Client Needs: Physiological Integrity
Integrated Process: Nursing Process/Evaluation
Content Area: Fundamental Skills: Medications/Blood & IV Therapy

References: Ignatavicius, Workman, p. 920. 2010.
Lewis, Dirksen, Heitkemper, Bucher, Camera, pp. 705–706. 2011.
Linton, p. 614. 2012.

86. 4

Rationale: The nurse should first clamp the tubing to prevent the solution from running freely through the tubing after it is attached to the IV bag. The nurse should next uncap the proximal (spike) portion of the tubing and attach it to the IV bag. The roller clamp is then opened slowly, and the fluid is allowed to flow through the tubing in a controlled fashion to prevent air from remaining in parts of the tubing.

Test-Taking Strategy: Use the process of elimination, and note the strategic word "first." This question tests a specific procedure related to IV therapy. Visualize this procedure to answer the question correctly. Review the intravenous infusion procedure if you had difficulty with this question.

Level of Cognitive Ability: Applying
Client Needs: Physiological Integrity
Integrated Process: Nursing Process/Implementation
Content Area: Fundamental Skills: Medications/Blood & IV Therapy
Reference: deWit, pp. 56–57. 2009.

87. 3

Rationale: An infiltrated IV is one that has dislodged from the vein and is lying in subcutaneous tissue. The pallor, coolness, and swelling are the result of IV fluid being deposited into the subcutaneous tissue. When the pressure in the tissues exceeds the pressure in the tubing, the flow of the IV solution will stop. The other three options identify complications that are likely to be accompanied by warmth at the site rather than coolness.

Test-Taking Strategy: Focus on the data in the question, and note the strategic word "cool." Recalling that coolness occurs at the site of IV infiltration will direct you to option 3. Review the signs of infiltration if you had difficulty with this question.

Level of Cognitive Ability: Analyzing
Client Needs: Physiological Integrity
Integrated Process: Nursing Process/Data Collection
Content Area: Fundamental Skills: Medications/Blood & IV Therapy
Reference: deWit, p. 59. 2009.

88. 2

Rationale: The tubing should not be removed from the IV catheter. With each break in the system, there is an increased chance of introducing bacteria into the system, which can lead to infection. Options 1 and 4 are appropriate. The flow rate should be checked immediately after changing the hospital gown, because the position of the roller clamp may have been affected during the change.

Test-Taking Strategy: Use the process of elimination, and note the strategic word "avoid." This word indicates a negative event query and asks you to select an incorrect action. Visualize this procedure, and use your knowledge of the basic principles related to IV therapy and asepsis to direct you to option 2. Review these principles if you had difficulty with this question.

Level of Cognitive Ability: Applying
Client Needs: Safe and Effective Care Environment
Integrated Process: Nursing Process/Implementation

Content Area: Fundamental Skills: Medications/Blood & IV Therapy
Reference: Christensen, Kockrow, p. 541. 2011. *Foundations and adult health nursing.*

89. 1

Rationale: Safe nursing practice includes monitoring an IV infusion at least once per hour for an adult client. Options 2, 3, and 4 do not provide time frames that are safe or acceptable.

Test-Taking Strategy: Use the process of elimination. To answer this question accurately, it is necessary to be familiar with the specific time frames indicated for this nursing procedure. For questions similar to this one, it is best to select the most frequently occurring time frame. Review the precautions related to the administration of IV fluid if you had difficulty with this question.

Level of Cognitive Ability: Applying
Client Needs: Physiological Integrity
Integrated Process: Nursing Process/Implementation
Content Area: Fundamental Skills: Medications/Blood & IV Therapy
Reference: deWit, p. 58. 2009.

90. 1

Rationale: Phlebitis at an IV site results in discomfort at the site and redness, warmth, and swelling proximal to the IV catheter. The IV catheter should be removed, and a new IV line should be inserted at a different site. The remaining options are incorrect; the signs and symptoms in the question are not associated with these conditions

Test-Taking Strategy: Use the process of elimination. Remember that comparable or alike options are not likely to be correct. In this case, options 3 and 4 are comparable or alike and are therefore eliminated. Recalling that warmth occurs at the site of phlebitis will direct you to option 1. Review the signs of phlebitis if you had difficulty with this question.

Level of Cognitive Ability: Analyzing
Client Needs: Physiological Integrity
Integrated Process: Nursing Process/Data Collection
Content Area: Fundamental Skills: Medications/Blood & IV Therapy
Reference: deWit, p. 59. 2009.

91. 4

Rationale: A dry, sterile dressing such as a sterile 2 × 2 gauze is used to apply pressure to the site while the catheter is discontinued and removed. This material is absorbent, sterile, and nonirritating to the site. A Band-Aid may be used to cover the site after hemostasis has occurred. An alcohol swab or Betadine would irritate the opened puncture site and would not stop the blood flow.

Test-Taking Strategy: Use the process of elimination. Visualize this procedure, and think about each of the items identified in the options to answer the question. Noting the word "sterile" in option 4 will assist with directing you to this option. Review the discontinuation of an IV line if you had difficulty with this question.

Level of Cognitive Ability: Applying
Client Needs: Safe and Effective Care Environment
Integrated Process: Nursing Process/Implementation
Content Area: Fundamental Skills: Medications/Blood & IV Therapy

References: Christensen, Kockrow, p. 554. 2011. *Foundations and adult health nursing.*
Potter, Perry, p. 541. 2009.

92. 1

Rationale: The nurse should change the IV tubing. The tubing has become contaminated, and, if used, it could result in a systemic infection in the client. Wiping or scrubbing the tubing is insufficient to prevent systemic infection.

Test-Taking Strategy: Use your knowledge of basic infection control measures and IV therapy concepts to answer this question. Note that options 2, 3, and 4 are comparable or alike, and eliminate these options. Review aseptic technique and IV therapy if you had difficulty with this question.

Level of Cognitive Ability: Applying
Client Needs: Safe and Effective Care Environment
Integrated Process: Nursing Process/Implementation
Content Area: Fundamental Skills: Medications/Blood & IV Therapy

Reference: Christensen, Kockrow, p. 553. 2011. *Foundations and adult health nursing.*

93. 2

Rationale: The nurse must remain with the client for the first 15 minutes of a transfusion, which is the most likely time that a transfusion reaction will occur. This enables the nurse to detect a reaction and intervene quickly. The nurse engages in safe nursing practice by obtaining coverage for the other clients during this time. Options 1 is too short of a time period. Options 3 and 4 are lengthy time periods.

Test-Taking Strategy: Use the process of elimination and your knowledge regarding blood transfusion procedures to answer this question. Remember, the client must be directly monitored for the first 15 minutes of the transfusion. Review the nursing responsibilities involved when beginning a blood transfusion if you had difficulty with this question.

Level of Cognitive Ability: Applying
Client Needs: Physiological Integrity
Integrated Process: Nursing Process/Implementation
Content Area: Fundamental Skills: Medications/Blood & IV Therapy

Reference: Christensen, Kockrow, pp. 547–548. 2011. *Foundations and adult health nursing.*

94. 2

Rationale: The client is told to report chills, itching, or rash immediately, because these could be signs of a possible transfusion reaction. Mild discomfort at the catheter site may be indicative of a problem, or it could result from the size of the IV catheter required to infuse the blood product. Sore throat, earache, sleepiness, and fatigue are unrelated to a transfusion reaction.

Test-Taking Strategy: Note the strategic words "most important" and "immediately." These tell you that more than one or all of the options may be partially or totally correct. With the knowledge that a transfusion reaction is of greatest concern to the nurse, prioritize and select the option that characterizes this problem. Review the signs of a transfusion reaction if you had difficulty with this question.

Level of Cognitive Ability: Applying
Client Needs: Physiological Integrity
Integrated Process: Nursing Process/Implementation
Content Area: Fundamental Skills: Medications/Blood & IV Therapy

Reference: Christensen, Kockrow, p. 548. 2011. *Foundations and adult health nursing.*

95. 1,2,3,6

Rationale: Clients with cardiac, respiratory, renal, or liver diseases and older and very young clients cannot tolerate an excessive fluid volume. The risk of fluid (circulatory) overload exists with these clients.

Test-Taking Strategy: Focus on the subject of fluid (circulatory) overload. Thinking about the physiology associated with each client described in the options will assist you with answering correctly. Review the concepts related to fluid overload if you had difficulty with this question.

Level of Cognitive Ability: Analyzing
Client Needs: Physiological Integrity
Integrated Process: Nursing Process/Data Collection
Content Area: Fundamental Skills: Medications/Blood & IV Therapy

Reference: Perry, Potter, p. 789. 2010.

UNIT 4

Fundamental Skills

Hygiene and Safety

PYRAMID TERMS

health care–associated (nosocomial) infections Previously referred to as "nosocomial" infections; infections acquired in the hospital or other health care facility that were not present or incubating at the time of the client's admission; also referred to as "hospital-acquired" infections.

home safety Removing items from the home environment and avoiding situations or events that place the client at risk for accident or injury

physical hazards Hazards that place clients at risk for accident, injury, or death

poison Any substance that impairs health or destroys life when ingested, inhaled, or otherwise absorbed by the body

restraints (safety devices) Physical devices (that the client is unable to remove) applied to restrict a client's movement are known as "physical restraints." Medications given to inhibit a specific behavior are known as "chemical restraints."

standard precautions Guidelines used by all health care providers with all clients to reduce the risk of infection for both clients and caregivers

transmission-based precautions Guidelines that are used in addition to standard precautions; used for specific syndromes that are highly suggestive of infection until a diagnosis is confirmed

warfare agent Substance that may be biological, chemical, or radioactive in nature that can cause mass destruction and fatality

PYRAMID TO SUCCESS

Safety and Infection Control is a subcategory of the Safe and Effective Care Environment component of the Client Needs section of the test plan for the NCLEX-PN. The pyramid points focus on maintaining environmental safety, preventing accidents, the medication reconciliation process, using restraints, priority nursing actions in the event of a disaster, and biological and chemical warfare agents. The pyramid points also focus on standard and transmission-based precautions and the measures required to handle hazardous or infectious materials.

CLIENT NEEDS

Safe and Effective Care Environment

- Following guidelines related to the emergency response plan and biological and chemical warfare agents
- Ensuring that clients' rights are upheld, including informed consent
- Establishing priorities
- Following guidelines regarding the use of restraints
- Handling hazardous and infectious materials safely
- Maintaining precautions to prevent errors, accidents, and injuries
- Using ergonomic principles
- Using standard, transmission-based, and other infection-control precautions

Health Promotion and Maintenance

- Assisting clients and families with identifying environmental hazards in the home
- Teaching clients and families about accident prevention
- Teaching clients and families about measures to be implemented during an emergency or disaster
- Teaching clients and families about preventing the spread of infection

Psychosocial Integrity

- Assessing the client for sensory or perceptual alterations
- Identifying cultural and religious lifestyles
- Identifying support systems

Physiological Integrity

- Assisting the client with activities of daily living
- Implementing priority nursing actions during an emergency or disaster
- Managing and providing care to clients with infectious diseases
- Providing comfort and assistance to the client
- Using assistive devices to prevent injury

I. HYGIENE

A. Description
1. The activity of providing care or promoting self-care, which includes bathing and grooming
2. Includes care of the skin, hair, nails, mouth, teeth, eyes, ears, nasal cavities, and perineal and genital areas
3. Personal hygiene is the activity of self-care, including bathing and grooming

B. General principles
1. Wash hands and wear gloves
2. Ensure privacy
3. Explain procedures to the client
4. Determine and treat pain
5. Determine the client's health status and readiness for hygiene procedures
6. Determine the client's routine hygiene practices
7. Use proper body mechanics during bathing and hygiene activities
8. Use time spent with client as an opportunity to determine the client's mental health status and implement communication and teaching
9. Maintain and encourage independence as much as possible

II. ENVIRONMENTAL SAFETY

A. Fire safety (See Priority Nursing Actions)
1. Keep open spaces free of clutter.
2. Clearly mark fire exits.
3. Know the locations of all fire alarms, exits, and extinguishers (Table 14-1).
4. Know the telephone number for reporting fires.
5. Know the agency's fire drill and evacuation plan.
6. Never use the elevator in the event of a fire.
7. Turn off oxygen and appliances in the vicinity of the fire.
8. In the event of a fire, if a client is on life support, maintain the client's respiratory status manually with an Ambu bag (resuscitation bag) until the client is moved away from the threat of the fire and placed back on life support.
9. In the event of a fire, ambulatory clients can be directed to walk by themselves to a safe area. In some cases, they may be able to assist with moving clients who are in wheelchairs.
10. Bedridden clients are generally moved from the scene of a fire by stretcher, bed, or wheelchair.
11. If a client must be carried from the area of a fire, appropriate transfer techniques should be used, ergonomic principles and good body mechanics should be instituted to prevent injury.
12. If fire department personnel are at the scene of the fire, they can help evacuate clients.

⚠ Remember the mnemonic RACE to set priorities in the event of a fire and the mnemonic PASS to use a fire extinguisher.

■■■ PRIORITY NURSING ACTIONS! ■■■

Actions to Take in the Event of a Fire
1. Rescue clients who are in immediate danger.
2. Activate the fire alarm.
3. Confine the fire.
4. Extinguish the fire: obtain the fire extinguisher.
5. Pull the pin on the fire extinguisher.
6. Aim at the base of the fire.
7. Squeeze the extinguisher handle.
8. Sweep extinguisher from side to side to coat the area of the fire evenly.

Remember the mnemonic *RACE* to prioritize in the event of a fire. *R* is rescue clients in immediate danger, *A* is alarm (sound the alarm), *C* is confine the fire by closing all doors, and *E* is extinguish or evacuate. To properly use the fire extinguisher, remember the mnemonic *PASS* to prioritize in the use of a fire extinguisher. *P* is pull the pin, *A* is aim at the base of the fire, *S* is squeeze the handle, and *S* is sweep from side to side to coat the area evenly.

Reference: Potter, P., & Perry, A. (2009). *Fundamentals of nursing* (7th ed., pp. 839–841). St. Louis: Mosby.

TABLE 14-1 Types of Fire Extinguishers

Type	Class of Fires
A	Wood, cloth, upholstery, paper, rubbish, and plastic
B	Flammable liquids or gases, grease, tar, and oil-based paint
C	Electrical equipment

Note: Certain extinguishers may be appropriate for more than one type of fire.

B. Electrical safety
1. Electrical equipment must be maintained in good working order and should be grounded.
2. Use a three-pronged electrical cord.
3. In a three-pronged electrical cord, the third, longer prong of the cord is the ground. The other two prongs carry the power to the piece of electrical equipment.
4. Any electrical equipment that the client brings into the health care facility must be inspected for safety before use.
5. Check electrical cords and outlets for exposed, frayed, or damaged wires.
6. Avoid overloading any circuit.
7. Read warning labels on all equipment. Never operate unfamiliar equipment.
8. Use safety extension cords only when absolutely necessary, and tape them to the floor with electrical tape.
9. Never run electrical wiring under carpets.
10. Never pull a plug by using the cord. Always grasp the plug itself.

11. Never use electrical appliances near sinks, bathtubs, or other water sources.
12. Always disconnect a plug from the outlet before cleaning equipment or appliances.
13. If a client receives an electrical shock, turn off the electricity before touching the client.

⚠ Any electrical equipment that the client brings into the health care facility must be inspected for safety before use.

C. Radiation safety
1. Know the health care agency's protocols and guidelines.
2. Label potentially radioactive material.
3. To reduce exposure to radiation:
   a. The time spent near the source should be limited (30 minutes per care provider per shift).
   b. The distance from the source should be as great as possible.
   c. A shielding device such as a lead apron should be used.
   d. A pregnant person and children younger than 16 years should not enter the room
   e. Limit visits from visitors to 30 minutes. Visitors should be at least 6 feet from the client.
4. Monitor radiation exposure with a film (dosimeter) badge.
5. Place the client who has a radiation implant in a private room.
6. Keep all linens and dressings in the client's room until the implant is removed.
7. Never touch dislodged implants.

D. Disposal of infectious wastes
1. Handle all infectious materials as a hazard.
2. Dispose of waste in designated areas only, and use proper containers for disposal.
3. Ensure that infectious material is properly labeled.
4. Dispose of all sharps immediately after use in closed, puncture-resistant disposal containers that are leakproof and labeled or color coded.

⚠ Needles (sharps) should not be recapped, bent, or broken because of the risk of accidental injury (needle-stick).

E. Physiological changes in the older client that increase the risk of accidents (Box 14-1)
F. Falls (Box 14-2 lists measures to prevent falls)
G. Medication errors (Box 14-3)
H. **Restraints (safety devices)**
1. Protective devices used to limit the physical activity of a client or immobilize a client or an extremity; state and agency policy must be followed with regard to their use

2. Guidelines for protective devices applied to clients with a mental health diagnosis may be governed by state mental health code standards.
3. Physical restraints: Restrict client movement through the application of a device.
4. Chemical restraints: Medications given to inhibit a specific behavior or movement

---

Box 14-1 Physiological Changes in the Older Client That Increase the Risk of Accidents

Musculoskeletal Changes
- Strength and function of muscles decrease.
- Joints become less mobile and bones become brittle.
- Postural changes and limited range of motion occur.

Nervous System Changes
- Voluntary and autonomic reflexes become slower.
- Decreased ability to respond to multiple stimuli occurs.
- Decreased sensitivity to touch occurs.

Sensory Changes
- Decreased vision and lens accommodation and cataracts develop.
- Delayed transmission of hot and cold impulses occurs.
- Impaired hearing develops, with high-frequency tones less perceptible.

Genitourinary Changes
- Increased nocturia and occurrences of incontinence may occur.

Adapted from Potter, A., & Perry, P. (2009). *Fundamentals of nursing* (7th ed., p. 816). St. Louis: Mosby. (Modified from Ebersole, P., Hess, P., & Luggen, A. (2004). *Toward healthy aging* (6th ed.). St. Louis: Mosby.

Box 14-2 Measures to Prevent Falls

- Determine the client's risk for falling.
- Ensure that the client at risk for falling is in a room near the nurses' station.
- Be alert to clients who are at risk for falling.
- Check to see if there is a notation on the door to the room indicating a fall risk.
- Orient the client to his or her physical surroundings.
- Instruct the client to seek assistance when getting up.
- Explain the use of the call-bell system.
- Keep the bed in the low position; the use of siderails is based on state and agency policies and procedures and must be followed
- Lock all beds, wheelchairs, and stretchers.
- Keep personal items within reach.
- Eliminate clutter and obstacles in the client's room.
- Provide adequate lighting, including subdued lighting at night.
- Reduce bathroom hazards.
- Maintain the client's toileting schedule throughout the day.

5. Interventions
    a. When restraints are necessary, the health care provider's (HCP's) prescriptions should state the type of restraint, identify specific client behaviors for which restraints are to be used, and identify a limited time frame for use.
    b. Prescriptions for restraints should be renewed within a specific time frame, according to agency policy.
    c. Restraints are not to be prescribed on an as-needed basis or PRN basis.
    d. The reason for the restraints should be given to the client and family, and their permission should be sought.
    e. Restraints should not interfere with any treatments or affect the client's health problem.
    f. Make sure that restraints are applied appropriately and according to the manufacturer's instructions.
    g. Use a half-bow or safety knot to secure the device to the bed frame or chair and not to the side rails. (This provides for quick release.)
    h. Because there are several different types of restraints, ensure that there is enough slack on the straps to allow some movement of the body part.
    i. Restraints with plastic quick-release buckles should not be knotted.
    j. Assess skin integrity and neurovascular and circulatory status every 30 minutes, and remove the restraint at least every 2 hours to permit muscle exercise and promote circulation.
    k. Continually assess and document the need for the restraints (Box 14-4).

⚠️ A HCP's prescription for use of a safety device is needed. Alternative measures for safety devices should always be used first.

6. Alternatives to restraints
    a. Orient the client and family to surroundings
    b. Explain all procedures and treatments to the client and family.
    c. Encourage family and friends to stay with the client, and use sitters for clients who need supervision.
    d. Assign confused and disoriented clients to rooms near the nurses' station.
    e. Provide appropriate visual and auditory stimuli to the client (e.g., clock, calendar, television, radio).
    f. Place familiar items (e.g., family pictures) near the client's bedside.
    g. Maintain toileting routines.
    h. Eliminate bothersome treatments (e.g., tube feedings) as soon as possible.
    i. Evaluate all medications that the client is receiving.
    j. Use relaxation techniques with the client.
    k. Institute exercise and ambulation schedules as the client's condition allows.

I. Poisons
    1. Any substance that impairs health or destroys life when ingested, inhaled, or otherwise absorbed by the body
    2. Specific antidotes or treatments are available for only some types of poisons.
    3. The capability of body tissue to recover from a poison determines the reversibility of the effect.
    4. Poison can impair the respiratory, circulatory, central nervous, hepatic, gastrointestinal, and renal systems of the body.
    5. Toddlers, preschoolers, and young school-age children must be protected from accidental poisoning.
    6. In older adults, diminished eyesight and impaired memory may result in the accidental ingestion of poisonous substances or an overdose of prescribed medications.
    7. A poison control center phone number should be visible on the telephone in homes with small children. In all cases of suspected poisoning, the number should be called immediately.
    8. Interventions
        a. Remove any obvious materials from the mouth, eye, or body area immediately.

Box 14-3 National Patient Safety Goals

- Improve the accuracy of patient identification.
- Improve the effectiveness of communication among caregivers.
- Improve the safety of using medications.
- Reduce the risk of health care–associated infections.
- Identify safety risk inherent in its patient population.

From The Joint Commission. http://www.jointcommission.org/assets/1/6/2011_NPSGs_HAP.pdf.

Box 14-4 Documentation Points with the Use of a Restraint (Security Device)

- Reason for restraint
- Method of restraint
- Date and time of the application of restraint
- Duration of use of restraint and the client's response
- Release from restraint with periodic exercise and circulatory, neurovascular, and skin assessment
- Determination of the continued need for restraint
- Evaluation of the client's response

b. Identify the type and amount of substance ingested.

c. Call the poison control center before attempting an intervention.

d. If the victim vomits or vomiting is induced, save the vomitus if requested to do so, and deliver it to the poison control center.

e. If instructed by the poison control center to take the poisoned person to the emergency department, call an ambulance.

f. Vomiting is never induced after the ingestion of lye, household cleaners, grease, or petroleum products.

g. Vomiting is never induced in an unconscious victim.

⚠ The Poison Control Center should be called first before attempting an intervention.

III. HEALTH CARE–ASSOCIATED INFECTIONS (Box 14-5)

A. **Health care–associated (nosocomial) infections** also are referred to as hospital-acquired infections.

B. Such infections are infections acquired in a hospital or other health care facility that were not present or incubating at the time of a client's admission.

C. Illness impairs the normal defense mechanisms of the body.

D. The hospital environment provides exposure to a variety of virulent organisms that the client has not been exposed to in the past; therefore, the client has not developed resistance to these organisms.

E. Infections can be transmitted by health care personnel who fail to practice proper hand washing procedures or fail to change gloves between client contacts.

F. Many health care agencies have dispensers containing an alcohol-based solution for hand rubs mounted at the entrance to each client's room.

IV. STANDARD PRECAUTIONS

A. Description
  1. Must be practiced with all clients in any setting, regardless of the diagnosis or presumed infectiousness
  2. Promote handwashing and the use of gloves, masks, eye protection, and gowns, when appropriate, during client contact.

Box 14-5 Common Drug-Resistant Health Care–Associated Infections

- Vancomycin-resistant enterococci
- Methicillin-resistant *Staphylococcus aureus*
- Multidrug-resistant tuberculosis

---

3. These precautions apply to blood, all body fluids, secretions, and excretions, regardless of whether they contain blood, nonintact skin, or mucous membranes.

B. Interventions
  1. Handle all blood and body fluids from all clients as if they were contaminated.
  2. An alcohol-based hand rub or a soap-and-water hand wash to decontaminate the hands is necessary before having direct contact with a client.
  3. The hands are also washed between client contacts; after contact with blood, body fluids, secretions, or excretions and after contact with equipment or articles contaminated by them; and immediately after gloves are removed.
  4. Gloves are worn when blood, body fluids, secretions, excretions, nonintact skin, mucous membranes, or contaminated items are touched. Gloves should be removed and hands washed between client care contacts.
  5. Masks, eye protection, or face shields are worn if client care activities may generate splashes or sprays of blood or body fluid.
  6. Gowns are worn if the soiling of clothing is likely from contact with blood or body fluid. Wash hands after removing a gown.
  7. Client care equipment is properly cleaned and reprocessed, and single-use items are discarded.
  8. Contaminated linens are placed in leakproof bags and handled to prevent skin and mucous membrane exposure.
  9. All sharp instruments and needles are discarded in a puncture-resistant container. Needles are disposed of uncapped.
  10. Use needleless devices or special needle safety devices whenever possible to reduce the risk to health care workers of needle sticks and sharps injuries.
  11. Spills of blood or body fluids are cleaned with a solution of bleach and water (diluted 1:10) or an agency-approved disinfectant.
  12. A private room is unnecessary unless the client's hygiene is unacceptable. The nurse should consult with an infection-control professional.

⚠ Handle all blood and body fluids from all clients as if they were contaminated.

V. TRANSMISSION-BASED PRECAUTIONS

A. Airborne precautions
  1. Diseases
     a. Measles
     b. Chickenpox (varicella)
     c. Disseminated varicella zoster
     d. Tuberculosis

2. Barrier protection for airborne precautions
   a. Single room maintained under negative pressure; door kept closed except when someone is entering or exiting the room
   b. Negative airflow pressure in the room, with a minimum of 6 to 12 air exchanges per hour, depending on the health care agency
   c. Use of ultraviolet germicide irradiation or a high-efficiency particulate air filter in the room
   d. Use of a mask or a personal respiratory protection device
   e. Place a mask on the client when the client needs to leave the room. The client leaves the room only if necessary.

B. Droplet precautions
   1. Diseases
      a. Adenovirus
      b. Diphtheria (pharyngeal)
      c. Epiglottitis
      d. Influenza, including H1N1 influenza
      e. Meningitis
      f. Mumps
      g. Mycoplasma pneumonia or meningococcal pneumonia
      h. Parvovirus B19
      i. Pertussis
      j. Pneumonia
      k. Rubella
      l. Scarlet fever
      m. Sepsis
      n. Streptococcal pharyngitis
   2. Barrier protection
      a. Private room or cohort client
      b. Use of a mask
      c. Place a mask on the client when the client is out of the room. The client leaves the room only if necessary.

C. Contact precautions
   1. Diseases
      a. Colonization or infection with a multidrug-resistant organism
      b. Enteric infections such as *Clostridium difficile*
      c. Respiratory infections such as respiratory syncytial virus
      d. Wound infections
      e. Skin infections such as cutaneous diphtheria, herpes simplex, impetigo, pediculosis, scabies, *Staphylococcus*, varicella zoster
      f. Eye infections such as conjunctivitis
      g. H1N1 influenza: Infection can occur by touching something with flu viruses on it and then touching the mouth or nose
   2. Barrier protection
      a. Private room or cohort client
      b. Use of gloves and a gown when in contact with the client

VI. EMERGENCY RESPONSE PLAN AND DISASTERS

A. Know the agency's disaster plan.
B. Internal disasters are those in which the agency is in danger.
C. External disasters occur in the community, and victims will be brought to the health care facility for care.
D. When the health care agency is notified of a disaster, the nurse should follow the guidelines specified in the agency's disaster plan.
E. See Chapter 8 for additional information about disaster planning.

⚠ In the event of a disaster, the emergency response plan is immediately activated.

VII. BIOLOGICAL WARFARE AGENTS

A. A **warfare agent** is a biological or chemical substance that can cause mass destruction or fatality.
B. Anthrax
   1. Caused by *Bacillus anthracis*; can be contracted through the digestive system, abrasions in the skin, or inhalation
   2. Transmitted by direct contact with the bacteria and its spores; spores are dormant encapsulated bacteria that become active when they enter a living host (no person-to-person spread; Box 14-6)

Box 14-6 Transmission and Symptoms of Anthrax

Skin

Spores enter the skin through cuts and abrasions and are contracted by handling contaminated animal skin products.
The infection starts with an itchy bump like a mosquito bite that progresses to a small, liquid-filled sac.
The sac becomes a painless ulcer with an area of black, dead tissue in the middle.
Toxins destroy the surrounding tissue.

Gastrointestinal System

Infection occurs after the ingestion of contaminated, undercooked meat.
Symptoms begin with nausea, loss of appetite, and vomiting.
The infection progresses to severe abdominal pain, the vomiting of blood, and severe diarrhea.

Inhalation

Infection is caused by the inhalation of bacterial spores, which multiply in the alveoli.
Symptoms begin with the same symptoms as influenza, including fever, muscle aches, and fatigue.
Symptoms suddenly become more severe with the development of breathing problems and shock.
Toxins cause hemorrhage and the destruction of lung tissue.

3. Carried to the lymph nodes and then spread to the rest of the body via the blood and lymph; high levels of toxins lead to shock and death

4. In the lungs, anthrax can cause a buildup of fluid, tissue decay, and death. It is fatal if untreated.

5. A blood test is available to detect anthrax. This test magnifies DNA from the blood sample and matches it with anthrax DNA.

6. Treated with ciprofloxacin (Cipro), doxycycline, or penicillin

7. Vaccine has limited availability

⚠ Anthrax is transmitted by direct contact with bacteria and spores and can be contracted through the digestive system, abrasions in the skin, or inhalation through the lungs.

C. Smallpox
1. Transmitted in air droplets and by handling contaminated materials
2. Highly contagious
3. Symptoms include fever, back pain, vomiting, malaise, and headache
4. Papules develop 2 days after symptoms develop and progress to pustular vesicles, which are initially abundant on the face and extremities
5. A vaccine is available to those at risk for exposure to smallpox

D. Botulism
1. Serious paralytic illness caused by a nerve toxin that is produced by the bacterium *Clostridium botulinum*. An infected client can die within 24 hours.
2. Spores are found in the soil and can spread through the air or food (particularly improperly canned food) or via a contaminated wound.
3. Cannot be spread from person to person
4. Symptoms include abdominal cramps, diarrhea, nausea, vomiting, double vision, blurred vision, drooping eyelids, difficulty swallowing or speaking, dry mouth, and muscle weakness.
5. Can progress to paralysis of the arms, legs, trunk, or respiratory muscles; mechanical ventilation becomes necessary
6. If diagnosed early, foodborne and wound botulism can be treated with an antitoxin that blocks the action of the toxin circulating in the blood.
7. Other treatments include the induction of vomiting, enemas, and penicillin.
8. No available vaccine

E. Plague
1. Caused by *Yersinia pestis*, which is a bacteria found in rodents and fleas

2. Contracted by being bitten by a rodent or flea carrying the plague bacterium, the ingestion of contaminated meat, or the handling of an animal infected with the bacteria
3. Transmitted by direct person-to-person spread
4. Forms include bubonic (most common), pneumonic, and septicemic (most deadly)
5. Begins with a fever, chest pain, lymph node swelling, and productive cough (hemoptysis)
6. Rapidly progresses to dyspnea, stridor, and cyanosis; death occurs as a result of respiratory failure, shock, and bleeding
7. Antibiotics are only effective if administered immediately. Medications of choice include streptomycin and gentamicin
8. Vaccine is available

F. Tularemia
1. Infectious disease of animals caused by the bacillus *Francisella tularensis*; also called deerfly fever or rabbit fever
2. Transmitted by ticks, deerflies, or contact with an infected animal
3. Symptoms include fever, headache, ulcerated skin lesion with localized lymph node enlargement, eye infection, gastrointestinal ulceration, and pneumonia.
4. Treated with antibiotics
5. Recovery produces lifelong immunity

G. Hemorrhagic fever
1. Caused by several viruses, including Marburg, Lassa, Junin, and Ebola
2. Virus is carried by rodents and mosquitoes
3. Can be transmitted by direct person-to-person spread via body fluids
4. Symptoms include fever, headache, malaise, conjunctivitis, nausea, vomiting, hypotension, hemorrhage of tissues and organs, and organ failure.
5. No known specific treatment is available; treatment is symptomatic

VIII. CHEMICAL WARFARE AGENTS

A. Sarin
1. A highly toxic nerve gas that can cause death within minutes of exposure
2. Enters the body through the eyes and skin; acts by paralyzing the respiratory muscles

B. Phosgene: Colorless gas normally used in chemical manufacturing; if inhaled at high concentrations for a long enough period, leads to severe respiratory distress, pulmonary edema, and death

C. Mustard gas: Yellow to brown in color and has a garlic-like odor that irritates the eyes and causes skin burns and blisters

D. Ionizing radiation
1. Acute radiation poisoning develops after substantial exposure to radiation

2. Can occur from external radiation or internal absorption

3. Symptoms depend on the amount of exposure to the radiation; range from nausea and vomiting, diarrhea, fever, electrolyte imbalances, and neurological and cardiovascular impairment to leukopenia, purpura, hemorrhage, and death

IX. NURSING RESPONSIBILITIES FOR EXPOSURE TO WARFARE AGENTS

A. Be aware that, at first, a bioterrorism attack may resemble a naturally occurring outbreak.

B. Nurses and other health care workers must be prepared to determine what happened, the number of clients who may be affected, and how and when clients will be expected to arrive.

C. It is essential to recognize any changes to the microorganism that may increase its virulence or make it resistant to conventional antibiotics or vaccines.

MORE QUESTIONS ON EVOLVE!

Practice Questions

96. A mother calls a neighborhood nurse and tells the nurse that her 3-year-old child has just ingested liquid furniture polish. The nurse would direct the mother to immediately:
    1. Induce vomiting.
    2. Call an ambulance.
    3. Call the poison control center.
    4. Bring the child to the emergency department.

97. An emergency department nurse receives a telephone call and is informed that a tornado has hit a local residential area and numerous casualties have occurred. The victims will be brought to the emergency department. Which of the following would be the initial nursing action?
    1. Prepare the triage rooms.
    2. Activate the agency disaster plan.
    3. Obtain additional supplies from the central supply department.
    4. Obtain additional nursing staff to assist with treating the casualties.

98. A nurse is caring for a client with a health care–associated infection caused by methicillin-resistant *Staphylococcus aureus* who is on contact precautions. The nurse prepares to provide colostomy care to the client. Which of the following protective items will be required to perform this procedure?
    1. Gloves and a gown
    2. Gloves and goggles
    3. Gloves, a gown, and goggles
    4. Gloves, a gown, and shoe protectors

99. The nurse would institute which precautions for a client diagnosed with *Clostridium difficile?*
    1. Droplet
    2. Contact
    3. Airborne
    4. Neutropenic

100. A nurse enters a client's room and finds that the wastebasket is on fire. The nurse immediately assists the client out of the room. The next nursing action would be to:
    1. Call for help.
    2. Extinguish the fire.
    3. Activate the fire alarm.
    4. Confine the fire by closing the room door.

101. A nurse enters the nursing lounge and discovers that a chair is on fire. The nurse activates the alarm, closes the lounge door, and obtains the fire extinguisher to extinguish the fire. The nurse pulls the pin on the fire extinguisher. The next action would be to:
    1. Aim at the base of the fire.
    2. Squeeze the handle on the extinguisher.
    3. Sweep the fire from side to side with the extinguisher.
    4. Sweep the fire from top to bottom with the extinguisher.

102. A nurse obtains a prescription from the physician to restrain a client using a jacket (security) restraint and instructs the nursing assistant to apply the restraint to the client. Which of the following observations, if made by the nurse, would indicate the inappropriate application of the restraint?
    1. A safety knot in the restraint strap
    2. The restraint straps are safely secured to the side rails.
    3. The jacket restraint strap does not tighten when force is applied against it.
    4. The jacket restraint is secure, and two fingers can easily slide between the restraint and the client's skin.

103. A nurse is caring for a client who has hand restraints. The nurse assesses the skin integrity of the restrained hands:
    1. Every 2 hours
    2. Every 3 hours
    3. Every 4 hours
    4. Every 30 minutes

104. A nurse is assisting with planning care for a client with an internal radiation implant. Which of the following should be included in the plan of care? **Select all that apply.**

- ❏ 1. Wearing gloves when emptying the client's bedpan
- ❏ 2. Keeping all linens in the room until the implant is removed
- ❏ 3. Wearing a film (dosimeter) badge when in the client's room
- ❏ 4. Wearing a lead apron when providing direct care to the client
- ❏ 5. Placing the client in a semiprivate room at the end of the hallway

105. A community health nurse is conducting a teaching session about terrorism with members of the community and discussing information regarding anthrax. The nurse tells those attending that anthrax can be transmitted via which route(s)? **Select all that apply.**

- ❏ 1. Skin
- ❏ 2. Kissing
- ❏ 3. Inhalation
- ❏ 4. Gastrointestinal
- ❏ 5. Direct contact with an infected individual
- ❏ 6. Sexual contact with an infected individual

ANSWERS

96. 3

Rationale: If a poisoning occurs, the poison control center should be contacted immediately. Vomiting should not be induced without instructions to do so, if the victim is unconscious, or the substance ingested is a strong corrosive or petroleum product. Bringing the child to the emergency department or calling an ambulance would not be the initial action, because this would delay treatment. The poison control center may advise the mother to bring the child to the emergency department; if this is the case, the mother should call an ambulance.

Test-Taking Strategy: Use the process of elimination. Note the strategic word "immediately" in the question. Eliminate options 2 and 4, because these options will delay treatment. Recalling that vomiting should not be induced if a corrosive substance was ingested will assist you with eliminating option 1. Review poison control measures if you had difficulty with this question.

Level of Cognitive Ability: Applying
Client Needs: Physiological Integrity
Integrated Process: Nursing Process/Implementation
Content Area: Fundamental Skills: Safety/Infection Control
Reference: deWit, p. 1081. 2009.

97. 2

Rationale: During a widespread disaster, many people will be brought to the emergency department for treatment. Although options 1, 3, and 4 may be components of preparing for the casualties, the initial nursing action must be to activate the disaster plan.

Test-Taking Strategy: Note the strategic word "initial," and note that option 2 is the umbrella option. Review the procedures related to the management of a disaster if you had difficulty with this question.

Level of Cognitive Ability: Applying
Client Needs: Safe and Effective Care Environment
Integrated Process: Nursing Process/Implementation
Content Area: Fundamental Skills: Safety/Infection Control
References: Christensen, Kockrow, pp. 361–362. 2011. *Foundations of nursing.*
deWit, pp. 1053–1054. 2009.

98. 3

Rationale: Goggles are worn to protect the mucous membranes of the eye during interventions that may produce splashes of blood, body fluids, secretions, and excretions. In addition, contact precautions require the use of gloves, and a gown should be worn if direct client contact is anticipated. Shoe protectors are not necessary.

Test-Taking Strategy: Note the strategic words "contact precautions" and "colostomy." Visualize the procedure for performing colostomy care and use the process of elimination to determine the items required to care for this client. Review contact precautions if you had difficulty with this question.

Level of Cognitive Ability: Applying
Client Needs: Safe and Effective Care Environment
Integrated Process: Nursing Process/Implementation
Content Area: Fundamental Skills: Safety/Infection Control
Reference: Christensen, Kockrow, p. 286. 2011. *Foundations of nursing.*

99. 2

Rationale: Contact precautions are necessary for colonization or infection with a multi-drug resistant organism. This includes enteric infection with *Clostridium difficile*. Droplet or airborne precautions are not necessary because the organism is not transferred via the respiratory route. Neutropenic precautions are used when the client needs protection from contracting an infection from others.

Test-Taking Strategy: Use the process of elimination and eliminate options 1 and 3 first because they are comparable or alike. To select from the remaining options think about the route of transmission of this infection to answer correctly. Review care of a client with *Clostridium difficile* if you had difficulty with this question.

Level of Cognitive Ability: Applying
Client Needs: Safe and Effective Care Environment
Integrated Process: Nursing Process/Implementation
Content Area: Fundamental Skills: Safety/Infection Control
Reference: Christensen, Kockrow, p. 286. 2011. *Foundations of nursing.*

100. 3

Rationale: The order of priority in the event of a fire is to rescue the clients who are in immediate danger. The next step is to

activate the fire alarm. The fire is then confined by closing all doors. Finally, the fire is extinguished.
Test-Taking Strategy: Note the strategic word "next." Remember the mnemonic *RACE* to help you to prioritize in the event of a fire: R = Rescue clients who are in immediate danger; A = Alarm, sound the alarm; C = Confine the fire by closing all doors; E = Extinguish or evacuate. Review fire safety procedures if you had difficulty with this question.
Level of Cognitive Ability: Applying
Client Needs: Safe and Effective Care Environment
Integrated Process: Nursing Process/Implementation
Content Area: Fundamental Skills: Safety/Infection Control
Reference: Christensen, Kockrow, pp. 357–359. 2011. *Foundations of nursing.*

101. 1

Rationale: A fire can be extinguished by using a fire extinguisher. To use the extinguisher, the pin is pulled first. The extinguisher should then be aimed at the base of the fire. The handle of the extinguisher is squeezed, and the fire is extinguished by sweeping from side to side to coat the area evenly.
Test-Taking Strategy: Note the strategic word "next." Remember the mnemonic *PASS* to prioritize in the use of a fire extinguisher: P = Pull the pin; A = Aim at the base of the fire; S = Squeeze the handle; S = Sweep from side to side to coat the area evenly. Review the procedures related to the use of a fire extinguisher if you had difficulty with this question.
Level of Cognitive Ability: Applying
Client Needs: Safe and Effective Care Environment
Integrated Process: Nursing Process/Implementation
Content Area: Fundamental Skills: Safety/Infection Control
Reference: Christensen, Kockrow, pp. 358–359. 2011. *Foundations of nursing.*

102. 2

Rationale: A half-bow or safety knot should be used when applying a restraint, because it does not tighten when force is applied against it, and it allows for the quick and easy removal of the restraint in case of an emergency. The restraint strap is secured to the bed frame (never to the side rail) to avoid accidental injury in case the side rail is released. The jacket restraint should be secure, and one to two fingers should easily slide between the restraint and the client's skin.
Test-Taking Strategy: Note the strategic word "inappropriate." This indicates that you are looking for an option that identifies an inaccurate measure related to the application of restraints. The words "secured to the side rails" in option 2 should direct you to this option as an inappropriate action. Review the guidelines related to the application of restraints if you had difficulty with this question
Level of Cognitive Ability: Evaluating
Client Needs: Safe and Effective Care Environment

Integrated Process: Teaching and Learning
Content Area: Fundamental Skills: Safety/Infection Control
References: Christensen, Kockrow, pp. 350–351. 2011. *Foundations of nursing.*
Linton, pp. 324–326. 2012.

103. 4

Rationale: The nurse needs to assess restraints and skin integrity every 30 minutes. Therefore options 1, 2, and 3 are incorrect. Agency guidelines regarding the use of restraints should always be followed.
Test-Taking Strategy: Use the process of elimination. In this situation, it is best to select the option that identifies the most frequent time frame. Review the guidelines related to the use of restraints if you had difficulty with this question.
Level of Cognitive Ability: Applying
Client Needs: Safe and Effective Care Environment
Integrated Process: Nursing Process/Implementation
Content Area: Fundamental Skills: Safety/Infection Control
Reference: deWit, p. 198. 2009.

104. 1, 2, 3, 4

Rationale: A private room with a private bath is essential if a client has an internal radiation implant. This is necessary to prevent the accidental exposure of other clients to radiation. The remaining options identify interventions that are necessary for a client with a radiation device.
Test-Taking Strategy: Focus on the subject, interventions to be included in the plan of care for a client with an internal radiation implant. Read each option carefully and think about the concerns related to exposure. Noting the word "semi-private" will assist in eliminating this option as a safe one. Review radiation safety principles if you had difficulty with this question.
Level of Cognitive Ability: Applying
Client Needs: Safe and Effective Care Environment
Integrated Process: Nursing Process/Planning
Content Area: Fundamental Skills: Safety/Infection Control
Reference: deWit, p. 175. 2009.

105. 1, 3, 4

Rationale: Anthrax is caused by *Bacillus anthracis*, and it can be contracted through the digestive system, abrasions in the skin, or inhalation. It cannot be spread from person to person.
Test-Taking Strategy: Knowledge regarding the methods of contracting anthrax is needed to answer this question. Remember that it is not spread by person-to-person contact. Review information related to anthrax infection if you had difficulty with this question.
Level of Cognitive Ability: Applying
Client Needs: Safe and Effective Care Environment
Integrated Process: Teaching and Learning
Content Area: Fundamental Skills: Safety/Infection Control
Reference: deWit, pp. 1065–1067. 2009.

15

Medication and Intravenous Administration

PYRAMID TERMS

conversion The first step in the calculation of a medication problem.

generic name Also known as the non–brand name of the medication or the U.S. adopted name; each medication has only one generic name

medication reconciliation An organized process to avoid medication errors by comparing the client's medication prescriptions with all the medications that the client was previously taking

milliequivalent(s) An expression of the number of grams of a medication contained in 1 mL of a solution; abbreviated mEq

parenteral Given by injection; may be intravenous, intramuscular, subcutaneous, or intradermal

reconstitution Dissolving a powder in a sterile diluent before use; usually sterile water or normal saline is used

trade name Also called the brand name; usually printed on the label in large, bold letters

unit A measurement of a medication in terms of its action rather than its physical weight

PYRAMID TO SUCCESS

When a medication or intravenous (IV) calculation question is presented, a nurse should always use the appropriate formula to solve the problem. Shortcuts should not be used when making these calculations. The problem and the answer should be expressed in the correct units of measure. Be careful with decimal points. It is important to place the decimal points in the correct places, or the answer will be incorrect. When solving a medication calculation problem, the nurse determines whether the answer is within reason and makes sense. In the clinical setting, the nurse should always seek assistance if he or she is unsure about the accuracy of a calculation.

On the NCLEX-PN, the fill-in-the-blank questions may require that you calculate a medication dose or an IV flow rate. You will be provided with an optional on-screen calculator for these medication and IV

problems. Even if you use the calculator to calculate dosages and flow rates, it is important to check the calculation before selecting an option or typing in the answer. Follow the formula, place the decimal points in the correct places, and check the accuracy of the calculation. Remember, practice makes perfect!

CLIENT NEEDS

Safe and Effective Care Environment

- Calculating medication doses and IV flow rates
- Maintaining clients' rights
- Handling hazardous or infectious materials
- Maintaining medical and surgical asepsis
- Maintaining standard and other precautions
- Preventing errors

Health Promotion and Maintenance

- Collecting physical data
- Preventing disease
- Respecting lifestyle choices
- Teaching the client about prescribed medication(s) or IV therapy

Psychosocial Integrity

- Identifying support systems
- Identifying the cultural, religious, and spiritual influences on health
- Interacting therapeutically with the client and family
- Identifying the use of coping mechanisms

Physiological Integrity

- Administering medications and IV therapy
- Identifying the adverse effects of and contraindications to medication or IV therapy
- Monitoring for the expected and unexpected effects of pharmacological therapy
- Monitoring laboratory values

I. MEDICATION ADMINISTRATION (Box 15-1)

II. DRUG-MEASUREMENT SYSTEMS

A. Metric system (Box 15-2)
1. The basic units of metric measurement are meter, liter, and gram
2. Meter measures length
3. Liter measures volume
4. Gram measures weight

B. Aothecary and household systems (Box 15-3)
1. Apothecary measures such as dram, grains, and minim are not commonly used in the clinical setting.
2. Commonly used household measures include drop, teaspoon, tablespoon, ounce, pint, and cup.

C. Additional common drug measures
1. Milliequivalent (mEq)
   a. The milliequivalent is an expression of the number of grams of a medication contained in 1 mL of a solution.
   b. For example: the measure of potassium is given in milliequivalents such as 5 mEq of potassium
2. Unit
   a. Measures a medication in terms of its action rather than its physical weight
   b. For example: Penicillin, heparin sodium, and insulin are measured in units

III. CONVERSIONS

A. Conversion between metric units (Box 15-4)
1. The metric system is a decimal system; therefore conversions between the units in this system can be done by either dividing or multiplying by 1000 or by moving the decimal point three places to the right or three places to the left.
2. In the metric system, to convert larger to smaller, multiply by 1000 or move the decimal point three places to the right; for example, 1 g = 1000 mg.
3. In the metric system, to convert smaller to larger, divide by 1000 or move the decimal point three places to the left; for example, 1000 mg = 1 g.

B. Conversion between household and metric systems
1. Conversions between the metric and household systems are equivalent—not equal—measures.
2. Conversion to equivalent measures between systems is necessary when a medication prescription is written in one system but the medication label is given in another.

Box 15-1 Medication Administration

Check the medication prescription.
Compare the client's medication prescription with all the medications that the client was previously taking (medication reconciliation)
Ask the client about a history of allergies.
Determine the client's current condition and the purpose of the prescribed medication or intravenous solution.
Determine the client's understanding regarding the purpose of the prescribed medication or intravenous solution.
Plan to teach the client about the medication and about self-administration at home.
Identify and address social, cultural, and religious concerns that the client may have about taking the medication.
Determine the need for conversion when preparing a dose of medication for administration to the client.
Check the six rights: right medication, right dose, right client, right route, right time and frequency, and right documentation.
Check the client's vital signs before administering the medication.
Identify any food or medication interactions before administering the medication
Document the administration of the prescribed therapy and client's response to the therapy.

Box 15-2 Metric System

Abbreviations	Equivalents
meter: m	1 mcg = 0.000001 g
liter: L	1 mg = 1000 mcg or 0.001 g
milliliter: mL	1 g = 1000 mg
kilogram: kg	1 kg = 1000 g
gram: g	1 kg = 2.2 lb
milligram: mg	1 mL = 0.001 L
microgram: mcg	

Box 15-3 Apothecary and Household Systems

Abbreviations	Equivalents
Apothecary (Weight)	1 gr = 60 or 65 mg
grain: gr	5 gr = 300 or 325 mg
ounce: oz	15 gr = 1000 mg or 1 g
	$^1/_{150}$ gr = 0.4 mg
Household (Volume)	1 fl oz = 30 mL
drops: gtt	1 T = 15 mL or 3 tsp
teaspoon: t or tsp	1 t or tsp = 5 mL
tablespoon: T or tbs	1 C = 8 fl oz
fluid ounce: fl oz	1 qt = 946 mL or 0.946 L
cup: C	1 qt = 2 pt or 32 fl oz
pint: pt	1 pt = 16 fl oz
quart: qt	16 oz = 1 lb
	2.2 lb = 1 kg
Household (Weight)	
pound: lb	

3. Medications are not always prescribed and prepared in the same system of measurement. Therefore it is necessary to convert units from one system to another.
4. Calculating equivalents between two systems may be done by using the method of ratio and proportion (Boxes 15-5 and 15-6).

⚠ Conversion is the first step in the calculation of dosages.

IV. CELSIUS AND FAHRENHEIT TEMPERATURES (Box 15-7)

A. To convert Fahrenheit to Celsius, first subtract 32, and then divide the result by 1.8.
B. To convert Celsius to Fahrenheit, first multiply by 1.8, and then add 32.

V. MEDICATION LABELS

A. A medication label will contain both the generic name and the trade name of the medication.
B. Always check the expiration dates on medication labels.

VI. MEDICATION PRESCRIPTIONS (Box 15-8)

A. In a medication prescription, the name of the medication is written first, followed by the dosage, route, and frequency.
B. Medication prescriptions are written according to the accepted abbreviations identified by The Joint Commission while also following the agency guidelines.

⚠ If the nurse has any questions about or sees inconsistencies in the written prescription, the nurse must contact the person who wrote the prescription immediately and must verify the prescription.

Box 15-4 Conversion between Metric Units

Problem 1
Convert 2 g to milligrams.

Solution
Change a larger unit to a smaller unit.
2 g = 2000 mg (moving decimal three places to right)

Problem 2
Convert 250 mL to liters.

Solution
Change a smaller unit to a larger unit.
250 mL = 0.25 L (moving decimal three places to left)

Box 15-6 Calculating Equivalents between Two Systems by Ratio and Proportion

Calculating equivalents between two systems may be done by using the method of ratio and proportion.

Problem
The physician prescribes nitroglycerin, grain (gr) $^1/_{150}$. The medication label reads 0.4 milligram (mg) per tablet. The nurse prepares to administer how many tablets to the client?

Ratio and Proportion Formula
H (on hand) :V (vehicle) :: (=) (desired dose) : X
1 gr : 60 mg :: $^1/_{150}$ gr : X mg
$60 \times ^1/_{150} = X$
X = 0.4 mg (1 tablet)

Box 15-5 Ratio and Proportion

Ratio: The relationship between two numbers, separated by a colon; for example, 1:2 (1 to 2).
Proportion: The relationship between two ratios, separated by a double colon (::) or an equal sign (=).
Formula: H (on hand) : V (vehicle) :: (=) (desired dose) : X (unknown)
To solve a ratio and proportion problem: The middle numbers (means) are multiplied and the end numbers (extremes) are multiplied.

Sample Problem
H = 1
V = 2
Desired dose = 3
X = unknown
Set up the formula: 1 : 2 :: 3 : X
Solve: Multiply means and extremes.
1X = 6
X = 6

Box 15-7 Celsius and Fahrenheit Temperature

Fahrenheit to Celsius
To convert Fahrenheit to Celsius, subtract 32 and divide the result by 1.8.
Formula:

$$C = \frac{(F - 32)}{1.8}$$

Celsius to Fahrenheit
To convert Celsius to Fahrenheit, multiply by 1.8 and add 32.
Formula:

$$F = (1.8 \times C) + 32$$

VII. ORAL MEDICATIONS

A. Scored tablets contain an indented mark to be used for breaking the tablet into partial dosages. When necessary, scored tablets (those marked for division) can be divided into halves or quarters.

B. Enteric-coated tablets and sustained-released capsules delay absorption until the medication reaches the small intestine. These medications should not be crushed.

C. Capsules contain a powdered or oily medication in a gelatin cover.

D. Oral liquids are supplied in solution form and contain a specific amount of medication in a given amount of solution, as stated on the label.

E. The medicine cup (Figure 15-1)
1. Has a capacity of 30 mL or 1 ounce
2. Used for oral liquids
3. Calibrated to measure teaspoons, tablespoons, and ounces
4. To pour accurately, hold the medication cup at eye level, and then line up the measure that is needed and pour.

F. Volumes of less than 5 mL are measured by using a syringe with the needle removed.

⚠ A calibrated dropper is used for giving medicine to children or for adding small amounts of liquid medication to water or juice. Calibrations are in milliliters or drops.

Box 15-8 Medication Prescriptions

Name of client
Date and time when prescription is written
Name of medication to be given
Dosage of medication
Medication route
Time and frequency of administration
Signature of person who wrote the prescription

▲ **FIGURE 15-1** Medicine cup. (From Kee, J., & Marshall, S. [2009]. *Clinical calculations: With applications to general and specialty areas* [6th ed.]. Philadelphia: Saunders.)

VIII. PARENTERAL MEDICATIONS

A. *Parenteral* always means injection route, and parenteral medications are administered by IV, intramuscular, intradermal, or subcutaneous routes

B. Parenteral medications are packaged in single-use ampules, single- and multiple-use rubber-stoppered vials, and premeasured syringes and cartridges.

C. The nurse should not administer more than 3 mL per intramuscular injection site or 1 mL per subcutaneous injection site. Larger volumes are difficult for an injection site to absorb and, if prescribed, need to be verified.

D. Always question and verify excessively large or small volumes of medication.

E. The standard 3-mL syringe is used to measure most injectable medications. It is calibrated in tenths (0.1) of a milliliter.

F. The calibrations on a syringe are read from the top of the rubber stopper on the syringe (i.e., not the middle section and not the bottom ring) (Figure 15-2).

G. Prefilled medication cartridge
1. The medication cartridge slips into the cartridge holder, which provides a plunger for the injection of the medication.
2. Designed to provide sufficient capacity to allow for the addition of a second medication when combined dosages are prescribed
3. The prefilled medication cartridge is to be used once and discarded. If a nurse is to give less than the full single dose provided, he or she needs to discard the extra amount before giving the client the injection, in accordance with agency policies and procedures.

⚠ Always question and verify excessively large or small volumes of medication.

H. Standard medication doses for adults are to be rounded to the nearest tenth (0.1) of a milliliter and measured on the milliliter scale; for example, 1.26 mL is rounded to 1.3 mL.

I. When volumes of more than 3 mL are required, a 5-mL syringe may be used. These syringes are calibrated in fifths (Figure 15-3). Other syringes that may be

▲ **FIGURE 15-2** Parts of a syringe. (From Kee, J., & Marshall, S. [2009]. *Clinical calculations: With applications to general and specialty areas* [6th ed.]. Philadelphia: Saunders.)

available are 10-, 20-, and 50-mL and may be used for medication administration requiring dilution.

J. Syringes larger than 10 mL are calibrated in full milliliter measures.

K. Tuberculin syringe (Figure 15-4)

1. Holds a total capacity of 1 mL; used to measure small or critical amounts of medication, such as allergen extract, vaccine, or a child's medication

2. It is calibrated in hundredths (0.01) of a milliliter, with each one tenth (0.1) marked on the metric scale.

L. Insulin syringe (Figure 15-5)

1. The standard unit-100 insulin syringe is used to measure unit-100 insulin only. It is calibrated for a total of 100 units or 1 mL. Low-dose insulin syringes (½-mL sizes) may be used when administering smaller doses.

2. Insulin should not be measured in any other type of syringe.

3. When the insulin prescription states to combine regular and neutral protamine Hagedorn (NPH) insulin, remember to draw regular insulin first and then to draw the NPH insulin.

M. Safety needles: Contain shielding devices that are attached to the syringe and slipped over the needle; their use reduces the incidence of needle stick injuries (Figure 15-6).

IX. INJECTABLE MEDICATIONS IN POWDER FORM

A. Some medications become unstable when stored in solution form and are therefore packaged in powder form.

B. Powders must be dissolved with a sterile diluent before use. Usually sterile water or normal saline is used. The dissolving procedure is called "reconstitution" (Box 15-9).

X. CALCULATING THE CORRECT DOSAGE (Box 15-10)

A. When calculating dosages of oral medications, check the calculation, and question the prescription if the calculation calls for more than three tablets.

B. When calculating dosages of parenteral medications, check the calculation, and question the prescription if the amount to be given is too large a dose.

C. Be sure that all measures are in the same system and that all units are in the same size, converting them when necessary. Carefully consider the reasonable amount of the medication that should be administered.

D. Round standard injection doses to tenths, and measure in a 3-mL syringe.

E. Round small, critical, or children's doses to hundredths, and measure in a 1-mL tuberculin syringe.

⚠ Regardless of the source of the error, if a nurse gives an incorrect dose, he or she is legally responsible for the action.

XI. INTRAVENOUS FLOW RATES (Box 15-11)

A. Monitor IVs frequently, even when being administered via an electronic infusion device and according to the agency's policy.

▲ **FIGURE 15-3** Five-milliliter syringe. (From Kee, J., & Marshall, S. [2009]. *Clinical calculations: With applications to general and specialty areas* [6th ed.]. Philadelphia: Saunders.)

▲ **FIGURE 15-4** Tuberculin syringe. (From Kee, J., & Marshall, S. [2009]. *Clinical calculations: With applications to general and specialty areas* [6th ed.]. Philadelphia: Saunders.)

▲ **FIGURE 15-5** Insulin syringe. (From Kee, J., & Marshall, S. [2009]. *Clinical calculations: With applications to general and specialty areas* [6th ed.]. Philadelphia: Saunders.)

B. If an IV is running behind schedule, collaborate with the health care provider (HCP) to determine the client's ability to tolerate an increased flow rate, particularly if the client has cardiac, pulmonary, renal, or neurological conditions.

▲ **FIGURE 15-6** BD SafetyGlide needle. (From Kee, J., & Marshall, S. [2009]. *Clinical calculations: With applications to general and specialty areas* [6th ed.]. Philadelphia: Saunders. Courtesy and © Becton, Dickinson, and Company; Franklin Lakes, NJ.)

Box 15-9 Reconstitution

When reconstituting a medication, locate the instructions on the label or in the vial package insert, and read and follow the directions carefully.

The instructions will state the volume of diluent to be used and the resulting volume of the reconstituted medication.

Often a powdered medication adds volume to the solution in addition to the amount of diluent added.

When reconstituting a multiple-dose vial, label the medication vial with the date and time of preparation, your initials, and the date of expiration.

It is also important to label the strength per volume.

The total volume of the prepared solution will always exceed the volume of the diluent added.

Box 15-10 Standard Formula for Calculating a Medication Dosage

$$\frac{D}{A} \times Q = X$$

D (desired) is the dosage that the HCP prescribed.

A (available) is the dosage strength as stated on the medication label.

Q (quantity) is the volume or form in which the dosage strength is available, such as tablets, capsules, or milliliters.

C. Whenever a prescribed IV rate is increased, the nurse should assess the client for increased heart rate, increased respirations, or increased lung congestion, which could indicate fluid overload.

D. IV fluids are most frequently prescribed on the basis of milliliters (mL) per hour to be administered.

E. The volume per hour prescribed is administered by adjusting the rate at which the IV infuses, which is counted in drops (gtt) per minute.

F. Most flow-rate calculations involve changing mL/ hour into gtt/minute.

⚠ The nurse should never increase the rate (speed up) of an IV infusion to catch up if the infusion is running behind schedule.

G. IV tubing
1. Calibrated in gtt/mL. This calibration is needed for calculating flow rates.
2. A standard or macrodrip set is used for routine adult IV administrations. Depending on the manufacturer and type of tubing, it requires 10, 15, or 20 gtt to equal 1 mL.
3. A minidrip or microdrip set is used when more exact measurements are needed, such as in intensive care and pediatric units.
4. In a minidrip or microdrip set, 60 gtt is equal to 1 mL.
5. The calibration, in gtt/mL, is written on the IV tubing package.

XII. ELECTRONIC INTRAVENOUS FLOW-RATE REGULATORS

A. Pump (Figure 15-7)
1. A pump is different from a controller in that it physically pumps fluids against resistance.

Box 15-11 Formulas for Intravenous Calculations

Flow Rates

$$\frac{\text{Total volume} \times \text{drop factor}}{\text{Time in minutes}} = \text{drops per minute}$$

Infusion Time

$$\frac{\text{Total volume to infuse}}{\text{Milliliters per hour being infused}} = \text{infusion time}$$

Number of Milliliters per Hour

$$\frac{\text{Total volume in milliliters}}{\text{Number of hours}} = \text{number of milliliters per hour}$$

▲ **FIGURE 15-7** Infusion pump. (From Kee, J., & Marshall, S. [2009]. *Clinical calculations: With applications to general and specialty areas* [6th ed.]. Philadelphia: Saunders.)

2. Gravity is not a factor in the use of a pump, and the height of the IV solution container is not a critical factor.
3. The flow rate on a pump is set in mL/hour.
4. The nurse should continue to assess the amount of IV solution in the IV container and monitor the pump to ensure the proper functioning of the machine.

MORE QUESTIONS ON EVOLVE!

Practice Questions

❖ **106.** The medication prescribed is hydromorphone hydrochloride (Dilaudid), 3 mg intramuscular every 4 hours as needed. The medication label reads hydromorphone hydrochloride (Dilaudid), 4 mg/1 mL. The nurse prepares to administer how many mL to the client?
Answer: _____ mL

❖ **107.** The medication prescribed is digoxin (Lanoxin), 0.25 mg orally daily. The medication label reads digoxin (Lanoxin), 0.125 mg/tablet. The nurse prepares how many tablet(s) to administer the dose?
Answer: _____ tablet(s)

❖ **108.** The medication prescribed is heparin sodium 650 units subcutaneously every 12 hours. The medication vial reads heparin sodium (Liquaemin), 1000 units/mL. The nurse prepares how many milliliters to administer one dose?
Answer: _____ mL

❖ **109.** The medication prescribed is metoclopramide hydrochloride (Reglan) 10 mg intramuscularly times one dose. The medication label reads metoclopramide hydrochloride (Reglan), 5 mg/mL. The nurse prepares how much medication to administer the dose?
Answer: _____ mL

❖ **110.** The medication prescribed is meperidine hydrochloride (Demerol), 35 mg intramuscularly. The medication label states meperidine hydrochloride (Demerol), 50 mg/mL. The nurse plans to prepare how much medication to administer the dose?
Answer: _____ mL

❖ **111.** The medication prescribed is prochlorperazine (Compazine), 20 mg intramuscular every 4 hours as needed. The medication label states prochlorperazine 10 mg/mL. The nurse prepares how much medication to administer the dose?
Answer: _____ mL

❖ **112.** The medication prescribed is atropine sulfate, 0.4 mg intramuscularly, immediately. The medication label states atropine sulfate, 0.3 mg/0.5 mL. The nurse prepares how much medication to administer the dose? (Round to the nearest tenth position.)
Answer: _____ mL

❖ **113.** The medication prescribed is levodopa (Larodopa), 1 g orally, twice daily. The medication label states levodopa, 500-mg tablets. The nurse prepares to administer how many tablets at the evening dose?
Answer: _____ tablet(s)

❖ **114.** The medication prescribed is zidovudine (AZT), 0.2 g orally every 4 hours. The medication label states zidovudine (AZT), 100-mg tablets. The nurse prepares to administer how many tablets for one dose?
Answer: _____ tablet(s)

❖ **115.** The medication prescribed is atropine sulfate, 0.4 mg. The medication label states atropine sulfate, 0.5 mg/0.5 mL. How many milliliters will the nurse prepare to administer to the client?
Answer: _____ mL

❖ **116.** The medication prescription states to administer Tylenol (acetaminophen) 650 mg orally for a temperature of more than 38° C. The medication bottle states Tylenol (acetaminophen), 325 mg tablets. The nurse takes the client's temperature and notes that it is 101° F. The nurse plans to take which of the following actions?
1. Administer two Tylenol tablets.
2. Administer three Tylenol tablets.

3. Do not administer the Tylenol at this time.
4. Check the client's temperature in 30 minutes.

117. The medication prescription reads phenytoin (Dilantin) 0.2 g orally twice daily. The medication label states 100-mg capsules. A nurse prepares how many capsule(s) to administer one dose?
Answer: _____ mL

118. The intravenous prescription is 1000 mL of 0.9% NaCl (normal saline) to run over 12 hours. The drop factor is 15 gtt/1 mL. The nurse plans to adjust the flow rate to how many gtt/minute? (Round answer to the nearest whole number.)
Answer: _____ gtt/minute

119. The medication is an intramuscular dose of 400,000 units of penicillin G benzathine (Bicillin). The label on the 10-mL ampule sent from the pharmacy reads penicillin G benzathine (Bicillin) 300,000 units/mL. The nurse prepares how much medication to administer the correct dose? (Round answer to the nearest tenth position.)
Answer: _____ mL

120. The intravenous prescription is 3000 mL of 5% dextrose (D5W) to run over a 24-hour period. The drop factor is 10 gtt/1 mL. The nurse plans to adjust the flow rate to how many gtt/minute? (Round answer to the nearest whole number.)
Answer: _____ gtt/minute

ANSWERS

106. 0.75
Rationale: Follow the formula for dosage calculation.
Formula:
$$\frac{\text{Desired} \times \text{mL}}{\text{Available}} = \text{mL per dose}$$
$$\frac{3 \text{ mg} \times 1 \text{ mL}}{4 \text{ mg}} = 0.75 \text{ mL per dose}$$

Test-Taking Strategy: Follow the formula for the calculation of the correct dose. Focus on the strategic information: the dose prescribed and the dose available. After you have performed the calculation, verify your answer using a calculator. Review medication calculations if you had difficulty with this question.
Level of Cognitive Ability: Applying
Client Needs: Physiological Integrity
Integrated Process: Nursing Process/Planning
Content Area: Fundamental Skills: Medications/Blood & IV Therapy
Reference: Kee, p. 86. 2009.

107. 2
Rationale: Follow the formula for dosage calculation.
Formula:
$$\frac{\text{Desired} \times \text{tablet(s)}}{\text{Available}} = \text{tablet(s) per dose}$$
$$\frac{0.25 \text{ mg} \times 1 \text{ tablet}}{0.125 \text{ mg}} = 2 \text{ tablets}$$

Test-Taking Strategy: Follow the formula for the calculation of the correct dose. Focus on the strategic information: the dose prescribed and the dose available. After you have performed the calculation, verify your answer using a calculator. Review medication calculations if you had difficulty with this question.
Level of Cognitive Ability: Applying
Client Needs: Physiological Integrity
Integrated Process: Nursing Process/Planning
Content Area: Fundamental Skills: Medications/Blood & IV Therapy
Reference: Ogden, p. 204. 2012.

108. 0.65
Rationale: Follow the formula for dosage calculation.
Formula:
$$\frac{\text{Desired} \times \text{mL}}{\text{Available}} = \text{mL per dose}$$
$$\frac{650 \text{ units} \times 1 \text{ mL}}{1000 \text{ units}} = 0.65 \text{ mL}$$

Test-Taking Strategy: Follow the formula for the calculation of the correct dose. Focus on the strategic information: the dose prescribed and the dose available. After you have performed the calculation, verify your answer using a calculator. Review medication calculations if you had difficulty with this question.
Level of Cognitive Ability: Applying
Client Needs: Physiological Integrity
Integrated Process: Nursing Process/Planning
Content Area: Fundamental Skills: Medications/Blood & IV Therapy
Reference: Kee, p. 86. 2009.

109. 2
Rationale: Follow the formula for dosage calculation.
Formula:
$$\frac{\text{Desired} \times \text{mL}}{\text{Available}} = \text{mL per dose}$$
$$\frac{10 \text{ mg} \times 1 \text{ mL}}{5 \text{ mg}} = 2 \text{ mL}$$

Test-Taking Strategy: Follow the formula for the calculation of the correct dose. Focus on the strategic information: the dose prescribed and the dose available. After you have performed the calculation, verify your answer using a calculator. Review medication calculations if you had difficulty with this question.
Level of Cognitive Ability: Applying
Client Needs: Physiological Integrity
Integrated Process: Nursing Process/Planning
Content Area: Fundamental Skills: Medications/Blood & IV Therapy
Reference: Ogden, p. 204. 2012.

❖ **110. 0.7**

Rationale: Follow the formula for dosage calculations.

Formula:

$$\frac{\text{Desired} \times \text{mL}}{\text{Available}} = \text{mL per dose}$$

$$\frac{35 \text{ mg} \times 1 \text{ mL}}{50 \text{ mg}} = 0.7 \text{ mL}$$

Test-Taking Strategy: Follow the formula for the calculation of the correct dose. Focus on the strategic information: the dose prescribed and the dose available. After you have performed the calculation, verify your answer using a calculator. Review medication calculations if you had difficulty with this question.

Level of Cognitive Ability: Applying
Client Needs: Physiological Integrity
Integrated Process: Nursing Process/Planning
Content Area: Fundamental Skills: Medications/Blood & IV Therapy
Reference: Kee, p. 86. 2009.

❖ **111. 2**

Rationale: Follow the formula for dosage calculation.

Formula:

$$\frac{\text{Desired} \times \text{mL}}{\text{Available}} = \text{mL per dose}$$

$$\frac{20 \text{ mg} \times 1 \text{ mL}}{10 \text{ mg}} = 2 \text{ mL}$$

Test-Taking Strategy: Follow the formula for the calculation of the correct dose. Focus on the strategic information: the dose prescribed and the dose available. After you have performed the calculation, verify your answer using a calculator. Review medication calculations if you had difficulty with this question.

Level of Cognitive Ability: Applying
Client Needs: Physiological Integrity
Integrated Process: Nursing Process/Planning
Content Area: Fundamental Skills: Medications/Blood & IV Therapy
Reference: Ogden, p. 204. 2012.

❖ **112. 0.7**

Rationale: Follow the formula for dosage calculation.

Formula:

$$\frac{\text{Desired} \times \text{mL}}{\text{Available}} = \text{mL per dose}$$

$$\frac{0.4 \text{ mg} \times 0.5 \text{ mL}}{0.3 \text{ mg}} = 0.66, \text{ or } 0.7 \text{ mL}$$

Test-Taking Strategy: Follow the formula for the calculation of the correct dose. Focus on the strategic information: the dose prescribed and the dose available. After you have performed the calculation, verify your answer using a calculator, and remember to round to the nearest tenth. Review medication calculations if you had difficulty with this question.

Level of Cognitive Ability: Applying
Client Needs: Physiological Integrity
Integrated Process: Nursing Process/Planning
Content Area: Fundamental Skills: Medications/Blood & IV Therapy
Reference: Kee, p. 86. 2009.

❖ **113. 2**

Rationale: Convert 1 g to milligrams. In the metric system, to convert larger to smaller, multiply by 1000, or move the decimal three places to the right; therefore 1 g = 1000 mg.

Formula:

$$\frac{\text{Desired} \times \text{tablet(s)}}{\text{Available}} = \text{tablet(s) per dose}$$

$$\frac{1000 \text{ mg} \times 1 \text{ tablet}}{500 \text{ mg}} = 2 \text{ tablets}$$

Test-Taking Strategy: For this medication calculation problem, it is necessary to first convert grams to milligrams. Follow the formula for conversion, and read the question carefully. After you have performed the calculation, verify your answer using a calculator. Review medication calculations and conversions if you had difficulty with this question.

Level of Cognitive Ability: Applying
Client Needs: Physiological Integrity
Integrated Process: Nursing Process/Planning
Content Area: Fundamental Skills: Medications/Blood & IV Therapy
Reference: Ogden, p. 204. 2012.

❖ **114. 2**

Rationale: Convert 0.2 g to mg. In the metric system, to convert larger to smaller, multiply by 1000, or move the decimal three places to the right; therefore 0.2 g = 200 mg.

Formula:

$$\frac{\text{Desired} \times \text{tablet(s)}}{\text{Available}} = \text{tablet(s) per dose}$$

$$\frac{200 \text{ mg} \times 1 \text{ tablet}}{100 \text{ mg}} = 2 \text{ tablets}$$

Test-Taking Strategy: For this medication calculation problem, it is necessary to first convert grams to milligrams. Follow the formula for conversion, and read the question carefully. After you have performed the calculation, verify your answer using a calculator. Review medication calculations and conversions if you had difficulty with this question.

Level of Cognitive Ability: Applying
Client Needs: Physiological Integrity
Integrated Process: Nursing Process/Planning
Content Area: Fundamental Skills: Medications/Blood & IV Therapy
Reference: Kee, p. 86. 2009.

❖ **115. 0.4**

Rationale: Follow the formula for dosage calculation.

Formula:

$$\frac{\text{Desired} \times \text{mL}}{\text{Available}} = \text{mL per dose}$$

$$\frac{0.4 \text{ mg} \times 0.5 \text{ mL}}{0.5 \text{ mg}} = 0.4 \text{ mL}$$

Test-Taking Strategy: Follow the formula for the calculation of the correct dose. Focus on the strategic information: the dose prescribed and the dose available. After you have performed the calculation, verify your answer using a calculator. Review medication calculations if you had difficulty with this question.

Level of Cognitive Ability: Applying
Client Needs: Physiological Integrity
Integrated Process: Nursing Process/Planning
Content Area: Fundamental Skills: Medications/Blood & IV Therapy
Reference: Ogden, p. 204. 2012.

116. 1

Rationale: Convert Fahrenheit to Celsius, and then calculate the dose to be administered.
Step 1: Conversion of Fahrenheit to Celsius
Formula: To convert Fahrenheit to Celsius, subtract 32, and divide the result by 1.8:

   C = (101 − 32) = 69, divided by 1.8 = 38.3°

Step 2: Dosage calculation
Formula:

$$\frac{Desired \times tablet(s)}{Available} = tablet(s)\ per\ dose$$

$$\frac{650\ mg \times 1\ tablet}{325\ mg} = 2\ tablets;\ therefore\ option\ 1\ is\ the\ correct\ answer.$$

Test-Taking Strategy: Focus on what the question is asking you to determine. For this medication calculation problem, it is necessary to convert Fahrenheit to Celsius. Follow the formula for conversion, and then perform the medication calculation. After you have performed the calculation, verify your answer using a calculator. Review these formulas if you had difficulty with this question.
Level of Cognitive Ability: Applying
Client Needs: Physiological Integrity
Integrated Process: Nursing Process/Planning
Content Area: Fundamental Skills: Medications/Blood & IV Therapy
Reference: Ogden, p. 135. 2012.

❖ 117. 2

Rationale: You must convert 0.2 g to milligrams. In the metric system, to convert larger to smaller, multiply by 1000 or move the decimal three places to the right. Therefore, 0.2 g equals 200 mg. After conversion from grams to milligrams, use the formula to calculate the correct dose.
Formula:

$$\frac{Desired \times capsule(s)}{Available} = capsule(s)\ per\ dose$$

$$\frac{200\ mg \times 1\ capsule}{100\ mg} = 2\ capsules$$

Test-Taking Strategy: In this medication calculation problem, first you must convert grams to milligrams. Once you have done the conversion and reread the medication calculation problem, you will know that 2 capsules is the correct answer. Recheck your work using a calculator and make sure that the answer makes sense. If you had difficulty with this question, review the formula for calculating medication doses.
Level of Cognitive Ability: Applying
Client Needs: Physiological Integrity
Integrated Process: Nursing Process/Planning

Content Area: Fundamental Skills: Medications/Blood & IV Therapy
Reference: Kee, Marshall, p. 86. 2009.

118. 21 ❖

Rationale: Use the intravenous (IV) flow rate formula.
Formula:

$$\frac{Total\ volume \times drop\ factor}{Time\ in\ minutes} = drops\ per\ minute$$

$$\frac{1000\ mL \times 15\ gtt}{720\ minutes} = \frac{15,000}{720} = 20.8,\ or\ 21\ drops\ per\ minute$$

Test-Taking Strategy: Follow the formula for calculating an infusion rate for an IV. Be sure to change 12 hours to minutes. After you have performed the calculation, verify your answer using a calculator and remember to round the answer to the nearest whole number. Review the formula for calculating infusion rates if you had difficulty with this question.
Level of Cognitive Ability: Applying
Client Needs: Physiological Integrity
Integrated Process: Nursing Process/Planning
Content Area: Fundamental Skills: Medications/Blood & IV Therapy
Reference: Kee, p. 223. 2009.

119. 1.3 ❖

Rationale: Follow the formula for dosage calculation.
Formula:

$$\frac{Desired \times mL}{Available} = mL\ per\ dose$$

$$\frac{400,000\ units \times 1\ mL}{300,000\ units} = 1.3\ mL$$

Test-Taking Strategy: Follow the formula for the calculation of the correct dose. Focus on the strategic information: the dose prescribed and the dose available. After you have performed the calculation, verify your answer using a calculator. Review medication calculations if you had difficulty with this question.
Level of Cognitive Ability: Applying
Client Needs: Physiological Integrity
Integrated Process: Nursing Process/Planning
Content Area: Fundamental Skills: Medications/Blood & IV Therapy
Reference: Kee, p. 86. 2009.

120. 21 ❖

Rationale: Use the intravenous (IV) flow rate formula.
Formula:

$$\frac{Total\ volume \times drop\ factor}{Time\ in\ minutes} = drops\ per\ minute$$

$$\frac{3000\ mL \times 10\ gtt}{1440\ minutes} = \frac{30,000}{1440}$$

$$= 20.8,\ or\ 21\ drops\ per\ minute$$

Test-Taking Strategy: Follow the formula for calculating the infusion rate for an IV. Be sure to change 24 hours to minutes.

After you have performed the calculation, verify your answer using a calculator, and remember to round the answer to the nearest whole number. Review the formula for calculating infusion rates if you had difficulty with this question.

Level of Cognitive Ability: Applying

Client Needs: Physiological Integrity

Integrated Process: Nursing Process/Planning

Content Area: Fundamental Skills: Medications/Blood & IV Therapy

Reference: Kee, p. 223. 2009.

16

Basic Life Support

PYRAMID TERMS

abdominal thrusts A method to relieve a foreign-body airway obstruction

automated external defibrillator (AED) A machine that converts ventricular fibrillation into a perfusing rhythm and that allows for early defibrillation by first responders

basic life support (BLS) A method that provides oxygen to the brain, heart, and other vital organs until help arrives

cardiopulmonary resuscitation (CPR) Another term for basic life support

head tilt–chin lift The preferred method for opening a victim's airway

jaw thrust maneuver The method used to open a victim's airway if a neck injury is suspected

PYRAMID TO SUCCESS

The Pyramid to Success focuses on emergency care guidelines and procedures performed by the health care provider (HCP). These include cardiopulmonary resuscitation (CPR), the abdominal thrust maneuver, and use of the automated external defibrillator. In addition to CPR guidelines for the HCP, the American Heart Association has also developed CPR guidelines for the lay rescuer. For additional information, access the American Heart Association Web site at www. americanheart.org.

CLIENT NEEDS

Safe and Effective Care Environment

- Acting as an advocate for the client's wishes
- Considering ethical and legal responsibilities
- Establishing priorities
- Following advance directives regarding the client's documented requests
- Implementing standard, transmission-based, and other precautions
- Upholding the client's rights

Health Promotion and Maintenance

- Performing the techniques of data collection
- Providing health promotion programs
- Teaching significant others about how to perform CPR and how to relieve choking (foreign-body airway obstruction)

Psychosocial Integrity

- Considering the client's cultural, religious, and spiritual preferences
- Discussing end-of-life, grief, and loss issues
- Providing emotional support to significant others

Physiological Integrity

- Administering emergency treatments
- Documenting the client's response to BLS measures
- Handling medical emergencies
- Identifying alterations in the cardiopulmonary system
- Performing CPR or foreign-body airway obstruction measures
- Using special equipment

I. BASIC LIFE SUPPORT (Box 16-1)

A. BLS provides oxygen to the brain, heart, and other vital organs until help arrives.

B. It is also known as **CPR**

II. GENERAL CAB GUIDELINES (Table 16-1)

A. Description: Cardiopulmonary resuscitation, known by most as CPR, is the process of providing oxygen to the brain, heart, and other vital organs in a victim who cannot do so for him- or herself.

B. Rescuers should follow the C-A-B formula:
1. C: compressions
2. A: airway
3. B: breathing

C. Basic steps include immediate recognition of the sudden cardiac arrest (unresponsiveness and absence of normal breathing) and activation of the emergency response system, early CPR, and rapid defibrillation with an AED.

D. Chest compressions (Figures 16-1 and 16-2)

1. Description: Chest compressions are used to keep blood moving through the victim's body, delivering oxygen to crucial areas, such as the brain.

Box 16-1 The CABs of Basic Life Support for the Health Care Provider

C: Compressions
A: Airway
B: Breathing

Note: Each step of the CABs of basic life support begins with assessment.

▲ **FIGURE 16-1** Chest compressions: Proper hand position for an adult. (From Potter, A., & Perry, P. [2010]. *Clinical nursing skills & techniques* [7th ed.]. St. Louis: Mosby.)

TABLE 16-1 Health Care Providers' CAB Maneuvers for Adults, Children, and Infants

Maneuver	Adult	Child	Infant
CIRCULATION			
Pulse check (10 seconds or less)	Carotid artery	Femoral artery	Brachial artery
Compression landmarks	Lower half of sternum	Center of chest, between nipples	Just below nipple line
Compression method: Push hard and fast, and allow for complete recoil.	Two hands: Heel of one hand, other hand on top	Two hands: Heel of one hand with second on top *or* One hand: Heel of one hand only	Two fingers or two thumbs/encircling hands technique
Compression depth	2 inches	2 inches	1.5 inches
Compression rate	Approximately 100/min	Approximately 100/min	Approximately 100/min
Compression-to-ventilation ratio (single rescuer)	30:2	30:2	30:2
AIRWAY BREATHS			
	Head tilt–chin lift (If trauma is suspected, use jaw thrust) Two effective breaths at 1 sec/breath	Head tilt–chin lift (If trauma is suspected, use jaw thrust) Two effective breaths at 1 sec/breath	Head tilt–chin lift (If trauma is suspected, use jaw thrust) Two effective breaths at 1 sec/breath
Rescue breathing without chest compressions	1 breath every 6-8 sec	1 breath every 6-8 sec	1 breath every 6-8 sec
Foreign-body airway obstruction	Abdominal thrusts	Abdominal thrusts	Back blows and chest thrusts
DEFIBRILLATION			
Automatic external defibrillator (AED)	Use adult pads; do not use child pads or a child system. For out-of-hospital response, provide five cycles (2 min) of CPR before shock if response time is longer than 4-5 min and arrest was not witnessed.	Use AED as soon as possible for sudden and in-hospital collapse. All: Use AED after five cycles of CPR (out of hospital); use child pads and system for child 1-8 years old, if available; if child pads and system are not available, use adult AED and pads	Use manual defibrillator if available or a pediatric dose attenuator system. If neither is available, use an AED

⚠️ When performing chest compressions, push hard and fast and avoid interrupted compressions.

2. Nursing considerations
    a. Stand or kneel beside the victim's chest; ensure that the victim is lying supine on a firm surface (if possible); air-filled mattresses should be deflated before performing CPR.
    b. Place the heel of one hand on the lower half of the sternum, which is the center or middle part of the victim's chest, with the heel of the other hand on top of the first so that the hands are overlapped and parallel.
    c. The adult chest is compressed to a depth of at least 2 inches and compressions should be hard and fast at a rate of at least 100 per minute.
    d. Allow complete recoil of the chest after each compression to allow the heart to fill completely before the next compression.
    e. A compression to ventilation ratio of 30:2 is recommended.
    f. If two rescuers are present, to prevent rescuer fatigue, rescuers may switch positions (compressor and ventilator) after approximately 2 minutes (or after 5 cycles of compression and ventilation at a ratio of 30:2).
    g. Interruptions in chest compressions need to be minimized.
    h. Chest compressions and ventilations are continued until spontaneous circulation returns or resuscitative efforts are terminated.

⚠️ To produce as much blood flow as possible, allow the chest to recoil (return to normal position) completely after delivery of each breath and each compression.

E. Airway
    1. Description: Before effective rescue breathing can be administered, a patent airway must be confirmed or, if it is not present, opened manually.
    2. Nursing considerations
        a. After delivering 30 compressions, the rescuer opens the victim's airway (after donning gloves and a face shield, if they are available).
        b. The head tilt–chin lift is the preferred method of opening the airway
        c. To perform the head tilt–chin lift, one hand is placed on the client's forehead, and firm pressure is applied to tilt the head backwards; using the first and second fingers of the other hand, pressure is applied under the bony part of the jaw, taking care not to block the airway and ensuring that the tongue is not obstructing the airway (Figure 16-3).
        d. If the victim has sustained a head, neck, or spinal cord injury, the jaw-thrust maneuver is used to open the airway.
        e. The jaw-thrust maneuver is performed by placing the first and second fingers of both hands on the corner-point of the mandible and both thumbs on the chin, then pushing the mandible upwards; this prevents obstruction of the airway by the tongue (Figure 16-4)

⚠️ If a neck injury is suspected, the jaw thrust maneuver is used to open the victim's airway.

F. Breathing
    1. Description: Once the airway has been secured, the rescuer delivers breaths to keep oxygen moving through the victim's body.

▲ **FIGURE 16-2** Positioning for proper compression techniques. (From Christensen, B., & Kockrow, E. [2006]. *Foundations of adult health nursing* [5th ed.]. St. Louis: Mosby.)

Upstroke
Downstroke
Effort arm (back)
Piston (arm)
Fulcrum (hip joints)
Resistance (lower half of sternum)

▲ **FIGURE 16-3** Opening the airway using the head tilt–chin lift maneuver. (From Lewis, S. M., Heitkemper, M. M., & Dirksen, S. R. [2007]. *Medical-surgical nursing: Assessment and management of clinical problems* [7th ed.]. St. Louis: Mosby.)

2. Nursing considerations
   a. A victim who is breathing is log-rolled onto his or her side as a unit (without twisting) with the lower arm in front of the body (recovery position) to help maintain an open airway; if a spinal cord injury is suspected, however, the victim should not be moved.
   b. Occasional gasps from a victim may not result in adequate ventilation and this victim should be treated as if he or she is not breathing.
   c. In the victim is not breathing give two ventilations (breaths) of 1 second per breath (mouth-to-mouth, mouth-to-barrier device, or bag mask if available, ensuring an adequate air seal); allow the victim to exhale between breaths (avoid excessive ventilation).
   d. Each rescue breath is delivered over 1 second; ventilations are delivered at a rate of 1 breath every 6 to 8 seconds (8 to 10 ventilations per minute).

⚠ When performing CPR, if you are unsuccessful at giving a breath, reposition the victim's head and try again (improper chin and head position is a common cause of difficulty in ventilating a victim)

   e. While giving ventilations watch for a visible chest rise; be alert to gastric distention, which indicates that the airway has not been properly opened and air from ventilations is entering the stomach rather than the lungs; this can result in regurgitation and aspiration.
   f. A sufficient tidal volume is needed when delivering breaths to produce a visible chest rise.
   g. A compression to ventilation ratio of 30:2 is recommended until an advanced airway is placed.
   h. In special situations, an alternative breathing method may be used (Box 16-2).

▲ **FIGURE 16-4** Opening the airway using the jaw thrust maneuver. (From Harkreader, H., & Hogan, M. A. [2004]. *Fundamentals of nursing: Caring and clinical judgment* [2nd ed.]. Philadelphia: W.B. Saunders. Used with permission of the American Heart Association. [1992]. Guidelines for cardiopulmonary resuscitation and emergency cardiac care: An international consensus on science and circulation. *Circulation, 102* [Suppl], 217–222.)

III. GUIDELINES FOR THE ADULT

A. Description: Adult CPR consists of life-support measures that include early recognition of cardiac arrest and activation of the emergency response system, early CPR using C-A-B procedure, rapid defibrillation if necessary, advanced life support, and postcardiac arrest care.
B. Nursing considerations
   1. The rescuer should ensure that the scene is safe before approaching the victim.
   2. The HCP should first determine if the victim is unresponsive with no breathing or normal breathing (by tapping the victim at the shoulder and shouting "Are you OK?"); activate the emergency response system; obtain the AED if alone and if one is easily accessible, attach and use the AED; and then begin CPR (using C-A-B procedures). If two rescuers are present then one can obtain the AED while the other begins CPR.
   3. Checking for a pulse: If a pulse is not felt within 10 seconds, the rescuer should start CPR, beginning with chest compressions at a ratio of 30:2 (compressions to ventilations).
   4. If a pulse is definitely felt, the rescuer should give 1 breath every 6 to 8 seconds if the victim is not breathing and recheck the pulse every 2 minutes.

IV. VARIATIONS IN CPR

A. Child
   1. Description
      a. A child is defined as a person between 1 and 8 years of age.
      b. The procedure is basically the same as that done for an adult; variations are listed below under nursing considerations.
   2. Nursing considerations
      a. If the rescuer is alone, 5 cycles of compressions and breaths (which will take about 2 minutes) are done before activating the emergency response system and obtaining an AED.

Box 16-2 Alternative Breathing Methods

■ Mouth-to-nose breathing may be used when it is impossible to ventilate a victim through the mouth (e.g., the mouth cannot be opened, the mouth is seriously injured, or a tight mouth-to-mouth seal is difficult to achieve).

■ Mouth-to-stoma breathing is used for the victim who has undergone a tracheal stoma; a round pediatric face mask is used to create an adequate seal.

b. One hand is used for chest compressions and ventilations are delivered more gently than in an adult.

c. Adjust chest compressions to the child's age and size; compression-breath ratio is 30:2.

d. If the child is breathing, ensure that the airway stays open.

e. If the child is not breathing, take the appropriate measures (mouth-to-mouth ventilation).

f. After 5 cycles of CPR, if there is no response and an AED is available, apply it and follow the AED prompts; use pediatric pads if available, if pediatric pads are not available, use adult pads.

g. Continue CPR until the child moves or help arrives.

B. Infant

1. Description: A person who is less than one year of age.

2. Nursing considerations

a. Determine unresponsiveness; stroke the infant and watch for a response, such as movement, but don't shake the infant

b. If there is no response, follow the C-A-B procedures.

c. If the rescuer is alone, 5 cycles of compressions and breaths (which will take about 2 minutes) are done before activating emergency response system and obtaining an AED.

If a second rescuer is present, that person activates the emergency response system while the first attends to the infant.

d. Compression-breath ratio is 30:2.

e. Use the brachial pulse to assess circulation.

f. The breastbone is compressed 1.5 inches at a rate of 100 times per minute with the use of two or three fingers.

g. In an infant, provide mouth-to-nose ventilation when delivering breaths.

⚠ The chest compression landmark for a child is in the center of the chest between the nipples. For the infant the landmark is just below the nipple line.

V. AUTOMATED EXTERNAL DEFIBRILLATOR

A. Description

1. This device, known by many as an AED, is used to convert ventricular fibrillation into a perfusing rhythm.

2. The AED differentiates nonventricular fibrillation rhythms and also permits early defibrillation by laypersons and first responders.

B. Nursing considerations

1. Attach the AED leads to the victim per AED instructions.

2. Turn on the AED and follow the AED prompts.

3. Ensure that no one is touching the victim when the shock is delivered.

4. Shockable rhythm: resume CPR immediately for 2 minutes after the shock so as to minimize interruptions.

5. Nonshockable rhythm: resume CPR immediately for 2 minutes and check rhythm every 2 minutes.

VI. FOREIGN-BODY AIRWAY OBSTRUCTION

A. Description: A variety of foreign bodies may become lodged in a person's airway, but the type most frequently encountered is food.

B. Nursing considerations for the adult

1. Ask the victim, "Are you choking?" The victim will not be able to speak or cough if he or she is choking and may place both hands on the neck (the universal sign for choking).

2. If the victim's airway is partially obstructed, a crowing sound is heard; encourage the victim to cough.

3. If the victim is having difficulty breathing, activate the emergency response system.

4. Relieve the obstruction with the use of the abdominal thrust maneuver (Figure 16-5 and Box 16-3).

5. Perform the abdominal thrust maneuver in rapid sequence until the object is dislodged or victim becomes unconscious.

6. If the victim becomes unconscious, place in a supine position, and begin CPR for 2 minutes and then activate emergency response system; if a second rescuer is present, that person should immediately activate the emergency response system.

7. Each time the airway is opened during CPR, the rescuer should look in the victim's mouth for an object and if found, remove it.

▲ **FIGURE 16-5** Abdominal thrusts. (From Christensen, B., & Kockrow, E. [2006]. *Foundations of adult health nursing* [5th ed.]. St. Louis: Mosby.)

C. Nursing considerations for the child
1. Choking is suspected in an child or infant experiencing acute respiratory distress associated with coughing, gagging, or stridor (high-pitched, noisy breathing)
2. Allow the victim to continue coughing if the cough is forceful.
3. If the cough is ineffective or the victim demonstrates increased respiratory difficulty accompanied by a high-pitched noise while inhaling, help is needed.
4. In a conscious child, the abdominal thrust maneuver should be performed until the obstruction is dislodged.

D. Nursing considerations for the infant
1. Assess the victim for obstruction and note breathing problems.
2. Place the infant over an arm or on the lap, position the head lower than the trunk, and support the head firmly, holding the jaw.
3. Deliver five back blows with the heel of the hand between the shoulder blades. (Figure 16-6).
4. Turn the infant over, positioning the head lower than the trunk.

▲ **FIGURE 16-6** Clearing airway obstruction in an infant. (From Christensen, B., & Kockrow, E. [2006]. *Foundations of adult health nursing* [5th ed.]. St. Louis: Mosby.)

Box 16-3 Abdominal Thrusts

1. Stand behind the victim.
2. Place your arms around the victim's waist.
3. Make a fist.
4. Place the thumb side of your fist just above the umbilicus (belly button) and well below the xiphoid process.
5. Perform five quick in and up abdominal thrusts (between the umbilicus and the xiphoid process).
6. Use chest thrusts for the obese victim or for the victim in the late stages of pregnancy.

---

5. Deliver five chest thrusts at the same location used for chest compressions
6. Check for a foreign object and remove it, only if one is seen; blind finger sweeps are avoided because the object can be forced back further into the throat.
7. Repeat the sequence until the object has been removed.

E. Pregnant or obese victim
1. Chest thrusts are used for obese victims or a victim in the late stage of pregnancy.
2. The rescuer places his or her arms under the axillae and across the chest.
3. The thumb side of a clenched fist is placed against the middle of the sternum, and the other hand is placed over the fist.
4. Backward chest thrusts are performed until the foreign body is expelled or the victim loses consciousness.
5. If a pregnant victim loses consciousness, the rescuer places her on her back, and then inserts a wedge (e.g., a pillow or rolled blanket) under the woman's right flank and hip to displace the uterus to the right side of the abdomen.
6. The rescuer then attempts ventilations; if ventilation is unsuccessful, the rescuer positions the hands as for chest compressions and delivers firm chest thrusts to remove the obstruction.
7. If defibrillation is needed in a pregnant victim, the paddles are placed one rib interspace higher than usual because the heart is displaced slightly by the enlarged uterus.

⚠ If the victim of a foreign body airway obstruction is pregnant, remember to place a wedge, such as a pillow or rolled blanket, under the right abdominal flank and hip to displace the uterus to the left side of the abdomen. This will prevent supine hypotension.

MORE QUESTIONS ON EVOLVE!

Practice Questions

121. A nursing instructor asks a nursing student to describe the procedure for relieving an airway obstruction on an unconscious pregnant woman at 8 months' gestation. The student describes the procedure correctly if the student states to:
1. Place the hands in the pelvis to perform the thrusts.
2. Perform abdominal thrusts until the object is dislodged.
3. Perform left lateral abdominal thrusts until the object is dislodged.
4. Place a rolled blanket under the right abdominal flank and hip area.

122. A nurse on the day shift walks into a client's room and finds the client unresponsive. The client is not breathing and does not have a pulse, and the nurse immediately calls out for help. The next nursing action is which of the following?
1. Deliver breaths.
2. Give the client oxygen.
3. Start chest compressions.
4. Ventilate with a mouth-to-mask device.

123. A nurse witnesses a neighbor's husband sustain a fall from the roof of his house. The nurse rushes to the victim and determines the need to open the airway. The nurse opens the airway in this victim with the use of which method?
1. Flexed position
2. Head tilt–chin lift
3. Jaw thrust maneuver
4. Modified head tilt–chin lift

124. A nurse understands that which of the following is a correct guideline for adult cardiopulmonary resuscitation (CPR) for a health care provider?
1. One breath should be given for every five compressions.
2. Two breaths should be given for every 15 compressions.
3. Initially, two quick breaths should be given as rapidly as possible.
4. Each rescue breath should be given over 1 second and should produce a visible chest rise.

125. A nurse attempts to relieve an airway obstruction on a 6-year-old conscious child. The nurse performs this maneuver by placing the hands between:
1. The groin and the abdomen
2. The umbilicus and the groin
3. The lower abdomen and the chest
4. The umbilicus and the xiphoid process

126. A nurse is performing cardiopulmonary resuscitation (CPR) on an adult. The nurse delivers how many breaths per minute to the client?

1. 6
2. 10
3. 18
4. 20

127. A nurse is performing cardiopulmonary resuscitation (CPR) on an infant. When performing chest compressions, the nurse understands that the compression rate is at least:
1. 60 times per minute
2. 80 times per minute
3. 100 times per minute
4. 160 times per minute

128. Which of the following is the most appropriate location for assessing the pulse of an infant who is less than 1 year old?
1. Radial
2. Carotid
3. Brachial
4. Popliteal

129. A nurse is teaching cardiopulmonary resuscitation to a group of nursing students. The nurse asks a student to describe the reason why blind finger sweeps are avoided in infants. The nurse determines that the student understands the reason if the student makes which statement?
1. "The object may have been swallowed."
2. "The infant may bite down on the finger"
3. "The mouth is too small to see the object."
4. "The object may be forced back further into the throat."

130. A nurse is performing cardiopulmonary resuscitation (CPR) on an adult client. The nurse understands that when performing chest compressions, one should depress the sternum:
1. 1 inch
2. ¾ inch
3. 2 inches
4. 3 inches

ANSWERS

121. 4

Rationale: To relieve an airway obstruction on an unconscious woman in an advanced stage of pregnancy, the woman is placed on her back. A wedge, such as a pillow or rolled blanket, is placed under the right abdominal flank and hip to displace the uterus to the left side of the abdomen. Options 1, 2, and 3 are incorrect and can cause harm to the woman and the fetus.
Test-Taking Strategy: Use the process of elimination, and note that the client is an unconscious pregnant woman at 8 months' gestation. Recall the concepts associated with hypotension and vena cava syndrome to assist with directing you to option 4. Review the principles associated with relieving an airway obstruction on a pregnant woman if you had difficulty with this question.
Level of Cognitive Ability: Evaluating
Client Needs: Physiological Integrity
Integrated Process: Nursing Process/Evaluation
Content Area: Maternity/Antepartum
References: Christensen, Kockrow, p. 908. [2011]. *Foundations of nursing.*
Leifer, p. 53. 2011.

122. 3

Rationale: The nurse would follow C-A-B, compressions, airway, and breathing. Therefore the next nursing action would be to start chest compressions.

Test-Taking Strategy: Visualize the steps of basic life support (BLS) to answer the question. Recalling CAB—compressions, airway, breathing—will assist with directing you to option 3. Also note that options 1, 2, and 4 are comparable or alike and address airway. Review the steps of BLS if you had difficulty with this question.

Level of Cognitive Ability: Applying
Client Needs: Physiological Integrity
Integrated Process: Nursing Process/Implementation
Content Area: Critical Care
Reference: Christensen, Kockrow, pp. 740–741. 2011. *Foundations of nursing.*

123. 3

Rationale: If a neck injury is suspected, the jaw thrust maneuver is used to open the airway. The head tilt–chin lift produces hyperextension of the neck and could cause complications if a neck injury is present. A flexed position is an inappropriate position for opening the airway.

Test-Taking Strategy: Use the process of elimination. Eliminate options 2 and 4 first, because they are comparable or alike. Next, eliminate option 1, because this position would not open the airway. If you had difficulty with this question, review the appropriate methods for opening an airway.

Level of Cognitive Ability: Applying
Client Needs: Physiological Integrity
Integrated Process: Nursing Process/Implementation
Content Area: Critical Care
References: Christensen, Kockrow, p. 740. 2011. *Foundations of nursing.*
deWit, p. 93. 2009.

124. 4

Rationale: During adult CPR, each rescue breath should be given over 1 second and should produce a visible chest rise. Excessive ventilation (too many breaths per minute or breaths that are too large or forceful) may be harmful and should not be performed. Health care providers should employ a 30-compression-to-2-ventilation ratio for the adult victim. Options 1, 2, and 3 are incorrect.

Level of Cognitive Ability: Understanding
Client Needs: Physiological Integrity
Integrated Process: Nursing Process/Implementation
Content Area: Adult Health/Cardiovascular
References: Berg, Hemphill, Abella, et al. (2010). pp. S685–S705. Christensen, Kockrow, pp. 742–743. 2011. *Foundations of nursing.*

125. 4

Rationale: To relieve an airway obstruction in a child, the rescuer stands behind the victim and places the arms directly under the victim's axillae and around the victim. The rescuer places the thumb side of one fist against the victim's abdomen in the midline slightly above the umbilicus and well below the tip of the xiphoid process. The rescuer grasps the fist with the other hand and delivers up to five thrusts. One must take care to not touch the xiphoid process or the lower margins of the rib cage, because force applied to these structures may damage the internal organs. Options 1, 2, and 3 are incorrect hand placements.

Test-Taking Strategy: Use the process of elimination, and note the age of the child. Eliminate options 1 and 2 first, because they are comparable or alike. From the remaining options, considering the anatomic location and the effect of the maneuver for dislodging an obstruction will direct you to option 4. If you had difficulty with this question, review the correct hand placement for relieving an airway obstruction.

Level of Cognitive Ability: Applying
Client Needs: Physiological Integrity
Integrated Process: Nursing Process/Implementation
Content Area: Critical Care
References: Christensen, Kockrow, p. 744. 2011. *Foundations of nursing.*

126. 2

Rationale: Each rescue breath is delivered over 1 second at a rate of 1 breath every 6 to 8 seconds (8 to 10 ventilations per minute). Options 1, 3, and 4 are incorrect.

Test-Taking Strategy: Focus on the subject, breaths per minute. It is necessary to know that the client receives 8 to 10 ventilations per minute. If you had difficulty with this question, review the CPR guidelines.

Level of Cognitive Ability: Applying
Client Needs: Physiological Integrity
Integrated Process: Nursing Process/Implementation
Content Area: Critical Care
Reference: Perry, Potter, p. 731. 2010.

127. 3

Rationale: For an infant, the rate of chest compressions is at least 100 per minute. Options 1 and 2 identify rates that are too low, and option 4 identifies a rate that is too high.

Test-Taking Strategy: Use the process of elimination, and consider the normal heart rate of an infant. Eliminate options 1 and 2 because of the low rates identified in the options. Eliminate option 4, because this rate would be much too rapid for an infant. Review the CPR guidelines for an infant if you had difficulty with this question.

Level of Cognitive Ability: Applying
Client Needs: Physiological Integrity
Integrated Process: Nursing Process/Implementation
Content Area: Critical Care
Reference: Christensen, Kockrow, p. 744. 2011. *Foundations of nursing.*

128. 3

Rationale: To assess a pulse in an infant (i.e., a child <1 year old), the pulse is checked at the brachial artery. The infant's relatively short, fat neck makes palpation of the carotid artery difficult. The popliteal and radial pulses are also difficult to palpate in an infant.

Test-Taking Strategy: Use the process of elimination and your knowledge regarding circulatory assessment in an infant. Considering the body structure of an infant will assist with directing you to option 3. Review cardiac assessment and basic life support for an infant if you had difficulty with this question.

Level of Cognitive Ability: Applying
Client Needs: Physiological Integrity
Integrated Process: Nursing Process/Data Collection

Content Area: Child Health: Eye/Ear/Throat/Respiratory/Cardiovascular
Reference: Christensen, Kockrow, p. 743. 2011. *Foundations of nursing.*

129. 4

Rationale: Blind finger sweeps are not recommended for infants and children because of the risk of forcing the object further down into the airway. Options 1, 2, and 3 are not related directly to the subject of the question.
Test-Taking Strategy: Focus on the subject, the reason for avoiding blind finger sweeps. Note that option 4, the correct option, addresses airway. Review the management of an obstructed airway in an infant or a child if you had difficulty with this question.
Level of Cognitive Ability: Understanding
Client Needs: Physiological Integrity
Integrated Process: Teaching and Learning
Content Area: Child Health: Eye/Ear/Throat/Respiratory/Cardiovascular
Reference: Christensen, Kockrow, p. 746. 2011. *Foundations of nursing.*

130. 3

Rationale: When performing CPR on an adult client, the sternum is depressed 2 inches. Options 1 and 2 identify compression depths that would be ineffective for an adult, and option 4 identifies a depth that could cause injury to the client.
Test-Taking Strategy: Note the strategic word "adult" in the question. Consider the normal body structure of an adult to assist with directing you to option 3. Review the procedure for performing adult CPR if you had difficulty with this question.
Level of Cognitive Ability: Applying
Client Needs: Physiological Integrity
Integrated Process: Nursing Process/Implementation
Content Area: Critical Care
Reference: Perry, Potter, p. 731. 2010.

17

Perioperative Nursing Care

PYRAMID TERMS

extended postoperative stage The period of at least 1 to 4 days after surgery

immediate postoperative stage The period of 1 to 4 hours after surgery

intermediate postoperative stage The period of 4 to 24 hours after surgery

perioperative nursing Nursing care given before (preoperative), during (intraoperative), and after (postoperative) surgery

 ## PYRAMID TO SUCCESS

The pyramid points focus on reinforcing instructions to the client, family, and significant others during the preoperative stage; medication reconciliation; preparing the client for the operative procedure; and ensuring that prescribed preoperative procedures have been performed, the results are within the expected range, and they have been documented. During the postoperative stage, the pyramid points focus on monitoring for surgical complications and implementing initial nursing measures if a complication arises. They also focus on preparing the client for discharge, reinforcing instructions related to the prescribed treatments, and identifying the need for home-care support services.

CLIENT NEEDS

Safe and Effective Care Environment

- Ensuring that advance directive documents are in the client's medical record
- Establishing priorities
- Informing the client about the surgical process
- Maintaining confidentiality
- Maintaining standard and other precautions
- Maintaining surgical asepsis
- Obtaining informed consent for the surgical procedure
- Preventing a surgical infection
- Providing safety to the medicated client
- Upholding the client's rights

Health Promotion and Maintenance

- Discussing expected body-image changes
- Identifying lifestyle choices
- Performing techniques of data collection
- Providing client and family teaching related to the prescribed discharge plan
- Providing health and wellness teaching to prevent complications

Psychosocial Integrity

- Assessing psychosocial concerns
- Assisting the client with the development of coping methods
- Communicating therapeutically
- Identifying support systems
- Identifying unexpected body-image changes
- Promoting an environment that will allow the client to express concerns

Physiological Integrity

- Administering preoperative and postoperative medications safely
- Initiating nursing interventions when surgical complications arise
- Monitoring for unexpected responses to treatments and procedures
- Monitoring for surgical complications
- Monitoring for wound infection
- Providing basic care and comfort
- Providing respiratory therapy

I. PREOPERATIVE CARE

⚠ A client may return home shortly after having a surgical procedure because many surgical procedures are done through ambulatory care or one-day stay surgical units. Perioperative care procedures apply even if the client returns home the same day of the surgical procedure.

A. Obtaining informed consent
1. The surgeon is responsible for obtaining the informed consent for surgery.
2. No sedation should be administered to the client before he or she signs the informed consent form.
3. Minors (<18 years old) may need a parent or legal guardian to sign the informed consent form.
4. Older clients may need a legal guardian to sign the informed consent form.
5. The nurse may witness the client signing the informed consent form.
6. The nurse needs to document the witnessing of the signing of the operative consent form after the client acknowledges understanding the procedure.

B. Nutrition
1. Check the surgeon's prescriptions regarding nothing by mouth (NPO) status before surgery.
2. Solid foods and liquids are generally withheld for 6 to 8 hours before general anesthesia and for 3 hours before surgery with local anesthesia to avoid aspiration.
3. Monitor intravenous (IV) fluids, if prescribed.
4. Note that parenteral nutrition may be prescribed for clients who are malnourished, have protein or metabolic deficiencies, or cannot ingest foods.

C. Elimination
1. If the client is to have intestinal or abdominal surgery, an enema, laxative, or both may be prescribed the night before surgery.
2. The client should void immediately before surgery.
3. Prepare to insert a Foley catheter, if prescribed.
4. If there is a Foley catheter in place, it should be emptied immediately before surgery, and the amount and quality of urine output should be documented.

D. Surgical site
1. Prepare to clean the surgical site with a mild antiseptic soap the night before surgery, as prescribed.
2. Inform the client about the procedure for shaving the operative site.

⚠ The hair on the head or face is shaved only if it will interfere with the surgical procedure and only if prescribed.

E. Reinforcing preoperative instructions
1. Inform the client about what to expect postoperatively.
2. Tell the client to notify the nurse if he or she experiences any postoperative pain, and that pain medication will be prescribed to be given as the client requests.
3. Instruct the client to use noninvasive pain relief techniques such as relaxation or guided imagery before the pain occurs and as soon as the pain is noticed.
4. Reinforce instructions about the use of a patient-controlled analgesia pump if its use is prescribed.
5. Inform the client that requesting an opioid after surgery will not make the client a drug addict, and explain the difference between analgesic need and psychological dependence.
6. The client should be instructed to not smoke for at least 24 hours before surgery and to refrain from taking daily prescribed medications, aspirin, selected vitamins, and herbal products unless they are approved by the surgeon.
7. Instruct the client in deep-breathing and coughing techniques, the use of incentive spirometry, and the importance of performing the techniques after surgery to prevent the development of pneumonia and atelectasis (Box 17-1 and Figure 17-1).

Box 17-1 Preoperative Instructions

Deep-Breathing and Coughing Exercises

Instruct the client that a sitting position provides the best lung expansion for coughing and deep-breathing exercises.

Instruct the client to breathe deeply three times by inhaling through the nostrils and exhaling slowly through pursed lips.

Instruct the client that the third breath should be held for 3 seconds; then the client should cough deeply three times splinting the operative site if necessary.

The client should perform this exercise every 2 hours.

Incentive Spirometry

Instruct the client to assume a sitting or upright position.

Instruct the client to place the mouth tightly around the mouthpiece.

Instruct the client to inhale slowly to raise and maintain the flow rate indicator between the 600 and 900 marks.

Instruct the client to hold his or her breath for 5 seconds and then to exhale through pursed lips.

Instruct the client to repeat this process 10 times every hour.

Leg and Foot Exercises

Gastrocnemius (calf) pumping: Instruct the client to move both ankles by pointing the toes up and then down.

Quadriceps (thigh) setting: Instruct the client to press the back of the knees against the bed and then to relax the knees. This contracts and relaxes the thigh and calf muscles to prevent thrombus formation.

Foot circles: Instruct the client to rotate each foot in a circle.

Hip and knee movements: Instruct the client to flex the knee and thigh, straighten the leg, and hold the position for 5 seconds before lowering. (This should not be performed if the client is having abdominal surgery or has a back problem.)

Splinting the Incision

If the surgical incision is abdominal or thoracic, instruct the client to place a pillow or one hand with the other hand on top over the incisional area.

During deep breathing and coughing, the client presses gently against the area of the incision to splint or support it.

▲ FIGURE 17-1 Incentive spirometer. (From Monahan, F., Sands, J., Neighbors, M., Marek, J., & Green, C. [2007]. *Phipps' medical-surgical nursing: Health and illness perspectives* [8th ed.]. St. Louis: Mosby.)

8. Instruct the client in leg and foot exercises to prevent venous stasis of blood and facilitate venous blood return (Figure 17-2; also see Box 17-1).
9. Instruct the client about how to splint an incision and how to turn and reposition (Figure 17-3; also see Box 17-1).
10. Inform the client of any invasive devices that may be needed after surgery, such as tubes, drains, Foley catheters, or IV lines.
11. Tell the client to not pull on any of the invasive devices. They will be removed as soon as possible.

F. Psychosocial preparation
1. Be alert to the client's anxiety level.
2. Ask the client about questions or concerns that he or she may have regarding surgery.
3. Allow time for privacy for the client to prepare psychologically for surgery.
4. Provide support and assistance as needed
5. Consider any cultural aspects when providing care. (Box 17-2).

G. Preoperative checklist
1. Ensure that the client is wearing an identification bracelet.
2. Check for client allergies (see Chapter 61 for information about latex allergy).
3. Review the preoperative checklist to be sure that each item is addressed before the client is transported to surgery.
4. Ensure that consent forms have been signed for the operative procedure, anesthesia, any blood transfusions, the disposal of a limb, or surgical sterilization procedures.
5. Ensure that a history and physical examination were completed and documented in the client's record (Box 17-3).
6. Ensure that any consultation reports that were prescribed are completed and documented in the client's record.

▲ FIGURE 17-2 Postoperative leg exercises. (From Lewis, S., Heitkemper, M., & Dirksen, S. [2004]. *Medical-surgical nursing: Assessment and management of clinical problems* [6th ed.]. St. Louis: Mosby.)

7. Ensure that the prescribed laboratory test results are documented in the client's record.
8. Ensure that any prescribed electrocardiography and chest radiography reports are noted in the client's record.
9. Ensure that blood type and screen or type and crossmatch are noted in the client's record.
10. Document that the client has voided before surgery.
11. Remove according to the agency's policy, the client's jewelry, makeup, dentures, hairpins, nail polish, and any prostheses.
    a. Hearing aids or glasses may be removed at the last possible moment before surgery.
    b. Clients with language or hearing concerns need to have access to translators until anesthesia induction.
12. Document that valuables were given to the client's family members or locked in the hospital safe.
13. Document that the prescribed preoperative medication was given (Box 17-4).
14. Monitor and document the client's vital signs.
15. Document the last time that the client ate or drank.

▲ **FIGURE 17-3** Techniques for splinting a wound when coughing. (From Lewis, S., Heitkemper, M., & Dirksen, S. [2004]. *Medical-surgical nursing: Assessment and management of clinical problems* [6th ed.]. St. Louis: Mosby.)

Box 17-2 Cultural Aspects of Perioperative Nursing Care

Cultural assessment includes questions related to:
- Primary language spoken and cultural practices
- Feelings related to surgery and pain
- Pain management
- Expectations
- Support systems
- Feelings toward self

Allow a family member to be present, if appropriate.

Secure the help of a professional interpreter to communicate with non–English speaking clients.

Use pictures or phrase cards to communicate and assess the non–English speaking client's perception of pain or other feelings.

Provide preoperative and postoperative educational materials in the appropriate language.

Adapted from Potter, P., & Perry, A. (2009). *Fundamentals of nursing* (7th ed.). St. Louis: Mosby.

H. Preoperative medications
1. Prepare to administer preoperative medications as prescribed or to have them be administered in the operating room immediately before the surgery.

Box 17-3 Medical Conditions That Increase the Risk of Surgery

- Bleeding disorders, such as thrombocytopenia and hemophilia
- Diabetes mellitus
- Chronic pain
- Heart disease, such as a recent myocardial infarction, dysrhythmia, congestive heart failure, and peripheral vascular disease
- Obstructive sleep apnea
- Upper respiratory infection
- Liver disease
- Fever
- Chronic respiratory disease, such as emphysema, bronchitis, or asthma
- Immunological disorders, such as leukemia, acquired immunodeficiency syndrome, bone marrow depression, and the use of chemotherapy or immunosuppressive agents
- The abuse of street drugs

Adapted from Potter, P., & Perry, A. (2009). *Fundamentals of nursing* (7th ed.). St. Louis: Mosby.

---

2. Instruct the client that he or she will feel drowsy after the medications are given.

⚠ After administering the preoperative medications, keep the client in bed with the side rails up. Place the call bell next to the client; instruct the client not to get out of bed and to call for assistance if needed.

I. Arrival at the operating room
1. When the client arrives to the operating room, the operating room nurse will verify the identification bracelet with the client's verbal response and review the client's chart (Boxes 17-5 and 17-6).
2. The client's chart will be checked for completeness.
3. The client's chart will be reviewed for informed consent forms, history and physical examination, and allergic reaction information.
4. The surgeon's prescriptions will be reviewed and their completion verified.
5. The IV line may be initiated at this time, or in the preoperative holding area if prescribed.
6. The anesthesia team will administer the prescribed anesthesia.

⚠ Verification of the client and the surgical operative site is critical.

II. POSTOPERATIVE CARE

A. Description:
1. **Immediate postoperative stage:** The period of 1 to 4 hours after surgery.
2. **Intermediate postoperative stage:** The period of 4 to 24 hours after surgery.
3. **Extended postoperative stage:** The period of at least 1 to 4 days after surgery.

B. Respiratory system

⚠ Monitor breath sounds—stridor, wheezing, or a crowing sound can indicate partial obstruction, bronchospasm, or laryngospasm; crackles or rhonchi may indicate pulmonary edema.

1. Monitor vital signs.
2. Monitor airway patency and ensure adequate ventilation (prolonged mechanical ventilation during anesthesia may affect postoperative lung function).
3. Remember that extubated clients who are lethargic may not be able to maintain an airway.

Box 17-4 Substances That Can Affect the Surgical Client

Antibiotics
These potentiate the action of anesthetic agents.

Anticholinergics
Medications with anticholinergic effects increase the potential for confusion.

Anticoagulants
These alter normal clotting factors and increase the risk of hemorrhage.
Aspirin (acetylsalicylic acid) and nonsteroidal anti-inflammatory drugs are commonly used medications that can alter clotting mechanisms.
Complementary remedies such as garlic and ginseng may also alter normal clotting factors.
These medications should be discontinued at least 48 hours before surgery or as prescribed.

Anticonvulsants
The long-term use of certain anticonvulsants can alter the metabolism of anesthetic agents.

Antidepressants
These may lower the blood pressure during anesthesia.
Complementary remedies such as St. John's wort may also lower blood pressure.

Antidysrhythmics
These reduce cardiac contractility and impair cardiac conduction during anesthesia.

Antihypertensives
These can interact with anesthetic agents and cause bradycardia, hypotension, and impaired circulation.

Corticosteroids
These cause adrenal atrophy and reduce the body's ability to withstand stress.
Before and during surgery, dosages may be temporarily increased.

Diuretics
These potentiate electrolyte imbalances after surgery.

Herbal Substances
These can interact with anesthesia and cause a variety of adverse effects. These substances may need to be stopped at a specific time before surgery. During the preoperative period, the client needs to be asked if he or she is taking any herbal substances.

Insulin
The need for insulin after surgery in a diabetic client may either be reduced, because the client's nutritional intake is decreased, or be increased, because of the stress response and the intravenous administration of glucose solutions.

Adapted from Potter, P., & Perry, A. (2009). *Fundamentals of nursing* (7th ed.). St. Louis: Mosby.

Box 17-5 The Joint Commission's Protocol for Preventing Wrong-Site, Wrong-Procedure, and Wrong-Person Surgery

Preoperative Client Verification
At least two client identifiers must be used to verify the client's identity (e.g., full name, date of birth).
 Confirm and verify the following:
■ Client's name on the identification band
■ Date of birth
■ Medical record number
■ Consent forms
■ Scheduled procedure and marked surgical site
■ Availability of implant, if needed
■ Availability of blood
■ Radiological examinations

Site Marking
Site verification is required for all procedures that involve laterality, multiple structures, or multiple levels.

The site is marked with a permanent marker that is visible after the skin is prepped and draped.
The operating surgeon marks the site with his or her initials before the client enters the operating suite.
The site is marked in accordance with client participation (i.e., verbal confirmation or pointing).
The client has the right to refuse marking of the site. Each institution will determine the policy for these situations.

Adapted from The Joint Commission. National Patient Safety Goals. Effective July 1, 2011, Hospital Accreditation Program. http://www.jointcommission.org/assets/1/6/NPSG_EPs_Scoring_HAP_20110706.pdf.

4. Monitor for secretions; if the client is unable to clear the airway by coughing, suction the secretions from the client's airway.
5. Observe chest movement for symmetry and the use of accessory muscles.
6. Monitor oxygen administration if prescribed.
7. Monitor pulse oximetry.
8. Encourage deep breathing and coughing exercises and the use of the incentive spirometer as soon as possible after surgery.
9. Note the rate, depth, and quality of respirations; the respiratory rate should be higher than 10 and lower than 30 breaths/min.
10. Monitor for signs of respiratory distress, atelectasis, or other respiratory complications.

C. Cardiovascular system
1. Monitor circulatory status, such as skin color, peripheral pulses, capillary refill, and the absence of edema, numbness, and tingling.
2. Monitor for bleeding.
3. Check the pulse for rate and rhythm (a bounding pulse may indicate hypertension, fluid overload, or client anxiety).
4. Monitor for cardiac dysrhythmias.
5. Monitor for signs of thrombophlebitis, particularly in clients who were in the lithotomy position during surgery.
6. Encourage the use of antiembolism stockings, if prescribed, to promote venous return, strengthen muscle tone, and prevent pooling of blood in the extremities.

D. Musculoskeletal system
1. Monitor the client for movement of the extremities.
2. Review surgeon's prescriptions regarding client positioning or restrictions.

Box 17-6 Time-Out Procedure

A time-out occurs in the operating room after the client has been prepped and draped. The entire team must verbally verify their agreement about the following:
- The client's name
- The procedure to be performed
- The surgical site
- Laterality, implants, and radiological examinations, if applicable

The documentation of the time-out should indicate that the following were verified:
- Correct client
- Correct site and side
- Agreement to proceed
- Correct client position
- Availability of implants or special equipment

Adapted from The Joint Commission. National Patient Safety Goals. Effective July 1, 2011, Hospital Accreditation Program. http://www.jointcommission.org/assets/1/6/NPSG_EPs_Scoring_HAP_20110706.pdf.

---

3. Encourage ambulation if prescribed; before ambulation, instruct the client to sit at the edge of the bed with his or her feet supported to assume balance.
4. Unless contraindicated, place the client in a low Fowler's position after surgery to increase the size of the thorax for lung expansion.
5. Avoid positioning the postoperative client in a supine position until pharyngeal reflexes have returned; if the client is comatose or semicomatose, position on the side (additionally, an oral airway may be needed).
6. If the client is unable to get out of bed, turn the client every 1 to 2 hours.

E. Neurological system
1. Monitor level of consciousness.
2. Frequent periodic attempts to awaken the client should continue until the client awakens.
3. Orient the client to the environment.
4. Speak in a soft tone; filter out extraneous noises in the environment.
5. Maintain body temperature and prevent heat loss by providing the client with warm blankets and raising the room temperature as necessary.

F. Temperature control
1. Monitor temperature.
2. Monitor for signs of hypothermia that may result from anesthesia, a cool operating room, or exposure of the skin and internal organs during surgery.
3. Apply warm blankets and continue oxygen as prescribed if the client experiences shivering.

G. Integumentary system
1. Check the surgical site, drains, and wound dressings (serous drainage may occur from an incision but if excessive bleeding occurs from the site notify the physician). (Figure 17-4)
2. Check the skin for redness, abrasions, or breakdown that may have resulted from surgical positioning.
3. Monitor body temperature and wound for signs of infection.
4. Maintain a dry, intact dressing.
5. Change dressings as prescribed, noting the amount of bleeding or drainage, odor, and intactness of sutures or staples.
6. Wound drains should be patent; prepare to assist with the removal of drains (as prescribed by the surgeon) when the drainage amount becomes insignificant.
7. An abdominal binder may be prescribed for obese and debilitated individuals to prevent dehiscence of the incision (Figure 17-5)

H. Fluid and electrolyte balance
1. Monitor IV fluid administration as prescribed.
2. Record intake and output.
3. Monitor for signs of fluid or electrolyte imbalances.

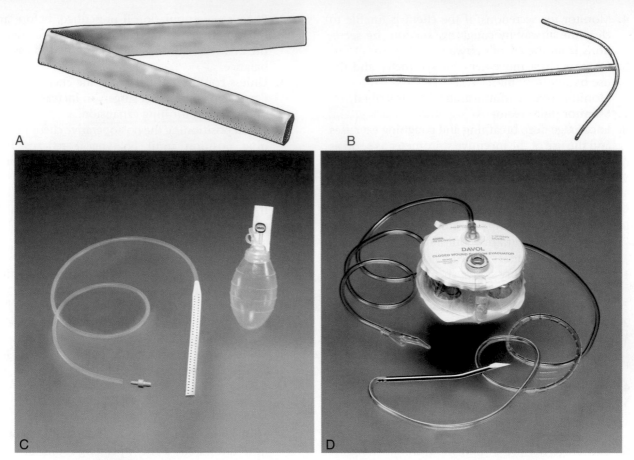

▲ **FIGURE 17-4** Types of surgical drains. Gravity drains drain directly through a tube from the surgical area. **A,** Penrose. **B,** T-tube. With closed-wound drains, drainage collects in a collecting vessel by means of the compression and reexpansion of the system. **C,** Jackson-Pratt. **D,** Hemovac. (**A** and **B,** From Ignatavicius, D., & Workman, L. [2010]. *Medical-surgical nursing: Patient-centered collaborative care* [6th ed.]. St. Louis: Saunders. **C** and **D,** Courtesy of C. R. Bard, Inc., Covington GA.)

▲ **FIGURE 17-5** Abdominal binders. **A,** Scultetus: Binder with flaps that wrap over each other. **B,** Straight binder with Velcro. (From Elkin, M., Perry, A., & Potter, P. [2008]. *Nursing interventions and clinical skills* [4th ed.]. St. Louis: Mosby.)

I. Gastrointestinal system
   1. Monitor intake and output and for nausea and vomiting.
   2. Maintain patency of the nasogastric tube if present.
   3. Monitor for abdominal distention.
   4. Monitor for passage of flatus and return of bowel sounds.
   5. Administer frequent oral care, at least every 2 hours.
   6. Maintain the NPO status until the gag reflex and peristalsis return.
   7. When oral fluids are permitted, start with ice chips and water.
   8. Ensure that the client advances to clear liquids and then to a regular diet, as prescribed and as the client can tolerate.

⚠ To prevent aspiration, turn the client to a side-lying position if vomiting occurs and have suctioning equipment available and ready to use.

J. Renal system
1. Assess the bladder for distention.
2. Monitor urine output (urinary output should be at least 30 mL/hr).
3. If the client does not have a Foley catheter, the client is expected to void within 6 to 8 hours postoperatively depending on the type of anesthesia administered; ensure that the amount is at least 200 mL.

K. Pain management
1. Assess the type of anesthetic used and preoperative medication that the client received, and note whether the client received any pain medications in the postanesthesia period.
2. Assess for pain and inquire about the type and location of pain; ask the client to rate the degree of pain on a scale of 1 to 10, with 10 being the most severe.
3. If the client is unable to rate the pain with a numerical pain scale, then use a descriptor scale that lists words that describe different levels of pain intensity, such as *no pain, mild pain, moderate pain,* and *severe pain.*
4. Monitor for objective data related to pain, such as facial expressions, body gestures, increased pulse rate, increased blood pressure, and increased respirations.
5. Inquire about the effectiveness of the last pain medication.
6. Administer pain medication as prescribed.
7. Ensure that the client with a patient-controlled analgesia pump understands how to use it.
8. If an opioid has been prescribed, during the initial administration, assess the client every 30 minutes for respiratory rate and pain relief.
9. Use noninvasive measures to relieve postoperative pain, including distraction, comfort measures, positioning, backrubs, and providing a quiet and restful environment.
10. Document effectiveness of the pain medication and noninvasive pain relief measures.

⚠ Consider cultural practices and beliefs when planning pain management.

III. PNEUMONIA AND ATELECTASIS (Figure 17-6 and Box 17-7)

A. Description
1. Pneumonia, which is an inflammation of the alveoli caused by an infectious process, may develop 3 to 5 days after the surgical procedure because of infection, aspiration, or immobility.
2. Atelectasis, which is a collapse of the alveoli with retained mucous secretions, is the most common postoperative complication. It usually occurs 1 to 2 days after the surgical procedure.

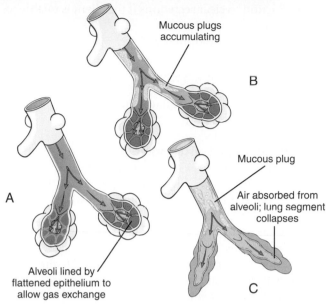

▲ **FIGURE 17-6** Postoperative atelectasis. **A,** Normal bronchiole and alveoli. **B,** Mucous plug in bronchiole. **C,** Collapse of alveoli as a result of atelectasis after the absorption of air. (From Lewis, S., Heitkemper, M., & Dirksen, S. [2004]. *Medical-surgical nursing: Assessment and management of clinical problems* [6th ed.]. St. Louis: Mosby.)

Box 17-7 Postoperative Complications

- Constipation
- Hemorrhage
- Hypoxia
- Paralytic ileus
- Pneumonia and atelectasis
- Pulmonary embolism
- Shock
- Thrombophlebitis
- Urinary retention
- Wound dehiscence
- Wound evisceration
- Wound infection

Note: The licensed practical/vocational nurse always notifies the registered nurse and/or the surgeon if signs of complications are noted.

B. Data collection
1. Dyspnea and increased respiratory rate
2. Elevated temperature
3. Productive cough and chest pain
4. Crackles over involved lung area

C. Interventions
1. Monitor lung and breath sounds and temperature.
2. Encourage ambulation.
3. Reposition the client every 1 to 2 hours.
4. Encourage the client to use an incentive spirometer and to cough and deep breathe.

5. Suction to clear secretions if the client is unable to cough.
6. Encourage fluid intake.

IV. HYPOXIA (see Box 17-7)

A. Description: An inadequate concentration of oxygen in the arterial blood
B. Data collection
   1. Restlessness and agitation
   2. Confusion
   3. Dyspnea
   4. Increased heart rate and blood pressure
   5. Diaphoresis
   6. Cyanosis
C. Interventions
   1. Monitor for signs of hypoxia, eliminate the cause of hypoxia, and notify the registered nurse and/or surgeon immediately.
   2. Monitor pulse oximetry.
   3. Administer oxygen, as prescribed.
   4. Encourage coughing, deep breathing, and the use of incentive spirometry.
   5. Turn and reposition the client frequently.
   6. Encourage ambulation.

V. PULMONARY EMBOLISM (see Box 17-7)

A. Description: An embolus blocking the pulmonary artery and disrupting the blood flow to one or more lobes of the lung
B. Data collection
   1. Dyspnea
   2. Sudden sharp chest or upper abdominal pain
   3. Increased heart rate and a decrease in blood pressure
   4. Cyanosis
C. Interventions
   1. Notify the registered nurse and/or surgeon immediately.
   2. Monitor vital signs.
   3. Administer oxygen, as prescribed.

VI. HEMORRHAGE (see Box 17-7)

A. Description: The loss of a large amount of blood externally or internally during a short period of time
B. Data collection
   1. Restlessness
   2. Weak, rapid pulse and hypotension
   3. Cool, clammy skin
   4. Tachypnea
   5. Reduced urine output
C. Interventions
   1. Apply pressure to the site of bleeding.
   2. Notify the registered nurse and/or surgeon immediately.
   3. Administer oxygen, as prescribed.

VII. SHOCK (see Box 17-7)

A. Description: A loss of circulatory fluid volume that is usually caused by hemorrhage
B. Data collection: Similar to data collection findings of hemorrhage
C. Interventions
   1. If shock develops, elevate the legs.
   2. If the client has had spinal anesthesia, do not elevate the legs any higher than placing them on a pillow; otherwise, diaphragm muscles could be impaired.
   3. Notify the registered nurse and/or surgeon immediately.
   4. Administer oxygen, as prescribed.
   5. Monitor the level of consciousness.
   6. Monitor vital signs for an increased pulse and decreased blood pressure.
   7. Monitor skin color and mucous membranes for moistness.

VIII. THROMBOPHLEBITIS (see Box 17-7)

A. Description
   1. An inflammation of a vein, often accompanied by clot formation
   2. Veins in the legs are most commonly affected
B. Data collection
   1. Aching or cramping leg pain
   2. Vein inflammation; vein feels hard and cord-like and is tender to touch
   3. Elevated temperature
C. Interventions
   1. Monitor legs for swelling, inflammation, cyanosis, pain, tenderness, and venous distention.
   2. Elevate the extremity 30 degrees without allowing any pressure on the popliteal area.
   3. Encourage the client to perform "foot pumps" while on bedrest.
   4. Encourage early ambulation, as prescribed.
   5. Encourage the use of antiembolism stockings, as prescribed, removing them twice a day to wash and inspect the legs.
   6. Use a sequential compression device (SCD), as prescribed (Figure 17-7).
   7. Perform passive range of motion every 2 hours if the client is on bedrest.
   8. Do not allow the client's legs to dangle.
   9. Instruct the client to not sit in one position for an extended period of time.
   10. Heparin sodium or warfarin (Coumadin) may be prescribed.

IX. URINARY RETENTION (see Box 17-7)

A. Description
   1. The involuntary accumulation of urine in the bladder from a loss of muscle tone

2. Occurs as a result of the effects of anesthetics and opioid analgesics
3. Appears 6 to 8 hours after surgery

B. Data collection
   1. Restlessness and diaphoresis
   2. Lower abdominal pain
   3. Inability to void and a distended bladder
   4. Elevated blood pressure
   5. On percussion, the bladder sounds like a drum

C. Interventions
   1. Monitor for voiding, and check for a distended bladder with an ultrasound bladder scanner, if available.
   2. Encourage fluid intake unless contraindicated.
   3. Assist the client to void by helping him or her to stand.
   4. Provide privacy.
   5. Pour warm water over the perineum or allow the client to hear running water to promote voiding.
   6. Catheterize the client, as prescribed, after all non-invasive techniques have been attempted.

X. CONSTIPATION (see Box 17-7)

A. Description
   1. The abnormal and infrequent passage of stool
   2. When the client resumes a solid diet after surgery, failure to pass stool within 48 hours is a cause for concern.

B. Data collection
   1. Abdominal distention
   2. Absence of bowel movements
   3. Anorexia, headache, and nausea

C. Interventions
   1. Check bowel sounds.
   2. Encourage fluid intake up to 3000 mL/day unless contraindicated.
   3. Encourage early ambulation.

▲ **FIGURE 17-7** Intermittent pulsatile compression device. (From Monahan, F., Sands, J., Neighbors, M., Marek, J., & Green, C. [2007]. *Phipps' medical-surgical nursing: Health and illness perspectives* [8th ed.]. St. Louis: Mosby.)

4. Encourage the consumption of fiber-rich foods unless contraindicated.
5. Administer stool softeners and laxatives, as prescribed.
6. Provide privacy and adequate time for bowel elimination.

XI. PARALYTIC ILEUS (see Box 17-7)

A. Description
   1. A failure of the appropriate forward movement of bowel contents
   2. May occur as a result of anesthetic medications or the manipulation of the bowel during the surgical procedure

B. Data collection
   1. Postoperative nausea and vomiting
   2. Abdominal distention
   3. Absence of bowel sounds, bowel movement, or flatus

C. Interventions
   1. Maintain NPO status until bowel sounds return.
   2. Maintain the patency of the nasogastric tube, if present.
   3. Encourage ambulation.
   4. Monitor IV fluids, as prescribed.
   5. Administer medications, as prescribed, to increase gastrointestinal motility and secretions.
   6. If ileus occurs, it is first treated nonsurgically with bowel decompression by the insertion of a nasogastric tube attached to intermittent or constant suction.

XII. WOUND INFECTION (see Box 17-7)

A. Description
   1. Often caused by poor aseptic technique or a wound that was contaminated before surgical exploration
   2. Usually occurs 3 to 6 days after surgery
   3. Purulent material may exit from the drains or separated wound edges.

B. Data collection
   1. Fever and chills
   2. Warm, tender, painful, and inflamed incision site
   3. Edematous skin at the incision and tight skin sutures
   4. Elevated white blood cell count

C. Interventions
   1. Monitor the temperature.
   2. Monitor the incision site for approximation of the suture line, edema, bleeding, and signs of infection (*REEDA: Redness, Edema, Ecchymosis, Drainage,* and *Approximation* of the wound edges).
   3. Maintain the patency of any drains, and keep drains and tubes away from the incision line.

4. Monitor drains, and assess drainage amount, color, and consistency.
5. Change dressings, as prescribed.
6. Administer antibiotics, as prescribed.

 XIII. WOUND DEHISCENCE (Figure 17-8; also see Box 17-7)

A. Description
1. The separation of the wound edges at the suture line
2. Usually occurs 6 to 8 days after surgery
B. Data collection
1. Increased drainage
2. Opened wound edges
3. The appearance of underlying tissues through the wound
C. Interventions
1. Notify the registered nurse and/or surgeon immediately.
2. Place the client in a low Fowler's position with the knees bent to prevent abdominal tension on abdominal wounds.
3. Cover the wound with a sterile normal saline dressing.
4. Prevent wound infection.

 XIV. WOUND EVISCERATION (see Box 17-7 and Figure 17-8)

A. Description
1. The protrusion of the internal organs and tissues through an opening in the wound edges

2. Most common among obese clients, clients who have had abdominal surgery, or those who have poor wound-healing ability
3. Usually occurs 6 to 8 days after surgery
4. Wound evisceration is an emergency.
B. Data collection
1. The discharge of serosanguineous fluid from a previously dry wound
2. The appearance of loops of bowel or other abdominal contents through the wound
3. The client may report feeling a popping sensation after coughing or turning.
C. Interventions (see Priority Nursing Actions)
1. Notify the registered nurse and/or surgeon immediately.
2. Place the client in a low Fowler's position with the knees bent to prevent abdominal tension.
3. Cover the wound with a sterile normal saline dressing.
4. Prevent wound infection.

■■■■■■■■ Priority Nursing Actions! ■■■■■

Steps to Take if Evisceration Occurs
1. Call for help; ask that the surgeon be notified and that needed supplies be brought to the client's room.
2. Stay with the client.
3. While waiting for supplies to arrive, place the client in a low Fowler's position with the knees bent.
4. Cover the wound with a sterile normal saline dressing and keep the dressing moist.
5. Take vital signs and monitor the client closely for signs of shock
6. Prepare the client for surgery as necessary.
7. Document the occurrence, the actions taken, and the client's response.

Wound evisceration is protrusion of the internal organs through an incision; it usually occurs 6 to 8 days after surgery. Evisceration is most common among obese clients, clients who have had abdominal surgery, or those who have poor wound-healing ability. Wound evisceration is an emergency. The nurse immediately calls for help and asks that the surgeon be notified and that needed supplies (vital sign measurement devices, sterile normal saline and dressings) be brought to the client's room. The nurse stays with the client and while waiting for supplies to arrive places the client in a low Fowler's position with the knees bent to prevent abdominal tension on an abdominal suture line. The nurse covers the wound with a sterile normal saline dressing as soon as supplies are available and keeps the dressing moist. Vital signs are monitored closely, and the client is monitored for signs of shock. The client is prepared for surgery if prescribed. The nurse also documents the occurrence, the actions taken, and the client's response.

Reference: Ignatavicius, D., & Workman, M. (2010). *Medical-surgical nursing: Patient-centered collaborative care* (6th ed., p. 296). St. Louis: Saunders.

A   B

▲ **FIGURE 17-8** **A,** Wound dehiscence. **B,** Wound evisceration. (From Ignatavicius, D., & Workman, L. [2010]. *Medical-surgical nursing: Critical thinking for collaborative care* [6th ed.]. St. Louis: Saunders.)

XV. AMBULATORY SURGERY

A. Criteria for client discharge
1. Is alert and oriented
2. Has voided
3. Has no respiratory distress
4. Vital signs and oxygen saturation are within normal limits
5. Is able to ambulate, swallow, and cough
6. Has minimal pain
7. Is not vomiting
8. Has minimal (if any) bleeding from the incision site
9. A responsible adult is available to drive the client home.
10. The surgeon has signed a release form.

B. Reinforcing discharge instructions (Box 17-8)
1. Should be performed before the date of the scheduled procedure
2. Provide written instructions to the client and family regarding the specifics of care.

Box 17-8 Reinforcing Discharge Instructions

Determine the client's readiness to learn, educational level, and desire to change or modify his or her lifestyle.

Determine the need for resources for home care.

Demonstrate the care of the incision and how to change the dressing.

Instruct the client to cover the incision with plastic as prescribed if showering is allowed.

Be sure that the client is provided with a 48-hour supply of dressings for home use.

Instruct the client about the importance of returning to the surgeon's office for follow-up visits.

Instruct the client that sutures and staples are usually removed in the surgeon's office 7 to 10 days after surgery and that the skin may become slightly reddened when they are ready to be removed.

Steri-Strips may be applied to provide extra support after the sutures are removed. Instruct the client to not remove the Steri-strips until they are close to falling off.

Instruct the client regarding the use of medications and their purposes, doses, administration, and side effects.

Instruct the client regarding proper diet and to drink 6 to 8 glasses of liquid per day.

Instruct the client regarding activity levels and to resume normal activities gradually.

Instruct the client to avoid lifting for 6 weeks if a major surgical procedure was performed.

Instruct the client with an abdominal incision to not lift anything weighing 10 lb or more and to not engage in any activities that involve pushing or pulling.

Clients usually can return to work after 6 to 8 weeks, as prescribed by the surgeon.

Instruct the client regarding the signs and symptoms of complications and when to call a surgeon.

3. Instruct the client and family about postoperative complications that can occur.
4. Suggest appropriate resources for home-care support.
5. Instruct the client to not drive for 24 hours if he or she has had a general anesthetic.
6. Inform the client to call the surgeon, ambulatory center, or emergency department if postoperative problems occur.
7. Instruct the client to keep follow-up appointments with the surgeon.

MORE QUESTIONS ON EVOLVE!

Practice Questions

131. A nurse is developing a plan of care for a client who is scheduled for surgery. The nurse would include which of the following activities in the nursing care plan for the client on the day of surgery?
    1. Have the client void immediately before surgery.
    2. Avoid oral hygiene and rinsing with mouthwash.
    3. Verify that the client has not eaten for the last 24 hours.
    4. Report immediately any slight increase in blood pressure or pulse.

132. A nurse is caring for a client who is scheduled for surgery. The client is concerned about the surgical procedure. To alleviate the client's fears and misconceptions about surgery, the nurse should:
    1. Tell the client that preoperative fear is normal.
    2. Explain all nursing care and possible discomfort that may result.
    3. Ask the client to discuss information known about the planned surgery.
    4. Provide explanations about the procedures involved in the planned surgery.

133. A nurse is collecting data from a client who is scheduled for surgery in 1 week in the ambulatory care surgical center. The nurse notes that the client has a history of arthritis and has been taking acetylsalicylic acid (aspirin). The nurse reports the information to the surgeon and anticipates that the surgeon will prescribe which of the following?
    1. Discontinue the aspirin immediately.
    2. Continue to take the aspirin as prescribed.
    3. Discontinue the aspirin 48 hours before the scheduled surgery.
    4. Decrease the dose of the aspirin to half of what is normally taken.

134. A nurse obtains the vital signs on a postoperative client who just returned to the nursing unit. The client's blood pressure (BP) is 100/60 mm Hg, the pulse is 90 beats per minute, and the respiration rate is 20 breaths per minute. On the basis of these findings, which of the following nursing actions should be performed?
1. Shake the client gently to arouse.
2. Continue to monitor the vital signs.
3. Call the registered nurse immediately.
4. Cover the client with a warm blanket.

135. A client arrives to the surgical nursing unit after surgery. The initial nursing action is to check the:
1. Patency of the airway
2. Dressing for bleeding
3. Tubes or drains for patency
4. Vital signs to compare with preoperative measurements

136. A nurse is monitoring an adult client for postoperative complications. Which of the following would be the most indicative of a potential postoperative complication that requires further observation?
1. A urinary output of 20 mL/hour
2. A temperature of 37.6° C (99.6° F)
3. A blood pressure of 100/70 mm Hg
4. Serous drainage on the surgical dressing

137. A nurse monitors the postoperative client frequently for the presence of secretions in the lungs, knowing that accumulated secretions can lead to:
1. Pneumonia
2. Fluid imbalance
3. Pulmonary edema
4. Carbon dioxide retention

138. A nurse is caring for a postoperative client who has a drain inserted into the surgical wound. Which of the following actions would the nurse avoid in the care of the drain?
1. Check the drain for patency.
2. Observe for bright red, bloody drainage.
3. Maintain aseptic technique when emptying.
4. Secure the drain by curling or folding it and taping it firmly to the body.

139. A nurse checks the client's surgical incision for signs of infection. Which of the following would be indicative of a potential infection?
1. The presence of serous drainage
2. The presence of purulent drainage
3. A temperature of 98.8° F (37.1° C)
4. The client complaining of feeling cold

140. A nurse is checking a client's surgical incision and notes an increase in the amount of drainage, a separation of the incision line, and the appearance of underlying tissue. Which of the following is the initial action?
1. Cover the wound with a Betadine-soaked dressing.
2. Apply a sterile dressing soaked with normal saline to the wound.
3. Leave the incision open to the air to assist with drying the drainage.
4. Clean the wound using aseptic technique, and apply a sterile, dry dressing.

ANSWERS

131. 1

Rationale: The nurse would assist the client with voiding immediately before surgery so that the bladder will be empty. Oral hygiene is allowed, but the client should not swallow any water. The client usually has a restriction of food and fluids for 8 hours before surgery rather than 24 hours. A slight increase in blood pressure and pulse is common during the preoperative period; this is generally the result of anxiety.

Test-Taking Strategy: Use the process of elimination, and read each option carefully. Eliminate option 3, knowing that the client should receive nothing by mouth for 8 hours before surgery. Eliminate option 4 because of the words "immediately" and "slight." There is no useful reason for option 2; in fact, oral hygiene may make the client feel more comfortable. Review general preoperative care if you had difficulty with this question.

Level of Cognitive Ability: Applying
Client Needs: Physiological Integrity
Integrated Process: Nursing Process/Planning

Content Area: Fundamental Skills: Perioperative Care
References: deWit, pp. 77, 81, 83. 2009.

132. 3

Rationale: Explanations should begin with the information that the client knows. Option 1 is a block to communication, and options 2 and 4 may produce additional anxiety in the client.

Test-Taking Strategy: Use the process of elimination. Remember to always focus on the client's feelings first; this will direct you to option 3. Additionally, option 3 is the only option that addresses data collection, which is the first step of the Nursing Process. Review the psychosocial aspects related to the preoperative client if you had difficulty with this question.

Level of Cognitive Ability: Applying
Client Needs: Psychosocial Integrity
Integrated Process: Caring
Content Area: Fundamental Skills: Perioperative Care
References: Christensen, Kockrow, pp. 20–21, 24. 2011. *Adult health nursing.*
deWit, p. 72. 2009.
Linton, pp. 266–267. 2012.

133. 3
Rationale: Anticoagulants alter normal clotting factors and increase the risk of hemorrhage. Aspirin has properties that can alter the clotting mechanism and should thus be discontinued at least 48 hours before surgery.
Test-Taking Strategy: Use the process of elimination. Remembering that aspirin has properties that can alter normal clotting factors and that it should be discontinued at least 48 hours before surgery will assist with directing you to option 3. Review the medications that affect the preoperative client if you had difficulty with this question.
Level of Cognitive Ability: Analyzing
Client Needs: Physiological Integrity
Integrated Process: Nursing Process/Planning
Content Area: Fundamental Skills: Perioperative Care
Reference: Christensen, Kockrow, p. 38. 2011. *Adult health nursing.*

134. 2
Rationale: A slightly lower-than-normal BP and an increased pulse rate are common after surgery. The level of consciousness can be determined by checking the client's response to light touch and verbal stimuli rather than by shaking the client. Warm blankets are applied to maintain the client's body temperature. There is no reason to contact the registered nurse immediately.
Test-Taking Strategy: Focus on the data in the question. Noting that the vital signs are within normal limits will direct you to option 2. Review expected postoperative findings if you had difficulty with this question.
Level of Cognitive Ability: Applying
Client Needs: Physiological Integrity
Integrated Process: Nursing Process/Implementation
Content Area: Fundamental Skills: Perioperative Care
References: Christensen, Kockrow, pp. 45–46. 2011. *Adult health nursing.*
deWit, p. 96. 2009.

135. 1
Rationale: If the airway is not patent, immediate measures must be taken for the survival of the client. After checking the client's airway, the nurse would then check the client's vital signs, and this would be followed by checking the dressings, tubes, and drains.
Test-Taking Strategy: Use the ABCs—airway, breathing, and circulation. Maintaining the airway patency is the first action to be taken. Options 2, 3, and 4 are all nursing actions that should be performed after a patent airway has been established. Review the care of the postoperative client if you had difficulty with this question.
Level of Cognitive Ability: Applying
Client Needs: Physiological Integrity
Integrated Process: Nursing Process/Implementation
Content Area: Fundamental Skills: Perioperative Care
Reference: Christensen, Kockrow, p. 45. 2011. *Adult health nursing.*

136. 1
Rationale: Urine output is maintained at a minimum of at least 30 mL/hour for an adult. An output of less than 30 mL/hour for each of two consecutive hours should be reported to the surgeon. A temperature more than 37° C (100° F) or less than 36.1° C (97° F) and a falling systolic blood pressure less than 90 mm Hg are to be reported. The client's preoperative or baseline blood pressure is used to make informed postoperative comparisons. Moderate or light serous drainage from the surgical site is considered normal.
Test-Taking Strategy: Knowledge of the normal ranges for temperature, blood pressure, urinary output, and wound drainage is necessary to determine the correct option. Use the process of elimination to determine that the urinary output is the only observation that is not within the normal range. Review expected postoperative findings if you had difficulty with this question.
Level of Cognitive Ability: Analyzing
Client Needs: Physiological Integrity
Integrated Process: Nursing Process/Data Collection
Content Area: Fundamental Skills: Perioperative Care
Reference: Christensen, Kockrow, p. 50. 2011. *Adult health nursing.*

137. 1
Rationale: The most common postoperative respiratory problems are atelectasis, pneumonia, and pulmonary emboli. Pneumonia is the inflammation of lung tissue that causes a productive cough, dyspnea, and crackles. Fluid imbalance can be a deficit or excess related to fluid loss or overload. Pulmonary edema usually results from left-sided heart failure, and it can be caused by medications, fluid overload, and smoke inhalation. Carbon dioxide retention results from the inability to exhale carbon dioxide in clients with conditions such as chronic obstructive pulmonary disease.
Test-Taking Strategy: Use the process of elimination, and note the strategic words "presence of secretions in the lungs." Focus on the subject of the postoperative client to direct you to option 1. Options 2, 3, and 4 most commonly occur with other conditions. Review postoperative complications if you had difficulty with this question.
Level of Cognitive Ability: Understanding
Client Needs: Physiological Integrity
Integrated Process: Nursing Process/Data Collection
Content Area: Fundamental Skills: Perioperative Care
References: Christensen, Kockrow, p. 49. 2011. *Adult health nursing.*
deWit, p. 103. 2009.

138. 4
Rationale: Aseptic technique must be used when emptying the drainage container or changing the dressing to avoid contamination of the wound. Usually drainage from the wound is pale, red, and watery, whereas active bleeding will be bright red in color. The drain should be checked for patency to provide an exit for the fluid or blood to promote healing. The nurse needs to ensure that drainage flows freely and that there are no kinks in the drains. Curling or folding the drain prevents the flow of the drainage.
Test-Taking Strategy: Use the process of elimination, and note the strategic word "avoid." Remember that the nurse needs to ensure that drainage flows freely from a drain. Review the care of the surgical client with a drain if you had difficulty with this question.

Level of Cognitive Ability: Applying
Client Needs: Physiological Integrity
Integrated Process: Nursing Process/Implementation
Content Area: Fundamental Skills: Perioperative Care
References: Christensen, Kockrow, p. 55. 2011. *Adult health nursing.*
deWit, pp. 100–101. 2009.

139. 2

Rationale: Signs and symptoms of a wound infection include warm, red, and tender skin around the incision. The client may have fever and chills. Purulent material may exit from drains or from separated wound edges. Infection may be caused by poor aseptic technique or a wound that was contaminated before surgical exploration; it appears 3 to 6 days after surgery. Serous drainage is not indicative of a wound infection. A temperature of 98.8° F is not an abnormal finding in a postoperative client. The fact that a client feels cold is not indicative of an infection, although chills and fever are signs of infection.

Test-Taking Strategy: Use the process of elimination. Noting the word "purulent" in option 2 will direct you to this option. Review the signs of a wound infection if you had difficulty with this question.

Level of Cognitive Ability: Understanding
Client Needs: Physiological Integrity
Integrated Process: Nursing Process/Data Collection
Content Area: Fundamental Skills: Perioperative Care

References: Christensen, Kockrow, p. 49. 2011. *Adult health nursing.*
deWit, pp. 100–101. 2009.
Linton, p. 283. 2012.

140. 2

Rationale: Wound dehiscence is the separation of the wound edges at the suture line. Signs and symptoms include increased drainage and the appearance of underlying tissues. It usually occurs as a complication 6 to 8 days after surgery. The client should be instructed to remain quiet and avoid coughing or straining, and he or she should be positioned to prevent further stress on the wound. Sterile dressings soaked with sterile normal saline should be used to cover the wound. The surgeon needs to be notified.

Test-Taking Strategy: Use the process of elimination. Eliminate option 3 first, because this action would expose the open wound and the underlying tissues to infection. Eliminate options 1 and 4 next, because a dressing soaked with Betadine and a dry dressing will irritate the exposed body tissues. Review emergency care when dehiscence or evisceration occurs if you had difficulty with this question.

Level of Cognitive Ability: Applying
Client Needs: Physiological Integrity
Integrated Process: Nursing Process/Implementation
Content Area: Fundamental Skills: Perioperative Care
Reference: Christensen, Kockrow, p. 48. 2011. *Adult health nursing.*

Positioning Clients

PYRAMID TERMS

Body mechanics The coordinated efforts of the musculoskel-etal and nervous systems to maintain balance, posture, and body alignment during lifting, bending, and moving to perform activities safely

ergonomic principles The anatomical, physiological, psycho-social, and mechanical principles affecting the efficient and safe use of an individual's energy.

Fowler's position The client is supine, and the head of the bed is elevated to 45 to 60 degrees

high Fowler's position The client is supine, and the head of the bed is elevated to 90 degrees

lateral (side-lying) position The client is lying on the side, and the head and shoulders are aligned with the hips and the spine parallel to the edge of the mattress. The head, neck, and upper arm are supported by a pillow; the lower shoulder is pulled forward slightly. The elbow is flexed at 90 degrees. The legs are flexed or extended, and a pillow is placed to support the back.

lithotomy position The client is lying on his or her back with the hips and knees flexed at right angles and the feet in stirrups

prone position The client is lying on his or her abdomen with the head turned to the side

reverse Trendelenburg's position The bed is tilted so that the foot of the client's bed is lower than the head of the bed

semi-Fowler's position (low Fowler's position) The client is supine, and the head of the bed is elevated approximately 30 degrees

Sims' position The client is lying on his or her side with the body turned prone at 45 degrees. The lower leg is extended with the upper leg flexed at the hip and knee at a 45- to 90-degree angle.

supine position The client is lying on his or her back. The head and shoulders are usually slightly elevated with a small pillow. The arms and legs are extended, and the legs are slightly abducted.

Trendelenburg's position The bed is tilted so that the head of the client's bed is lower than the foot of the bed. This position is contraindicated for clients with head injuries, increased intracranial pressure, spinal cord injuries, and certain cardiac and respiratory disorders.

PYRAMID TO SUCCESS

Nursing responsibilities include positioning clients in a safe and appropriate manner to provide safety and com-fort. Knowledge regarding the client's position required for a certain procedure or condition is expected. It is the nurse's responsibility to reduce the likelihood and pre-vent the development of complications related to an existing condition, a prescribed treatment, or a medical or surgical procedure. It is imperative that the nurse re-view the health care provider's (HCP's) prescriptions after treatments or procedures and that he or she take note of instructions regarding positioning and mobility (Figures 18-1 and 18-2). The nurse must also be aware of the various body pressure points when clients are positioned in lying or sitting positions (Figure 18-3).

CLIENT NEEDS

Safe and Effective Care Environment

- Preventing accidents and injuries
- Positioning the client appropriately and safely
- Ensuring environmental and personal safety
- Establishing priorities
- Providing protective measures
- Using equipment safely
- Using ergonomic principles and body mechanics when moving a client

Health Promotion and Maintenance

- Providing information regarding the need for prescribed therapies
- Performing the techniques of data collection

Psychosocial Integrity

- Assisting the client with the use of coping mechanisms
- Keeping the family informed about the client's progress
- Providing support to the client

Physiological Integrity

- Monitoring airway patency
- Providing comfort measures for rest and sleep
- Preventing the complications of immobility
- Providing nutrition and oral intake
- Providing personal hygiene to the client as needed
- Using assistive devices

Trendelenburg's

Fowler's

Reverse Trendelenburg's

Semi-Fowler's

Flat

▲ **FIGURE 18-1** Common bed positions. (From Potter, P., & Perry, A. [2010]. *Fundamentals of nursing* [7th ed.]. St. Louis: Mosby.)

I. GUIDELINES FOR POSITIONING

A. Principles of body movement for clients
 1. Body movement and alignment are important for clients. Many clients are unable to change position or move in bed independently.
 2. Basic principles include maintaining correct anatomical position and changing the position frequently.

B. Position in a safe and appropriate manner to provide safety, alignment, and comfort.

C. Select a position that will prevent the development of complications related to an existing condition, a prescribed treatment, or a medical or surgical procedure.

⚠ Always review the HCP's prescription, especially after treatments or procedures, and take note of instructions regarding positioning and mobility.

II. ERGONOMIC PRINCIPLES RELATED TO BODY MECHANICS (Box 18-1)

III. POSITIONS TO ENSURE SAFETY AND COMFORT

A. Integumentary system
 1. Autograft: After surgery, the site is immobilized for approximately 3 to 7 days to provide the time

Lateral (side-lying) position

Semiprone (Sims' or forward side-lying) position

Supine position

Prone position. The client's arms and shoulders may be positioned in internal or external rotation.

▲ **FIGURE 18-2** Common client positions. (From Harkreader, H. & Hogan, M. [2004]. *Fundamentals of nursing: Caring and clinical judgment* [2nd ed.]. Philadelphia: Saunders.)

needed for the graft to adhere and attach to the wound bed.

2. Burns of the face and head: Elevate the head of the bed to prevent or reduce facial, head, and tracheal edema.

3. Circumferential burns of the extremities: Elevate the extremities above the level of the heart to prevent or reduce dependent edema.

4. Skin graft: Elevate and immobilize the graft site to prevent the movement and shearing of the graft and the disruption of tissue; avoid weight bearing.

B. Reproductive system

1. Mastectomy

a. Position the client with the head of the bed elevated at least 30 degrees (semi-Fowler's position), with the affected arm elevated on a pillow to promote lymphatic fluid return after the removal of axillary lymph nodes.

b. Turn the client only to the back and the unaffected side.

2. Perineal and vaginal procedures: Place the client in the **lithotomy position** (Figure 18-4).

C. Endocrine system

1. Hypophysectomy: Elevate the head of the bed to prevent increased intracranial pressure.

2. Thyroidectomy

a. Place the client in **semi-Fowler's** or **Fowler's position** to reduce swelling and edema in the neck area.

b. Sandbags or pillows may be used to support the client's head or neck.

D. Gastrointestinal system

1. Hemorrhoidectomy: Assist the client to a **lateral (side-lying) position** to prevent pain and bleeding.

Box 18-1 Body Mechanics for Health Care Workers

1. When planning to move a client, arrange for adequate help. Use mechanical aids as much as possible.
2. Encourage the client to assist as much as possible.
3. Keep your back, neck, pelvis, and feet aligned. Avoid twisting.
4. Flex your knees, and keep your feet wide apart.
5. Position yourself close to the client or to the object being lifted.
6. Use your arms and legs rather than your back.
7. Slide the client toward yourself using a pull sheet. When transferring a client onto a stretcher, a slide board is more appropriate.
8. Set (tighten) your abdominal and gluteal muscles in preparation for the move.
9. The person with the heaviest load should coordinate the efforts of the team involved by counting to three.

Adapted from Potter, P., & Perry, A. (2009). *Fundamentals of nursing* (7th ed.). St. Louis: Mosby.

▲ **FIGURE 18-3** Pressure points of lying and sitting positions. (From Elkin, M., Perry, A., & Potter, P. [2008]. *Nursing interventions and clinical skills* [4th ed.]. St. Louis: Mosby.)

▲ **FIGURE 18-4** Lithotomy position for examination. (From Potter, P., & Perry, A. [2010]. *Fundamentals of nursing* [7th ed.]. St. Louis: Mosby.)

2. Gastroesophageal reflux disease: **Reverse Trendelenburg's position** may be prescribed to promote gastric emptying and prevent esophageal reflux.
3. Liver biopsy
   a. During the procedure
      (1) Position the client supine with the right side of the upper abdomen exposed.
      (2) The client's right arm is raised and extended over the left shoulder behind the head.
      (3) The liver is located on the right side, and this position provides for maximal exposure of the right intercostal spaces.
   b. After the procedure
      (1) Assist the client into a right **lateral (side-lying) position.**
      (2) Place a small pillow or folded towel under the puncture site for at least 3 hours to provide pressure to the site and prevent bleeding.
4. Paracentesis: The client is positioned in a semi-Fowler's position in bed, or sitting upright on the side of the bed or in a chair with the feet supported. The client is assisted to a position of comfort following the procedure.
5. Nasogastric tube
   a. Insertion
      (1) Position the client in a **high Fowler's position** with the head tilted forward.
      (2) This position will help close the trachea and open the esophagus.

⚠ If the client receiving a continuous tube feeding needs to be placed in a supine position when providing care, such as when giving a bed bath or changing linens, shut the feeding off to prevent aspiration. Remember to turn the feeding back on and check the rate of flow when the client is placed back into the semi-Fowler's or Fowler's position.

   b. Irrigations and tube feedings
      (1) Keep the head of the bed elevated 30 degrees (**semi-Fowler's position**) to prevent aspiration.

      (2) Maintain head elevation for 1 hour after an intermittent feeding.
      (3) The head of the bed should remain elevated for continuous feedings.
6. Rectal enemas or irrigations: Place the client in left **Sims' position** to allow the solution to flow by gravity in the natural direction of the colon.
7. Sengstaken-Blakemore tube and Minnesota tubes: May be used to control bleeding from esophageal varices when medication is ineffective; maintain elevation of the head of the bed to increase lung expansion and reduce portal blood flow, thereby permitting the effective compression of the esophageal varices.

E. Respiratory system
   1. Chronic obstructive pulmonary disease: For the client with advanced disease, place the client in a sitting position, leaning forward, with the arms over several pillows or on an overbed table. This position will help the client to breathe easier.
   2. Laryngectomy (radical neck dissection): Place the client in a **semi-Fowler's** or **Fowler's position** to maintain a patent airway and minimize edema.
   3. Bronchoscopy postprocedure: Place the client in a **semi-Fowler's position** to prevent choking or aspiration resulting from an impaired ability to swallow.
   4. Postural drainage: The lung segment to be drained should be in the uppermost position. **Trendelenburg's position** may be used.
   5. Thoracentesis
      a. During the procedure: To facilitate the removal of fluid from the pleural space, position the client sitting on the edge of the bed and leaning over the bedside table with the feet supported on a stool or lying in bed on the unaffected side with the head of the bed elevated approximately 45 degrees (**Fowler's position**).
      b. After the procedure: Assist the client to a position of comfort.
   6. Thoracotomy: Check the HCP's prescriptions regarding positioning.

⚠ Always check the HCP's prescription regarding positioning for the client who had a thoracotomy, lung wedge resection, lobectomy of the lung, or pneumonectomy.

F. Cardiovascular system
   1. Abdominal aneurysm resection
      a. After surgery, limit the elevation of the head of the bed to 45 degrees (**Fowler's position**) to avoid flexion of the graft.
      b. The client may be turned from side to side.

2. Amputation of the lower extremity
   a. During the first 24 hours after amputation, elevate the foot of the bed to reduce edema. The stump is supported with pillows but not elevated because of the risk of flexion contractures.
   b. Consult with the HCP and then position the client prone twice a day for a 20- to 30-minute period to stretch muscles and prevent flexion contractures of the hip.
3. Arterial vascular grafting of an extremity
   a. To promote graft patency after the procedure, bedrest is usually maintained for approximately 24 hours, and the client's affected extremity is kept straight.
   b. Limit movement and avoid flexion of the client's hip and knee.
4. Cardiac catheterization
   a. If the femoral artery was used, the client is maintained on bedrest for approximately 3 to 4 hours. The client may turn from side to side.
   b. The client's affected extremity is kept straight and the head elevated no more than 30 degrees until hemostasis is adequately achieved.
5. Congestive heart failure and pulmonary edema: Position the client upright (**high Fowler's position**), preferably with the bed in a chair-sitting position, to decrease venous return and lung congestion.

   ⚠ Most often, clients with respiratory and cardiac disorders should be positioned with the head of the bed elevated.

6. Peripheral arterial disease
   a. Obtain the HCP's prescription for positioning.
   b. Because swelling can prevent arterial blood flow, clients may be advised to elevate their feet when at rest. They should not raise their legs above the level of the heart, because extreme elevation slows arterial blood flow. Some clients may be advised to maintain a slightly dependent position to promote perfusion.
7. Deep vein thrombosis
   a. If the extremity is red, edematous, and painful and traditional heparin therapy is initiated, bedrest with leg elevation may be prescribed for the client.
   b. Clients receiving low-molecular-weight heparin can usually be out of bed after 24 hours, if the pain level permits.
8. Varicose veins: Leg elevation above the level of the heart is usually prescribed. The client is also advised to minimize prolonged sitting or standing during daily activities.
9. Venous insufficiency and leg ulcers: Leg elevation is usually prescribed.

G. Sensory system
1. Cataract surgery: Postoperatively, elevate the head of the bed (**semi-Fowler's** to **Fowler's position**), and position the client on the back or the non-operative side to prevent the development of edema at the operative site.
2. Retinal detachment
   a. If the detachment is large, bedrest and bilateral eye patching may be prescribed to minimize eye movement and prevent the extension of the detachment.
   b. Restrictions in activity and positioning after the repair of the detachment depend on the HCP's preference and the surgical procedure performed.

H. Neurological system
1. Autonomic dysreflexia: Elevate the head of the bed to a **high Fowler's position** to help with adequate ventilation and prevent hypertensive stroke.

   ⚠ If autonomic dysreflexia occurs, immediately place the client in a high-Fowler's position.

2. Cerebral aneurysm: Bedrest is maintained with the head of the bed elevated 30 to 45 degrees (**semi-Fowler's** to **Fowler's position**) to prevent pressure on the aneurysm site.
3. Cerebral angiography
   a. Maintain bedrest for the length of time, as prescribed.
   b. The extremity into which the contrast medium is injected is kept straight and immobilized for approximately 8 hours.
4. Brain attack (stroke)
   a. In clients with hemorrhagic strokes, the head of the bed is usually elevated to 30 degrees to reduce intracranial pressure and facilitate venous drainage.
   b. For clients with ischemic strokes, the head of the bed is usually kept flat.
   c. Maintain the client's head in a midline, neutral position to facilitate venous drainage from the head.
   d. Avoid extreme hip and neck flexion; extreme hip flexion may increase intrathoracic pressure, whereas extreme neck flexion prohibits venous drainage from the brain.
5. Craniotomy
   a. The client should not be positioned on the site that was operated on, especially if the bone flap has been removed, because the brain has no bony covering over the affected site.
   b. Elevate the head of the bed 30 to 45 degrees (**semi-Fowler's** to **Fowler's position**), and maintain the head in a midline, neutral position to facilitate venous drainage from the head.
   c. Avoid extreme hip and neck flexion.
6. Traumatic head injury: Elevate the head of the bed.

7. Laminectomy
   a. Logroll the client.
   b. When the client is out of bed, the client's back is kept straight (the client is placed in a straight-backed chair) with the feet resting comfortably on the floor.
8. Increased intracranial pressure
   a. Elevate the head of the bed 30 to 45 degrees (**semi-Fowler's** to **Fowler's position**), and maintain the head in a midline, neutral position to facilitate venous drainage from the head.
   b. Avoid extreme hip and neck flexion.

⚠ Do not place a client with a head injury in a flat or Trendelenburg position because of the risk of increased intracranial pressure.

9. Lumbar puncture
   a. During the procedure: Assist the client to the **lateral (side-lying) position,** with the back bowed at the edge of the examining table, the knees flexed up to the abdomen, and the head bent so that the chin is resting on the chest.
   b. After the procedure: Place the client in the **supine position** for 4 to 12 hours, as prescribed.
10. Spinal cord injury
    a. Immobilize the client on a spinal backboard with the head in a neutral position to prevent an incomplete injury from becoming complete.
    b. Prevent head flexion, rotation, or extension. The head is immobilized with a firm, padded cervical collar.
    c. Logroll the client. No part of the body should be twisted or turned, and the client should not be allowed to assume a sitting position.

I. Musculoskeletal system
   1. Total hip replacement
      a. Positioning depends on the surgical techniques used, the method of implantation, and the prosthesis. Also follow agency policy.
      b. Avoid extreme internal and external rotation.
      c. Avoid adduction. A side-lying position on the operative side is not usually allowed (unless specifically prescribed by the surgeon).
      d. Maintain abduction when the client is in a **supine position** or positioned on the non-operative side.
      e. Place a pillow between the client's legs to maintain abduction. Instruct the client to not cross the legs.
      f. Check the surgeon's prescriptions regarding the elevation of the head of the bed. Flexion is usually limited to 60 degrees during the first postoperative week and then to 90 degrees for 2 to 3 months thereafter.
   2. Devices used for proper positioning (Box 18-2)

Box 18-2 Devices Used for Proper Positioning

Pillows
Pillows provide support, elevate body parts, splint incisional areas, and reduce postoperative pain during activity, coughing, or deep breathing. They should be the appropriate size for the body part to be positioned.

Foot Boots
Foot boots are made of rigid plastic or heavy foam, and they keep the foot flexed at the proper angle. They should be removed two or three times a day to assess skin integrity and joint mobility.

Trochanter Rolls
These rolls prevent the external rotation of the legs when the client is in the supine position. To form a roll, use a cotton bath blanket or a sheet folded lengthwise to a width that extends from the greater trochanter of the femur to the lower border of the popliteal space.

Sandbags
Sandbags are filled plastic tubes that can be shaped to body contours to provide support. They immobilize the extremities and maintain specific body alignment.

Hand Rolls
Hand rolls maintain the fingers in a slightly flexed and functional position, and they keep the thumb slightly adducted in opposition to the fingers.

Hand–Wrist Splints
These splints are individually molded for the client to maintain the proper alignment of the thumb in slight adduction and the wrist in slight dorsiflexion.

Trapeze Bar
This bar descends from a securely fastened overhead bar attached to the bed frame. It allows the client to use the upper extremities to raise the trunk off of the bed, to assist with transfer from the bed to a wheelchair, and to perform upper-arm strengthening exercises.

Side Rails
These bars, which are positioned along the sides of the length of the bed, ensure client safety and are useful for increasing mobility. They also provide assistance to the client with rolling from side to side or sitting up in bed.

Bed Boards
These plywood boards are placed under the entire surface area of the mattress. They are useful for increasing back support and body alignment.

Wedge Pillow
This triangular-shaped pillow is made of heavy foam, and it is used to maintain the legs in abduction after total hip replacement surgery.

Adapted from Potter, P., & Perry, A. (2009). *Fundamentals of nursing* (7th ed.). St. Louis: Mosby.

MORE QUESTIONS ON EVOLVE!

Practice Questions

141. A nurse is preparing to reposition a dependent client who weighs more than 250 pounds. What intervention is best for the nurse to consider when moving this client?
1. Get help.
2. Keep elbows close and work close to the body.
3. First, place the client in Trendelenburg's position
4. Administer oral pain medication 5 minutes before moving the client.

142. A nurse is assigned to assist with caring for a client after cardiac catheterization. The nurse plans to maintain bedrest with:
1. High Fowler's position
2. Bathroom privileges only
3. Head elevation of 45 degrees
4. Head elevation of no more than 30 degrees

143. A nurse is reinforcing home-care instructions to a client and family regarding care after cataract removal from the right eye. Which of the following statements, if made by the client, would indicate an understanding of the instructions?
1. "I will not sleep on my left side."
2. "I will not sleep on my right side."
3. "I will take aspirin if I have any pain."
4. "I will not wear my glasses until my surgeon says it is okay."

144. After a liver biopsy, the nurse places the client in which of the following positions?
1. Prone
2. Supine
3. A left side-lying position with a small pillow or folded towel under the puncture site
4. A right side-lying position with a small pillow or folded towel under the puncture site

145. A nurse is administering a cleansing enema to a client with a fecal impaction. Before administering the enema, the nurse assists the client to which of the following positions?
1. Left Sims' position
2. Right Sims' position
3. On the left side of the body with the head of the bed elevated 45 degrees

4. On the right side of the body with the head of the bed elevated 45 degrees

146. A client is being prepared for a thoracentesis. The nurse assigned to care for the client assists the client to which of the following positions for the procedure?
1. Sims' position with the head of the bed flat
2. Prone with the head turned to the side supported by a pillow
3. Lying in bed on the affected side with the head of the bed elevated 45 degrees
4. Lying in bed on the unaffected side with the head of the bed elevated 45 degrees

147. A nurse is assisting with the insertion of a nasogastric tube into a client. The nurse places the client in which position for insertion?
1. Right side
2. Low Fowler's position
3. High Fowler's position
4. Supine with the head flat

148. A nurse is assisting with caring for a client after a craniotomy. The nurse plans to position the client in a:
1. Prone position
2. Supine position
3. Semi-Fowler's position
4. Dorsal recumbent position

149. A nurse is turning a postoperative client who had extensive back surgery yesterday. What turning intervention or position would be best for repositioning this client?
1. Logrolling
2. Semi-Fowler's
3. Sims' (semi-prone)
4. 30-degree lateral (side-lying)

150. The nurse is caring for a client after a supratentorial craniotomy in which a large tumor was removed from the left side. Choose the positions in which the nurse can safely place the client. **Select all that apply.**
- ❏ 1. On the left side
- ❏ 2. With the neck flexed
- ❏ 3. Supine on the left side
- ❏ 4. With extreme hip flexion
- ❏ 5. In a semi-Fowler's position
- ❏ 6. With the head in a midline position

ANSWERS

141. 1

Rationale: Although it is possible to move and position clients independently, getting help first is the best intervention. Lower back strain is a common injury among health care workers. In addition, the shearing of the client's skin over bony prominences may occur when health care workers move clients independently. Administering oral pain medication is necessary, but oral medications need to be given at least 30 to 45 minutes before clients are moved. Keeping the elbows close and working close to the body are useful techniques, but they would not be enough when independently moving a 250-pound client. This client is dependent, so he or she is probably not able to help much, if any.

Test-Taking Strategy: Focus on the data in the question. This client's dependent condition and weight make him or her too difficult for one person to move. Review the procedures and interventions for moving and positioning clients if you had difficulty with this question.

Level of Cognitive Ability: Applying
Client Needs: Physiological Integrity
Integrated Process: Nursing Process/Planning
Content Area: Fundamental Skills: Safety/Infection Control
Reference: deWit, p. 774. 2009.

142. 4

Rationale: After cardiac catheterization, the extremity into which the catheter was inserted is kept straight for the prescribed time period. The client may turn from side to side. The head of the bed is not elevated to more than 30 degrees to keep the affected leg straight at the groin and prevent arterial occlusion. Bathroom privileges are not allowed during the immediate postcatheterization period. For the high Fowler's position, the head of the bed is elevated 90 degrees.

Test-Taking Strategy: Use the process of elimination. Recalling that concerns after this procedure are bleeding and arterial occlusion will direct you to option 4. Review the care of the client after cardiac catheterization if you had difficulty with this question.

Level of Cognitive Ability: Applying
Client Needs: Physiological Integrity
Integrated Process: Nursing Process/Planning
Content Area: Adult Health/Cardiovascular
References: Christensen, Kockrow, p. 1544. 2011. *Adult health nursing.*
Ignatavicius, Workman, p. 724. 2010.

143. 2

Rationale: After cataract surgery, the client should not sleep on the side of the body that was operated on. Clients should be instructed not to take aspirin or any medications that contain aspirin. Acetaminophen (Tylenol) can be taken as needed for pain. Clients may wear their glasses.

Test-Taking Strategy: Use the process of elimination. If you can remember to instruct clients to stay off of the operative side, this will assist you with answering questions related to cataract surgery. Review the care of the client after cataract surgery if you had difficulty with this question.

Level of Cognitive Ability: Evaluating
Client Needs: Physiological Integrity

Integrated Process: Nursing Process/Evaluation
Content Area: Adult Health/Eye
Reference: deWit, p. 643. 2009.

144. 4

Rationale: After a liver biopsy, the client is assisted with assuming a right side-lying position with a small pillow or folded towel under the puncture site for at least 3 hours. Options 1, 2, and 3 are incorrect positions.

Test-Taking Strategy: Knowledge regarding the anatomy of the body will assist you with answering this question. Remember that the liver is on the right side of the body and that the application of pressure on the right side will minimize the escape of blood or bile through the puncture site. Review the care of the client after a liver biopsy if you had difficulty with this question.

Level of Cognitive Ability: Applying
Client Needs: Physiological Integrity
Integrated Process: Nursing Process/Implementation
Content Area: Adult Health/Gastrointestinal
Reference: Pagana, Pagana, p. 604. 2009.

145. 1

Rationale: When administering an enema, the client is placed in a left Sims' position so that the enema solution can flow by gravity in the natural direction of the colon. The head of the bed is not elevated.

Test-Taking Strategy: Recalling the anatomy of the bowel will assist you with eliminating options 2 and 4. Also, options 3 can be eliminated because the head of the bed should be flat during enema administration. Review the procedure for enema administration if you had difficulty with this question.

Level of Cognitive Ability: Applying
Client Needs: Physiological Integrity
Integrated Process: Nursing Process/Implementation
Content Area: Adult Health/Gastrointestinal
Reference: Christensen, Kockrow, p. 593. 2011. *Foundations of nursing.*

146. 4

Rationale: To facilitate the removal of fluid from the chest, the client is positioned sitting on the edge of the bed, leaning over a bedside table, with the feet supported on a stool or lying in bed on the unaffected side with the head of the bed elevated 45 degrees (Fowler's position). Options 1, 2, and 3 are incorrect.

Test-Taking Strategy: Visualize this procedure. Option 3 can be eliminated, because if the client was lying on the affected side, it would be very difficult to perform the procedure. Option 1 can be eliminated, because, the Sims' position is primarily used for rectal enemas or irrigations. In the prone position, the client is lying on his or her abdomen, which is not an appropriate position for this procedure. Review the procedure for the removal of fluid from the chest if you had difficulty with this question.

Level of Cognitive Ability: Applying
Client Needs: Physiological Integrity
Integrated Process: Nursing Process/Implementation
Content Area: Adult Health/Respiratory
Reference: Pagana, Pagana, pp. 898–900. 2009.

147. 3

Rationale: During the insertion of a nasogastric tube, the client is placed in a sitting or high Fowler's position to reduce the risk of pulmonary aspiration if the client should vomit. Options 1, 2, and 4 do not facilitate the insertion of the tube or prevent aspiration.

Test-Taking Strategy: Visualize this procedure. Recalling that a concern with the insertion of a nasogastric tube is pulmonary aspiration will direct you to option 3. Review the procedure for inserting a nasogastric tube if you had difficulty with this question.

Level of Cognitive Ability: Applying
Client Needs: Physiological Integrity
Integrated Process: Nursing Process/Implementation
Content Area: Adult Health/Gastrointestinal
Reference: Christensen, & Kockrow. (2011). *Foundations of nursing* (p. 586).

148. 3

Rationale: After a craniotomy, the head of the bed is elevated 30 to 45 degrees (semi-Fowler's to Fowler's position), and the client's head is maintained in a midline, neutral position to facilitate venous drainage. Options 1, 2, and 4 are incorrect positions.

Test-Taking Strategy: Focus on the surgical procedure. Recalling that a goal of care after this surgery is to facilitate venous drainage will direct you to option 3. Review the care of the client after a craniotomy if you had difficulty with this question.

Level of Cognitive Ability: Applying
Client Needs: Physiological Integrity
Integrated Process: Nursing Process/Planning
Content Area: Adult Health/Neurological
Reference: deWit, p. 544. 2009.

149. 1

Rationale: Logrolling is used to maintain neck and spinal alignment after injury or surgery. A minimum of three to four staff members is recommended to prevent injury to the client, and a draw or pull sheet is also suggested. Options 2, 3, and 4 do not maintain proper spinal alignment and could be harmful.

Test-Taking Strategy: Focus on the type of surgery performed and the need to maintain proper spinal alignment. This will direct you to option 1. Review the care of the client after spinal surgery or injury if you had difficulty with this question.

Level of Cognitive Ability: Applying
Client Needs: Physiological Integrity
Integrated Process: Nursing Process/Implementation
Content Area: Adult Health/Neurological
Reference: deWit, p. 559. 2009.

150. 5, 6

Rationale: Clients who have undergone supratentorial surgery should have the head of the bed elevated 30 degrees to promote venous drainage from the head. The client is positioned to avoid extreme hip or neck flexion, and the head is maintained in a midline, neutral position. If a large tumor has been removed, the client should be placed on the nonoperative side to prevent the displacement of the cranial contents.

Test-Taking Strategy: Focus on the data in the question. Remember that a primary concern is the risk for increased intracranial pressure. Therefore, use concepts related to preventing increased intracranial pressure to answer this question. In addition, remember that, with "supra" tentorial surgery, the head is kept "up," and the client is placed on the nonoperative side. Review the positioning of a client after craniotomy if you had difficulty with this question.

Level of Cognitive Ability: Applying
Client Needs: Physiological Integrity
Integrated Process: Nursing Process/Implementation
Content Area: Adult Health/Neurological
Reference: deWit, pp. 544–546. 2009.

Care of a Client with a Tube

PYRAMID TERMS

chest tube A tube that returns negative pressure to the intra-pleural space. It is used to remove abnormal accumulations of air and fluid from the pleural space.

endotracheal tube A tube used to maintain a patent airway that is indicated when the client needs mechanical ventilation.

tracheostomy An artificial opening created in the trachea to establish an airway. A tracheostomy tube is inserted into the opening and the tube attaches to the mechanical ventilator or another type of oxygen delivery device.

 ## PYRAMID TO SUCCESS

The Pyramid to Success focuses on the common types of tubes used in the clinical setting. The NCLEX-PN examination is likely to address content areas related to the appropriate care of certain tubes and the immediate interventions required if a complication arises. Focus on the specific data-collection points related to the specific type of tube. Review the procedures for verifying the correct placement of a tube and the procedures for administering medications or feedings through a tube, if appropriate. The pyramid points also focus on interventions associated with complications or emergencies that may occur.

CLIENT NEEDS

Safe and Effective Care Environment

- Acting as a client advocate
- Collaborating with members of the health care team
- Ensuring that advance directives are in the client's medical record
- Ensuring client's rights
- Establishing priorities
- Handling infectious materials
- Maintaining medical and surgical asepsis
- Maintaining standard and other precautions
- Obtaining informed consent for invasive procedures

Health Promotion and Maintenance

- Assisting the client with accepting lifestyle changes
- Preventing disease
- Providing client and family education regarding care at home
- Performing techniques of data collection

Psychosocial Integrity

- Discussing situational role changes
- Discussing unexpected body-image changes
- Identifying support systems
- Monitoring for sensory/perceptual alterations
- Providing home-care services

Physiological Integrity

- Administering medications
- Initiating emergency interventions for complications
- Implementing measures to ensure basic care and comfort
- Monitoring for potential complications associated with the tube
- Monitoring laboratory values
- Preparing for diagnostic tests to confirm the accurate placement of the tube
- Providing nutrition and oral hydration
- Providing respiratory care

I. **NASOGASTRIC TUBES**

A. Description
   1. Short tubes used to intubate the stomach
   2. Inserted from the nose to the stomach
B. Purpose
   1. To decompress the stomach by removing fluids or gas to promote abdominal comfort
   2. To allow surgical anastomoses to heal without distention
   3. To decrease the risk of aspiration
   4. To administer medications in clients who are unable to swallow
   5. To provide nutrition by acting as a temporary feeding tube
   6. To irrigate the stomach and remove toxic substances, such as in poisonings

C. Types of tubes and routes (Figure 19-1)
1. Levin: Single-lumen nasogastric (NG) tube used to remove gastric contents via intermittent suction or to provide tube feedings
2. Salem sump tube: A Salem sump is a double-lumen nasogastric tube with air vent (pigtail) used for decompression with intermittent continuous suction.

⚠ The air vent on a Salem sump tube is not to be clamped and is to be kept above the level of the stomach. If leakage occurs through the air vent, instill 30 mL of air into the air vent and irrigate the main lumen with normal saline (NS).

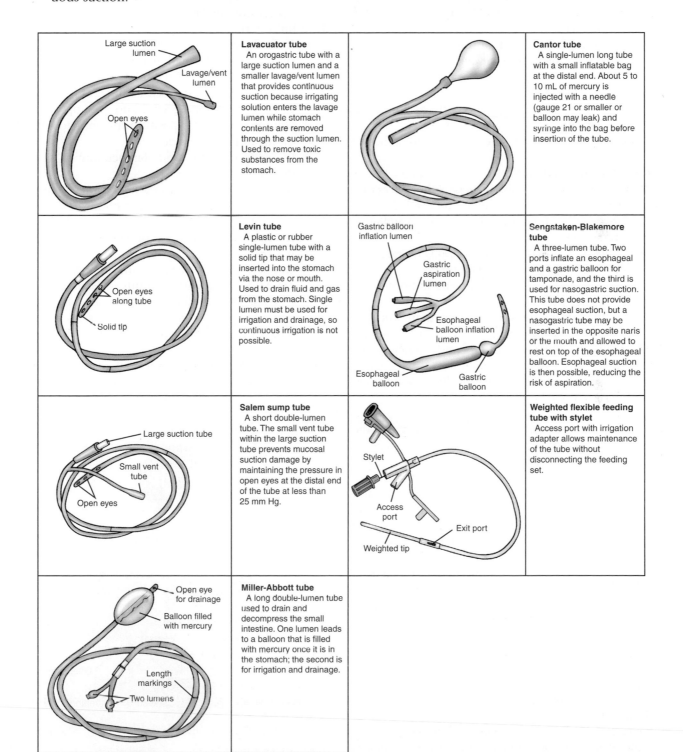

Lavacuator tube
An orogastric tube with a large suction lumen and a smaller lavage/vent lumen that provides continuous suction because irrigating solution enters the lavage lumen while stomach contents are removed through the suction lumen. Used to remove toxic substances from the stomach.

Cantor tube
A single-lumen long tube with a small inflatable bag at the distal end. About 5 to 10 mL of mercury is injected with a needle (gauge 21 or smaller or balloon may leak) and syringe into the bag before insertion of the tube.

Levin tube
A plastic or rubber single-lumen tube with a solid tip that may be inserted into the stomach via the nose or mouth. Used to drain fluid and gas from the stomach. Single lumen must be used for irrigation and drainage, so continuous irrigation is not possible.

Sengstaken-Blakemore tube
A three-lumen tube. Two ports inflate an esophageal and a gastric balloon for tamponade, and the third is used for nasogastric suction. This tube does not provide esophageal suction, but a nasogastric tube may be inserted in the opposite naris or the mouth and allowed to rest on top of the esophageal balloon. Esophageal suction is then possible, reducing the risk of aspiration.

Salem sump tube
A short double-lumen tube. The small vent tube within the large suction tube prevents mucosal suction damage by maintaining the pressure in open eyes at the distal end of the tube at less than 25 mm Hg.

Weighted flexible feeding tube with stylet
Access port with irrigation adapter allows maintenance of the tube without disconnecting the feeding set.

Miller-Abbott tube
A long double-lumen tube used to drain and decompress the small intestine. One lumen leads to a balloon that is filled with mercury once it is in the stomach; the second is for irrigation and drainage.

▲ **FIGURE 19-1** Examples of tubes used in the digestive tract. (From Linton, A. [2007]. *Introduction to medical-surgical nursing* [4th ed.]. Philadelphia: Saunders.)

D. Determining placement
1. Note that the most reliable method for determining placement is by x-ray study, which should be performed after initial placement.
2. Determine tube placement every 4 hours and before administering feedings or medications.
3. Determine tube placement by aspirating gastric contents and measuring the pH, which should be lower than 4 (pH values >6 indicate intestinal placement).
4. Inserting 5 to 10 mL of air into the NG tube and listening for the rush of air over the stomach with a stethoscope is an alternative method for determining placement, but it should not be the sole method of determining placement as a result of unreliability.
5. Secure the tube to the client's nose with adhesive tape.

E. Checking the residual
1. Check residual volumes every 4 hours, before each feeding, or before giving medications.
2. Aspirate all stomach contents (residual) and measure amount.
3. Re-instill residual feeding to prevent excessive fluid and electrolyte losses unless the residual volume exceeds 100 mL, appears abnormal, or per agency policy.
4. Usually, if the residual is less than 100 mL, the feeding is administered (the health care provider's [HCP's] prescriptions and agency policy are followed).
5. Aspiration from some small-caliber, soft-walled tubes may not be possible.

F. Irrigating
1. Perform irrigation every 4 hours to check the patency of the tube.
2. Check placement before irrigating.
3. Gently instill 30 to 50 mL of water or NS (depending on agency policy) with an irrigation syringe.
4. Pull back on the syringe plunger to withdraw the fluid to check patency. Repeat if the tube remains sluggish.

G. Removal of an NG tube: Ask the client to take a deep breath and hold. Remove the tube slowly and evenly over the course of 3 to 6 seconds (coil the tube around the hand as it is being removed).

II. GASTROINTESTINAL TUBE FEEDINGS

A. Tubes (Figure 19-2)
B. Types of administration
1. Bolus
   a. Resembles normal meal feeding patterns
   b. Approximately 300 to 400 mL of formula is administered over a 30- to 60-minute period every 3 to 6 hours

2. Continuous
   a. Administered continuously for 24 hours
   b. An infusion pump regulates the flow
3. Cyclical
   a. Administered either during the day- or nighttime for 8 to 16 hours
   b. An infusion pump regulates the flow.
   c. Feedings at night allow for more freedom during the day.

C. Administering feedings
1. If feedings are prescribed, x-ray confirmation should be performed before initiating feedings after the insertion of the tube.
2. Keep the head of the bed elevated at least 30 degrees at all times, even if no feeding is being administered. Also, position the comatose client on his or her right side.
3. Warm feeding to room temperature to prevent diarrhea and cramps.
4. Aspirate all stomach contents (residual), measure the amount, and return the contents to the stomach to prevent electrolyte imbalances (unless the residual exceeds 100 mL or as defined by agency policy).
5. Check the HCP's prescriptions and agency policy regarding residual amounts. Usually, if the residual is less than 100 mL, the feeding is administered. Large-volume aspirates indicate delayed gastric emptying and place the client at risk for aspiration.
6. Check tube placement by aspirating gastric contents and measuring the pH (should be 4 or lower).

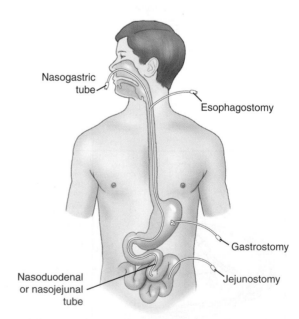

▲ **FIGURE 19-2** Diagram of the placement of enteral feeding tubes. (From Leonard, P. [2009]. *Building a medical vocabulary: With Spanish translations* [7th ed.]. St. Louis: Mosby.)

7. Check the bowel sounds. The feeding may be held and the HCP may be notified if bowel sounds are absent.
8. Use a feeding pump for continuous or cyclical feedings.
9. For a bolus feeding, leave the client in a high Fowler's position for 30 minutes after feeding, followed by a semi-Fowler's position (30 to 45 degrees).
10. For a continuous feeding, keep the client in a semi-Fowler's position at all times.

D. Precautions

⚠ Always check the placement of a gastrointestinal tube before instilling feeding solutions, medications, or any other solution. If the tube is incorrectly placed, the client is at risk for aspiration.

1. Change the feeding container and tubing every 24 hours.
2. Do not allow the solution to hang for more than 4 hours to prevent bacterial growth in the solution, per agency policy.
3. Check the expiration date on the formula before administering it.
4. Shake the formula well before pouring it into the feeding bag.
5. Always check the placement of the tube before a feeding.
6. Always check the bowel sounds. Feedings cannot be administered if bowel sounds are absent.
7. Administer the feeding at the prescribed rate or via gravity flow (bolus feedings) with a 60-mL syringe with the plunger removed.
8. Gently flush with 30 to 50 mL water or NS (depending on agency policy) with an irrigation syringe after the feeding.

⚠ If the client vomits, stop the tube feeding and place the client in a side-lying position; suction the client as needed.

E. Administration of medications (see Priority Nursing Actions)

III. INTESTINAL TUBES

A. Description
  1. Passed nasally into the small intestine
  2. Used to decompress the bowel or to remove intestinal contents
  3. Designed to enter the small intestine through the pyloric sphincter with the use of the weight of a small bag containing a special substance (tungsten) at the end
B. Types of tubes (see Figure 19-1)
  1. Cantor or Harris tube (single lumen)
  2. Miller-Abbott tube (double lumen)

▬▬▬■ PRIORITY NURSING ACTIONS! ■▬▬▬

Steps for Administering Medications Via a Nasogastric or Gastrostomy Tube
1. Check the HCP's prescription.
2. Prepare the medication for administration.
3. Ensure that the medication prescribed can be crushed or (if it is a capsule) that it can be opened; use elixir forms of medications if available.
4. Dissolve crushed medication or capsule contents in 15 to 30 mL of water.
5. Verify the client's identity and explain the procedure to the client.
6. Check tube placement and residual contents before instilling the medication; check for bowel sounds.
7. Draw up the medication into a catheter tip syringe, clear excess air from the syringe, and insert the medication into the tube.
8. Flush with 30 to 50 mL of water or NS (depending on agency policy).
9. Clamp the tube for 30 to 60 minutes (depending on medication and agency policy).
10. Document the administration of the medication and any other appropriate information.

The nurse always checks the HCP's prescription before administering any medication to a client. Once the prescription is verified, the medication is prepared for administration. The nurse determines the reason for administration and checks for any contraindications to administering the medication and for any potential interactions. When preparing medications for administration through a nasogastric or gastrostomy tube, the nurse needs to ensure that the medication prescribed can be crushed or (if it is a capsule) that it can be opened. Whole tablets or capsules cannot be administered through a tube because they can cause a tube blockage. Elixir forms of medications can also be used if available. The nurse then dissolves the crushed medication or capsule contents in 15 to 30 mL of water. Client identity is always verified before medication administration, and the procedure is explained to the client. The nurse checks tube placement and residual contents before instilling the medication and checks for bowel sounds. The nurse also performs any additional data collection procedures, such as checking the apical heart rate for cardiac medications or checking the blood pressure for antihypertensives. The medication is drawn up into a catheter tip syringe, excess air is removed from the syringe, and the medication is inserted into the tube. The tube is flushed with 30 to 50 mL of water or NS (depending on agency policy) to ensure that all medication has been instilled. The tube is then clamped for 30 to 60 minutes (depending on medication and agency policy) to ensure it is absorbed. (If the tube is not clamped and is reattached to suction then the medication will be aspirated out with the suction.) The nurse then documents the administration of the medication and any other appropriate information.

Reference: Potter, P., & Perry, A. (2009). *Fundamentals of nursing* (7th ed., p. 719). St. Louis: Mosby.

C. Interventions
1. Position the client on the right side to facilitate the passage of the small bag within the tube through the pylorus of the stomach and into the small intestine.
2. Do not secure the tube to the client's face with tape until it has reached its final placement in the intestines. This may take several hours.
3. An x-ray study is performed to verify desired placement.
4. Monitor drainage from the tube
5. If the tube becomes blocked, the registered nurse and HCP are notified. A small amount of air injected into the lumen may be prescribed to clear the tube.
6. Check the abdomen and measure the abdominal girth.

IV. ESOPHAGEAL AND GASTRIC TUBES

A. Description
1. Used to apply pressure against the esophageal veins to control bleeding; not commonly used but may be considered for use if medication therapy is ineffective.
2. Not used if the client has ulceration or necrosis of the esophagus or has had previous esophageal surgery
3. Types include Sengstaken-Blakemore tube and Minnesota tube (see Figure 19-1)

B. Interventions
1. The patency and integrity of all balloons are checked before insertion, and each lumen is labeled.
2. The client is placed in an upright or Fowler's position for insertion.
3. Prepare the client for an x-ray study immediately after insertion to verify placement.
4. Maintain head elevation after the tube is in place.
5. The balloon ports are double-clamped to prevent air leaks.
6. Scissors are kept at the bedside at all times.
7. The client is monitored for respiratory distress. If it occurs, notify the registered nurse immediately. The tubes will be cut to deflate the balloons.
8. Monitor for increased bloody drainage that may indicate persistent bleeding.
9. Monitor for signs of esophageal rupture, including a drop in blood pressure, increased heart rate, and back and upper abdominal pain. (Esophageal rupture is an emergency and must be reported immediately.)

V. URINARY AND RENAL TUBES

A. Types: Straight, indwelling, and triple lumen (Figure 19-3)

B. Routine urinary catheter care
1. Use gloves, and wash the perineal area with warm soapy water.
2. With the nondominant hand, pull back the labia or foreskin to expose the meatus (in the adult male, return the foreskin to its normal position).
3. Clean along the catheter with soap and water.
4. Anchor the catheter to the thigh according to agency policy.
5. Maintain the catheter bag below the level of the bladder.

C. Ureteral and nephrostomy tubes
1. Never clamp the tubes.
2. Maintain patency.
3. Monitor output closely.

⚠ If the client has a ureteral or nephrostomy tube, monitor output closely. Urine output of less than 30 mL/hour or lack of output for more than 15 minutes should be reported to the HCP immediately.

VI. RESPIRATORY SYSTEM TUBES

A. Endotracheal tubes (Figure 19-4)
1. Description
   a. Used to maintain a patent airway
   b. Indicated when the client needs mechanical ventilation
   c. If the client requires an artificial airway for longer than 10 to 14 days, a tracheostomy may be created to avoid the mucosal and vocal cord damage that can be caused by the endotracheal tube.
2. Orotracheal
   a. Inserted through the mouth; allows for the use of a larger-diameter tube and reduces the work of breathing
   b. Indicated when the client has a nasal obstruction or a predisposition to epistaxis
   c. Uncomfortable and can be manipulated by the tongue, thus causing airway obstruction; an oral airway may be needed to prevent the client from biting on the tube
3. Nasotracheal
   a. Inserted through the nose; requires the use of a smaller-sized tube, which increases both resistance and the client's work of breathing
   b. Discouraged for clients with bleeding disorders
   c. More comfortable for the client; he or she is unable to manipulate the tube with the tongue
4. Interventions
   a. Placement is confirmed by a chest x-ray study (correct placement is 1 to 2 cm above the carina) and by auscultating both sides of

A Straight catheter (cross-section)

Urine drainage

B Indwelling retention catheter
(cross-section)

Catheter tip

5-10 cc inflated
balloon

Balloon inflation

Urine drainage

C Triple-lumen catheter (cross-section)

30 cc inflated balloon

Balloon inflation

Urine drainage flows out

Irrigation solution flows in

▲ **FIGURE 19-3** Types of urinary catheters: **A,** Straight catheter (cross-section). **B,** Indwelling retention catheter (cross-section). **C,** Triple-lumen catheter (cross-section). (From Elkin, M., Perry, A., & Potter, P. [2008]. *Nursing interventions and clinical skills* [4th ed.]. St. Louis: Mosby.)

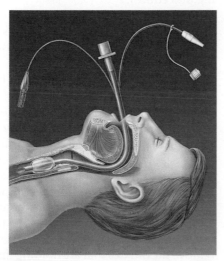

▲ **FIGURE 19-4** Endotracheal tube with inflated cuff. (From Perry, A., & Potter, P. [2004]. *Clinical nursing skills and nursing techniques* [5th ed.]. St. Louis: Mosby.)

chest while manually ventilating with resuscitation (Ambu) bag. If breath sounds and chest wall movement are absent on the left side, the tube may be in the right main stem bronchus.

b. If the tube is in the stomach, louder breath sounds will be heard over the stomach than over the chest, and abdominal distention will be present.

c. The tube is secured immediately after intubation with adhesive tape.

d. Monitor the position of the tube at the lip or nose.

e. Monitor the skin and mucous membranes.

f. Suction the tube only when needed.

g. The oral tube needs to be moved to the opposite side of the mouth daily to prevent pressure and necrosis of the lip and mouth area, prevent nerve damage, and facilitate the inspection and cleaning of the mouth. Moving the tube to the opposite side of the mouth should be done by two health care providers.

h. To prevent dislodgment, prevent pulling or tugging on the tube. Suction, coughing, and speaking attempts by the client place extra stress on the tube and can cause dislodgment.

i. Cuff inflation is maintained to create a seal and to allow for the complete mechanical control of respirations.

⚠ A resuscitation (Ambu) bag needs to be kept at the bedside of a client with an endotracheal tube or tracheostomy tube at all times.

5. Extubation
   a. Hyperoxygenate the client, and suction the endotracheal tube and the oral cavity.
   b. Place the client in semi-Fowler's position.
   c. The cuff is deflated. The client is asked to inhale. At peak inspiration, the tube is removed and the airway is suctioned through the tube as it is pulled out.
   d. After removal, instruct the client to cough and deep breathe to assist with the removal of accumulated secretions from the throat.
   e. Apply oxygen therapy, as prescribed.
   f. Monitor for respiratory difficulty. Contact the registered nurse and HCP if respiratory difficulty occurs.
   g. Inform the client that hoarseness or a sore throat is normal and that he or she should limit talking if it occurs.

B. Tracheostomy
   1. Description
      a. A tracheotomy is a surgical incision into the trachea for the purpose of establishing an airway.
      b. The tracheostomy is the stoma or opening that results from the tracheotomy. It can be temporary or permanent.
   2. Single-cannula tube: Has an outer but no inner cannula; used for a client with a thick neck or longer trachea in whom a standard tube will not enter the trachea
   3. Cuffed tube: Has an outer and inner cannula, an obturator, and a cuff
   4. Cuffless tube
      a. Has an outer cannula, an open and plugged inner cannula, and an obturator
      b. Used long term for the client who is no longer at risk for aspiration
   5. Fenestrated tube (Figure 19-5)
      a. Has an opening along the posterior wall of the outer cannula
      b. When the tube is capped, the client can breathe through the upper airway and speak.
      c. The cuff is always deflated before the tube is capped.
   6. Interventions
      a. Monitor the respirations and for bilateral breath sounds.
      b. Monitor the pulse oximetry.
      c. Encourage coughing and deep breathing.
      d. Maintain a semi-Fowler's to high Fowler's position.

Air movement through upper nasal and oral air passages

Air moves through fenestrations and around tube

Decannulation cap/button plugs airway

Cuff deflated

▲ **FIGURE 19-5** Breathing through a fenestrated tracheostomy tube with a cap in place and the cuff deflated. (From Ignatavicius, D., & Workman, M. [2010]. *Medical-surgical nursing: Patient-centered collaborative care* [6th ed.]. St. Louis: Saunders.)

   e. Monitor for bleeding, difficulty breathing (pneumothorax), and crepitus (subcutaneous emphysema).
   f. Monitor respiratory treatments, as prescribed.
   g. Suction as needed; hyperoxygenate the client before suction (see Chapter 49 for the suctioning procedure).
   h. If the client is allowed to eat, sit him or her up for meals, and ensure that the cuff is inflated (if the tube is not capped) for meals and for 1 hour after meals.
   i. Assess the stoma and secretions for blood or purulent drainage.
   j. Follow the HCP's prescriptions and agency policy for cleaning the tracheostomy site and the inner cannula. Half-strength hydrogen peroxide is usually used.
   k. Administer humidified oxygen, as prescribed. The normal humidification process is bypassed in a client with a tracheostomy.
   l. Obtain assistance with changing the tracheostomy ties. After placing the new ties, cut and remove the old ties that are holding the tracheostomy tube in place (some securing devices are soft and made with Velcro to hold the tube in place).
   m. Keep a resuscitation (Ambu) bag, an obturator, clamps, and a spare tracheotomy set at the bedside.
   n. Provide frequent mouth care, to reduce the risk of pneumonia.

TABLE 19-1 Complications of a Tracheostomy

Complications and Description	Manifestations	Management	Prevention
Tracheomalacia: Consistent pressure exerted by the cuff causes tracheal dilation and the erosion of cartilage	An increased amount of air is required in the cuff to maintain the seal. A larger tracheostomy tube is required to prevent an air leak at the stoma Food particles are seen in tracheal secretions The client does not receive the set tidal volume on the ventilator.	No special management is needed unless bleeding occurs.	Use an uncuffed tube as soon as possible. Monitor the cuff pressure and air volumes closely to detect changes.
Tracheal stenosis: A narrowed tracheal lumen is the result of scar formation from irritation of the tracheal mucosa by the cuff.	Stenosis is usually seen after the cuff is deflated or the tracheostomy tube is removed. The client has increased coughing, an inability to expectorate secretions, or difficulty breathing or talking.	Tracheal dilation or surgical intervention is used.	Prevent the pulling of and traction on the tracheostomy tube. Properly secure the tube in the midline position. Maintain proper cuff pressure.
Tracheoesophageal fistula: Excessive cuff pressure causes erosion of the posterior wall of the trachea. A hole is created between the trachea and the anterior esophagus. The client at highest risk also has a nasogastric tube present.	Similar to tracheomalacia: • Food particles are seen in the tracheal secretions. • Increased air is needed in the cuff to achieve a seal. • The client has increased coughing and choking while eating. • The client does not receive the set tidal volume on the ventilator.	Manually administer oxygen by mask to prevent hypoxemia. Use of a small, soft feeding tube instead of a nasogastric tube for tube feedings. A gastrostomy or jejunostomy may be performed. Monitor the client with a nasogastric tube closely; assess for tracheoesophageal fistula and aspiration.	Maintain cuff pressure. Monitor the amount of air needed for inflation and detect changes. Progress to a deflated cuff or a cuffless tube as soon as possible.
Trachea-innominate artery fistula: A malpositioned tube causes its distal tip to push against the lateral wall of the tracheostomy. Continued pressure causes the necrosis and erosion of the innominate artery. **This is a medical emergency.**	The tracheostomy tube pulsates in synchrony with the heartbeat. There is heavy bleeding from the stoma. **This is a life-threatening complication.**	Remove the tracheostomy tube immediately. Apply direct pressure to the innominate artery at the stoma site. Prepare the client for immediate surgical repair.	Correct the tube size, length, and midline position. Prevent the pulling of or tugging on the tracheostomy tube. Immediately notify the registered nurse and HCP regarding the pulsating tube.

Adapted from Ignatavicius, D., & Workman, M. (2010). *Medical-surgical nursing* (6th ed.). St. Louis: Saunders.

7. Complications of a tracheostomy (Table 19-1 and Box 19-1)

 Never insert a decannulation plug into a tracheostomy tube until the cuff is deflated and the inner cannula is removed. Prior insertion prevents airflow to the client.

 VII. CHEST-TUBE DRAINAGE SYSTEM (Figure 19-6)

A. Description

1. Returns negative pressure to the intrapleural space
2. Used to remove abnormal accumulations of air and fluid from the pleural space
3. **Chest-tube** placement (Figure 19-7)

B. Collection chamber
1. Where the **chest tube** from the client connects to the system
2. Drainage from the tube drains into and collects in a series of calibrated columns in this chamber.

C. Water-seal chamber
1. Allows fluid and air to drain from the pleural space and prevents air from entering the pleural space.
2. Water oscillates (i.e., moves up as the client inhales and moves down as the client exhales).
3. Continuous bubbling indicates an air leak in the **chest-tube** system.

D. Suction-control chamber
1. Provides suction, which can be controlled to provide negative pressure to the chest.

Box 19-1 Complications of a Tracheostomy

Tube Obstruction

Data Collection

Difficulty breathing
Noisy respirations
Difficulty inserting the suction catheter
Thick, dry secretions
Unexplained peak pressures if the client is on a mechanical ventilator

Prevention and Interventions

Assist the client to cough and deep breathe.
Provide humidification and suctioning.
Clean the inner cannula regularly.
The HCP repositions or replaces the tube if obstruction occurs as a result of cuff prolapse over the end of the tube.

Tube Dislodgment

Prevention and Interventions

Secure the tube in place.
Minimize the manipulation of and traction on the tube.
Ensure that the client does not pull on the tube.
Ensure that a tracheostomy tube of the same type and size is at the client's bedside.

Be familiar with facility policy regarding the replacement of a tracheostomy tube as a nursing procedure.
During the first 72 hours after the surgical placement of the tracheostomy:

- The nurse manually ventilates the client with the use of a manual resuscitation (Ambu) bag while another nurse calls the resuscitation team for help.

More than 72 hours after the surgical placement of the tracheostomy:

- Extend the client's neck and open the tissues of the stoma to secure the airway.
- Grasp the retention sutures (if they are present) to spread the opening.
- Use a tracheal dilator (curved clamp) to hold the stoma open.
- Prepare to assist with the insertion of the tracheostomy tube. Place an obturator into tracheostomy tube, replace the tube, and remove the obturator.
- Maintain ventilation with the use of a resuscitation (Ambu) bag.
- Check the airflow, and check for bilateral breath sounds.
- If unable to secure an airway, call the resuscitation team and the anesthesiologist.

2. Filled with various levels of water to achieve the desired level of suction; without this control, lung tissue could be sucked into the **chest tube**
3. Gentle bubbling indicates that there is suction. It does not indicate that air is escaping from the pleural space.

E. Dry-suction system
   1. Because this is a dry-suction system, the absence of bubbling is noted in the suction-control chamber.
   2. A knob on the collection device is used to set the prescribed amount of suction. Then the wall-suction source dial is turned until a small orange floater valve appears in the window on the device. When the orange floater valve is in the window, the correct amount of suction has been applied.

F. Interventions
   1. Collection chamber
      a. Monitor the drainage. The HCP is notified if the drainage is more than 70 to 100 mL/hr or the drainage becomes bright red or increases suddenly.
      b. Mark the **chest-tube** drainage in the collection chamber at 1- to 4-hour intervals with the use of a piece of tape.

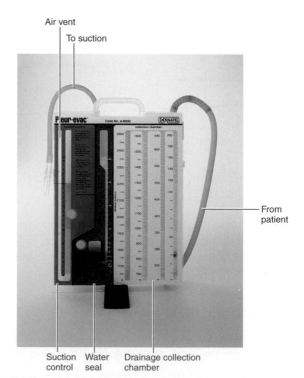

▲ **FIGURE 19-6** The Pleur-Evac drainage system, a commercial three-bottle chest drainage device. (From Ignatavicius, D., & Workman, M. [2010]. *Medical-surgical nursing: Patient-centered collaborative care* [6th ed.]. St. Louis: Saunders.)

▲ **FIGURE 19-7** Chest tube placement. (From Ignatavicius, D., & Workman, M. [2010]. *Medical-surgical nursing: Patient-centered collaborative care* [6th ed.]. St. Louis: Saunders.)

2. Water-seal chamber
   a. Monitor for the fluctuation of the fluid level in the water-seal chamber.
   b. Fluctuation in the water-seal chamber stops if the tube is obstructed, a dependent loop exists, the suction is not working properly, or the lung has re-expanded.
   c. If the client has a known pneumothorax, intermittent bubbling in the water-seal chamber is expected as air is drained from the chest. Continuous bubbling indicates an air leak in the system.
   d. Notify the registered nurse and HCP if there is continuous bubbling in the water-seal chamber.
3. Suction-control chamber: Gentle bubbling should be noted in the suction-control chamber. Vigorous bubbling indicates an air leak, and the registered nurse and physician should be notified.
4. An occlusive sterile dressing is maintained at the insertion site.

5. A chest radiograph assesses the position of the tube and determines whether the lung has re-expanded.
6. Monitor the respiratory status and listen to the lung sounds.
7. Monitor for signs of an extended pneumothorax or hemothorax.
8. Keep the drainage system below the level of the chest and the tubes free of kinks, dependent loops, or other obstructions.
9. Ensure that all connections are secure.
10. Encourage coughing and deep breathing.
11. Change the client's position frequently to promote drainage and ventilation.
12. Stripping or milking a **chest tube** is not done unless specifically prescribed by a HCP and agency policy allows.
13. Keep a clamp and a sterile occlusive dressing at the bedside at all times.
14. A **chest tube** is never clamped without a written prescription from the health care provider. Also, determine agency policy for clamping **chest tubes.**
15. If the drainage system cracks or breaks, insert the **chest tube** into a bottle of sterile water. The cracked or broken system is removed and replaced with a new system.
16. When the **chest tube** is removed, the client is asked to take a deep breath and hold it, and the tube is removed. A dry sterile dressing, petroleum gauze dressing, or Telfa dressing (depending on the HCP's preference) is taped in place after the removal of the **chest tube.**
17. Depending on the HCP's preference, when the **chest tube** is removed, the client may be asked to take a deep breath, exhale, and bear down (i.e., Valsalva's maneuver).

⚠ If the chest tube is pulled out of the chest accidentally, pinch the skin opening together, apply an occlusive sterile dressing, cover the dressing with overlapping pieces of 2-inch tape, and call the registered nurse and health care provider immediately.

MORE QUESTIONS ON EVOLVE!

Practice Questions

151. A nurse is preparing to administer an intermittent tube feeding to a client. The nurse aspirates 90 mL of residual tube feeding. What should the nurse do with the aspirated feeding?
   1. Hold the feeding.
   2. Contact the health care provider (HCP).
   3. Re-instill the residual and administer the feeding.
   4. Deduct the amount of the residual from the new feeding and administer that amount to the client.

152. A nurse is providing endotracheal suctioning to a client who is mechanically ventilated when the client becomes restless and tachycardic. What should the nurse do?
1. Notify the health care provider (HCP) immediately.
2. Finish the suctioning as quickly as possible.
3. Contact the respiratory department to suction the client.
4. Discontinue suctioning until the client is stabilized and monitor vital signs.

153. A nurse is checking a client for the correct placement of a nasogastric (NG) tube. The nurse aspirates the client's stomach contents and checks their pH level. Which of the following pH values indicates the correct placement of the tube?
1. 4.0
2. 7.0
3. 7.5
4. 7.35

154. A licensed practical nurse (LPN) is preparing to assist a registered nurse (RN) with removing a nasogastric (NG) tube from the client. The LPN would instruct the client to do which of the following?
1. Exhale.
2. Inhale and exhale quickly.
3. Take and hold a deep breath.
4. Perform Valsalva's maneuver.

155. A nurse is preparing to administer medication through a nasogastric (NG) tube that is connected to suction. Which of the following indicates the accurate procedure for medication administration?
1. Position the client supine to assist with medication absorption.
2. Clamp the NG tube for 30 minutes after medication administration.
3. Aspirate the NG tube after medication administration to maintain patency.
4. Change the suction setting to low intermittent suction for 30 minutes after medication administration.

156. A nurse is assigned to assist with caring for a client with esophageal varices who has a Sengstaken-Blakemore tube inserted. The nurse checks the client's room to ensure that which priority item is at the bedside?
1. An obturator
2. A Kelly clamp
3. An irrigation set
4. A pair of scissors

157. A nurse is inserting an indwelling urinary catheter into a male client. As the catheter is inserted into the urethra, urine begins to flow into the tubing. At this point, the nurse:
1. Immediately inflates the balloon
2. Inserts the catheter 2.5 to 5 cm and inflates the balloon
3. Inserts the catheter until resistance is met and inflates the balloon
4. Withdraws the catheter approximately 1 inch and inflates the balloon

158. A nurse is assigned to assist with caring for a client who has a chest tube. The nurse notes fluctuations of the fluid level in the water-seal chamber. Based on this observation, which action would be appropriate?
1. Empty the drainage.
2. Encourage the client to deep breathe.
3. Continue to monitor, because this is an expected finding.
4. Encourage the client to hold his or her breath periodically.

159. A nurse is assigned to assist the physician with the removal of a chest tube. The nurse instructs the client to do which of the following during this process?
1. Stay very still.
2. Exhale forcefully.
3. Inhale and exhale quickly.
4. Perform Valsalva's maneuver.

160. A nurse is preparing to begin a continuous tube feeding on a client with a nasogastric tube. The nurse positions the client:
1. Supine
2. Supine on the right side
3. With the head elevated 15 degrees
4. With the head elevated 45 degrees

161. A nurse is preparing to administer an intermittent tube feeding to a client with a nasogastric tube. The nurse checks the residual and obtains an amount of 200 mL. The nurse would:
1. Hold the feeding.
2. Administer the feeding.
3. Flush the tubing with 30 mL of water.
4. Elevate the head of the bed to 90 degrees and administer the feeding.

162. A nurse is assisting in caring for a client with a chest tube. The nurse understands that which of the following is an incorrect action for the care of the client?
1. Pin the tubing to the bed linens.
2. Be sure all connections are taped.

3. Be sure all connections remain airtight.
4. Do not allow the tubing to become kinked or obstructed by the weight of the client.

163. A nurse is assigned to care for a client who has a chest tube. The nurse is told to monitor the client for crepitus (subcutaneous emphysema). The nurse monitors the client for this complication by:
   1. Monitoring for pain
   2. Monitoring respirations hourly
   3. Checking the blood pressure every 2 hours
   4. Palpating for the leakage of air into the subcutaneous tissues

164. A nurse is told that an assigned client will have a fenestrated tracheostomy tube inserted. The nurse prepares the client for the procedure, knowing that this type of tube:
   1. Enables the client to speak
   2. Prevents the client from speaking
   3. Is necessary for mechanical ventilation

4. Prevents air from being inhaled through the tracheostomy opening

165. A nurse is assisting with monitoring the functioning of a chest-tube drainage system in a client who just returned from the recovery room after a thoracotomy with wedge resection. Which findings would the nurse expect to note? **Select all that apply.**
   ❑ 1. Excessive bubbling in the water-seal chamber
   ❑ 2. Vigorous bubbling in the suction-control chamber
   ❑ 3. 50 mL of drainage in the drainage-collection chamber
   ❑ 4. The drainage system is maintained below the client's chest.
   ❑ 5. An occlusive dressing is in place over the chest-tube insertion site.
   ❑ 6. Fluctuation of water in the tube of the water-seal chamber during inhalation and exhalation

ANSWERS

151. 3
Rationale: Unless otherwise instructed, an amount of less than 100 mL may be reinstituted; then a normal amount of tube feeding is administered. It is important to return the contents to the stomach to prevent electrolyte imbalances.
Test-Taking Strategy: Use the process of elimination. Option 1 could cause an electrolyte and nutritional imbalance. The HCP does not need to be notified for this normal occurrence. To prevent dehydration, clients need to get the correct amount of feeding prescribed. Review tube-feeding administration if you had difficulty with this question.
Level of Cognitive Ability: Applying
Client Needs: Physiological Integrity
Integrated Process: Nursing Process/Implementation
Content Area: Fundamental Skills: Nutrition
Reference: Christensen, Kockrow, pp. 648–649. 2011. *Foundations of nursing.*

152. 4
Rationale: If a client becomes cyanotic or restless or develops tachycardia, bradycardia, or another abnormal heart rhythm, the nurse must discontinue suctioning until the client is stabilized. It is also important to monitor the vital signs and the pulse oximetry. If the client's condition continues to deteriorate, then the respiratory department and HCP may need to be notified.
Test-Taking Strategy: Use the process of elimination. Focusing on the data in the question will direct you to option 4. Review endotracheal suctioning if you had difficulty with this question.
Level of Cognitive Ability: Applying
Client Needs: Physiological Integrity
Integrated Process: Nursing Process/Implementation
Content Area: Adult Health/Respiratory

References: deWit, pp. 310–312. 2009.
Lewis, Dirksen, Heitkemper, Bucher, Camera, pp. 1701–1702. 2011.

153. 1
Rationale: If the NG tube is in the stomach, the pH of the contents will be acidic. Option 2 indicates a slightly acidic pH. Option 3 indicates an alkaline pH. Option 4 indicates a neutral pH.
Test-Taking Strategy: Use the process of elimination. Recalling that gastric contents are acidic will direct you to option 1. Review the procedure for checking NG tube placement if you had difficulty with this question.
Level of Cognitive Ability: Understanding
Client Needs: Physiological Integrity
Integrated Process: Nursing Process/Data Collection
Content Area: Adult Health/Gastrointestinal
Reference: Christensen, Kockrow, p. 587. 2011. *Foundations of nursing.*

154. 3
Rationale: When the RN removes the NG tube, the client is instructed to take and hold a deep breath. This will close the epiglottis, and the airway will be temporarily obstructed during the tube removal. This allows for the easy withdrawal of the tube through the esophagus into the nose. The RN removes the tube with one very smooth, continuous pull. Options 1, 2, and 4 are incorrect.
Test-Taking Strategy: Use the process of elimination, and focus on the subject of removing an NG tube. Visualize the procedure, and consider what each client action identified in the options would produce. Review the removal of an NG tube if you had difficulty with this question.
Level of Cognitive Ability: Applying
Client Needs: Physiological Integrity
Integrated Process: Nursing Process/Implementation

Content Area: Adult Health/Gastrointestinal
Reference: Christensen, Kockrow, p. 590. 2011. *Foundations of nursing.*

155. 2
Rationale: If a client has an NG tube connected to suction, the nurse should wait up to 30 minutes before reconnecting the tube to the suction apparatus to allow adequate time for medication absorption. Aspirating the NG tube will remove the medication that has just been administered. Low intermittent suction will also remove the medication. The client should not be placed in the supine position because of the risk for aspiration.
Test-Taking Strategy: Use the process of elimination. Eliminate options 3 and 4 first, because these actions are comparable or alike and will produce the same effect. Recalling that the client should not be placed in a supine position will assist you with eliminating option 1. Review the administration of medications through an NG tube if you had difficulty with this question.
Level of Cognitive Ability: Applying
Client Needs: Physiological Integrity
Integrated Process: Nursing Process/Implementation
Content Area: Fundamental Skills: Medications/Blood & IV Therapy
References: Christensen, Kockrow, p. 706. 2011. *Foundations and adult health nursing.*
Perry, Potter, pp. 537, 539. 2010.

156. 4
Rationale: When the client has a Sengstaken-Blakemore tube, a pair of scissors must be kept at the client's bedside at all times. The client needs to be observed for sudden respiratory distress, which occurs if the gastric balloon ruptures and the entire tube moves upward. If this occurs, the registered nurse is notified immediately and the balloon lumens will be cut. An obturator and a Kelly clamp are kept at the bedside of a client with a tracheostomy. An irrigation set may also be kept at the bedside, but it is not the priority item.
Test-Taking Strategy: Use your knowledge of the structure, function, and placement of a Sengstaken-Blakemore tube to answer this question. Note the strategic word "priority" in the question; this should assist you with eliminating options 1, 2, and 3. Review the care of a client with a Sengstaken-Blakemore tube if you had difficulty with this question.
Level of Cognitive Ability: Applying
Client Needs: Safe and Effective Care Environment
Integrated Process: Nursing Process/Implementation
Content Area: Fundamental Skills: Safety/Infection Control
References: Black, Hawks. p. 1156. 2009.
Ignatavicius, Workman. p. 1353. 2010.

157. 2
Rationale: The catheter's balloon is behind the opening at the insertion tip. The catheter is inserted 2.5 to 5 cm after urine begins to flow to provide sufficient space to inflate the balloon. Inserting the catheter the extra distance will ensure that the balloon is inflated inside the bladder and not in the urethra, which could produce trauma.

Test-Taking Strategy: Visualize the proper procedure for inserting an indwelling urinary catheter to assist you with answering this question. Note the strategic words "urine begins to flow." Options 3 and 4 can easily be eliminated. Eliminate option 1 next because of the word "immediately." Review bladder catheterization if you had difficulty with this question.
Level of Cognitive Ability: Applying
Client Needs: Physiological Integrity
Integrated Process: Nursing Process/Implementation
Content Area: Adult Health/Renal
Reference: Potter, Perry, p. 1158. 2009.

158. 3
Rationale: The presence of fluctuations in the fluid level in the water-seal chamber indicates a patent drainage system. With normal breathing, the water level rises with inspiration and falls with expiration. The apparatus and all connections must remain airtight at all times, and the drainage is never emptied. Encouraging the client to deep breathe is unrelated to this observation. The client is not told to hold his or her breath.
Test-Taking Strategy: Focus on the subject of the question—the fluctuation of the fluid level in the water-seal chamber. This will assist you with eliminating options 1, 2, and 4. Review the expected and unexpected findings when caring for a client with a chest tube if you had difficulty with this question.
Level of Cognitive Ability: Applying
Client Needs: Physiological Integrity
Integrated Process: Nursing Process/Implementation
Content Area: Adult Health/Respiratory
Reference: Christensen, Kockrow, p. 1646. 2011. *Foundations and adult health nursing.*

159. 4
Rationale: When the chest tube is removed, the client is asked to perform Valsalva's maneuver (i.e., take a deep breath, exhale, and bear down), the tube is quickly withdrawn, and an airtight dressing is taped in place. An alternative instruction is to ask the client to take a deep breath and hold the breath while the tube is removed. Options 1, 2, and 3 are incorrect client instructions.
Test-Taking Strategy: Use the process of elimination. Visualize the procedure and the client instructions given in each option as you answer the question. This will direct you to option 4. Review the procedure for the removal of a chest tube if you had difficulty with this question.
Level of Cognitive Ability: Applying
Client Needs: Physiological Integrity
Integrated Process: Nursing Process/Implementation
Content Area: Adult Health/Respiratory
References: deWit, p. 348. 2009.
Lewis, Dirksen, Heitkemper, Bucher, Camera, p. 571. 2011.

160. 4
Rationale: When a tube feeding is administered, the client is placed in a high Fowler's position for a bolus feeding and in a semi-Fowler's position (30 to 45 degrees) for a continuous feeding to allow gravity to help the flow of formula and to prevent reflux and aspiration. Options 1, 2, and 3 are inappropriate positions during a tube feeding.

Test-Taking Strategy: Use the process of elimination. Elimi-nate options 1 and 2 first, because they are comparable or alike. Recalling the risks associated with the administration of a tube feeding will direct you to option 4. Review the administration of tube feedings if you had difficulty with this question.
Level of Cognitive Ability: Applying
Client Needs: Physiological Integrity
Integrated Process: Nursing Process/Implementation
Content Area: Fundamental Skills: Safety/Infection Control
Reference: Christensen, Kockrow, p. 648. 2011. *Foundations of nursing.*

161. 1
Rationale: When 200 mL of residual formula are obtained, the feeding is held and the health care provider (HCP) is notified, because this is an indication that the feeding is not being absorbed. If the residual is less than 100 mL, the feeding is usu-ally administered. Large-volume aspirates indicate delayed gas-tric emptying and place the client at risk for aspiration. Always check the HCP's prescriptions and agency policy regarding re-sidual amounts. Elevating the head of the bed to 90 degrees and flushing the tubing are not appropriate actions.
Test-Taking Strategy: Use the process of elimination. Elimi-nate options 2 and 4 first, because they are comparable or alike. Recalling that the feeding is held when more than 100 mL of residual are obtained will direct you to option 1. Review the procedure for administering intermittent tube feedings if you had difficulty with this question.
Level of Cognitive Ability: Applying
Client Needs: Physiological Integrity
Integrated Process: Nursing Process/Implementation
Content Area: Adult Health/Gastrointestinal
Reference: Christensen, Kockrow, p. 649. 2011. *Foundations of nursing.*

162. 1
Rationale: Chest-tube tubing is never pinned to the bed linens, because this presents the risk of accidental dislodgment of the tube when the client moves. Options 2, 3, and 4 are appropriate interventions for the plan of care for a client with a chest tube.
Test-Taking Strategy: Note the strategic word "incorrect" in the question. This word indicates a negative event query and asks you to select an incorrect action. Use the process of elim-ination, and recall the complications associated with a chest tube. Review the care of the client with a chest tube if you had difficulty with this question.
Level of Cognitive Ability: Applying
Client Needs: Physiological Integrity
Integrated Process: Nursing Process/Implementation
Content Area: Adult Health/Respiratory
Reference: Christensen, Kockrow, p. 1645. 2011. *Foundations and adult health nursing.*

163. 4
Rationale: Subcutaneous emphysema is also known as crepi-tus. It presents as a "puffed-up" appearance that is caused by the leakage of air into the subcutaneous tissues. It is monitored by palpating, and it feels like bubble wrap when palpated. Although options 1, 2, and 3 may be components of the plan of care for a client with a chest tube, these actions will not identify subcutaneous emphysema.

Test-Taking Strategy: Use the process of elimination. Note the similarity between the words "subcutaneous emphysema" in the question and "subcutaneous tissues" in the correct option. Review subcutaneous emphysema if you had difficulty with this question.
Level of Cognitive Ability: Applying
Client Needs: Physiological Integrity
Integrated Process: Nursing Process/Data Collection
Content Area: Adult Health/Respiratory
References: Black, Hawks, p. 1546. 2009.

164. 1
Rationale: A fenestrated tube has a small opening in the outer cannula that allows some air to escape through the larynx; this type of tube enables the client to speak. Options 2, 3, and 4 are incorrect with regard to this type of tube.
Test-Taking Strategy: Knowledge regarding the design and purpose of a fenestrated tracheostomy tube will direct you to option 1. Review the purpose of a fenestrated tube if you had difficulty with this question.
Level of Cognitive Ability: Understanding
Client Needs: Physiological Integrity
Integrated Process: Nursing Process/Planning
Content Area: Adult Health/Respiratory
References: deWit, p. 306. 2009.
Lewis, Dirksen, Heitkemper, Bucher, Camera, pp. 529, 534. 2011.

165. 3, 4, 5, 6
Rationale: The bubbling of water in the water-seal chamber indicates air drainage from the client. This is usually seen when intrathoracic pressure is greater than atmospheric pressure, and it may occur during exhalation, coughing, or sneezing. Exces-sive bubbling in the water-seal chamber may indicate an air leak, which is an unexpected finding. The fluctuation of water in the tube in the water-seal chamber during inhalation and exhalation is expected. An absence of fluctuation may indicate that the chest tube is obstructed, the lung has re-expanded, or no more air is leaking into the pleural space. Gentle (not vig-orous) bubbling should be noted in the suction-control cham-ber. A total of 50 mL of drainage is not excessive in a client returning to the nursing unit from the recovery room; however, drainage of more than 70 to 100 mL/hr is considered excessive and requires physician notification. The chest-tube insertion site is covered with an occlusive (airtight) dressing to prevent air from entering the pleural space. Positioning the drainage system below the client's chest allows gravity to drain the pleu-ral space.
Test-Taking Strategy: Thinking about the physiology associ-ated with the functioning of a chest-tube drainage system will help you to answer this question. The words "excessive bub-bling" and "vigorous bubbling" will assist you with eliminating options 1 and 2. Review the care of the client with a chest-tube drainage system if you had difficulty with this question.
Level of Cognitive Ability: Analyzing
Client Needs: Physiological Integrity
Integrated Process: Nursing Process/Data Collection
Content Area: Adult Health/Respiratory
References: Christensen, Kockrow, p. 1646. 2011. *Foundations and adult health nursing.*
Lewis, Dirksen, Heitkemper, Bucher, Camera, p. 572. 2011.

Maternity Nursing

Female Reproductive System

PYRAMID TERMS

amniotic fluid The pale, straw-colored fluid that surrounds and protects the fetus. The fetus floats in the amniotic fluid, which serves as a cushion against injury from sudden blows or movements. It also helps maintain a constant body temperature for the fetus. The fetus modifies the amniotic fluid through the processes of swallowing, urinating, and movement through the respiratory tract.

ballottement The rebounding of the fetus against the examiner's finger on palpation. When the cervix is tapped, the fetus floats upward in the amniotic fluid. A rebound is felt by the examiner when the fetus falls back.

Chadwick's sign The violet coloration of the vaginal mucous membranes that is visible from about 4 weeks' gestation and presents as a result of increased vascularity. This is considered a probable sign of pregnancy.

delivery The actual event of birth. The expulsion or extraction of the neonate and the fetal membranes at birth.

fertilization The union of an ovum and sperm. Fertilization occurs within 12 hours of ovulation and within 2 to 3 days of insemination, the average duration of viability of the ovum and the sperm.

Goodell's sign The softening of the cervix. This occurs at the beginning of the second month of gestation and is considered a probable sign of pregnancy.

gravida A pregnant woman. The woman is called gravida I (or primigravida) during the first pregnancy, gravida II during the second, and so on.

Hegar's sign The compressibility and softening of the lower uterine segment. This occurs at about 6 weeks' gestation, and it is considered a probable sign of pregnancy.

implantation The embedding of the fertilized ovum in the uterine mucosa, which occurs 6 to 10 days after conception.

infant A human born alive; also, a human from 28 days of age until the first birthday,

labor A coordinated sequence of rhythmic, involuntary uterine contractions that result in the effacement and dilation of cervix. This is followed by the expulsion of the products of conception.

lochia Vaginal discharge from the uterus that consists of blood from the vessels of the placental site, tissue debris from the decidua, and mucus. Lochia lasts for 2 to 6 weeks postpartum, and is differentiated by color: rubra, serosa, or alba.

Nägele's rule A way to determine the estimated date of birth that works on the premise that the woman has a 28-day menstrual cycle. Subtract 3 months from the first day of last menstrual period, add 7 days, and then adjust the year.

newborn A human offspring from the time of birth to day 28 of life; also called a neonate.

parity The number of pregnancies that have reached viability, regardless of whether the infants were alive or stillborn.

placenta The organ that provides for the exchange of nutrients and waste products between the fetus and the mother and that produces hormones to maintain pregnancy. It develops by the third month of gestation, and is also called the afterbirth.

quickening The maternal perception of fetal movement, which usually appears around 16 to 20 weeks' gestation.

PYRAMID TO SUCCESS

The Pyramid to Success focuses on the physiological and psychosocial aspects related to the experience of pregnancy. The pyramid points begin with instructing the pregnant client with regard to measures that will promote a healthy environment for both the mother and fetus. Focus on the importance of antenatal follow-up care, nutrition, and the interventions for common discomforts that occur during pregnancy. Review the purpose of the commonly prescribed diagnostic tests and procedures during the antenatal period. Focus on disorders that can occur during pregnancy, particularly gestational hypertension and diabetes. Review the labor and delivery process and the immediate interventions when the mother or fetal status is compromised, such as prolapsed cord or altered fetal heart rate. Review the fetal effects that result from the mother with acquired immunodeficiency syndrome or the mother who abuses substances. Focus on the normal expectations of the postpartum period and the complications that can occur. The pyramid points also focus on the normal physical assessment findings of the newborn and the early identification of disorders of the newborn. The last pyramid point focuses on maternity and newborn medications.

CLIENT NEEDS

Safe and Effective Care Environment

- Collaborating with other members of the health care team
- Establishing priorities of care
- Handling infectious materials safely
- Maintaining asepsis
- Maintaining confidentiality
- Obtaining informed consent for procedures
- Providing continuity of care
- Upholding parent rights
- Using standard, transmission-based, and other precautions when delivering care

Health Promotion and Maintenance

- Monitoring growth and development
- Ensuring health and wellness
- Discussing expected body-image changes
- Identifying high-risk behaviors
- Identifying lifestyle choices
- Performing techniques of data collection
- Providing antepartum, intrapartum, postpartum, and newborn care

Psychosocial Integrity

- Considering cultural, spiritual, and religious influences regarding birth and motherhood
- Discussing situational role changes
- Ensuring therapeutic interactions within the family
- Identifying available support systems
- Identifying coping mechanisms

Physiological Integrity

- Identifying at-risk clients during pregnancy
- Instructing the client about prescribed diagnostic tests and procedures
- Monitoring for expected outcomes and effects related to pharmacological and parenteral therapies
- Monitoring for normal expectations during pregnancy
- Monitoring the client during the labor and delivery process
- Providing interventions for unexpected events during the pregnancy
- Providing nonpharmacological and pharmacological comfort interventions during pregnancy
- Teaching the client about nutrition during pregnancy and the postpartum period
- Teaching the client about the physiological changes that occur during pregnancy

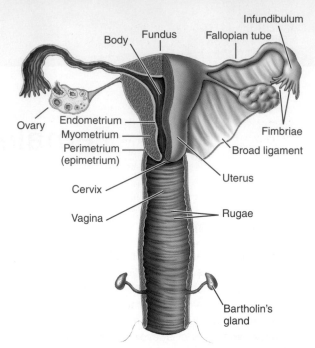

▲ **FIGURE 20-1** Female reproductive organs. (From Herlihy, B., & Maebius, N. [2007]. *The human body in health and illness* [3rd ed.]. Philadelphia: Saunders.)

I. FEMALE REPRODUCTIVE STRUCTURES (Figure 20-1)

A. Ovaries
  1. Form and expel ova
  2. Primary source of estrogen and progesterone

B. Fallopian tubes
  1. Muscular tubes (oviducts) that are approximate to the ovaries and that connect into the uterus
  2. Provide transportation for the ova from the ovaries to the uterus

C. Uterus
  1. Muscular organ shaped like an upside-down pear in which the fetus develops.
  2. Cavity from which menstruation occurs

D. Cervix
  1. Internal os of the cervix opens into the body of the uterine cavity.
  2. Cervical canal is located between the internal cervical os and the external cervical os.
  3. External cervical os opens into the vagina.

E. Vagina
  1. A muscular tube that extends from the cervix to the vaginal opening in the perineum
  2. Known as the birth canal
  3. Passage between the cervical os and the external environment
    a. Passageway for menstrual blood flow
    b. Passageway for fetus
    c. Passageway for penis for intercourse

Box 20-1 Menstrual Cycle

Ovarian Changes

Preovulatory Phase

- The hypothalamus releases gonadotropin-releasing hormone through the portal system to the anterior pituitary system.
- Secretion of follicle-stimulating hormone (FSH) by the anterior lobe of the pituitary gland stimulates growth of follicles.
- Most follicles die, leaving one to mature into a large graafian follicle.
- Estrogen produced by the follicle stimulates increased secretions of luteinizing hormone (LH) by the anterior lobe of the pituitary gland.
- The follicle ruptures and releases an ovum into the peritoneal cavity.

Luteal Phase

- The luteal phase begins with ovulation.
- Body temperature drops and then rises by 0.5° to 1° F around the time of ovulation.
- Corpus luteum is formed from follicle cells that remain in the ovary following ovulation.
- Corpus luteum secretes estrogen and progesterone during the remaining 14 days of the cycle.
- Corpus luteum degenerates if the ovum is not fertilized, and secretion of estrogen and progesterone declines.
- The decline of estrogen and progesterone stimulates the anterior pituitary to secrete more FSH and LH, initiating a new reproductive cycle.

Uterine Changes

Menstrual Phase

- The menstrual phase consists of 4 to 6 days of bleeding as the endometrium breaks down because of the decreased levels of estrogen and progesterone.
- The level of FSH increases, enabling the beginning of a new cycle.

Proliferative Phase

- The proliferative phase lasts about 9 days.
- Estrogen stimulates proliferation and growth of the endometrium.
- As estrogen increases, it suppresses secretion of FSH and increases secretion of LH.
- Secretion of LH stimulates ovulation and the development of the corpus luteum.
- Ovulation occurs between days 12 and 16.
- The estrogen level is high and the progesterone level is low.

Secretory Phase

- The secretory phase lasts about 12 days and follows ovulation.
- This phase is initiated in response to the increase in LH level.
- The graafian follicle is replaced by the corpus luteum.
- The corpus luteum secretes progesterone and estrogen.
- Progesterone prepares the endometrium for pregnancy if a fertilized ovum is implanted.

II. MENSTRUAL CYCLE (Box 20-1)

A. Menstrual cycle: The regularly recurring physiological changes in the endometrium that culminate in its shedding; may vary in duration, with average of approximately 28 days; ovarian and uterine changes occur

B. Ovarian hormones
1. Ovarian hormones include the follicle-stimulating hormone (FSH) and luteinizing hormone (LH).
2. The hormones are released by the anterior pituitary gland.
3. The hormones produce changes in the ovaries.
4. Secretion of ovarian hormones leads to changes in the endometrium.

C. Ovarian and uterine phases (see Box 20-1)

III. FEMALE PELVIS

A. True pelvis
1. Lies below the pelvic brim (the lower, curved, bony canal)
2. Consists of the pelvic inlet, the mid pelvis, and the pelvic outlet

B. False pelvis
1. Shallow portion above the pelvic brim
2. Supports the abdominal viscera

C. Types of pelvis
1. Gynecoid
   a. Normal female pelvis
   b. Transversely rounded or blunt

⚠ The gynecoid pelvis is most favorable for successful labor and birth.

2. Android
   a. Heart-shaped or angulated
   b. Resembles a male pelvis
   c. Not favorable for **labor**
   d. Narrow pelvic planes can cause slow descent and mid-pelvis arrest
3. Anthropoid
   a. Oval shape
   b. The outlet is adequate, with a normal or moderately narrow pubic arch
4. Platypelloid
   a. Flat shape with an oval inlet
   b. The transverse diameter is wide, but the anteroposterior diameter is short, thus making **labor** and birth difficult

IV. FERTILIZATION AND IMPLANTATION

A. Fertilization
1. **Fertilization** occurs in the ampulla of the fallopian (uterine) tube.
2. It occurs within 12 hours of ovulation and within 2 to 3 days of insemination, the average durations of viability for the ovum and sperm.
3. It takes place when sperm and ovum unite.
4. Once fertilized, the membrane of the ovum undergoes changes that prevent entry of other sperm.
5. Each reproductive cell carries 23 chromosomes.
6. Sperm carry an X or a Y chromosome—XY, male; XX, female.

B. Implantation
1. Zygote (fertilized ovum) is propelled toward the uterus
2. The zygote implants 6 to 8 days after **fertilization**
3. Blastocyst (embryonic form) secretes chorionic gonadotropin to ensure that the corpus luteum remains viable. It secretes estrogen and progesterone for the first 2 to 3 months of gestation.

V. FETAL DEVELOPMENT (Box 20-2)

A. Preembryonic period: First 2 weeks after conception
B. Embryonic stage: Begins on day 15 and continues through approximately the eighth week after conception
C. Fetal period: Begins the ninth week after conception and ends with birth

VI. FETAL ENVIRONMENT

A. Amnion
1. Encloses the amniotic cavity
2. Inner cell membrane that forms about the second week of embryonic development
3. Forms a fluid-filled sac that surrounds the embryo and later the fetus

B. Chorion
1. Outer membrane
2. Becomes vascularized and forms the fetal part of the **placenta**

C. Amniotic fluid
1. Consists of 800 to 1200 mL by the end of pregnancy
2. Surrounds, cushions, and protects the fetus and allows for fetal movement
3. Maintains the body temperature of the fetus
4. Consists largely of fetal urine and is therefore a measure of fetal kidney function
5. The fetus modifies the **amniotic fluid** through the processes of swallowing, urinating, and movement through the respiratory tract.

D. Placenta
1. The **placenta** provides for exchange of nutrients and waste products between the fetus and mother.
2. Begins to form at **implantation**; structure is complete by week 12.
3. It produces hormones to maintain pregnancy and assumes full responsibility for the production of these hormones by the twelfth week of gestation.
4. In the third trimester, transfer of maternal immunoglobulin provides the fetus with passive immunity to certain diseases for the first few months after birth.
5. By week 10 and 12, genetic testing can be done via chorionic villus sampling (CVS).

⚠ Large particles such as bacteria cannot pass through the placenta, but nutrients, drugs, antibodies, and viruses can pass through the placenta.

VII. FETAL CIRCULATION (Figure 20-2)

A. Umbilical cord
1. Contains two arteries and one vein
2. Arteries carry deoxygenated blood and waste products from the fetus
3. Vein carries oxygenated blood and provides oxygen and nutrients to the fetus

B. Fetal heart rate (FHR)
1. Depends on gestational age: may be 160 to 170 beats per minute during the first trimester, but slows with fetal growth to 110 to 120 (low end) to 160 (high end) beats per minute near or at term.
2. The FHR is approximately twice the maternal heart rate

C. Fetal circulation bypass
1. Present as a result of nonfunctioning lungs
2. Bypasses must close after birth to allow blood to flow through the lungs and the liver
3. Ductus arteriosus connects the pulmonary artery to the aorta, bypassing the lungs
4. Ductus venosus connects the umbilical vein and the inferior vena cava, bypassing the liver
5. Foramen ovale is the opening between the right and left atria of heart, bypassing the lungs

⚠ The fetal heart is 160 to 170 beats/min in the first trimester, but slows with fetal growth to 120 to 160 beats/min near or at term. The health care provider (HCP) must be notified if the fetal heart rate is outside these parameters.

VIII. FAMILY PLANNING

A. Description
1. Involves choosing when to have children
2. Includes contraception, prevention of pregnancy, and methods to achieve pregnancy

Box 20-2 Fetal Development

Preembryonic Period
First 2 weeks after conception

Embryonic Period
Beginning day 15 through approximately week 8 after
  conception

Fetal Period
Week 9 after conception to birth

Week 1
Blastocyst is free-floating.

Weeks 2 to 3
Embryo is 1.5 to 2 mm in length.
Lung buds appear
Blood circulation begins.
Heart is tubular and begins to beat.
Neural plate becomes brain and spinal cord

Week 5
Embryo is 0.4 to 0.5 cm in length.
Embryo is 0.4 g.
Double heart chambers are visible.
Heart is beating.
Limb buds form.

Week 8
Embryo is 3 cm in length.
Embryo is 2 g.
Eyelids begin to fuse.
Circulatory system through umbilical cord is well established.
Every organ system is present.

Week 12
Fetus is 6 to 9 cm in length.
Fetus is 19 g.
Face is well formed
Limbs are long and slender.
Kidneys begin to form urine.
Spontaneous movements occur.
Heartbeat is detected by Doppler transducer between 10 and
  12 weeks.
Sex is visually recognizable.

Week 16
Fetus is 11.5 to 13.5 cm in length.
Fetus is 100 g.
Active movements are present.
Fetal skin is transparent.
Lanugo hair begins to develop.
Skeletal ossification occurs.

Week 20
Fetus is 16 to 18.5 cm in length.
Fetus is 300 g.
Lanugo covers the entire body.
Fetus has nails.
Muscles are developed.
Enamel and dentin are depositing.
Heartbeat is detected by regular (nonelectronic) fetoscope.

Week 24
Fetus is 23 cm in length.
Fetus is 600 g.
Hair on head is well formed.
Skin is reddish and wrinkled.
Reflex hand grasp functions.
Vernix caseosa covers entire body.
Fetus has ability to hear.

Week 28
Fetus is 27 cm in length.
Fetus is 1100 g.
Limbs are well flexed.
Brain is developing rapidly.
Eyelids open and close.
Lungs are developed sufficiently to provide gas exchange
  (lecithin forming).
If born, neonate can breathe at this time.

Week 32
Fetus is 31 cm in length.
Fetus is 1800 to 2100 g.
Bones are fully developed.
Subcutaneous fat has collected.
The L/S (lecithin-to-sphingomyelin) ratio is 1.2:1.

Week 36
The fetus is 35 cm in length.
The fetus is 2200 to 2900 g.
The skin is pink and the body is rounded.
The skin is less wrinkled.
Lanugo is disappearing.
The L/S ratio is higher than 2:1.

Week 40
The fetus is 40 cm in length.
The fetus is 3200+ g.
The skin is pinkish and smooth.
Lanugo is present on upper arms and shoulders.
Vernix caseosa decreases.
Fingernails extend beyond fingertips.
Sole (plantar) creases run down to the heel.
The testes are in the scrotum.
The labia majora are well developed.

B. Birth control
  1. Woman and partner should consider effectiveness, safety, and personal preference when choosing a contraceptive method
  2. Woman's preferences are most important and cultural practices and beliefs and religious or other personal beliefs may affect the choice of contraceptive
  3. Other factors that may affect contraceptive choice include family-planning goals, age, frequency of intercourse, and the individual's capacity for compliance with chosen method

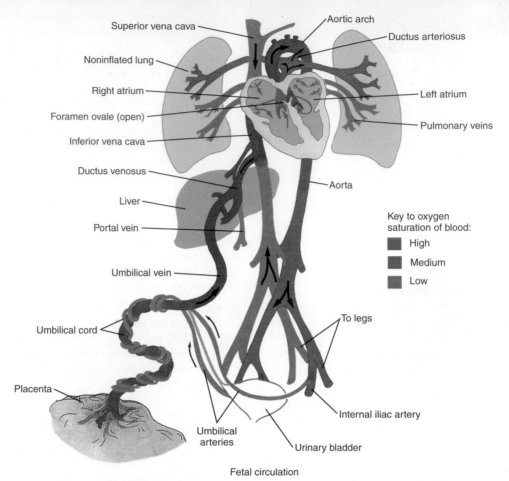

Key to oxygen saturation of blood:

■ High
■ Medium
■ Low

Fetal circulation

▲ **FIGURE 20-2** Schematic illustration of the fetal circulation. (From Lowdermilk, D., Perry, S., Cashion, K., & Alden, K.R. [2011]. *Maternity & women's health care* [10th ed.]. St. Louis: Mosby.)

4. If family-planning goals are already met, sterilization of either the male or female partner may be an option
5. For women who frequently engage in coitus, oral contraceptives or a long-term method, such as an intrauterine device (IUD) may be considered
6. Use of spermicide, condoms, or a diaphragm may be desirable when sexual activity is limited
7. Some methods of contraception may have adverse effects and thus the nurse may need to initiate an informed consent

C. Infertility
1. Involuntary inability to conceive when desired
2. Some contributing factors in men include abnormalities of the sperm, abnormal erections or ejaculations, or abnormalities of seminal fluid
3. Some contributing factors in women include disorders of ovulation or abnormalities of fallopian tubes or cervix
4. Diagnostic tests may be helpful in determining cause of infertility
5. Infertility options may include medication, surgical procedures, therapeutic insemination, in vitro fertilization, surrogate mothers, and/or embryo hosts

MORE QUESTIONS ON EVOLVE!

Practice Questions

166. The nurse is collecting data from a pregnant client when the client asks the nurse about the purpose of the fallopian tubes. The nurse responds to the client, knowing that the fallopian tubes:
1. Are the organ of copulation
2. Are where the fetus develops
3. Are where fertilization occurs
4. Secrete estrogen and progesterone

167. A nursing student is assigned to care for an adolescent female client in the health care clinic, and the instructor reviews the menstrual cycle with the student. The instructor determines that the student understands the process of the secretion of follicle-stimulating hormone (FSH) and luteinizing hormone (LH) if the student states:
1. "FSH and LH are secreted by the adrenal glands."
2. "FSH and LH are released from the anterior pituitary gland."

3. "FSH and LH are secreted by the corpus luteum of the ovary."
4. "FSH and LH stimulate the formation of milk during pregnancy."

168. The nurse working in a prenatal clinic reviews a client's chart and notes that the health care provider documents that the client has a gynecoid pelvis. The nurse understands that this type of pelvis is:
1. Not favorable for labor
2. Not normally a female pelvis type
3. A wide pelvis with a short diameter
4. The most favorable for labor and birth

169. The client asks the nurse about the purpose of the placenta. The nurse plans to respond to the client, knowing that the placenta:
1. Cushions and protects the fetus
2. Maintains the body temperature of the fetus
3. Surrounds the fetus and allows for fetal movement
4. Provides an exchange of nutrients and waste products between the mother and the fetus

170. The nurse is describing the process of fetal circulation to a client during a prenatal visit. The nurse tells the client that fetal circulation consists of:
1. Two umbilical veins and one umbilical artery
2. Two umbilical arteries and one umbilical vein
3. Arteries that carry oxygenated blood to the fetus
4. Veins that carry deoxygenated blood to the fetus

171. A nursing student is assigned to a client in labor. The nursing instructor asks the student to describe fetal circulation, specifically the ductus venosus. The instructor determines that the student understands the structure of the ductus venosus if the student states that it:
1. Connects the pulmonary artery to the aorta
2. Is an opening between the right and left atria
3. Connects the umbilical vein to the inferior vena cava
4. Connects the umbilical artery to the inferior vena cava

172. During a prenatal visit, the nurse checks the fetal heart rate (FHR) of a client in the third trimester of pregnancy. The nurse determines that the FHR is normal if which of the following heart rates is noted?
1. 80 beats per minute
2. 100 beats per minute
3. 150 beats per minute
4. 180 beats per minute

173. The nurse is teaching a pregnant woman about the physiological effects and hormone changes that occur during pregnancy. The woman asks the nurse about the purpose of estrogen. The nurse bases the response on which of the following purposes of estrogen?
1. It maintains the uterine lining for implantation.
2. It stimulates the metabolism of glucose, and converts glucose to fat.
3. It prevents the involution of the corpus luteum, and maintains the production of progesterone until the placenta is formed.
4. It stimulates uterine development to provide an environment for the fetus, and stimulates the breasts to prepare for lactation.

174. A nursing student is asked to describe the size of the uterus in a nonpregnant client. Which of the following responses, if made by the student, indicates an understanding of the anatomy of this structure?
1. "The uterus weighs about 2 ounces."
2. "The uterus weighs about 2.2 pounds."
3. "The uterus has a capacity of about 50 milliliters."
4. "The uterus is round in shape and weighs approximately 1000 grams."

175. The nursing instructor asks a nursing student to ❖ list the functions of the amniotic fluid. The student responds correctly by stating that which of the following are functions of amniotic fluid? **Select all that apply.**
❑ 1. Allows for fetal movement
❑ 2. Is a measure of kidney function
❑ 3. Surrounds, cushions, and protects the fetus
❑ 4. Maintains the body temperature of the fetus
❑ 5. Prevents large particles such as bacteria from passing to the fetus
❑ 6. Provides an exchange of nutrients and waste products between the mother and the fetus

ANSWERS

166. 3
Rationale: Each fallopian tube is a hollow muscular tube that transports a mature oocyte for final maturation and fertilization. Fertilization typically occurs near the boundary between the ampulla and the isthmus of the tube. The vagina is the organ of copulation, and the fetus develops in the uterus. Estrogen is a hormone that is produced by the ovarian follicles, the corpus luteum, the adrenal cortex, and the placenta during pregnancy. Progesterone is a hormone that is secreted by the corpus luteum of the ovary, the adrenal glands, and the placenta during pregnancy.

Test-Taking Strategy: Recalling the anatomy and physiology of the female reproductive system will direct you to the correct option. Remember that fertilization occurs in the fallopian tube. Review the female reproductive system if you had difficulty with this question.
Level of Cognitive Ability: Understanding
Client Needs: Physiological Integrity
Integrated Process: Nursing Process/Implementation
Content Area: Maternity/Antepartum
Reference: Leifer, p. 25. 2011.

167. 2
Rationale: FSH and LH are released from the anterior pituitary gland to stimulate follicular growth and development, growth of the Graafian follicle, and production of progesterone. Options 1, 3, and 4 are incorrect.
Test-Taking Strategy: Use the process of elimination. Option 4 can be eliminated because the case of the question does not address pregnancy. Use your knowledge related to anatomy and physiology of the reproductive system and the menstrual cycle to select the correct option. Review the menstrual cycle if you had difficulty with this question.
Level of Cognitive Ability: Understanding
Client Needs: Physiological Integrity
Integrated Process: Teaching and Learning
Content Area: Maternity/Antepartum
Reference: Leifer, p. 27. 2011.

168. 4
Rationale: A gynecoid pelvis is a normal female pelvis, and it is the most favorable for successful labor and birth. An android pelvis would not be favorable for labor because of the narrow pelvic planes. An anthropoid pelvis has an outlet that is adequate, with a normal or moderately narrow pubic arch. The platypelloid pelvis has a wide transverse diameter, but the anteroposterior diameter is short, thus making the outlet inadequate.
Test-Taking Strategy: Knowledge regarding pelvic types is required to answer this question. Remember that the gynecoid pelvis is the normal female pelvis. Review pelvic types if you had difficulty with this question.
Level of Cognitive Ability: Understanding
Client Needs: Physiological Integrity
Integrated Process: Nursing Process/Data Collection
Content Area: Maternity/Antepartum
Reference: Leifer, pp. 25–26. 2011.

169. 4
Rationale: The placenta provides an exchange of nutrients and waste products between the mother and the fetus. The amniotic fluid surrounds, cushions, and protects the fetus and allows for fetal movement. The amniotic fluid also maintains the body temperature of the fetus.
Test-Taking Strategy: Knowledge regarding the purpose of the placenta and amniotic fluid is required to answer this question. Remember that the placenta provides nutrients. Review the structure and function of the placenta and the amniotic fluid if you had difficulty with this question.
Level of Cognitive Ability: Understanding
Client Needs: Physiological Integrity
Integrated Process: Nursing Process/Planning

Content Area: Maternity/Antepartum
Reference: Leifer, pp. 38–39. 2011.

170. 2
Rationale: Blood pumped by the fetus' heart leaves the fetus through two umbilical arteries. After the blood is oxygenated, it is then returned by one umbilical vein. Arteries carry deoxygenated blood and waste products from the fetus, and veins carry oxygenated blood and provide oxygen and nutrients to the fetus.
Test-Taking Strategy: Recall the anatomy of fetal circulation to answer this question. Remember that there are three umbilical vessels within an umbilical cord (two arteries and one vein). Review the fetal circulation if you had difficulty with this question.
Level of Cognitive Ability: Applying
Client Needs: Physiological Integrity
Integrated Process: Teaching and Learning
Content Area: Maternity/Antepartum
Reference: Leifer, pp. 39–40. 2011.

171. 3
Rationale: The ductus venosus connects the umbilical vein to the inferior vena cava. The foramen ovale is a temporary opening between the right and left atria. The ductus arteriosus joins the aorta and the pulmonary artery.
Test-Taking Strategy: Recall the anatomy of the fetal circulation to answer this question. Remember that the ductus venosus connects the umbilical vein to the inferior vena cava. Review the fetal circulation if you had difficulty with this question.
Level of Cognitive Ability: Understanding
Client Needs: Physiological Integrity
Integrated Process: Teaching and Learning
Content Area: Maternity/Antepartum
Reference: Leifer, pp. 39–40. 2011.

172. 3
Rationale: Fetal heart rate depends on gestational age. It is normally 160 to 170 beats per minute during the first trimester, but it slows with fetal growth to 110 or 120 (low end) to 160 (high end) beats per minute near or at term.
Test-Taking Strategy: Noting the strategic words "third trimester" will direct you to the correct option. Review the fetal heart rate if you had difficulty with this question.
Level of Cognitive Ability: Understanding
Client Needs: Physiological Integrity
Integrated Process: Nursing Process/Data Collection
Content Area: Maternity/Antepartum
Reference: Leifer, p. 133. 2011.

173. 4
Rationale: Estrogen stimulates uterine development to provide an environment for the fetus, and it stimulates the breasts to prepare for lactation. Progesterone maintains the uterine lining for implantation and relaxes all smooth muscle. Human placental lactogen stimulates the metabolism of glucose and converts the glucose to fat. Human chorionic gonadotropin prevents the involution of the corpus luteum and maintains the production of progesterone until the placenta is formed.

Test-Taking Strategy: Recalling the functions of various hormones related to pregnancy will direct you to the correct option. Remember that estrogen stimulates uterine development to provide an environment for the fetus and that it stimulates the breasts to prepare for lactation. Review these various hormones if you had difficulty with this question.
Level of Cognitive Ability: Understanding
Client Needs: Physiological Integrity
Integrated Process: Teaching and Learning
Content Area: Maternity/Antepartum
Reference: Leifer, p. 39. 2011.

174. 1
Rationale: Before conception, the uterus is a small, pear-shaped organ that is contained entirely in the pelvic cavity. Before pregnancy, the uterus weighs approximately 60 g (2 oz), and it has a capacity of about 10 mL (⅓ oz). At the end of pregnancy, the uterus weighs approximately 1000 g (2.2 lb), and it has a capacity that is sufficient for the fetus, the placenta, and the amniotic fluid.
Test-Taking Strategy: Note the strategic word "nonpregnant." Visualizing each of the items identified in the options will direct you to the correct option. Review the anatomy of the uterus if you had difficulty with this question.

Level of Cognitive Ability: Understanding
Client Needs: Physiological Integrity
Integrated Process: Teaching and Learning
Content Area: Maternity/Antepartum
Reference: Leifer, p. 24. 2011.

175. 1, 2, 3, 4
Rationale: The amniotic fluid surrounds, cushions, and protects the fetus. It allows the fetus to move freely, it maintains the body temperature of the fetus, and it helps to measure kidney function, because the amount of fluid is based on the amount of urination from the fetus. The placenta prevents large particles such as bacteria from passing to the fetus, and it provides an exchange of nutrients and waste products between the mother and the fetus.
Test-Taking Strategy: Focus on the subject of the question: the functions of the amniotic fluid. Visualizing the anatomical location of the amniotic fluid will direct you to the correct options. Review the function of the amniotic fluid if you had difficulty with this question.
Level of Cognitive Ability: Understanding
Client Needs: Physiological Integrity
Integrated Process: Teaching and Learning
Content Area: Maternity/Antepartum
Reference: Leifer, p. 35. 2011.

Obstetrical Assessment

I. GESTATION

A. Time from the **fertilization** of the ovum until the estimated date of birth

B. Lasts approximately 280 days or 40 weeks

C. First trimester lasts from week 1 through 13; second trimester last from weeks 14 through 26; third trimester lasts from weeks 27 through 40

D. **Nägele's rule** for estimating date of birth: To be accurate, the woman must have a regular 28-day menstrual cycle. The rule must be adjusted if woman's cycle is longer or shorter than 28 days (Box 21-1).

II. GRAVIDITY AND PARITY

A. Gravidity
1. **Gravida:** A woman who is pregnant
2. Gravidity: Number of pregnancies
3. Nulligravida: A woman who has never been pregnant
4. Primigravida: A woman who is pregnant for the first time
5. Multigravida: A woman who has had two or more pregnancies

B. Parity
1. **Parity:** The number of births (not the number of fetuses [e.g., twins]) carried past 20 weeks' gestation, whether or not the fetus was born alive
2. Nullipara: A woman who has not had a birth at more than 20 weeks' gestation
3. Primipara: A woman who has had one birth that occurred after 20 weeks' gestation
4. Multipara: A woman who has had two or more pregnancies that resulted in viable offspring

C. Use of GTPAL: Pregnancy outcomes can be described with the GTPAL acronym (Box 21-2)
1. G = Gravidity; number of pregnancies, including the present one
2. T = Term births; number of children born at term (i.e., longer than 37 weeks' gestation)
3. P = Preterm births; number of children born before 37 weeks' gestation
4. A = Abortions or miscarriages; number of abortions/miscarriages (included in **gravida** if before 20 weeks' gestation; included in **parity** if past 20 weeks' gestation). Note that a termination of the pregnancy after 20 weeks is referred to as a "therapeutic termination."
5. L = Live births; number of live births or living children

III. PREGNANCY SIGNS

A. Presumptive signs
1. Amenorrhea
2. Nausea and vomiting
3. Increased size and fullness in breasts; pronounced nipples
4. Urinary frequency
5. Fatigue
6. **Quickening:** First perception of fetal movement appearing usually in the sixteenth to twentieth week of gestation
7. Discoloration of vaginal mucosa

B. Probable signs
1. Uterine enlargement
2. **Goodell's sign:** Softening of the cervix that occurs at the beginning of the second month of pregnancy
3. **Chadwick's sign:** Violet coloration of the mucous membranes of the cervix, vagina, and vulva that occurs at about week 4
4. **Hegar's sign:** Compressibility and softening of the lower uterine segment that occurs at about week 6
5. Braxton Hicks contractions: Irregular contractions that occur intermittently throughout pregnancy and do not increase in intensity or duration or cause cervical dilation
6. **Ballottement:** The rebounding of the fetus against the examiner's fingers on palpation
7. Positive pregnancy test for determination of human chorionic gonadotropin

C. Positive signs (diagnostic)
1. Outline of the fetus via radiography or ultrasound
2. Fetal heart rate (approximately 120 to 160 beats per minute) detected by electronic devices at 10 to 12 weeks' gestation, and by nonelectronic device (fetoscope) at 20 weeks' gestation
3. Fetal movements palpated by the examiner

Box 21-1 Nägele's Rule for Determining the Estimated Date of Birth

Take the first day of the last menstrual period: September 12, 2013
- Subtract 3 months: June 12, 2013
- Add 7 days: June 19, 2013
- Adjust the year: June 19, 2014

Estimated date of birth: June 19, 2014

Box 21-2 GTPAL Acronym

G = Gravidity
T = Term births
P = Preterm births
A = Abortions/miscarriages
L = Live births

Example: A woman is pregnant for the fourth time. She had one elective abortion during the first trimester, a daughter who was born at 40 weeks' gestation, and a son who was born at 36 weeks' gestation. Therefore, she is gravida (G) = 4; term (T) = 1 (the daughter born at 40 weeks' gestation). She is also preterm (P) = 1 (the son born at 36 weeks' gestation); abortion (A) = 1 (the abortion is counted in the gravida because it occurred before 20 weeks' gestation); and live births (L) = 2. Therefore, she would be considered GTPAL = 4, 1, 1, 1, 2.

Box 21-3 Measuring Fundal Height

1. Place the client in a supine position.
2. Place the end of the tape measure at the level of the symphysis pubis.
3. Stretch the tape to the top of the uterine fundus.

▲ **FIGURE 21-1** Measurement of fundal height. (From Perry, S., Hockenberry, M., Lowdermilk, D., & Wilson, D. [2009]. *Maternal-child nursing care* [4th ed.]. St. Louis: Mosby. Courtesy of Chris Rozales, San Francisco, CA.)

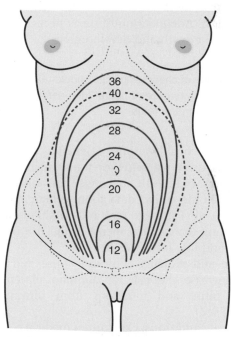

▲ **FIGURE 21-2** Height of fundus by weeks of normal gestation with a single fetus. *Dashed line,* Height after lightening. (From Perry, S., Hockenberry, M., Lowdermilk, D., & Wilson, D. [2009]. *Maternal-child nursing care* [4th ed.]. St. Louis: Mosby.)

IV. FUNDAL HEIGHT (Box 21-3)

A. Measured to evaluate the gestational age of the fetus (Figure 21-1)

B. During the second and third trimesters (weeks 18 to 30), the fundal height in centimeters approximately equals the fetus' age in weeks, plus or minus 2 cm (Figure 21-2).

C. At approximately 14 to 16 weeks, the fundus can be found above the symphysis pubis.

D. At approximately 20 to 22 weeks, the fundus rises to the level of the umbilicus.

E. At term, the fundus nearly reaches the xiphoid process.

 When assessing fundal height, monitor the client closely for supine hypotension when placed in the supine position.

V. MATERNAL RISK FACTORS

A. Maternal age
   1. Women younger than 20 years and older than 35 years are at risk for adverse perinatal outcomes.

B. Adolescent pregnancy
1. Factors that result in adolescent pregnancy include the early onset of menarche, changing sexual behaviors in this age group, problems with family relationships, poverty, and a lack of knowledge of reproduction and birth control.
2. Major concerns related to adolescent pregnancy include poor nutritional status, emotional and behavioral difficulties, lack of support systems, increased risk of stillbirth, low birth weight, fetal mortality, cephalopelvic disproportion, and increased risks of maternal complications (hypertension, anemia, prolonged labor, and infections).
3. The role of the nurse in reducing the risks and consequences of adolescent pregnancy is twofold: first, to encourage early and continued prenatal care, and second, to refer the adolescent, if necessary, for appropriate assistance, which can help counter the effects of a negative socioeconomic environment.

C. Nutrition: Adequate nutrition is necessary for normal fetal growth and development.

⚠️ Women of childbearing age should take folic acid supplements to prevent neural tube defects and orofacial clefts in the fetus.

D. Genetic considerations: Genetic abnormalities such as defective genes or transmissible inherited disorders can result in congenital anomalies; the nurse should collect data about genetic risks

E. Health care: Failure to seek and obtain prenatal care, including dental care, increases the risk of preterm birth and low-birth weight

F. Abuse and violence: Physical abuse and violence can increase the risk for abruptio placentae, preterm birth, and infections from unwanted and forced sex.

G. Medical conditions: Concurrent medical conditions, such as but not limited to diabetes mellitus, hypertensive disorder, or cardiac disease, increase the risks in pregnancy.

H. German measles (rubella): Maternal infection during the first 8 weeks of gestation carries the highest rate of fetal infection.

I. Sexually transmitted infections
1. Syphilis
   a. Organism may cross the **placenta**
   b. Infection usually leads to spontaneous abortions and increases the incidence of mental subnormality and physical deformities
2. Condylomata acuminata (human papillomavirus)
   a. Transmission may occur during vaginal birth.

b. Infection is associated with the development of epithelial tumors of the mucous membranes of the larynx in children.
3. Gonorrhea
   a. Fetus is contaminated at the time of delivery.
   b. Maternal infection may result in postpartum infection in the **newborn**.
   c. Risks to the neonate include ophthalmia neonatorum, pneumonia, and sepsis.
4. Chlamydial infection
   a. Transmission may occur during vaginal birth and can result in neonatal conjunctivitis or pneumonitis
   b. Infection can cause premature rupture of the membranes, premature labor, and postpartum endometritis
5. Trichomoniasis: associated with premature rupture of the membranes and postpartum endometritis

J. Human immunodeficiency virus (HIV)
1. HIV is transmitted via blood, blood products, and other body fluids such as urine, semen, vaginal secretions; the virus is also transmitted through exposure to infected secretions during birth and via breast milk.
2. Repeated exposure to the virus during pregnancy through unsafe sex practices and/or intravenous drug use can increase the risk of transmission to the fetus.
3. Perinatal administration of zidovudine may be recommended to decrease risk of transmission of HIV from mother to fetus.

K. Substance abuse
1. Substance abuse threatens normal fetal growth and the successful term completion of the pregnancy.
2. Substance abuse places the pregnancy at risk for fetal growth restriction, abruption placentae, and fetal bradycardia.
3. Many substances cross the **placenta** and can be teratogenic; no drugs, including tobacco and over-the-counter medications, should be taken unless prescribed by the health care provider.
4. Smoking (tobacco) can lead to low birth weight, a higher incidence of birth defects, and stillbirths.
5. Physical signs of drug abuse may include dilated or contracted pupils, fatigue, track (needle) marks, skin abscesses, inflamed nasal mucosa, and inappropriate behavior by the mother.
6. The consumption of alcohol during pregnancy may lead to fetal alcohol syndrome and can cause jitteriness, physical abnormalities, congenital anomalies, and growth deficits.

L. Viral hepatitis (see Chapter 22 for information regarding hepatitis B infection)

MORE QUESTIONS ON EVOLVE!

Practice Questions

176. The client arrives at the prenatal clinic for her first prenatal assessment. The client tells the nurse that the first day of her last menstrual period was October 20, 2012. Using Nägele's rule, the nurse determines the estimated date of birth to be:
1. July 12, 2013
2. July 27, 2013
3. August 12, 2013
4. August 27, 2013

177. A pregnant client asks the nurse in the clinic when she will be able to start feeling the fetus move. The nurse responds by telling the mother that fetal movements will be noted between:
1. 6 and 8 weeks' gestation
2. 8 and 10 weeks' gestation
3. 10 and 12 weeks' gestation
4. 16 and 20 weeks' gestation

178. The nurse is collecting data during the admission assessment of a client who is pregnant with twins. The client has a healthy 5-year-old child who was delivered at 38 weeks, and she tells the nurse that she does not have a history of any type of abortion or fetal demise. The nurse would document the GTPAL for this client as:
1. G = 3, T = 2, P = 0, A = 0, L = 1
2. G = 2, T = 1, P = 0, A = 0, L = 1
3. G = 1, T = 1, P = 1, A = 0, L = 1
4. G = 2, T = 0, P = 0, A = 0, L = 1

179. The nurse is collecting data during the admission assessment of a client who is pregnant with triplets. The client also has a 3-year-old child who was born at 39 weeks' gestation. The nurse would document which gravida and para status on this client?
1. Gravida I, para I
2. Gravida II, para I
3. Gravida II, para II
4. Gravida III, para II

180. The nurse is reviewing the record of a client who has just been told that her pregnancy test is positive. The nurse notes that the physician has documented the presence of Goodell's sign. The nurse determines that this sign is indicative of:
1. A softening of the cervix
2. The presence of fetal movement
3. The presence of human chorionic gonadotropin in the urine
4. A soft blowing sound that corresponds with the maternal pulse that is heard while auscultating the uterus

181. A primipara is being evaluated in the clinic during her second trimester of pregnancy. Which of the following would indicate an abnormal physical finding that necessitates further testing?
1. Quickening
2. Braxton Hicks contractions
3. Consistent increase in fundal height
4. Fetal heart rate of 180 beats per minute

182. The nurse is collecting data from a pregnant client who is at 28 weeks' gestation. The nurse measures the fundal height in centimeters and expects the findings to be which of the following?
1. 22 cm
2. 28 cm
3. 36 cm
4. 40 cm

183. A pregnant client is seen in the health care clinic for a regular prenatal visit. The client tells the nurse that she is experiencing irregular contractions. The nurse determines that the client is experiencing Braxton Hicks contractions. Based on this finding, which nursing action is appropriate?
1. Contact the health care provider.
2. Instruct the client to maintain bedrest for the remainder of the pregnancy.
3. Tell the client that these are common and they may occur throughout the pregnancy.
4. Call the maternity unit and inform them that the client will be admitted in a prelabor condition.

184. The nursing instructor asks a nursing student to describe the process of quickening. Which of the following statements, if made by the student, indicates an understanding of this term?
1. "It is the fetal movement that is felt by the mother."
2. "It is the compressibility of the lower uterine segment."
3. "It is the irregular, painless contractions that occur throughout pregnancy."
4. "It is the soft blowing sound that can be heard when the uterus is auscultated."

185. The nurse is collecting data from a client who suspects she is pregnant. The nurse is checking the client for probable signs of pregnancy. What are the probable sign(s) of pregnancy that the nurse should recognize? **Select all that apply.**
- ❑ 1. Ballottement
- ❑ 2. Chadwick's sign
- ❑ 3. Uterine enlargement
- ❑ 4. Braxton Hicks contractions
- ❑ 5. Outline of fetus via radiography or ultrasound
- ❑ 6. Fetal heart rate detected by a nonelectronic device

ANSWERS

176. 2

Rationale: The accurate use of Nägele's rule requires that the woman have a regular 28-day menstrual cycle. Subtract 3 months from the first day of the last menstrual period, add 7 days, and then adjust the year as appropriate. In this case, the first day of the LMP was October 20, 2012. When you subtract 3 months, you get July 20, 2012. If you add 7 days, you get July 27, 2012. Add 1 year to this, and you get the estimated date of birth: July 27, 2013.

Test-Taking Strategy: Follow Nägele's rule to answer this question. Read all of the options carefully and note the dates and years in the options before selecting an answer. Review Nägele's rule if you had difficulty with this question.

Level of Cognitive Ability: Understanding
Client Needs: Health Promotion and Maintenance
Integrated Process: Nursing Process/Data Collection
Content Area: Maternity/Antepartum
Reference: Christensen, Kockrow, p. 787. 2011. *Foundations of nursing.*

177. 4

Rationale: Quickening is fetal movement that usually first occurs between 16 and 20 weeks' gestation. The expectant mother first notices subtle fetal movements during this time, and these gradually increase in intensity. Options 1, 2, and 3 are incorrect; these gestational time frames are too early for quickening.

Test-Taking Strategy: Use the process of elimination and your knowledge regarding the occurrence of quickening. In this situation, it is best to select the option that indicates the greatest length of gestational time. Review the process of quickening if you had difficulty with this question.

Level of Cognitive Ability: Applying
Client Needs: Health Promotion and Maintenance
Integrated Process: Teaching and Learning
Content Area: Maternity/Antepartum
Reference: Christensen, Kockrow, p. 786. 2011. *Foundations of nursing.*

178. 2

Rationale: Pregnancy outcomes can be described with the GTPAL acronym: G = gravidity (number of pregnancies); T = term births (number born after 37 weeks); P = preterm births (number born before 37 weeks' gestation); A = abortions/miscarriages (number of abortions/miscarriages); L = live births (number of live births or living children). Therefore, a woman who is pregnant with twins and who already has a child has a gravida of 2. Because the child was delivered at 38 weeks, the number of preterm births is 0, and the number of term births is 1. The number of abortions is 0, and the number of live births is 1.

Test-Taking Strategy: Specific knowledge about GTPAL is needed to answer this question. Your knowledge and understanding will direct you to option 2. Review the GTPAL method of describing pregnancy outcomes if you had difficulty answering this question.

Level of Cognitive Ability: Understanding
Client Needs: Health Promotion and Maintenance
Integrated Process: Nursing Process/Data Collection
Content Area: Maternity/Antepartum

References: Leifer, pp. 47–48. 2011.
McKinney, James, Murray, Ashwill, pp. 262–263. 2009.

179. 2

Rationale: Gravida is a term that refers to a woman who is or who has been pregnant, regardless of the duration of the pregnancy. *Parity* is a term that means the number of births after 20 weeks' gestation; it does not reflect the number of fetuses or infants. Options 1, 3, and 4 are incorrect on the basis of these definitions.

Test-Taking Strategy: Knowledge of the terms *gravida* and *parity* is necessary to answer this question correctly. Remember that *gravida* refers to a woman who is or has been pregnant, regardless of the duration of the pregnancy. *Parity* means the number of births past 20 weeks' gestation. Review the definitions of these terms if you had difficulty with this question.

Level of Cognitive Ability: Applying
Client Needs: Physiological Integrity
Integrated Process: Nursing Process/Implementation
Content Area: Maternity/Antepartum
Reference: Leifer, pp. 47–48. 2011.

180. 1

Rationale: During the early weeks of pregnancy, the cervix becomes softer as a result of pelvic vasoconstriction, which causes Goodell's sign. Cervical softening is noted by the examiner during a pelvic examination. Goodell's sign does not indicate the presence of fetal movement. Human chorionic gonadotropin is noted in maternal urine with a positive urine pregnancy test. A soft blowing sound that corresponds with the maternal pulse may be auscultated over the uterus; it is the result of blood circulating through the placenta.

Test-Taking Strategy: Use the process of elimination and your knowledge regarding the physiological findings of Goodell's sign to answer this question. Remember that Goodell's sign refers to a softening of the cervix. Review the changes in the cervix that occur during pregnancy if you had difficulty with this question.

Level of Cognitive Ability: Understanding
Client Needs: Health Promotion and Maintenance
Integrated Process: Nursing Process/Data Collection
Content Area: Maternity/Antepartum
Reference: Leifer, p. 49. 2011.

181. 4

Rationale: The fetal heart rate depends on the gestational age. It is 160 to 170 beats per minute during the first trimester, and it slows with fetal growth to approximately 120 to 160 beats per minute. Options 1, 2, and 3 are normal expected findings.

Test-Taking Strategy: Note the strategic words "indicate an abnormal physical finding." Recalling the normal fetal heart rate will direct you to the correct option. Review the normal assessment findings of pregnancy if you had difficulty with this question.

Level of Cognitive Ability: Understanding
Client Needs: Physiological Integrity
Integrated Process: Nursing Process/Data Collection
Content Area: Maternity/Antepartum
Reference: Christensen, Kockrow, p. 822. 2011. *Foundations of nursing.*

182. 2

Rationale: During the second and third trimesters (18 to 30 weeks' gestation), the fundal height in centimeters approximately equals the fetus' age in weeks plus or minus 2 cm. At 14 to 16 weeks' gestation, the fundus can be located halfway between the symphysis pubis and the umbilicus. At 20 to 22 weeks' gestation, the fundus is at the umbilicus, and, at term, the fundus is at the xiphoid process.

Test-Taking Strategy: Use the process of elimination. Remember that, during the second and third trimesters, the fundal height in centimeters approximately equals the fetus' age in weeks plus or minus 2 cm. Review fundal height if you had difficulty with this question.

Level of Cognitive Ability: Understanding
Client Needs: Health Promotion and Maintenance
Integrated Process: Nursing Process/Data Collection
Content Area: Maternity/Antepartum
References: Christensen, Kockrow, p. 782. 2011. *Foundations of nursing.*
Perry, Hockenberry, Lowdermilk, Wilson, p. 214. 2010.

183. 3

Rationale: Braxton Hicks contractions are irregular, painless contractions that may occur intermittently throughout pregnancy. Because Braxton Hicks contractions may occur and are normal in some pregnant women during pregnancy, options 1, 2, and 4 are unnecessary and inappropriate actions.

Test-Taking Strategy: Use the process of elimination. Options 1 and 4 are comparable or alike and can thus be eliminated first. From the remaining options, knowing that Braxton Hicks contractions are common and can occur throughout pregnancy will assist with directing you to the correct option. Review the physiology associated with Braxton Hicks contractions if you had difficulty with this question.

Level of Cognitive Ability: Applying
Client Needs: Health Promotion and Maintenance
Integrated Process: Nursing Process/Implementation
Content Area: Maternity/Antepartum
Reference: Leifer, pp. 50, 126. 2011.

184. 1

Rationale: Quickening is fetal movement that appears usually at week 16 to 20, when the expectant mother first notices subtle fetal movements that gradually increase in intensity. A compressibility of the lower uterine segment occurs at about 6 weeks' gestation and is called *Hegar's sign*. Braxton Hicks contractions are irregular, painless contractions that may occur throughout pregnancy. A soft blowing sound that corresponds with the maternal pulse may be auscultated over the uterus; this is known as *uterine souffle*. This sound is the result of blood circulation to the placenta, and it corresponds with the maternal pulse.

Test-Taking Strategy: Use the process of elimination and your knowledge regarding the term *quickening* to answer this question. Review quickening if you had difficulty with this question.

Level of Cognitive Ability: Understanding
Client Needs: Health Promotion and Maintenance
Integrated Process: Teaching and Learning
Content Area: Maternity/Antepartum
Reference: Leifer, p. 49. 2011.

185. 1, 2, 3, 4

Rationale: The probable signs of pregnancy include uterine enlargement, Hegar's sign (the compressibility and softening of the lower uterine segment that occurs at about week 6), Goodell's sign (the softening of the cervix that occurs at the beginning of the second month of pregnancy), Chadwick's sign (the violet coloration of the mucous membranes of the cervix, vagina, and vulva that occurs at about week 4), ballottement (the rebounding of the fetus against the examiner's fingers on palpation), Braxton Hicks contractions, and a positive pregnancy test that measures for human chorionic gonadotropin. Positive signs of pregnancy include a fetal heart rate that is detected by an electronic device (Doppler transducer) at 10 to 12 weeks' gestation and by a nonelectronic device (fetoscope) at 20 weeks' gestation; active fetal movements that are palpable by the examiner; and an outline of the fetus via radiography or ultrasound.

Test-Taking Strategy: Focusing on the subject of the probable signs of pregnancy will assist you with answering this question. Remember that the detection of the fetal heart rate and an outline of the fetus via radiography or ultrasound are positive signs of pregnancy. Review the probable signs of pregnancy if you had difficulty with this question.

Level of Cognitive Ability: Understanding
Client Needs: Health Promotion and Maintenance
Integrated Process: Nursing Process/Data Collection
Content Area: Maternity/Antepartum
Reference: Leifer, p. 48. 2011.

Prenatal Period and Risk Conditions

I. PHYSIOLOGICAL MATERNAL CHANGES

A. Cardiovascular system
 1. Circulating blood volume increases by approximately 40% to 50%; physiological anemia may occur as the plasma increase exceeds the increase in the production of red blood cells.
 2. Heart is elevated upward and to the left because of displacement of the diaphragm as the uterus enlarges (Figure 22-1).
 3. There is an increase in the body's demand for iron.
 4. Sodium and water retention may occur, which can lead to weight gain.

B. Respiratory system
 1. Oxygen consumption increases as a result of an increase in metabolic rate and tissue mass.
 2. Diaphragm is elevated as a result of the enlarged uterus (see Figure 22-1).
 3. Shortness of breath may be experienced.

⚠ During pregnancy, a woman's pulse rate may increase about 10 to 15 beats/minute, the blood pressure slightly decreases in the second trimester, and the respiratory rate remains unchanged or slightly increases.

C. Gastrointestinal (GI) system
 1. Nausea and vomiting may occur as a result of the secretion of human chorionic gonadotropin (hCG), which usually subsides by the third month.
 2. An increase in the body's nutritional requirements (i.e., vitamins, minerals, calories, protein, and iron) is needed.
 3. Constipation may occur as a result of decreased GI motility or pressure of the uterus.
 4. Changes in appetite, flatulence, and heartburn may occur as a result of decreased GI motility and slow emptying of the stomach.
 5. Alterations in taste and smell may occur.
 6. Hemorrhoids may occur as a result of increased venous pressure.
 7. Gum tissue may become swollen and easily bleed because of increasing levels of estrogen.
 8. Ptyalism (excessive secretion of saliva) may occur because of increasing levels of estrogen.

D. Renal system
 1. Frequency of urination occurs during the first and third trimesters as a result of the pressure of the enlarging uterus on the bladder, which causes decreased bladder capacity.
 2. Decreased bladder tone and bladder capacity occurs as a result of hormonal changes.
 3. The renal threshold for glucose may be reduced.

E. Endocrine system
 1. Basal metabolic rate and metabolic function increases.
 2. Anterior lobe of pituitary gland enlarges.
 3. Thyroid gland enlarges slightly and thyroid activity increases.
 4. Parathyroid gland increases in size.
 5. Aldosterone levels gradually increase.
 6. Body weight increases.
 7. Water retention is increased, which can contribute to weight gain.

F. Reproductive system
 1. Uterus
     a. Uterus enlarges from 60 to 1000 g secondary to hyperplasia and hypertrophy.
     b. Size and number of blood vessels and lymphatics increase.
     c. Irregular contractions occur.
 2. Cervix
     a. Cervix becomes shorter, more elastic, and larger in diameter.
     b. Endocervical glands secrete a thick mucus plug, which is expelled from the canal when dilation begins.
     c. Increased vascularization and an increase in estrogen causes a softening and a violet discoloration (**Chadwick's sign**), which occurs at about week 4.
 3. Ovaries
     a. Secrete progesterone for first 6 to 7 weeks of pregnancy
     b. Block maturation of new follicles
     c. Cease ovum production
 4. Vagina
     a. Hypertrophy and thickening of the muscle occurs

▲ **FIGURE 22-1** Changes in position of the heart, lungs, and thoracic cage in pregnancy. *Broken line*, nonpregnant state; *solid line*, change that occurs during pregnancy. (From Perry, S., Hockenberry, M., Lowdermilk, D., & Wilson, D. [2010]. *Maternal child nursing care* [4th ed.]. St. Louis: Mosby).

▲ **FIGURE 22-2** Striae gravidarum and linea nigra in a dark-skinned person. (From Perry, S., Hockenberry, M., Lowdermilk, D., & Wilson, D. [2010]. *Maternal-child nursing care* [4th ed.]. St. Louis: Mosby. Courtesy Shannon Perry, Phoenix, AZ).

H. Musculoskeletal system: Changes in center of gravity begin in the second trimester and are caused by the hormones relaxin and progesterone.

⚠ During pregnancy, postural changes occur as the increased weight of uterus causes a forward pull of the bony pelvis. It is important for the nurse to encourage the client to implement measures that maintain correct posture to prevent a backache.

II. PSYCHOLOGICAL MATERNAL CHANGES

A. Ambivalence
1. May occur even when the pregnancy is planned
2. Mother may experience a dependence–independence conflict and ambivalence related to role changes, changes in body image, and fear of the unknown
3. Partner may experience ambivalence related to assuming a new role, increased financial responsibilities, and having to share attention with the child

B. Acceptance: Factors that may be related to the acceptance of the pregnancy are the woman's readiness for the experience and her identification with the motherhood role.

C. Emotional lability
1. Manifested by frequency in the change of emotional states or extremes in emotional states caused by hormone changes
2. These emotional changes are common, but the mother may believe that these changes are abnormal.

D. Body image changes
1. Perception of her image during pregnancy occurs gradually and may be either positive or negative.
2. Physical changes and symptoms that the woman experiences during pregnancy contribute to her body image.

b. Increase in vaginal secretions occurs; secretions are usually thick, white, and acidic
5. Breasts
  a. Breast size increases
  b. Increase in blood flow to the breasts; swelling, tingling, and tenderness are common
  c. Nipples become more pronounced and the areolae become darker, with an increase in ductal growth
  d. Superficial veins become prominent
  e. Montgomery's follicles become hypertrophied
  f. Colostrum may leak from the breasts.

G. Skin
1. Changes in skin occur secondary to increased levels of melanocyte-stimulating hormone, which increase secondary to increases in estrogen and progesterone.
  a. A dark streak down the midline of the abdomen may appear (linea nigra; Figure 22-2).
  b. Chloasma (mask of pregnancy), which is a blotchy, brownish hyperpigmentation, may occur over the forehead, cheeks, and nose.
  c. Reddish-purple stretch marks (striae) may occur on the abdomen, breasts, thighs, and upper arms.
2. Vascular spider nevi may occur on neck, chest, face, arms, and legs.
3. The rate of hair growth may increase.

E. Relationship with the fetus
1. The woman may daydream to prepare for motherhood and think about the maternal qualities she would like to possess.
2. The woman first accepts the biological fact that she is pregnant.
3. The woman next accepts the growing fetus as distinct from herself and a person to nurture.
4. Finally, the woman prepares realistically for the birth and parenting of the child.

III. DISCOMFORTS OF PREGNANCY

A. Nausea and vomiting
1. Occurs during the first trimester
2. Caused by elevated hCG levels and changes in carbohydrate metabolism
3. Interventions
   a. Eat dry crackers before rising.
   b. Avoid brushing the teeth immediately after rising.
   c. Eat small, frequent, low-fat meals during the day.
   d. Drink liquids between meals rather than at meals.
   e. Avoid fried and spicy foods.
   f. Undergo acupressure if approved by the health care provider (HCP). (Some types may require a prescription.)
   g. Take herbal remedies, only if approved by a HCP.

B. Syncope
1. Usually occurs during the first trimester; supine hypotension occurs, particularly during the second and third trimesters
2. May be hormonally triggered or caused by increased blood volume, anemia, fatigue, sudden position changes, or lying supine
3. Interventions
   a. Sit with the feet elevated.
   b. Change positions slowly.

⚠ The nurse needs to instruct the pregnant client to avoid lying in the supine position, particularly in the second and third trimesters. The supine position places the woman at risk for supine hypotension, which occurs as a result of pressure of the uterus on the inferior vena cava.

C. Urinary urgency and frequency
1. Usually occurs during the first and third trimesters
2. Caused by the pressure of the uterus on the bladder
3. Interventions
   a. Drink 2 quarts of fluid during the day.
   b. Limit fluid intake during the evening.
   c. Void at regular intervals.
   d. Sleep on the side at night.
   e. Wear perineal pads, if necessary.
   f. Perform Kegel exercises.

D. Breast tenderness
1. Can occur from the first through the third trimesters
2. Caused by increased levels of estrogen and progesterone
3. Interventions
   a. Encourage the use of a supportive bra with nonelastic straps.
   b. Avoid the use of soap on the nipples and areolae to prevent drying.

E. Increased vaginal discharge
1. Can occur from the first through the third trimesters
2. Caused by hypertrophy and thickening of the vaginal mucosa and increased mucus production
3. Interventions
   a. Wear cotton underwear.
   b. Avoid douching.
   c. Use proper cleansing and hygiene techniques.
   d. Advise the client to consult the HCP if an infection is suspected.

F. Nasal stuffiness or nosebleeds
1. Occurs during the first through the third trimesters
2. Occurs as a result of increased estrogen that causes swelling of the nasal tissues and dryness
3. Interventions
   a. Encourage the use of a humidifier.
   b. Avoid the use of nasal sprays or antihistamines (the HCP should always be consulted regarding their use).

G. Fatigue
1. Occurs usually during the first and third trimesters
2. Is usually the result of hormonal changes
3. Interventions
   a. Arrange frequent rest periods throughout the day.
   b. Use correct body mechanics.
   c. Engage in regular exercise with HCP approval.
   d. Perform muscle relaxation and strengthening exercises for the legs and hip joints.
   e. Avoid eating and drinking foods that contain stimulants throughout the pregnancy.

H. Heartburn
1. Occurs during the second and third trimesters
2. Results from increased progesterone levels, decreased GI motility, esophageal reflux, and the displacement of the stomach by the enlarging uterus
3. Interventions
   a. Eat small, frequent meals and avoid fatty and spicy food.
   b. Sit upright for 30 minutes after a meal.

c. Drink milk between meals.

d. Perform tailor-sitting exercises.

e. Take antacids, only if recommended by the HCP.

I. Ankle edema

1. Usually occurs during the second and third trimesters

2. Occurs as a result of vasodilation, venous stasis, and increased venous pressure below the uterus

3. Interventions

a. Elevate the legs during the day.

b. Sleep on the left side.

c. Wear supportive stockings.

d. Avoid sitting or standing in one position for long periods.

J. Varicose veins

1. Usually occur during the second and third trimesters

2. Occur because of weakening walls of the veins or valves and venous congestion

3. Interventions

a. Wear support hose.

b. Elevate the feet when sitting.

c. Lie with the feet and hips elevated.

d. Avoid long periods of standing or sitting.

e. Move about while standing to improve circulation.

f. Avoid leg crossing.

g. Avoid constricting articles of clothing such as knee-high stockings.

K. Headaches

1. Usually occur during the second and third trimesters

2. Occur as a result of changes in blood volume and vascular tone

3. Interventions

a. Change position slowly.

b. Apply a cool cloth to the forehead.

c. Eat a small snack.

d. Use acetaminophen (Tylenol) only if prescribed by the HCP.

L. Hemorrhoids

1. Usually occur during the second and third trimesters

2. Occur as a result of increased venous pressure and/or constipation

3. Interventions

a. Soak in a warm sitz bath.

b. Sit on a soft pillow.

c. Eat high-fiber foods and avoid constipation.

d. Drink sufficient fluids.

e. Increase exercise, such as walking, with HCP approval.

f. Apply ointments, suppositories, or compresses as prescribed by the HCP.

M. Constipation

1. Usually occurs during the second and third trimesters

2. Occurs as a result of decreased intestinal motility, the displacement of the intestines, and the ingestion of iron supplements

3. Interventions

a. Eat high-fiber foods.

b. Drink sufficient fluids.

c. Exercise regularly with HCP approval.

d. Avoid laxatives and enemas unless their use is approved by the HCP.

N. Backache

1. Usually occurs during the second and third trimesters

2. Occurs as a result of the exaggerated lumbosacral curve, which is caused by the enlarged uterus

3. Interventions

a. Encourage rest.

b. Use correct body mechanics and improve posture.

c. Wear low-heeled shoes.

d. Perform pelvic rocking and abdominal breathing exercises.

e. Sleep on a firm mattress.

O. Leg cramps

1. Usually occur during the second and third trimesters

2. Occur as a result of an altered calcium–phosphorus balance, the pressure of the uterus on nerves, or fatigue

3. Interventions

a. Get regular exercise, especially walking, with HCP approval.

b. Dorsiflex the foot while extending the knee of the affected leg.

c. Increase calcium intake.

P. Shortness of breath

1. Can occur during the second and third trimesters

2. Occurs as a result of pressure on the diaphragm

3. Interventions

a. Allow frequent rest periods and avoid overexertion.

b. Sleep with the head elevated or on the side.

IV. ANTEPARTUM DIAGNOSTIC TESTING

⚠ The usual schedule for antepartum health care visits is every 4 weeks for the first 28 to 32 weeks, every 2 weeks from 32 to 36 weeks, and every week from 36 to 40 weeks.

A. Blood type and Rh factor

1. ABO typing is performed to determine the woman's blood type in the ABO antigen system.

2. Rh typing is done to determine the woman's blood type in the rhesus antigen system (Rh positive indicates the presence of the antigen; Rh negative indicates the absence of the antigen).

3. If the client is Rh negative and has a negative antibody screen, the client will need repeat antibody screens and should receive Rh$_0$ (D) immune globulin (RhoGAM) at 28 weeks' gestation.

B. Rubella titer

1. If the client has a negative titer (less than 1:8), this indicates susceptibility to the rubella virus. The client should receive the appropriate immunization postpartum.
2. The client must be using effective birth control at the time of the immunization. She must be counseled not to become pregnant for 1 to 3 months after immunization (as specified by the HCP) and to avoid contact with anyone who is immunocompromised.
3. If the rubella vaccine is administered at the same time as the Rh immunoglobulin, it may not be effective.

⚠ Rubella vaccine is not given during pregnancy because the live attenuated virus may cross the placenta and present a risk to the developing fetus.

C. Hemoglobin and hematocrit levels

1. Hemoglobin and hematocrit levels will drop during gestation as a result of increased plasma volume.
2. A decrease in the hemoglobin level below 10 g/dL or a decrease in the hematocrit level below 30% indicates anemia.

D. Papanicolaou (Pap) smear: Done during the initial prenatal examination to screen for cervical neoplasia

E. Sexually transmitted infections (Table 22-1)

TABLE 22-1 Monitoring for Sexually Transmitted Infections

Disease	Laboratory Test
Gonorrhea	A vaginal culture is performed during the initial prenatal examination to screen for gonorrhea; it may be repeated during the third trimester for high-risk clients.
Syphilis	A culture of lesions (if present) is performed during the initial prenatal examination to screen for syphilis. Diagnosis is dependent on the microscopic examination of primary and secondary lesion tissue and serology (Venereal Disease Research Laboratory or rapid plasma reagin test). The culture may be repeated during the third trimester for high-risk clients.
Herpes virus	A culture is indicated for clients with an infection and/or positive history and for those with active lesions. Testing is performed to determine the route of delivery; weekly cultures may be performed from 35 or 36 weeks' gestation until delivery.
Chlamydia	A vaginal culture is indicated if the client is in a high-risk group or if infants from previous pregnancies have developed neonatal conjunctivitis or pneumonia.

F. Sickle cell screening

1. Indicated for clients who are at risk for sickle cell disease
2. A positive test result may indicate a need for further screening.

G. Tuberculin skin test

1. The HCP may prefer to perform this skin test after **delivery**.
2. A positive skin test indicates the need for a chest radiograph (using an abdominal lead shield) to rule out active disease. In a pregnant client, a chest radiograph will not be performed until after 20 weeks' gestation (i.e., after the fetal organs are formed).
3. Those who convert to positive may be referred for treatment with medication after **delivery**.

H. Hepatitis B surface antigen

1. Recommended for all women because of the prevalence of the disease in the general population
2. Vaccination for hepatitis B antigen may be specifically indicated for the following:
   a. Health care workers
   b. Clients born in Asia, Africa, Haiti, or the Pacific islands
   c. Clients with previously undiagnosed jaundice or chronic liver disease
   d. Intravenous (IV) drug abusers
   e. Clients with tattoos
   f. Clients with histories of blood transfusions
   g. Clients with histories of multiple episodes of sexually transmitted infections
   h. Clients who have been previously rejected as blood donors
   i. Clients with histories of dialysis or renal transplantation
   j. Clients from households having hepatitis B–infected members or hemodialysis clients
3. Hepatitis B vaccine is not contraindicated during pregnancy and may be recommended by the HCP.
4. See Unit 15 for additional information about hepatitis.

I. Urinalysis and urine culture

1. A urine specimen for glucose and protein determinations should be obtained at every prenatal visit.
2. Glycosuria is a common result of decreased renal threshold that occurs during pregnancy.
3. If glycosuria persists, this may indicate diabetes mellitus.
4. White blood cells in the urine may indicate infection.
5. Ketonuria may result from insufficient food intake or vomiting.
6. Protein levels of 2+ to 4+ in the urine may indicate infection or gestational hypertension.

J. Ultrasonography
1. Outlines and identifies fetal and maternal structures
2. Helps confirm gestational age and estimated date of **delivery**
3. May be done abdominally or transvaginally during pregnancy
4. Interventions
   a. If an abdominal ultrasound is being performed, the woman may need to drink water to fill the bladder before the procedure to obtain a better image of the fetus.
   b. If a transvaginal ultrasound is being performed, a lubricated probe is inserted into the vagina.
   c. Inform the client that the test presents no known risks to the client or the fetus.

K. Biophysical profile
1. Noninvasive assessment of the fetus that includes fetal breathing movements, fetal movements, fetal tone, **amniotic fluid** index, and fetal heart rate patterns via a nonstress test
2. Normal fetal biophysical activities indicate that the central nervous system is functional and the fetus is not hypoxemic.

L. Doppler blood flow analysis; noninvasive (ultrasonography) method of studying blood flow in the fetus and **placenta**

M. Percutaneous umbilical blood sampling
1. Performed if fetal blood sampling is necessary
2. Involves insertion of needle directly into fetal umbilical vessel under ultrasound guidance
3. Fetal heart rate monitoring is necessary for 1 hour after procedure and a follow-up ultrasound to check for bleeding or hematoma formation is done 1 hour after the procedure

N. Alpha-fetoprotein (AFP) screening
1. Assesses the quantity of fetal serum proteins. If the AFP level is elevated, it is associated with open neural tube and abdominal wall defects.
2. Can detect spina bifida and Down syndrome
3. Interventions
   a. Explain that the AFP level is determined by a maternal blood sample that is drawn at 15 to 18 weeks' gestation.
   b. If the level is elevated and the gestation is less than 18 weeks, a second sample is drawn and screened.
   c. Ultrasonography is performed if the AFP level is elevated to rule out fetal abnormalities and multiple gestations.

O. Chorionic villus sampling (CVS)
1. The HCP aspirates a small sample of chorionic villus tissue at 10 to 13 weeks' gestation.
2. CVS is performed to detect genetic abnormalities.
3. Interventions

   a. The client may need to drink water to fill the bladder before the procedure to aid in visualizing the uterus for catheter insertion.
   b. Obtain baseline vital signs and fetal heart rate; monitor frequently after the procedure.
   c. Rh-negative women may be given Rh_0 (D) immune globulin (RhoGAM), because CVS increases the risk of Rh sensitization.

P. Amniocentesis
1. Aspiration of **amniotic fluid**; best performed between 15 and 20 weeks of pregnancy because **amniotic fluid** volume is adequate and many viable fetal cells are present in the fluid by this time.
2. Performed to determine genetic disorders, metabolic defects, and fetal lung maturity
3. Risks
   a. Maternal hemorrhage
   b. Infection
   c. Rh isoimmunization
   d. Abruptio placentae
   e. **Amniotic fluid** emboli
   f. Premature rupture of the membranes
4. Interventions
   a. If less than 20 weeks' gestation, the woman should have a full bladder to support the uterus. If more than 20 weeks' gestation, the woman should have an empty bladder to minimize the chance of puncture.
   b. Prepare the client for ultrasonography, which is performed to locate the **placenta** and avoid puncture.
   c. Obtain baseline vital signs and fetal heart rate. Monitor every 15 minutes.
   d. Position the client supine during the exam and on the left side after the exam.

⚠ After chorionic villus sampling and amniocentesis, instruct the client that if chills, fever, bleeding, leakage of fluid at the needle insertion site, decreased fetal movement, uterine contractions, or cramping occurs, she must notify the HCP.

Q. Kick counts (fetal movement counting)
1. The mother sits quietly or lies down on her left side and counts fetal kicks for a period of time, as instructed.
2. By gestational week 28, if fewer than 10 kicks in a 2-hour period are felt, the mother needs to contact the HCP.

R. Fern test
1. A microscopic slide test to determine the presence of **amniotic fluid** leakage
2. Using sterile technique, a specimen is obtained from the external os of the cervix and vaginal pool and examined on a slide under a microscope

3. A fernlike pattern that results from the salts of **amniotic fluid** indicates the presence of **amniotic fluid**.
4. Interventions
   a. Place the client in the dorsal lithotomy position.
   b. Instruct the client to cough. This causes the fluid to leak from the uterus if the membranes are ruptured.

S. Nitrazine test
1. A Nitrazine test strip is used to detect the presence of **amniotic fluid** in vaginal secretions.
2. Vaginal secretions have a pH of 4.5 to 5.5. They do not affect the yellow color of the Nitrazine strip or swab.
3. **Amniotic fluid** has a pH of 7.0 to 7.5 and turns the yellow Nitrazine strip or swab blue in color.
4. Interventions
   a. Place the client in the dorsal lithotomy position.
   b. Touch the test tape to the fluid.
   c. Assess the test tape for a blue-green, blue-gray, or deep blue color, which indicates that the membranes are probably ruptured.

T. Nonstress test (Box 22-1)
U. Contraction stress test (Box 22-2)

V. NUTRITION

A. General guidelines
1. The MyPlate Web site (www.choosemyplate.gov) provides unique, individualized nutrition guidance to meet the needs of the pregnant woman and breast-feeding mothers. The woman should be assisted to prepare a nutritional plan.
2. The average expected weight gain during pregnancy is 25 to 35 pounds for women with a normal pre-pregnancy weight, depending on HCP preference.
3. An increase of about 300 calories per day is needed during pregnancy.
4. Calorie needs are greater during the last two trimesters than in the first.
5. An increase of about 500 calories per day is needed during lactation.
6. Encourage a diet high in folic acid and nutrient-dense foods, with prenatal supplements, as prescribed.
7. A diet high in folic acid is necessary for all women of childbearing age to prevent neural tube defects and orofacial clefts in the fetus during the first trimester of pregnancy.
8. Encourage the consumption of at least 8 to 10 (8-oz) glasses of fluid each day, of which 4 to 6 glasses should be water.
9. Sodium is not restricted unless specifically prescribed by the HCP.
10. Alcohol-containing beverages should not be consumed.

B. Vegetarianism (Box 22-3)
1. Ensure that the client eats a sufficient amount of varied foods to meet normal nutrient and energy needs.
2. Protein consumption can be increased by consuming a variety of vegetable protein sources that are based on whole grains, legumes, seeds, nuts, and vegetables combined to provide all essential amino acids.

Box 22-1 Nonstress Test

Description
- Performed to assess placental function and oxygenation
- Determines fetal well-being
- Evaluates fetal heart rate (FHR) in response to fetal movement

Interventions
An external ultrasound transducer and tocodynamometer are applied to the mother, and a tracing of at least 20 minutes' duration is obtained so that the FHR and the uterine activity can be observed.
Obtain a baseline blood pressure reading, and monitor the blood pressure frequently.
Position the mother in the left lateral position to avoid vena cava compression.
The mother may be asked to press a button every time she feels fetal movement. The monitor records a mark at each point of fetal movement, and this is used as a reference point to assess FHR response.

Results

Reactive Nonstress Test (Normal, Negative)
"Reactive" indicates a healthy fetus.
The result requires two or more FHR accelerations of at least 15 beats per minute and lasting at least 15 seconds from the beginning of the acceleration to the end, in association with fetal movement, during a 20-minute period.

Nonreactive Nonstress Test (Abnormal)
No accelerations or accelerations of less than 15 beats per minute or lasting less than 15 seconds in duration during a 40-minute observation

Unsatisfactory
Cannot be interpreted because of the poor quality of the FHR tracing

3. Potential deficiencies in vegetarian diets include energy, protein, vitamin B_{12}, zinc, iron, calcium, omega-3 fatty acids, and vitamin D (if limited exposure to sunlight).
4. Protein intake can be increased by consumption of a variety of vegetable protein sources based on whole grains, legumes, seeds, nuts, and vegetables combined to provide essential amino acids.
5. To enhance absorption of iron, vegetarians should include a good source of iron and vitamin C with each meal.
6. Foods commonly eaten include tofu, tempeh, soy milk and soy products, meat analogues, legumes, nuts, seeds, sprouts, and a variety of fruits and vegetables.

C. Lactose intolerance
1. Lactose consumed by an individual with lactose intolerance can cause abdominal distention, discomfort, nausea, vomiting, cramps, and loose stools.
2. Clients who experience lactose intolerance need to regularly incorporate sources of calcium (other than dairy products) into their dietary patterns.
3. Milk may be tolerated in cooked form (e.g., custards, fermented dairy products).
4. Cheese and yogurt are sometimes tolerated.
5. Lactase, which is an enzyme, may be prescribed and taken before ingesting milk or milk products.
6. Lactase-treated milk and lactose-free products are also available commercially.

Box 22-2 Contraction Stress Test

Description
- Assesses placental oxygenation and function
- Determines fetal ability to tolerate labor
- Determines fetal well-being
- Fetus is exposed to the stressor of contractions to assess the adequacy of placental perfusion under simulated labor conditions
- Performed if the nonstress test is abnormal

Interventions
The external fetal monitor is applied to the mother, and a 20- to 30-minute baseline strip is recorded.

The uterus is stimulated to contract, either by the administration of a dilute dose of oxytocin (Pitocin) or by having the mother use nipple stimulation, until three palpable contractions with a duration of 40 seconds or more during a 10-minute period have been achieved.

Frequent maternal blood pressure readings are obtained, and the mother is monitored closely while increasing doses of oxytocin are given.

Results

Negative Contraction Stress Test (Normal)
Represented by no late decelerations of the fetal heart rate (FHR)

Positive Contraction Stress Test (Abnormal)
Represented by late decelerations of the FHR with 50% or more of the contractions in the absence of hyperstimulation of the uterus

Equivocal
Contains decelerations but with less than 50% of the contractions, or uterine activity shows a hyperstimulated uterus

Unsatisfactory
Adequate uterine contractions cannot be achieved or the FHR tracing is not of sufficient quality for adequate interpretation

Box 22-3 Types of Semi-Vegetarian and Vegetarian Diets

Pescatarian
Abstains from eating all meat and animal flesh with the exception of fish.

Flexitarian/Semi-Vegetarian
Consumes mostly a vegetarian diet, but occasionally eats meat.

Vegetarian (Lacto-Ovo-Vegetarian)
Does not consume beef, pork, poultry, fish, shellfish, or animal flesh of any kind, but does eat eggs and dairy products.
- A lacto-vegetarian does not eat eggs, but does eat dairy products.
- An ovo-vegetarian does not eat meat or dairy products, but does eat eggs.

Vegan
Does not consume meat of any kind and also does not eat eggs, dairy products, or processed foods containing these or other animal-derived ingredients such as gelatin.

Raw Vegan/Raw Food Diet
Consumes unprocessed vegan foods that have not been heated above 115° F (46° C).

Macrobiotic
Consumes unprocessed vegan foods, such as whole grains and fruits and vegetables, and occasionally consumes fish; also consumes Asian vegetables, such as daikon, and sea vegetables, such as seaweed.

Box 22-4 Types of Abortions

Spontaneous	Pregnancy ends because of natural causes
Induced	Therapeutic or elective reasons exist for terminating pregnancy
Threatened	Spotting and cramping without cervical change occur
Inevitable	Spotting and cramping occur and cervix begins to dilate and efface
Incomplete	Loss of some of the products of conception occurs, with part of the products retained (most often placenta is retained)
Complete	Loss of all products of conception occurs
Missed	Products of conception are retained in utero after fetal death
Habitual	Spontaneous abortions occur in three or more successive pregnancies

D. Pica
   1. Definition: Eating nonfood substances such as dirt, clay, starch, and freezer frost
   2. The cause is unknown. Cultural values, such as beliefs regarding a material's effect on the mother or fetus, may make pica a common practice.
   3. Iron-deficiency anemia may occur as a result of pica.
E. Cultural considerations: See Chapter 6 for information about cultural considerations and nutrition.

VI. ABORTION

A. Description: A pregnancy that ends before 20 weeks' gestation, either spontaneously or electively
B. Types (Box 22-4)
C. Data collection
   1. Spontaneous vaginal bleeding with the passage of clots and tissue through the vagina
   2. Low uterine cramping and contractions
   3. Hemorrhage and shock can occur.
D. Interventions
   1. Maintain bedrest.
   2. Monitor the vital signs.
   3. Monitor for cramping and bleeding.
   4. Count perineal pads to evaluate blood loss. Save expelled tissues and clots.
   5. Maintain IV fluids as prescribed. Monitor for the signs of shock.
   6. Prepare the client for dilation and curettage, as prescribed, for incomplete abortion.
   7. Prepare to administer Rh_0 (D) immune globulin (RhoGAM) to appropriate Rh-negative women.

VII. ANEMIA

A. Description
   1. Develops as a result of iron deficiency
   2. Predisposes the client to postpartum infection and hemorrhage
B. Data collection
   1. Fatigue
   2. Headache
   3. Pallor
   4. Tachycardia
   5. Hemoglobin value usually less than 10 g/dL and hematocrit value usually less than 30%
C. Interventions
   1. Monitor hemoglobin and hematocrit levels every 2 weeks.
   2. Administer and instruct the client about iron and folic acid supplements.
   3. Teach the client to monitor for signs and symptoms of infection.
   4. Prepare to administer parenteral iron, which may be prescribed for severe anemia.
   5. Prepare to administer transfusions if prescribed for severe anemia.
   6. Prepare for the administration of oxytocic medications during the postpartum period if excessive bleeding is a concern.

VIII. CARDIAC DISEASE

A. Description: A pregnant client with cardiac disease may be unable physiologically to cope with the added plasma volume and increased cardiac output that occur during pregnancy; blood volume is at a maximum during the last weeks of the second trimester.
B. Data collection
   1. Signs and symptoms of cardiac decompensation
      a. Cough
      b. Dyspnea and fatigue
      c. Palpitations and tachycardia
      d. Peripheral edema
      e. Chest pain
   2. Signs of respiratory infection
   3. Signs of heart failure and pulmonary edema
C. Interventions
   1. Monitor the vital signs, fetal heart rate, and condition of fetus.
   2. Limit physical activities, and stress the need for sufficient rest.
   3. Monitor for signs of cardiac stress and decompensation
   4. Encourage adequate nutrition to prevent anemia and fluids and fiber to prevent constipation; additionally, a low sodium diet may be prescribed to prevent fluid retention and heart failure.
   5. Avoid excessive weight gain.

6. During **labor**, prepare to do the following:
   a. Monitor the vital signs frequently.
   b. Place the client on a cardiac monitor and an external fetal monitor.
   c. Maintain bedrest with the mother lying on her side and her head and shoulders elevated.
   d. Administer oxygen and pain medication, as prescribed.

⚠ Excessive weight gain places stress on the heart. Additionally, obesity places the client at increased risk for complications of pregnancy.

IX. CHORIOAMNIONITIS

A. Description
   1. A bacterial infection of the amniotic cavity that can result from the premature rupture of the membranes, vaginitis, amniocentesis, or intra-uterine procedures.
   2. It may result in the development of postpartum endometritis.
B. Data collection
   1. Uterine tenderness
   2. Elevated temperature
   3. Maternal or fetal tachycardia
   4. Foul odor to **amniotic fluid**
   5. Leukocytosis
C. Interventions
   1. Monitor maternal vital signs and fetal heart rate.
   2. Monitor for uterine tenderness, contractions, and fetal activity.
   3. Monitor the results of blood cultures. Prepare for amniocentesis to obtain **amniotic fluid** for analysis (Gram stain and leukocyte count).
   4. Administer antibiotics, as prescribed, after cultures are obtained.
   5. Oxytocic medications may be prescribed to increase uterine tone.
   6. Prepare to obtain neonatal cultures after **delivery**, as prescribed.

X. DIABETES MELLITUS

A. Description
   1. Pregnancy places demands on carbohydrate metabolism and causes insulin requirements to change.
   2. Maternal glucose crosses the **placenta**, but insulin does not.
   3. During the first trimester, maternal insulin needs decrease.
   4. During the second and third trimesters, increases in placental hormones cause an insulin-resistant state that requires an increase in the woman's insulin dose.

5. After placental **delivery**, placental hormone levels drop abruptly, and insulin requirements decrease.
6. The fetus produces its own insulin and pulls glucose from the mother, which predisposes the mother to hypoglycemic reactions.
7. The newborn **infant** of a diabetic mother may be large in size but will have functions related to gestational age rather than size.
8. The newborn **infant** of a diabetic mother is subject to hypoglycemia, hyperbilirubinemia, respiratory distress syndrome, hypocalcemia, and congenital anomalies.

B. Gestational diabetes mellitus
   1. Occurs during pregnancy (during the second or third trimester) among clients not previously diagnosed as diabetic. Occurs when the pancreas cannot respond to the demand for more insulin.
   2. Pregnant women should be screened for gestational diabetes between 24 and 28 weeks' gestation.
   3. An oral glucose tolerance test may be prescribed to confirm gestational diabetes mellitus.
   4. Gestational diabetes frequently can be treated by diet alone; however, some clients may need insulin.
   5. Most gestational diabetics convert to a euglycemic state after **delivery**; however, these individuals have an increased risk for developing diabetes mellitus during their lifetimes.

⚠ Many oral hypoglycemic agents are unsafe for use during pregnancy; usually insulin is prescribed.

C. Predisposing conditions for gestational diabetes
   1. Older than 35 years old
   2. Obese
   3. Multiple gestations
   4. Family history of diabetes mellitus
D. Data collection
   1. Excessive thirst
   2. Hunger
   3. Weight loss
   4. Blurred vision
   5. Frequent urination
   6. Recurrent urinary tract infections and vaginal yeast infections
   7. Glycosuria and ketonuria
   8. Signs of gestational hypertension
   9. Polyhydramnios
   10. Fetus may be large for gestational age
E. Interventions
   1. Include diet, insulin (if diet cannot control blood glucose levels), exercise, and blood glucose determinations to maintain blood glucose levels between 65 and 130 mg/dL.
   2. Observe for signs of hyperglycemia, glycosuria, ketonuria, and hypoglycemia.

3. Monitor weight.
4. Increase calorie intake, as prescribed, with adequate insulin therapy so that glucose will move into the cells.
5. Monitor for signs of maternal complications, such as preeclampsia (hypertension, proteinuria, and edema).
6. Monitor for signs of infection.
7. Instruct the client to report burning and pain on urination, vaginal discharge or itching, or any other signs of infection to the HCP.
8. Monitor the fetal status and for signs of fetal compromise.

 F. Interventions during **labor**
1. Monitor the fetal status continuously for signs of distress; if noted, prepare the client for immediate cesarean section.
2. Carefully regulate insulin and provide IV glucose, as prescribed, because **labor** depletes glycogen.

 G. Interventions during the postpartum period
1. Observe the client closely for a hypoglycemic reaction, because a precipitous drop in insulin requirements normally occurs. The client may not require insulin for the first 24 hours.
2. Reregulate insulin needs, as prescribed, after the first day, according to blood glucose testing and HCP's prescriptions.
3. Determine dietary needs on the basis of blood glucose and insulin requirements.
4. Monitor for signs of infection or postpartum hemorrhage.

XI. DISSEMINATED INTRAVASCULAR COAGULATION (DIC)

A. Description: A condition in the mother's body that results in an exaggerated clotting process, which increases the formation of clots in the microcirculation

⚠ The rapid and extensive formation of clots that occurs in DIC causes the platelets and clotting factors to be depleted. This results in bleeding and the potential vascular occlusion of organs from thromboembolus formation.

B. Predisposing conditions (Box 22-5)
C. Data collection
1. Uncontrolled bleeding
2. Bruising, purpura, petechiae, and ecchymosis
3. Hematuria, hematemesis, or vaginal bleeding
4. Presence of occult blood in excretions, such as stool (melena)
5. Signs of shock
6. Decreased fibrinogen level, platelet count, and hematocrit level

7. Increased prothrombin time, partial thromboplastin time, clotting time, and fibrin degradation products
D. Interventions
1. Remove the underlying cause.
2. Monitor the vital signs and for bleeding and signs of shock.
3. Assist in preparing to administer oxygen therapy, volume replacement, blood-component therapy, and possibly heparin therapy.
4. Monitor for complications associated with fluid and blood replacement and heparin therapy.
5. Monitor the urine output, and maintain it at 30 mL/hr. (Renal failure is a complication of this condition.)

XII. ECTOPIC PREGNANCY

A. Description: Pregnancy that occurs in a site other than a uterine site, with **implantation** usually occurring in the ampulla of the fallopian tube (Figure 22-3)
B. Data collection
1. Missed period
2. Abdominal pain
3. Vaginal spotting to bleeding that is dark red or brown
4. Rupture: Increased pain, referred shoulder pain, and signs of shock

---

Box 22-5 Predisposing Conditions for Disseminated Intravascular Coagulation

- Abruptio placentae
- Amniotic fluid embolism
- Gestational hypertension
- Intrauterine fetal death
- Liver disease
- Sepsis

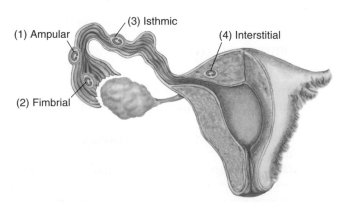

▲ **FIGURE 22-3** Sites of tubal ectopic pregnancy. The numbers indicate the order of prevalence. (From Murray, S., & McKinney, E. [2010], *Foundations of maternal newborn nursing* [5th ed.]. Philadelphia: Saunders).

C. Interventions
1. Obtain vital signs.
2. Monitor bleeding and initiate measures to prevent rupture and shock.
3. Methotrexate (a folic acid antagonist) may be prescribed to inhibit cell division in the developing embryo.
4. Prepare the client for laparotomy and the removal of the pregnancy and tube, if necessary, or repair of the tube.
5. Administer antibiotics. Rh_0 (D) immune globulin (RhoGAM) is given to appropriate Rh-negative women.

XIII. ENDOMETRITIS

A. Description
1. Infection of the lining of the uterus occurring in the postpartum period; caused by bacteria that invade the uterus at the placental site
2. The infection may spread, involve the entire endometrium, and cause peritonitis, pelvic thrombophlebitis, or cellulitis
B. Data collection
1. Chills and fever
2. Increased pulse
3. Decreased appetite
4. Headache
5. Backache
6. Prolonged, severe afterpains
7. Tender, large uterus
8. Foul odor to **lochia** or reddish-brown **lochia**
9. Ileus
10. Elevated white blood cell count
C. Interventions
1. Monitor the vital signs.
2. Place the mother in Fowler's position to facilitate the drainage of **lochia**.
3. Provide a private room for the mother.
4. Inform the mother that it is not necessary to isolate the newborn **infant** from the mother.
5. Instruct the mother in proper handwashing techniques.
6. Initiate contact precautions, as necessary.
7. Monitor intake and output (I&O), and encourage fluid intake.
8. IV antibiotics may be prescribed.
9. Administer comfort measures, such as back rubs, position changes, and pain medications, as prescribed.
10. Oxytocic medications may be prescribed to improve uterine tone.

XIV. FETAL DEATH IN UTERO

A. Description
1. Death of a fetus after 20 weeks' gestation and before birth

2. Disseminated intravascular coagulation can develop if the dead fetus is retained in the uterus for 3 to 4 weeks or longer.
B. Data collection
1. Absence of fetal movement
2. Absence of fetal heart tones
3. Maternal weight loss
4. Lack of fetal growth or decrease in fundal height
5. Lack of cardiac activity and other characteristics suggestive of fetal death noted on the ultrasound
C. Interventions
1. Prepare for the **delivery** of the fetus.
2. Support the client's decision about **labor**, birth, and the postpartum period.
3. Facilitate the grieving process as appropriate considering cultural practices and beliefs.
4. Accept behaviors such as anger and hostility from the parents.
5. Refer parents to an appropriate support group.

⚠ Cultural and religious practices and beliefs are important to consider when caring for the parents of a fetus who has died. Be aware of the cultural and religious practices and beliefs of the client.

XV. HEPATITIS B

A. Description
1. The risks of prematurity, low birth weight, and neonatal death increase if the mother has hepatitis B infection.
2. It is transmitted through blood, saliva, vaginal secretions, semen, breast milk, and across the placental barrier.
B. Interventions
1. Minimize the risk for intrapartum ascending infections by limiting the number of vaginal examinations.
2. Remove the maternal blood from the neonate immediately after birth.
3. Suction the neonate immediately after birth.
4. Bathe the neonate before any invasive procedures.
5. Clean and dry the face and eyes of the neonate before instilling eye prophylaxis.
6. Infection of the neonate can be prevented by the administration of hepatitis B immune globulin and hepatitis B vaccine soon after birth.
7. Discourage the mother from kissing the neonate until the neonate has received the vaccine.
8. Inform the mother that the hepatitis B vaccine will be administered to the neonate and that the second dose will be administered at 1 month. The third dose is administered at 6 months.

⚠ Support breast-feeding after neonatal treatment for hepatitis B; breast-feeding is not contraindicated if the neonate has been vaccinated.

XVI. HEMATOMA

A. Description
   1. Occurs after the escape of blood into the maternal tissue after the **delivery**
   2. Predisposing conditions include operative **delivery** with forceps or injury to a blood vessel
B. Data collection (Box 22-6)
C. Interventions
   1. Monitor the vital signs.
   2. Monitor the client for abnormal pain, especially when forceps **delivery** has occurred.
   3. Apply ice to the hematoma site.
   4. Administer analgesics, as prescribed.
   5. Monitor I&O.
   6. Encourage fluids and voiding. Prepare for urinary catheterization if the client is unable to void.
   7. Prepare to administer blood replacements, as prescribed.
   8. Monitor for signs of infection, such as increased temperature, pulse rate, and white blood cell count.
   9. Administer antibiotics, as prescribed, because infection is common after hematoma formation.
   10. Prepare for the incision and evacuation of the hematoma, if necessary.

XVII. HUMAN IMMUNODEFICIENCY VIRUS (HIV) AND ACQUIRED IMMUNODEFICIENCY SYNDROME (AIDS)

A. Description
   1. The human immunodeficiency virus (HIV) is the causative factor of the development of acquired immunodeficiency syndrome.
   2. Women infected with the HIV virus may first demonstrate symptoms at the time of pregnancy or possibly develop life-threatening infections, because normal pregnancy involves some suppression of the maternal immune system.
   3. Zidovudine (Retrovir) is recommended for the prevention of maternal–fetal HIV transmission. It is administered orally beginning after 14 weeks' gestation, intravenously during **labor**, and in the form of syrup to the neonate for 6 weeks after birth.

B. Transmission
   1. Sexual exposure to genital secretions of an infected person
   2. Parenteral exposure to infected blood and tissue
   3. Perinatal exposure of an **infant** to infected maternal secretions through the birth process or breast-feeding
C. Risks to the mother: The mother with HIV is managed as high risk because she is vulnerable to infections.
D. Diagnosis
   1. Tests used to determine the presence of antibodies to HIV include enzyme-linked immunosorbent assay (ELISA), Western blot (WB), and immunofluorescence assay (IFA)
   2. A single reactive ELISA test result by itself cannot be used to diagnose HIV and should be repeated in duplicate with the same blood sample. If the result is repeatedly reactive, follow-up tests using WB or IFA should be performed.
   3. A positive WB or IFA is considered confirmatory for HIV.
   4. A positive ELISA that fails to be confirmed by WB or IFA should not be considered negative for HIV. Repeat testing should take place in 3 to 6 months.
   5. See Chapter 11 for additional laboratory tests.
E. Data collection (Box 22-7)

Box 22-7 Stages of Acquired Immunodeficiency Syndrome

Stage 1
- Fever
- Myalgia
- Lymphadenopathy
- Headache

Stage 2
- Active infection but asymptomatic; may remain so for years
- May experience an outbreak of herpes zoster (shingles)
- May experience a transient thrombocytopenia

Stage 3
- Symptomatic
- Evidence of immune dysfunction
- All body systems can present with signs of immune dysfunction
- Integumentary and gynecological problems are common

Stage 4
- Advanced human immunodeficiency virus infection
- Vulnerable to common bacterial infections
- Development of opportunistic infections
- Serious immune compromise

Box 22-6 Hematoma: Data Collection Findings

Abnormal, severe pain
Pressure in perineal area (client states that she feels like she has to have a bowel movement)
Palpable, sensitive swelling in the perineal area, with discolored skin
Inability to void
Decreased hemoglobin and hematocrit levels
Signs of shock, such as pallor, tachycardia, and hypotension, if significant blood loss has occurred

F. Interventions
1. Prenatal period
   a. Prevent opportunistic infections.
   b. Avoid procedures that increase the risk of perinatal transmission, such as amniocentesis and fetal scalp sampling.
2. Intrapartum period
   a. If the fetus has not been exposed to HIV in utero, the highest risk exists during **delivery** through the birth canal.
   b. Avoid the use of scalp electrodes.
   c. Avoid episiotomy to decrease the amount of maternal blood in and around the birth canal.
   d. Avoid the administration of oxytocin (Pitocin), because oxytocin contractions can be strong, thus inducing vaginal tears or necessitating the need for an episiotomy.
   e. Place heavy absorbent pads under the mother's hips to absorb **amniotic fluid** and maternal blood.
   f. Minimize the neonate's exposure to maternal blood and body fluids. Promptly remove the neonate from the mother's blood after **delivery**.
   g. Suction the **infant** promptly.
   h. Prepare to administer zidovudine as prescribed to the mother during **labor** and **delivery**.
3. Postpartum period
   a. Monitor for signs of infection.
   b. Place the mother in protective isolation if she is immunosuppressed.
   c. Restrict breast-feeding.
   d. Instruct the mother to monitor for signs of infection and report any signs if they occur.
G. The neonate and HIV
1. Description
   a. Neonates born to HIV-positive clients may test positive, because the mother's positive antibodies may persist for as long as 18 months after birth. All neonates acquire maternal antibody to HIV infection, but not all acquire infection.
   b. The use of antiviral medication, the reduction of neonate exposure to maternal blood and body fluids, and the early identification of HIV during pregnancy reduce the risk of transmission to the neonate.
2. Interventions
   a. Bathe the neonate carefully before any invasive procedure, such as the administration of vitamin K, heel sticks, or venipunctures. The umbilical cord stump is cleaned meticulously every day until it is healed.
   b. The neonate can room with the mother.
   c. Prepare to administer zidovudine to the newborn **infant**, as prescribed, for the first 6 weeks of life.

   d. All HIV-exposed newborn **infants** should be treated with medication to prevent infection with *Pneumocystis jiroveci*.
   e. Note that an HIV culture is recommended at the age of 1 month and after 4 months of age. **Infants** at risk for HIV infection should be seen by the HCP at birth and at 1 week, 2 weeks, 1 month, 2 months, and 4 months of age.
   f. The neonate may be asymptomatic for the first several years of life. He or she needs to be monitored for early signs of immunodeficiency.

   ⚠ Infants at risk for HIV infection need to receive all recommended immunizations at the regular schedule; however, no live vaccines should be administered.

XVIII. HYDATIDIFORM MOLE

A. Description
1. A form of gestational trophoblastic disease that occurs when the trophoblasts, which are the peripheral cells that attach the fertilized ovum to the uterine wall, develop abnormally.
2. Presents as an edematous, grapelike cluster that may be nonmalignant or may develop into choriocarcinoma
B. Data collection
1. Fetal heart rate not detectable
2. Vaginal bleeding, which may occur as early as the fourth week or as late as the second trimester; it is usually bright red or dark brown in color, and it may be slight, profuse, or intermittent
3. Signs of gestational hypertension such as an elevated blood pressure, edema, and proteinuria, may be present before gestational week 20
4. Fundal height is greater than expected for date
5. Elevated hCG levels
6. Ultrasound shows a characteristic snowstorm pattern
C. Interventions
1. Prepare the mother for uterine evacuation (before evacuation, diagnostic tests are done to detect metastatic disease).
2. Evacuation of the mole is done by vacuum aspiration. Oxytocin (Pitocin) is administered after evacuation to contract the uterus.
3. Tissue is sent to the laboratory for evaluation. Follow-up is important to detect changes that are suggestive of malignancy.
4. Monitor for postprocedure hemorrhage and infection.
5. hCG levels are monitored every 1 to 2 weeks until normal prepregnancy levels are attained. The levels are then checked every 1 to 2 months for 1 year.

6. Instruct the parents regarding birth control measures so that pregnancy can be prevented during the 1-year follow-up.

XIX. HYPEREMESIS GRAVIDARUM

A. Description: Intractable nausea and vomiting that persists beyond the first trimester and causes disturbances in nutrition, electrolytes, and fluid balance
B. Data collection
   1. Nausea is most pronounced on arising; however, it can occur at other times during the day
   2. Persistent vomiting and weight loss
   3. Signs of dehydration and electrolyte imbalances
C. Interventions
   1. Measures to alleviate nausea, including medication therapy, are initiated. If this is unsuccessful and weight loss and electrolyte imbalances occur, the administration of IV fluid and electrolyte replacement or parenteral nutrition may be necessary.
   2. Monitor the vital signs, intake, output, weight, and calorie count.
   3. Monitor the laboratory data and for signs of dehydration and electrolyte imbalances.
   4. Monitor the urine for ketones.
   5. Monitor the fetal heart rate, fetal activity, and fetal growth.
   6. Encourage the intake of small portions of food (low-fat, easily digestible carbohydrates, such as cereals, rice, and pasta).
   7. Liquids should be taken between meals to avoid distending the stomach and triggering vomiting.
   8. Encourage the client to sit upright after meals.

XX. GESTATIONAL HYPERTENSION (GH)

A. Description and types (Table 22-2): Hypertension can be mild or severe, leading to preeclampsia and then eclampsia (seizures).

⚠ Signs of preeclampsia are hypertension, generalized edema, and proteinuria.

B. Data collection (Table 22-3)
C. Predisposing conditions
   1. Primigravida
   2. Age younger than 19 years or older than 40 years
   3. Chronic renal disease
   4. Chronic hypertension
   5. Diabetes mellitus
   6. Rh incompatibility
   7. History of or family history of gestational hypertension (GH)
D. Complications of GH
   1. Abruptio placentae
   2. Disseminated intravascular coagulation
   3. Thrombocytopenia
   4. Placental insufficiency

TABLE 22-2 Classification of Hypertensive States of Pregnancy

Type	Description
Gestational Hypertensive Disorders	
Gestational hypertension	Development of mild hypertension during pregnancy in previously normotensive woman without proteinuria or pathologic edema
Gestational proteinuria	Development of proteinuria after 20 weeks' gestation in a previously nonproteinuric woman without hypertension
Preeclampsia	Development of hypertension and proteinuria in a previously normotensive woman after 20 weeks' gestation or during the early postpartum period; in the presence of trophoblastic disease, it can develop before 20 weeks' gestation
Eclampsia	Development of seizures or coma in a preeclamptic woman
Chronic Hypertensive Disorders	
Chronic hypertension	Hypertension and/or proteinuria in pregnant woman with chronic hypertension before 20 weeks' gestation and persistent for 12 weeks after delivery
Superimposed preeclampsia or eclampsia	Development of preeclampsia or eclampsia in a woman with chronic hypertension before 20 weeks' gestation

Adapted from Lowdermilk, D., & Perry, S. (2009). *Maternity nursing* (8th ed.). St. Louis: Mosby.

5. Intrauterine growth restriction
6. Intrauterine fetal death
E. Interventions for mild hypertension
   1. Monitor blood pressure.
   2. Monitor fetal activity and fetal growth.
   3. Encourage frequent rest periods. Instruct the client to lie in the lateral position.
   4. Administer antihypertensive medications, as prescribed. Teach the client about the importance of the medications.
   5. Monitor I&O.
   6. Evaluate renal function through prescribed studies such as blood urea nitrogen, serum creatinine, and 24-hour urine levels for creatinine clearance and protein.
F. Interventions for mild preeclampsia
   1. Provide bedrest, and place the client in a lateral position.
   2. Monitor the blood pressure and weight.
   3. Monitor the neurological status, because changes can indicate cerebral hypoxia or impending seizure.
   4. Monitor the deep tendon reflexes and for the presence of clonus, because hyperreflexia indicates increased central nervous system irritability (Box 22-8)
   5. Provide adequate fluids.

TABLE 22-3 Mild versus Severe Preeclampsia

Parameter Evaluated	Mild	Severe
Systolic blood pressure	≥140 but <160 mm Hg	≥160 mm Hg (two readings, 6 hours apart, while on bedrest)
Diastolic blood pressure	≥90 but <110 mm Hg	≥110 mm Hg
Proteinuria (a 24-hour specimen is preferred to eliminate hour-to-hour variations)	≥0.3 g but <2 g in a 24-hour specimen (1+ on a random dipstick test)	≥5 g in a 24-hour specimen (≥3+ on a random dipstick test)
Creatinine, serum (renal function)	Normal	Elevated (>1.2 mg/dL)
Platelets	Normal	Decreased (<100,000 cells/mm³)
Liver enzymes (alanine aminotransferase or aspartate aminotransferase)	Normal or minimal increase in levels	Elevated levels
Urine output	Normal	Oliguria common, often <500 mL/day
Severe, unrelenting headache not attributable to other cause; mental confusion (cerebral edema)	Absent	Often present
Persistent right upper quadrant or epigastric pain or pain penetrating to the back (distention of the liver capsule); nausea and vomiting	Absent	May be present and often precedes seizure
Visual disturbances (spots or "sparkles," temporary blindness; photophobia)	Absent to minimal	Common
Pulmonary edema, heart failure, and cyanosis	Absent	May be present
Fetal growth restriction	Normal growth	Growth restriction and reduced amniotic fluid volume

Adapted from Murray, S., & McKinney, E. (2010). *Foundations of maternal-newborn nursing* (5th ed.). St. Louis: Saunders.

Box 22-8 Checking Reflexes

Biceps Reflex

The thumb is placed over the client's biceps tendon, and the client's elbow is supported with the palm of the hand.

The examiner strikes a downward blow over the thumb with the percussion hammer.

Normal Response: Flexion of the arm at the elbow

Patellar Reflex

The client is positioned with the legs dangling over the edge of the examining table, or lying on her back, with the legs slightly flexed.

The examiner strikes the patellar tendon just below the kneecap with the percussion hammer.

Normal Response: Extension or kicking out of the leg

Clonus Reflex

The client is positioned with the legs dangling over the edge of the examining table.

The leg is supported with one hand, and the client's foot is sharply dorsiflexed with the other hand.

The dorsiflexed position is maintained for a few seconds; then the foot is released.

Normal Response (Negative Clonus Response):

The foot will remain steady in the dorsiflexed position.

No rhythmic oscillations or jerking of the foot will be felt.

When released, the foot will drop to a plantarflexed position, with no oscillations.

Abnormal Response (Positive Clonus Response):

Rhythmic oscillations will occur when the foot is dorsiflexed.

Similar oscillations will be noted when the foot drops to the plantarflexed position.

Grading the Response

0 = Reflex absent
1+ = Reflex present but hypoactive
2+ = Normal reflex
3+ = Hyperactive reflex
4+ = Hyperactive reflex with clonus present

6. Monitor I&O. A urinary output of 30 mL/hour indicates adequate renal perfusion.
7. Increase dietary protein and carbohydrates with no added salt.
8. Administer medications, as prescribed, to lower the blood pressure. Blood pressure should not be lowered drastically, because placental perfusion can be compromised.
9. Monitor for HELLP syndrome: a laboratory diagnosis for severe preeclampsia characterized by *h*emolysis (H), *e*levated *l*iver enzymes (EL), and *l*ow *p*latelets (LP).

G. Interventions for severe preeclampsia
  1. Maintain bedrest.
  2. Magnesium sulfate (use a controlled infusion device) may be prescribed to prevent seizures. This may be continued for 24 to 48 hours postpartum.
  3. Monitor for signs of magnesium toxicity, including flushing, sweating, hypotension, depressed deep tendon reflexes, and central nervous system depression, including respiratory depression. Keep the antidote (calcium gluconate) at the client's bedside.
  4. Assist to administer antihypertensives, as prescribed.
  5. Prepare for the induction of **labor**.
H. Eclampsia
  1. Data collection: Characterized by generalized seizures (Box 22-9)
  2. Interventions (see Priority Nursing Actions)

XXI. INCOMPETENT CERVIX

> ### ▬▬▬ PRIORITY NURSING ACTIONS! ▬▬▬
>
> **Actions to Take in the Event of Eclampsia**
> 1. Remain with the client and call for help.
> 2. Ensure an open airway, turn the client on her side, and administer oxygen by face mask at 8 to 10 L/minute.
> 3. Monitor fetal heart rate patterns.
> 4. Assist in administering medications to control the seizures as prescribed.
> 5. After the seizure, insert an oral airway and suction the client's mouth as needed.
> 6. Prepare for the delivery of the fetus after stabilization of the client, if warranted.
> 7. Document the occurrence, the client's response, and outcome.
>
> Eclampsia refers to the occurrence of a seizure. It is a potentially preventable extension of severe preeclampsia; early identification of preeclampsia in a pregnant client allows intervention before the condition reaches the seizure state. If eclampsia occurs, the nurse remains with the client and calls for help. The nurse ensures an open airway. If the client is not on her side already, the nurse attempts to turn the client on her side. The side-lying position permits greater circulation through the placenta and may help prevent aspiration. The nurse administers oxygen by face mask at 8 to 10 L/minute to ensure adequate placental oxygenation. The nurse also notes the time the seizure began and the duration of the seizure and protects the client from injury during the event. The nurse monitors fetal heart rate patterns closely and assists to administer medications as prescribed (magnesium sulfate may be prescribed). After the seizure, the nurse inserts an oral airway to maintain airway patency and suctions the client's mouth as needed. If warranted, the nurse prepares for the delivery of the fetus after stabilization of the client. The nurse documents the occurrence, the client's response, and the outcome.
>
> *References:* McKinney, E., James, S., Murray, S., & Ashwill, J. (2009). *Maternal-child nursing* (3rd ed., p. 629). St. Louis: Saunders; and Perry, S., Hockenberry, M., Lowdermilk, D., & Wilson, D. (2010). *Maternal child nursing care* (4th ed., p. 347). St. Louis: Mosby.

> ### Box 22-9 Eclampsia
>
> An eclampsia seizure typically begins with twitching around the mouth. The body then becomes rigid in a state of tonic muscular contractions, which last 15 to 20 seconds. The facial muscles and then all of the body muscles alternatively contract and relax in rapid succession; this is the clonic phase, which may last about 1 minute. Respiration ceases during the seizure, because the diaphragm tends to remain fixed. Breathing resumes shortly after the seizure, and postictal sleep occurs.

A. Description
  1. Premature dilation of the cervix, which occurs most often during the fourth or fifth month of pregnancy and is associated with structural or functional defects of the cervix
  2. Treatment involves surgical placement of a cervical cerclage.
B. Data collection
  1. Vaginal bleeding
  2. Fetal membranes visible through the cervix
C. Interventions
  1. Provide bedrest, hydration, and tocolysis, as prescribed, to inhibit uterine contractions.
  2. Prepare for cervical cerclage (at 10 to 14 weeks' gestation), in which a band of fascia or nonabsorbable ribbon is placed around the cervix beneath the mucosa to constrict the internal os of the cervix.
  3. After cervical cerclage, the woman is told to refrain from intercourse and avoid prolonged standing and heavy lifting.
  4. The cervical cerclage is removed at 37 weeks' gestation or left in place and a cesarean **delivery** is performed. If removed, the cerclage must be repeated with each successive pregnancy.
  5. After the procedure, monitor for contractions, rupture of the membranes, and signs of infection.
  6. Instruct the woman to report any postprocedure vaginal bleeding or increased uterine contractions immediately to the HCP.

XXII. INFECTIONS

A. Toxoplasmosis
  1. Caused by infection with the protozoan intracellular parasite *Toxoplasma gondii*
  2. Produces a rash and symptoms of acute, flulike infection in the mother
  3. Transmitted to the mother through raw meat or the handling of the cat litter of infected cats
  4. Organism is transmitted to the fetus across the **placenta**
  5. Can cause spontaneous abortion in the first trimester

B. Rubella (German measles)
1. Extremely teratogenic during the first trimester
2. Transmitted to the fetus across the **placenta**
3. Causes congenital defects of the eyes, heart, ears, and brain
4. If not immune (titer of 1:8 or less), the mother should be vaccinated during the postpartum period. She must then wait 1 to 3 months (as specified by HCP) before becoming pregnant again.

C. Cytomegalovirus
1. The organism is transmitted through close personal contact or across the **placenta** to the fetus, or the fetus may be infected through the birth canal
2. The mother may be asymptomatic, and most **infants** are asymptomatic at birth.
3. Cytomegalovirus causes low birth weight, intrauterine growth retardation, enlarged liver and spleen, jaundice, mental retardation, blindness, hearing loss, and seizures.
4. Antiviral medications may be prescribed for severe infections in the mother, but these medications are toxic and may only temporarily suppress the shedding of the virus.

D. Herpes simplex virus
1. Affects the external genitalia, vagina, and cervix
2. Causes draining, painful vesicles
3. Virus is usually transmitted to the fetus during birth through the infected vagina or via an ascending infection after rupture of the membranes
4. No vaginal examinations are done in the presence of active vaginal herpetic lesions.
5. Can cause death or severe neurological impairment in the newborn
6. **Delivery** of the fetus is usually by cesarean section if active lesions are present in the vagina. **Delivery** may be performed vaginally if the lesions are in the anal, perineal, or inner thigh area. (Strict precautions are necessary to protect the fetus during **delivery**.)
7. Maintain contact precautions

E. Group B *Streptococcus* (GBS)
1. A leading cause of life-threatening perinatal infections
2. The gram-positive bacterium colonizes the rectum, vagina, cervix, and urethra of pregnant and nonpregnant women.
3. Meningitis, fasciitis, and intraabdominal abscess can occur in the pregnant client if she is infected at the time of birth.
4. Transmission occurs during vaginal **delivery**.
5. Early-onset newborn GBS occurs within the first week after birth, usually within 48 hours. It can include infections such as sepsis, pneumonia, or meningitis, and permanent neurological disability can result.

6. Diagnosis of the mother is done via vaginal and rectal cultures between 35 and 37 weeks' gestation.
7. Antibiotics such as penicillin may be prescribed for the mother during **labor** and birth. IV antibiotics may be prescribed for infected **infants.**

XXIII. MULTIPLE GESTATION

A. Description
1. Results from the **fertilization** of two ova (fraternal or dizygotic) or a splitting of one of the fertilized ovum (identical or monozygotic)
2. Complications include spontaneous abortion, anemia, congenital anomalies, hyperemesis gravidarum, intrauterine growth restriction, gestational hypertension, polyhydramnios, postpartum hemorrhage, premature rupture of membranes, and preterm **labor** and **delivery**

B. Data collection
1. Excessive fetal activity
2. Uterus large for gestational age
3. Palpation of three or four large fetal parts in the uterus
4. Auscultation of more than one fetal heart rate
5. Excessive weight gain

C. Interventions
1. Monitor the vital signs.
2. Monitor the fetal heart rates, fetal activity, and fetal growth.
3. Monitor for cervical changes.
4. Prepare the client for ultrasound, as prescribed.
5. Monitor for anemia. Administer supplemental vitamins, as prescribed.
6. Monitor for preterm **labor** and treat it promptly.
7. Prepare for cesarean section for abnormal presentations.
8. Prepare to administer oxytocic medications after **delivery** to prevent postpartum hemorrhage from uterine overdistention.

XXIV. SEXUALLY TRANSMITTED INFECTIONS

A. Chlamydia
1. Description
   a. Sexually transmitted pathogen associated with an increased risk of premature birth, stillbirth, neonatal conjunctivitis, and newborn chlamydial pneumonia
   b. Can cause salpingitis, pelvic abscesses, ectopic pregnancy, chronic pelvic pain, and infertility
   c. Diagnostic test is culture for *Chlamydia trachomatis*
2. Data collection
   a. Usually asymptomatic
   b. Bleeding between periods or after coitus
   c. Mucoid or purulent cervical discharge
   d. Dysuria and pelvic pain

3. Interventions
    a. Screen the client to determine whether the client is at high risk. A vaginal culture is indicated for all pregnant clients if the client is in a high-risk group or **infants** from previous pregnancies have developed neonatal conjunctivitis or pneumonia.
    b. Instruct the client about the importance of rescreening, because reinfection can occur as the client nears term.
    c. Ensure that the sexual partner is treated.

B. Syphilis
  1. Description
    a. Chronic infectious disease caused by the organism *Treponema pallidum*
    b. Transmission is by intimate physical contact with syphilitic lesions, which are usually found on the skin, mucous membranes of the mouth, and genitals
    c. Infection may cause abortion or premature **labor**. Passed to the fetus after the fourth month of pregnancy as congenital syphilis.
  2. Data collection (Box 22-10)
  3. Interventions
    a. Obtain a serum test (Venereal Disease Research Laboratory or rapid plasma reagin) for syphilis on the first prenatal visit. Prepare to repeat the test at 36 weeks' gestation, because the disease may be acquired after the initial visit.
    b. If the test result is positive, treatment with an antibiotic such as penicillin may be necessary.
    c. Instruct the client that the treatment of her partner is necessary if an infection is present.

Box 22-10 Stages of Syphilis

Primary Stage
- Most infectious stage
- Appearance of ulcerative, painless lesions produced by spirochetes at the point of entry into the body

Secondary Stage
- Highly infectious stage
- Lesions appear about 3 weeks after the primary stage and may occur anywhere on the skin and mucous membranes
- Generalized lymphadenopathy occurs

Tertiary Stage
- Spirochetes enter the internal organs and cause permanent damage; symptoms may occur 10 to 30 years after the occurrence of an untreated primary lesion
- Disease invades the central nervous system, causing meningitis, ataxia, general paresis, and progressive mental deterioration
- Affects the aortic valve and the aorta

C. Gonorrhea
  1. Description
    a. An infection caused by *Neisseria gonorrhoeae*, which causes inflammation of the mucous membranes of the genital and urinary tracts
    b. Transmission of the organism is by sexual intercourse.
    c. Infection may be transmitted to the newborn's eyes during **delivery**, causing blindness (ophthalmia neonatorum).
  2. Data collection: Usually asymptomatic. Vaginal discharge, urinary frequency, and lower abdominal pain are possible
  3. Interventions
    a. Obtain a vaginal culture for gonorrhea on the first prenatal visit. Prepare to repeat the culture during the third trimester in high-risk clients.
    b. Instruct the client that the treatment of her partner is necessary if infection is present.

D. Condylomata acuminata (human papillomavirus)
  1. Description
    a. Caused by human papilloma virus (HPV). Affects the cervix, urethra, anus, penis, and scrotum.
    b. A culture is indicated for clients with a positive history or with active lesions, and weekly cultures may be done at weeks 35 or 36 of pregnancy until **delivery**. The test is performed to determine the route of **delivery**.
  2. Data collection
    a. Small to large wartlike growths on the genitals
    b. Cervical cell changes may be noted, because HPV is associated with cervical malignancies
  3. Interventions
    a. Lesions are removed with the use of cytotoxic agents, cryotherapy, electrocautery, and laser.
    b. Encourage a yearly Papanicolaou (Pap) smear.
    c. Sexual contact is avoided until the lesions are healed. (Condoms reduce transmission.)

E. Trichomoniasis
  1. Description
    a. Caused by *Trichomonas vaginalis*.
    b. Normal saline wet smear of vaginal secretions indicates the presence of protozoa
    c. Infection is associated with premature rupture of membranes and postpartum endometritis.
  2. Data collection
    a. Yellowish to greenish, frothy, mucopurulent, copious, and malodorous vaginal discharge
    b. Inflammation of the vulva, vagina, or both may be present
  3. Interventions
    a. Metronidazole (Flagyl) may be prescribed.
    b. Sexual partner may need to be treated.

F. Bacterial vaginosis
  1. Description
    a. Caused by *Haemophilus vaginalis* (*Gardnerella vaginalis*)
    b. Associated with premature **labor** and birth

2. Data collection
   a. Client complains of "fishy odor" to vaginal secretions and increased odor after intercourse.
   b. Microscopic examination of vaginal secretions identifies the infection.
3. Interventions
   a. Treatment with oral metronidazole (Flagyl) may be prescribed.
   b. Sexual partner may need to be treated

G. Vaginal candidiasis
   1. Description
      a. *Candida albicans* is the most common causative organism
      b. Predisposing factors include the use of antibiotics, diabetes mellitus, and obesity
      c. Diagnosis is by identifying the spores of *Candida albicans*
   2. Data collection
      a. Vulvar and vaginal pruritus
      b. White, lumpy, and cottage-cheese–like discharge from the vagina
   3. Interventions
      a. An antifungal vaginal preparation such as miconazole (Monistat) may be prescribed.
      b. For extensive irritation and swelling, sitz baths may be prescribed.
      c. Sexual partner may need to be treated.

XXV. TUBERCULOSIS

A. Description
   1. A highly communicable disease caused by *Mycobacterium tuberculosis*
   2. Transmitted by the airborne route
   3. A multidrug-resistant strain can exist as a result of improper compliance, noncompliance with treatment programs, and the development of mutations in the tubercle bacilli
B. Transmission
   1. Transplacental transmission is rare.
   2. Can occur during birth through the aspiration of infected **amniotic fluid**
   3. Newborn can become infected from contact with infected individuals
C. Risk to mother: Active disease during pregnancy has been associated with an increase in hypertensive disorders of pregnancy.
D. Diagnosis: If a chest radiograph is required for the mother, it is obtained only after 20 weeks' gestation, and a lead shield for the abdomen is required.

⚠ Tuberculin skin testing is safe during pregnancy; however the HCP may want to delay testing until after delivery.

E. Data collection
   1. Mother
      a. May be asymptomatic
      b. Fever and chills
      c. Night sweats
      d. Weight loss
      e. Fatigue
      f. Cough, hemoptysis, or green or yellow sputum
      g. Dyspnea
      h. Pleural pain
   2. Neonate
      a. Fever
      b. Lethargy
      c. Poor feeding
      d. Failure to thrive
      e. Respiratory distress
      f. Hepatosplenomegaly
      g. Meningitis
      h. Disease may spread to all major organs
F. Interventions
   1. Pregnant client
      a. Administer isoniazid (INH), pyrazinamide, and rifampin (Rifadin) daily for 9 months, as prescribed. Ethambutol (Myambutol) is added if medication resistance is probable.
      b. Pyridoxine (vitamin B_6) should be administered along with INH to pregnant women to prevent fetal neurotoxicity caused by the INH.
      c. Promote breast-feeding only if the mother is noninfectious.
   2. Newborn **infant**
      a. Management focuses on preventing disease and treating early infection.
      b. The **infant** is skin tested at birth and may be placed on INH therapy. The skin test is repeated in 3 to 4 months, and the INH may be stopped if the skin test results remain negative.
      c. If the skin test result is positive, the **infant** should receive INH for at least 6 months.
      d. If the mother's sputum is free of organisms, the **infant** does not need to be isolated from the mother while in the hospital.

XXVI. UNINARY TRACT INFECTION AND PYELONEPHRITIS (refer to Chapter 53)

MORE QUESTIONS ON EVOLVE!

Practice Questions

186. The client is undergoing an amniocentesis at 16 weeks' gestation to detect the presence of biochemical or chromosomal abnormalities. The nurse instructs the client:
   1. That the bladder must be full during the exam
   2. That the bladder must be empty during the exam

3. She will be given RhoGAM because she is Rh positive

4. Not to eat or drink anything 4 to 6 hours before the exam

187. The client at 28 weeks' gestation is Rh negative and Coombs antibody negative. The nurse determines that the client understands what the nurse has taught her about Rh sensitization when the client states:
1. "I know I can never have another child."
2. "I am glad I won't have to have these shots if I have another child."
3. "I will have to have an injection once a month until the baby is born."
4. "I will tell the nurse at the hospital that I had RhoGAM during pregnancy."

188. While assisting with the measurement of fundal height, the client at 36 weeks' gestation states that she is feeling lightheaded. On the basis of the nurse's knowledge of pregnancy, the nurse determines that this is most likely a result of:
1. A full bladder
2. Emotional instability
3. Insufficient iron intake
4. Compression of the vena cava

189. A contraction stress test is scheduled for the client. The woman asks the nurse about the test. The most accurate description of the test includes which of the following?
1. "Uterine contractions are stimulated by Leopold's maneuvers."
2. "An internal fetal monitor is attached, and you will walk on a treadmill until contractions begin."
3. "The uterus is stimulated to contract by either small amounts of oxytocin (Pitocin) or by nipple stimulation."
4. "Small amounts of oxytocin (Pitocin) are administered during internal fetal monitoring to stimulate uterine contractions."

190. The client at 38 weeks' gestation is admitted to the birthing center in early labor. The client is carrying twins, and one of the fetuses is in a breech presentation. The nurse assists with planning care for the client and identifies which of the following as the lowest priority for the care of this client?
1. Measuring the fundal height
2. Attaching electronic fetal monitoring
3. Preparing the client for a possible cesarean section

4. Gathering equipment for starting an intravenous line

191. The perinatal client is admitted to the obstetric unit during an exacerbation of a heart condition. When planning for the nutritional requirements of the client, the nurse would consult with the dietitian to ensure which of the following?
1. A low-calorie diet to ensure the absence of weight gain
2. A diet that is high in fluids and fiber to decrease constipation
3. A diet that is low in fluids and fiber to decrease blood volume
4. Unlimited sodium intake to increase the circulating blood volume

192. The nurse caring for a client with abruptio placentae is monitoring the client for signs of disseminated intravascular coagulopathy (DIC). The nurse would suspect DIC if he or she observes:
1. Rapid clotting times
2. Pain and swelling of the calf of one leg
3. Laboratory values that indicate increased platelets
4. Petechiae, oozing from injection sites, and hematuria

193. The nurse has a teaching session with a malnourished client regarding iron supplementation to prevent anemia during pregnancy. Which of the following statements, if made by the client, would indicate successful learning?
1. "Iron supplements will give me diarrhea."
2. "The iron is needed for the red blood cells."
3. "Meat does not provide iron and should be avoided."
4. "My body has all the iron it needs, and I don't need to take supplements."

194. During a prenatal visit, the nurse is explaining dietary management to a client with diabetes mellitus. The nurse determines that the teaching has been effective when the client states:
1. "I can eat more sweets now, because I need more calories."
2. "I need more fat in my diet so that the baby can gain enough weight."
3. "I need to eat a high-protein, low-carbohydrate diet now to control my blood glucose."
4. "I need to increase the fiber in my diet to control my blood glucose and prevent constipation."

195. The nurse is assigned to assist with caring for a client who is at risk for eclampsia. If the client progresses from preeclampsia to eclampsia, the nurse's first action should be to:
1. Administer oxygen by face mask.
2. Clear and maintain an open airway.
3. Check the blood pressure and the fetal heart tones.
4. Prepare for the administration of intravenous magnesium sulfate.

196. The client is in her second trimester of pregnancy. She complains of frequent low back pain and ankle edema at the end of the day. The nurse recommends which measure to help relieve both discomforts?
1. Lie on the left side with the feet dorsiflexed.
2. Soak the feet in hot water after performing 10 pelvic tilt exercises.
3. Lie on the right side with the feet elevated on a pillow and a heating pad on the back.
4. Lie on the floor with the legs elevated onto a couch or padded chair, with the hips and knees at a right angle.

197. The pregnant woman complains of being awakened frequently by leg cramps. The nurse reinforces instructions to the client's partner and tells the partner to:
1. Dorsiflex the client's foot while flexing the knee.
2. Plantarflex the client's foot while flexing the knee.
3. Dorsiflex the client's foot while extending the knee.

4. Plantarflex the client's foot while extending the knee.

198. The nurse is providing instructions to a pregnant client with heartburn regarding measures that will alleviate the discomfort. The nurse instructs the client to:
1. Eliminate between-meal snacks.
2. Drink decaffeinated coffee and tea.
3. Lie down for 30 minutes after eating.
4. Substitute salt in cooking for other spices.

199. The nurse is doing a 48-hour postpartum check on a client with mild gestational hypertension (GH). Which of the following data indicate that the GH is not resolving?
1. Urinary output has increased.
2. There is no evidence of dependent edema.
3. The client complains of a headache and blurred vision.
4. The blood pressure reading has returned to the prenatal baseline.

200. The nurse is monitoring a pregnant client with gestational hypertension who is at risk for preeclampsia. The nurse checks the client for which classic signs of preeclampsia? **Select all that apply.**
☐ 1. Proteinuria
☐ 2. Hypertension
☐ 3. Low-grade fever
☐ 4. Generalized edema
☐ 5. Increased pulse rate
☐ 6. Increased respiratory rate

ANSWERS

186. 1
Rationale: Before 20 weeks' gestation, the bladder must be kept full during amniocentesis to support the weight of the uterus. After 20 weeks' gestation, the bladder should be emptied to minimize the chance of puncturing the placenta or fetus. Rh₀ (D) immune globulin (RhoGAM) is administered to Rh-negative woman because of the risk of contact with the fetal blood during the exam. There are no fluid or food restrictions. Monitoring the fetal heart tones and the vital signs throughout and after the exam is an important intervention.
Test-Taking Strategy: Focus on the strategic words "16 weeks' gestation." Remember that before 20 weeks' gestation, the bladder must be kept full to support the weight of the uterus. Review client instructions for amniocentesis if you had difficulty with this question.
Level of Cognitive Ability: Applying
Client Needs: Physiological Integrity
Integrated Process: Nursing Process/Implementation
Content Area: Maternity/Antepartum
References: Leifer, p. 81. 2011.

Pagana, Pagana, p. 51. 2009. *Mosby's diagnostic and laboratory test reference.*

187. 4
Rationale: As described in the question, it is accepted practice to administer Rh₀ (D) immune globulin (RhoGAM) to an Rh-negative woman at 28 weeks' gestation, with a second injection within 72 hours of delivery. This prevents sensitization, which could jeopardize a future pregnancy. For subsequent pregnancies or abortions, the injections must be repeated, because the immunity is passive. Options 1, 2, and 3 are inaccurate information.
Test-Taking Strategy: Note the strategic words "that the client understands." Recalling the guidelines regarding the administration of RhoGAM will direct you to the correct option. Review Rh sensitization if you had difficulty with this question.
Level of Cognitive Ability: Evaluating
Client Needs: Physiological Integrity
Integrated Process: Nursing Process/Evaluation
Content Area: Maternity/Antepartum

References: Christensen, Kockrow, pp. 855–856. 2011. *Foundations of nursing.*
Leifer, p. 81. 2011.

188. 4
Rationale: Compression of the inferior vena cava and aorta by the uterus may cause supine hypotension syndrome during pregnancy. Having the woman turn onto her left side or elevating the right buttock during fundal height measurement will prevent or correct the problem. Options 1, 2, and 3 are not the cause of the problem described in the question.
Test-Taking Strategy: Focus on the data in the question, and recall the complications associated with pregnancy. Use the ABCs—airway, breathing, and circulation—to direct you to the correct option. Review the interventions for supine hypotension syndrome if you had difficulty with this question.
Level of Cognitive Ability: Understanding
Client Needs: Physiological Integrity
Integrated Process: Nursing Process/Data Collection
Content Area: Maternity/Antepartum
Reference: Leifer, p. 53. 2011.

189. 3
Rationale: A contraction stress test assesses placental oxygenation and function and determines the fetus' ability to tolerate labor as well as its well-being. The test is performed if the nonstress test result is abnormal. During the stress test, the fetus is exposed to the stressor of contractions to assess the adequacy of placental perfusion under simulated labor conditions. An external fetal monitor is applied to the mother, and a 20- to 30-minute baseline strip is recorded. The uterus is stimulated to contract, either by the administration of a dilute dose of oxytocin (Pitocin) or by having the mother use nipple stimulation, until three palpable contractions with a duration of 40 seconds or more during a 10-minute period have occurred. Frequent maternal blood pressure readings are performed, and the client is monitored closely while increasing doses of oxytocin are given. Leopold's maneuvers are performed to locate the position of the fetus.
Test-Taking Strategy: Knowledge regarding the contraction stress test is required to answer the question. Remember that during both the nonstress test and the contraction stress test, external monitoring is performed. Review the contraction stress test if you had difficulty with this question.
Level of Cognitive Ability: Understanding
Client Needs: Physiological Integrity
Integrated Process: Nursing Process/Implementation
Content Area: Maternity/Antepartum
Reference: Leifer, p. 81. 2011.

190. 1
Rationale: Option 1 is a low priority, because fundal height should be measured at each antepartal clinic visit; it is not a priority of care during the intrapartum period. Options 2, 3, and 4 are all high priorities. The twins should be monitored by dual electronic fetal monitoring, and any signs of distress should be reported. Many health care providers choose to perform a cesarean birth if either of the twins is breech. The mother should have an intravenous line in place in case fluid or blood replacement is required.

Test-Taking Strategy: Note the strategic words "lowest priority." Use Maslow's Hierarchy of Needs theory and the ABCs—airway, breathing, and circulation—to prioritize and direct you to the correct option. Review the care of the pregnant client with a breech presentation if you had difficulty with this question.
Level of Cognitive Ability: Analyzing
Client Needs: Physiological Integrity
Integrated Process: Nursing Process/Planning
Content Area: Maternity/Intrapartum
References: Christensen, Kockrow, pp. 809–810. 2011. *Foundations of nursing.*
Leifer, pp. 189–190. 2011.

191. 2
Rationale: Constipation causes the client to use Valsalva's maneuver. This causes blood to rush to the heart and overload the cardiac system. The absence of weight gain is not recommended during pregnancy. Diets that are low in fluid and fiber cause a decrease in blood volume, which in turn deprives the fetus of nutrients. Too much sodium could cause an overload to the circulating blood volume and contribute to the cardiac condition.
Test-Taking Strategy: Use the process of elimination, and try to relate the situation to something with which you are familiar. Look for options that would apply to any heart condition, think about the needs of a pregnant client, and use the process of elimination. Review dietary measures for the client with cardiac disease if you had difficulty with this question.
Level of Cognitive Ability: Applying
Client Needs: Physiological Integrity
Integrated Process: Nursing Process/Planning
Content Area: Maternity/Antepartum
Reference: Leifer, pp. 65, 101–102. 2011.

192. 4
Rationale: DIC is a state of diffuse clotting in which clotting factors are consumed, which leads to widespread bleeding. Platelet counts are decreased, because they are consumed by the process. Coagulation studies show no clot formation (clotting times are thus prolonged), and fibrin plugs may clog the microvasculature diffusely rather than in an isolated area.
Test-Taking Strategy: Use the process of elimination. Eliminate option 2 on the basis of the knowledge that DIC is a widespread problem rather than a localized one. Eliminate options 1 and 3 next, because they are comparable or alike. Review the signs related to DIC if you had difficulty with this question.
Level of Cognitive Ability: Analyzing
Client Needs: Physiological Integrity
Integrated Process: Nursing Process/Data Collection
Content Area: Maternity/Antepartum
References: Christensen, Kockrow, pp. 893–894. 2011. *Foundations of nursing.*
Leifer, p. 90. 2011.

193. 2
Rationale: A nutritional supplement that is commonly needed during pregnancy for the red blood cells is iron. Anemia of pregnancy is primarily caused by iron deficiency. Iron supplements usually cause constipation. Meats are an excellent

source of iron. Iron for the fetus comes from the maternal serum.

Test-Taking Strategy: Use the process of elimination. Note the strategic word "malnourished." Eliminate options 3 and 4 because of the closed-ended words "not" and "all." Knowledge regarding the effects of iron supplements will assist you with eliminating option 1. Review the relationship of nutrition to anemia if you had difficulty with this question.

Level of Cognitive Ability: Evaluating
Client Needs: Physiological Integrity
Integrated Process: Nursing Process/Evaluation
Content Area: Maternity/Antepartum
Reference: Christensen, Kockrow, p. 622. 2011. *Foundations of nursing.*

194. 4

Rationale: An increase in calories is needed during pregnancy, but concentrated sugars should be avoided, because they may cause hyperglycemia. The fat intake should be 20% to 30% of the total calories. The client with diabetes needs about 50% to 60% of her caloric intake from carbohydrates and about 12% to 20% from protein. High-fiber foods will control blood glucose levels and prevent constipation.

Test-Taking Strategy: Note the strategic words "teaching has been effective." Use the process of elimination and your knowledge regarding diabetes mellitus and diet therapy to direct you to the correct option. Review the components of the diabetic diet if you had difficulty with this question.

Level of Cognitive Ability: Evaluating
Client Needs: Health Promotion and Maintenance
Integrated Process: Nursing Process/Evaluation
Content Area: Maternity/Antepartum
References: Christensen, Kockrow, pp. 905–907. 2011. *Foundations of nursing.*
Leifer, pp. 99–100. 2011.

195. 2

Rationale: The first actions are to maintain an open airway and to prevent injuries to the client. The client should be turned to the side and monitored for airway compromise. Options 1, 3, and 4 may be components of care, but they are not the first actions.

Test-Taking Strategy: Note the strategic word "first." Use the ABCs—airway, breathing, and circulation—to answer this question. Airway is the first priority. Review the care of the client with eclampsia if you had difficulty with this question.

Level of Cognitive Ability: Applying
Client Needs: Physiological Integrity
Integrated Process: Nursing Process/Implementation
Content Area: Critical Care
Reference: Perry, Hockenberry, Lowdermilk, Wilson, pp. 346–347. 2010.

196. 4

Rationale: The position described in option 4 will produce the posture of the pelvic tilt while countering gravity as the force that leads to the edema of the lower extremities. Although the other options may seem useful, options 2 and 3 identify heat, which should be prescribed by the health care provider (HCP). Option 1 will not relieve back pain and ankle edema.

Test-Taking Strategy: Use the process of elimination. Focus on the subject of the question, back pain and ankle edema.

Eliminate options 2 and 3, because the application of heat needs to be prescribed by the HCP. From the remaining options, focus on the subject to direct you to the correct option. Review the measures that will reduce these discomforts if you had difficulty with this question.

Level of Cognitive Ability: Applying
Client Needs: Physiological Integrity
Integrated Process: Nursing Process/Implementation
Content Area: Maternity/Antepartum
Reference: Leifer, p. 65. 2011.

197. 3

Rationale: Leg cramps often occur when the pregnant woman stretches her leg and plantarflexes her foot. Dorsiflexion of the foot while extending the knee stretches the gastrocnemius muscle, prevents the muscle from contracting, and halts the cramping. Therefore, the remaining options are incorrect.

Test-Taking Strategy: Use the process of elimination. Knowledge regarding the actions that will alleviate muscle cramps will assist you with answering the question. Visualize each of the descriptions in the options to help direct you to the correct option. Review the measures to alleviate muscle cramps if you had difficulty with this question.

Level of Cognitive Ability: Applying
Client Needs: Health Promotion and Maintenance
Integrated Process: Teaching and Learning
Content Area: Maternity/Antepartum
Reference: Leifer, p. 66. 2011.

198. 2

Rationale: Spices tend to trigger heartburn. Caffeine, like spices, may cause heartburn and needs to be avoided. Eating smaller, more frequent portions is preferable to eating three large meals to control heartburn. Lying down after meals is likely to lead to the reflux of stomach contents and cause heartburn. Salt leads to the retention of fluid..

Test-Taking Strategy: Use the process of elimination, focus on the subject, and recall those items that cause heartburn. This will direct you to option 2. Review the measures that alleviate heartburn if you had difficulty with this question.

Level of Cognitive Ability: Applying
Client Needs: Health Promotion and Maintenance
Integrated Process: Teaching and Learning
Content Area: Maternity/Antepartum
Reference: Leifer, p. 66. 2011.

199. 3

Rationale: Options 1, 2, and 4 are all signs that the GH is being resolved. Option 3 is a symptom of the worsening of the GH.

Test-Taking Strategy: Note the strategic words "not resolving." These words indicate a negative event query and the need to select a manifestation of GH. Recalling the signs of worsening GH will direct you to the correct option. Review these signs if you had difficulty with this question.

Level of Cognitive Ability: Evaluating
Client Needs: Physiological Integrity
Integrated Process: Nursing Process/Evaluation
Content Area: Maternity/Antepartum
Reference: Leifer, pp. 94–95. 2011.

❖ **200. 1, 2, 4**

Rationale: The three classic signs of preeclampsia are hypertension, generalized edema, and proteinuria. A low-grade fever, increased pulse rate, and increased respiratory rate are not associated with preeclampsia.

Test-Taking Strategy: Focus on the subject—the classic signs of preeclampsia. Thinking about the pathophysiology associated with this disorder will direct you to the correct options. Remember that the classic signs of preeclampsia are hypertension, generalized edema, and proteinuria. Review the signs of preeclampsia if you had difficulty with this question.

Level of Cognitive Ability: Applying
Client Needs: Physiological Integrity
Integrated Process: Nursing Process/Data Collection
Content Area: Maternity/Antepartum
Reference: Christensen, Kockrow, pp. 622, 896. 2011. *Foundations of nursing.*

Labor and Delivery and Associated Complications

I. THE PROCESS OF LABOR: "THE FOUR Ps" (Box 23-1)

A. Description
1. **Labor**: A coordinated sequence of rhythmic involuntary uterine contractions
2. **Delivery**: The actual event of birth

B. Four major factors—the four Ps—interact during normal childbirth; all four Ps are interrelated

C. Powers: Uterine and abdominal contractions
1. The forces acting to expel the fetus and **placenta**
2. Effacement: The shortening and thinning of the cervix during the first stage of **labor**
3. Dilation: The enlargement of the cervical os and cervical canal during the first stage of **labor**
4. Pushing efforts of the mother during the second stage

D. Passageway: Composed of the mother's rigid bony pelvis and the soft tissues of the cervix, pelvic floor, vagina, and introitus

E. Passenger: The fetus, membranes, and **placenta**

F. Psyche: A woman's emotional structure that can determine her entire response to **labor** and influence physiological and psychological functioning

G. Attitude
1. The relationship of the fetal body parts with one another
2. The normal intrauterine attitude is flexion, in which the fetal back is rounded, the head is forward on the chest, and the arms and legs are flexed in against the body. The other attitude, extension, tends to present larger fetal diameters.

H. Lie
1. Relationship of the spine of the fetus to the spine of the mother
2. Longitudinal or vertical: Fetal spine is parallel to the mother's spine. The fetus is in either a cephalic or breech presentation (Figure 23-1).
3. Transverse or horizontal: Fetal spine is at a right angle, or perpendicular, to the mother's spine. The presenting part is usually the shoulder, and **delivery** is by cesarean section (see Figure 23-1).

I. Presentation
1. Portion of the fetus that enters the pelvis first
2. Cephalic: The most common presentation; fetal head presents first
3. Breech: Buttocks present first.
   a. **Delivery** by cesarean section may be required, although vaginal birth is often possible
   b. Breech presentation has three variations: frank, full (complete), and footling.
4. Shoulder: Fetus is in a transverse lie; the arm, back, abdomen, or side could present. If the fetus does not spontaneously rotate or it is not possible to turn the fetus manually, a cesarean section may be performed.

Box 23-1 The Four Ps

- Powers
- Passageway
- Passenger
- Psyche

A Longitudinal lie   B Transverse lie

▲ **FIGURE 23-1** Fetal lie. **A,** In a longitudinal lie, the long axis of the fetus is parallel to the long axis of the mother. **B,** In a transverse lie, the long axis of the fetus is at a right angle to the long axis of the mother. The mother's abdomen has a wide, short appearance. (From McKinney, E., James, S., Murray, S., & Ashwill, J. [2009]. *Maternal-child nursing* [3rd ed.]. St. Louis: Saunders).

J. Presenting part: The specific fetal structure lying nearest to the cervix

K. Position: The relationship of the assigned area of the presenting part or landmark to the maternal pelvis (Box 23-2)

L. Station
1. The measurement of the progress of descent in centimeters above or below the midplane from the presenting part to the ischial spine
2. Station 0: At the ischial spine
3. Minus station: Above the ischial spine
4. Plus station: Below the ischial spine
5. Engagement: When the widest part of the presenting part has passed the inlet; usually corresponds to a 0 station

II. MECHANISMS OF LABOR (Box 23-3)

A. Data collection
1. Lightening or dropping: Is also known as engagement and occurs when the fetus descends into the pelvis about 2 weeks before **delivery**. Lightening or dropping is first noticeable in first pregnancies.
2. Braxton Hicks contractions increase.
3. Vaginal mucosa congested. Vaginal mucus increases.
4. Appearance of bloody show (brownish or blood-tinged cervical mucus is passed).
5. Cervix ripens and becomes soft and partly effaced; it may begin to dilate.
6. Sudden burst of energy experienced by the mother. This is also known as "nesting" and occurs 24 to 48 hours before the onset of **labor**.
7. Loss of 1 to 3 pounds from water loss resulting from fluid shifts produced by changes in progesterone and estrogen levels.
8. Spontaneous rupture of the membranes occurs.

B. True **labor** and false **labor** (Box 23-4)

Box 23-2 Fetal Positions

- ROA: Right occipitoanterior
- LOA: Left occipitoanterior
- ROP: Right occipitoposterior
- LOP: Left occipitoposterior
- ROT: Right occipitotransverse
- LOT: Left occipitotransverse
- RMA: Right mentoanterior
- LMA: Left mentoanterior
- RMP: Right mentoposterior
- LSA: Left sacroanterior
- LSP: Left sacroposterior

Box 23-4 True Labor and False Labor

True Labor

Contractions occur regularly. They become stronger, last longer, and occur closer together.

Cervical dilation and effacement are progressive.

The fetus usually becomes engaged in the pelvis and begins to descend.

False Labor

False labor does not produce dilation, effacement, or descent.

Contractions are irregular and without progression.

Walking has no effect on contractions and often relieves the condition.

For example, consider a woman who has been sleeping and who wakes up with contractions. If she gets up and moves around and her contractions become stronger and closer together, this is true labor. If the contractions go away when she does this, it is false labor.

Box 23-3 Mechanisms of Labor

Engagement

Engagement is the mechanism by which the fetus nestles into the pelvis. It also is called *lightening* or *dropping*.

Descent

Descent is the process that the fetal head undergoes as it begins its journey through the pelvis. It is a continuous process from the time of engagement until birth, and is assessed by the measurement called *station*.

Flexion

Flexion is the process of the fetal head's nodding forward toward the fetal chest.

Internal Rotation

The internal rotation of the fetus occurs most commonly from the occipitotransverse position, which is assumed at engagement into the pelvis, to the occipitoanterior position while continuously descending.

Extension

Extension enables the head to emerge when the fetus is in a cephalic position, and it begins after the head crowns. Extension is complete when the head passes under the symphysis pubis and occiput and the anterior fontanel, brow, face, and chin pass over the sacrum and coccyx and are over the perineum.

Restitution

Restitution is the realignment of the fetal head with the body after the head emerges.

External Rotation

The shoulders externally rotate after the head emerges and restitution occurs, so that the shoulders are in the anteroposterior diameter of the pelvis.

Expulsion

Expulsion is the birth of the entire body.

1. True **labor**: Contractions may manifest as back pain in some women. Contractions often resemble menstrual cramps during early **labor**.
2. False **labor**: Also known as prodromal **labor**, contractions are felt in abdomen and groin, and may be more annoying than painful

⚠️ In true labor, contractions increase in duration and intensity. In false labor, contractions are irregular and do not produce dilation, effacement, or descent.

III. LEOPOLD'S MANEUVERS

A. Description: A method of palpation for determining the presentation and position of the fetus; an aid for locating fetal heart sounds.
B. If the head is in the fundus, a hard, round, movable object is felt. The buttocks feel soft and have an irregular shape, and they are more difficult to move.
C. The fetus' back, which is a smooth, hard surface, should be felt on one side of the abdomen.
D. Irregular knobs and lumps, which may be the hands, feet, elbows, and knees, are felt on the opposite side of the abdomen.

IV. BREATHING TECHNIQUES (Box 23-5)

Box 23-5 Breathing Techniques

First-Stage Breathing

Cleansing Breath
- Each contraction begins and ends with a deep inspiration and expiration.

Slow-Paced Breathing
- A slow, deep breathing that promotes relaxation
- Used as long as possible during labor

Modified-Paced Breathing
- Used when slow-paced breathing is no longer effective
- Shallow, fast breathing

Pattern-Paced Breathing
- Sometimes called *pant-blow*
- After a certain number of breaths (modified-paced breathing), the woman exhales with a slight blow and then begins the modified-paced breathing again.

Breathing to Prevent Pushing
- The woman blows repeatedly using short puffs when the urge to push is strong.

Second-Stage Breathing
Several variations of breathing can be used in the pushing stage of labor, and the woman may grunt, groan, sigh, or moan as she pushes. Prolonged breath-holding while pushing with a closed glottis may result in a decrease in cardiac output. Therefore, if breath-holding while pushing is used, the open glottis method (limiting breath-holding to less than 6 to 8 seconds) should be done.

A. Provide a focus during contractions, thus interfering with pain sensory transmission
B. Promote relaxation and oxygenation
C. Begin with simple breathing patterns and progress to more complex ones as needed

V. FETAL MONITORING

A. Description
1. Displays fetal heart rate (FHR) and uterine activity
2. Monitors the uterine activity, frequency, and duration of contractions.
3. Monitors the FHR in relation to maternal contractions.
4. Baseline FHR is measured between contractions. The normal FHR at term is 120 to 160 beats per minute.
B. External fetal monitoring
1. Noninvasive; performed with the use of a tocotransducer or a Doppler ultrasonic transducer
2. Leopold's maneuvers are performed to determine on which side the fetal back is located, and the ultrasound transducer is then placed over this area and fastened with a belt.
3. The tocotransducer is placed over the fundus of the uterus, where contractions feel the strongest, and fastened with a belt.
4. Allow the client to assume a comfortable position, avoiding vena cava compression (maternal supine hypotensive syndrome).
5. The preferred maternal position is to have her lie on her side to increase perfusion.
C. Internal fetal monitoring
1. Invasive; requires rupturing the membranes and attaching an electrode to the presenting part of the fetus
2. Mother must be dilated 2 to 3 cm before internal monitoring can be performed
D. Periodic patterns in the FHR
1. Fetal bradycardia and tachycardia
   a. Bradycardia: FHR is less than 120 beats per minute for 10 minutes or longer.
   b. Tachycardia: FHR is greater than 160 beats per minute for 10 minutes or longer.

⚠️ If fetal bradycardia or tachycardia occurs, change the position of the mother, administer oxygen, and assess the mother's vital signs. Notify the health care provider (HCP) as soon as possible.

2. Variability
   a. Fluctuations in the baseline FHR
   b. Absence of variability or undetected variability is considered nonreassuring.
   c. Decreased variability can result from fetal hypoxemia, acidosis, or certain medications.

d. A temporary decrease in variability can occur when the fetus is in a sleep state. (Sleep states do not usually last more than 30 minutes.)

3. Accelerations
   a. Brief, temporary increases in the FHR of at least 15 beats above the baseline and lasting at least 15 seconds
   b. Usually a reassuring sign that reflects a responsive, nonacidotic fetus
   c. Usually occur with fetal movement or stimulation
   d. May be nonperiodic (having no relation to contractions) or periodic
   e. May occur with uterine contractions, vaginal examinations, mild cord compression, or when the fetus is in a breech presentation

4. Early decelerations
   a. Decreases in FHR below baseline. The rate at the lowest point of the deceleration usually remains greater than 100 beats/min.
   b. Occur during contractions as the fetal head is pressed against the woman's pelvis or soft tissues, such as the cervix, and return to baseline FHR by the end of the contraction.
   c. Tracing shows a uniform shape and mirror image of uterine contractions.
   d. Not associated with fetal compromise and requires no intervention.

5. Late decelerations
   a. Nonreassuring patterns that reflect impaired placental exchange or uteroplacental insufficiency.
   b. Patterns look similar to early decelerations but begin well after the contraction begins and return to baseline after the contraction ends.
   c. Degree of the fall in the heart rate from baseline is not related to the amount of uteroplacental insufficiency.

⚠ Interventions for late decelerations include improving placental blood flow and fetal oxygenation.

6. Variable decelerations
   a. Variable decelerations are caused by conditions that restrict flow through the umbilical cord.
   b. Variable decelerations do not have the uniform appearance of early and late decelerations.
   c. Their shape, duration, and degree of fall below baseline heart rate are variable. They fall and rise abruptly with the onset and relief of cord compression.
   d. Variable decelerations also may be nonperiodic, occurring at times that are unrelated to contractions.
   e. One considers the baseline rate and variability when evaluating variable decelerations.

f. Variable decelerations are significant when the FHR repeatedly decreases to less than 70 beats per minute and persists at that level for at least 60 seconds before returning to baseline.

7. Hypertonic uterine activity
   a. Checking uterine activity includes frequency, duration, intensity of contractions, and uterine resting tone
   b. Uterus should relax between contractions for 60 seconds or more
   c. Uterine contraction intensity is about 50 to 75 mm Hg (with intrauterine catheter) during **labor** and may reach 110 mm Hg with pushing during the second stage.
   d. Average resting tone is 5 to 15 mm Hg
   e. In hypertonic uterine activity, reduced uterine blood flow and decreased fetal oxygen supply occur.

8. Nonreassuring FHR patterns (Box 23-6)
9. Interventions for nonreassuring patterns (see Priority Nursing Actions)

VI. FOUR STAGES OF LABOR (Table 23-1)

▰▰▰▰ PRIORITY NURSING ACTIONS! ▰▰▰▰

Actions to Take for a Nonreassuring Fetal Heart Rate Pattern

1. Call the registered nurse and stay with the client.
2. Identify the cause.
3. Stop the oxytocin (Pitocin) infusion.
4. Change the mother's position.
5. Administer oxygen by face mask at 8 to 10 L/min and infuse intravenous fluids as prescribed.
6. Prepare to initiate continuous electronic fetal monitoring with internal devices if not contraindicated.
7. Prepare for cesarean delivery if necessary.
8. Document the event, actions taken, and the mother's response.

Nonreassuring fetal heart rate patterns include bradycardia, tachycardia, late decelerations, prolonged decelerations, hypertonic uterine activity, decreased or absent variability, or variable decelerations falling to less than 70 beats/min for longer than 60 seconds. If a nonreassuring fetal heart rate pattern is noted, the registered nurse is called who will then contact the HCP as soon as possible. (The nurse stays with the client and asks another nurse to contact the registered nurse.) The nurse needs to identify the cause of the pattern immediately. This includes checking for a prolapsed umbilical cord and checking maternal vital signs to identify hypotension, hypertension, or fever that can contribute to the fetal response associated with the nonreassuring pattern. If the mother is receiving an oxytocin (Pitocin) infusion, it is stopped because oxytocin causes uterine stimulation, which can worsen the nonreassuring pattern. A tocolytic may be prescribed. The mother is repositioned because this may improve placental perfusion (avoid the supine position). Oxygen is administered by face mask at 8 to 10 L/min to increase maternal blood oxygen saturation making more oxygen available to the fetus, and intravenous fluids are infused to expand the mother's blood volume and improve placental perfusion. If not contraindicated, the nurse prepares to initiate continuous electronic fetal monitoring with internal devices. Cesarean delivery may be necessary, and the nurse should prepare for this procedure. Birth preparation should also include neonatal resuscitation. The nurse documents the event, actions taken, the mother's response, and any other pertinent data.

Reference: McKinney, E., James, S., Murray, S., & Ashwill, J. (2009). *Maternal-child nursing* (3rd ed., p. 397). St. Louis: Saunders.

A. Stage 1: Latent phase
   1. Description: Stage 1 is the longest.
   2. Data collection
      a. Cervical dilation of up to 1 to 4 cm
      b. Uterine contractions every 15 to 30 minutes, 15 to 30 seconds in duration, and of mild intensity
   3. Interventions
      a. Encourage the mother and partner to participate in care.
      b. Assist with comfort measures, changes of position, and ambulation.
      c. Keep the mother and partner informed of progress.
      d. Offer fluids and ice chips.
      e. Encourage voiding every 1 to 2 hours.

Box 23-6 Nonreassuring FHR Patterns

Bradycardia
Tachycardia
Late decelerations
Prolonged decelerations
Hypertonic uterine activity
Decreased or absent variability
Variable decelerations falling to less than 70 beats/min for longer than 60 seconds

B. Stage 1: Active phase
   1. Data collection
      a. Cervical dilation of 4 to 7 cm
      b. Uterine contractions every 3 to 5 minutes, 30 to 60 seconds in duration, and of moderate intensity
   2. Interventions
      a. Encourage the maintenance of effective breathing patterns. Assist the woman to cope with contractions.
      b. Provide a quiet environment.
      c. Keep the mother and partner informed of progress.
      d. Promote comfort with back rubs, sacral pressure, pillow support, frequent position changes, and oral care; fluids, food, and ice chips, as prescribed; and ointment for dry lips.
      e. Instruct the partner in effleurage (light stroking of abdomen).
      f. Encourage voiding every 1 to 2 hours.
C. Stage 1: Transition phase
   1. Data collection
      a. Cervical dilation of 8 to 10 cm
      b. Uterine contractions every 2 to 3 minutes, 45 to 90 seconds in duration, and of strong intensity
   2. Interventions
      a. Encourage rest between contractions.
      b. Remind the woman to begin her breathing pattern before the contraction becomes too intense.
      c. Keep the mother and partner informed of progress.
      d. Provide privacy but also constant support.
      e. Offer fluids, ice chips, and ointment for dry lips.
      f. Encourage voiding every 1 to 2 hours.
D. Interventions throughout stage 1
      a. Monitor maternal vital signs.
      b. Monitor FHR via ultrasound Doppler, fetoscope, or electronic fetal monitor.
      c. Assess FHR before, during, and after a contraction, noting that the normal FHR is 120 to 160 beats per minute.

TABLE 23-1 Four Stages of Labor

First Stage	Second Stage	Third Stage	Fourth Stage
Effacement and dilation of the cervix	Expulsion of the fetus	Separation of the placenta	Physical recovery
Divided into three stages: latent, active, and transition	Pushing stage	Expulsion of the placenta	1-4 hours after the expulsion of the placenta
Woman is sociable, talkative, and excited in the latent phase, becoming tired, restless, and anxious as labor intensifies and contractions become stronger	Woman has intense concentration on pushing with contractions; may fall asleep between contractions	Woman is excited and relieved after baby's birth; usually very tired	Woman is tired but may find it difficult to rest because of excitement; eager to become acquainted with her newborn

d. Monitor uterine contractions by palpation or tocodynamometer, and determine frequency, duration, and intensity.

e. Assist with monitoring the status of cervical dilation and effacement.

f. Assist with monitoring fetal station, presentation, and position by Leopold's maneuvers.

g. Assist with pelvic examinations and prepare for a Nitrazine or fern test to assess for the rupture of membranes.

⚠ If the membranes rupture, the priority is to check the fetal heart rate. Then, check the color of the amniotic fluid because meconium-stained fluid can indicate fetal distress.

E. Stage 2

1. Data collection
   a. Cervical dilation is complete.
   b. Progress of **labor** is measured by the descent of the fetal head through the birth canal (change in fetal station).
   c. Uterine contractions occur every 2 to 3 minutes and last 60 to 75 seconds, and the intensity is strong.
   d. Increase in bloody show occurs.
   e. The mother feels the urge to bear down. Assist the mother with pushing efforts.

2. Interventions
   a. Perform assessments every 5 minutes.
   b. Monitor maternal vital signs.
   c. Monitor FHR via ultrasound Doppler, fetoscope, or electronic fetal monitor.
   d. Monitor the FHR before, during, and after a contraction, noting that normal FHR is 120 to 160 beats per minute.
   e. Monitor the uterine contractions with palpation or monitoring, determining the frequency, duration, and intensity.
   f. Provide the mother with encouragement and praise, and provide for rest between contractions.
   g. Keep the mother and partner informed of progress.
   h. Maintain privacy.
   i. Provide ice chips and ointment for dry lips.
   j. Assist the mother into a position that promotes comfort and that assists with pushing efforts.
   k. Monitor for signs of approaching birth, such as perineal bulging or visualization of the fetal head.
   l. Prepare for birth (expulsion of fetus).

F. Stage 3

1. Data collection
   a. Contractions occur until the **placenta** is expelled.
   b. Placental separation and expulsion occur.

c. Expulsion of the **placenta** occurs 5 to 30 minutes after the birth of the baby.

d. Schultze mechanism: Center portion of **placenta** separates first, and its shiny fetal surface emerges from vagina

e. Duncan mechanism: Margin of the **placenta** separates, and the dull, red, rough maternal surface emerges from the vagina first.

2. Interventions
   a. Monitor maternal vital signs and uterine status.
   b. Provide the parents with explanation regarding expulsion of the **placenta**.
   c. After the expulsion of the **placenta**, the uterine fundus remains firm and is located approximately two fingerbreadths below the umbilicus.
   d. Examine the **placenta** for cotyledons and membranes to verify that it is intact. Examine the umbilical cord for the presence of one vein and two arteries.
   e. Monitor the mother for a shivering reaction. Provide warmth.
   f. Promote parental–neonatal attachment.

G. Stage 4

1. Description: The period of time from 1 to 4 hours after **delivery**

2. Data collection
   a. Blood pressure returns to prelabor level.
   b. Pulse is slightly lower than during **labor**.
   c. Fundus contracted and midline after delivery; the fundus is usually at the umbilicus.

⚠ Monitor lochia discharge. Lochia may be moderate in amount and red in color in stage 4.

3. Interventions
   a. Maternal assessments are performed every 15 minutes for 1 hour, every 30 minutes for 1 hour, and hourly for 2 hours (or as per agency policy).
   b. Provide warm blankets.
   c. Apply ice packs to the perineum.
   d. Massage the fundus, if needed, if the fundus is flaccid (boggy).
   e. Provide breast-feeding support, as needed.
   f. See Chapter 25 for information about caring for the **newborn**.

VII. ANESTHESIA

A. Local anesthesia
   1. Used for blocking the pain during episiotomy
   2. Administered just before the birth of the baby
   3. No effect on the fetus

B. Pudendal block
   1. Administered just before the birth of the baby
   2. Injection site is at the pudendal nerve through a transvaginal route

3. Blocks the perineal area for episiotomy
4. Effect lasts about 30 minutes
5. No effect on contractions or the fetus

C. Lumbar epidural block
1. Injection site in the epidural space at L3-L4
2. Administered after **labor** is established or just before a scheduled cesarean birth
3. Relieves pain from contractions and numbs the vagina and perineum
4. May cause hypotension, bladder distention, and a prolonged second stage.
5. Does not cause headache, because the dura mater is not penetrated
6. Monitor maternal blood pressure.
7. IV fluids are administered, as prescribed. Increase fluids, as prescribed, if hypotension occurs.
8. Observe for any adverse effects from opioid epidurals, such as nausea and vomiting, pruritus, or respiratory depression.

D. Intrathecal opioid analgesics
1. Medication is injected into the subarachnoid space and has a rapid onset of action.
2. May be used in combination with a lumbar epidural block

E. Subarachnoid (spinal) block
1. Injection site is in the spinal subarachnoid space at L3-L5
2. The block is administered just before birth
3. Relieves uterine and perineal pain and numbs the vagina, perineum, and lower extremities
4. Usually causes maternal hypotension
5. May cause postpartum headache
6. The mother must lie flat 8 to 12 hours after spinal injection.
7. IV fluids are administered, as prescribed

F. General anesthesia
1. May be used for some surgical interventions
2. The mother is not awake.

⚠ General anesthesia presents a danger of respiratory depression, vomiting, and aspiration.

VIII. OBSTETRICAL PROCEDURES

A. Bishop score (Table 23-2)
1. Used to determine maternal readiness for **labor** induction and evaluates cervical status and fetal position
2. Indicated before the induction of **labor**
3. The five factors are assigned a score of 0 to 3, and the total score is calculated.
4. A score of 6 or more indicates a readiness for **labor** induction.

B. Induction
1. Induction is a deliberate initiation of uterine contractions that stimulates **labor**.

TABLE 23-2 Factors of the Bishop Score

Score	0	1	2	3
Dilation of cervix (cm)	0	1-2 cm	3-4 cm	>5 cm
Effacement of cervix (%)	0%-30%	40%-50%	60%-70%	>80%
Consistency of cervix	Firm	Medium	Soft	
Position of cervix	Posterior	Midposition	Anterior	
Station of presenting part	−3	−2	−1	+1, +2

2. Elective induction may be accomplished by oxytocin (Pitocin) infusion.
3. Baseline tracing of uterine contractions and FHR is obtained.
4. IV dosage of oxytocin may be increased, as prescribed, only after assessing contractions, FHR, and maternal blood pressure and pulse.
5. The rate of oxytocin is not increased when the desired contraction pattern is obtained (contraction frequency of 2 to 3 minutes and lasting 60 seconds).

⚠ An oxytocin (Pitocin) infusion is discontinued if uterine contraction frequency is less than 2 minutes or duration is longer than 90 seconds, or if fetal distress is noted.

C. Amniotomy
1. Artificial rupture of membranes (AROM); performed by the HCP to stimulate **labor**
2. Performed if the fetus is at 0 or a plus station
3. Increases the risk of prolapsed cord and infection
4. Monitor the FHR before and after amniotomy.
5. Record the time of amniotomy, FHR, and characteristics of the fluid.
6. Meconium-stained **amniotic fluid** may be associated with fetal distress.
7. Bloody **amniotic fluid** may indicate abruptio placentae or fetal trauma.
8. An unpleasant odor to the **amniotic fluid** is associated with infection.
9. Polyhydramnios is associated with maternal diabetes and certain congenital disorders.
10. Oligohydramnios is associated with intrauterine growth restriction and congenital disorders.
11. More variable decelerations are likely to occur after the rupture of the membranes as a result of cord compression during contractions.
12. Limit client activity, if prescribed.

D. External version
1. External manipulation of the fetus from an abnormal presentation into a normal presentation
2. Indicated for an abnormal presentation that exists after 34 weeks' gestation
3. Monitor vital signs.
4. Women who are Rh-negative should receive Rh_0 (D) immunoglobulin (RhoGAM)at 28 weeks' gestation.
5. Prepare for nonstress test to evaluate fetal well-being
6. IV fluids and tocolytic therapy may be administered to relax the uterus and permit easier manipulation of the fetus.
7. Ultrasound is used during the procedure to evaluate fetal position and placental placement and guide direction of the fetus
8. Accomplished by the exertion of gentle, constant pressure on the abdomen to direct the fetus into a cephalic presentation, if possible
9. Monitor blood pressure to identify vena cava syndrome.
10. Monitor for unusual pain.
11. After the procedure
    a. Perform a nonstress test to evaluate fetal well-being.
    b. Monitor for uterine activity, bleeding, ruptured membranes, and decreased fetal activity.
    c. With Rh-negative clients, perform Kleihauer-Betke test as prescribed to detect the presence and amount of fetal blood in the maternal circulation and to identify clients who need additional Rh_0 (D) immunoglobulin

E. Episiotomy
1. Incision made into the perineum to enlarge the vaginal outlet and facilitate **delivery**
2. Check episiotomy site.
3. Institute measures to relieve pain.
4. Provide an ice pack during the first 24 hours.
5. Instruct the client regarding the use of sitz baths.
6. Apply analgesic spray or ointment, as prescribed.
7. Provide perineal care with the use of clean technique.
8. Instruct the client regarding the proper care of the incision.
9. Instruct the client to dry the perineal area from front to back and to blot the area rather than wipe it.
10. Instruct the client to shower rather than bathe in a tub.
11. Apply a perineal pad without touching the inside surface of the pad.
12. Report any bright red bleeding to the HCP.

F. Forceps **delivery**
1. Two double-crossed, spoonlike articulated blades are used to assist in the **delivery** of the fetal head

2. Reassure the mother and explain the need for the forceps.
3. Monitor the mother and fetus during **delivery**.
4. Check the neonate and mother after **delivery** for any possible injury.
5. Assist with the repair of any lacerations.

G. Vacuum extraction
1. A cap-like suction device is applied to the fetal head to facilitate extraction.
2. Suction is used to assist with the **delivery** of the fetal head.
3. Traction is applied during uterine contractions until the descent of the fetal head is achieved.
4. The suction device should not be kept in place any longer than 25 minutes.
5. Monitor the FHR every 5 minutes if external fetal monitoring is not used.
6. Check the **newborn** at birth and monitor him or her throughout the postpartum period for signs of cerebral trauma.
7. Monitor for developing cephalhematoma.
8. Caput succedaneum is normal and will resolve in 24 hours.

H. Cesarean **delivery**
1. Birth of the fetus usually through a transabdominal incision of the uterus
2. Preoperative
    a. If planned, prepare the mother and partner.
    b. If an emergency, quickly explain the need and procedure to the mother and partner.
    c. Obtain informed consent.
    d. Make sure that the preoperative diagnostic tests are done, including testing for the Rh factor.
    e. Prepare the mother for the insertion of an IV line and a Foley catheter.
    f. Prepare the abdomen, as prescribed.
    g. Monitor the mother and fetus continuously.
    h. Provide emotional support.
    i. Administer preoperative medications, as prescribed.
3. Postoperative
    a. Monitor the vital signs.
    b. Provide pain relief.
    c. Encourage turning, coughing, and deep breathing.
    d. Encourage ambulation.
    e. Monitor for signs of infection and bleeding.
    f. Burning and pain on urination may indicate a bladder infection.
    g. A tender uterus and foul-smelling **lochia** may indicate endometritis.
    h. A productive cough or chills may indicate pneumonia.
    i. Pain, tenderness, or edema of the extremity may indicate thrombophlebitis.

IX. ABRUPTIO PLACENTAE (Figure 23-2)

A. Description: Premature separation of the **placenta** (the detachment of part or all of the **placenta** from its **implantation** site) after 20 weeks' gestation and before the birth of the baby

B. Data collection
1. Dark red vaginal bleeding; however, if the bleeding is high in the uterus or minimal, there can be an absence of visible blood
2. Uterine pain and/or tenderness
3. Uterine rigidity
4. Severe abdominal pain
5. Signs of fetal distress
6. Signs of maternal shock if bleeding is excessive

C. Interventions
1. Monitor maternal vital signs and FHR.
2. Assess for excessive vaginal bleeding, abdominal pain, and an increase in fundal height.

Marginal abruption
with external bleeding

Partial abruption
with concealed bleeding

Complete abruption
with concealed bleeding

▲ **FIGURE 23-2** Types of abruptio placentae. (From Murray, S., & McKinney, E. [2010]. *Foundations of maternal-newborn nursing* [5th ed.]. Philadelphia: Saunders).

3. Maintain bedrest; administer oxygen, IV fluids, and blood products, as prescribed.
4. Place the mother in Trendelenburg's position, if indicated, to decrease the pressure of the fetus on the **placenta** or in the lateral position with the head of the bed flat if there are signs of hypovolemic shock caused by blood loss.
5. Monitor and report any uterine activity.
6. Prepare for the **delivery** of the fetus as quickly as possible, with vaginal **delivery** preferable if the fetus is healthy and stable and the presenting part is in the pelvis. Emergency cesarean section is performed if the fetus is alive but shows signs of distress.
7. Monitor for signs of disseminated intravascular coagulopathy (DIC) during the postpartum period.

⚠ Know the differences between placenta previa and abruptio placentae. In placenta previa, there is painless, bright red vaginal bleeding and the uterus is soft, relaxed, and nontender. In abruptio placentae, there is dark red vaginal bleeding, uterine pain or tenderness or both, and uterine rigidity.

X. AMNIOTIC FLUID EMBOLISM

A. Description
1. Occurs when **amniotic fluid** containing particles of debris (e.g., vernix, hair, skin, cells, meconium) enters the maternal circulation.
2. The debris deposits in the pulmonary arterioles and is usually fatal to the mother.

B. Data collection
1. Abrupt onset of respiratory distress and chest pain
2. Cyanosis
3. Seizures
4. Heart failure and pulmonary edema
5. Fetal bradycardia and distress if **delivery** has not occurred at the time of the embolism

C. Interventions
1. Institute or assist with cardiopulmonary resuscitation.
2. Administer oxygen at 8 to 10 L/min by face mask or resuscitation bag delivering 100% oxygen, as prescribed.
3. Prepare the client for intubation and mechanical ventilation.
4. Position the woman on her side.
5. IV fluids, blood products, and medications may be prescribed to correct coagulation failure.
6. Monitor the fetal status.
7. Prepare for emergency **delivery** after the woman is stabilized.
8. Provide emotional support to the woman, the partner, and the family.

XI. DYSTOCIA

A. Description
1. Difficult **labor** that is prolonged or more painful
2. Occurs as a result of problems caused by uterine contractions, the fetus, or the bones and tissues of the maternal pelvis
3. The fetus may be excessively large, malpositioned, or in an abnormal position.
4. Contractions may be hypotonic or hypertonic.
5. Hypotonic contractions are short, irregular, and weak. Amniotomy and oxytocin (Pitocin) infusion may be treatment measures.
6. Hypertonic contractions are painful, occur frequently, and are uncoordinated. Treatment depends on cause and includes pain relief measures and rest.
7. Dystocia can result in maternal dehydration, infection, fetal injury, or death.

B. Data collection
1. Excessive abdominal pain
2. Abnormal contraction pattern
3. Fetal distress
4. Maternal or fetal tachycardia
5. Lack of progress of **labor**

C. Interventions
1. Check FHR; monitor for fetal distress.
2. Monitor uterine contractions.
3. Monitor maternal temperature and heart rate.
4. Assist with pelvic examination, measurements, ultrasound, and other procedures.
5. Prophylactic antibiotics may be prescribed to prevent infection.
6. IV fluids may be prescribed.
7. Monitor intake and output.
8. Monitor for dehydration.
9. Instruct the mother in breathing techniques and relaxation exercises.
10. Fetal monitoring is needed if oxytocin (Pitocin) is prescribed (oxytocin is not prescribed for hypertonic uterine contractions).
11. Monitor the color of the **amniotic fluid**.
12. Provide rest and comfort as with a normal **delivery**, such as back rubs and position changes.
13. Assess the mother's fatigue and pain. Administer sedatives and pain medications, as prescribed.
14. Monitor for prolapse of the cord after the rupture of the membranes.

XII. FETAL DISTRESS

A. Data collection
1. FHR of less than 120 or more than 160 beats per minute
2. Meconium-stained **amniotic fluid**
3. Fetal hyperactivity
4. Progressive decrease in baseline variability

5. Severe variable decelerations
6. Late decelerations

B. Interventions
1. Place the mother in a lateral position.
2. Administer oxygen at 8 to 10 L/min via face mask, as prescribed.
3. Oxytocin (Pitocin) infusion is discontinued.
4. Monitor the maternal and fetal status.

⚠ In the event of fetal distress, prepare the client for emergency cesarean delivery.

XIII. INTRAUTERINE FETAL DEMISE

A. Data collection
1. Loss of fetal movement
2. Absence of fetal heart tones
3. DIC screen (Monitor for coagulation abnormalities, because DIC is a complication that is related to intrauterine fetal demise.)
4. Low hemoglobin and hematocrit levels; low platelet count; prolonged bleeding and clotting times
5. Bleeding from puncture sites (which could be indicative of DIC)

B. Interventions
1. Encourage the mother and her family to verbalize their feelings; provide emotional support.
2. Incorporate religious and cultural health care beliefs and practices into the plan of care.
3. Allow the mother choices related to **labor** and **delivery**.
4. Administer blood and blood products, as prescribed, if DIC occurs.

XIV. PLACENTAL ABNORMALITIES

A. Description: **Placenta** accreta is an abnormally adherent **placenta**. **Placenta** increta occurs when the **placenta** penetrates the uterine muscle itself. **Placenta** percreta occurs when the **placenta** goes all the way through the uterus.

B. Data collection: May cause hemorrhage immediately after birth because the **placenta** does not separate cleanly

C. Intervention
1. Monitor for hemorrhage and shock.
2. Prepare the client for a hysterectomy if a large portion of the **placenta** is abnormally adherent.

XV. PLACENTA PREVIA (Figure 23-3)

A. Description
1. The **placenta** is improperly implanted in the lower uterine segment near or over the internal cervical os.

Marginal
Placenta is implanted in lower uterus but its lower border is >3 cm from internal cervical os.

Partial
Lower border of placenta is within 3 cm of internal cervical os but does not fully cover it.

Total
Placenta completely covers internal cervical os.

▲ **FIGURE 23-3** The three classifications of placenta previa. (From Murray, S., & McKinney, E. [2006]. *Foundations of maternal-newborn nursing* [4th ed.]. Philadelphia: Saunders).

2. Management depends on the classification of the previa and the gestational age of the fetus.
B. Data collection
   1. Sudden onset of painless, bright-red vaginal bleeding during the last half of pregnancy; suspect **placenta** previa whenever vaginal bleeding occurs after 24 weeks' gestation
   2. Soft, relaxed, nontender uterus
   3. Fundal height may be greater than expected for gestational age
C. Interventions
   1. Monitor maternal vital signs, FHR, and fetal activity.
   2. Prepare for ultrasound to confirm diagnosis.
   3. Vaginal examination or any other action that would stimulate uterine activity is avoided.
   4. Maintain bedrest in a side-lying position as prescribed.
   5. Monitor the amount of bleeding. (Treat signs of shock.)
   6. IV fluids, blood products, or tocolytic medications may be prescribed.
   7. If bleeding is heavy, a cesarean section may be performed.

XVI. PRECIPITOUS LABOR AND DELIVERY

A. Description: **Labor** that lasts less than 3 hours from the onset of contractions to birth
B. Interventions
   1. Have a precipitous **delivery** tray available (hemostats, scissors, and cord clamp).
   2. Stay with the mother at all times.
   3. Provide emotional support and keep the mother calm.
   4. Encourage the mother to pant between contractions.
   5. Prepare for the rupturing of the membranes when the head crowns if they are not already ruptured.
   6. Do not try to keep the fetus from being delivered.
   7. If **delivery** is necessary before the arrival of the HCP:
      a. Apply gentle pressure to the fetal head upward toward the vagina to prevent damage to the fetal head and vaginal lacerations.
      b. Support the **infant's** body during **delivery**.
      c. Deliver the **infant** between contractions, checking for the cord around the neck.
      d. Restitution is used to deliver the posterior shoulder.
      e. Gentle downward pressure is used to move the anterior shoulder under the pubic symphysis.
      f. Clear the **infant's** mouth.
      g. Dry and cover the **infant** to keep the body warm.
      h. Allow the **placenta** to separate naturally.
      i. Place the **infant** on the mother's abdomen or breast to induce uterine contractions.

XVII. PREMATURE RUPTURE OF THE MEMBRANES

A. Description
   1. The spontaneous rupture of the amniotic membrane before the onset of **labor**
   2. Gestational age usually determines the plan and intervention
   3. When the rupture of membranes is before term and **delivery** will be delayed, infection becomes a risk.
B. Data collection
   1. Evidence of fluid pooling in the vaginal vault. The Nitrazine test is positive.
   2. Amount, color, consistency, and odor of fluid needs to be assessed.
   3. Vital signs are monitored; elevated temperature may indicate the presence of infection
   4. Fetal monitoring is necessary; tachycardia may indicate infection
C. Interventions
   1. Assist with tests to assess gestational age.
   2. Avoid vaginal examinations because of the risk of infection.

3. Monitor maternal and fetal status for signs of compromise or infection.
4. Administer antibiotics, as prescribed.

XVIII. PRETERM LABOR

A. Description
  1. Cervical changes and uterine contractions occurring between 20 and 37 weeks' gestation.
  2. Risk factors include a history of medical conditions; present and past obstetric problems; infection; and social and environmental factors, including substance abuse.
  3. Additional risk factors include a multifetal pregnancy, which contributes to overdistention of uterus; anemia, which decreases oxygen supply to uterus; and age younger than 18 years, or first pregnancy and older than 40 years
B. Data collection
  1. Uterine contractions (painful or painless)
  2. Abdominal cramping (may be accompanied by diarrhea)
  3. Low back pain
  4. Pelvic pressure or heaviness
  5. Change in the character and amount of usual discharge; may be thicker or thinner, bloody, brown or colorless, or odorous
  6. Rupture of amniotic membranes
C. Interventions
  1. Focus is on stopping the **labor**: identify and treat infection, restrict activity, and ensure hydration.
  2. Maintain bedrest and a lateral position.
  3. Monitor the fetal status.
  4. Administer fluids.
  5. Tocolytic medications may be prescribed to suppress **labor**.

XIX. PROLAPSED UMBILICAL CORD (Figure 23-4)

A. Description: The umbilical cord is displaced between the presenting part and the amnion, or it is protruding through the cervix, causing compression of the cord and compromising fetal circulation.
B. Data collection
  1. The client has a feeling that something is coming through the vagina.
  2. The umbilical cord is visible or palpable.
  3. The FHR is irregular and slow.
  4. The fetal heart monitor will show variable deceleration or bradycardia after the rupture of the membranes.
  5. If fetal hypoxia is severe, violent fetal activity may occur and then cease.
C. Interventions (see Priority Nursing Actions)

■■■■■ PRIORITY NURSING ACTIONS! ■■■■■

Steps to Take if Umbilical Cord Prolapse Is Suspected

1. Call the registered nurse and stay with the client.
2. Elevate the fetal presenting part that is lying on the cord by applying finger pressure on the fetal part with a gloved hand.
3. Place the client into extreme Trendelenburg's or modified Sims' position or a knee-chest position.
4. Administer oxygen, 8 to 10 L/min, by face mask to the client.
5. Monitor the fetal heart rate and assess the fetus for hypoxia.
6. Prepare to start intravenous fluids or increase the rate of an existing solution.
7. Prepare for immediate birth.
8. Document the event, actions taken, and the client's response.

If umbilical cord prolapse occurs, the cord is lying alongside or below the presenting part of the fetus and can be seen or felt in or protruding from the vagina. The nurse stays with the client and asks another nurse to call the registered nurse, who will contact the HCP immediately. The nurse must relieve cord pressure immediately so that the fetus receives adequate oxygenation. The nurse can relieve cord pressure by elevating the fetal presenting part that is lying on the cord. The nurse does this by quickly gloving the hand and inserting two fingers into the vagina to the cervix and exerting upward pressure on the presenting part. The nurse also relieves cord pressure by placing the client into extreme Trendelenburg's or modified Sims' position or a knee-chest position (a rolled towel is placed under the client's hip). The nurse administers oxygen, 8 to 10 L/min, by face mask to the client, monitors the fetal heart rate and fetal heart rate patterns, and assesses the fetus for hypoxia. The client is prepared for immediate birth (vaginal or cesarean). The nurse documents the event, actions taken, the client's response, and any additional pertinent information. The nurse never attempts to push the cord into the uterus. If the umbilical cord is protruding from the vagina, the cord is wrapped loosely in a sterile towel saturated with warm sterile normal saline.

Reference: Perry, S., Hockenberry, M., Lowdermilk, D., & Wilson, D. (2010). *Maternal child nursing care* (4th ed., p. 467). St. Louis: Mosby.

XX. RUPTURE OF THE UTERUS

A. Description
  1. Separation of the uterine tissue from the stress of **labor**; classified as complete or incomplete
  2. Complete: Extends through the entire uterine wall into the peritoneal cavity or the broad ligament
  3. Incomplete: Extends into the peritoneum but not into the peritoneal cavity or the broad ligament
  4. Manifestations vary with the extent of the rupture.

A   B   C   D

▲ **FIGURE 23-4** Prolapse of the umbilical cord. Note the pressure of the presenting part on the umbilical cord; this endangers fetal circulation. **A,** Occult (hidden) prolapse of the cord. **B,** Complete prolapse of the cord. **C,** Cord presenting in front of the fetal head may be seen in the vagina. **D,** Frank breech presentation with prolapsed cord. (From Lowdermilk, D., & Perry, S. [2007]. *Maternity & women's health care* [9th ed.]. St. Louis: Mosby).

B. Data ollection
1. Abdominal pain or tenderness
2. Chest pain
3. Contractions may stop or fail to progress
4. Rigid abdomen
5. Absent fetal heart rate
6. Signs of maternal shock
7. Fetus palpated outside of the uterus (complete rupture)

C. Interventions
1. Monitor for and assist with treating signs of shock (oxygen, IV fluids, and blood products may be prescribed)
2. Prepare the client for cesarean section (hysterectomy may be necessary).
3. Provide emotional support for the mother and partner

XXI. SUPINE HYPOTENSION (VENA CAVA SYNDROME)

A. Description
1. Occurs when the venous return to the heart is impaired by the weight of the uterus
2. Results from the partial occlusion of the vena cava and the descending aorta and causes reduced cardiac return, cardiac output, and blood pressure

B. Data collection
1. Faintness, lightheadedness, dizziness, and breathlessness
2. Pallor, clammy (damp, cool) skin, and sweating
3. Hypotension and tachycardia
4. Nausea
5. Fetal distress

C. Interventions
1. Position the client on her side to shift the weight of the fetus off the inferior vena cava until signs and symptoms subside and vital signs stabilize.

2. Monitor the vital signs and the FHR.

⚠ Place a pillow or wedge under the client's hip to displace the gravid uterus off the vena cava. Avoid the supine position.

XXII. UTERINE INVERSION

A. Description
1. Uterus turns inside out; may be partial or complete
2. Usually occurs during **delivery** or after the **delivery** of the **placenta**

B. Data collection
1. A depression in the fundal area of the uterus is noted
2. Interior of the uterus may be seen through the cervix or protruding through the vagina
3. Severe pain
4. Hemorrhage
5. Signs of shock

C. Interventions
1. Monitor for hemorrhage and signs of shock, and treat shock.
2. Prepare the client for a return of the uterus to the correct position via the vagina. If unsuccessful, laparotomy with replacement to the correct position is done.

MORE QUESTIONS ON EVOLVE!

Practice Questions

201. The nurse is assigned to care for a client who is in early labor. When collecting data from the client, it is **most** important for the nurse to first determine which of the following?

1. Baseline fetal heart rate
2. Intensity of contractions
3. Maternal blood pressure
4. Frequency of contractions

202. Leopold's maneuvers will be performed on a pregnant client. The client asks the nurse about the procedure. The nurse responds, knowing that this procedure:
1. Measures the height of the maternal fundus
2. Determines the "lie" and "attitude" of the fetus
3. Is a systematic method for palpating the fetus through the maternal back
4. Is a systematic method for palpating the fetus through the maternal abdominal wall

203. The nurse is caring for a client who is in labor. The nurse rechecks the client's blood pressure and notes that it has dropped. To decrease the incidence of supine hypotension, the nurse should encourage the client to remain in which position?
1. Squatting
2. Left lateral
3. Tailor sitting
4. Semi-Fowler's

204. After a precipitous delivery, the nurse notes that the new mother is passive and only touches her newborn infant briefly with her fingertips. The nurse would do which of the following to help the woman process what has happened?
1. Encourage the mother to breast-feed soon after birth.
2. Support the mother in her reaction to the newborn infant.
3. Tell the mother that it is important to hold the newborn infant.
6. Document a complete account of the mother's reaction in the birth record.

205. A primigravida's membranes rupture spontaneously. The nurse's first action is to:
1. Determine the fetal heart rate.
2. Prepare for immediate delivery.
3. Monitor the contraction pattern.
4. Note the amount, color, and odor of the amniotic fluid.

206. After the client vaginally delivers a viable newborn, the nurse sees the umbilical cord lengthen and observes a spurt of blood from the vagina. The nurse recognizes these findings as signs of:
1. Uterine atony
2. Placenta previa

3. Abruptio placentae
4. Placental separation

207. The nurse is assigned to assist with caring for a client who has been admitted to the labor unit. The client is 9 cm dilated and is experiencing precipitous labor. A priority nursing action is to:
1. Prepare for an oxytocin infusion.
2. Keep the client in a side-lying position.
3. Prepare the client for epidural anesthesia.
4. Encourage the client to start pushing with the contractions.

208. The client is admitted to the labor suite complaining of painless vaginal bleeding. The nurse assists with the examination of the client, knowing that a routine labor procedure that is contraindicated with this client's situation is:
1. Leopold's maneuvers
2. A manual pelvic examination
3. Hemoglobin and hematocrit evaluation
4. External electronic fetal heart rate monitoring

209. The nurse is assigned to assist with caring for a client with abruptio placentae who is experiencing vaginal bleeding. The nurse collects data from the client, knowing that abruptio placenta is accompanied by which additional finding?
1. Soft abdomen on palpation
2. Uterine tenderness on palpation
3. No complaints of abdominal pain
4. Lack of uterine irritability or tetanic contractions

210. The nurse is assigned to work in the delivery room and is assisting with caring for a client who has just delivered a newborn infant. The nurse is monitoring for signs of placental separation, knowing that which of the following indicates that the placenta has separated?
1. A change in the uterine contour
2. Sudden and sharp abdominal pain
3. A shortening of the umbilical cord
4. A decrease in blood loss from the introitus

211. The nurse is assisting with caring for a client with abruptio placenta. While caring for the client, the nurse notes that the client begins to develop signs of shock. The nurse would first:
1. Monitor the urinary output.
2. Monitor the maternal pulse.
3. Turn the client onto her side.
4. Monitor the maternal blood pressure.

212. The client who is being prepared for a cesarean delivery is brought to the delivery room. To

maintain the optimal perfusion of oxygenated blood to the fetus, the nurse places the client in the:
1. Prone position
2. Semi-Fowler's position
3. Trendelenburg's position
4. Supine position with a wedge under the right hip

213. A woman in active labor has contractions every 2 to 3 minutes that last for 45 seconds. The fetal heart rate between contractions is 100 beats per minute. On the basis of these findings, the priority nursing intervention is to:
1. Monitor the maternal vital signs.
2. Notify the registered nurse (RN) immediately.
3. Continue monitoring labor and the fetal heart rate.
4. Encourage relaxation and breathing techniques between contractions.

214. The nurse is assigned to assist with caring for a client who is being admitted to the birthing center in early labor. On admission, the nurse would initially:
1. Estimate the fetal size.
2. Check pelvic adequacy.
3. Administer an analgesic.
4. Determine the maternal and fetal vital signs.

215. The nurse is collecting data from a client who has been diagnosed with placenta previa. Choose the findings that the nurse would expect to note. **Select all that apply.**
❏ 1. Uterine rigidity
❏ 2. Uterine tenderness
❏ 3. Severe abdominal pain
❏ 4. Bright red vaginal bleeding
❏ 5. Soft, relaxed, nontender uterus

ANSWERS

201. 1
Rationale: The nurse should first determine the baseline fetal heart rate. Although options 2, 3, and 4 are components of the data collection process, the fetal heart rate is the priority.
Test-Taking Strategy: Note the strategic word "first." Use the ABCs—airway, breathing, and circulation—when selecting an answer. Fetal heart rate reflects the use of the ABCs. Review the care of the client in labor if you had difficulty with this question.
Level of Cognitive Ability: Applying
Client Needs: Physiological Integrity
Integrated Process: Nursing Process/Implementation
Content Area: Maternity/Intrapartum
References: Christensen, Kockrow, p. 819. 2011. *Foundations of nursing.*
Leifer, 2011. pp. 132–133, 140.

202. 4
Rationale: Leopold's maneuvers comprise a systematic method for palpating the fetus through the maternal abdominal wall. Options 1, 2, and 3 are incorrect.
Test-Taking Strategy: Knowledge of the purpose of and procedure for Leopold's maneuvers is required to answer this question. Visualizing this procedure will assist with directing you to the correct option. Review Leopold's maneuvers if you had difficulty with this question.
Level of Cognitive Ability: Understanding
Client Needs: Physiological Integrity
Integrated Process: Nursing Process/Data Collection
Content Area: Maternity/Intrapartum
Reference: Leifer, pp. 47, 131. 2011.

203. 2
Rationale: Pressure from the enlarged uterus on the aorta and the vena cava when the woman is supine can result in hypotension. This can be relieved by having the woman lie on her left side. Options 1, 3, and 4 are incorrect because they would not prevent hypotension.
Test-Taking Strategy: Use the process of elimination and your knowledge of the anatomy of the pregnant uterus and the physiological response caused by pressure on the large abdominal vessels. Note that options 1, 3, and 4 are all comparable or alike in that the client would be upright. Review nursing measures for the hypotensive pregnant client if you had difficulty with this question.
Level of Cognitive Ability: Applying
Client Needs: Physiological Integrity
Integrated Process: Nursing Process/Implementation
Content Area: Maternity/Intrapartum
Reference: Leifer, p. 53. 2011.

204. 2
Rationale: Women who have experienced precipitous labor and delivery often describe feelings of disbelief that their labor has progressed so rapidly. To assist the woman with understanding what has happened, it is best to support the mother in her reaction to the newborn infant. Options 1, 3, and 4 do not acknowledge the mother's feelings.
Test-Taking Strategy: Use therapeutic communication techniques. Option 2 is the only choice that acknowledges the mother's feelings. Review the care of the mother after a precipitous birth if you had difficulty with this question.
Level of Cognitive Ability: Applying
Client Needs: Psychosocial Integrity
Integrated Process: Caring
Content Area: Maternity/Intrapartum
Reference: Christensen, Kockrow, pp. 834–836. 2011. *Foundations of nursing.*

205. 1
Rationale: When the membranes rupture, the nurse immediately assesses the fetal heart rate to detect changes associated

with prolapse or the compression of the umbilical cord. Monitoring the contraction pattern and noting the amount, color, and odor of the amniotic fluid may be performed, but these would not be the first actions. There is no information in the question that indicates the need to prepare the client for immediate delivery.

Test-Taking Strategy: Note the strategic word "first." Use the ABCs—airway, breathing, and circulation. Fetal heart rate is associated with fetal circulation. Review the initial nursing interventions when the membranes rupture if you had difficulty with this question.

Level of Cognitive Ability: Applying
Client Needs: Physiological Integrity
Integrated Process: Nursing Process/Implementation
Content Area: Maternity/Intrapartum
References: Christensen, Kockrow, p. 835. 2011. *Foundations of nursing.*
Leifer, p. 129. 2011.

206. 4

Rationale: As the placenta separates, it settles downward into the lower uterine segment, the umbilical cord lengthens, and a sudden trickle or spurt of blood appears. The clinical manifestations identified in the question are not related to options 1, 2, and 3.

Test-Taking Strategy: Use the process of elimination. Note that options 1, 2, and 3 are comparable or alike in that they represent complications associated with pregnancy. Option 4 indicates a normal finding after the vaginal delivery of the newborn. Review this stage of labor if you had difficulty with this question.

Level of Cognitive Ability: Understanding
Client Needs: Physiological Integrity
Integrated Process: Nursing Process/Data Collection
Content Area: Maternity/Intrapartum
Reference: Leifer, p. 146. 2011.

207. 2

Rationale: Precipitous labor progresses quickly, with frequent contractions and short periods of relaxation between them. This does not allow for the maximal reperfusion of the placenta with oxygenated blood. Priority care of this client includes the promotion of fetal oxygenation. A side-lying position can assist with providing blood flow to the uterus by preventing vena cava and abdominal aorta compression. Further stimulation with oxytocin is contraindicated. There may not be enough time to administer epidural anesthesia before delivery with such quick progression. Pushing with contractions is not indicated, especially with this type of labor. The controlled delivery of the fetus is essential to prevent maternal and fetal injury.

Test-Taking Strategy: Note the strategic words "precipitous" and "priority." Use the ABCs—airway, breathing, and circulation—and consider the baby's as well as the mother's needs. Option 2 will promote fetal oxygenation. Review the care of the client with precipitous labor if you had difficulty with this question.

Level of Cognitive Ability: Applying
Client Needs: Physiological Integrity
Integrated Process: Nursing Process/Implementation
Content Area: Maternity/Intrapartum
Reference: Leifer, pp. 53, 137. 2011.

208. 2

Rationale: Painless vaginal bleeding is a sign of possible placenta previa. Digital examination of the cervix is contraindicated because it can lead to maternal and fetal hemorrhage. Leopold's maneuvers can reveal a nonengaged presenting part or malpresentation, both of which often accompany placenta previa because of the placenta filling the lower uterine segment. Hemoglobin and hematocrit values help estimate the amount of blood loss. External electronic fetal monitoring is crucial for evaluating the status of the fetus, which is at risk for severe hypoxia. Options 1, 3, and 4 are procedures that would not place the client at further risk.

Test-Taking Strategy: Use the process of elimination, and note the strategic word "contraindicated." Option 2 is the only procedure that is invasive to the pregnancy and that endangers the physiological safety of the client and fetus. Review the care of the client with placenta previa if you had difficulty with this question.

Level of Cognitive Ability: Analyzing
Client Needs: Physiological Integrity
Integrated Process: Nursing Process/Data Collection
Content Area: Maternity/Intrapartum
Reference: Leifer, pp. 88–90. 2011.

209. 2

Rationale: Vaginal bleeding in a pregnant client is most often caused by placenta previa or a placental abruption. Uterine tenderness accompanies abruptio placentae, especially with a central abruption and trapped blood behind the placenta. The abdomen will feel hard and boardlike on palpation as the blood penetrates the myometrium and causes uterine irritability. A sustained tetanic contraction can occur if the client is in labor and the uterine muscle cannot relax.

Test-Taking Strategy: Note the subject of the question, abruptio placentae. It can be easy to confuse a placenta previa and abruption. Remember, the difference involves the presence of uterine pain and tenderness with an abruptio placenta as opposed to painless bleeding with a placenta previa. Options 1, 3, and 4 describe the absence of a sign or symptom of abruptio placentae, whereas option 2 is the only one that describes the presence of one. Review the signs of abruptio placentae if you had difficulty with this question.

Level of Cognitive Ability: Understanding
Client Needs: Physiological Integrity
Integrated Process: Nursing Process/Data Collection
Content Area: Maternity/Intrapartum
References: Christensen, Kockrow, pp. 892–893. 2011. *Foundations of nursing.*
Leifer. p. 90. 2011.

210. 1

Rationale: Signs of placental separation include the lengthening of the umbilical cord, a sudden gush of dark blood from the introitus, a firmly contracted uterus, and the uterus changing from a discoid to a globular shape. The client may experience vaginal fullness but not sudden and sharp abdominal pain.

Test-Taking Strategy: Use the process of elimination. Thinking about what one would expect to occur when the placenta separates will assist you to eliminate options 3 and 4. Option 2 is eliminated because of the words "sudden and sharp." Review

the signs of placental separation if you had difficulty with this question.
Level of Cognitive Ability: Understanding
Client Needs: Physiological Integrity
Integrated Process: Nursing Process/Data Collection
Content Area: Maternity/Intrapartum
Reference: Leifer, p. 146. 2011.

211. 3
Rationale: With a pregnant client who is in shock, the nurse would want to increase perfusion to the placenta. A simple way to do this that requires no equipment is to turn the mother on her side. This would increase blood flow to the placenta by relieving pressure from the gravid uterus on the great vessels. The nurse would immediately contact the registered nurse, who would then contact the health care provider. The other options would follow quickly.
Test-Taking Strategy: Note the strategic word "first." Eliminate options 2 and 4, because they are comparable or alike. Recalling that positioning will affect the status of blood flow will assist with directing you to option 3 from the remaining options. Review the care of the pregnant client in shock if you had difficulty with this question.
Level of Cognitive Ability: Applying
Client Needs: Physiological Integrity
Integrated Process: Nursing Process/Implementation
Content Area: Critical Care
Reference: McKinney, James, Murray, Ashwill, p. 692. 2009.

212. 4
Rationale: Vena cava and descending aorta compression by the pregnant uterus impede blood return from the lower trunk and extremities, thereby decreasing cardiac return, cardiac output, and blood flow to the uterus and subsequently to the fetus. The best position to prevent this would be side-lying, with the uterus displaced off the abdominal vessels. Positioning for abdominal surgery necessitates a supine position; however, a wedge placed under the right hip provides for the displacement of the uterus. A prone or semi-Fowler's position is not practical for this type of abdominal surgery. Trendelenburg's position places pressure from the pregnant uterus on the diaphragm and lungs, thus decreasing respiratory capacity and oxygenation.
Test-Taking Strategy: Note the strategic words "maintain the optimal perfusion." Use the process of elimination, and visualize each of the positions and their effect on the fetus. Review client positioning if you had difficulty with this question.
Level of Cognitive Ability: Applying
Client Needs: Physiological Integrity
Integrated Process: Nursing Process/Implementation
Content Area: Maternity/Intrapartum
References: Leifer, p. 209. 2011.
McKinney, James, Murray, Ashwill, pp. 400, 448. 2009.

213. 2
Rationale: Fetal bradycardia between contractions may indicate the need for immediate medical management. The nurse

would immediately contact the RN, who would then contact the health care provider. Options 1, 3, and 4 will delay necessary and immediate interventions.
Test-Taking Strategy: Use the ABCs—airway, breathing, and circulation. Note that the woman is in active labor and the fetal heart rate is below normal. It is imperative that the circulation in the fetus be restored to normal limits. Review the care of the client in active labor if you had difficulty with this question.
Level of Cognitive Ability: Applying
Client Needs: Physiological Integrity
Integrated Process: Nursing Process/Implementation
Content Area: Maternity/Intrapartum
References: Christensen, Kockrow, p. 822. 2011. *Foundations of nursing.*
Leifer. p. 133. 2011.
McKinney, James, Murray, Ashwill, p. 398. 2009.

214. 4
Rationale: To evaluate a woman's physical well-being, her temperature, pulse, respirations, and blood pressure (as well as the fetal heartbeat) are checked. Option 3 is incorrect, because it would be too premature for an analgesic; medication given too early tends to slow or stop labor contractions. Options 1 and 2 are incorrect. These assessments should be performed by the health care provider during prenatal visits.
Test-Taking Strategy: Note the strategic word "initially," and use the ABCs—airway, breathing, and circulation; this will direct you to the correct option. Remember, measuring the vital signs is the priority. Review the care of the client in labor if you had difficulty with this question.
Level of Cognitive Ability: Applying
Client Needs: Physiological Integrity
Integrated Process: Nursing Process/Implementation
Content Area: Maternity/Intrapartum
Reference: McKinney, James, Murray, Ashwill, pp. 355, 361. 2009.

215. 4, 5
Rationale: Painless bright red vaginal bleeding during the second or third trimester of pregnancy is a sign of placenta previa. The client will have a soft and relaxed nontender uterus. In clients with abruptio placentae, severe abdominal pain is present. Uterine tenderness accompanies placental abruption. Additionally, with abruptio placentae, the abdomen will feel hard and boardlike on palpation as the blood penetrates the myometrium and causes uterine irritability.
Test-Taking Strategy: Remember that the difference between placenta previa and abruptio placentae involves the presence of uterine pain and tenderness with an abruption as opposed to painless bleeding with a previa. Review the signs of placenta previa and abruptio placentae if you had difficulty with this question.
Level of Cognitive Ability: Analyzing
Client Needs: Physiological Integrity
Integrated Process: Nursing Process/Data Collection
Content Area: Maternity/Intrapartum
Reference: Leifer, pp. 89–90. 2011.

The Postpartum Period and Associated Complications

I. POSTPARTUM

A. Description: Period when the reproductive tract returns to the normal, nonpregnant state

B. Postpartum period: Starts immediately after **delivery** and is usually completed by week 6 after **delivery**

II. PHYSIOLOGICAL MATERNAL CHANGES

A. Involution (Figure 24-1)

1. Description
   a. The rapid decrease in the size of the uterus as it returns to the nonpregnant state
   b. Clients who breast-feed may experience a more rapid involution due to the release of oxytocin during breast-feeding.
2. Data collection
   a. Weight of the uterus decreases from 2 lb to 2 oz in 6 weeks
   b. Endometrium regenerates
   c. Fundus steadily descends into the pelvis. The fundal height decreases about one fingerbreadth (1 cm) per day.
   d. By 10 days postpartum, the uterus cannot be palpated abdominally.
   e. A flaccid fundus indicates uterine atony and should be massaged until firm.
   f. A tender fundus indicates an infection.
   g. Afterpains decrease in frequency after the first few days.

B. **Lochia** (Figure 24-2)

1. Description: Discharge from the uterus that consists of blood from the vessels of the placental site and debris from the decidua
2. Data collection
   a. Rubra: Bright red discharge that occurs from **delivery** day to day 3 postpartum
   b. Serosa: Brownish-pink discharge that occurs from days 4 to 10 postpartum
   c. Alba: White discharge that occurs from days 11 to 14 postpartum
   d. Normally the discharge smells like normal menstrual flow

   e. Discharge decreases daily in amount
   f. Discharge increases with ambulation

⚠ To determine most accurately the amount of lochial flow, weigh the perineal pad before and after use and identify the amount of time between pad changes.

C. Cervix: Cervical involution occurs. After 1 week, the muscle begins to regenerate.

D. Vagina: Vaginal distention decreases, although muscle tone is never restored completely to the pregravid state.

E. Ovarian function and menstruation
1. Ovarian function depends on the rapidity with which pituitary function is restored.
2. Menstrual flow resumes within 1 to 2 months in non–breast-feeding mothers.
3. Menstrual flow usually resumes within 3 to 6 months in breast-feeding mothers.
4. Breast-feeding mothers may experience amenorrhea during the entire period of lactation.

⚠ Woman may ovulate without menstruating, so breast-feeding should not be considered a form of birth control.

F. Breasts
1. Breasts continue to secrete colostrum for the first 48 to 72 hours after **delivery**.
2. A decrease of estrogen and progesterone levels after **delivery** stimulates increased prolactin levels, which promote breast milk production.
3. Breasts become distended with milk on the third day.
4. Engorgement occurs on approximately day 4 in non–breast-feeding mothers; breast-feeding will relieve engorgement.
5. The non–breast-feeding mother should avoid nipple stimulation. She can also apply a breast binder, wear a tight-fitting bra, apply ice packs, or take a mild analgesic to relieve the discomfort of engorgement, which usually resolves within 24 to 36 hours after it begins.
6. Breast-feeding relieves engorgement.

▲ **FIGURE 24-1** Involution of the uterus. The height of uterine fundus decreases by approximately 1 cm/day. (From McKinney, E., James, S., Murray, S., & Ashwill, J. [2009]. *Maternal-child nursing* [3rd ed.]. Philadelphia: Saunders).

Scant: <2.5-cm (1-inch) stain

Light: 2.5- to 10-cm (1- to 4-inch) stain

Moderate: 10- to 15-cm (4- to 6-inch) stain

Heavy: Saturated in 1 hour

▲ **FIGURE 24-2** Guidelines for assessing the amount of lochia on the perineal pad. (From McKinney, E., James, S., Murray, S., & Ashwill, J. [2009]. *Maternal-child nursing* [3rd ed.]. Philadelphia: Saunders).

G. Urinary tract
  1. May have urinary retention because of a loss of elasticity, tone, and sensation in the bladder from trauma, medications, anesthesia, and lack of privacy
  2. Diuresis usually begins within the first 12 hours after **delivery**.

H. Gastrointestinal tract
  1. Women are usually very hungry after **delivery**.
  2. Constipation can occur (bowel movement usually occurs by the second or third postpartum day).
  3. Hemorrhoids are common.

I. Vital signs (Table 24-1)

TABLE 24-1 Normal Postpartum Vital Signs

Vital Sign	Description
Temperature	May rise to 100.4° F as a result of the dehydrating effects of labor; any higher elevation may be caused by infection and must be reported
Pulse	May decrease to 50 beats per minute (normal puerperal bradycardia); a pulse rate of >100 beats per minute may indicate excessive blood loss or infection
Blood pressure	Should be normal; suspect hypovolemia if it decreases
Respirations	Rarely changes; if respirations increase significantly, suspect pulmonary embolism, uterine atony, or hemorrhage

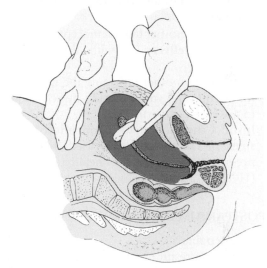

▲ **FIGURE 24-3** Palpating the fundus of the uterus during the fourth stage of labor. Note that the upper hand is cupped over the fundus; the lower hand dips in above the symphysis pubis and supports the uterus while it is massaged gently. (From Lowdermilk, D., & Perry, S. [2009]. *Maternity nursing* [8th ed.]. St. Louis: Mosby).

III. POSTPARTUM INTERVENTIONS

A. Data collection
  1. Monitor the vital signs.
  2. Monitor pain level.
  3. Monitor the height, consistency, and location of the fundus (Figure 24-3).
  4. Monitor the color, amount, and odor of the **lochia**.
  5. Check the breasts for engorgement.
  6. Monitor the perineum for swelling or discoloration.
  7. Check the episiotomy for healing.
  8. Check the incisions or dressings of the cesarean birth client.
  9. Monitor the intake and output (I&O).
  10. Monitor the bowel status.

11. Encourage frequent voiding.
12. Encourage ambulation.
13. Check the extremities for thrombophlebitis (redness, tenderness, or warmth of legs).
14. $Rh_0(D)$ immune globulin (RhoGAM) is prescribed to be administered within 72 hours postpartum to the Rh-negative client who has given birth to an Rh-positive neonate.
15. Monitor parent–**newborn** bonding.
16. Monitor the mother's emotional status.

B. Client teaching
1. Demonstrate **newborn** care skills as necessary.
2. Provide the opportunity for the mother to bathe the **newborn**.
3. Instruct the mother regarding feeding technique.
4. Instruct the mother to avoid heavy lifting for at least 3 weeks.
5. Instruct the mother to plan at least one rest period per day.
6. Instruct the mother that contraception should begin after **delivery** or with the initiation of intercourse.
7. Instruct the mother regarding the importance of follow-up care, which should be scheduled at 4 to 6 weeks postpartum.
8. Instruct the mother to report immediately any signs of chills, fever, increased **lochia**, or depressed feelings to the health care provider (HCP).

IV. POSTPARTUM DISCOMFORTS

A. Afterbirth pains
1. Occur as a result of contractions of the uterus
2. Are more common among multiparas, breast-feeding mothers, clients treated with oxytocin (Pitocin), and clients who had an overdistended uterus during pregnancy (e.g., those who carried twins).

B. Perineal discomfort
1. Apply ice packs to the perineum, as prescribed, during the first 24 hours to reduce swelling.
2. After the first 24 hours, apply warmth by sitz baths, as prescribed.

C. Episiotomy
1. Instruct the client to administer perineal care after each voiding.
2. Encourage the use of analgesic spray, as prescribed.
3. Administer analgesics, as prescribed, if comfort measures are unsuccessful.

D. Perineal lacerations
1. Care as for an episiotomy. Administer perineal care and use analgesic spray and analgesics for comfort.
2. Rectal suppositories and enemas may be contraindicated (to avoid injury to sutures).

E. Breast discomfort from engorgement
1. Encourage the wearing of a support bra at all times, even while sleeping.
2. Encourage the use of ice packs if the client is not breast-feeding.
3. Encourage the use of warm soaks before feeding for the breast-feeding mother.
4. Administer analgesics, as prescribed, if comfort measures are unsuccessful.

F. Constipation
1. Encourage adequate intake of fluids (2000 mL/day).
2. Encourage a diet high in fiber.
3. Encourage ambulation.
4. Administer stool softener, laxative, enema, or suppository if needed and prescribed.

G. Postpartum depression (Box 24-1)
1. Acknowledge the client's feelings and demonstrate a caring attitude.
2. Determine availability of family support and other support systems and assist the client to verbalize her feelings.
3. Monitor the **newborn** for appropriate growth and development expectations.
4. Assist significant other and other appropriate family members to discuss feelings and identify ways to assist client.

⚠ All clients should be assessed for depression during pregnancy and in the postpartum period.

V. NUTRITIONAL COUNSELING

A. Discuss caloric intake for breast-feeding and non–breast-feeding mothers.
B. Nutritional needs depend on prepregnancy weight, ideal weight for height, and whether the mother is breast-feeding (check the HCP's prescription).

Box 24-1 Signs and Symptoms of Postpartum Depression

Anxiety
Appetite changes
Crying, sadness
Difficulty concentrating or making decisions
Fatigue, unable to sleep
Feelings of guilt
Irritability and agitation
Lack of energy
Less responsive to the infant
Loss of pleasure in normal activities
Suicide thoughts

Adapted from McKinney, E., James, S., Murray, S., & Ashwill, J. (2009). *Maternal-child nursing* (3rd ed., p. 712). St. Louis: Saunders.

C. If the mother is breast-feeding, calorie needs increase by approximately 200 to 500 cal/day, and the mother may require increased fluids and the continuance of prenatal vitamins and minerals.

VI. BREAST-FEEDING

A. Interventions
1. Put the baby to the mother's breast as soon as the mother's and baby's conditions are stable (on the **delivery** table, if possible).
2. Stay with the mother each time she nurses until she feels secure and confident with the baby and her feelings.
3. Monitor LATCH (L = latch achieved by **infant**; A = audible swallowing; T = type of nipple; C = comfort of mother; H = help given to mother with nursing).
4. Uterine cramping may occur during the first day after **delivery** while the mother is nursing, when oxytocin stimulation causes the uterus to contract.
5. Use general hygiene and wash the breasts once daily.
6. If engorgement occurs, have the mother breast-feed frequently, apply warm packs before feeding, apply ice packs after feedings, and massage the breasts.
7. The mother should not use soap on the breasts, because it tends to remove natural oils, which increases the chance of cracked nipples.
8. If cracked nipples develop, expose the nipples to air for 10 to 20 minutes after feeding, rotate the position of the baby for each feeding, and be sure that the baby is latched on to the areola and not just the nipple.
9. Bra should be well fitted, supportive, and non-underwire.
10. Breasts may leak between feedings or during coitus. Place a breast pad in the bra.
11. Calories should be increased by 200 to 500 cal/day, and the diet should include additional fluids. Prenatal vitamins should be taken, as prescribed.
12. Baby's stools are usually light yellow, seedy, watery, and frequent.
13. Medications, including over-the-counter medications, need to be avoided, unless prescribed because they may be unsafe when breast-feeding.
14. Gas-producing foods and caffeine should be limited.
15. Hormonal contraceptives may cause a decrease in the milk supply and are best avoided during the first 6 weeks after birth.
16. Oral contraceptives that contain estrogen are not recommended for breast-feeding mothers. Progestin-only birth control pills are less likely to interfere with the milk supply.
17. The baby will develop his or her own feeding schedule.

B. Breast-feeding procedure for mother (Box 24-2)

VII. CYSTITIS

A. Description: Infection of the bladder
B. Data collection and interventions: Refer to Chapter 53 for information.

⚠ If cystitis is suspected, obtain a urine specimen for culture and sensitivity before initiating antibiotic therapy.

VIII. HEMATOMA

A. Description
1. Localized collection of blood into the tissues of the reproductive sac after **delivery**. Vulvar hematomas are the most common.
2. Predisposing conditions include operative **delivery** with forceps or injury to a blood vessel.
3. Can be a life-threatening condition
B. Data collection
1. Abnormal severe pain
2. Pressure in the perineal area
3. Sensitive, bulging mass in the perineal area with discolored skin
4. Inability to void
5. Decreased hemoglobin and hematocrit levels
6. Signs of shock (e.g., pallor, tachycardia, hypotension) if significant blood loss has occurred
C. Interventions
1. Monitor the vital signs.
2. Monitor the client for abnormal pain, especially when a forceps **delivery** has occurred.
3. Place ice on the hematoma site.
4. Administer analgesics as prescribed.

Box 24-2 Breast-Feeding Procedure for the Mother

Wash the hands and assume a comfortable position.
Start with the breast with which the last feeding ended.
Brush the newborn infant's lower lip with the nipple.
Tickle the lips to have the infant open the mouth wide.
Guide the nipple and the surrounding areola into the infant's mouth.
Listen for audible sucking and swallowing.
After the baby has nursed, release suction by depressing the infant's chin or inserting a clean finger into the infant's mouth.
Burp the infant after the first breast.
Repeat the procedure on the second breast until the infant stops nursing.
Burp the infant again.

5. Monitor the I&O.
6. Encourage fluids and voiding.
7. Prepare for urinary catheterization if the client is unable to void.
8. Administer blood products as prescribed.
9. Monitor for signs of infection, such as increased temperature, pulse rate, and white blood cell (WBC) count.
10. Administer antibiotics as prescribed because infection is common after hematoma formation.
11. Prepare the client for the incision and evacuation of the hematoma, if necessary.

IX. HEMORRHAGE (Box 24-3)

A. Description
1. Bleeding of 500 mL or more after **delivery**
2. Primary cause of maternal mortality that demands prompt recognition and intervention

B. Data collection
1. Early: Hemorrhage occurs during the first 24 hours after **delivery**. Early signs include restlessness and increased pulse rate.
2. Late: Hemorrhage occurs more than 24 hours after **delivery**. A decrease in blood pressure is a later sign of hemorrhage.

C. Interventions
1. Massage the fundus, taking care to not overmassage (Figure 24-4).
2. Remain with the client and ask another nurse to notify the registered nurse (RN), who will then contact the HCP.

3. Monitor the vital signs and fundus every 5 to 15 minutes.
4. Assess and estimate blood loss by pad count.
5. Turn the client to check for pooled blood underneath her.
6. Monitor level of consciousness.
7. Administer fluids, as prescribed, and monitor the I&O.
8. Monitor hemoglobin and hematocrit levels.
9. Maintain asepsis because hemorrhage predisposes infection.

Box 24-3 Postpartum Hemorrhage

Causes
- Uterine atony (poor muscle tone)
- Laceration of the vagina
- Cervix, perineum, or labia hematoma development
- Retained placental fragments

Predisposing Factors
- High parity
- Dystocia
- Prolonged labor
- Operative delivery (cesarean or forceps delivery, intrauterine manipulation)
- Overdistention of the uterus (polyhydramnios, multiple gestation, large neonate)
- Abruptio placentae
- Previous history of postpartum hemorrhage
- Infection
- Placenta previa

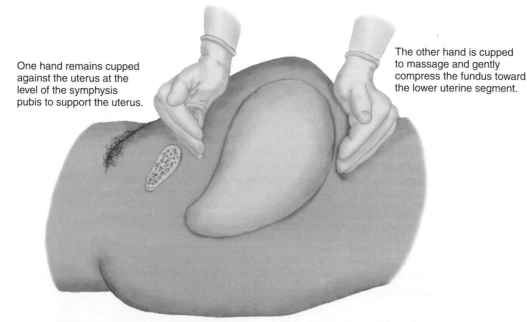

One hand remains cupped against the uterus at the level of the symphysis pubis to support the uterus.

The other hand is cupped to massage and gently compress the fundus toward the lower uterine segment.

▲ **FIGURE 24-4** Technique for fundal massage. One hand remains cupped against the uterus at the level of the symphysis pubis to support the uterus. The other hand is cupped to massage and compress the fundus gently toward the lower uterine segment. (From McKinney, E., James S., Murray, S., & Ashwill, J. [2009] *Maternal child nursing* [3rd ed., p. 697]. St. Louis: Saunders).

10. Prepare for administration of oxytocin (Pitocin) if prescribed.
11. Prepare for administration of IV fluids and blood transfusions if prescribed.

X. INFECTION

A. Description: Any infection of the reproductive organs that occurs within 28 days of **delivery** or abortion.

B. Data collection
   1. Fever
   2. Chills
   3. Anorexia
   4. Pelvic discomfort or pain
   5. Vaginal discharge that is malodorous. Normal vaginal discharge has a fleshy odor or an odor similar to a menstrual period.
   6. Elevated WBC count

⚠ A temperature of 100.4° F is normal during the first 24 hours postpartum because of dehydration; a temperature of 100.4° F or greater after 24 hours postpartum indicates infection.

C. Interventions
   1. Monitor the vital signs and temperature every 2 to 4 hours.
   2. Make the mother as comfortable as possible. Position her for comfort and to promote drainage.
   3. Keep the mother warmed if she is chilled.
   4. Isolate the baby from the mother only if the mother can infect the baby.
   5. Provide a nutritious, high-calorie, high-protein diet.
   6. Encourage fluids to 3000 to 4000 mL/day, if not contraindicated.
   7. Encourage frequent voiding; monitor the I&O.
   8. Monitor culture results if cultures were prescribed.
   9. Administer antibiotics, as prescribed.

XI. MASTITIS

A. Description
   1. Inflammation of the breast as a result of infection
   2. Primarily occurs in breast-feeding mothers 2 to 3 weeks after **delivery** but may occur at any time during lactation

B. Data collection
   1. Localized heat and swelling
   2. Pain; tender axillary lymph nodes
   3. Elevated temperature
   4. Complaints of flulike symptoms

C. Interventions
   1. Instruct the mother in good handwashing and breast hygiene techniques.

2. Promote comfort.
3. Apply heat or cold to the site, as prescribed.
4. Maintain lactation in breast-feeding mothers.
5. Encourage the manual expression of breast milk or the use of a breast pump every 4 hours.
6. Encourage the mother to support the breasts with a supportive, non-underwire bra.
7. Administer analgesics or antibiotics, as prescribed.

XII. PERINATAL LOSS

A. Description
   1. Perinatal loss is associated with miscarriage, neonatal death, stillbirth, and therapeutic abortion.
   2. Loss and grief may also coincide with the birth of a preterm **infant**, an **infant** who has suffered complications, or an **infant** with congenital anomalies. It may also occur within a family who is giving up a child for adoption.

B. Interventions

⚠ Not all interventions are appropriate for every woman and her significant family. It is crucial to consider religious and cultural health care practices and beliefs when planning care for a woman and family who have experienced perinatal loss.

   1. Communicate therapeutically and actively listen, providing parents with time to grieve.
   2. Notify the hospital chaplain or other religious person.
   3. Discuss with the parents about options such as seeing, holding, bathing, and/or dressing the deceased **infant**; visitation by other family members or friends; religious or cultural rituals; and funeral arrangements.
   4. Prepare a special memories box with keepsakes such as footprints, handprints, locks of hair, and pictures.
   5. Admit the mother to a private room. If possible, mark the door to the room with a special card (per agency procedure) that denotes to hospital staff that this family has experienced a loss. See Chapter 23 for additional information on fetal demise.

XIII. PULMONARY EMBOLISM

A. Description: The passage of a thrombus (often originates in one of the uterine or other pelvic veins) into the lungs, where it disrupts the circulation of blood

B. Data collection
   1. Dyspnea, tachypnea, and tachycardia
   2. Congested cough
   3. Hemoptysis

4. Pleuritic chest pain
5. Feeling of impending doom
C. Interventions
1. Administer oxygen, as prescribed.
2. Position the client with the head of the bed elevated.
3. Monitor the vital signs frequently, especially respiratory and heart rate and breath sounds.
4. Monitor for signs of respiratory distress and hypoxemia, such as tachypnea, tachycardia, restlessness, cool and clammy skin, cyanosis, and the use of accessory muscles.
5. Administer intravenous fluids as prescribed.
6. Administer anticoagulants as prescribed.
7. Prepare to assist the HCP to administer medications to dissolve the clot if prescribed.

XIV. SUBINVOLUTION

A. Description: Incomplete involution or the failure of the uterus to return to its normal size and condition
B. Data collection
1. Uterine pain on palpation
2. Uterus is larger than expected.
3. More vaginal bleeding than normal
C. Interventions
1. Monitor the vital signs.
2. Check the uterus and fundus.
3. Monitor for uterine pain and vaginal bleeding.
4. Elevate the legs to promote venous return.
5. Encourage frequent voiding.
6. Monitor the hemoglobin and hematocrit levels.
7. Methylergonovine maleate (Methergine), which provides sustained contraction of the uterus, may be prescribed.

XV. THROMBOPHLEBITIS

A. Description
1. A condition in which a clot forms in a vessel wall as a result of the inflammation of the vessel wall.
2. A partial obstruction of the vessel can occur.
3. Increased blood-clotting factors during the postpartum period place the client at risk.
4. Early ambulation in the postoperative period after cesarean section is a preventive action.
B. Types
1. Superficial thrombophlebitis
2. Femoral thrombophlebitis
3. Pelvic thrombophlebitis
C. Data collection (Box 24-4)
D. Interventions
1. Specific therapies may depend on the location of the thrombophlebitis.

2. Assess the lower extremities for edema, tenderness, varices, and increased skin temperature.
3. Maintain bedrest, if prescribed.
4. Elevate the affected leg.
5. Apply a bed cradle, and keep bedclothes off the affected leg.
6. Never massage the leg.
7. Monitor for manifestations of pulmonary embolism.
8. Apply hot packs or moist heat to the affected site as prescribed to alleviate discomfort.
9. Apply elastic stockings (support hose) if prescribed.
10. Administer analgesics and antibiotics as prescribed.
11. Heparin sodium IV may be prescribed for femoral or pelvic thrombophlebitis to prevent further thrombus formation.
E. Client teaching (Box 24-5)

Box 24-4 Data Collection: Types of Thrombophlebitis

Superficial
- Tenderness and pain in the affected lower extremity
- Warm and pinkish-red color over the thrombus area
- Palpable thrombus that feels bumpy and hard

Femoral
- Chills and fever
- Malaise
- Pain, stiffness, and swelling of the affected leg
- Shiny, white skin over the affected area
- Diminished peripheral pulses

Pelvic
- Severe chills
- Dramatic body temperature changes
- Occurrence of pulmonary embolism may be the first sign

Box 24-5 Client Education for Thrombophlebitis

Avoid crossing the legs.
Avoid prolonged sitting.
Avoid constrictive clothing.
Avoid pressure behind the knees.
Never massage the leg.
Know how to apply elastic stockings (support hose) if prescribed.
Understand the importance of anticoagulant therapy if prescribed.
Understand the importance of follow up with the HCP.

MORE QUESTIONS ON EVOLVE!

Practice Questions

216. The client received epidural anesthesia during labor and had a forceps delivery after pushing for 2 hours. At 6 hours postpartum, the client's systolic blood pressure (BP) dropped 20 points, the diastolic BP dropped 10 points, and her pulse is 120 beats per minute. The client is very anxious and restless. The nurse is told that the client has a vulvar hematoma. On the basis of this diagnosis, the nurse would plan to:
1. Reassure the client.
2. Apply perineal pressure.
3. Monitor the fundal height.
4. Prepare the client for surgery.

217. The nurse is assigned to care for the client after a cesarean section. To prevent thrombophlebitis, the nurse encourages the woman to take which priority action?
1. Ambulate frequently.
2. Wear support stockings.
3. Apply warm, moist packs to the legs.
4. Remain on bedrest, with the legs elevated.

218. A postpartum client is getting ready for discharge. The nurse suspects that the client is in need of further teaching related to breast-feeding when she states:
1. "I don't need birth control since I will be breast-feeding."
2. "I need to increase my caloric intake by 500 calories a day."
3. "I shouldn't use soap to wash my breasts since I will be breast-feeding."
4. "I need to be sure that I increase my fluid intake and take my prenatal vitamins while breast-feeding."

219. The nurse is caring for a postpartum client with a diagnosis of thrombophlebitis. The client suddenly complains of chest pain and dyspnea. The nurse would initially check the:
1. Vital signs
2. Fundal height
3. Presence of calf pain
4. Level of consciousness (LOC)

220. The nurse suspects that the client has a pulmonary embolism. The most important nursing action is to:
1. Monitor the vital signs.
2. Elevate the head of the bed.
3. Increase the intravenous flow rate.
4. Administer oxygen by face mask, as prescribed.

221. The nurse notes that the 4-hour postpartum client has cool, clammy skin and that she is restless and excessively thirsty. The nurse immediately notifies the registered nurse and then:
1. Checks the vital signs
2. Begins fundal massage
3. Encourages ambulation
4. Encourages the client to drink fluids

222. The nurse is assisting with caring for a postpartum client who is experiencing uterine hemorrhage. When planning to meet the psychosocial needs of the client, the nurse would:
1. Maintain strict bedrest.
2. Monitor the vital signs every 2 hours.
3. Perform firm fundal massage every 2 hours.
4. Keep the client and her family members informed of her progress.

223. The nurse palpates the fundus and checks the character of the lochia of a postpartum client who is in the fourth stage of labor. The nurse expects the lochia to be:
1. Red
2. Pink
3. White
4. Serosanguineous

224. After episiotomy and the delivery of a newborn, the nurse performs a perineal check on the mother. The nurse notes a trickle of bright red blood coming from the perineum. The nurse checks the fundus and notes that it is firm. The nurse determines that:
1. This is a normal expectation after episiotomy.
2. The mother should be allowed bathroom privileges only.
3. The bright red bleeding is abnormal and should be reported.
4. The perineal assessment should be performed more frequently.

225. The nurse is assigned to care for the client during the postpartum period. The client asks the nurse what the term *involution* means. The nurse responds to the client, knowing that involution is:
1. The inverted uterus returning to normal
2. The gradual reversal of the uterine muscle into the abdominal cavity
3. The descent of the uterus into the pelvic cavity, which occurs at a rate of 2 cm/day
4. The progressive descent of the uterus into the pelvic cavity, which occurs at a rate of approximately 1 cm/day

226. A mother is breast-feeding her newborn baby and experiences breast engorgement. The nurse

encourages the mother to do which of the following to provide relief of the engorgement?
1. Breast-feed only during the daytime hours.
2. Apply cold compresses to the breast before feeding.
3. Avoid the use of a bra while the breasts are engorged.
4. Massage the breasts before feeding to stimulate let-down.

227. After delivery, the nurse checks the height of the uterine fundus. The nurse expects that the position of the fundus would most likely be noted:
1. To the right of the abdomen
2. At the level of the umbilicus
3. About 4 cm above the level of the umbilicus
4. One fingerbreadth above the symphysis pubis

228. The nurse is caring for a postpartum client. At 4 hours postpartum, the client's temperature is 102° F (38.9° C). The appropriate nursing action would be to:
1. Apply cool packs to the abdomen.
2. Continue to monitor the temperature.
3. Remove the blanket from the client's bed.

4. Notify the registered nurse, who will then contact the health care provider (HCP).

229. The nurse is assisting with planning care for a postpartum woman who has small vulvar hematomas. To assist with reducing the swelling, the nurse should:
1. Check the vital signs every 4 hours.
2. Measure the fundal height every 4 hours.
3. Prepare a heat pack for application to the area.
4. Prepare an ice pack for application to the area.

230. The nurse is preparing a list of self-care instructions for a postpartum client who has been diagnosed with mastitis. Choose the instructions that would be included on the list. **Select all that apply.**
☐ 1. Wear a supportive, non-underwire bra.
☐ 2. Rest during the acute phase.
☐ 3. Maintain a fluid intake of at least 3000 mL.
☐ 4. Continue to breast-feed if the breasts are not too sore.
☐ 5. Take the prescribed antibiotics until the soreness subsides.
☐ 6. Avoid decompression of the breasts by breast-feeding or breast pump.

ANSWERS

216. 4

Rationale: The information provided in the question indicates that the client is experiencing blood loss. Surgery would be indicated for this complication to stop the bleeding. Options 1, 2, and 3 would not assist with controlling the bleeding in this emergency situation.
Test-Taking Strategy: Focus on the information provided in the question and note that the client has a vulvar hematoma. Note that the signs and symptoms in the question indicate the presence of bleeding; this should direct you to the correct option. Review the nursing interventions related to vulvar hematomas if you had difficulty with this question.
Level of Cognitive Ability: Analyzing
Client Needs: Physiological Integrity
Integrated Process: Nursing Process/Planning
Content Area: Maternity/Postpartum
References: Leifer, p. 239. 2011.
McKinney, James, Murray, Ashwill, p. 698. 2009.

217. 1

Rationale: Stasis is believed to be a major predisposing factor for the development of thrombophlebitis. Because cesarean delivery poses a risk factor, the client should ambulate early and frequently to promote circulation and prevent stasis. Options 2, 3, and 4 are implemented if thrombophlebitis occurs.
Test-Taking Strategy: Focus on the subject of the question, the prevention of thrombophlebitis, and note the strategic word "priority." Options 3 and 4 are implemented if thrombophlebitis occurs. Although wearing support stockings may be

prescribed in the postoperative period to promote venous return, ambulating frequently (option 1) is the priority preventive measure. Review the content related to the prevention of thrombophlebitis during the postoperative period if you had difficulty with this question.
Level of Cognitive Ability: Applying
Client Needs: Physiological Integrity
Integrated Process: Nursing Process/Implementation
Content Area: Maternity/Postpartum
Reference: Leifer, p. 210. 2011.

218. 1

Rationale: Amenorrhea may occur during breast-feeding, but the client can still ovulate without menstruating. The use of soap on the breasts is avoided because it tends to remove natural oils, which can lead to cracked nipples. The caloric intake should be increased by 200 to 500 cal/day (per health care provider's prescription), and the diet should include additional fluids and prenatal vitamins, as prescribed.
Test-Taking Strategy: Note the strategic words "need of further teaching." These words indicate a negative event query and the need to select the incorrect statement. Recalling the physiology related to amenorrhea and ovulation during breast-feeding will direct you to the correct option. Review teaching points for the woman who is breast-feeding if you had difficulty answering this question.
Level of Cognitive Ability: Evaluating
Client Needs: Health Promotion and Maintenance
Integrated Process: Teaching and Learning
Content Area: Maternity/Postpartum
Reference: Leifer, p. 266. 2011.

219. 1

Rationale: Pulmonary embolism is a complication of thrombophlebitis. Changes in the vital signs are one of the first things to occur with pulmonary embolism, because pulmonary blood flow is compromised. Fundal height is unrelated to the subject of the question. Calf pain is an indicator of thrombophlebitis. Level of consciousness may change as the condition worsens; worsening would indicate hypoxia.

Test-Taking Strategy: Note the strategic word "initially." Use the ABCs—airway, breathing, and circulation—to direct you to the correct option. Review the complications of thrombophlebitis if you had difficulty with this question.

Level of Cognitive Ability: Applying
Client Needs: Physiological Integrity
Integrated Process: Nursing Process/Data Collection
Content Area: Critical Care
References: Christensen, Kockrow, pp. 913–914. 2011. *Foundations of nursing.*
Leifer, pp. 240–241. 2011.

220. 4

Rationale: Because pulmonary circulation is compromised in the presence of an embolus, cardiorespiratory support is initiated by oxygen administration. Options 1 and 2 may be components of the plan of care, but they are not the most important actions. The nurse would not increase the intravenous rate without a prescription from the health care provider to do so.

Test-Taking Strategy: Note the strategic words "most important," and use the ABCs—airway, breathing, and circulation. This will direct you to the correct option – oxygen is the priority. Review the care of the client in the event of a pulmonary embolism if you had difficulty with this question.

Level of Cognitive Ability: Applying
Client Needs: Physiological Integrity
Integrated Process: Nursing Process/Implementation
Content Area: Critical Care
References: McKinney, James, Murray, Ashwill, p. 705. 2009. Swearingen, p. 127. 2012.

221. 1

Rationale: Symptoms of hypovolemia include cool, clammy, and pale skin; feelings of anxiety and restlessness; and thirst. The nurse would check the vital signs. The nurse would not ambulate the client or encourage fluids until specific prescriptions are given to do so. There is no information in the question to indicate the need for fundal massage.

Test-Taking Strategy: Focus on the symptoms in the question. Use the ABCs—airway, breathing, and circulation—to direct you to the correct option. Review the nursing care of the client with hypovolemia if you had difficulty with this question.

Level of Cognitive Ability: Applying
Client Needs: Physiological Integrity
Integrated Process: Nursing Process/Implementation
Content Area: Critical Care
References: Leifer, p. 236. 2011.
McKinney, James, Murray, Ashwill, p. 701. 2009.

222. 4

Rationale: Keeping the client and her family informed about her condition will help minimize fear and apprehension. Options 1, 2, and 3 identify physiological interventions.

Test-Taking Strategy: Use the process of elimination. Focus on the strategic words "meet the psychosocial needs." Option 4 is the only option that addresses psychosocial needs. Review the interventions that will meet the psychosocial needs of the client if you had difficulty with this question.

Level of Cognitive Ability: Applying
Client Needs: Psychosocial Integrity
Integrated Process: Caring
Content Area: Maternity/Postpartum
Reference: McKinney, James, Murray, Ashwill, p. 700. 2009.

223. 1

Rationale: The color of the lochia during the fourth stage of labor is bright red, and this may last from 1 to 3 days. The color of the lochia then changes to a pinkish brown, and occurs from day 4 to 10 postpartum. Finally, the lochia changes to a creamy white color that occurs from day 10 to 14 postpartum.

Test-Taking Strategy: Focus on the strategic words "fourth stage of labor"; this will direct you to the correct option. In the immediate postpartum period, the lochia is red in color. Review the expected postpartum findings if you had difficulty with this question.

Level of Cognitive Ability: Understanding
Client Needs: Physiological Integrity
Integrated Process: Nursing Process/Data Collection
Content Area: Maternity/Postpartum
Reference: Leifer, pp. 201–202. 2011.

224. 3

Rationale: Lochial flow should be distinguished from bleeding that originates from a laceration or an episiotomy, which is usually brighter red than lochia and presents as a continuous trickle of bleeding, even though the fundus of the uterus is firm. This bright red bleeding is abnormal and needs to be reported. Therefore, the other options are incorrect interpretations.

Test-Taking Strategy: Note the strategic words "trickle" and "bright red." This should be an indication that the flow is not normal. Review the lochial flow and the complications associated with episiotomy if you had difficulty with this question.

Level of Cognitive Ability: Analyzing
Client Needs: Physiological Integrity
Integrated Process: Nursing Process/Data Collection
Content Area: Maternity/Postpartum
References: Christensen, Kockrow, p. 849. 2011. *Foundations of nursing.*
Leifer, p. 202. 2011.

225. 4

Rationale: Involution is the progressive descent of the uterus into the pelvic cavity. After birth, descent occurs at a rate of approximately one fingerbreadth or 1 cm per day. The other options do not accurately describe involution.

Test-Taking Strategy: Use your knowledge of medical terminology to help you to define the word *involution.* This will assist with directing you to the correct option. Review the process of involution if you had difficulty with this question.

Level of Cognitive Ability: Understanding
Client Needs: Health Promotion and Maintenance
Integrated Process: Nursing Process/Implementation
Content Area: Maternity/Postpartum

References: Leifer, pp. 200, 244. 2011.
McKinney, James, Murray, Ashwill, p. 456. 2009.

226. 4

Rationale: Comfort measures for breast engorgement include massaging the breasts before feeding to stimulate let-down, wearing a supportive and well-fitting bra at all times, taking a warm shower or applying warm compresses just before feeding, and alternating breasts during feeding.

Test-Taking Strategy: Use the process of elimination to answer the question. Eliminate option 1 because of the closed-ended word "only." From the remaining options, recalling the self-care measures that promote the comfort of the mother with breast engorgement will direct you to the correct option. Review these measures if you had difficulty with this question.

Level of Cognitive Ability: Applying
Client Needs: Health Promotion and Maintenance
Integrated Process: Nursing Process/Implementation
Content Area: Maternity/Postpartum
References: Leifer, pp. 227–228. 2011.
Perry, Hockenberry, Lowdermilk, Wilson, pp. 696–697. 2010.

227. 2

Rationale: After delivery, the uterine fundus should be at the level of the umbilicus or one to three fingerbreadths below it and in the midline of the abdomen. If the fundus is 4 cm above the umbilicus, this may indicate that there are blood clots in the uterus that need to be expelled by fundal massage. If the fundus is noted to the right of the abdomen, it may indicate a full bladder. By about 10 days postpartum, the uterus will be in the symphysis pubis area.

Test-Taking Strategy: Note the strategic words "after delivery" and visualize the process of involution. Remember that after delivery, the uterine fundus should be at the level of the umbilicus or one to three fingerbreadths below it and in the midline of the abdomen. Review expected postdelivery findings if you had difficulty with this question.

Level of Cognitive Ability: Understanding
Client Needs: Physiological Integrity
Integrated Process: Nursing Process/Data Collection
Content Area: Maternity/Postpartum
Reference: Leifer, p. 201. 2011.

228. 4

Rationale: During the first 24 hours postpartum, the mother's temperature may be elevated as a result of dehydration. However, if the temperature is more than 2° F above normal, this may indicate infection, and the HCP will need to be notified. Applying cool packs to the abdomen is an inappropriate action and additionally, this action requires a prescription. The remaining options may be a component of care but are not the most appropriate based on the data in the question.

Test-Taking Strategy: Use the process of elimination. Focus on the strategic words "4 hours" and "102° F." Noting that this temperature is extreme as compared with the normal temperature will direct you to option 4. Review the expected postpartum findings if you had difficulty with this question.

Level of Cognitive Ability: Applying
Client Needs: Physiological Integrity
Integrated Process: Nursing Process/Implementation
Content Area: Maternity/Postpartum
Reference: Leifer, p. 232. 2011.

229. 4

Rationale: The application of ice will reduce the swelling caused by hematoma formation in the vulvar area. Options 1, 2, and 3 will not reduce swelling.

Test-Taking Strategy: Use the process of elimination. Focus on the subject of the question—the reduction of swelling. This will assist you with eliminating options 1 and 2. Recalling the principles related to heat and cold will direct you to option 4. Review the nursing care of the client with a hematoma if you had difficulty with this question.

Level of Cognitive Ability: Applying
Client Needs: Physiological Integrity
Integrated Process: Nursing Process/Implementation
Content Area: Maternity/Postpartum
Reference: Leifer, pp. 204, 239–240. 2011.

230. 1, 2, 3, 4

Rationale: Mastitis is an infection of the lactating breast. Client instructions include resting during the acute phase, maintaining a fluid intake of at least 3000 mL per day, and taking analgesics to relieve discomfort. Antibiotics may be prescribed and are taken until the complete prescribed course is finished. They are not stopped when the soreness subsides. Additional supportive measures include the use of moist heat or ice packs and the wearing of a supportive bra. Continued decompression of the breast by breast-feeding or breast pump is important to empty the breast and prevent the formation of an abscess.

Test-Taking Strategy: Think about the pathophysiology associated with mastitis. Recalling that supportive measures include rest, moist heat or ice packs, antibiotics, analgesics, increased fluid intake, breast support, and the decompression of the breasts will assist you with answering the question. Review the treatment of mastitis if you had difficulty with this question.

Level of Cognitive Ability: Applying
Client Needs: Physiological Integrity
Integrated Process: Teaching and Learning
Content Area: Maternity/Postpartum
References: Christensen, Kockrow, pp. 901–902. 2011. *Foundations of nursing.*
Leifer, pp. 242–244. 2011.

Care of the Newborn

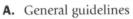

I. INITIAL CARE OF THE NEWBORN

A. Data collection
1. Observe or assist with the initiation of respirations.
2. Determine Apgar score.
3. Note characteristics of cry.
4. Monitor for nasal flaring, grunting, retractions, abnormal respirations, and cyanosis.
5. Obtain vital signs.
6. Observe for signs of hypothermia or hyperthermia.
7. Check for gross anomalies.

B. Interventions
1. Suction the mouth and then the nares with a bulb syringe.
2. Dry the baby and stimulate crying by rubbing.
3. Maintain temperature stability; wrap the baby in warm blankets and place a stockinette cap on the **newborn's** head.
4. Keep the baby with the mother to facilitate bonding.
5. Place the baby at the mother's breast if breast-feeding is planned, or place the baby on the mother's abdomen.
6. Place the baby in a preheated warmer after initial parent–**infant** acquaintance process.
7. Elevate the head of the crib to facilitate the drainage of mucus if mucus is a concern.
8. Ensure proper identification.
9. Footprint the **newborn** on an identification sheet per agency procedures; a security alarm tag may be placed on the newborn.
10. Place matching identification bracelets on the mother and the **newborn.**

C. Apgar scoring system
1. Assess each of the five items to be scored, and add the points assessed for each item to determine the **newborn's** total score.
2. Five vital indicators (Table 25-1)
3. Interventions: Apgar score (Table 25-2)

 The newborn's Apgar score is assessed and recorded at 1 minute and 5 minutes after birth

II. INITIAL PHYSICAL EXAMINATION

A. General guidelines
1. Keep the **newborn** warm during the examination.
2. Begin with general observations; then first perform the assessments that are the least disturbing to the **newborn.**
3. Initiate nursing interventions for abnormal findings and document findings.

B. Vital signs
1. Heart rate: 100 to 160 beats per minute (apical). Check for a full minute because of irregularities after birth, especially with crying.
2. Respirations: 30 to 60 breaths per minute. Check for a full minute.
3. Assess heart rate and respiratory rate first while the **newborn** is resting or sleeping.
4. Axillary temperature: 96.8° to 99° F (36° to 37.2° C)
5. Blood pressure: approximately 73/55 mm Hg

C. Body measurements (approximate)
1. Length: 45 to 55 cm (18 to 22 inches)
2. Weight: 2500 to 4300 g (5.5 to 9.5 pounds)
3. Head circumference: 33 to 35 cm (13.2 to 14 inches)

D. Head
1. One-fourth of the body length (cephalocaudal development)
2. Bones of the skull are not fused.
3. Palpable sutures (connective tissue between the skull bones)
4. Fontanels: Unossified membranous tissue at the junction of the sutures (Table 25-3)
5. Molding: Asymmetry of the head as a result of pressure in the birth canal; disappears in about 72 hours
6. Masses from birth trauma
   a. Caput succedaneum: Edema of the soft tissue over bone (crosses over the suture line); subsides within a few days
   b. Cephalhematoma: Swelling caused by bleeding into an area between the bone and its periosteum (does not cross over the suture line); usually absorbed within 6 weeks with no treatment

7. Head lag
   a. Common when pulling the **newborn** to a sitting position
   b. When prone, the **newborn** should be able to lift the head slightly and turn the head from side to side.
E. Eyes
   1. Slate gray (light skin) or brown gray (dark skin)
   2. Symmetrical and clear
   3. Pupils are equal and round; react to light by accommodation
   4. Blink reflex is present
   5. Eyes cross because of weak extraocular muscles

TABLE 25-1 The Five Vital Indicators of the Apgar Score

Indicator	0 Points	1 Point	2 Points
Heart rate	Absent	Less than 100 beats/minute	More than 100 beats/minute
Respiratory rate	Absent	Slow, irregular, weak cry	Good, vigorous cry
Muscle tone	Flaccid, limp	Minimal flexion of the extremities	Good flexion, active motion
Reflex irritability	No response	Minimal response (grimace) to suction or the gentle slap on the soles	Responds promptly with a cry or active movement
Skin color	Pallor or cyanosis	Body skin color normal, extremities blue	Body and extremity skin color normal

TABLE 25-2 Apgar Score Interventions

Score	Intervention
8-10	No intervention except support the infant's spontaneous efforts
4-7	Gently stimulate Rub the infant's back Administer oxygen to the infant
0-3	Infant requires resuscitation

Note: The newborn's Apgar score obtained at 5 minutes of age reflects the efficacy of any initial resuscitation efforts.

TABLE 25-3 Fontanels

Location	Characteristics	Closure
Anterior	Soft, flat, and diamond-shaped; 5 cm wide by 2-3 cm long	Between the ages of 12 and 18 months
Posterior	Triangular, 0.5-1 cm wide; located between the occipital and parietal bones	Between birth and the age of 2 or 3 months

6. Able to track and fixate momentarily
7. Red reflex is present
8. Eyelids often edematous as a result of pressure during the birth process and the effects of eye medication
F. Ears
   1. Symmetrical
   2. Firm cartilage with recoil
   3. Pinna should be on or above a line drawn from the canthus of the eye.
   4. Low-set ears are associated with Down syndrome
G. Nose
   1. Flat, broad, and located in the center of the face
   2. Obligatory nose breathing
   3. Occasional sneezing to remove obstructions
   4. Nares are patent and should not flare (flaring is an indication of respiratory distress)
H. Mouth
   1. Gums pink and moist
   2. Soft and hard palates intact
   3. Epstein's pearls (small, white cysts) may be present on the hard palate
   4. Uvula in midline
   5. Tongue symmetrical and moves freely, with a short frenulum
   6. Sucking and crying movements are symmetrical
   7. Able to swallow
   8. Root and gag reflexes present

⚠ When assessing the newborn's mouth, look for the presence of thrush [*Candida albicans*], which are white patchy areas on the tongue or gums that cannot be removed with a washcloth; these may be painful.

I. Neck
   1. Short and thick
   2. Head held in midline
   3. Trachea in midline
   4. Good range of motion with flexion and extension
   5. Check for torticollis (head inclined to one side as a result of contraction of muscles on that side of the neck).
J. Chest
   1. Appears circular because anteroposterior and lateral diameters are about equal
   2. Respirations are diaphragmatic—chest and abdomen should rise and fall in synchrony, not in a seesaw pattern.
   3. Bronchial sounds on auscultation
   4. Nipples prominent and often edematous
   5. Milky secretion (witch's milk) possible
   6. Breast tissue present
   7. Clavicles are palpated to check for fractures.
K. Skin
   1. Pinkish red (light-skinned **newborn**) to pinkish brown or pinkish yellow (dark-skinned **newborn**)

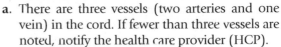

2. Vernix caseosa
3. Lanugo
4. Milia
5. Dry, peeling skin
6. Dark red color is common among premature **newborns**
7. Cyanosis is common with hypothermia, infection, and hypoglycemia and with cardiac, respiratory, or neurological abnormalities
8. Acrocyanosis (peripheral cyanosis) is normal during the first few hours after birth and if the **infant** becomes cold; it results from the poor perfusion of blood to the periphery of the body (Figure 25-1).
9. Check for ecchymosis and petechiae as a result of the trauma of birth.
10. Check the skin turgor over the abdomen to determine hydration status.
11. Observe for forceps marks.
12. Harlequin sign
    a. Deep pink or red color develops over one side of the **newborn's** body while the other side remains pale or of normal color.
    b. May indicate sepsis or a shunting of blood caused by a cardiac problem
13. Birthmarks (Table 25-4)

▲ **FIGURE 25-1** Acrocyanosis. (From McKinney, E., James, S., Murray, S., & Ashwill, J. [2009]. *Maternal-child nursing* [3rd ed.]. St. Louis: Saunders. Courtesy of Todd Shiros, Santa Fe Springs, CA).

L. Abdomen
1. Umbilical cord
    a. There are three vessels (two arteries and one vein) in the cord. If fewer than three vessels are noted, notify the health care provider (HCP).
    b. A small, thin cord may be associated with poor fetal growth
    c. Check for an intact cord, and ensure that the clamp is secured.
    d. The cord should be clamped for at least the first 24 hours after birth. The clamp can be removed when the cord is dried and occluded.
    e. Note any bleeding or drainage from the cord.
    f. Hospital protocol and HCP's preference determine the technique for cord care. Protocols may include antibiotic ointment, triple dye, or cleansing with sterile water or soap and water.
    g. If symptoms of infection (e.g., moistness, oozing, discharge, reddened base) occur, notify the HCP; usually an antibiotic treatment is prescribed.
2. Gastrointestinal
    a. Monitor the cord for meconium staining.
    b. The **newborn** will be checked for the presence of an umbilical hernia.
    c. Note abdominal depression that may be associated with diaphragmatic hernia, an obstruction, a mass, or sepsis.
    d. Check for bowel sounds, which should occur within 1 to 2 hours after birth.
3. Anus
    a. Anal opening is patent.
    b. First stool (meconium) should pass within the first 24 hours.

M. Genitals
1. Female
    a. Labia edematous and clitoris enlarged
    b. Smegma present (thick, white mucus discharge)

TABLE 25-4 Birthmarks

Birthmark	Characteristics	Location	Treatment	Length of Presence
Telangiectatic nevi (stork bites)	Pale pink or red; flat, dilated capillaries Blanch easily More noticeable during crying periods	Eyelids, nose, lower occipital bone, and nape of neck	None	Usually disappear by the age of 2 years
Nevus flammeus (port-wine stain)	Capillary angioma directly below the epidermis Nonelevated; sharply demarcated; red to purple; dense areas of capillaries	Commonly appears on the face	May require surgery in the future	Only removed by surgery; does not fade with time
Nevus vasculosus (strawberry mark)	Capillary hemangioma Raised; clearly delineated; dark red with rough surface	Common in the head region	None	Disappears by the age of 7 to 9 years
Mongolian spots	Bluish-black pigmentation common among Asian and dark-skinned individuals	Lumbar dorsal area and buttocks	None	Gradually fade during the first and second years of life

c. Pseudomenstruation possible (blood-tinged mucus)

d. Hymen tag may be visible.

e. First voiding should occur within 24 hours.

2. Male

a. Prepuce (foreskin) covers glans penis.

b. Scrotum edematous

c. Meatus at tip of penis

d. Testes descended but may retract with cold

e. Check for hernia or hydrocele.

f. First voiding should occur within 24 hours.

N. Spine

1. Straight

2. Posture flexed

3. Supports head momentarily when prone

4. Arms and legs flexed

5. Chin flexed on upper chest

6. Sporadic movements that are well coordinated

7. A degree of hypotonicity or hypertonicity is indicative of central nervous system damage and this finding needs to be reported.

8. Check for hair tufts and dimples along the spinal column (may be indicative of a possible opening).

O. Extremities

1. Flexed

2. Full range of motion and symmetrical movements

3. Fists clenched

4. Should be 10 fingers and 10 toes, all separate

5. Legs bowed

6. Major gluteal folds are even

7. Creases on soles of feet

8. The **newborn** will be checked for fractures (especially clavicle) or dislocations (hip).

9. The **newborn** will be checked for hip dysplasia; when the thighs are rotated outward, no clicks should be heard. (Ortolani's sign and Barlow's sign are two assessment tools that the HCP may use to assess for developmental dysplagia of hip.)

10. Pulses palpable (radial, brachial, and femoral)

⚠ Slight tremors in the newborn may be a common finding, but could also be a sign of hypoglycemia or drug withdrawal.

III. BODY SYSTEMS: DATA COLLECTION AND INTERVENTIONS

A. Cardiovascular system

1. Keep the **newborn** warm.

2. Take the apical heart rate for 1 full minute.

3. The HCP will listen for murmurs.

4. Palpate pulses.

5. Check for cyanosis; blanch the skin on the trunk and extremities to check circulation.

6. Observe for cardiac distress when the **newborn** is feeding.

B. Respiratory system

1. Suction the airway as necessary. Use a bulb syringe for upper airway suctioning (compress bulb before insertion) and a French catheter for deeper suctioning)

2. Observe for respiratory distress and hypoxemia.

a. Nasal flaring

b. Increasingly severe retractions

c. Grunting

d. Cyanosis

e. Bradycardia and periods of apnea that last more than 15 seconds

3. Administer oxygen via hood if necessary and as prescribed.

C. Hepatic system

1. Normal or physiological jaundice appears after the first 24 hours in full-term neonates and after the first 48 hours in premature neonates. Jaundice occurring before this time (pathological jaundice) may indicate the early hemolysis of red blood cells and must be reported to the HCP.

2. Physiological jaundice peaks about the fifth day of life (indirect bilirubin levels: 6 to 7 mg/dL).

3. Monitor the serum bilirubin levels.

4. Feed early to stimulate intestinal activity and to keep the bilirubin level low.

5. Prevent chilling, because hypothermia can cause acidosis, which interferes with bilirubin conjugation and excretion.

6. The **newborn's** liver stores iron that was passed from the mother for 5 to 6 months.

7. Glycogen storage occurs in the liver.

8. The neonate is at risk for hemorrhagic disorders. Coagulation factors synthesized in the liver are dependent on vitamin K, which is not synthesized until intestinal bacteria are present.

9. Handle the neonate carefully and monitor for any bruising or bleeding episodes.

10. Watch for meconium stool and subsequent stools.

11. Intramuscular vitamin K will be prescribed for the neonate to prevent hemorrhagic disorders; administer in the lateral aspect of the middle third of the vastus lateralis muscle.

12. Check the **newborn's** hemoglobin and blood glucose levels per facility protocol.

D. Renal system

1. The immature kidneys cannot concentrate urine.

2. A weight loss of approximately 5% to 10% during the first week of life occurs as a result of voiding and limited intake.

3. Weigh the **newborn** daily.

4. Monitor intake and output (I&O); weigh diapers, if necessary (1 g of diaper weight equals 1mL of urine).

5. If the diaper requires weighing, record the weight before putting it on the **newborn**; after the **newborn** voids, reweigh the diaper and subtract the pre-voided weight.
6. Measure the specific gravity of the urine, if necessary.
7. Monitor for signs of dehydration (dry mucous membranes, sunken eyeballs, poor skin turgor, sunken fontanels).

E. Immune system
1. The **newborn** receives passive immunity via the **placenta** (immunoglobulin G)
2. The **newborn** receives passive immunity from the colostrum (immunoglobulin A)
3. Elevations in immunoglobulin M indicate infection in utero
4. Use aseptic technique when caring for the **newborn.**
5. Observe standard precautions when handling the **newborn.**
6. Ensure meticulous handwashing.
7. Ensure that infection-free staff members care for the **newborn.**
8. Monitor the **newborn's** temperature.
9. Observe for any cracks or openings in the skin.
10. Administer eye medication within 1 hour after birth to prevent ophthalmia neonatorum.
   a. The agent used varies depending on agency protocols, but usually ophthalmic forms of erythromycin (0.5%) and tetracycline (1%) are prescribed, because both are bacteriostatic and bactericidal. They provide prophylaxis against infection by *Neisseria gonorrhoeae* and *Chlamydia trachomatis*
   b. Silver nitrate (1%) solution may be prescribed, but its use is minimal, because it does not protect against chlamydial infection and it can cause chemical conjunctivitis.
11. Provide cord care.
   a. The umbilical clamp can be removed after 24 hours.
   b. Teach the mother how to perform cord care.
   c. Keep the cord clean and dry; follow agency protocol and HCP prescription for cleaning the cord during a bath and/or with diaper changes.
   d. Keep the diaper from covering the cord; fold the diaper below the cord.
   e. Monitor the cord for odor, swelling, or discharge.
   f. Sponge bathe the **newborn** until the cord falls off (usually within 2 weeks).
12. Provide circumcision care.
   a. Apply petroleum jelly gauze to the penis, except when a PlastiBell is used.
   b. Remove the petroleum jelly gauze, if applied, after the first voiding following the circumcision.
   c. Observe for swelling, infection, or bleeding from the circumcision site.
   d. Teach the mother how to care for the circumcision site.
   e. Clean the penis after each voiding by squeezing warm water over it.
   f. A milky covering over the glans penis is normal and should not be disrupted.
   g. Monitor for urinary retention.

F. Thermal regulatory system
1. Prevent cold stress (Figure 25-2)
2. **Newborns** do not shiver to produce heat.
3. **Newborns** have brown fat deposits that produce heat.
4. Heat is dissipated through vasodilation.
5. Prevent heat loss that results from evaporation by keeping the **newborn** dry and well-wrapped with a blanket.
6. Prevent heat loss that results from radiation by keeping the **newborn** away from cold objects and outside walls.
7. Prevent heat loss that results from convection by shielding the **newborn** from drafts.
8. Prevent heat loss that results from conduction by performing all treatments on a warm, padded surface.
9. Keep the temperature in the room warm.
10. Take the **newborn's** axillary temperature every hour for the first 4 hours of life, every 4 hours for the remainder of the first 24 hours, and then every shift.

▲ **FIGURE 25-2** Effects of cold stress. When a newborn is stressed by cold, oxygen consumption increases, and pulmonary and peripheral vasoconstriction occur, decreasing oxygen uptake by the lungs and oxygen to the tissues; anaerobic glycolysis increases; and there is a decrease in PO_2 and pH, leading to metabolic acidosis. (From Perry, S., Hockenberry, M., Lowdermilk, D., & Wilson, D. [2010]. *Maternal child nursing care* [4th ed.]. St. Louis: Mosby).

Cold stress causes oxygen consumption and energy to be diverted from maintaining normal brain cell function and cardiac function, resulting in serious metabolic and physiological conditions.

G. Metabolic system and gastrointestinal system
1. **Newborns** can digest simple carbohydrates, but they cannot digest fats as a result of their lack of lipase.
2. Proteins may be only partially broken down, so they may serve as antigens and provoke an allergic reaction.
3. The **newborn** has a small stomach capacity (about 90 mL) with rapid intestinal peristalsis (bowel emptying time is 2.5 to 3 hours).
4. Breast-feeding can usually begin immediately after birth; based on the HCP's preference and agency protocols, bottle-fed **newborns** may be given sterile water or 5% dextrose before a feeding with formula.
5. Observe feeding reflexes, such as rooting, sucking, and swallowing.
6. Assist the mother with breast-feeding or formula feeding
7. Burp the **newborn** during and after feeding.
8. Monitor for regurgitation or vomiting.
9. Elevate the head of the crib if regurgitation or vomiting is a concern after a feeding.
10. Observe for normal stool and the passage of meconium.
    a. Meconium stool, which is greenish black with a thick, sticky, tar-like consistency, is usually passed within the first 24 hours of life.
    b. Transitional stool, which is the second type of stool excreted by the **newborn**, is greenish brown and of looser consistency than meconium.
    c. Seedy, yellow stools are noted in breast-fed **newborns**; pale yellow to light brown stools are seen in formula-fed **newborns**.
11. **Newborn**: A screening test is performed (includes the test for phenylketonuria) before discharge after sufficient protein intake occurs. The **newborn** should be on formula or breast milk for a minimum of 24 hours before screening.

 H. Neurological system
1. The **newborn's** head size is proportionally larger than that of adults as a result of cephalocaudal development.
2. Myelinization of the nerve fibers is incomplete, so primitive reflexes are present.
3. Fontanels are open to allow for brain growth.
4. Check for an abnormal head size and a bulging or depressed anterior fontanel.

5. Measure and graph the head circumference in relation to the chest circumference and length.
6. Check the **newborn's** movements, noting symmetry, posture, and abnormal movements.
7. Observe for jitteriness, marked tremors, and seizures.
8. The **newborn's** reflexes will be tested.
9. Check for lethargy.
10. Monitor the pitch of the cry. A high-shrill cry can indicate increased intracranial pressure.

I. Reflexes
1. Sucking and rooting
   a. The **newborn's** lip, cheek, or the corner of the mouth is touched with a nipple.
   b. The **newborn** turns his or her head toward the nipple, opens the mouth, takes hold of the nipple, and sucks.
   c. The rooting reflex usually disappears after 3 to 4 months but may persist for up to 1 year.
2. Swallowing reflex
   a. Occurs spontaneously after sucking and obtaining fluids
   b. The **newborn** swallows in coordination with sucking without gagging, coughing, or vomiting.
3. Tonic neck or fencing position
   a. While the **newborn** is falling asleep or sleeping, the head is turned gently and quickly to one side.
   b. As the **newborn** faces the left side, the left arm and leg extend outward while the right arm and leg flex.
   c. When the head is turned to the right side, the right arm and leg extend outward while the left arm and leg flex.
   d. Usually disappears within 3 to 4 months
4. Palmar–plantar grasp
   a. The examiner's finger is placed in the palm of the **newborn's** hand, and then another finger is placed at the base of the toes.
   b. The **newborn's** fingers curl around the examiner's fingers, and the **newborn's** toes curl downward.
   c. Palmar response lessens within 3 to 4 months.
   d. Plantar response lessens within 8 months.
5. Moro reflex
   a. The **newborn** is held in a semisitting position, and then the head and trunk are allowed to fall backward to at least a 30-degree angle.
   b. The **newborn** assumes sharp extension and abduction of the arms with the thumbs and forefingers in a "C" position; this is followed by flexion and adduction to an "embrace" position (legs following a similar pattern).

c. Present at birth and is absent by 6 months of age if neurological maturation is not delayed.

d. A body jerk motion may be the response between 8 to 18 weeks.

e. A persistent response lasting more than 6 months may indicate pregnancy neurological abnormality.

6. Startle reflex

a. The response is best elicited if the **newborn** is at least 24 hours old.

b. The examiner makes a loud noise or claps the hands to elicit the response.

c. The **newborn's** arms adduct while the elbows flex.

d. The hands stay clenched.

e. The reflex should disappear within 4 months.

7. Pull to sit response

a. The **newborn** is pulled up from the wrist while he or she is in the prone position.

b. The head will lag until the **newborn** is in an upright position; then the head will be level with the chest and shoulders momentarily before falling forward.

c. The head will then lift for a few minutes.

d. The response depends on the **newborn's** general muscle tone and condition as well as his or her maturity level.

8. Babinski sign (plantar reflex)

a. Beginning at the heel of the foot, the examiner will gently stroke upward along the lateral aspect of the sole. The examiner then moves the finger along the ball of the foot.

b. The **newborn's** toes hyperextend while the big toe dorsiflexes.

c. This reflex disappears after the **newborn** is 1 year old.

d. The absence of this reflex indicates the need for a neurological examination.

9. Stepping or walking

a. The **newborn** is held in a vertical position, allowing one foot to touch a table surface.

b. The **newborn** simulates walking, alternately flexing and extending the feet.

c. The reflex is usually present for 3 to 4 months.

10. Crawling

a. The **newborn** is placed on his or her abdomen.

b. The **newborn** begins making crawling movements with the arms and legs.

c. The reflex usually disappears after about 6 weeks.

IV. NEWBORN SAFETY

A. **Newborn** identification

1. Information bracelets are applied to the mother and the **newborn** immediately after birth and before the mother and the **newborn** are separated; additionally, identification pictures of the **newborn** and footprints from the **newborn** may be obtained before the **newborn** leaves the mother's side in the **delivery** room. (Agency policies and protocols are always followed.)

2. Identification bracelets include name, sex, date, time of birth, and identification numbers.

3. Some agencies use identification bracelets that have radiofrequency transmitters that set off alarms if the **newborn** is removed from a certain area.

4. Agencies also conduct unit- and hospital-wide drills to prevent **newborn** abductions.

B. **Newborn** abduction

1. The mother is taught to check the identification of any person who comes to remove the baby from her room and is taught other precautions to prevent **infant** abduction (nurses must be wearing photo identification or some other security badge) (Box 25-1).

2. Closed-circuit televisions, code-alert bands, or computer monitoring systems may be used on some units.

3. The **newborn** is wheeled in a bassinette rather than carried in a staff member's arms.

V. PARENT TEACHING

A. Formula feeding

1. Teach sterilization techniques if the water supply is from an area where the purification process of the water is questionable.

2. Remind the mother not to heat the bottle of formula in a microwave oven.

3. Inform the mother that formula is a sufficient diet for the first 4 to 6 months.

4. Assess the mother's ability to burp the **newborn**.

Box 25-1 Precautions to Prevent Infant Abductions

All personnel must wear identification that is easily visible at all times.

Teach the parents to only allow hospital staff with proper identification to take their infants from them.

Question anyone with a newborn near an exit or in an unusual part of the facility.

Never leave infants unattended.

Teach the parents that the infant must be observed at all times.

When the infant is in the mother's room, position the crib away from the doorway.

Teach the parents home safety precautions: suggest that the parents do not place announcements in the paper or signs in their yard that may alert an abductor that a new baby is in the home.

B. Breast-feeding
1. Monitor the **newborn's** ability to properly attach to the mother's breast and suck (Figure 25-3).
2. Teach the mother about engorgement.
3. Teach the mother how to pump her breasts and how to store breast milk properly.
4. Inform the mother that breast milk is a sufficient diet for the first 4 to 6 months.
5. Give the mother the phone numbers of local organizations that offer support to breast-feeding mothers.

C. Bathing
1. Bathe the **newborn** in a warm room before feeding.
2. Have all equipment for bathing available.
3. Use a mild soap (not on the face).
4. Proceed from the cleanest area to the dirtiest area.
5. Clean the eyes from the inner canthus outward.
6. Special care should be taken to clean under the folds of the neck, the underarms, groin, and genital area.
7. Make bath time enjoyable for both the **newborn** and the mother.

D. Clothing
1. Assess diaper and clothing needs for the **newborn** with the mother.
2. Instruct the mother that the **newborn's** head should be covered during cold weather to prevent heat loss.
3. Instruct the mother to layer the **newborn's** clothing in cooler weather.
4. To be comfortable, the **newborn** should be dressed in one more layer of clothing than what the parents are wearing.

E. Cord care: See cord care under Body Systems: Data Collection and Interventions.

F. Circumcision: See circumcision care under Body Systems: Data Collection and Interventions.

G. Uncircumcised **newborn**
1. Inform the mother that the foreskin and glans are two similar layers of cells that separate from each other and that the separation process is normally complete by 3 years of age, but can remain adhered until puberty.
2. Instruct the mother to not pull back the foreskin but rather to allow for the natural separation to occur.
3. Inform the mother that, as the process of separation occurs, sterile sloughed cells build up between the layers of the foreskin and the glans. When retraction occurs, daily gentle washing of the glans with soap and water is sufficient to maintain adequate cleanliness.

VI. PRETERM NEWBORN

A. Description
1. A neonate born before 37 weeks' gestation
2. The primary concern relates to the immaturity of all body systems.

B. Data collection
1. Respirations irregular with periods of apnea
2. Body temperature is below normal.
3. Poor suck and swallow reflexes
4. Bowel sounds are diminished.
5. Urinary output is increased or decreased
6. Extremities are thin, with minimal creasing on the soles and palms.
7. Extremities extend but do not maintain flexion.
8. Lanugo, on the skin and in the hair on the **newborn's** head, is present in woolly patches.
9. Skin is thin, with visible blood vessels and minimal subcutaneous fat pads.
10. Skin may appear jaundiced.
11. Testes are undescended in boys.
12. Labia are narrow in girls.

C. Interventions
1. Monitor the vital signs every 2 to 4 hours.
2. Maintain airway and cardiopulmonary function.
3. Administer oxygen and humidification, as prescribed.
4. Monitor I&O and electrolyte balance.
5. Monitor the weight daily.
6. Maintain the **newborn** in a warming device.
7. Position the **newborn** every 1 to 2 hours, and handle the **newborn** carefully.
8. Avoid exposing the **newborn** to infections.
9. Provide the **newborn** with appropriate stimulation, such as touch and cuddling.

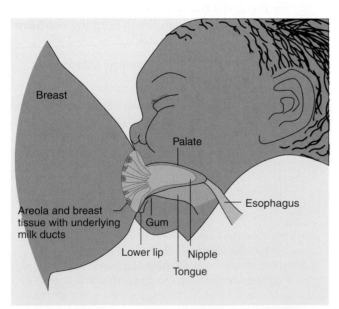

▲ **FIGURE 25-3** Correct attachment (latch-on) of an infant at the breast. (From Perry, S., Hockenberry, M., Lowdermilk, D., & Wilson, D. [2010] *Maternal child nursing care* [4th ed.]. St. Louis: Mosby).

VII. POSTTERM NEWBORN

A. Description: A neonate born after 42 weeks' gestation
B. Data collection
1. Hypoglycemia
2. Parchment-like skin (dry and cracked) without lanugo
3. Fingernails long and extended over the ends of the fingers
4. Profuse scalp hair
5. Long and thin body
6. Extremities show wasting of fat and muscle.
7. Meconium staining may be present on nails and umbilical cord.

C. Interventions
1. Provide normal **newborn** care, including stimulation such as touching and cuddling.
2. Monitor for hypoglycemia.
3. Maintain temperature.
4. Monitor for meconium aspiration.

VIII. SMALL FOR GESTATIONAL AGE

A. Description: A neonate who is plotted at or below the 10th percentile on the intrauterine growth curve
B. Data collection
1. Fetal distress
2. Lowered or elevated body temperature
3. Physical abnormalities
4. Hypoglycemia
5. Signs of polycythemia: ruddy appearance, cyanosis, jaundice
6. Signs of infection
7. Signs of meconium aspiration

C. Interventions
1. Maintain airway; observe for signs of respiratory distress.
2. Maintain body temperature
3. Monitor for infection; initiate measures to prevent sepsis.
4. Monitor the blood glucose levels and for signs of hypoglycemia.
5. Initiate early feedings. Monitor for signs of aspiration.
6. Provide stimulation, such as touch and cuddling.

IX. LARGE FOR GESTATIONAL AGE

A. Description: A neonate who is plotted at or above the 90th percentile on the intrauterine growth curve
B. Data collection
1. Respiratory distress
2. Birth trauma or injury
3. Hypoglycemia
C. Interventions
1. Maintain airway; observe for signs of respiratory distress.

2. Check for birth trauma or injury. Monitor the vital signs.
3. Monitor the blood glucose levels and for signs of hypoglycemia.
4. Initiate early feedings.
5. Monitor for infection; initiate measures to prevent sepsis.
6. Provide stimulation, such as touch and cuddling.

X. RESPIRATORY DISTRESS SYNDROME

A. Description: A serious lung disorder caused by immaturity and the inability to produce surfactant, resulting in hypoxia and acidosis
B. Data collection
1. Tachypnea, flaring nares, retractions, expiratory grunting, seesaw respirations
2. Decreased breath sounds
3. Apnea
4. Pallor and cyanosis
5. Hypothermia
6. Poor muscle tone
C. Interventions
1. Monitor respiratory status.
2. Maintain airway and cardiopulmonary function and support respirations as prescribed.
3. Monitor the arterial blood gases (ABGs) and the oxygen saturation levels (ABGs from umbilical artery) as prescribed.
4. Monitor the ABGs so that oxygen administered to the **newborn** is at the lowest possible concentration necessary to maintain adequate arterial oxygenation.
5. Before discharge, any premature **newborn** who has been given oxygen support will be scheduled for an eye examination to check for retinal damage.
6. Suction every 2 hours or more often, as necessary.
7. Position the **newborn** on his or her side or back, with the neck slightly extended.
8. Administer respiratory therapy (percussion and vibration), as prescribed. Use a padded small plastic cup or a small oxygen mask for percussion. Use a padded electric toothbrush for vibration.
9. Provide nutrition.
10. Support bonding.
11. Prepare parents for a short- to long-term period of oxygen dependency, if necessary.
12. Encourage the mother to pump her breasts for future breast-feeding, if she so desires.
13. Encourage as much parental participation in the **newborn's** care as the condition allows.

⚠ Prepare to assist to administer surfactant replacement (instilled into endotracheal tube) to a newborn with respiratory distress syndrome.

XI. MECONIUM ASPIRATION SYNDROME

A. Description
1. Occurs in term or postterm **infants**
2. Fetal distress increases intestinal peristalsis, relaxing the anal sphincter and releasing meconium into the **amniotic fluid**.
3. Aspiration can occur in utero or with the first breath.

B. Data collection
1. Respiratory distress is present at birth. Tachypnea, cyanosis, retractions, nasal flaring, grunting, crackles, and rhonchi may be present.
2. The **infant's** nails, skin, and umbilical cord may be stained a yellow-green color.

C. Interventions
1. Suctioning must be done immediately after the head is delivered before the first breath is taken; vocal cords should be viewed to see if the airway is clear before stimulation and crying.
2. **Infants** with severe meconium aspiration syndrome may benefit from extracorporeal membrane oxygenation, which is a therapy that uses a heart-lung machine to provide oxygen to the circulation, allowing the lungs to rest.

XII. BRONCHOPULMONARY DYSPLASIA

A. Description
1. A chronic pulmonary condition that affects **infants** who have experienced respiratory failure or who have been oxygen dependent for more than 28 days.
2. X-ray findings are abnormal and indicate areas of overinflation and atelectasis.

B. Data collection
1. Tachypnea and tachycardia
2. Retractions, nasal flaring, and labored breathing
3. Crackles, decreased air movement, and occasional expiratory wheezing

C. Interventions
1. Monitor airway and respiratory status and provide oxygen as prescribed.
2. Medications may include surfactant, diuretics, corticosteroids, and bronchodilators.

XIII. TRANSIENT TACHYPNEA OF THE NEWBORN

A. Description
1. Respiratory condition that results from the incomplete evacuation of the fetal lung fluid in full-term **infants**
2. Usually disappears within 24 to 48 hours

B. Data collection
1. Tachypnea
2. Nasal flaring, expiratory grunting, and retractions
3. Wet lung sounds heard during auscultation
4. Cyanosis

C. Interventions
1. Supportive care (based on manifestations)
2. Oxygen is administered as prescribed

XIV. INTRAVENTRICULAR HEMORRHAGE

A. Description
1. Bleeding within the ventricles of the brain
2. Risk factors include prematurity, respiratory distress syndrome, trauma, or asphyxia.

B. Data collection
1. Diminished or absent Moro reflex, lethargy, apnea, poor feeding, high-pitched and shrill cry, and seizure activity

C. Interventions: Treatment is supportive.

XV. RETINOPATHY OF PREMATURITY

A. Description
1. A vascular disorder that involves the gradual replacement of the retina by fibrous tissue and blood vessels.
2. Primarily caused by prematurity and the use of supplemental oxygen in the **newborn** for more than 30 days

B. Data collection: Leuckorrhea (white tissue on the retrolental space), vitreous hemorrhage, myopia, strabismus, and cataracts (check for red reflex)

C. Interventions: Laser photocoagulation surgery

XVI. NECROTIZING ENTEROCOLITIS

A. Description
1. An acute inflammatory disease of the gastrointestinal tract
2. Usually occurs 4 to 10 days after birth in a term baby

B. Data collection: Increased abdominal girth, decreased or absent bowel sounds, bowel loop distension, vomiting, bile-stained emesis, abdominal tenderness, and occult blood in the stools

C. Interventions
1. Oral feedings are held and a gastric tube is used to decompress the abdomen.
2. Intravenous antibiotics and intravenous fluids may be prescribed.
3. Surgery may be indicated

XVII. HYPERBILIRUBINEMIA

A. Description
1. Evaluation is indicated when serum bilirubin levels are more than 12 mg/dL in the term **newborn**.
2. Therapy is aimed at preventing kernicterus, which results in permanent neurological damage as a result of the deposition of bilirubin in the brain cells.

B. Data collection
1. Jaundice
2. Elevated serum bilirubin levels
3. Enlarged liver
4. Poor muscle tone
5. Lethargy
6. Poor sucking reflex

C. Interventions
1. Monitor for the presence of jaundice.
   a. Examine the **newborn's** skin color in natural light.
   b. Press a finger over a bony prominence or the tip of the **newborn's** nose to press out capillary blood from the tissues.
   c. Note that jaundice starts at the head first and then spreads to the chest, the abdomen, the arms and legs, and the hands and feet, which are the last to be jaundiced.
2. Keep the **newborn** well hydrated to maintain blood volume.
3. Facilitate early, frequent feeding to hasten the passage of meconium and to encourage the excretion of bilirubin.
4. Report any signs of jaundice that presents during the first 24 hours and any abnormal signs and symptoms to the HCP.
5. Prepare for phototherapy, and monitor the **newborn** closely during the treatment.

⚠ At any serum bilirubin level, the appearance of jaundice during the first day of life indicates a pathological process.

D. Phototherapy
1. Description
   a. Use of intense fluorescent lights to reduce serum bilirubin levels in the **newborn**
   b. Injury from treatment (e.g., eye damage, dehydration, sensory deprivation) can occur.
2. Interventions
   a. Expose as much of the **newborn's** skin as possible.
   b. Cover the genital area, and monitor the genital area for skin irritation or breakdown.
   c. Cover the **newborn's** eyes with shields or patches; make sure the eyelids are closed when shields or patches are applied.
   d. Remove the shields or patches at least once per shift (during a feeding) to inspect the eyes for infection or irritation and to allow for eye contact and bonding with the parents.
   e. Measure the lamp energy output to ensure efficacy of the treatment (done with a special device known as a photometer).
   f. Monitor the skin temperature closely.
   g. Increase fluids to compensate for water loss.
   h. Expect loose green stools and green urine.
   i. Monitor the **newborn's** skin color with the fluorescent light turned off every 4 to 8 hours.
   j. Monitor the skin for bronze baby syndrome, which is a grayish-brown discoloration of the skin.
   k. Reposition the **newborn** every 2 hours.
   l. Provide stimulation.
   m. After treatment, continue monitoring for signs of hyperbilirubinemia, because rebound elevations are normal after therapy is discontinued.
   n. Turn off phototherapy lights before drawing a blood specimen for serum bilirubin levels and do not leave blood specimen uncovered under the fluorescent lights (to prevent breakdown of bilirubin in blood specimen).

XVIII. ERYTHROBLASTOSIS FETALIS

A. Description
1. Destruction of the red blood cells that result from an antigen–antibody reaction.
2. Characterized by hemolytic anemia or hyperbilirubinemia
3. Exchange of fetal and maternal blood takes place primarily when the **placenta** separates at birth (Figure 25-4).
4. Antibodies are harmless to the mother but attach to the erythrocytes in the fetus and cause hemolysis.
5. Sensitization is rare with the first pregnancy.

B. Data collection
1. Anemia
2. Jaundice that develops rapidly after birth and before 24 hours
3. Edema

C. Interventions
1. Administer $Rh_0(D)$ immune globulin (RhoGAM) to the mother during the first 72 hours after **delivery** if the Rh-negative mother delivers an Rh-positive fetus but remains unsensitized.
2. Assist with exchange transfusion after birth or intrauterine transfusion, as prescribed.
3. The baby's blood is replaced with Rh-negative blood to stop the destruction of the baby's red blood cells. The Rh-negative blood is gradually replaced with the baby's own blood.
4. Reassure the mother that the **newborn** will experience no untoward effects as a result of the condition.

XIX. TORCH SYNDROME

A. Description
1. TORCH infections are infections that occur in the fetus or **newborn**

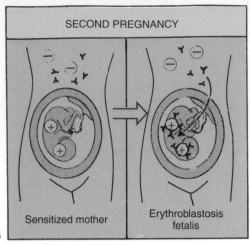

▲ **FIGURE 25-4** Development of maternal sensitization to Rh antigens. **A,** Fetal Rh-positive erythrocytes enter the maternal system. Maternal anti-Rh antibodies are formed. **B,** Anti-Rh antibodies cross placenta and attack fetal erythrocytes. (From Hockenberry, M., & Wilson, D. [2009]. *Wong's essentials of pediatric nursing* [8th ed.]. St. Louis: Mosby).

TABLE 25-5 Infections Included in TORCH Syndrome

Infection	Characteristics
Toxoplasmosis	• Caused by a protozoal infection • Produces no serious effects in the mother • Can be transmitted to the fetus • Can result in severe physical and developmental abnormalities • Common carriers include cat feces and raw beef
Other infections	• Can include syphilis, gonorrhea, varicella, hepatitis B, HIV, and human parvovirus B19
Rubella	• Systemic viral infection. • Causes congenital rubella syndrome, which includes congenital heart disease, cataracts, growth retardation, and pneumonia if the mother becomes infected within the first trimester • Deafness and some learning disabilities can occur if the mother becomes infected during the first trimester
Cytomegalovirus	• Viral infection that persists in the body indefinitely, with periods of reactivation without symptoms • Can infect the fetus or infant during delivery or after birth through breast milk, blood transfusions, or contact with infected secretions • May cause microcephaly, blindness, deafness, and mental and motor retardation.
Herpes simplex	• Sexually transmitted infection that is caused by a virus • Has periods of reactivation • Neonate commonly infected during delivery by direct contact with lesions in the genital tract • Can cause neurological impairment or death

2. Caused by one of the following:
   a. Toxoplasmosis
   b. Other infections
   c. Rubella
   d. Cytomegalovirus
   e. Herpes
B. Infections (Table 25-5)

 XX. SYPHILIS

A. Description
   1. Sexually transmitted infection
   2. Congenital syphilis can result in premature **delivery**, skin lesions, and abnormal skeletal development.

3. The organism *Treponema pallidum*, a spirochete, can cross the **placenta** throughout pregnancy and infect the fetus, usually after 18 weeks' gestation.
4. Risks include preterm birth, stillbirth, and low birth weight.
5. Congenital effects are irreversible and may include central nervous system damage and hearing loss.
B. Data collection
   1. Hepatosplenomegaly
   2. Joint swelling
   3. Palmar rash
   4. Anemia
   5. Jaundice

6. Snuffles (syphilitic rhinitis)
7. Ascites
8. Pneumonitis
9. Cerebrospinal fluid changes
C. Interventions
1. Monitor the **newborn** for signs of syphilis.
2. Monitor for palmar rash and snuffles.
3. Prepare the **newborn** for serological testing, if prescribed.
4. Administer antibiotic therapy, as prescribed.
5. Use standard precautions and drainage and secretion (contact) precautions with suspected congenital syphilis.
6. Wear gloves when handling the neonate until antibiotic therapy has been administered for 24 hours.
7. Provide psychological support to the mother, and provide instructions regarding follow-up care of the **newborn**.

XXI. ADDICTED NEWBORN

A. Description
1. A **newborn** who has become passively addicted to drugs that have passed through the **placenta**
2. Data collection findings and withdrawal times may vary depending on specific addicting drugs.
3. See also fetal alcohol syndrome.
B. Data collection
1. Irritability
2. Tremors
3. Hyperactivity and hypertonicity
4. Respiratory distress
5. Vomiting
6. High-pitched cry
7. Sneezing
8. Fever
9. Diarrhea
10. Excessive sweating
11. Poor feeding
12. Extreme sucking of fists
13. Seizures
C. Interventions
1. Monitor the respiratory and cardiac status frequently.
2. Monitor vital signs.
3. Hold the **newborn** firm and close to the body during feeding and when giving care. Swaddle the **newborn**.
4. Initiate seizure precautions (pad the sides of the crib).
5. Provide small frequent feedings and allow a longer period for feeding.
6. Monitor the I&O.
7. Administer intravenous hydration, as prescribed.

8. Protect the neonate's skin from injury, which can be caused by constant rubbing from hyperactive jitters.
9. Swaddle the newborn.
10. Place the **newborn** in a quiet room and reduce stimulation.
11. Allow the mother to express feelings such as anxiety and guilt.
12. Refer the mother for treatment of her substance abuse problem.

XXII. FETAL ALCOHOL SYNDROME

A. Description
1. Caused by maternal alcohol use during pregnancy
2. Most serious cause of teratogenesis
3. Causes mental and physical retardation
B. Data collection
1. Facial changes
   a. Short palpebral fissures
   b. Hypoplastic philtrum
   c. Short, upturned nose
   d. Flat midface
   e. Thin upper lip
   f. Low nasal bridge
2. Abnormal palmar creases
3. Respiratory distress (apnea, cyanosis)
4. Congenital heart disorders
5. Irritability and hypersensitivity to stimuli
6. Tremors
7. Poor feeding
8. Seizures
C. Interventions
1. Monitor for respiratory distress.
2. Position with the head elevated if secretions are a concern; have a nasal aspirator or suction available.
3. Keep resuscitation equipment at the bedside.
4. Monitor for hypoglycemia.
5. Check the suck and swallow reflex.
6. Administer small feedings and burp the baby well.
7. Suction as necessary.
8. Monitor the I&O.
9. Monitor the weight and head circumference.
10. Decrease environmental stimuli.

XXIII. NEWBORN WITH ACQUIRED IMMUNODEFICIENCY SYNDROME

A. Description
1. The fetus of a human immunodeficiency virus (HIV)-positive woman should be monitored closely throughout the pregnancy.
2. Serial ultrasound screenings should be done during pregnancy to identify intrauterine growth restriction.

3. Weekly nonstress testing after 32 weeks of gestation and biophysical profiles may be necessary during pregnancy.
4. Neonates born to HIV-positive clients may test positive because the mother's positive antibodies may persist for as long as 18 months after birth.
5. The use of antiviral medication, the reduction of neonate exposure to maternal blood and body fluids, and the early identification of HIV during pregnancy reduce the risk of transmission to the **newborn**.
6. All neonates born to HIV-positive mothers acquire maternal antibody to HIV infection, but not all acquire the infection.
7. The neonate may be asymptomatic for the first several years of life.

B. Transmission
1. Across placental barrier
2. During **labor** and **delivery**
3. Via breast milk

C. Data collection
1. Possibly no outward signs at birth
2. Signs of immunodeficiency
3. Hepatomegaly
4. Splenomegaly
5. Lymphadenopathy
6. Impairment in growth and development

D. Interventions
1. Cleanse the **newborn's** skin carefully before any invasive procedure, such as the administration of vitamin K, heel sticks, or venipunctures.
2. Circumcisions are not done on **newborns** with HIV-positive mothers until the **newborn's** status is determined.
3. **Newborn** can room with mother.
4. All HIV-exposed **newborns** should be treated with medication to prevent infection by *Pneumocystis jiroveci.*
5. Antiretroviral medication may be administered, as prescribed, for the first 6 weeks of life.
6. Monitor for early signs of immunodeficiency, such as hepatomegaly, splenomegaly, lymphadenopathy, and impairment in growth and development.
7. **Newborns** at risk for HIV infection should be seen by the HCP at birth and at 1 week, 2 weeks, 1 month, and 2 months of life.
8. Inform the mother that an HIV culture is recommended at the ages of 1 month and 4 months.

E. Immunizations
1. Immunizations with live vaccines, such as measles–mumps–rubella, should not be done until the **newborn's**, **infant's,** or child's HIV status is confirmed.
2. If a child is infected, live vaccine will not be given.

 Newborns at risk for HIV infection need to receive all recommended immunizations according to the regular schedule.

XXIV. NEWBORN OF A DIABETIC MOTHER

A. Description
1. A neonate born to an insulin-dependent or gestational diabetic mother
2. Hypoglycemia, hyperbilirubinemia, respiratory distress syndrome, hypocalcemia, and congenital anomalies may be present

B. Data collection
1. Excessive size and weight as a result of excess fat and glycogen in tissues
2. Edema or puffiness in the face and cheeks
3. Signs of hypoglycemia, such as twitching, difficulty feeding, lethargy, apnea, seizures, and cyanosis
4. Hyperbilirubinemia
5. Signs of respiratory distress, such as tachypnea, cyanosis, retractions, grunting, and nasal flaring

C. Interventions
1. Monitor for signs of respiratory distress.
2. Monitor the bilirubin and blood glucose levels.
3. Monitor the weight.
4. Feed the **infant** soon after birth with glucose in water, breast milk, or formula, as prescribed.
5. Prepare to assist in administering intravenous glucose to treat hypoglycemia, if necessary and as prescribed.
6. Monitor for edema.
7. Monitor for apnea, tremors, and seizures.

XXV. HYPOGLYCEMIA

A. Description
1. Abnormally low levels of glucose in the blood (<40 mg/dL during the first 72 hours or <45 mg/dL after the first 3 days of life)
2. Normal blood glucose level is 40 to 60 mg/dL in a 1-day-old neonate and 50 to 90 mg/dL in a neonate who is more than 1 day old.

B. Data collection
1. Increased respiratory rate
2. Twitching, nervousness, tremors, or poor muscle tone
3. Unstable temperature
4. Lethargy, apnea, seizures, or cyanosis

C. Interventions
1. Prevent low blood glucose through early feedings.
2. Administer glucose orally or intravenously, as prescribed.
3. Monitor the blood glucose levels, as prescribed.
4. Monitor for feeding problems.
5. Monitor for apneic periods.
6. Monitor for shrill or intermittent cries.
7. Evaluate lethargy and poor muscle tone.

MORE QUESTIONS ON EVOLVE!

Practice Questions

231. The nurse administers erythromycin ointment (0.5%) to the newborn's eyes, and the mother asks the nurse why this is done. The nurse tells the client that this is routinely done to:
1. Prevent cataracts in the neonate born to a woman who is susceptible to rubella.
2. Protect the neonate's eyes from possible infections acquired while hospitalized.
3. Minimize the spread of microorganisms to the neonate from invasive procedures during labor.
4. Prevent ophthalmia neonatorum from occurring after delivery to a neonate born to a woman with an untreated gonococcal infection.

232. A client asks the nurse why her newborn baby needs an injection of vitamin K. The nurse makes which statement to the client?
1. "Your newborn needs vitamin K to develop immunity."
2. "The vitamin K will protect your newborn from becoming jaundiced."
3. "Newborns are deficient in vitamin K. This injection prevents your baby from abnormal bleeding."
4. "Newborns have sterile bowels. The vitamin K will colonize the bowel with the necessary bacteria."

233. The nurse is assigned to assist with caring for a neonate born to a mother with acquired immunodeficiency syndrome (AIDS). The nurse understands that which of the following should be included in the plan of care?
1. Monitor the neonate's vital signs routinely.
2. Maintain standard precautions at all times while caring for the neonate.
3. Instruct breast-feeding mothers regarding the treatment of their nipples with an antifungal cream.
4. Initiate a referral to evaluate for blindness, deafness, learning, or behavioral problems in the neonate.

234. The nurse in the newborn nursery receives a telephone call to prepare for the admission of an infant born at 43 weeks' gestation with Apgar scores of 1 and 4. When planning for the admission of this infant, the nurse's highest priority should be to:
1. Turn on the apnea and cardiorespiratory monitor.

2. Connect the resuscitation bag to the oxygen outlet.
3. Set up the intravenous line with 5% dextrose in water.
4. Set the radiant warmer control temperature at 36.5° C (97.6° F).

235. The nurse is caring for a postterm neonate immediately after admission to the nursery. The priority nursing action would be to monitor:
1. Urinary output
2. Blood glucose levels
3. Total bilirubin levels
4. Hemoglobin and hematocrit level

236. The nurse is reinforcing instructions to a new mother about cord care and how to monitor for infection. The nurse tells the mother that which of the following is a sign of infection?
1. A darkened drying stump
2. A moist cord with discharge
3. A purple stump that shows pinkness around the base
4. A purple stump that shows some moistness at the base

237. The nurse is reinforcing measures regarding the care of the newborn with a mother. To bathe the newborn, the mother should be taught to:
1. Begin with the eyes and face.
2. Start with the dirtiest area first.
3. Begin with the feet and work upward.
4. Only wash the diaper area, because this is the only part of the baby that gets soiled.

238. After birth, the nurse prevents hypothermia as a result of evaporation in the newborn by:
1. Warming the crib pad
2. Closing the doors of the room
3. Drying the baby with a warm blanket
4. Turning on the overhead radiant warmer

239. The nurse is planning to teach cord care to a new mother. The nurse plans to tell the mother that:
1. Alcohol is the only agent used to clean the cord.
2. It takes 21 days for the cord to dry up and fall off.
3. Cord care is done only at birth to control bleeding.
4. The process of keeping the cord clean and dry will decrease bacterial growth.

240. A neonate has just been circumcised. The nurse would expect the surgical site to appear:
1. Pink, without drainage
2. Reddened, with a small amount of bloody drainage

3. Reddened, with a small amount of yellow exudate on the glans
4. Reddened, with a large amount of bloody drainage that requires a dressing change every 30 minutes

241. Preterm newborns are at risk for developing respiratory distress syndrome (RDS). The nurse monitors for the clinical signs associated with RDS, knowing that these signs include:
1. Tachypnea and retractions
2. Acrocyanosis and grunting
3. Hypotension and bradycardia
4. The presence of a barrel chest with acrocyanosis

242. The nurse notes hypotonia, irritability, and a poor sucking reflex in a full-term newborn infant after admission to the nursery. The nurse suspects fetal alcohol syndrome (FAS) and is aware that which of the following additional signs would be consistent with FAS?
1. A length of 19 inches
2. Abnormal palmar creases
3. A birth weight of 6 pounds and 14 ounces
4. A head circumference that is appropriate for gestational age

243. A pregnant human immunodeficiency virus (HIV)-positive woman delivers a baby. The nurse provides guidance to help the client make decisions regarding newborn care. The nurse determines that additional guidance is needed if the woman states that she will:

1. Be sure to wash her hands before feeding the newborn.
2. Breast-feed, especially for the first 6 weeks postpartum.
3. Be sure to wash her hands before and after bathroom use.
4. Administer the prescribed antiviral medication to the newborn for the first 6 weeks after delivery.

244. A pregnant woman has a positive history of genital herpes, but she has not had lesions during her pregnancy. The nurse plans to provide which of the following information to the client?
1. "You will be isolated from your newborn after delivery."
2. "There is little risk to your baby during your pregnancy, birth, and after delivery."
3. "Vaginal deliveries can reduce neonatal infection risks, even if you have an active lesion at birth."
4. "You will be evaluated at the time of delivery for herpetic genital tract lesions. If they are present, a cesarean delivery will be needed."

245. The nurse is preparing to care for a newborn who is receiving phototherapy. Choose the measures that would be implemented. **Select all that apply.**
☐ 1. Avoid stimulation.
☐ 2. Decrease fluid intake.
☐ 3. Expose all of the newborn's skin.
☐ 4. Monitor the skin temperature closely.
☐ 5. Reposition the newborn every 2 hours.
☐ 6. Cover the newborn's eyes with shields or patches.

ANSWERS

231. 4
Rationale: Erythromycin ophthalmic ointment 0.5% is used as a prophylactic treatment for ophthalmia neonatorum, which is caused by the bacteria *Neisseria gonorrhoeae*. The preventive treatment of gonorrhea is required by law. Options 1, 2, and 3 are not the purposes of administering this medication to the newborn infant.
Test-Taking Strategy: Use the process of elimination and your knowledge of the purpose of administering erythromycin ophthalmic ointment to the newborn infant. Remember that erythromycin ophthalmic ointment 0.5% is used as a prophylactic treatment of ophthalmia neonatorum in newborns. Review the initial care of the newborn infant if you had difficulty with this question.
Level of Cognitive Ability: Applying
Client Needs: Safe and Effective Care Environment

Integrated Process: Nursing Process/Implementation
Content Area: Newborn
Reference: Leifer, pp. 152–153. 2011.

232. 3
Rationale: Vitamin K is necessary for the body to synthesize coagulation factors, and it is administered to the newborn infant to prevent abnormal bleeding. It promotes the liver's formation of the clotting factors II, VII, IX, and X. Newborn infants are deficient in vitamin K, because the bowel does not have the bacteria necessary for synthesizing this fat-soluble vitamin. The normal flora in the intestinal tract produces vitamin K, but the newborn's bowel does not support the normal production of vitamin K until bacteria have adequately colonized it. The bowel becomes colonized by bacteria as food is ingested. Vitamin K does not promote the development of immunity or prevent the infant from becoming jaundiced.

Test-Taking Strategy: Use the process of elimination. Because jaundice and immunity are not related to the action of vitamin K, eliminate options 1 and 2. From the remaining options, recall the action of vitamin K to direct you to option 3. Review the purpose of vitamin K injection if you had difficulty with this question.
Level of Cognitive Ability: Applying
Client's Needs: Psychological Integrity
Integrated Process: Nursing Process/Implementation
Content Area: Newborn
Reference: Leifer, p. 153. 2011.

233. 2
Rationale: The neonate born to a mother with AIDS must be cared for with strict attention to standard precautions. This prevents the transmission of the infection from the neonate, if he or she is infected, to others, and it prevents the transmission of other infectious agents to the possibly immunocompromised neonate. A mother with AIDS should not breast-feed. Options 1 and 4 are not specifically associated with the care of a potentially AIDS-infected neonate.
Test-Taking Strategy: Use the process of elimination and your knowledge regarding the care of a neonate infant born to a woman with AIDS. Eliminate options 1 and 4 first, because they are not specifically associated with the care of a potentially infected neonate. Recalling that AIDS-infected mothers should not breast-feed will direct you to option 2. Review the care of a neonate born to a woman with AIDS if you had difficulty with this question.
Level of Cognitive Ability: Understanding
Client Needs: Safe and Effective Care Environment
Integrated Process: Nursing Process/Planning
Content Area: Newborn
References: Christensen, Kockrow, pp. 903–904. 2011. *Foundations of nursing.*
Leifer, pp. 733, 771. 2011.

234. 2
Rationale: The highest priority during the admission to the nursery of a newborn with low Apgar scores is airway support, which would involve preparing respiratory resuscitation equipment. The remaining options are also important, although they are of lower initial priority. The newborn infant will be placed on a cardiorespiratory monitor. Setting up an intravenous line with 5% dextrose in water would provide circulatory support and may be prescribed. The radiant warmer will provide an external heat source, which is necessary to prevent further respiratory distress.
Test-Taking Strategy: Use the process of elimination, and note the strategic words "highest priority." This question asks you to prioritize care on the basis of information about a newborn infant's condition. Use the ABCs—airway, breathing, and circulation. A method of planning for airway support is to have the resuscitation bag connected to an oxygen source. Review the care of the newborn infant with low Apgar scores if you had difficulty with this question.
Level of Cognitive Ability: Analyzing
Client Needs: Physiological Integrity
Integrated Process: Nursing Process/Planning
Content Area: Critical Care

Reference: Perry, Hockenberry, Lowdermilk, Wilson, pp. 644, 647. 2010.

235. 2
Rationale: The most common metabolic complication in the postterm newborn is hypoglycemia, which can produce central nervous system abnormalities and mental retardation if it is not corrected immediately. Urinary output, although important, is not the highest priority action. The polycythemia contributes to increased bilirubin levels, usually beginning on the second day after delivery. Hemoglobin and hematocrit levels are monitored, because the postterm neonate may exhibit polycythemia; however, this also does not require immediate attention.
Test-Taking Strategy: Use the process of elimination, and note the strategic word "priority." Recalling that hypoglycemia is a primary concern in the postterm newborn will direct you to the correct option. Review the care of the postterm newborn if you had difficulty with this question.
Level of Cognitive Ability: Analyzing
Client Needs: Physiological Integrity
Integrated Process: Nursing Process/Data Collection
Content Area: Newborn
Reference: Leifer, p. 318. 2011.

236. 2
Rationale: Signs of infection of the umbilical cord are moistness, oozing, discharge, and a reddened base. If signs of infection occur, the health care provider is notified. Antibiotic treatment may be necessary.
Test-Taking Strategy: Use the process of elimination. Options 1 and 3 identify normal signs and are eliminated first. From the remaining options, noting the word "discharge" in option 2 will direct you to this option. Review the signs and symptoms of infection if you had difficulty with this question.
Level of Cognitive Ability: Applying
Client Needs: Physiological Integrity
Integrated Process: Teaching and Learning
Content Area: Newborn
Reference: Leifer, pp. 218–219. 2011.

237. 1
Rationale: Bathing should start at the eyes and face, which are usually the cleanest areas. Next, the external ears and behind the ears are cleansed. The newborn's neck should be washed, because formula, breast milk, or lint will often accumulate in the folds of the neck. The hands and arms are then washed. The baby's legs are washed, with the diaper area being washed last.
Test-Taking Strategy: Use the basic techniques of bathing a client to answer the question. Remember, when bathing an adult or a baby, start with the cleanest part of the body and proceed to the dirtiest part. Options 2, 3, and 4 are incorrect. Review the techniques for bathing a newborn if you had difficulty with this question.
Level of Cognitive Ability: Applying
Client Needs: Health Promotion and Maintenance
Integrated Process: Teaching and Learning
Content Area: Newborn
References: Christensen, Kockrow, p. 965. 2011. *Foundations of nursing.*
Leifer, p. 296. 2011.

238. 3

Rationale: Evaporation occurs when moisture from the newborn's wet body surface dissipates heat along with moisture. By keeping the newborn dry (and by drying the wet newborn at birth), evaporation is prevented. Conduction occurs when the newborn is on a cold surface, such as a cold pad or mattress. Convection occurs as air moves across the newborn's skin from an open door and heat is transferred to the air. Radiation occurs when heat from the newborn radiates to a colder surface.

Test-Taking Strategy: Recalling the methods of preventing heat loss in a newborn and focusing on the subject of evaporation will direct you to the correct option. Review the methods of heat loss if you had difficulty with this question.

Level of Cognitive Ability: Applying
Client Needs: Physiological Integrity
Integrated Process: Nursing Process/Implementation
Content Area: Newborn
Reference: Leifer, pp. 150, 215. 2011.

239. 4

Rationale: The cord should be kept clean and dry to decrease bacterial growth; this includes keeping the diaper folded below the cord to keep urine away from the cord. The cord should be cleansed two to three times a day. It usually falls off within 7 to 14 days. Agents other than alcohol may be prescribed to clean the cord.

Test-Taking Strategy: Use the process of elimination. Eliminate options 1 and 3, noting the closed-ended word "only." Recall that cord care is required until the cord dries up and falls off, and that agents other than alcohol may be prescribed for cord care. Option 2 is incorrect, because the cord should fall off between 7 and 14 days after birth. Review the concepts of cord care if you had difficulty with this question.

Level of Cognitive Ability: Understanding
Client Needs: Physiological Integrity
Integrated Process: Teaching and Learning
Content Area: Newborn
Reference: Leifer, pp. 218–219. 2011.

240. 2

Rationale: The glans penis is normally dark red. After circumcision, a small amount of bloody drainage is expected. During the normal healing process, the glans becomes covered with a yellow exudate. If excessive bleeding is noted from the circumcision, the nurse applies gentle pressure to the site of bleeding with a sterile gauze pad. If the bleeding is not controlled, the health care provider is notified, because a blood vessel may need to be ligated.

Test-Taking Strategy: Use the process of elimination, and focus on the subject of the expected appearance. Remember that a small amount of bloody drainage is expected. Review the expected findings after circumcision if you had difficulty with this question.

Level of Cognitive Ability: Understanding
Client Needs: Physiological Integrity
Integrated Process: Nursing Process/Data Collection
Content Area: Newborn
References: Christensen, Kockrow, pp. 850, 875–876. 2011. *Foundations of nursing.*
Leifer, pp. 290–292. 2011,

241. 1

Rationale: The newborn infant with RDS may present with clinical signs of cyanosis, tachypnea, apnea, nasal flaring, chest wall retractions, or audible grunts. Acrocyanosis is a bluish discoloration of the hands and feet that is associated with immature peripheral circulation, and it is not uncommon during the first few hours of life. Options 2, 3, and 4 do not indicate clinical signs of RDS.

Test-Taking Strategy: Use the process of elimination. Recalling that acrocyanosis may be a normal sign in a newborn infant will assist you with eliminating options 2 and 4. From the remaining options, it is necessary to be familiar with the signs of RDS. In addition, note the relationship between the diagnosis and the signs noted in option 1. Review the signs of RDS if you had difficulty with this question.

Level of Cognitive Ability: Analyzing
Client Needs: Physiological Integrity
Integrated Process: Nursing Process/Data Collection
Content Area: Newborn
References: Christensen, Kockrow, p. 917. 2011. *Foundations of nursing.*
Leifer, pp. 307–308. 2011.

242. 2

Rationale: Features of newborn infants who are diagnosed with FAS include craniofacial abnormalities, intrauterine growth restriction, cardiac abnormalities, abnormal palmar creases, and respiratory distress. Options 1, 3, and 4 are normal findings in the full-term newborn infant.

Test-Taking Strategy: Use the process of elimination and your knowledge regarding the normal findings in the full-term newborn infant to answer this question. Note that options 1, 3, and 4 are comparable or alike and that they represent normal findings. Review the content related to normal newborn infant findings and FAS if you had difficulty with this question.

Level of Cognitive Ability: Analyzing
Client Needs: Physiological Integrity
Integrated Process: Nursing Process/Data Collection
Content Area: Newborn
Reference: Leifer, p. 109. 2011.

243. 2

Rationale: The mode of perinatal transmission of HIV to the fetus or neonate of an HIV-positive woman can occur during the antenatal, intrapartal, or postpartum periods. HIV transmission can occur during breast-feeding; thus, HIV-positive clients need to bottle-feed their neonates. Antiviral medications will be prescribed for the neonate for the first 6 weeks of life. The principles related to handwashing need to be taught to the mother.

Test-Taking Strategy: Use the process of elimination, and note the strategic words "additional guidance is needed." These words indicate a negative event query and ask you to select an option that is an incorrect statement. Options 1 and 3 can be eliminated first, because they are comparable or alike. From the remaining options, recalling the modes of transmission of HIV from the mother to the newborn will direct you to option 2. Review these modes of HIV transmission if you had difficulty with this question.

Level of Cognitive Ability: Evaluating
Client Needs: Safe and Effective Care Environment
Integrated Process: Teaching and Learning

Content Area: Fundamental Skills: Safety/Infection Control
Reference: Leifer, p. 222. 2011.

244. 4

Rationale: If herpetic genital lesions are present at the time of delivery, a cesarean delivery will be necessary to reduce the risk of infecting the neonate. In the absence of herpetic genital lesions, a vaginal delivery may be indicated, unless there are other reasons for performing a cesarean delivery. Maternal isolation is not necessary, but potentially exposed neonates should be cultured on the day of delivery.

Test-Taking Strategy: Use the process of elimination. Focusing on the subject of a positive history of genital herpes and recalling the risks to the neonate will direct you to the correct option. Review the methods of transmission of genital herpes to the neonate if you had difficulty with this question.

Level of Cognitive Ability: Applying
Client Needs: Safe and Effective Care Environment
Integrated Process: Nursing Process/Implementation
Content Area: Fundamental Skills: Safety/Infection Control
Reference: Perry, Hockenberry, Lowdermilk, Wilson, p. 106. 2010.

❖ 245. 4, 5, 6

Rationale: Phototherapy is the use of intense fluorescent lights to reduce serum bilirubin levels in the newborn. Injury from treatment (e.g., eye damage, dehydration, sensory deprivation) can occur. Interventions include exposing as much of the newborn's skin as possible; however, the genital area is covered. The newborn's eyes are also covered with shields or patches to ensure that the eyelids are closed. The shields or patches are removed at least once per shift to inspect the eyes for infection or irritation and to allow for eye contact. The nurse measures the quantity of light every 8 hours, monitors the skin temperature closely, and increases fluids to compensate for water loss. The newborn will have loose green stools and green-colored urine. The newborn's skin color is monitored with the fluorescent light turned off every 4 to 8 hours, and he or she is monitored for bronze baby syndrome, which is a grayish-brown discoloration of the skin. The newborn is repositioned every 2 hours, and stimulation is provided. After treatment, the newborn is monitored for signs of hyperbilirubinemia, because rebound elevations are normal after therapy is discontinued.

Test-Taking Strategy: Focus on the subject of phototherapy. Recalling that injury from treatment and sensory deprivation can occur will assist you with determining the correct interventions. Review the interventions for the newborn who is receiving phototherapy if you had difficulty with this question.

Level of Cognitive Ability: Applying
Client Needs: Safe and Effective Care Environment
Integrated Process: Nursing Process/Implementation
Content Area: Newborn
Reference: Leifer, pp. 341–342. 2011.

26

Maternity and Newborn Medications

 I. **Rh₀(D) IMMUNE GLOBULIN (RhoGAM)**

A. Description
1. Prevention of anti-Rh₀(D) antibody formation is most successful if the medication is administered twice, at 28 weeks of gestation and again within 72 hours after **delivery**.
2. The immune globulin also should be administered within 72 hours after potential or actual exposure to Rh-positive blood and must be given with each subsequent exposure or potential exposure to Rh-positive blood.

B. Use: To prevent isoimmunization in Rh-negative clients who are exposed or potentially exposed to Rh-positive red blood cells by transfusion, termination of pregnancy, amniocentesis, chorionic villus sampling (CVS), abdominal trauma, or bleeding during pregnancy or birth process

 C. Adverse effects and contraindications
1. Adverse effects include elevated temperature and tenderness at the injection site
2. Contraindicated for Rh-positive women and in clients with a history of systemic allergic reactions to preparations containing human immunoglobulins
3. Not administered to a **newborn**

D. Interventions
1. Administer to the mother by intramuscular injection at 28 weeks' gestation and within 72 hours after **delivery**; it is never administered by the intravenous (IV) route
2. Monitor for temperature elevation.
3. Monitor injection site for tenderness.

 ⚠ Rh₀(D) IMMUNE GLOBULIN (RhoGAM) is of no benefit once the client has developed a positive antibody titer to the Rh antigen.

II. **TOCOLYTICS**

A. Description: Tocolytics are medications that produce uterine relaxation and suppress uterine activity (Box 26-1 and Table 26-1).
B. Uses: To stop uterine contractions and prevent preterm birth

C. Adverse effects and contraindications
1. See Table 26-1 for a description of adverse effects.
2. Maternal contraindications include severe pre-eclampsia and eclampsia, active vaginal bleeding, intrauterine infection, cardiac disease, and a medical or obstetric condition that contraindicates continuation of pregnancy.
3. Fetal contraindications include estimated gestational age greater than 37 weeks, cervical dilation greater than 4 cm, fetal demise, lethal fetal anomaly, chorioamnionitis, acute fetal distress, and chronic intrauterine growth restriction.

D. Interventions for the client receiving tocolytic therapy
1. Position the client on her side to enhance placental perfusion and reduce pressure on the cervix.
2. Monitor maternal vital signs, fetal status, and **labor** status frequently according to agency protocol.
3. Monitor for signs of adverse effects to the medication.
4. Monitor daily weight and input and output (I&O) status and provide fluid intake as prescribed.
5. Offer comfort measures and provide psychosocial support to the client and family.
6. See Table 26-1 for interventions specific to each tocolytic medication.

III. **MAGNESIUM SULFATE**

A. Description (see Table 26-1)
1. Magnesium sulfate is a central nervous system depressant and anticonvulsant.
2. The medication causes smooth muscle relaxation.
3. The antidote is calcium gluconate.
B. Uses
1. Stopping preterm **labor** to prevent preterm birth
2. Preventing and controlling seizures in preeclamptic and eclamptic clients
C. Adverse effects and contraindications
1. Magnesium sulfate can cause respiratory depression, depressed reflexes, flushing, hypotension, extreme muscle weakness, decreased urine

output, pulmonary edema, and elevated serum magnesium levels.
2. Continuous IV infusion increases the risk of magnesium toxicity in the **newborn**.
3. Intravenous administration should not be used for 2 hours preceding **delivery**.
4. Magnesium sulfate may be prescribed for the first 12 to 24 hours postpartum if it is used for preeclampsia.

Box 26-1 Tocolytics

Indomethacin (Indocin): prostaglandin inhibitor
Magnesium sulfate
Nifedipine (Procardia, Adalat, Nifedical): calcium channel blocker
Terbutaline (Brethine): β_2 selective adrenergic agonist

5. High doses can cause loss of deep tendon reflexes, heart block, respiratory paralysis, and cardiac arrest.
6. The medication is contraindicated in the client with heart block, myocardial damage, or renal failure.
7. The medication is used with caution in the client with severe renal impairment.
D. Interventions
1. Monitor maternal vital signs, especially respirations, every 30 to 60 minutes.
2. Monitor renal function (output and renal function laboratory values) and cardiac function (electrocardiogram).
3. Monitor magnesium levels—the target range is 4 to 7.5 mEq/L (5 to 8 mg/dL); if a rise in the magnesium level occurs, the health care provider (HCP) is notified immediately.

TABLE 26-1 Tocolytics

Medication, Classification, and Actions	Adverse Effects	Nursing Interventions
Indomethacin (Indocin)—prostaglandin inhibitor; relaxes uterine smooth muscle	*Maternal*—Nausea and vomiting, dyspepsia, dizziness *Fetal*—Premature closure of ductus arteriosus *Newborn*—Bronchopulmonary dysplasia, respiratory distress syndrome, intracranial pressure, necrotizing enterocolitis, hyperbilirubinemia	Used when other methods fail, depending on gestational age. Not used in women with bleeding potential, peptic ulcer disease, or oligohydramnios. Agency protocol for administration is followed. Amniotic fluid volume and function of ductus arteriosus is determined before therapy and within 48 hours of discontinuing therapy.
Magnesium sulfate—central nervous system depressant; relaxes smooth muscle, including the uterus; used to stop preterm labor contractions; used for preeclamptic clients to prevent seizures	*Maternal*—Depressed respirations, depressed deep tendon reflexes (DTRs), hypotension, extreme muscle weakness, flushing, decreased urine output, pulmonary edema, serum magnesium levels >9 mg/dL *Newborn*—Hypotonia and sleepiness	An IV controller pump is used for administration. Agency protocol for administration is followed. Infusion is discontinued and the HCP is notified if adverse effects occur. Monitor for respirations <12/min, urine output <100 mL/4 hr (30 mL/hr). DTRs are monitored. Magnesium levels are monitored and values outside therapeutic range are reported (4 to 7.5 mEq/L or 5 to 8 mg/dL). Keep calcium gluconate available (antidote).
Nifedipine (Procardia, Adalat, Nifedical)—calcium channel blocker; relaxes smooth muscles, including the uterus, by blocking calcium entry	*Maternal*—Tachycardia, hypotension, dizziness, headache, nervousness, facial flushing, fatigue, nausea *Newborn*—Hypotension	Agency protocol for administration is followed. The use of this medication is avoided or used cautiously with magnesium sulfate because severe hypotension can occur. Monitor for adverse effects.
Terbutaline (Brethine)—β-adrenergic agonist; relaxes smooth muscles, inhibiting uterine activity and causing bronchodilation	*Maternal*—Tachycardia, palpitations, pulmonary edema, chest pain, myocardial ischemia, hypotension, tremors, hypokalemia, hyperglycemia *Newborn*—Tachycardia, hypotension, ileus, hypocalcemia, hyperbilirubinemia, hyperinsulinemia with hypoglycemia	Monitor for adverse effects and the HCP is notified if they occur. Teach woman and family to monitor for adverse effects and when to notify the HCP.

4. It is always administered by IV infusion via an infusion monitoring device such as a controller pump. The dose being administered is closely and carefully monitored and agency protocol for administration is always followed.
5. Calcium gluconate is always kept on hand in case of a magnesium sulfate overdose, because calcium gluconate antagonizes the effect of magnesium sulfate.
6. Deep tendon reflexes are monitored hourly for signs of developing toxicity.
7. The patellar reflex or knee jerk reflex is tested before administration of a repeat parenteral dose (used as an indicator of central nervous system depression); suppressed reflex may be a sign of impending respiratory arrest (Table 26-2).
8. Patellar reflex must be present and respiratory rate must be greater than 16 breaths/min (or as designated by agency protocol) before each parenteral dose.
9. Monitor I&O hourly; output should be maintained at 30 mL/hr because the medication is eliminated through the kidneys.

⚠ The client receiving magnesium sulfate intravenously is monitored closely for signs of toxicity. The HCP is contacted if respirations are less than 12 breaths/min, which indicate respiratory depression, or if any other adverse effects occur.

IV. BETAMETHASONE AND DEXAMETHASONE

A. Description: Corticosteroid that increases the production of surfactant to accelerate fetal lung maturity and reduce the incidence or severity of respiratory distress syndrome
B. Use: For the client in preterm **labor** between 28 and 32 weeks' gestation whose **labor** can be inhibited for 48 hours without jeopardizing the mother or fetus
C. Adverse effects and contraindications
   1. May decrease the mother's resistance to infection

2. Pulmonary edema secondary to sodium and fluid retention can occur
3. Elevated blood glucose levels in a woman with diabetes mellitus can occur
D. Interventions
   1. Monitor maternal vital signs, lung sounds, and for edema.
   2. Monitor mother for signs of infection.
   3. Monitor white blood cell count.
   4. Monitor blood glucose levels.

V. OPIOID ANALGESICS

A. Description
   1. Used to relieve moderate to severe pain associated with **labor**
   2. Administered by the intramuscular or intravenous (IV) route
   3. Regular use of opioids during pregnancy may produce withdrawal symptoms in the **newborn** (irritability, excessive crying, tremors, hyperactive reflexes, fever, vomiting, diarrhea, yawning, sneezing, and seizures).
   4. Antidotes for opioids
      a. Naloxone (Narcan) is usually the treatment of choice because it rapidly reverses the opioid toxicity; the dose may need to be repeated every few hours until opioid concentrations have dropped to nontoxic levels.
      b. Nalmefene (Revex) is a long-acting opioid antagonist that does not require repeat doses.
      c. These medications can cause withdrawal in opioid-dependent clients.
B. Meperidine hydrochloride (Demerol) and hydromorphone hydrochloride (Dilaudid)
   1. Can cause dizziness, nausea, vomiting, sedation, decreased blood pressure, decreased respirations, diaphoresis, flushed face, urinary retention
   2. May be prescribed to be administered with an antiemetic such as promethazine (Phenergan) to prevent nausea
   3. High dosages may result in respiratory depression, skeletal muscle flaccidity, cold clammy skin, cyanosis, extreme somnolence progressing to seizures, stupor, and coma.
   4. Used cautiously in clients delivering preterm **infants**
   5. Not administered in early **labor** because it may slow the **labor** process
   6. Not administered in advanced **labor** (within 1 hour of expected **delivery**); if the medication is not adequately removed from the fetal circulation respiratory depression can occur.
C. Fentanyl (Sublimaze) and sufentanil (Sufenta): Can cause respiratory depression, dizziness, drowsiness, hypotension, urinary retention, fetal narcosis and distress

TABLE 26-2 Assessing Deep Tendon Reflexes

Grade	Deep Tendon Reflex Response
0	No response
1	Sluggish or diminished
2	Active or expected response
3	More brisk than expected, slightly hyperactive
4	Brisk, hyperactive, with intermittent or transient clonus

From Seidel, H.M., Ball, J.W., Dains, J.E., & Benedict, G.W. (2006). *Mosby's guide to physical examination* (5th ed.). St. Louis: Mosby.

D. Butorphanol tartrate (Stadol) and nalbuphine (Nubain)
1. Can cause confusion, sedation, sweating, nausea, vomiting, hypotension, sinusoidal-like fetal heart rhythm
2. Use with caution in a woman with preexisting opioid dependency because these medications can precipitate withdrawal symptoms in the woman and **newborn**.
E. Interventions
1. Monitor vital signs, particularly respiratory status; if respirations are 12 breaths/min or fewer, withhold the medication and notify the registered nurse (RN).
2. Monitor the fetal heart rate and characteristics of uterine contractions.
3. Monitor for blood pressure changes (hypotension); maintain the woman in a recumbent position (elevate the hip with a wedge pillow or other device).
4. Record the woman's response and level of pain relief.
5. Monitor the bladder for distention and urinary retention.
6. The antidote naloxone (Narcan) should be available, especially if **delivery** is going to occur during peak drug absorption time.

⚠ A drug history is obtained before the administration of an opioid analgesic. Some medications may be contraindicated if the woman has a history of opioid dependency because these medications can precipitate withdrawal symptoms in the woman and newborn.

VI. PROSTAGLANDINS (Box 26-2)

A. Description
1. Ripen the cervix, making it softer and causing it to begin to dilate and efface
2. Stimulate uterine contractions
3. Administered vaginally
B. Uses
1. Preinduction cervical ripening (ripening of the cervix before the induction of **labor** when the Bishop score is 4 or less)
2. Induction of **labor**
3. Induction of abortion (abortifacient agent)
C. Adverse effects and contraindications
1. Gastrointestinal effects, including diarrhea, nausea, vomiting, and stomach cramps
2. Fever, chills, flushing, headache, hypotension

Box 26-2 Prostaglandins

Prostaglandin E$_2$: Dinoprostone (Cervidil vaginal insert, Prepidil gel)

---

3. Tachysystole (12 or more uterine contractions in 20 minutes without an alteration in the fetal heart rate pattern)
4. Hyperstimulation of the uterus
5. Fetal passage of meconium
6. Contraindications (Box 26-3)
D. Interventions
1. Maternal vital signs, fetal heart rate pattern, and status of pregnancy including indications for cervical ripening or the induction of **labor**, signs of **labor** or impending **labor**, and the Bishop score are monitored (see Table 23-2 for information about the Bishop score).
2. Monitor for adverse effects to the medication.
3. Have the woman void before administration of the medication and then have her maintain a supine with lateral tilt or side-lying position for 30 to 60 minutes (gel form) up to 2 hours (insert form) after administration, depending on the medication administered.
4. Treatment is discontinued when the Bishop score is 8 or more (cervix ripens) or an effective contraction pattern is established (3 or more contractions in a 10-minute period). Additionally, signs of adverse effects indicate that the treatment needs to be discontinued.
5. Agency protocol is followed for the induction of **labor** if cervical ripening has occurred and **labor** has not begun; oxytocin (Pitocin) may be prescribed if needed 6 to 12 hours after discontinuation of prostaglandin therapy.

VII. UTERINE STIMULANTS (OXYTOCICS): OXYTOCIN (PITOCIN)

A. Description
1. Oxytocin stimulates the smooth muscle of the uterus and increases the force, frequency, and duration of uterine contractions.
2. Oxytocin also promotes milk letdown.

Box 26-3 Contraindications to the Use of Prostaglandins

Active cardiac, hepatic, pulmonary, or renal disease
Acute pelvic inflammatory disease
Clients whom vaginal delivery is not indicated
Fetal malpresentation
History of cesarean section or major uterine surgery
History of difficult labor or traumatic labor
Hypersensitivity to prostaglandins
Maternal fever or infection
Nonreassuring fetal heart rate pattern
Placenta previa or unexplained vaginal bleeding
Regular progressive uterine contractions
Significant cephalopelvic disproportion

3. For the induction of **labor**, oxytocin is administered by the IV route (other routes of administration include intranasal and intramuscular).

4. Minimal cervical change usually is noted until the active phase of **labor** is achieved.

B. Uses

1. Induces or augments **labor**
2. Controls postpartum bleeding
3. Promotes milk letdown and facilitates breast-feeding (intranasal route)
4. Manages an incomplete abortion

C. Adverse effects and contraindications

1. Adverse effects may include allergies, dysrhythmias, changes in blood pressure, uterine rupture, and water intoxication; intranasal administration may cause nasal vasoconstriction.

2. Oxytocin may produce uterine hypertonicity, resulting in fetal or maternal adverse effects.

3. High doses may cause hypotension, with rebound hypertension.

4. Postpartum hemorrhage can occur and should be monitored for because the uterus may become atonic when the medication wears off.

5. Oxytocin should not be used in a client who cannot deliver vaginally or in a client with hypertonic uterine contractions; it is also contraindicated in a client with active genital herpes.

D. Interventions

1. Monitor maternal vital signs (every 15 minutes), especially the blood pressure and heart rate, weight, intake and output, level of consciousness, and lung sounds.

2. Frequency, duration, force of contractions, and resting uterine tone is monitored every 15 minutes.

3. The fetal heart rate is monitored every 15 minutes. The HCP is notified if significant changes occur; use of an internal fetal scalp electrode may be prescribed.

4. The medication is administered by IV infusion via an infusion monitoring device; the prescribed additive solution is piggybacked at the port nearest the point of venous insertion (prescribed additive solution may be normal saline, lactated Ringer's, or D5W)

5. The dose being administered is carefully monitored; the client is not left unattended while the oxytocin is infusing.

6. Administer oxygen if prescribed.

7. The client is monitored for hypertonic contractions or a nonreassuring fetal heart rate (FHR). The HCP is notified if these occur (see Priority Nursing Actions).

8. The medication is stopped if uterine hyperstimulation or a nonreassuring fetal heart rate occurs; the client is turned on her side, the IV rate of the normal saline will be increased,

---

◼◼◼ PRIORITY NURSING ACTIONS! ◼◼◼

Steps to Take if Hypertonic Contractions or a Nonreassuring FHR Occurs During Oxytocin (Pitocin) Infusion

1. Stop the oxytocin (Pitocin) infusion and notify the RN immediately, who in turn will contact the HCP.
2. Turn the woman on her side and stay with the woman.
3. Increase the flow rate of the IV additive solution as directed by the RN.
4. Administer oxygen by snug facemask at 8 to 10 L/min.
5. Monitor maternal vital signs; FHR and patterns; and frequency, duration, and force of contractions.
6. The event, actions taken, and the response are documented.

Oxytocin (Pitocin) is a uterine stimulant and stimulates the smooth muscle of the uterus and increases the force, frequency, and duration of uterine contractions. It is administered to induce or augment labor. The presence of hypertonic contractions or a nonreassuring FHR indicates the need to institute emergency measures to reduce uterine stimulation and increase fetal oxygenation. The nurse would always follow the agency's protocol regarding the procedure to take in this event. Keeping the emergency goals of care in mind (to reduce uterine stimulation and increase fetal oxygenation) will assist in guiding your actions. The oxytocin infusion needs to be stopped in order to reduce uterine contractions. The RN is notified immediately and will then contact the HCP. The nurse turns the woman to her side to increase placental oxygenation. The nurse never leaves a client if an emergency situation is present. The flow rate of the IV additive solution is increased and oxygen is administered. These actions will also facilitate the goals of care. Once these emergency actions are taken, the nurse continuously monitors maternal vital signs, FHR and patterns, and frequency, duration, and force of contractions. The nurse also assists in implementing any additional prescriptions and documents the event, actions taken, and the response.

---

and oxygen will be administered via face mask.

9. Monitor for signs of water intoxication.
10. Have emergency equipment available.
11. The dose of the medication and the time the medication was started, increased, maintained, and discontinued is documented. The client's response is documented.
12. Keep the client and family informed of the client's progress.

VIII. MEDICATIONS USED TO MANAGE POSTPARTUM HEMORRHAGE (Box 26-4)

A. Ergot alkaloids
1. Description

Box 26-4 Medications Used to Manage Postpartum Hemorrhage

Ergonovine maleate, ergometrine (Ergotrate Maleate)
Methylergonovine (Metherginc)
Oxytocin (Pitocin)
Prostaglandin F_{2a}: Carboprost tromethamine (Hemabate)

---

a. Ergonovine maleate or ergometrine and methylergonovine maleate (Methergine) are ergot alkaloids.
b. These medications directly stimulate uterine muscle, increase the force and frequency of contractions, and produce a firm tetanic contraction of the uterus
c. Can produce arterial vasoconstriction and vasospasm of the coronary arteries
d. Ergot alkaloids are administered postpartum and are not administered before the **delivery** of the **placenta**.

2. Uses
   a. Postpartum hemorrhage
   b. Postabortal hemorrhage resulting from atony or involution
3. Adverse effects and contraindications
   a. Can cause nausea, uterine cramping, bradycardia, dysrhythmias, myocardial infarction, and severe hypertension
   b. High doses are associated with peripheral vasospasm or vasoconstriction, angina, miosis, confusion, respiratory depression, seizures, or unconsciousness; uterine tetany can occur
   c. Contraindicated during pregnancy and in clients with significant cardiovascular disease, peripheral vascular disease, or hypertension
4. Interventions
   a. Monitor maternal vital signs, weight, intake and output, level of consciousness, and lung sounds.
   b. Monitor the blood pressure closely; the medication produces vasoconstriction and, if a rise in blood pressure is noted, withhold the medication and notify the RN.
   c. Uterine contractions are monitored (frequency, strength, and duration).
   d. Monitor for chest pain, headache, shortness of breath, itching, pale or cold hands or feet, nausea, diarrhea, or dizziness.
   e. Monitor the extremities for color, warmth, movement, and pain.
   f. Monitor for vaginal bleeding.
   g. Notify the RN, who will then notify the HCP, if chest pain or other adverse effects occur.
   h. Analgesics are administered as prescribed; they may be required because the medication produces painful uterine contractions.

⚠ The woman's blood pressure is checked before administration of an ergot alkaloid. These medications can cause severe hypertension and are therefore contraindicated in a client with hypertension.

B. Prostaglandin $F_{2\alpha}$ (carboprost tromethamine [Hemabate])
   1. Description: Contracts the uterus
   2. Uses: Postpartum hemorrhage
   3. Adverse effects and contraindications
      a. Can cause headache, nausea, vomiting, diarrhea, fever, tachycardia, hypertension
      b. Contraindicated if the client has asthma
   4. Interventions
      a. Monitor vital signs.
      b. Monitor for vaginal bleeding (uterine tone is also monitored).
C. Oxytocin (Pitocin): See section on uterine stimulants

IX. RUBELLA VACCINE

A. Given subcutaneously before hospital discharge to a nonimmune postpartum client
B. Administered if the rubella titer is less than 1:8
C. Adverse effects: Transient rash, hypersensitivity
D. Contraindicated in a client with an allergy to duck eggs
E. Interventions
   1. Ask the client about an allergy to duck eggs; the HCP is notified before administration if an allergy exists.
   2. The vaccine is not administered if the client or other family members are immunocompromised.
   3. If the rubella vaccine is administered at the same time as $Rh_o(D)$ immune globulin (RhoGAM), it may not be effective.

⚠ The client should avoid pregnancy for 1 to 3 months (or as prescribed) after immunization with rubella vaccine. Inform the client about the need for using a contraception method during this time.

X. LUNG SURFACTANTS (Box 26-5)

A. Description
   1. Lung surfactants replenish surfactant and restore surface activity to the lungs to prevent and treat respiratory distress syndrome.
   2. Lung surfactants are administered by the intratracheal route.
B. Use: To prevent or treat respiratory distress syndrome in premature **infants**
C. Adverse effects and contraindications

Box 26-5 Lung Surfactant Replacement Therapy

Beractant (Survanta)
Calfactant (Infasurf)
Poractant alfa (Curosurf)

1. Adverse effects include transient bradycardia and oxygen desaturation; pulmonary hemorrhage, mucus plugging, and endotracheal tube reflex can also occur.
2. Surfactants are administered with caution in those at risk for circulatory overload.

D. Interventions
1. The surfactant is instilled through the catheter inserted into the **newborn's** endotracheal tube; suctioning is avoided for at least 2 hours after administration.
2. Monitor for bradycardia and decreased oxygen saturation during administration.
3. Monitor respiratory status and lung sounds and for signs of adverse effects.

XI. EYE PROPHYLAXIS FOR THE NEWBORN

A. Description
1. Preventive eye treatment against ophthalmia neonatorum in the **newborn** is required by law in the United States.
2. The agent used varies depending on agency protocols but usually ophthalmic forms of erythromycin (0.5%) or tetracycline (1%) are prescribed because they are bacteriostatic and bactericidal and provide prophylaxis against *Neisseria gonorrhoeae* and *Chlamydia trachomatis*.
3. Silver nitrate (1%) solution may be prescribed, but its use is minimal because it does not protect against chlamydial infection and can cause chemical conjunctivitis.

B. Use: A prophylactic measure to protect against *Neisseria gonorrhoeae* and *Chlamydia trachomatis*

C. Adverse effect: Silver nitrate (1%) solution can cause chemical conjunctivitis.

D. Interventions
1. Cleanse the **newborn's** eyes before instilling the medication.
2. Do not flush the eyes after instillation.

⚠ Instillation of eye medication can be delayed for up to 1 hour after birth to facilitate eye contact and parent-newborn attachment and bonding.

XII. VITAMIN K

A. Description
1. The **newborn** is at risk for hemorrhagic disorders; coagulation factors synthesized in the liver depend on vitamin K, which is not synthesized until intestinal bacteria are present.
2. **Newborn**s are deficient in vitamin K for the first 5 to 8 days of life because of the lack of intestinal bacteria.

B. Use: Prophylaxis and treatment of hemorrhagic disease of the **newborn**

C. Adverse effect: Vitamin K can cause hyperbilirubinemia in the **newborn**.

D. Interventions
1. Protect the medication from light.
2. Administer during the early **newborn** period.
3. Administer in the lateral aspect of the middle third of the vastus lateralis muscle of the thigh.
4. Monitor for bruising at the injection site and for bleeding from the cord.
5. Monitor for jaundice and monitor the bilirubin level because the medication can cause hyperbilirubinemia in the **newborn**.

XIII. HEPATITIS B VIRUS (HBV) VACCINE

A. Description: Given intramuscularly to the **newborn** before discharge from the agency

B. Use: Recommended for all **newborns** to prevent hepatitis B

C. Adverse effect: Rash, fever, erythema, and pain at injection site

D. Interventions
1. Parental consent must be obtained.
2. Administer in the lateral aspect of the middle third of the vastus lateralis muscle:
3. If the **infant** was born to a HBsAg-positive mother, hepatitis B immune globulin (HBIG) is usually given within 12 hours of birth in addition to the hepatitis B vaccine. Then, the regularly scheduled HBV vaccination schedule is followed.
4. Document immunization administration on a vaccination card for the parents to have a record.

MORE QUESTIONS ON EVOLVE!

Practice Questions

246. Methylergonovine (Methergine) is prescribed for a woman to treat postpartum hemorrhage. Before the administration of methylergonovine, the priority nursing action is to check the:
  1. Uterine tone
  2. Blood pressure
  3. Amount of lochia
  4. Deep tendon reflexes

247. A nurse is caring for a client who is receiving oxytocin (Pitocin) to induce labor. The nurse discontinues the oxytocin infusion and notifies the

registered nurse if which of the following is noted on data collection of the client?
1. Fatigue
2. Drowsiness
3. Uterine hyperstimulation
4. Early decelerations of the fetal heart rate

248. A pregnant client is receiving magnesium sulfate for the management of preeclampsia. A nurse determines that the client is experiencing toxicity from the medication if which of the following is noted on data collection?
1. Proteinuria of 3+
2. Presence of deep tendon reflexes
3. Serum magnesium level of 6 mEq/L
4. Respirations of 10 breaths per minute

249. Epidural analgesia is administered to a woman for pain relief after a cesarean birth. The nurse assigned to care for the woman ensures that which medication is readily available if respiratory depression occurs?
1. Betamethasone
2. Morphine sulfate
3. Naloxone (Narcan)
4. Meperidine hydrochloride (Demerol)

250. $Rh_0(D)$ immune globulin (RhoGAM) is prescribed for a woman after the delivery of a newborn infant, and the nurse provides information to the woman about the purpose of the medication. The nurse determines that the woman understands the purpose of the medication if the woman states that it will protect her next baby from which of the following?
1. Having Rh-positive blood
2. Developing a rubella infection
3. Developing physiological jaundice
4. Being affected by Rh incompatibility

251. A woman with preeclampsia is receiving magnesium sulfate. The nurse assigned to care for the client determines that the magnesium sulfate therapy is effective if:
1. Scotomas are present.
2. Seizures do not occur.
3. Ankle clonus is noted.
4. The blood pressure decreases.

252. Methylergonovine (Methergine) is prescribed for a client with postpartum hemorrhage. Before administering the medication, a nurse contacts the health care provider who prescribed the medication if which of the following conditions is documented in the client's medical history?
1. Hypotension
2. Hypothyroidism
3. Diabetes mellitus
4. Peripheral vascular disease

253. A nursing instructor asks a nursing student to describe the procedure for administering erythromycin ointment to the eyes of a neonate. The instructor determines that the student needs to research this procedure further if the student states:
1. "I will flush the eyes after instilling the ointment."
2. "I will cleanse the neonate's eyes before instilling the ointment."
3. "The administration of the eye ointment is within 1 hour after delivery."
4. "I will instill the eye ointment into each of the neonate's conjunctival sacs."

254. A 31-week preterm labor client dilated to 4 centimeters has been started on magnesium sulfate. Her contractions have stopped. If the client's labor can be inhibited for the next 48 hours, what medication does the nurse anticipate will be prescribed?
1. Betamethasone
2. Nalbuphine (Nubain)
3. Misoprostol (Cytotec)
4. $Rh_0(D)$ immune globulin (RhoGAM)

255. A nurse is monitoring a preterm labor client who is receiving magnesium sulfate intravenously. The nurse monitors for which adverse effect(s) of this medication? **Select all that apply.**
☐ 1. Flushing
☐ 2. Hypertension
☐ 3. Increased urine output
☐ 4. Depressed respirations
☐ 5. Extreme muscle weakness
☐ 6. Hyperactive deep tendon reflexes

ANSWERS

246. 2
Rationale: Methylergonovine, which is an ergot alkaloid, is an agent that is used to prevent or control postpartum hemorrhage by contracting the uterus. Methylergonovine causes continuous uterine contractions and may elevate the blood pressure. A priority before the administration of the medication is to check the blood pressure. The health care provider should be notified if hypertension is present. Although options 1, 3, and 4 may be components of the postpartum data collection procedures, option 2 is related specifically to the administration of this medication.

Test-Taking Strategy: Use the process of elimination. Eliminate options 1 and 3 first, because they are comparable or alike and

related to one another. From the remaining options, use the ABCs—airway, breathing, and circulation. Obtaining the blood pressure is a method of checking circulation. Review the adverse effects of methylergonovine if you had difficulty with this question.
Level of Cognitive Ability: Analyzing
Client Needs: Physiological Integrity
Integrated Process: Nursing Process/Data Collection
Content Area: Maternity/Postpartum
Reference: Hodgson, Kizior, p. 744. 2011.

247. 3
Rationale: Oxytocin stimulates uterine contractions, and it is one of the common pharmacological methods used to induce labor. An adverse effect associated with the administration of the medication is the hyperstimulation of uterine contractions. Therefore, oxytocin infusion must be stopped when any signs of uterine hyperstimulation are present. Fatigue and drowsiness may be caused by the labor experience. Early decelerations of the fetal heart rate are a reassuring sign and do not indicate fetal distress.
Test-Taking Strategy: Use the process of elimination, and focus on the subject of an adverse effect to oxytocin. Options 1 and 2 can be eliminated first because they are comparable or alike. From the remaining options, recalling that early decelerations of the fetal heart rate are a reassuring sign will direct you to option 3. Review the nursing responsibilities associated with oxytocin if you had difficulty with this question.
Level of Cognitive Ability: Analyzing
Client Needs: Physiological Integrity
Integrated Process: Nursing Process/Implementation
Content Area: Maternity/Intrapartum
References: Hodgson, Kizior, pp. 879–880. 2011.
Kee, Hayes, McCuistion, p. 850. 2009.

248. 4
Rationale: Magnesium toxicity can occur as a result of magnesium sulfate therapy. Signs of magnesium sulfate toxicity relate to the central nervous system depressant effects of the medication and include respiratory depression (respiratory rate less than 12 breaths per minute), a loss of deep tendon reflexes, and a sudden drop in the fetal heart rate, maternal heart rate, and blood pressure. Therapeutic serum levels of magnesium are 4 to 7.5 mEq/L or 5 to 8 mg/dL. Proteinuria of 3+ is likely to be noted in a client with preeclampsia.
Test-Taking Strategy: Use the process of elimination. Eliminate option 2 first, because it is a normal finding. Next, eliminate option 3, knowing that the therapeutic serum level of magnesium is between 4 and 7.5 mEq/L. From the remaining options, recalling that proteinuria of 3+ would be noted in a client with preeclampsia will direct you to the correct option. Review the adverse effects of magnesium sulfate if you had difficulty with this question.
Level of Cognitive Ability: Analyzing
Client Needs: Physiological Integrity
Integrated Process: Nursing Process/Data Collection
Content Area: Maternity/Intrapartum
References: Lehne, pp. 511–512. 2010.
Leifer, p. 94. 2011.

249. 3
Rationale: Opioids are used for epidural analgesia. An adverse effect of epidural analgesia is a delayed respiratory depression.

Naloxone (Narcan) is an opioid antagonist, which reverses the effects of opioids and is given for respiratory depression. Morphine sulfate and meperidine hydrochloride are opioid analgesics. Betamethasone is a corticosteroid that is administered to enhance fetal lung maturity.
Test-Taking Strategy: Use the process of elimination, and focus on the subject of the question: the antidote for respiratory depression. Eliminate options 2 and 4 first, knowing that these medications are opioid analgesics. Next, eliminate option 1, knowing that this medication is a corticosteroid. Review the purposes and actions of these medications if you had difficulty with this question.
Level of Cognitive Ability: Applying
Client Needs: Physiological Integrity
Integrated Process: Nursing Process/Planning
Content Area: Maternity/Postpartum
Reference: Hodgson, Kizior, pp. 802–803. 2011.

250. 4
Rationale: Rh incompatibility can occur when an Rh-negative mother becomes sensitized to the Rh antigen. Sensitization may develop when an Rh-negative woman becomes pregnant with a fetus who is Rh positive. During pregnancy and at delivery, some of the baby's Rh-positive blood can enter the maternal circulation, thus causing the woman's immune system to form antibodies against the Rh-positive blood. The administration of $Rh_0(D)$ immune globulin prevents the woman from developing antibodies against Rh-positive blood by providing passive antibody protection against the Rh antigen.
Test-Taking Strategy: Use the process of elimination. Options 2 and 3 can be eliminated first. From the remaining options, note the relationship between the name of the medication, $Rh_0(D)$ immune globulin, and the word "incompatibility" in the correct option. Review the purpose of $Rh_0(D)$ immune globulin if you had difficulty with this question.
Level of Cognitive Ability: Analyzing
Client Needs: Physiological Integrity
Integrated Process: Teaching and Learning
Content Area: Maternity/Postpartum
References: Hodgson, Kizior, pp. 1007–1008. 2011.
Kee, Hayes, McCuistion, p. 867. 2009.

251. 2
Rationale: For a client with preeclampsia, the goal of care is directed at preventing eclampsia (seizures). Magnesium sulfate is an anticonvulsant rather than an antihypertensive agent. Although a decrease in blood pressure may be noted initially, this effect is usually transient. Scotomas are areas of complete or partial blindness. Visual disturbances, such as scotomas, often precede an eclamptic seizure. Ankle clonus indicates hyperreflexia and may precede the onset of eclampsia.
Test-Taking Strategy: Use the process of elimination. Knowing that magnesium sulfate is an anticonvulsant will direct you to option 2. Review the actions and uses of magnesium sulfate if you had difficulty with this question.
Level of Cognitive Ability: Evaluating
Client Needs: Physiological Integrity
Integrated Process: Nursing Process/Evaluation
Content Area: Maternity/Intrapartum
References: Hodgson, Kizior, p. 709. 2011.
Leifer, p. 94. 2011.

252. 4

Rationale: Methylergonovine is an ergot alkaloid that is used to treat postpartum hemorrhage. Ergot alkaloids are avoided in clients with significant cardiovascular disease, peripheral vascular disease, hypertension, eclampsia, or preeclampsia, because these conditions are worsened by the vasoconstrictive effects of the ergot alkaloids. Options 1, 2, and 3 are not contraindications related to the use of ergot alkaloids.

Test-Taking Strategy: Use the process of elimination. Recalling that ergot alkaloids produce vasoconstriction will direct you to option 4. Review the effects of ergot alkaloids and the associated contraindications if you had difficulty with this question.

Level of Cognitive Ability: Analyzing
Client Needs: Physiological Integrity
Integrated Process: Nursing Process/Implementation
Content Area: Maternity/Postpartum
Reference: Hodgson, Kizior, p. 743. 2011.

253. 1

Rationale: Eye prophylaxis protects the neonate against *Neisseria gonorrhoeae* and *Chlamydia trachomatis*. The eyes are not flushed after the instillation of the medication, because the flush will wash away the administered medication. Options 2, 3, and 4 are correct statements regarding the procedure for administering eye medication to the neonate.

Test-Taking Strategy: Use the process of elimination, and note the strategic words "needs to research." These words indicate a negative event query and ask you to select an option that is an incorrect statement. Visualize the effect of each statement. This will direct you to option 1. Review the procedure for administering eye medication to the neonate if you had difficulty with this question.

Level of Cognitive Ability: Evaluating
Client Needs: Physiological Integrity
Integrated Process: Teaching and Learning
Content Area: Newborn
References: Kee, Hayes, McCuistion, p. 439. 2009.
Lehne, p. 1136. 2010.

254. 1

Rationale: Betamethasone, which is a glucocorticoid, is given to stimulate fetal lung maturation. It is used for clients in preterm labor between 28 and 32 weeks' gestation if the labor can be inhibited for 48 hours. Nalbuphine (Nubain) is an opioid analgesic. Misoprostol (Cytotec) is a prostaglandin that is given to ripen and soften the cervix and to stimulate uterine contractions. Rh$_0$(D) immune globulin (RhoGAM) is given to RH-negative clients to prevent sensitization.

Test-Taking Strategy: Use the process of elimination. Noting the strategic words "31-week preterm labor client" and recalling that betamethasone is used to stimulate surfactant release will direct you to the correct option. Review the purpose and actions of the medications in the options if you had difficulty with this question.

Level of Cognitive Ability: Analyzing
Client Needs: Physiological Integrity
Integrated Process: Nursing Process/Planning
Content Area: Maternity/Intrapartum
Reference: Kee, Hayes, McCuistion, p. 823. 2009.

255. 1, 4, 5

Rationale: Magnesium sulfate is a central nervous system depressant, and it relaxes smooth muscle, including the uterus. It is used to stop preterm labor contractions, and it is used for preeclamptic clients to prevent seizures. Adverse effects include flushing, depressed respirations, depressed deep tendon reflexes, hypotension, extreme muscle weakness, decreased urine output, pulmonary edema, and elevated serum magnesium levels.

Test-Taking Strategy: Focus on the subject of adverse effects of magnesium sulfate. Recalling that this medication is a central nervous system depressant will assist you with answering correctly. Review the adverse effects of magnesium sulfate if you had difficulty with this question.

Level of Cognitive Ability: Analyzing
Client Needs: Physiological Integrity
Integrated Process: Nursing Process/Data Collection
Content Area: Maternity/Intrapartum
Reference: Hodgson, Kizior, p. 713. 2011.

Growth and Development Across the Life Span

PYRAMID TERMS

abuse The willful infliction of pain, injury, mental anguish, or unreasonable confinement. Abuse can include verbal assaults, the demand to perform demeaning tasks, theft, or the mismanagement of personal belongings (exploitation). Abuse inflicted can be physical, emotional, or sexual.

aging The biopsychosocial process of change that occurs between birth and death.

auscultation The physical assessment (data collection) technique that involves listening to sounds within the body. Special equipment such as a stethoscope may be needed to perform this technique.

dementia An organic syndrome identified by a gradual and progressive deterioration in intellectual functioning. Long- and short-term memory losses occur with impairment in judgment, abstract thinking, problem-solving ability, and behavior resulting in a self-care deficit. A common type of dementia is Alzheimer's disease.

depression A mood disorder that can be identified by feelings of sadness, hopelessness, worthlessness, and a decreased interest in activities.

ego One's "sense of self"; provides functions such as problem solving, the mobilization of defense mechanisms, reality testing, and the capability of functioning independently; it is the mediator between the id and the superego.

id Source of all primitive drives and instincts; considered to be the reservoir of all psychic energy.

inspection The first physical assessment (data collection) technique; begins the moment that the examiner meets the client. It involves a visual assessment of the client during the health history and making observations during the physical examination of specific body systems.

neglect The lack of providing the services necessary for physical or mental health, including a failure to prevent injury.

objective data Information about the client that is obtained by the examiner through the physical examination and review of the results of laboratory, radiological, or other diagnostic studies.

palpation A physical assessment (data collection) technique that involves using the hands to feel certain parts of the client's body, including some organs. The examiner uses this technique to collect data about texture, size, and consistency of the body part being examined.

percussion A physical assessment (data collection) technique that involves tapping the body to check the size, borders, and consistency of some organs as well as to check for the presence of fluid within body cavities. Direct percussion is performed by striking the fingers directly on the body surface. Indirect percussion is performed by striking a finger of one hand on a finger of the other hand as it is placed on the body surface, such as over an organ.

polypharmacy Taking multiple prescription and/or over-the-counter medications together.

play An activity that is spontaneous or organized and provides entertainment or diversion. It is a part of childhood that is necessary for the development of a normal personality and social, physical, and intellectual skills.

safety Instituting measures that ensure protection and the prevention of an accident or injury.

self-neglect The choice to avoid medical care or other services that could improve one's optimal function. Unless an individual has been declared legally incompetent, he or she has the right to refuse care.

subjective data Information obtained from the client during history-taking. It is what the client says about himself or herself.

superego The moral component of the personality, including internalization of the values, ideals, and moral standards of society.

PYRAMID TO SUCCESS

Normal growth and development proceed in an orderly, systematic, and predictable pattern that provides a basis for identifying and assessing an individual's abilities. Understanding the path of growth and development across the life span assists the nurse with identifying appropriate and expected human behavior. The Pyramid to Success focuses on Sigmund Freud's theory of psychosexual development, Jean Piaget's theory of cognitive development, Erik Erikson's psychosocial theory, and Lawrence Kohlberg's theory of moral development. Growth and development concepts also focus on the aging process and on physical characteristics, nutritional behaviors, skills, play, and specific safety measures that are relevant to a particular age group that will ensure a safe and hazard-free environment. Data collection techniques on the adult client are also a focus on the Pyramid to Success. When a question is presented on the NCLEX-PN, if an age is identified in the question, note the age, and think about the associated growth and developmental concepts to answer the question correctly.

CLIENT NEEDS

Safe and Effective Care Environment

- Acting as a client advocate
- Consulting with members of the health care team
- Ensuring home safety and security plans
- Establishing priorities
- Maintaining confidentiality
- Preventing accidents
- Providing care in accordance with ethical and legal standards
- Respecting client and family needs on the basis of their preferences
- Upholding client's rights

Health Promotion and Maintenance

- Discussing high-risk behaviors and lifestyle choices
- Discussing lifestyle choices
- Identifying changes that occur as a result of the aging process

- Identifying developmental stages and transitions
- Identifying expected body image changes
- Monitoring growth and development
- Performing the techniques associated with the health and physical assessment of the client
- Providing client and family education
- Respecting health care beliefs and preferences

Psychosocial Integrity

- Assessing for abuse and neglect
- Considering grief and loss issues and end-of-life care
- Identifying coping mechanisms
- Identifying cultural practices and beliefs of the client and appropriate support systems
- Identifying the loss of the quantity and quality of relationships with the older client
- Monitoring for adjustment to potential deteriorations in physical and mental health and well-being in the older client
- Monitoring for changes in and adjustment to role functioning in the older client (i.e., threats to independent functioning)
- Monitoring for sensory and perceptual alterations
- Providing resources for the client and family

Physiological Integrity

- Administering medications safely and teaching the client about prescribed medications
- Identifying practices or restrictions related to procedures and treatments
- Monitoring for alterations in body systems and the related risks of the aging process
- Providing basic care and comfort needs
- Providing interventions that are compatible with the client's age; cultural, religious, and health care beliefs; education level; and language

27

Theories of Growth and Development

I. PSYCHOSOCIAL DEVELOPMENT AND ERIK ERIKSON

A. The theory
   1. Erikson's theory of psychosocial development describes the human life cycle as a series of eight **ego** developmental stages from birth to death.
   2. Each stage presents a psychosocial crisis, the goal of which is to integrate physical, maturational, and societal demands.
   3. The theory focuses on psychosocial tasks that are accomplished throughout the life cycle.
   4. The **ego** is separate and liberated from the **id,** developed across the course of the complete life cycle.
   5. **Ego** development is influenced by familial, social, and developmental factors.

B. Psychosocial development: Occurs through a life-long series of crises affected by social and cultural factors.

⚠ According to Erikson's theory of psychosocial development, each psychosocial crisis must be resolved for the child or adult to progress emotionally. Unsuccessful resolution leaves the person emotionally disabled.

C. Stages of psychosocial development (Table 27-1)

II. COGNITIVE DEVELOPMENT AND JEAN PIAGET

A. The theory
   1. Piaget's theory defines cognitive acts as the ways in which the mind organizes and adapts to its environment (i.e., "mental mapping").
   2. Schema: Refers to an individual's cognitive structure or framework of thought.
   3. Schemata
      a. Schemata are categories that an individual forms in his or her mind to organize and understand the world.
      b. A young child has only a few schemata with which to understand the world; gradually these are increased.
      c. Adults use a wide variety of schemata to understand the world.
   4. Assimilation
      a. Assimilation is the ability to incorporate new ideas, objects, and experiences into the framework of one's thoughts.
      b. The growing child will perceive and give meaning to new information according to what is already known and understood.
   5. Accommodation
      a. Accommodation is the ability to change a schema to introduce new ideas, objects, or experiences.
      b. Accommodation changes the mental structure so that new experiences can be added.

B. Stages of cognitive development
   1. Sensorimotor stage
      a. 0 to 2 years
      b. Development proceeds from reflex activity to imagining and solving problems through the senses and movement.
      c. The infant or toddler learns about reality and how it works.
      d. The infant or toddler does not recognize that objects continue to exist, even if out of the visual field.
   2. Preoperational stage
      a. 2 to 7 years
      b. The child learns to think in terms of past, present, and future.
      c. The child moves from knowing the world through sensation and movement to prelogical thinking and finding solutions to problems.
      d. The child is egocentric.
      e. The child is unable to conceptualize and requires concrete examples.
   3. Concrete operational
      a. 7 to 11 years
      b. The child is able to classify, order, and sort facts.
      c. The child moves from prelogical thought to solving concrete problems through logic.
   4. Formal operations
      a. 11 years to adulthood
      b. The person is able to think abstractly and logically.

TABLE 27-1 Erik Erikson's Stages of Psychosocial Development

Age	Psychosocial Crisis	Task	Resolution of Crisis	
			Successful	**Unsuccessful**
Infancy (birth to 18 months)	Trust vs. mistrust	Attachment to the mother	Trust in other people; faith and hope about the environment and the future	General difficulties relating to others effectively; suspicion; trust/fear conflict; fear of the future
Early childhood (18 months to 3 years)	Autonomy vs. shame and doubt	Gaining some basic control over the self and the environment	Sense of self-control and adequacy; will power	Independence/fear conflict; severe feelings of self-doubt
Late childhood (3-6 years)	Initiative vs. guilt	Becoming purposeful and directive	Ability to initiate one's own activities; sense of purpose	Aggression/fear conflict; sense of inadequacy or guilt
School age (6-12 years)	Industry vs. inferiority	Developing social, physical, and learning skills	Competence; ability to learn and work	Sense of inferiority; difficulty learning and working
Adolescence (12-20 years)	Identity vs. role confusion	Developing a sense of identity	Sense of personal identity	Confusion about who one is; identity submerged in relationships or group memberships
Early adulthood (20-35 years)	Intimacy vs. isolation	Establishing intimate bonds of love and friendship	Ability to love deeply and commit oneself	Emotional isolation; egocentricity
Middle adulthood (35-65 years)	Generativity vs. stagnation	Fulfilling life goals that involve family, career, and society	Ability to give and care for others	Self-absorption; inability to grow as a person
Later (65 years to death)	Integrity vs. despair	Looking back over one's life and accepting its meaning	Sense of integrity and fulfillment	Dissatisfaction with life

Adapted from Varcarolis, E. (2010). *Foundations of psychiatric mental health nursing* (6th ed.). Philadelphia: Saunders.

c. Logical thinking is expanded to include solving abstract and concrete problems.

III. MORAL DEVELOPMENT AND LAWRENCE KOHLBERG

A. Moral development
   1. Moral development is a complicated process involving the acceptance of the values and rules of society in a way that shapes behavior.
   2. Moral development is classified into a series of levels and behaviors.
B. Levels of moral development (Box 27-1)

IV. PSYCHOSEXUAL DEVELOPMENT AND SIGMUND FREUD

A. Components of the theory (Box 27-2)
   1. Levels of awareness
   2. Agencies of the mind (**id, ego, superego**)
   3. Concept of anxiety and defense mechanisms
   4. Psychosexual stages of development
B. Levels of awareness
   1. Conscious level of awareness
      a. The conscious mind is logical and regulated by the reality principle.
      b. Consciousness includes all experiences that are within an individual's awareness and that the individual is able to control.
      c. Consciousness includes all information that is easily remembered and immediately available to an individual.
   2. Preconscious level of awareness
      a. The preconscious is also called the *subconscious.*
      b. Preconscious includes experiences, thoughts, feelings, or desires that might not be in an individual's immediate awareness but that can be recalled to consciousness.
      c. The subconscious can help repress unpleasant thoughts or feelings and examine and censor certain wishes and thinking.
   3. Unconscious level of awareness
      a. The unconscious is not logical and is governed by the pleasure principle, which refers to seeking immediate tension reduction.
      b. Memories, feelings, thoughts, and wishes are repressed and not available to the conscious mind.
      c. These repressed memories, thoughts, or feelings, if made prematurely conscious, can cause anxiety.
C. Agencies of the mind: Id, ego, and superego

Box 27-1 Moral Development and Lawrence Kohlberg

Level One: Preconventional Morality

Stage 0 (Birth-2 Years): Egocentric Judgment
The infant has no awareness of right or wrong.

Stage 1 (2-3 Years): Punishment–Obedience Orientation
At this stage, children cannot reason as mature members of society.

Children view the world in a selfish way, with no real understanding of right or wrong.

The child obeys rules and demonstrates acceptable behavior to avoid punishment and to avoid displeasing those who are in power, and because he or she fears punishment from a superior force, such as a parent.

A toddler typically is at the first substage of the preconventional stage. This involves a punishment–obedience orientation in which the toddler makes judgments on the basis of avoiding punishment or obtaining a reward.

Physical punishment and withholding privileges tend to give the toddler a negative view of morals.

Withdrawing love and affection as punishment leads to feelings of guilt in the toddler.

Appropriate discipline includes providing simple explanations of why certain behaviors are not acceptable, praising appropriate behavior, and using distractions when the toddler is headed for danger.

Stage 2 (4-7 Years): Instrumental Relativist Orientation
The child conforms to rules to obtain rewards or have favors returned.

The child's moral standards are those of others, and the child observes them to avoid punishment or obtain rewards.

A preschooler is in the preconventional stage of moral development.

During this stage, the conscience emerges, and the emphasis is on external control.

Level Two: Conventional Morality
The child conforms to rules to please others.
The child has an increased awareness of others' feelings.
A concern for social order begins to emerge.
A child views good behavior as that of which those in authority will approve.
If the behavior is not acceptable, the child feels guilty.

Stage 3 (7-10 Years): Good Boy–Nice Girl Orientation
Conformity occurs to avoid disapproval or dislike by others.
This stage involves living up to what is expected by individuals close to the child or what individuals generally expect of others in their roles as son, brother, friend, and so on.

Being good is important and is interpreted as having good motives and showing concern about others.

It also means maintaining mutual relationships with the use of such characteristics as trust, loyalty, respect, and gratitude.

Stage 4 (10-12 Years): Law and Order Orientation
The child has more concern with society as a whole.

The emphasis is on obeying laws to maintain social order.

Moral reasoning develops as the child shifts the focus of living to society.

The school-age child is at the conventional level of the role-conformity stage and has an increased desire to please others.

The child observes and to some extent internalizes the standards of others.

The child wants to be considered "good" by those individuals whose opinions matter to him or her.

Level Three: Postconventional Morality
The individual focuses on individual rights and principles of conscience.
The focus is a concern regarding what is best for all.

Stage 5 (12 Years and Older): Social Contract and Legalistic Orientation
The adolescent is aware that people hold a variety of values and opinions and most values and rules are relative to the group.

The adolescent in this stage gives as well as takes and does not expect to get something without paying for it.

Stage 6: Universal Ethical Principles Orientation
Conformity is based on universal principles of justice and occurs to avoid self-condemnation.

This stage involves following self-chosen ethical principles.

The development of the postconventional level of morality occurs in the adolescent at about the age of 13 years. It is marked by the development of an individual conscience and a defined set of moral values.

The adolescent can now acknowledge a conflict between two socially accepted standards and try to decide between them.

The control of conduct is now internal, both in standards observed and in reasoning about right and wrong.

Box 27-2 Psychosexual Development and Sigmund Freud: Components of the Theory

- Levels of awareness
- Agencies of the mind: id, ego, and superego
- Concept of anxiety and defense mechanisms
- Psychosexual stages of development

⚠ The id, ego, and superego are the three systems of personality. These psychological processes follow different operating principles. In a mature and well-adjusted personality, they work together as a team under the leadership of the ego.

1. The **id**
   a. Source of all drives
   b. Present at birth
   c. Includes genetic inheritance, reflexes, capacities to respond, instincts, basic drives, needs, and wishes that motivate an individual
   d. Operates according to the pleasure principle
   e. Does not tolerate uncomfortable states and seeks to discharge tension and return to a more comfortable, constant level of energy
   f. Acts immediately in an impulsive, irrational way; pays no attention to the consequences of its actions; and therefore often behaves in ways that are harmful to the self and others
   g. The primary process is a psychological activity in which the **id** attempts to reduce tension.
   h. The primary process can include hallucinating or forming an image of the object that will satisfy needs and remove tension.
   i. The primary process by itself is not capable of reducing tension; therefore, a secondary psychological process must develop if the individual is to survive. When this occurs, the structure of the second system of the personality, the **ego,** begins to take form.

2. The **ego**
   a. Functions include reality testing and problem solving
   b. Begins its development during the fourth or fifth month of life
   c. Emerges out of the **id** and acts as an intermediary between the **id** and the external world
   d. Emerges because the needs, wishes, and demands of the **id** require appropriate exchanges with the outside world of reality
   e. Distinguishes between things in the mind and things in the external world
   f. Reality testing is a function of the **ego,** and the **ego** uses realistic thinking
   g. The **ego** follows the reality principle and operates by means of the secondary process of realistic thinking.
   h. The aim of the reality principle is to satisfy the **id's** impulses in the external world with an object that is suitable. The reality principle determines whether an experience is true or false and whether it has external existence.
   i. The **ego** devises a plan and tests the plan by some kind of action to see if it will work.

3. The superego
   a. Necessary part of socialization that develops during the phallic stage of 3 to 6 years of age
   b. Develops from the interactions with one's parents during the extended period of childhood dependency
   c. Includes the internalization of the values, ideals, and moral standards of society
   d. Child internalizes the moral standards of the parents and society
   e. The **superego** consists of the conscience and the **ego** ideal.
   f. The conscience refers to the capacity for self-evaluation and criticism. When moral codes are violated, the conscience punishes the individual by instilling guilt.
   g. What parents approve of and what they reward the child for doing become incorporated as the **ego** ideal by the mechanism of introjection.
   h. The **superego** strives for perfection rather than pleasure and represents the ideal rather than the real.
   i. Living up to one's **ego** ideal results in the individual feeling proud and increases self-esteem.

D. Anxiety and defense mechanisms
   1. The **ego** develops defenses or defense mechanisms to fight off anxiety.
   2. Defense mechanisms operate on an **unconscious** level (except for suppression), so the individual is not aware of their operation.
   3. Defense mechanisms deny, falsify, or distort reality to make it less threatening.
   4. An individual cannot survive without defense mechanisms; however, if they become too extreme in distorting reality, then interference in healthy adjustment and personal growth may occur.

E. Psychosexual stages of development (Box 27-3)
   1. Human development proceeds through a series of stages from infancy to adulthood.
   2. Each stage is characterized by the inborn tendency of all individuals to reduce tension and seek pleasure.
   3. Each stage is associated with a particular conflict that must be resolved before the child can move successfully to the next stage.
   4. Experiences during the early stages determine an individual's adjustment patterns and the personality traits that the individual has as an adult.

Box 27-3 Freud's Psychosexual Stages of Development

Oral Stage (Birth-1 Year)

During this stage, the infant is concerned with his or her own gratification.

The infant is all id, operating on the pleasure principle and striving for the immediate gratification of his or her needs.

When the infant experiences the gratification of basic needs, a sense of trust and security begins.

The ego begins to emerge as the infant begins to see himself or herself as separate from the mother. This marks the beginning of the development of a sense of self.

Anal Stage (1-3 Years)

Toilet training occurs during this period, and the child gains pleasure from both the elimination and retention of feces.

The conflict of this stage is between demands from society and parents and the sensations of pleasure associated with the anus.

The child begins to gain a sense of control over instinctive drives and learns to delay immediate gratification to gain a future goal.

Phallic Stage (3-6 Years)

The child experiences both pleasurable and conflicting feelings associated with the genital organs.

The pleasures of masturbation and the fantasy life of children set the stage for the Oedipus complex.

The child's unconscious sexual attraction to and wish to possess the parent of the opposite sex, the hostility toward and desire to remove the parent of the same sex, and the subsequent guilt regarding these wishes comprise the conflict that the child faces.

The conflict is resolved when the child identifies with the parent of the same sex.

The emergence of the superego is both the solution to and the result of these intense impulses.

Latency Stage (6-12 Years)

During this stage, there is a tapering off of conscious biological and sexual urges.

The sexual impulses are channeled and elevated into a more culturally accepted level of activity.

The growth of ego functions and the ability to care about and relate to others outside of the home are the tasks of this stage of development.

Genital Stage (12 Years and Beyond)

This emerges at adolescence with the onset of puberty, when the genital organs mature.

The individual gains gratification from his or her own body.

During this stage, the individual develops satisfying sexual and emotional relationships with members of the opposite sex.

The individual plans life goals and gains a strong sense of personal identity.

MORE QUESTIONS ON EVOLVE!

Practice Questions

256. A nursing instructor asks a nursing student about Kohlberg's theory of moral development. The instructor determines that the student needs to further research this theory if the student states that a component of the theory includes which of the following?
1. Individuals move through all six stages in a sequential fashion.
2. Moral development progresses in relation to cognitive development.
3. A person's ability to make moral judgments develops over a period of time.
4. It provides a framework for understanding how individuals determine a moral code to guide their behavior.

257. The parent of an 8-year-old child tells the nurse that she is concerned about the child because the child seems to be more attentive to friends than anything else. The appropriate nursing response would be which of the following?
1. "You need to be concerned."

2. "You need to monitor the child's behavior closely."
3. "At this age, the child is developing his or her own personality."
4. "You need to provide more praise to the child to stop this behavior."

258. A parent of a 4-year-old child tells the nurse that she is concerned because the child has been masturbating. The appropriate response by the nurse is which of the following?
1. "This is a normal behavior at this age."
2. "Children usually begin this behavior at the age of 8 years."
3. "This is not normal behavior. The child should be brought to the mental health clinic."
4. "The child is very young to begin this behavior and should be brought to the mental health clinic."

259. A nurse is providing instructions to a new parent regarding the psychosocial development of the infant. Using Erikson's psychosocial development theory, the nurse would instruct the parent to:
1. Allow the infant to signal a need.
2. Anticipate all of the needs of the infant.

3. Attend to the crying infant immediately.
4. Avoid the infant during the first 10 minutes of crying.

260. The parent of a 3-year-old tells the nurse that the child is constantly rebelling and having temper tantrums. Which instruction should the nurse provide to the parent?
1. Set limits on the child's behavior.
2. Ignore the child when this behavior occurs.
3. Allow the behavior, because this is normal at this age period.
4. Punish the child every time the child says "no" to change the behavior.

261. The nurse is caring for an older client who is reminiscing about past life experiences in a positive manner. The nurse understands that this behavior indicates which of the following?
1. A mental status alteration.
2. A normal psychosocial response.
3. Requiring a psychiatric consultation.
4. A sensory deficit requiring social activities.

262. A nursing student is preparing a conference on Freud's psychosocial stages of development, specifically the anal stage. Which of the following appropriately relates to this stage?
1. Gratification of self.
2. Beginning of toilet training.
3. Tapering off of conscious biological and sexual urges.
4. Association with pleasurable and conflicting feelings about the genital organs.

263. A nursing instructor asks a nursing student to describe the formal operations stage of Piaget's cognitive developmental theory. The appropriate response by the nursing student is: "The child:
1. has the ability to think abstractly."
2. develops logical thought patterns."
3. begins to understand the environment."
4. has difficulty separating fantasy from reality."

264. According to Kohlberg's theory of moral development, at the preconventional level, moral development is thought to be motivated by which of the following?
1. Peer pressure
2. Social pressures
3. The parents' behavior
4. Punishment and reward

265. Which of the following are components of ❖ Kohlberg's theory of moral development? **Select all that apply.**
☐ 1. Individuals move through all six stages in a sequential fashion.
☐ 2. Moral development progresses in relation to cognitive development.
☐ 3. A person's ability to make moral judgments develops over a period of time.
☐ 4. The theory provides a framework for understanding how individuals determine a moral code to guide their behavior.
☐ 5. In stage 1 (punishment–obedience orientation), children are expected to reason as mature members of society.
☐ 6. In stage 2 (instrumental relativist orientation), the child conforms to rules to obtain rewards or to have favors returned.

ANSWERS

256. 1
Rationale: Kohlberg's theory states that individuals move through the six stages of development in a sequential fashion but that not everyone reaches stages 5 or 6 as part of their development of personal morality. Options 2, 3, and 4 are correct statements regarding Kohlberg's theory.
Test-Taking Strategy: Note the strategic words "needs to further research." These words indicate a negative event query and ask you to select an option that is an incorrect statement. Also, note the closed-ended word "all" in option 1. Review Kohlberg's theory if you had difficulty with this question.
Level of Cognitive Ability: Understanding
Client Needs: Health Promotion and Maintenance
Integrated Process: Teaching and Learning
Content Area: Fundamental Skills: Developmental Stages
References: Leifer, pp. 365–366. 2011.
McKinney, James, Murray, Ashwill, pp. 56–57. 2009.

257. 3
Rationale: According to Erikson, from the ages of 7 to 12 years, the child begins to move toward receiving support from peers and friends and away from that of parents. The child also begins to develop special interests that reflect his or her own developing personality instead of those of the parents. Therefore, the other options identify incorrect responses.
Test-Taking Strategy: Use Erikson's psychosocial development theory related to school-age children to assist with eliminating options 1 and 2. Eliminate option 4 next; although praising the child for accomplishments is important at this age, the behavior that the child is exhibiting is normal. Review Erikson's psychosocial development theory if you had difficulty with this question.
Level of Cognitive Ability: Applying
Client Needs: Health Promotion and Maintenance
Integrated Process: Teaching and Learning
Content Area: Fundamental Skills: Developmental Stages
References: Hockenberry, Wilson, p. 80. 2009.
Perry, Hockenberry, Lowdermilk, Wilson, p. 850. 2010.

258. 1

Rationale: According to Freud's psychosexual stages of development, the child is in the phallic stage between the ages of 3 and 6 years. At this time, the child devotes much energy to examining his or her genitalia, masturbating, and expressing interest in sexual concerns. Therefore, the other options are incorrect.

Test-Taking Strategy: Use the process of elimination. Eliminate options 3 and 4, because they are comparable or alike. From the remaining options, use Freud's psychosexual stages of development to direct you to option 1. Review Freud's psychosexual stages of development if you had difficulty with this question.

Level of Cognitive Ability: Applying
Client Needs: Health Promotion and Maintenance
Integrated Process: Nursing Process/Implementation
Content Area: Fundamental Skills: Developmental Stages
Reference: Leifer, p. 436. 2011.

259. 1

Rationale: According to Erikson, the caregiver should not try to anticipate the infant's needs at all times, but rather must allow the infant to signal his or her needs. If an infant is not allowed to signal a need, he or she will not learn how to control the environment. Erikson believed that a delayed or prolonged response to an infant's signal would inhibit the development of trust and lead to the mistrust of others. Therefore, the remaining options are incorrect.

Test-Taking Strategy: Use the process of elimination. Eliminate options 3 and 4 first because of the words "immediately" and "avoid." Additionally, option 2 can be eliminated because of the closed-ended word "all." Review Erikson's psychosocial development theory if you had difficulty with this question.

Level of Cognitive Ability: Applying
Client Needs: Health Promotion and Maintenance
Integrated Process: Teaching and Learning
Content Area: Fundamental Skills: Developmental Stages
References: Hockenberry, Wilson, p. 79. 2009.
McKinney, James, Murray, Ashwill, pp. 56–57. 2009.

260. 1

Rationale: According to Erikson, the child focuses on independence between the ages of 1 and 3 years. Gaining independence often means that the child has to rebel against the parents' wishes. Saying things like "no" and "mine" and having temper tantrums are common during this period of development. Being consistent and setting limits on the child's behavior are necessary elements. Punishing the child every time the child says "no" is likely to produce a negative response.

Test-Taking Strategy: Use the process of elimination. Options 2 and 3 can be eliminated first, because they are comparable or alike. Eliminate option 4 next, because this action is likely to produce a negative response during this normal developmental pattern. Review the psychosocial development of the toddler according to Erikson if you had difficulty with this question.

Level of Cognitive Ability: Applying
Client Needs: Health Promotion and Maintenance
Integrated Process: Teaching and Learning
Content Area: Fundamental Skills: Developmental Stages
Reference: McKinney, James, Murray, Ashwill, p. 56. 2009.

261. 2

Rationale: According to Erikson, the later years of life are from 65 years of age until death. The adult reminisces about past life experiences, often viewing them in a positive way. The adult needs to feel good about his or her accomplishments, see successes in his or her life, and feel that he or she has made a contribution to society.

Test-Taking Strategy: Use your knowledge regarding Erikson's theory of psychosocial development of late adulthood to answer the question. Note that options 1, 3, and 4 are comparable or alike; this will direct you to option 2. Review Erikson's theory of psychosocial development if you had difficulty with this question.

Level of Cognitive Ability: Understanding
Client Needs: Psychosocial Integrity
Integrated Process: Nursing Process/Planning
Content Area: Fundamental Skills: Developmental Stages
Reference: Touhy, Jett, pp. 43–45. 2010.

262. 2

Rationale: Toilet training generally occurs during this period. According to Freud, the child gains pleasure from both the elimination and retention of feces. Option 1 relates to the oral stage. Option 3 relates to the latency period. Option 4 relates to the phallic stage.

Test-Taking Strategy: Use the process of elimination. Note the relationship between the words "anal" in the question and "toilet training" in the correct option. Review Freud's psychosocial stages of development if you had difficulty with this question.

Level of Cognitive Ability: Understanding
Client Needs: Health Promotion and Maintenance
Integrated Process: Nursing Process/Planning
Content Area: Fundamental Skills: Developmental Stages
References: Leifer, p. 411. 2011.
Hockenberry, Wilson, p. 78. 2009.

263. 1

Rationale: In the formal operations stage, the child has the abilities to think abstractly and solve problems. Option 2 identifies the concrete operations stage. Option 3 identifies the sensorimotor stage. Option 4 identifies the preoperational stage.

Test-Taking Strategy: Knowledge regarding the characteristics of Piaget's cognitive developmental theory is required to answer this question. Remember, in the formal operations stage, the child has the abilities to think abstractly and solve problems. Review Piaget's cognitive developmental theory if you had difficulty with this question.

Level of Cognitive Ability: Understanding
Client Needs: Health Promotion and Maintenance
Integrated Process: Teaching and Learning
Content Area: Fundamental Skills: Developmental Stages
Reference: Hockenberry, Wilson, pp. 80–81. 2009.

264. 4

Rationale: In the preconventional level, morals are thought to be motivated by punishment and reward. If the child is obedient and not punished, then he or she is being moral. The child sees actions as either good or bad. If the child's actions are good, then the child is praised. If the child's actions are bad, then the child is punished.

Test-Taking Strategy: Use the process of elimination. Eliminate options 1 and 2, because they are comparable or alike. Knowledge that the preconventional stage occurs between the ages of 2 and 7 years will assist with directing you to option 4. Review Kohlberg's theory of moral development if you had difficulty with this question.

Level of Cognitive Ability: Understanding
Client Needs: Psychosocial Integrity
Integrated Process: Nursing Process/Planning
Content Area: Fundamental Skills: Developmental Stages
Reference: McKinney, James, Murray, Ashwill, pp. 58–59. 2009.

❖　**265. 2, 3, 4, 6**
Rationale: Kohlberg's theory states that individuals move through the six stages of development in a sequential fashion, but not everyone reaches stages 5 and 6 during his or her development of personal morality. The theory provides a framework for understanding how individuals determine a moral code to guide their behavior. It also states that moral development progresses in relation to cognitive development and a person's ability to make moral judgments develops over a period of time. In stage 1 (ages 2-3 years; punishment–obedience orientation), children cannot reason as mature members of society because they are too young to do so. In stage 2 (ages 4-7 years; instrumental relativist orientation), the child conforms to rules to obtain rewards or have favors returned.

Test-Taking Strategy: Read each option carefully. Recalling the ages associated with each stage and that the theory provides a framework for understanding how individuals determine a moral code to guide their behavior will assist you with answering the question. Review Kohlberg's theory if you had difficulty with this question.

Level of Cognitive Ability: Understanding
Client Needs: Psychosocial Integrity
Integrated Process: Nursing Process/Planning
Content Area: Fundamental Skills: Developmental Stages
Reference: Hockenberry, Wilson, p. 81. 2009.

Developmental Stages

I. THE HOSPITALIZED INFANT AND TODDLER

A. Separation anxiety
1. Protest
   a. Cries, screams, searches for a parent; avoids and rejects contact with strangers
   b. Verbal attacks on others
   c. Physical fighting: kicks, fights, hits, and pinches
2. Despair
   a. Withdrawn, depressed, and uninterested in the environment
   b. Loss of newly learned skills
3. Detachment
   a. Detachment is uncommon and occurs only after lengthy separations from the parent.
   b. Superficially, the toddler appears to have adjusted to the loss.
   c. During the detachment phase, the toddler again becomes more interested in the environment, **plays** with others, and seems to form new relationships. This behavior is a form of resignation and is not a sign of contentment.
   d. The toddler detaches from the parents in an effort to escape the emotional pain of desiring the parent's presence.
   e. The toddler copes by forming shallow relationships with others, becoming increasingly self-centered, and attaching primary importance to material objects.
   f. Detachment is the most serious phase, because the reversal of the potential adverse effects is less likely to occur after detachment is established. In most situations, the temporary separation imposed by hospitalization does not cause such prolonged parental absence that the toddler enters into detachment.

B. Fear of injury and pain: Affected by previous experiences, separation from parents, and preparation for the experience

C. Loss of control
1. Hospitalization with its own set of rituals and routines can severely disrupt the life of a toddler

2. The lack of control is often exhibited in behaviors related to feeding, toileting, playing, and bedtime.
3. The toddler may demonstrate regression.

D. Interventions
1. Provide cuddling and touch and talk softly to the infant.
2. Provide opportunities for sucking and oral stimulation for the infant using a pacifier if the infant is not to receive anything by mouth.
3. Provide stimulation for the infant, if appropriate, with the use of objects of contrasting colors and textures.
4. Provide routines and rituals that are as close as possible to what the toddler is used to at home.
5. Provide as many choices to the toddler as possible to enable him or her to have some control.
6. Approach the toddler with a positive attitude.
7. Allow the toddler to express feelings of protest.
8. Encourage the toddler to talk about parents or others in his or her life.
9. Accept regressive behavior without ridiculing the toddler.
10. Provide the toddler with favorite and comforting objects.
11. Allow the toddler as much mobility as possible.
12. Anticipate temper tantrums from the toddler, and maintain a safe environment for physical acting out.
13. Employ pain-reduction techniques, as appropriate.

⚠ For the hospitalized toddler, provide routines and rituals as close to possible to what he or she is used to at home.

II. THE HOSPITALIZED PRESCHOOLER

A. Separation anxiety
1. Separation anxiety is generally less obvious and less serious than in the toddler.
2. As stress increases, the preschooler's ability to separate from the parents decreases.

3. Protest
    a. Protest is less direct and aggressive than seen in the toddler.
    b. The preschooler may displace feelings onto others.
4. Despair
    a. The preschooler reacts in a manner similar to the toddler.
    b. The preschooler is quietly withdrawn, depressed, and uninterested in the environment.
    c. The child exhibits loss of newly learned skills.
    d. The preschooler becomes generally uncooperative, refusing to eat or take medication.
    e. The preschooler repeatedly asks when the parents will be visiting.
5. Detachment: Similar to the toddler
B. Fear of injury and pain
    1. The preschooler has a general lack of understanding of body integrity.
    2. The child fears invasive procedures and mutilation.
    3. The child imagines things to be much worse than they are.
    4. Preschoolers believe that they are ill because of something they did or thought.
C. Loss of control
    1. The preschooler likes familiar routines and rituals, and may show regression if not allowed to maintain some control.
    2. The child has attained a good deal of independence and self-care at home. He or she may expect that to continue in the hospital.
D. Interventions
    1. Provide a safe and secure environment.
    2. Take time for communication.
    3. Allow the preschooler to express anger.
    4. Acknowledge fears and anxieties.
    5. Accept regressive behavior. Assist the preschooler to move from regressive to appropriate behaviors according to age.
    6. Encourage rooming-in or leaving a favorite toy.
    7. Allow mobility, and provide **play** and diversional activities.
    8. Place the preschooler with other children of the same age if possible.
    9. Encourage the preschooler to be independent.
    10. Explain procedures simply, on the preschooler's level.
    11. Avoid intrusive procedures when possible.
    12. Allow for the wearing of underpants.

III. THE HOSPITALIZED SCHOOL-AGE CHILD

A. Separation anxiety
    1. The school-age child is accustomed to periods of separation from the parents, but as stressors are added, the separation becomes more difficult.

2. The child is more concerned with missing school and the fear that friends will forget him or her.
3. Usually, the stages of behavior of protest, despair, and detachment do not occur with the school-age child.
B. Fear of injury and pain
    1. The school-age child fears bodily injury and pain.
    2. The child fears illness itself, disability, death, and intrusive procedures in genital areas.
    3. The child is uncomfortable with any type of sexual examination.
    4. The child groans or whines, holds rigidly still, and communicates about pain.
C. Loss of control
    1. The child is usually highly social, independent, and involved with activities.
    2. The child seeks information and asks relevant questions about tests, procedures, and the illness.
    3. The child associates his or her actions with the cause of the illness.
    4. The child may feel helpless and dependent if physical limitations occur.
D. Interventions
    1. Encourage rooming-in.
    2. Focus on the school-age child's abilities and needs.
    3. Encourage the school-age child to become involved with his or her own care.
    4. Accept regression but encourage independence.
    5. Provide choices to the school-age child.
    6. Allow for the expression of feelings, both verbally and nonverbally.
    7. Acknowledge fears and concerns and allow for discussion.
    8. Explain all procedures with the use of body diagrams or outlines.
    9. Provide privacy.
    10. Avoid intrusive procedures, if possible.
    11. Allow the school-age child to wear underpants.
    12. Involve the school-age child in activities that are appropriate to his or her developmental level and illness.
    13. Encourage the school-age child to contact friends.
    14. Provide for educational needs.
    15. Employ appropriate interventions to relieve pain.

IV. THE HOSPITALIZED ADOLESCENT

A. Separation anxiety
    1. Adolescents are not sure whether they want their parents with them when they are hospitalized.
    2. Separation from friends is a source of anxiety.
    3. Adolescents become upset if friends go on with their lives, excluding them.

⚠ For the hospitalized adolescent, separation from friends is a source of anxiety.

B. Fear of injury and pain
1. Adolescents fear being different from others and their peers.
2. Adolescents may give the impression that they are not afraid, although they are terrified.
3. Adolescents become guarded when any areas related to sexual development are examined.

C. Loss of control
1. Behaviors exhibited include anger, withdrawal, and uncooperativeness.
2. Adolescents seek help and then reject it.

D. Interventions
1. Encourage questions about appearance and the effects of the illness on the future.
2. Explore feelings about the hospital and the significance that the illness might have with regard to relationships.
3. Encourage the adolescent to wear his or her own clothes and perform normal grooming activities.
4. Allow favorite foods to be brought in to the hospital, if possible.
5. Provide privacy.
6. Use body diagrams to prepare for procedures.
7. Introduce to other adolescents in the nursing unit.
8. Encourage the maintenance of contact with peer groups.
9. Provide for educational needs.
10. Identify the formation of future plans.
11. Help develop positive coping mechanisms.

V. COMMUNICATION APPROACHES

A. General guidelines (Box 28-1)

B. Infant
1. Infants respond to the nonverbal communication behaviors of adults, such as holding, rocking, patting, and touching.
2. Use a slow approach; allow the infant to get to know the nurse.
3. Use a calm, soft, soothing voice.
4. Be responsive to cries.
5. Talk and read to infants.
6. Allow security objects such as blankets and pacifiers, if the infant has them.

Box 28-1 General Guidelines for Communication

Allow the child time to feel comfortable with the nurse.
Communicate through the use of objects.
Allow the child to express fears and concerns.
Speak clearly and in a quiet, unhurried voice.
Offer choices when possible.
Be honest with the child.
Set limits with the child as appropriate.

C. Toddler
1. Approach the toddler cautiously.
2. Remember that toddlers accept the verbal communications of others literally.
3. Learn the toddler's words for common items and use them in conversations.
4. Use short, concrete terms.
5. Prepare the toddler for procedures immediately before the event.
6. Repeat explanations and descriptions.
7. Use **play** for demonstrations.
8. Use visual aids such as picture books, puppets, and dolls.
9. Allow the toddler to handle the equipment or instruments. Explain what the equipment or instrument does and how it feels.
10. Encourage the use of comfort objects.

D. Preschooler
1. Seek opportunities to offer choices.
2. Speak in simple sentences.
3. Be concise. Limit the length of explanations.
4. Allow for the asking of questions.
5. Describe the procedures as they are about to be performed.
6. Use **play** to explain procedures and activities.
7. Allow the handling of equipment or instruments, which will ease fear and help answer questions.

E. School-age child
1. Establish limits.
2. Provide reassurance to help with alleviating fears and anxieties.
3. Engage in conversations that encourage thinking.
4. Use medical **play** techniques.
5. Use photographs, books, dolls, and videos to explain procedures.
6. Explain in clear terms.
7. Allow time for composure and privacy.

F. Adolescent
1. Remember that the adolescent may be preoccupied with body image.
2. Encourage and support independence.
3. Provide privacy.
4. Use photographs, books, CDs, DVDs, videos, and the Internet to explain procedures.
5. Engage in conversations about the adolescent's interests.
6. Avoid becoming too abstract, too detailed, and too technical.
7. Avoid responding to less-than-desirable social behaviors by prying, confrontation, or judgmental attitudes.

VI. DEVELOPMENTAL CHARACTERISTICS

A. Infant
1. Physical
   a. Height increases by ¾ inch per month.

b. Weight is doubled at 5 to 6 months and tripled at 12 months.

c. At birth, head circumference is 2 to 3 cm greater than chest circumference.

d. By 1 to 2 years of age, head circumference and chest circumference are equal.

e. The anterior fontanel (soft and flat in a normal infant) closes by 12 to 18 months.

f. The posterior fontanel (soft and flat in a normal infant) closes by 2 to 3 months.

g. There are 10 upper and 10 lower deciduous teeth by the age of 2½ years.

h. Lower central incisors are present by 6 to 8 months.

i. The infant sleeps most of the time.

2. Vital signs (Box 28-2)

3. Nutrition

a. The infant may breast-feed or bottle-feed (with iron-fortified formula), depending on the mother's choice; however, human milk is the preferred form of nutrition for all infants, especially during the first 6 months.

b. All infants should receive daily vitamin D supplementation (200 IU) starting in the first 2 months of life to prevent rickets and vitamin D deficiency.

c. Iron stores from birth are depleted by 4 months; if the infant is being only breast-fed, iron supplementation usually with iron-fortified cereal is needed.

d. Whole milk, low-fat milk, skim milk, other animal milk, or imitation milk should not be given to infants as a primary source of nutrition because these food sources lack the necessary components needed for growth and have limited digestibility.

e. Fluoride supplementation may be needed at about 6 months of age, depending on the infant's intake of fluoridated tap water.

f. Solid foods (strained, pureed, or finely mashed) are introduced at about 5 to 6 months of age.

Introduce solid foods one at a time, usually at intervals of 4 to 5 days, to identify food allergens.

g. The sequence of introduction of solid foods varies depending on the health care provider's preference and usually is as follows: iron-fortified rice cereal; fruits, vegetables, and then meats.

h. At 12 months of age, eggs can be given (introduce egg whites in small quantities to detect an allergy); cheese may be used as a substitute for meat.

i. Avoid solid foods that place the infant at risk for choking, such as nuts, foods with seeds, raisins, popcorn, grapes, and pieces of hot dog.

j. Avoid microwaving baby bottles and baby food.

k. Never mix food and/or medications with formula.

l. Avoid adding honey to formula, water, or other fluids (risk of botulism).

m. Offer fruit juice from a cup (12 to 13 months or at a prescribed age) rather than a bottle to prevent nursing (bottle mouth) caries; fruit juice is limited because of its high sugar content.

4. Skills (Box 28-3)

5. **Play**

a. Solitary

b. Birth to 3 months: Verbal, visual, and tactile stimuli

c. 4 to 6 months: Initiates actions and recognizes new experiences

d. 6 to 12 months: Aware of self, imitates, and repeats pleasurable actions

e. Enjoys soft stuffed animals, crib mobiles with contrasting colors, squeeze toys, rattles, musical toys, water toys during the bath, large picture books, and push toys after he or she begins to walk

6. **Safety**

⚠ The parents need to be instructed to keep the poison control number available and to contact the poison control center immediately in the event of a poisoning.

a. Parents must baby-proof the home.

b. Guard the infant when on a bed or changing table.

c. Use gates to protect the infant from stairs.

d. Be sure that bath water is not hot. Do not leave the infant unattended in the bath.

e. Do not hold the infant while drinking or working near hot liquids.

f. Cool vaporizers should be used rather than steam vaporizers to prevent burn injuries.

g. Avoid offering food that is round and similar in size to the airway to prevent choking.

h. Be sure that toys have no small pieces.

Box 28-2 Vital Signs: The Newborn and 1-Year-Old Infant

Newborn
Temperature: Axillary, 97.9° to 98° F
Apical rate: 120 to 140 beats per minute
Respirations: 30 to 60 breaths per minute (average, 40) breaths per minute
Blood pressure: Average, 73/55 mm Hg

1-Year-Old Infant
Temperature: Axillary, 97° to 99° F
Apical rate: 90 to 130 beats per minute
Respirations: 20 to 40 breaths per minute
Blood pressure: Average, 90/56 mm Hg

i. Hanging toys or mobiles over the crib should be well out of reach to prevent strangulation.

j. Avoid placing large toys in the crib. An older infant may use them as steps to climb out.

k. Cribs should be positioned away from curtains and blind cords.

l. Cover electrical outlets.

m. Remove hazardous objects from low, reachable places.

n. Remove chemicals, medications, poisons, and plants from the infant's reach.

Box 28-3 Infant Skills

2 to 3 Months
- Smiles
- Turns head from side to side
- Cries
- Follows objects
- Holds head in midline

4 to 5 Months
- Grasps objects
- Switches objects from hand to hand
- Rolls over for the first time
- Enjoys social interaction
- Begins to show memory
- Aware of unfamiliar surroundings

6 to 7 Months
- Creeps
- Sits with support
- Imitates
- Exhibits fear of strangers
- Holds arms out
- Frequent mood swings
- Waves "bye-bye"

8 to 9 Months
- Sits steadily unsupported
- Crawls
- May stand while holding on
- Begins to stand without help

10 to 11 Months
- Can change from a prone to a sitting position
- Walks while holding onto furniture
- Stands securely
- Entertains self for periods of time

12 to 13 Months
- Walks with one hand held
- Can take a few steps without falling
- Can drink from a cup

14 to 15 Months
- Walks alone
- Can crawl up stairs
- Shows emotions such as anger and affection
- Will explore away from his or her mother in familiar surroundings

---

⚠️ Never shake an infant because of the risk of causing a closed head injury known as shaken baby syndrome.

B. Toddler
1. Physical
   a. Height and weight increase in a steplike fashion that reflects growth spurts and lags.
   b. The head circumference increases about 1 inch between the ages of 1 and 2 years. Thereafter, head circumference increases about ½ inch per year until the age of 5 years.
   c. Anterior fontanel closes between ages 12 and 18 months.
   d. Weight gain is slower than in infancy. By 2 years of age, the average weight is 22 to 27 pounds.
   e. Normal height changes include a growth of about 3 inches per year. The average height of a toddler is 34 inches at 2 years old.
   f. Lordosis, also known as a pot belly, is evident.
   g. The toddler should see a dentist soon after the first teeth erupt (usually around 1 year of age), and oral hygiene measures should be instituted. Regular dental care is essential, and the toddler will require assistance with brushing and flossing the teeth. (Fluoride supplements may be necessary if the water is not fluoridated.)
   h. A toddler should never be allowed to fall asleep with a bottle containing milk, juice, soda, or sweetened water because of the risk of nursing (bottle-mouth) caries.
   i. A toddler typically sleeps through the night. He or she has one daytime nap, which is usually discontinued at about the age of 3.
   j. A consistent bedtime ritual helps prepare the toddler for sleep.
   k. Security objects at bedtime may assist in sleep.
2. Vital signs (Box 28-4)
3. Nutrition

⚠️ Refer to the following web site for the current dietary guidelines for kids: http://www.choosemyplate.gov/specificaudiences.html.

   a. Most toddlers prefer to feed themselves.
   b. The toddler generally does best by eating several small nutritious meals each day rather than three large meals.
   c. Offer a limited number of foods at any one time.

Box 28-4 The Toddler's Vital Signs

Temperature: Axillary, 97.5° to 98.6° F
Apical rate: 80 to 120 beats per minute
Respirations: 20 to 30 breaths per minute
Blood pressure: Average, 92/55 mm Hg

d. Offer finger foods. Avoid concentrated sweets and empty calories.

e. Toddlers are at risk for aspiration of small foods that are not easily chewed, such as nuts, foods with seeds, raisins, popcorn, grapes, and pieces of hot dog.

f. Physiological anorexia is normal as a result of the alternating periods of fast and slow growth.

g. Sit the toddler in a high chair at the family table for meals.

h. Allow sufficient time to eat, but remove food when the toddler begins to **play** with it.

i. The toddler drinks well from a cup that is held with both hands.

j. Avoid using food as a reward or punishment.

4. Skills

a. The toddler begins to walk with one hand held by the age of 12 to 13 months.

b. The toddler runs by the age of 2 years, and walks backward and hops on one foot by the age of 3 years.

c. The toddler usually cannot alternate feet when climbing stairs.

d. The toddler begins to master fine motor skills for building, undressing, and drawing lines.

e. The young toddler often uses the word "no," even when he or she means "yes," to assert independence.

f. The toddler begins to use short sentences and has a vocabulary of about 300 words by the age of 2 years.

5. Bowel and bladder control

a. Certain signs indicate a toddler is ready for toilet training (Box 28-5).

b. Bowel control develops before bladder control.

c. By age 3, the toddler achieves fairly good bowel and bladder control.

d. The toddler may stay dry during the day but may need a diaper at night until about age 4.

6. **Play**

a. The major socializing mechanism is parallel **play**. Therapeutic **play** can begin at this age.

Box 28-5 Signs of Readiness for Toilet Training

- Able to stay dry for 2 hours
- Waking dry from a nap
- Able to sit, squat, and walk
- Able to remove clothing
- Recognizes urge to defecate or urinate
- Expresses willingness to please parent
- Able to sit on toilet for 5 to 10 minutes without fussing or getting off

Adapted from Hockenberry, M., & Wilson, D. (2009). *Wong's essentials of pediatric nursing* (8th ed., p. 417). St. Louis: Mosby.

---

b. The toddler has a short attention span that causes him or her to change toys often.

c. The toddler explores the body parts of self and others.

d. Typical toys include push-pull toys, blocks, sand, finger paints, bubbles, large balls, crayons, trucks, dolls, Play-Doh, toy telephones, cloth books, and wooden puzzles.

7. **Safety**

⚠ Toddlers are eager to explore the world around them. They need to be supervised at play to ensure safety.

a. Use back burners on the stove to prepare a meal, and turn pot handles inward and toward the middle of the stove.

b. Keep dangling cords from small appliances away from the toddler.

c. Place inaccessible locks on windows and doors, and keep furniture away from windows.

d. Secure screens on all windows.

e. Place **safety** gates at stairways.

f. Do not allow the toddler to sleep or **play** in an upper bunk bed.

g. Never leave the toddler alone near a bathtub, pail of water, swimming pool, or any other body of water.

h. Keep toilet lids closed.

i. Keep all medicines, poisons, household plants, and toxic products high and locked out of reach.

C. Preschooler

1. Physical

a. Grows 2½ to 3 inches per year

b. Average height is 37 inches at age 3, 40½ inches at age 4, and 43 inches at age 5

c. Gains 5 pounds per year; average weight of 35 to 40 pounds at age 5

d. Requires about 12 hours of sleep each day

e. A security object and a nightlight help with sleeping.

f. At the beginning of the preschool period, the eruption of the deciduous (primary) teeth is complete.

g. Regular dental care is essential, and the preschooler requires assistance with the brushing and flossing of teeth. Fluoride supplements may be necessary if the water is not fluoridated.

2. Vital signs (Box 28-6)

Box 28-6 The Preschooler's Vital Signs

Temperature: Axillary, 97.5° to 98.6° F
Apical rate: 70 to 110 beats per minute
Respirations: 16 to 22 breaths per minute
Blood pressure: Average, 95/57 mm Hg

3. Nutrition
   a. Exhibits food fads and strong taste preferences
   b. By 5 years old, tends to focus on social aspects of eating, table conversations, manners, and willingness to try new foods
4. Skills
   a. Has good posture
   b. Develops fine motor coordination
   c. Can hop, skip, and run more smoothly
   d. Athletic abilities begin to develop.
   e. Demonstrates increased balancing skills
   f. Alternates feet when climbing stairs
   g. Can tie shoelaces
   h. May talk continuously and ask many "why" questions
   i. Vocabulary increases to about 900 words by age 3 and to about 2100 words by age 5.
   j. By age 3, the preschooler usually talks in three- or four-word sentences and speaks in short phrases.
   k. By age 4, the preschooler uses five- or six-word sentences. By age 5, the preschooler speaks in longer sentences that contain all parts of speech.
   l. The preschooler can be readily understood by others and can clearly understand what others are saying.
5. Bowel and bladder control
   a. By age 4, the preschooler has daytime control of bowel and bladder, but may experience bed-wetting accidents at night.
   b. By age 5, the preschooler achieves both bowel and bladder control, although accidents may occur in stressful situations.
6. **Play**
   a. Cooperative
   b. Imaginary playmates
   c. Likes to build and create things; **play** is simple and imaginative
   d. Understands sharing and is able to interact with peers
   e. Requires regular socialization with children of the same age
   f. **Play** activities include a large space for running and jumping
   g. Likes dress-up clothes, paints, paper, and crayons for creative expression
   h. Swimming and sports aid with growth and development
   i. Puzzles and toys aid with fine motor development
7. **Safety**
   a. Preschoolers are active and inquisitive.
   b. Because of their magical thinking, they may believe that daring feats seen in cartoons are possible and may attempt them.

   c. Preschoolers can learn simple **safety** practices, because they can follow simple and verbal directions, and their attention span is longer.
   d. Teach the preschooler basic **safety** rules to ensure **safety** when playing in a playground near swings and ladders.
   e. Never allow the preschooler to **play** with matches or lighters.
   f. The preschooler should be taught what to do in the event of a fire or if his or her clothes catch fire. Fire drills should be practiced with the preschooler.
   g. Guns should be stored unloaded and secured under lock and key. The preschooler should be taught to leave an area immediately if a gun is seen and to tell an adult.
   h. Teach the preschooler his or her full name, address, parents' names, and telephone number.
   i. Teach the preschooler how to dial 911 in an emergency situation.

   ⚠ Teach a preschooler and school-age child to leave an area immediately if a gun is visible and to tell an adult. The child should also be taught never to point a toy gun at another person.

D. School-age child
   1. Physical
      a. Girls usually grow faster than boys.
      b. Growth of about 2 inches per year between the ages of 6 and 12 years
      c. Height ranges from 45 inches at age 6 to 59 inches at age 12
      d. Weight gain of 4½ to 6½ pounds per year
      e. Average weight of 46 pounds at age 6 and 88 pounds at age 12
      f. The first permanent (secondary) teeth erupt around age 6, and the deciduous teeth are gradually lost.
      g. Regular dentist visits are necessary, and the school-age child needs to be supervised during the brushing and flossing of teeth. Fluoride supplements may be necessary if the water is not fluoridated.
      h. Sleep requirements range from 10 to 12 hours per night.
   2. Vital signs (Box 28-7)
   3. Nutrition
      a. School-age children have increased growth needs.

Box 28-7 The School-Age Child's Vital Signs

Temperature: Oral, 97.5° to 98.6° F
Apical rate: 60 to 100 beats per minute
Respirations: 18 to 20 breaths per minute
Blood pressure: Average, 107/64 mm Hg

b. School-age children may still be picky eaters but are willing to try new foods.

4. Skills
   a. School-age children exhibit refinement of fine motor skills.
   b. Development of gross motor skills continues.
   c. Strength and endurance increase.

5. **Play**
   a. **Play** is more competitive.
   b. Rules and rituals are important aspects of **play** and games.
   c. The school-age child enjoys drawing, collecting items, dolls, pets, guessing games, board games, listening to the radio, television, reading, videos or DVDs, and computer games.
   d. The child participates in team sports.
   e. The child participates in secret clubs, peer-group activities, and scout organizations.

6. **Safety**
   a. The school-age child experiences less fear during **play** activities. He or she frequently imitates real life with the use of tools and household items.
   b. Major causes of injuries include bicycles, skateboards, and team sports as the child increases motor abilities and independence.
   c. Children should always wear a helmet when riding a bike or using inline skates or skateboards.
   d. Teach the school-age child water **safety** rules.
   e. Instruct the school-age child to avoid teasing or playing roughly with animals.
   f. Never allow the school-age child to **play** with matches or lighters.
   g. The school-age child should be taught what to do in the event of a fire or if clothes catch fire. Fire drills should be practiced with the school-age child.
   h. Guns should be stored unloaded and secured under lock and key. The school-age child should be taught to leave an area immediately if a gun is seen and to tell an adult.
   i. Teach the school-age child traffic **safety** rules.
   j. Teach the school-age child how to dial 911 in an emergency situation.

⚠ Teach the preschooler and school-age child that if another person touches his or her body in an inappropriate way, an adult should be told. Also teach the child to avoid speaking to strangers and never to accept a ride, toys, or gifts from a stranger.

E. Adolescent
   1. Physical
      a. Puberty: The maturational, hormonal, and growth process that occurs when the reproductive organs begin to function and the secondary sex characteristics develop.

b. Body mass increases to adult size.
c. Sebaceous and sweat glands become active and fully functional.
d. Body hair distribution occurs.
e. Increase in height, weight, breast development, and pelvic girth occur in girls.
f. Menstrual periods usually occur about 2½ years after the onset of puberty.
g. In boys, an increase in height, weight, muscle mass, and penis and testicle size occur.
h. The voice deepens in boys.
i. Normal weight gain during puberty: Girls gain 15 to 55 pounds and boys gain 15 to 65 pounds.
j. Careful brushing and care of the teeth are important, and many adolescents need to wear braces.
k. Sleep patterns include a tendency to stay up late; therefore, in an attempt to catch up on missed sleep, adolescents sleep late whenever possible. An overall average of 8 hours per night is recommended.

2. Vital signs (Box 28-8)
3. Nutrition
   a. Adolescents typically eat whenever they have a break in activities.
   b. Calcium, zinc, iron, folic acid, and protein are especially important nutritional needs.
   c. Adolescents tend to snack on empty calories and the importance of adequate and healthy nutrition needs to be stressed.
   d. Body image is important.

4. Skills
   a. Gross and fine motor skills are well developed.
   b. Strength and endurance increase.

5. **Play**
   a. Games and athletics are the most common forms of **play**.
   b. Competition and strict rules are important.
   c. Adolescents enjoy activities such as sports, videos, movies, reading, parties, dancing, hobbies, computer games, music, communicating via the Internet and other social media platforms and experimenting, such as with makeup, hairstyles, tattoos, and piercings.
   d. Friends are important. Adolescents like to gather in small groups.

6. **Safety**
   a. Adolescents are risk takers.
   b. Adolescents have a natural urge to experiment and be independent.

Box 28-8 The Adolescent's Vital Signs

Temperature: Oral, 97.5° to 98.6° F
Apical rate: 55 to 90 beats per minute
Respirations: 12 to 20 breaths per minute
Blood pressure: Average, 121/70 mm Hg

c. Instruct adolescents regarding the dangers related to drugs, alcohol, cigarettes, caffeine, suntanning, and motor vehicles of any type.

d. Help adolescents to recognize that there are choices when difficult or potentially dangerous situations arise.

e. Advocate the use of seat belts.

f. Instruct adolescents regarding the consequences of the injuries that motor vehicle crashes can cause.

g. Instruct adolescents regarding water **safety**. Emphasize that they should enter the water feet first, as opposed to diving, especially when the depth of the water is unknown.

h. Instruct adolescents about the dangers associated with guns, violence, and gangs.

i. Instruct adolescents about the complications associated with body piercing, tattooing, and suntanning.

⚠ Discuss issues such as date rape, sexual relationships, and transmission of sexually transmitted infections with the adolescent. Also discuss the dangers of the Internet and other social media platforms related to communicating and setting up meetings (dates) with unknown persons.

F. Early adulthood

1. Description: Period between the late teens and the mid to late thirties

2. Physical changes
   a. The person has completed physical growth by the age of 20 years.
   b. The person is quite active.
   c. Severe illnesses are less common than those seen among older age groups.
   d. The person tends to ignore physical symptoms and postpones seeking health care.
   e. Lifestyle habits such as smoking, stress, lack of exercise, poor personal hygiene, and family history of disease increase the risk of future illness.

3. Cognitive changes
   a. The person has rational thinking habits.
   b. Conceptual, problem-solving, and motor skills increase.
   c. The person identifies preferred occupational areas.

4. Psychosocial changes
   a. The person separates from the family of origin.
   b. The person gives much attention to occupational and social pursuits to improve socioeconomic status.
   c. The person makes decisions regarding career, marriage, and parenthood.
   d. The person needs to adapt to new situations.

5. Sexuality
   a. The person has the emotional maturity to develop mature sexual relationships.
   b. The person is at risk for sexually transmitted infections.

G. Middle adulthood

1. Description: Period between the mid to late thirties and the mid sixties

2. Physical changes
   a. Occur between the ages of 40 and 65 years
   b. The individual becomes aware that changes in reproductive and physical abilities signify the beginning of another stage in life.
   c. Menopause occurs in women; climacteric occurs in men.
   d. Physiological changes often have an impact on self-concept and body image.
   e. Physiological concerns include stress, level of wellness, and the formation of positive health habits.

3. Cognitive changes
   a. The person may be interested in learning new skills.
   b. The person may become involved with educational or vocational programs for entering the job market or changing careers.

4. Psychosocial changes
   a. These may include expected events, such as children moving away from home (postparental family stage), or unexpected events, such as the death of a close friend.
   b. Time and financial demands decrease as children move away from home and the couple face redefining their relationship.
   c. Adults may become grandparents.
   d. Adults are achieving generativity.

5. Sexuality
   a. Many couples renew their relationships and find increased marital and sexual satisfaction.
   b. The onset of menopause and climacteric may affect sexual health.
   c. Stress, health, and medications can affect sexuality.

H. Later adulthood (period between 65 years to death): refer to Chapter 30.

VII. CAR SAFETY SEATS AND GUIDELINES

A. The safest place for all children to ride, regardless of age, is in the back seat of the car.

B. There are different types of car **safety** seats and the manufacturer's guidelines need to be followed.

C. A rear-facing car **safety** seat is never placed in the front seat of a vehicle because if the air bag inflates it will hit the back of the car **safety** seat (where the child's head is) and cause serious injury.

D. Make sure that the **safety** seat is installed tightly and that the seat is at the correct angle so that the infant's head does not fall forward.

E. Lock the car doors; four-door cars should be equipped with child **safety** locks on the back doors.

F. For specific information on types of car **safety** seats for different age groups and the child's size and weight, refer to the American Academy of Pediatrics *Car Safety Seats: Information for Families for 2011* at www.healthychildren.org/English/safety-prevention/on-the-go/Pages/Car-Safety-Seats-Information-for-Families.aspx

MORE QUESTIONS ON EVOLVE!

Practice Questions

266. The parent of a 16-year-old child tells the nurse that she is concerned because the child sleeps until noon every weekend and whenever there is a day off from school. Which of the following is the appropriate nursing response?
    1. "Adolescents love to sleep late in the morning."
    2. "The child shouldn't be staying up so late at night."
    3. "If the child eats properly, that shouldn't be happening."
    4. "The child should have a blood test to check for anemia."

267. A 16-year-old child is admitted to the hospital for acute appendicitis, and an appendectomy is performed. Which of the following interventions is most appropriate to facilitate normal growth and development?
    1. Encourage the child to rest and read.
    2. Encourage the parents to room in with the child.
    3. Allow the family to bring in favorite computer games.
    4. Allow the child to participate in activities with other individuals in the same age group when the condition permits.

268. The emergency room nurse is providing discharge teaching to the parents of a 2-year-old child who sustained burns from a hot cup of coffee that had been left on the kitchen counter. The nurse evaluates that the parents have correctly understood the teaching when they state which of the following?
    1. "We will be sure to not leave hot liquids unattended."
    2. "I guess my child needs to understand what the word 'hot' means."
    3. "We will be sure that our child stays in his room when we work in the kitchen."
    4. "We will install a safety gate as soon as we get home so that our child can't get into the kitchen."

269. The parent of a 4-year-old child expresses concern because her hospitalized child has started sucking his thumb. The mother states that this behavior began 2 days after hospital admission. Which of the following is the appropriate nursing response?
    1. "It is best to ignore the behavior."
    2. "Your child is acting like a baby."
    3. "The doctor will need to be notified."
    4. "A 4-year-old is too old for this type of behavior."

270. The parent of a toddler asks a nurse when it is safe to place the car safety seat in a face-forward position. Which of the following is the best nursing response?
    1. When the toddler weighs 20 lb and is 1 year old
    2. When the weight of the toddler is more than 40 lb
    3. The seat should not be placed in a face-forward position unless there are safety locks in the car.
    4. The seat should never be placed in a face-forward position because of the risk of the child unbuckling the harness.

271. The parents of a 2-year-old arrive at the hospital to visit the child. The child is in the play room and ignores the parents during the visit. The nurse tells the parents that this behavior in a 2-year-old child indicates which of the following?
    1. That the child is withdrawn
    2. That the child is exhibiting a normal pattern
    3. That the child has adjusted to the hospitalized setting
    4. That the child is more interested in playing with other children

272. When caring for a 3-year-old child, the nurse should provide which toy for this child?
    1. A puzzle
    2. A wagon
    3. A golf set
    4. A farm set

273. Upon palpation of the fontanel of a 3-month-old newborn, the nurse notes that the anterior fontanel has not closed and is soft and flat. Which of the following actions should the nurse take?
    1. Increase oral fluids.
    2. Document the findings.
    3. Notify the registered nurse.
    4. Elevate the head of the bed to 90 degrees.

274. A nurse is caring for a 5-year-old child who has been placed in traction after a fracture of the femur. Which of the following is the most appropriate activity for this child?
1. Blocks
2. A puzzle
3. A music video
4. Large picture books

❖ **275.** Select the interventions that are appropriate for the care of an infant. **Select all that apply.**

☐ 1. Provide swaddling.
☐ 2. Talk in a loud voice.
☐ 3. Provide the infant with a bottle of juice at naptime.
☐ 4. Hang mobiles with black-and-white contrast designs.
☐ 5. Caress the infant while bathing or during diaper changes.
☐ 6. Allow the infant to cry for at least 10 minutes before responding.

ANSWERS

266. 1
Rationale: The sleep patterns of the adolescent vary according to individual needs. Adolescents love to sleep late in the morning, but they should be encouraged to be responsible for waking themselves, particularly in time to get ready for school. Options 2, 3, and 4 are incorrect.
Test-Taking Strategy: Use the process of elimination. Options 2 and 3 can be eliminated first, because they are inappropriate responses. From the remaining options, there is no indication that a physiological alteration is present; therefore, option 1 is most appropriate. Review adolescent sleep patterns if you had difficulty with this question.
Level of Cognitive Ability: Applying
Client Needs: Physiological Integrity
Integrated Process: Nursing Process/Implementation
Content Area: Fundamental Skills: Developmental Stages
References: Leifer, p. 203. 2011.
McKinney, James, Murray, Ashwill, p. 161. 2009.

267. 4
Rationale: Adolescents often are not sure whether they want their parents with them when they are hospitalized. Because of the importance of the peer group, separation from friends is a source of anxiety. Ideally, the peer group will support the ill friend. Options 1, 2, and 3 isolate the child from the peer group.
Test-Taking Strategy: Consider the psychosocial needs of the adolescent when answering the question. Options 1, 2, and 3 are comparable or alike in that they isolate the child from their own peer group. Review the psychosocial needs of the adolescent if you had difficulty with this question.
Level of Cognitive Ability: Applying
Client Needs: Psychosocial Integrity
Integrated Process: Nursing Process/Implementation
Content Area: Fundamental Skills: Developmental Stages
Reference: Leifer, p. 484. 2011.

268. 1
Rationale: Toddlers, with their increased mobility and developing motor skills, can reach hot water, open fires, or hot objects placed on counters and stoves above their eye level. Parents should be encouraged to remain in the kitchen when preparing a meal and reminded to use the back burners on the stove. Pot handles should be turned inward and toward the middle of the stove. Hot liquids should never be left

unattended, and the toddler should always be supervised. Options 2, 3, and 4 do not reflect an adequate understanding of the principles of safety.
Test-Taking Strategy: Use the process of elimination. Option 2 can be easily eliminated. Options 3 and 4 are comparable or alike in that they isolate the child from the environment. Review safety principles for the toddler if you had difficulty with this question.
Level of Cognitive Ability: Evaluating
Client Needs: Safe and Effective Care Environment
Integrated Process: Nursing Process/Evaluation
Content Area: Fundamental Skills: Safety/Infection Control
Reference: Leifer, p. 415. 2011.

269. 1
Rationale: In the hospitalized preschooler, it is best to accept regression if it occurs, because it is most often caused by the stress of the hospitalization. Parents may be overly concerned about regression and should be told that their child may continue the behavior at home. There is no need to call the physician. Options 2 and 4 are inappropriate.
Test-Taking Strategy: Use the process of elimination. Options 2, 3, and 4 will cause additional stress and concern in the parent. Review the psychosocial issues related to the hospitalized preschool child if you had difficulty with this question.
Level of Cognitive Ability: Applying
Client Needs: Psychosocial Integrity
Integrated Process: Nursing Process/Implementation
Content Area: Fundamental Skills: Developmental Stages
Reference: Leifer, pp. 475, 483. 2011.

270. 1
Rationale: The transition point for switching to the forward-facing position is defined by the manufacturer of the convertible car safety seat, but it is generally at a body weight of 9 kg (20 lb) and an age of 1 year. Options 2, 3, and 4 are incorrect.
Test-Taking Strategy: Use the process of elimination, and focus on the subject of the question. Eliminate options 3 and 4 first because of the closed-ended words "not" and "never." From the remaining options, use your knowledge regarding car safety and the toddler to answer the question. Review these safety principles if you had difficulty with this question.
Level of Cognitive Ability: Applying
Client Needs: Safe and Effective Care Environment
Integrated Process: Teaching and Learning
Content Area: Fundamental Skills: Safety/Infection Control

References: American Academy of Pediatrics. *Car Safety Seats: Information for Families for 2011.* www.healthychildren.org/English/safety-prevention/on-the-go/Pages/Car-Safety-Seats-Information-for-Families.aspx.
Leifer, pp. 403, 417. 2011.

271. 2
Rationale: The toddler is particularly vulnerable to separation. A toddler often shows anger at being left by ignoring the parent or pretending to be more interested in play than in going home. The parents of hospitalized toddlers are frequently distressed by such behavior. The toddler normally engages in parallel play and plays alongside (but not with) other children. Options 2, 3, and 4 are incorrect.
Test-Taking Strategy: Use the concepts of growth and development. Option 3 can be easily eliminated first. There is no information in the question to support option 1. From the remaining options, knowledge regarding separation anxiety in the toddler will direct you to option 2. Review these concepts if you had difficulty with this question.
Level of Cognitive Ability: Understanding
Client Needs: Psychosocial Integrity
Integrated Process: Nursing Process/Implementation
Content Area: Fundamental Skills: Developmental Stages
Reference: Leifer, pp. 472–473. 2011.

272. 2
Rationale: Toys for the toddler must be strong, safe, and too large to swallow or place in the ear or nose. Toddlers need supervision at all times. Push-pull toys, large balls, large crayons, trucks, and dolls are some appropriate toys. A puzzle with large pieces only may be appropriate. A farm set and a golf set may contain items that the child could swallow.
Test-Taking Strategy: Use the process of elimination. Options 3 and 4 can be easily eliminated, because they contain items that could be swallowed by the child. From the remaining options, the most appropriate toy is a wagon. Remember that large and strong toys are safest for the toddler. Review safety measures for the toddler if you had difficulty with this question.
Level of Cognitive Ability: Understanding
Client Needs: Safe and Effective Care Environment
Integrated Process: Nursing Process/Implementation
Content Area: Fundamental Skills: Developmental Stages
Reference: Leifer, pp. 403–404, 417–418. 2011.

273. 2
Rationale: The anterior fontanel is diamond shaped and located on the top of the head. It should be soft and flat in a normal infant, and it normally closes by 12 to 18 months of age. The posterior fontanel closes by 2 to 3 months of age. Therefore, because the findings are normal, the nurse would document the findings
Test-Taking Strategy: Use the process of elimination. Note the strategic words "soft and flat." These should provide you with the clue that this is a normal finding. A bulging or tense fontanel may result from crying or increased intracranial pressure. Review normal findings in the infant if you had difficulty with this question.

Level of Cognitive Ability: Applying
Client Needs: Physiological Integrity
Integrated Process: Nursing Process/Implementation
Content Area: Fundamental Skills: Developmental Stages
Reference: Leifer, pp. 280–281, 556. 2011.

274. 2
Rationale: In the preschooler, play is simple and imaginative, and it includes activities such as dressing up, paints, crayons, and simple board and card games. Puzzles are also appropriate and aid with fine motor development. Blocks are most appropriate for the toddler. A music video is most appropriate for the adolescent. Large picture books are most appropriate for the infant.
Test-Taking Strategy: Note the age of the child, and think about the age-related activity that would be appropriate. Eliminate option 3, knowing that it is most appropriate for the adolescent. From the remaining options, the word "blocks" in option 1 and "large" in option 4 should provide you with the clue that these activities would be more appropriate for a child who is less than 5 years old. Review the appropriate activities for a preschooler if you had difficulty with this question.
Level of Cognitive Ability: Applying
Client Needs: Psychosocial Integrity
Integrated Process: Nursing Process/Implementation
Content Area: Fundamental Skills: Developmental Stages
Reference: Leifer, pp. 432–433. 2011.

275. 1, 4, 5
Rationale: Holding, caressing, and swaddling provide warmth and tactile stimulation for the infant. To provide auditory stimulation, the nurse should talk to the infant in a soft voice and should instruct the mother to do so also. Additional interventions include playing a music box, radio, or television or having a ticking clock or metronome nearby. Hanging a bright, shiny object within 20 to 25 cm of the infant's face in the midline and hanging mobiles with contrasting colors (e.g., black and white) provide visual stimulation. Crying is an infant's way of communicating; therefore, the nurse would respond to the infant's crying. The mother is taught to do so also. An infant or child should never be allowed to fall asleep with a bottle containing milk, juice, soda, or sweetened water because of the risk of nursing (bottle-mouth) caries.
Test-Taking Strategy: Focus on the subject of the care of the infant. Noting the word "loud" in option 2 and the words "at least 10 minutes before responding" in option 6 will assist you with eliminating these interventions. Recalling the concerns related to dental caries will assist you with eliminating option 3. Review the guidelines related to the care of an infant if you had difficulty with this question.
Level of Cognitive Ability: Applying
Client Needs: Psychosocial Integrity
Integrated Process: Nursing Process/Implementation
Content Area: Fundamental Skills: Developmental Stages
References: McKinney, James, Murray, Ashwill, pp. 487, 556. 2009.
Perry, Hockenberry, Lowdermilk, Wilson, pp. 560–561. 2010.

Health and Physical Assessment of the Adult Client

This chapter provides a comprehensive review of health and physical assessment techniques of the adult client.

⚠ Health and physical assessment techniques that can be performed by the licensed practical nurse/licensed vocational nurse may vary depending on the scope of practice defined by the agency and state board of nursing practice act.

I. ENVIRONMENT/SETTING

A. Establish a relationship and explain the procedure to the client.

B. Ensure privacy and make the client feel comfortable (provide a comfortable room temperature and sufficient lighting; remove distractions such as noise or objects; avoid interruptions).

C. Sit down for the interview (avoid barriers such as a desk), maintain an appropriate social distance, and maintain eye level.

D. Use therapeutic communication techniques and open-ended questions to obtain information about the client's symptoms and concerns. Allow time for the client to ask questions.

E. Consider religious and cultural characteristics such as language (the need for an interpreter), values and beliefs, health practices, eye contact, and touch.

F. Keep note-taking to a minimum so the client is the focus of attention.

G. Types of health and physical assessments (Box 29-1)

II. HEALTH HISTORY

A. General state of health: body features and physical characteristics, body movements, body posture, level of consciousness, nutritional status, speech

B. Chief complaint and history of present illness (direct client quotes) that directs the client to seek care

C. Family history: the health status of direct blood relatives as well as the client's spouse

D. Social history
   1. Data about the client's lifestyle with a focus on factors that may affect health

   2. Information about alcohol, drug, and tobacco use; sexual practices; tattoos; body piercing; travel history; and work setting to identify occupational hazards

E. Domestic violence screening
   1. Done to determine if the client is experiencing any form of domestic violence
   2. Conducted during a one-to-one interview with client while obtaining the health history.

III. MENTAL STATUS EXAM

A. The mental status can be checked while obtaining **subjective data** from the client during the health history interview.

B. Appearance
   1. Note appearance, including posture, body movements, dress, hygiene, and grooming.
   2. An inappropriate appearance and poor hygiene may be indicative of **depression**, manic disorder, **dementia**, organic brain disease, or another disorder.

C. Behavior
   1. Level of consciousness: Check alertness and awareness and the client's ability to interact appropriately with the environment.
   2. Facial expression and body language: Check for appropriate eye contact and determine whether facial expression and body language are appropriate to the situation. This data collection technique also provides information regarding the client's mood and affect.
   3. Speech: Check speech pattern for articulation and appropriateness of conversation.

D. Cognitive level of functioning (Box 29-2)

IV. PHYSICAL EXAM

A. Overview
   1. Gather equipment needed for the examination.
   2. Use the senses of sight, smell, touch, and hearing to collect data.
   3. Data collection includes **inspection**, **palpation**, **percussion**, and **auscultation**. These skills are

Box 29-1 Types of Health and Physical Data Collections

Complete data collection: Includes a complete health history and physical examination and forms a baseline database

Focused data collection: Focuses on a limited or short-term problem, such as the client's complaint

Episodic/follow-up data collection: Focuses on evaluating a client's progress

Emergency data collection: Involves the rapid collection of data, often during the provision of lifesaving measures

Adapted from Jarvis, C. (2012). *Physical examination & health assessment* (6th ed., p. 8). St. Louis: Saunders.

Box 29-2 The Mental-Status Examination: Cognitive Level of Functioning

Orientation: Assess the client's orientation to person, place, and time.

Attention span: Assess the client's ability to concentrate.

Recent memory: This is assessed by asking the client to recall a recent occurrence (e.g., the means of transportation used to get to the health care agency for the physical assessment).

Remote memory: This is assessed by asking the client about a verifiable past event (e.g., a vacation).

New learning: This is used to assess the client's ability to recall unrelated words identified by the examiner. The examiner selects four words and asks the client to recall the words 5, 10, and 30 minutes later.

Judgment: This determines whether the client's actions or decisions regarding discussions during the interview are realistic.

Thought processes and perceptions: The way the client thinks and what the client says should be logical, coherent, and relevant. The client should be consistently aware of reality.

performed one at a time, in this order (except for the abdominal assessment).

B. Data collection techniques

⚠ Data collection techniques primarily used by the licensed practical nurse/licensed vocational nurse include inspection, some palpation procedures, and auscultation.

1. **Inspection**
   a. The first data collection technique uses vision and smell senses while observing the client.
   b. Requires good lighting, adequate exposure, and possibly the use of certain instruments by the registered nurse (RN) or health care provider (HCP) (examiners), such as an otoscope or ophthalmoscope

2. **Palpation**
   a. Uses the sense of touch
   b. Warm the hands before touching the client.
   c. Identify tender areas and palpate them last.
   d. The examiner will start with light **palpation** to detect surface characteristics, and then perform deeper **palpation**.
   e. Check texture, temperature, and moisture of the skin, as well as organ location and size.
   f. Check for swelling, vibration or pulsation, rigidity or spasticity, and crepitation.
   g. Check for the presence of lumps or masses, as well as the presence of tenderness or pain.

3. **Percussion**
   a. The examiner will tap the client's skin to check underlying structures and determine vibrations and sounds related to intensity, duration, pitch, quality, and location.
   b. Provides information related to the presence of air, fluid, or solid masses as well as organ size, shape, and position.

4. **Auscultation**: Involves listening to sounds produced by the body, such as heart, lung, or bowel sounds

C. Vital signs
   1. Includes temperature, radial pulse (apical pulse may be measured during the cardiovascular data collection process), respirations, blood pressure, pulse oximetry, and presence of pain
   2. Height and weight and nutritional status are also checked.

V. BODY SYSTEMS DATA: COLLECTION PROCESS

A. Integumentary system: involves **inspection** and **palpation** of skin, hair, and nails.
   1. **Subjective data**: Self-care behaviors, history of skin disease, medications being taken, environmental or occupational hazards and exposure to toxic substances, changes in skin color or pigmentation, change in a mole or a sore that does not heal, presence of tattoos
   2. **Objective data**: Color, temperature (hypothermia or hyperthermia); excessive dryness or moisture; skin turgor; texture (smoothness, firmness); excessive bruising, itching, rash; hair loss (alopecia) or nail abnormalities such as pitting; lesions (may be inspected by the examiner with a magnifier and light or with the use of a wood's light [ultraviolet light used in a darkened room]); scars or birthmarks; edema; capillary filling time (Box 29-3, Box 29-4, and Table 29-1)

⚠ To test skin turgor, gently pinch a large fold of skin and check the ability of the skin to return to its place when released. (Poor turgor occurs in severe dehydration or extreme weight loss.)

3. Client teaching
   a. Provide information about factors that can be harmful to the skin such as the sun.
   b. Encourage performing self-examination of the skin monthly.

B. Head, neck, and lymph nodes: involves **inspection** and **palpation** of the head, neck, and lymph nodes.
   1. Ask the client about headaches, episodes of dizziness (lightheadedness) or vertigo (spinning sensation), history of head injury, loss of consciousness, seizures, episodes of neck pain, limitations of range of motion, numbness or tingling in the shoulders, arms, or hands, lumps or swelling in the neck, difficulty swallowing, medications being taken, history of surgery in the head/neck region.
   2. Head
      a. Inspect and palpate: Size, shape, masses or tenderness, and symmetry of the skull
      b. The temporal arteries, located above the cheekbone between the eye and the top of the ear will be palpated.
      c. Temporomandibular joint: The client is asked to open his or her mouth. The examiner will look for any crepitation, tenderness, or limited range of motion.

Box 29-3 Characteristics of Skin Color

Cyanosis: Mottled bluish coloration
Erythema: Redness
Pallor: Pale, whitish coloration
Jaundice: Yellow coloration

Box 29-4 Assessing Capillary Filling Time

Depress the nail bed to produce blanching.
Release and observe for the return of color.
Color will return within 3 seconds if arterial capillary perfusion is normal.

---

   d. Face: Inspect facial structures for shape, symmetry, involuntary movements, or swelling such as periorbital edema (swelling around the eyes).
3. Neck
   a. Inspected for symmetry of accessory neck muscles.
   b. Check the range of motion.
   c. Cranial nerve XI (spinal accessory nerve) is tested to check muscle strength. The client is asked to rotate the head forcibly against resistance applied to the side of the chin. Also is asked to shrug the shoulders against resistance.
   d. The trachea is palpated: It should be midline, without any deviations.
   e. Thyroid gland: The neck is inspected as the client takes a sip of water and swallows (thyroid tissue moves up with a swallow). **Palpation** is done using an anterior-and-posterior approach. (Usually the normal adult thyroid cannot be palpated. If it is enlarged, the examiner will auscultate for a bruit.)
4. Lymph nodes
   a. The examiner will palpate using a gentle pressure and a circular motion of the finger pads.
   b. The examiner will begin with the preauricular lymph nodes (in front of the ear). Then, the examiner moves to the posterior auricular lymph nodes and then downward toward the supraclavicular lymph nodes.
   c. Palpated with both hands, comparing the two sides for symmetry.
   d. If nodes are palpated, their size, shape, location, mobility, consistency, and tenderness are noted.
5. Client teaching: The client is instructed to notify the HCP if persistent headache, dizziness, or neck pain occurs, swelling or lumps are noted in the head/neck region, or a neck or head injury occurs.

⚠ Neck movements are never performed if the client has sustained a neck injury or a neck injury is suspected.

TABLE 29-1 Pitting Edema Scale

Scale	Description	"Measurement"*	
1+	A barely perceptible pit	2 mm (3/32 in)	
2+	A deeper pit, rebounds in a few seconds	4 mm (6/32 in)	
3+	A deep pit, rebounds in 10-20 seconds	6 mm (1/4 in)	
4+	A deeper pit, rebounds in >30 seconds	8 mm (5/16 in)	

*"Measurement" is in quotation marks because depth of edema is rarely actually measured but is included as a frame of reference.
From Wilson, A., & Giddens, J. (2009). *Health assessment for nursing practice* (4th ed., p. 255). St. Louis: Mosby. Description column data from Kirton, C. Assessing edema, *Nursing 96* 26(7):54, 1996. Illustrations from Canobblo, M. (1990). *Cardiovascular disorders*. St. Louis: Mosby.

C. Eyes: Includes **inspection**, **palpation**, vision-testing procedures, and the use of an ophthalmoscope.
1. **Subjective data**: Difficulty with vision (e.g., decreased acuity, double vision, blurring, blind spots); pain, redness, swelling, watery or other discharge from the eye; use of glasses or contact lenses; medications being taken; history of eye problems
2. **Objective data**
   a. The external eye structures are inspected, including eyebrows, for symmetry; eyelashes for even distribution; eyelids for ptosis (drooping); eyeballs for exophthalmos (protrusion) or enophthalmos (sunken).
   b. Structures inspected include the conjunctiva (should be clear), sclera (should be white), and lacrimal apparatus (check for excessive tearing, redness, tenderness, or swelling), cornea and lens (should be smooth and clear), iris (should be flat, with a round regular shape and even coloration), eyelids, and pupils (Box 29-5).
3. Snellen eye chart
   a. The client is positioned in a well-lit spot 20 feet from the chart, with the chart at eye level, and asked to read the smallest line he or she can discern. (The client is instructed to leave glasses on or contact lenses in.) If the glasses are for reading only, they are removed because they blur distant vision.)
   b. One eye at a time is tested.
   c. Results are recorded using the fraction at the end of the last line successfully read on the chart. Normal visual acuity is 20/20 (distance in feet at which the client is standing from the chart/ distance in feet at which a normal eye could have read that particular line).

Box 29-5 Assessing and Documenting Pupillary Responses

Pupillary Light Reflex
Darken the room (to dilate the client's pupils) and ask the client to look forward.
Test each eye.
Advance a light in from the side to note constriction of the same-side pupil (direct light reflex) and simultaneous constriction of the other pupil (consensual light reflex).

Accommodation
Ask the client to focus on a distant object (dilates the pupil).
Ask the client to shift gaze to a near object held about 3 inches from the nose.
Normal response includes pupillary constriction and convergence of the axes of the eye.

Documenting Normal Findings: PERRLA
P = pupils
E = equal
R = round
RL = reactive to light
A = reactive to accommodation

4. Near vision
   a. Tested using a hand-held vision screener (held about 14 inches from the eye) that contains various sizes of print or the client is asked to read from a magazine.
   b. Each eye is tested separately with the client's glasses on or contact lenses in; normal result is 14/14 (distance in inches at which the subject holds the card from the eye/distance in inches at which a normal eye could have read that particular line)
5. Confrontation test
   a. Used to measure peripheral vision and compare the client's peripheral vision with the examiner's (under the assumption that the examiner's peripheral vision is normal)
   b. The client covers one eye and looks straight ahead. The examiner, positioned 2 feet away, covers his or her eye opposite the client's covered eye.
   c. The examiner advances a finger or other small object in from the periphery from several directions. The client should see the object at the same time the examiner does.
6. Corneal light reflex
   a. Used to check for parallel alignment of the axes of the eye
   b. The client is asked to gaze straight ahead as the examiner holds a light about 12 inches from the client.
   c. The examiner looks for reflection of the light on the corneas in exactly the same spot in each eye.
7. Cover test
   a. Used to check for slight degrees of deviated alignment
   b. Each eye is tested separately.
   c. The examiner asks the client to gaze straight ahead and cover one eye.
   d. The examiner observes the uncovered eye, expecting to note a steady, fixed gaze.
8. Six cardinal positions of gaze
   a. Used to check for muscle weakness in the eyes
   b. The client is asked to hold the head steady, and then follow movement of an object through the positions of gaze.
   c. The client should follow the object in a parallel manner with the two eyes.
   d. The client is checked for nystagmus, an oscillating movement of the eye, best noted around the iris.
9. Color vision
   a. The Ishihara chart is a tool used to check color vision. It determines the client's ability to distinguish a pattern of color (a number) in a series of color plates.
   b. The examiner tests each eye separately and asks the client to identify the number that he or she sees on the chart.

c. The ability to read the number correctly depends on the normal functioning of color vision.

10. Examination of the internal structures
    a. An ophthalmoscope is used to inspect the fundus, including the retina, choroids, optic-nerve disc, macula, fovea centralis, and retinal vessels.
    b. The examiner inspects the size, color, and clarity of the disc, the integrity of the vessels, and the appearance of the macula and fovea and looks for retinal lesions.
    c. Performed in a darkened room
    d. The client's eye glasses are removed (contact lenses are left in place).

11. Client teaching
    a. Instruct the client to notify the HCP if alterations in vision occur or any redness, swelling, or drainage from the eye is noted.
    b. Inform the client of the importance of regular eye examinations.

D. Ears: Includes **inspection**, **palpation**, hearing tests, and the use of an otoscope
   1. **Subjective data**: Difficulty hearing, earaches, drainage from the ears, dizziness, ringing in the ears, exposure to environmental noise, use of a hearing aid, medications being taken, history of ear problems or infections
   2. **Objective data**
      a. Inspect and palpate the external ear, noting size, shape, symmetry, skin color, and the presence of pain
      b. Inspect the external auditory meatus for size, swelling, redness, discharge, and foreign bodies. Some cerumen (ear wax) may be present.
   3. Conductive and sensorineural hearing loss
      a. Conductive hearing loss occurs as a result of a physical obstruction to the transmission of sound waves.
      b. Sensorineural hearing loss occurs as a result of a pathological process in the inner ear or of the sensory fibers that lead to the cerebral cortex.
   4. Voice test
      a. Used to determine whether hearing loss has occurred
      b. One ear is tested at a time. (The ear not being tested is occluded by the client.)
      c. The examiner stands 1 to 2 feet from the client, covers his or her mouth so that the client cannot read the lips, exhales fully, and softly whispers two-syllable words in the direction of the unoccluded ear. The client points a finger up during the test when the examiner's voice is heard. (A ticking watch may also be used to test hearing acuity.)
   5. Pure-tone audiometry testing: provides a precise quantitative measure of hearing by checking the client's ability to hear sounds of varying frequencies (done by a person skilled in performing audiometry testing)

   6. Tuning-fork tests
      a. Used to measure hearing on the basis of air conduction or bone conduction; includes the Weber and Rinne test
      b. To activate the tuning fork, the examiner holds the base and lightly taps the tines against the other hand, setting the fork in vibration.
   7. Weber test
      a. The stem of the vibrating tuning fork is placed in the midline of the client's skull and the client is asked if the tone sounds the same in both ears or better in one ear.
      b. The client hears the tone by bone conduction and the sound should be heard equally in both ears.
   8. Rinne test
      a. The stem of the vibrating tuning fork is placed on the client's mastoid process.
      b. When the client no longer hears the sound, the tuning fork is quickly inverted and placed near the ear canal. The client should still hear a sound.
      c. Normally the sound is heard twice as long by way of air conduction (near the ear canal) than by way of bone conduction (at the mastoid process).
   9. Otoscopic exam
      a. An otoscope is used. For best visualization, the largest speculum that fits comfortably into the client's ear canal should be used.
      b. The examiner asks the client to tilt the head slightly away, to the opposite shoulder. Next the nurse pulls the pinna up and back (on an adult or older child), holds the otoscope upside down, and inserts the speculum slightly down and forward, approximately half an inch, into the ear canal.
      c. The normal tympanic membrane is translucent, shiny, and pearly gray.

   ⚠ Before performing an otoscopic exam and inserting the speculum, the examiner checks the auditory canal for foreign bodies. The client is instructed not to move the head during the examination to avoid damage to the canal and tympanic membrane.

   10. Client teaching
       a. Instruct the client to notify the HCP if an alteration in hearing or ear pain or ringing in the ears occurs, or redness, swelling, or drainage from the ear is noted.
       b. Instruct the client in the proper method of cleaning the ear canal.
       c. The client should cleanse the ear canal with the corner of a moistened washcloth and should

never insert sharp objects or cotton-tipped applicators into the ear canal.

E. Nose, mouth, and throat: Includes **inspection** and **palpation**

1. **Subjective** data

   a. Nose: Check for discharge or nosebleed (epistaxis), facial or sinus pain, history of frequent colds, altered sense of smell, allergies, medications being taken, history of nose trauma or surgery.

   b. Mouth and throat: Check for the presence of sores or lesions, bleeding from the gums or elsewhere, altered sense of taste, toothaches, use of dentures or other appliances, tooth- and mouth-care hygiene habits, at-risk behaviors (e.g., smoking, alcohol consumption), history of infection, trauma, or surgery

2. **Objective data**

   a. External nose should be midline and in proportion to other facial features

   b. Patency of the nostrils can be tested by pushing each nasal cavity closed and asking the client to sniff inward through the other nostril

   c. Use of a nasal speculum and penlight or a short, wide-tipped speculum attached to an otoscope head is used by the examiner to inspect for redness, swelling, discharge, bleeding, or foreign bodies. The nasal septum is checked for deviation.

   d. The examiner presses the frontal sinuses (below the eyebrows) and over the maxillary sinuses (below the cheekbones). The client should feel firm pressure but no pain.

   e. The external and inner surfaces of the lips are checked for color, moisture, cracking, or lesions.

   f. The teeth are inspected for condition and number (should be white, spaced evenly, straight, and clean, free of debris and decay).

   g. The alignment of the upper and lower jaw is checked by having the client bite down.

   h. The gums are inspected for swelling, bleeding, discoloration, and retraction of gingival margins (gums normally appear pink).

   i. The tongue is inspected for color, surface characteristics, moisture, white patches, nodules, and ulcerations (dorsal surface is normally rough; ventral surface is smooth and glistening, with visible veins).

   j. The examiner retracts the cheek with a tongue depressor to check the buccal mucosa and checks the color and for the presence of nodules or lesions. Normal mucosa is glistening, pink, soft, moist, and smooth.

   k. Using a penlight and tongue depressor, the examiner inspects the hard and soft palates for color, shape, texture, and defects. The

hard palate (roof of the mouth), which is located anteriorly, should be white and dome-shaped; and the soft palate, which extends posteriorly, should be light pink and smooth. The pharyngeal (gag) reflex can also be tested.

   l. The uvula is inspected for midline location. The examiner asks the client to say "ahhh" and watches for the soft palate and uvula to rise in the midline. (This tests one function of cranial nerve X, the vagus nerve.)

   m. Using a penlight and tongue depressor, the examiner inspects the throat for color, presence of tonsils, and the presence of exudate or lesions; cranial nerve XII is tested (the hypoglossal nerve) by asking the client to stick out the tongue (should protrude in the midline)

3. Client teaching

   a. Emphasize the importance of hygiene and tooth care, as well as regular dental examinations and the use of fluoridated water or fluoride supplements.

   b. Encourage the client to avoid at-risk behaviors (e.g., smoking, alcohol consumption).

   c. Stress the importance of reporting pain or abnormal occurrence (e.g., nodules, lesions, signs of infection).

F. Lungs

1. **Subjective data**: Cough; expectoration of sputum; shortness of breath or dyspnea; chest pain on breathing; environmental exposure to pollution or chemicals; medications being taken; history of respiratory disease or infection; last tuberculosis test, chest x-ray, pneumonia and any influenza immunizations including the H1N1 vaccine (H and N refer to hemagglutinin and neuroaminidase, respectively, which are surface antigens; and the number 1 refers to the specific subtype of those antigens); smoking history and formula for pack years (number of packs smoked per day × number of years of smoking)

2. **Objective data**: Includes **inspection, palpation, percussion**, and **auscultation**

3. **Inspection** of the anterior and posterior chest: note skin color and condition and the rate and quality of respirations, look for lumps or lesions, note the shape and configuration of the chest wall, note the position the client takes to breathe.

4. **Palpation**: The examiner will palpate the entire chest wall, noting skin temperature and moisture and looking for areas of tenderness and lumps, lesions, masses, or tenderness; chest excursion and tactile or vocal fremitus are assessed.

5. **Percussion**

   a. The examiner starts at the apices, percusses across the top of the shoulders, moving to the interspaces, making a side-to-side comparison all the way down the lung area (Fig. 29-1)

▲ FIGURE 29-1 Landmarks for chest auscultation and percussion. **A,** Posterior view. **B,** Anterior view. **C,** Lateral view. (From Wilson, A. F., & Giddens, J. F. [2009]. *Health assessment for nursing practice* [4th ed.]. St. Louis: Mosby).

b. The examiner will determine the predominant note. Resonance is noted in healthy lung tissue.

c. Hyperresonance is noted when excessive air is present, and a dull note indicates lung density.

6. Auscultation

   a. Use the flat diaphragm end piece of the stethoscope and hold it firmly against the chest wall and listen to at least one full respiration in each location (anterior, posterior, and lateral).

   b. Posterior: Start at the apices and move side to side for comparison (see Fig. 29-1)

   c. Anterior: Auscultate the lung fields from the apices in the supraclavicular area down to the sixth rib. Avoid **auscultation** over female breast tissue (displace this tissue), because sounds will not be heard clearly (see Fig. 29-1).

   d. Compare findings on each side

7. Normal breath sounds: Three types of breath sounds are considered normal in certain parts of the thorax. These include vesicular, bronchovesicular, and bronchial. Breath sounds should be clear to **auscultation** (Fig. 29-2).

8. Abnormal breath sounds: Also known as adventitious sounds (Table 29-2)

9. Voice sounds (Box 29-6)

   a. Performed when a pathological lung condition is suspected

   b. The examiner will auscultate the spoken word over the chest wall.

   c. The client is asked to repeat a phrase while the examiner listens to the chest.

   d. Normal voice transmission is soft and muffled. The examiner can hear the sound but is unable to distinguish exactly what is being said.

 When auscultating breath sounds, instruct the client to breathe through the mouth and monitor the client for dizziness.

10. Client teaching

    a. Encourage the client to avoid exposure to environmental hazards, including smoking. (Discuss smoking cessation programs as appropriate.)

KEY: ▢ Bronchovesicular over main bronchi   ▢ Vesicular over lesser bronchi, bronchioles, and lobes   ▢ Bronchial over trachea

▲ **FIGURE 29-2** Auscultatory sounds. **A,** Anterior thorax. **B,** Posterior thorax. (From Wilson, A. F., & Giddens, J. F. [2009]. *Health assessment for nursing practice* [4th ed.]. St. Louis: Mosby).

TABLE 29-2 Characteristics of Adventitious Sounds

Adventitious Sounds	Characteristics	Clinical Examples
Crackles (previously called *rales*) fine crackles	Fine: high-pitched crackling and popping noises (discontinuous sounds) heard during the end of inspiration. Not cleared by cough. Medium: medium-pitched moist sound heard about halfway through inspiration; not cleared by cough. Coarse: Low-pitched, bubbling or gurgling sounds that start early in inspiration and extend into the first part of expiration.	Fine: May be heard in pneumonia, heart failure, asthma, and restrictive pulmonary diseases. Medium: same as fine but condition is worse. Coarse: same as fine and medium as noted above; may be heard in terminally ill clients with diminished gag reflex and in individuals with pulmonary edema or pulmonary fibrosis.
Wheeze (also called *sibilant* wheeze)	High-pitched, musical sound similar to a squeak. Heard more commonly during expiration, but may also be heard during inspiration. Occurs in small airways.	Heard in narrowed airway diseases such as asthma.
Rhonchi (also called *sonorous* wheeze)	Low-pitched, coarse, loud, low snoring or moaning tone. Actually sounds like snoring. Heard primarily during expiration, but may also be heard during inspiration. Coughing may clear.	Heard in disorders causing obstruction of the trachea or bronchus, such as chronic bronchitis.
Pleural friction rub	A superficial, low-pitched, coarse rubbing or grating sound. Sounds like two surfaces rubbing together. Heard throughout inspiration and expiration. Loudest over the lower anterolateral surface. Not cleared by cough.	Heard in individuals with pleurisy (inflammation of the pleural surfaces).

Data from Wilson, A. F., & Giddens, J. F. (2009). *Health assessment for nursing practice* (4th ed., p. 221). St. Louis: Mosby.

Box 29-6 Voice Sounds on Lung Auscultation

Bronchophony
Ask the client to repeat the words "ninety-nine."
Normal voice transmission is soft, muffled, and indistinct.

Egophony
Ask the client to repeat a long "ee-ee-ee" sound.
Normally the nurse would hear the "ee-ee-ee" sound.

Whispered Pectoriloquy
Ask the client to whisper the word "ninety-nine."
Normal voice transmission is faint, muffled, and almost inaudible.

b. The client should undergo periodic examinations as prescribed (e.g., chest x-ray, tuberculosis skin testing).
c. Encourage the client to obtain pneumonia and influenza immunizations.
d. The HCP should be notified if the client experiences persistent cough, shortness of breath, or other respiratory symptoms.

G. The heart and peripheral vascular system
1. **Subjective data**: Chest pain, dyspnea, cough, fatigue, edema, nocturia, leg pain or cramps (claudication), changes in skin color, obesity, medications being taken, cardiovascular risk factors, family

history of cardiac or vascular problems, personal history of cardiac or vascular problems.

2. **Objective data**: May include **inspection**, **palpation**, **percussion**, and **auscultation**.

3. **Inspection**: The examiner will inspect the anterior chest for pulsations (apical impulse) created as the left ventricle rotates against the chest wall during systole; not always visible.

4. **Palpation**
   a. The examiner will palpate the apical impulse at the fourth or fifth interspace, or medial to the midclavicular line (not palpable in obese clients or clients with thick chest walls).
   b. The examiner will palpate the apex, left sternal border, and base for pulsations; normally none are present.

5. **Percussion**: This may be performed by the examiner to outline the heart's borders and check for cardiac enlargement (denoted by resonance over the lung and dull notes over the heart).

6. **Auscultation**
   a. **Auscultation** areas of the heart (Fig. 29-3)
   b. Auscultate heart rate and rhythm. Check for a pulse deficit (auscultate the apical heart beat while palpating an artery) if an irregularity is noted.
   c. Check for S1 ("lub") and S2 ("dub") sounds. If abnormalities such as irregularities in the beat, extra heart sounds, or the presence of gentle blowing or swooshing noises (murmurs) are noted, the RN or HCP are notified.

7. Peripheral vascular system
   a. Check for adequacy of blood flow to the extremities by palpating arterial pulses for equality and symmetry and checking the condition of the skin and nails
   b. Check for pretibial edema and measure calf circumference (see Table 29-1)
   c. Measure blood pressure
   d. The examiner will palpate superficial inguinal nodes (using firm but gentle pressure), beginning in the inguinal area and moving down toward the inner thigh
   e. An ultrasonic stethoscope may be needed to amplify the sounds of a pulse wave if the pulse cannot be palpated.
   f. Carotid artery: Located in the groove between the trachea and sternocleidomastoid muscle, medial to and alongside the muscle
   g. The examiner will palpate one carotid artery at a time to avoid compromising blood flow to the brain. The examiner will also auscultate each carotid artery for the presence of a bruit (a blowing, swishing sound, which indicates blood-flow turbulence). Normally a bruit is not present.
   h. Palpate the arteries in the extremities (Box 29-7)

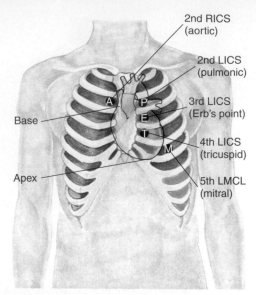

▲ **FIGURE 29-3** Auscultation areas of the heart. (From Wilson, A. F., & Giddens, J. F. [2009]. *Health assessment for nursing practice* [4th ed.]. St. Louis: Mosby).

Box 29-7 Arterial Pulse Points and Grading the Force of Pulses

Arteries in the Arms and Hands
Radial pulse: Located at the radial side of the forearm at the wrist
Ulnar pulse: Located on the opposite side of the location of the radial pulse at the wrist
Brachial pulse: Located above the elbow at the antecubital fossa, between the biceps and triceps muscles

Arteries in the Legs
Femoral pulse: Located below the inguinal ligament, midway between the symphysis pubis and the anterosuperior iliac spine
Popliteal pulse: Located behind the knee
Dorsalis pedis pulse: Located at the top of the foot, in line with the groove between the extensor tendons of the great and first toes
Posterior tibial pulse: Located inside of the ankle, behind and below the medial malleolus (ankle bone)

Grading the Force
4+ = strong and bounding
3+ = full pulse, increased
2+ = normal, easily palpable
1+ = weak, barely palpable

8. Client teaching
   a. Advise the client to modify lifestyle for risk factors associated with heart and vascular disease
   b. Encourage the client to seek regular physical examinations.
   c. Client should seek medical assistance for signs of heart or vascular disease

H. The breasts
1. **Subjective data**: Pain or tenderness, lumps or thickening, swollen axillary lymph nodes, nipple discharge, rash or swelling, medications being taken, personal or family history of breast disease, trauma or injury to the breasts, previous surgery on the breasts, breast self-examination compliance, mammograms as prescribed
2. **Objective data**: Includes **inspection** and **palpation**

⚠ An important role of the nurse is to teach the client how to perform the breat self-examination (BSE), which involves inspection and palpation.

3. **Inspection**
   a. Performed with the client's arms raised above the head, the hands pressed against the hips, and the arms extended straight ahead while the client sits and leans forward
   b. The client is taught to check size and symmetry (one breast is often larger than the other); masses, flattening, retraction, or dimpling; color and venous pattern; size, color, shape, and discharge in the nipple and areola; and the direction in which nipples point
4. **Palpation**
   a. Client lies supine, with the arm on the side being examined behind the head and a small pillow under the shoulder
   b. The client is taught to use the pads of the first three fingers to compress the breast tissue gently against the chest wall, noting tissue consistency.
   c. **Palpation** is performed systematically, ensuring that the entire breast and tail are palpated
   d. The client is taught to note the consistency of the breast tissue, which normally feels dense, firm, and elastic.
   e. The client is taught to gently palpate the nipple and areola and compresse the nipple, noting any discharge.
5. Axillary lymph nodes
   a. The examiner faces the client and stands on the side being examined, supporting the client's arm in a slightly flexed position, and abducts the arm away from the chest wall.
   b. The examiner places the free hand against the client's chest wall and high in the axillary hollow, then, with the fingertips, gently presses down, rolling soft tissue over the surface of the ribs and muscles
   c. Lymph nodes are normally not palpable.
6. Client teaching
   a. Encourage and teach the client to perform breast self-examination (BSE). (Refer to Chapter 43 for information on performing the BSE.)

b. Breast self-examination should be performed 7 to 10 days after the menses. Postmenopausal clients or those who have had a hysterectomy should select a specific day of the month and perform BSE monthly on that day.
c. Regular physical examinations and mammograms should be obtained as prescribed.
d. The client should report lumps or masses to the HCP immediately.

I. The abdomen
1. **Subjective data**: Changes in appetite or weight, difficulty swallowing, dietary intake, intolerance to certain foods, nausea or vomiting, pain, bowel habits, medications being taken, history of abdominal problems or abdominal surgery
2. **Objective data**
   a. The client is asked to empty the bladder.
   b. Be sure to warm the hands and the end piece of the stethoscope.
   c. Painful areas are examined last.

⚠ When performing an abdominal assessment, the specific order for assessment techniques is inspection, auscultation, percussion, and palpation.

3. Inspection
   a. Contour: The examiner will look down at the abdomen and then across the abdomen from the rib margin to the pubic bone; described as flat, rounded, concave, or protuberant.
   b. Symmetry: Note any bulging or masses.
   c. Umbilicus: Should be midline and inverted.
   d. Skin surface: Should be smooth and even.
   e. Pulsations from the aorta may be noted in the epigastric area, and peristaltic waves may be noted across the abdomen.
4. Auscultation
   a. The examiner will perform auscultation before **percussion** and **palpation**, which can increase peristalsis.
   b. Hold the stethoscope lightly against the skin and listen for bowel sounds in all four quadrants. Begin in the right lower quadrant (as bowel sounds are normally heard here).
   c. Note the character and frequency of normal bowel sounds: high-pitched gurgling sounds occurring irregularly from 5 to 30 times a minute
   d. Identify as normal, hypoactive, or hyperactive (borborygmus)
   e. Absent sounds: Auscultate for 5 minutes before determining that sounds are absent.
5. **Percussion**
   a. All four quadrants are percussed lightly by the examiner.
   b. Borders of the liver and spleen are percussed.
   c. Tympany should predominate over the abdomen with dullness over the liver and spleen.

d. **Percussion** over the kidney at the 12th rib (costovertebral angle) should produce no pain.

6. **Palpation**
   a. The examiner will begin with light **palpation** of all four quadrants, using the fingers to depress the skin about 1 cm. Next deep **palpation is performed.**
   b. The examiner will palpate the liver and spleen (which may not be palpable).
   c. The aortic pulsation is palpated in the upper abdomen slightly to the left of midline. Normally it pulsates in a forward direction. (Pulsation expands laterally if an aneurysm is present.)

7. Client teaching
   a. Encourage the client to consume a balanced diet.
   b. Substances that can cause gastric irritation should be avoided.
   c. The regular use of laxatives is discouraged.
   d. Lifestyle behaviors that can cause gastric irritation (e.g., smoking, spicy foods) should be avoided.
   e. Regular physical examinations are important.
   f. The client should report gastrointestinal problems to the HCP.

J. Musculoskeletal system
   1. **Subjective data**: Joint pain or stiffness; redness, swelling, or warm joints; limited motion of joints; muscle pain, cramps, or weakness; bone pain; limitations in activities of daily living; exercise patterns; exposure to occupational hazards (e.g., heavy lifting, prolonged standing or sitting); medications being taken; history of joint, muscle, or bone injuries; history of surgery of the joints, muscles, or bones
   2. **Objective data**: Can include **inspection** and **palpation**
   3. **Inspection**: Inspect gait and posture and for cervical, thoracic, and lumbar curves (Box 29-8).
   4. **Palpation**: The examiner will palpate all bones, joints, and surrounding muscles.
   5. Range of motion
      a. The examiner will perform active and passive range-of-motion exercises of each major joint.
      b. Check for pain, limited mobility, spastic movement, joint instability, stiffness, and contractures.

c. Normally joints are nontender, without swelling, and move freely.

6. Muscle tone and strength
   a. This will be checked during measurement of range of motion
   b. The client is asked to flex the muscle to be examined and then to resist while applying opposing force against the flexion.
   c. Check for increased tone (hypertonicity) or little tone (hypotonicity).

7. Grading muscle strength (Table 29-3)
8. Client teaching
   a. The client should consume a balanced diet, including foods high in calcium and vitamin D.
   b. Activities that cause muscle strain or stress to the joints should be avoided.
   c. Encourage the client to maintain a normal weight.
   d. Participation in a regular exercise program is beneficial.
   e. The client should contact the HCP if joint or muscle pain or problems occur or if limitations in range of motion or muscle strength develop.

K. Neurological system (refer to Chapter 57 for additional information)
   1. **Subjective data:** Headaches, dizziness or vertigo, tremors, weakness, incoordination, numbness or tingling in any area of the body, difficulty speaking or swallowing, medications being taken, history of seizures, history of head injury or surgery, exposure to environmental or occupational hazards (e.g., chemicals, alcohol, drugs)

Box 29-8 **Common Postural Abnormalities**

Lordosis (swayback): Increased lumbar curvature
Kyphosis (hunchback): Exaggeration of the posterior curvature of the thoracic spine
Scoliosis: Lateral spinal curvature

TABLE 29-3 Criteria for Grading and Recording Muscle Strength

Functional Level	Lovett Scale	Grade	Percent of Normal
No evidence of contractility	Zero (0)	0	0
Evidence of slight contractility	Trace (T)	1	10
Complete range of motion with gravity eliminated	Poor (P)	2	25
Complete range of motion with gravity	Fair (F)	3	50
Complete range of motion against gravity with some resistance	Good (G)	4	75
Complete range of motion against gravity with full resistance	Normal (N)	5	100

Data from Wilson, A., & Giddens, J. (2009). *Health assessment for nursing practice* (4th ed., p. 330). St. Louis: Mosby.

2. **Objective data**: Include assessment of cranial nerves, level of consciousness, pupils, motor function, cerebellar function, coordination, sensory function, and reflexes
3. Note mental and emotional status, behavior and appearance, language ability, and intellectual functioning, including memory, knowledge, abstract thinking, association, and judgment
4. Vital signs: Check temperature, pulse, respirations, and blood pressure; monitor for blood pressure or pulse changes, which may indicate increased intracranial pressure (ICP). (See Chapter 57 for abnormal respiratory patterns.)
5. Cranial nerves: Assessed by the examiner (Table 29-4)
6. Level of consciousness
   a. Check the client's behavior to determine level of consciousness (e.g., alertness, confusion, delirium, unconsciousness, stupor, coma). The data collection process becomes increasingly invasive as the client is less responsive.
   b. Speak to client
   c. Determine appropriateness of behavior and conversation.
   d. Lightly touch the client (as culturally appropriate).
7. Pupils
   a. Check size, equality, and reaction to light (brisk, slow, or fixed) and note any unusual eye movements (check direct light and consensual light reflex).
   b. This component of the neurological examination may be performed during the data collection process of the eye.
8. Motor function
   a. Check muscle tone, including strength and equality.
   b. Monitor for voluntary and involuntary movements and purposeful and nonpurposeful movements.
   c. This component of the neurological examination may be performed during the data collection process of the musculoskeletal system.

TABLE 29-4 Assessment of the Cranial Nerves

Cranial Nerve	Testing the Nerve
Cranial nerve I: Olfactory Sensory Controls the sense of smell	The client is asked to close the eyes and occlude one nostril with a finger. Then, the client is asked to identify nonirritating and familiar odors (e.g., coffee, tea, cloves, soap, chewing gum, peppermint). The test is repeated on the other nostril.
Cranial nerve II: Optic Sensory Controls vision	Visual acuity is assessed with a Snellen chart and an ophthalmoscopic exam. Peripheral vision is checked by confrontation. Color vision is checked.
Cranial nerve III: Oculomotor Motor Controls pupillary constriction, upper-eyelid elevation, and most eye movement. Cranial nerve IV: Trochlear Motor Controls downward and inward eye movement. Cranial nerve VI: Abducens Motor Controls lateral eye movement	The motor functions of these nerves overlap; therefore they should be tested together. The eyelids are inspected for ptosis (drooping), then ocular movements are assessed noting any eye deviation. Accommodation and direct and consensual light reflexes are tested.
Cranial nerve V: Trigeminal Sensory and motor Controls sensation in the cornea, nasal and oral mucosa, and facial skin, as well as mastication	To test motor function, the client is asked to clench the teeth and the muscles of mastication are assessed; then the examiner tries to open the client's jaws after asking client to keep them tightly closed. The corneal reflex is tested by lightly touching the client's cornea with a cotton wisp. (This test may be omitted if the client is alert and blinking normally.) Sensory function is checked by asking the client to close the eyes; the examiner lightly touches forehead, cheeks, and chin, noting whether the touch is felt equally on the two sides.
Cranial nerve VII: Facial Sensory and motor Controls movement of the face and taste sensation	Taste perception is tested on the anterior two thirds of the tongue; the client should be able to taste salty and sweet tastes. The client is asked to smile, frown, and show the teeth, and asked to puff out the cheeks. The examiner attempts to close the client's eyes against resistance.

Continued

TABLE 29-4 Assessment of the Cranial Nerves—cont'd

Cranial Nerve	Testing the Nerve
Cranial nerve VIII: Acoustic Sensory Controls hearing and vestibular function	Assessing the client's ability to hear tests the cochlear portion. Assessing the client's sense of equilibrium tests the vestibular portion. The client's hearing is checked using acuity tests. Observe the client's balance and watch for swaying when he or she is walking or standing. Assessment of sensorineural hearing loss may be done by the examiner with the Weber or Rinne test.
Cranial nerve IX: Glossopharyngeal Sensory and motor Controls swallowing ability, sensation in the pharyngeal soft palate and tonsillar mucosa, taste perception on the posterior third of the tongue, and salivation Usually cranial nerves IX and X are tested together	The client's taste perception is tested on the posterior one third of the tongue or pharynx; the client should be able to taste bitter and sour tastes. The soft palate is inspected and the examiner watches for symmetrical elevation when the client says "aaah." The posterior pharyngeal wall is touched with a tongue depressor to elicit the gag reflex.
Cranial nerve X: Vagus Sensory and motor Controls swallowing and phonation, sensation in the exterior ear's posterior wall, and sensation behind the ear Controls sensation in the thoracic and abdominal viscera Usually cranial nerves IX and X are tested together	Refer to cranial nerve IX.
Cranial nerve XI: Spinal accessory Motor Controls strength of neck and shoulder muscles	The examiner palpates and inspects the sternocleidomastoid muscle as the client pushes the chin against the examiner's hand. The examiner palpates and inspects the trapezius muscle as the client shrugs the shoulders against the examiner's resistance.
Cranial nerve XII: Hypoglossal Motor Controls tongue movements involved in swallowing and speech	The examiner observes the tongue for asymmetry, atrophy, deviation to one side, and fasciculations (uncontrollable twitching). The client is asked to push the tongue against a tongue depressor, and then the client is asked to move the tongue rapidly in and out and from side to side.

9. Cerebellar function
   a. Monitor gait as the client walks in a straight line, heel to toe (tandem walking)
   b. Romberg test: The client is asked to stand with the feet together and the arms at the sides and to close the eyes and hold the position. Normally the client can maintain posture and balance.
   c. If appropriate, the client is asked to perform a shallow knee bend or hop in place on one leg and then the other.
10. Coordination
   a. This is checked by asking the client to perform rapid alternating movements of the hands (e.g., turning the hands over and patting the knees continuously).
   b. The examiner asks the client to touch the examiner's finger, then his or her own nose. The client keeps the eyes open, and the examiner moves the finger to different spots to ensure that the client's movements are smooth and accurate.

   c. Heel-to-shin test: The client is assisted into a supine position, then asked to place the heel on the opposite knee and run it down the shin. Normally the client moves the heel down the shin in a straight line.
11. Sensory function
   a. Pain: Checked by applying an object with a sharp point and one with a dull point to the client's body in random order; the client is asked to identify the sharp and dull feelings.
   b. Light touch: A piece of cotton is brushed over the client's skin at various locations in a random order and the client is asked to say when the touch is felt.
   c. Vibration: A tuning fork is used to test the client's ability to feel vibrations over bony prominences. The client is asked to announce when the vibration starts and stops.
   d. Position sense (kinesthesia): The client's finger or toe is moved up or down and the client is asked which way it has been moved. This tests the client's ability to perceive passive movement.

e. Stereognosis: Tests the client's ability to recognize objects placed in his or her hand

f. Graphesthesia: Tests the client's ability to
identify a number traced on the client's hand

g. Two-point discrimination: Tests the client's
ability to discriminate two simultaneous pin-
pricks on the skin

12. Deep tendon reflexes

   a. Includes testing the following reflexes: biceps,
   triceps, brachioradialis, patella, Achilles

   b. Limb should be relaxed

   c. The tendon is tapped quickly with a reflex
   hammer, which should cause contraction
   of muscle.

   d. Scoring deep tendon reflex activity (Box 29-9)

13. Plantar reflex

   a. A cutaneous (superficial) reflex; is tested with
   a pointed but not sharp object

   b. The sole of the client's foot is stroked from
   the heel, up the lateral side, and then across
   the ball of the foot to the medial side.

   c. The normal response is plantar flexion of
   all toes.

⚠ Dorsiflexion of the great toe and fanning of the
other toes (Babinski's sign) is abnormal in anyone
older than 2 years and indicates the presence of central nervous system disease.

14. Client teaching

   a. The client should avoid exposure to environmental hazards (e.g., insecticides, lead).

   b. High-risk behaviors that can result in head
   and spinal cord injuries should be avoided.

   c. Protective devices (e.g., a helmet, body pads)
   should be worn during participating in high-
   risk behaviors.

L. Female genitalia and reproductive tract

   1. **Subjective data**: Urinary difficulties or symptoms
   such as frequency, urgency, or burning, vaginal
   discharge, pain, menstrual and obstetric histories,
   onset of menopause, medications being taken,
   sexual activity and the use of contraceptives, history of sexually transmitted infections

   2. **Objective data**

      a. Use a calm and relaxing approach. The exami-
      nation is embarrassing for many women and
      may be a difficult experience for an adolescent.

      b. Consider the client's cultural background and
      her beliefs with regard to examination of the
      genitalia.

      c. A complete examination will include the exter-
      nal genitalia and a vaginal examination.

      d. The nurse's role is to prepare the client for the
      examination and assist the HCP.

      e. The client is asked to empty her bladder before
      the examination.

Box 29-9 Scoring Deep Tendon Reflex Activity

0 = No response
1+ = Sluggish or diminished
2+ = Active or expected response
3+ = Slightly hyperactive, more brisk than normal; not necessarily pathologic
4+ = Brisk, hyperactive with intermittent clonus associated with disease

Adapted from Wilson, A. F., & Giddens, J. F. (2009). *Health assessment for nursing practice* (4th ed., p. 387, Box 16-3) St. Louis:
Mosby.

   f. The client is placed in the lithotomy position,
   and a drape is placed across the client.

3. External genitalia

   a. Quantity and distribution of hair

   b. Characteristics of labia majora and minora
   (no inflammation, edema, lesions, or lacerations should be noted)

   c. Urethral orifice is observed for color and
   position

   d. Vaginal orifice (introitus) is inspected for
   inflammation, edema, discoloration, discharge, and lesions

   e. The examiner may check Skene's and Bartho-
   lin's glands for tenderness or discharge (if discharge is present, color, odor, and consistency
   are noted and a culture of the discharge is
   obtained)

   f. The client is checked for the presence of a
   cystocele (a portion of the vaginal wall and
   bladder prolapse or fall into the orifice anteriorly); or a rectocele (bulging of the posterior
   wall of the vagina caused by prolapse of the
   rectum)

4. Speculum examination of the internal genitalia

   a. Performed by the HCP

   b. Permits visualization of the cervix and vagina

   c. Papanicolaou smear: A painless screening test
   for cervical cancer is done; the specimen is
   obtained during the speculum examination,
   and the nurse helps prepare the specimen for
   laboratory analysis

5. Client teaching

   a. Stress the importance of personal hygiene.

   b. Explain the purpose and recommended
   frequency of Papanicolaou (Pap) tests.

   c. Explain the signs of sexually transmitted
   infections.

   d. Educate the client on the measures to prevent a
   sexually transmitted infection.

   e. Inform the client with a sexually transmitted
   infection that she must inform her sexual partner of the need for an examination.

M. Male genitalia
1. **Subjective data**: Urinary difficulty (e.g., frequency, urgency, hesitancy or straining, dysuria, nocturia), pain, lesions, or discharge on or from the penis, pain or lesions in the scrotum, medications being taken, sexual activity and the use of contraceptives, history of sexually transmitted infections
2. **Objective data**
   a. Includes assessment (**inspection** and **palpation**) by the examiner of the external genitalia and inguinal ring and canal
   b. The client may stand or lie down for this examination.
   c. Genitalia are manipulated gently to avoid causing erection or discomfort.
   d. Sexual maturity is checked by noting the size and shape of the penis and testes, the color and texture of the scrotal skin, and the character and distribution of pubic hair.
   e. The penis is checked for the presence of lesions or discharge. A culture is obtained if a discharge is present.
   f. The scrotum is inspected for size, shape, and symmetry (normally the left testicle hangs lower than the right) and palpated for the presence of any lumps.
   g. Inguinal ring and canal. **Inspection** (asking the client to bear down) and **palpation** are performed by the HCP to check for the presence of a hernia.
3. Client teaching
   a. Stress the importance of personal hygiene.
   b. Teach the client how to perform testicular self-examination (TSE). A day of the month is selected and the exam is performed on the same day each month after a shower or bath when the hands are warm and soapy and the scrotum is warm. (Refer to Chapter 43 for information on performing the TSE.)
   c. Explain the signs of sexually transmitted infections.
   d. Educate the client on measures to prevent sexually transmitted infections.
   e. Inform the client with a sexually transmitted infection that he must inform his sexual partner of the need for an examination.
N. Rectum and anus
1. **Subjective data**: Usual bowel pattern; any change in bowel habits; rectal pain, bleeding from the rectum, or black or tarry stools; dietary habits; problems with urination; previous screening for colorectal cancer; medications being taken; history of rectal or colon problems; family history of rectal or colon problems

2. **Objective data**
   a. Examination can detect colorectal cancer in its early stages. In men, the rectal examination can also detect prostate tumors.
   b. Women may be examined in the lithotomy position after examination of the genitalia.
   c. A man is best examined by having the client bend forward with his hips flexed and upper body resting over the examination table.
   d. A nonambulatory client may be examined in the left lateral (Sims') position.
   e. The external anus is inspected for lumps or lesions, rashes, inflammation or excoriation, scars, or hemorrhoids.
   f. Digital examination is performed by the HCP to assess sphincter tone; check for tenderness, irregularities, polyps, masses, or nodules in the rectal wall; and assess the prostate gland.
   g. The prostate gland is normally firm, without bogginess, tenderness, or nodules. (Hardness or nodules may indicate the presence of a cancerous lesion.)
3. Client teaching
   a. The diet should include high-fiber and low-fat foods and plenty of liquids.
   b. The client should obtain regular digital examinations.
   c. Identify the symptoms of colorectal cancer or prostatic cancer (men).
   d. The client should follow the American Cancer Society's guidelines for screening for colorectal cancer.

VI. DOCUMENTING HEALTH AND PHYSICAL ASSESSMENT FINDINGS

A. Documentation findings may be recorded either written or electronically (depending on agency protocol).
B. Whether written or electronic, the documentation is a legal document and permanent record of the client's health status.
C. Principles of documentation need to be followed and data need to be recorded accurately, concisely, completely, legibly, and objectively without bias or opinions. Also, always follow agency protocol for documentation.
D. Documentation findings serve as a source of client information for other HCPs.
E. Record findings about the client's health history and physical examination as soon as possible after completion of the health assessment.
F. Refer to Chapter 7 for additional information about documentation guidelines.

MORE QUESTIONS ON EVOLVE!

Practice Questions

276. A Spanish-speaking client arrives at the triage desk in the emergency department and states to the nurse, "No speak English, need interpreter." What is the best action for the nurse to take?
1. Have one of the client's family members interpret.
2. Have the Spanish-speaking triage receptionist interpret.
3. Seek an interpreter from the hospital's interpreter services.
4. Obtain a Spanish-English dictionary and attempt to triage the client.

277. A client with a diagnosis of asthma is admitted to the hospital with respiratory distress. What type of adventitious lung sounds would the nurse expect to hear when collecting data related to the respiratory system for this client?
1. Stridor
2. Wheezes
3. Diminished
4. Pleural friction rub

278. The nurse is reviewing the client's health record and notes that the client elicited a positive Romberg sign. The nurse understands that this indicates which of the following?
1. An involuntary rhythmic, rapid, twitching of the eyeballs
2. A dorsiflexion of the ankle and great toe with fanning of the other toes
3. A significant sway when the client stands erect with feet together, arms at the side, and the eyes closed
4. A lack of normal sense of position when the client is unable to return extended fingers to a point of reference

279. The nurse notes documentation that a client is exhibiting Cheyne-Stokes respirations. On data collection of the client, the nurse expects to note which of the following?
1. Rhythmic respirations with periods of apnea
2. Regular rapid and deep, sustained respirations
3. Totally irregular respiration in rhythm and depth
4. Irregular respirations with pauses at the end of inspiration and expiration

280. The nurse notes documentation that a client has conductive hearing loss. The nurse understands that this type of hearing loss is caused by which of the following?

1. A defect in the cochlea
2. A defect in the 8th cranial nerve
3. A physical obstruction to the transmission of sound waves
4. A defect in the sensory fibers that lead to the cerebral cortex

281. While collecting data related to the cardiac system on a client diagnosed with an incompetent heart valve, the nurse auscultates a murmur. Which of the following best describes the sound of a heart murmur?
1. Lubb-dubb sounds
2. Scratchy, leathery heart noise
3. Gentle, blowing or swooshing noise
4. Abrupt, high-pitched snapping noise

282. The nurse is preparing to assist the health care provider test the extraocular movements in a client to check for muscle weakness in the eyes. The nurse anticipates that which physical assessment technique will be done to assess for muscle weakness in the eye?
1. Testing the corneal reflexes
2. Testing the six cardinal positions of gaze
3. Testing visual acuity using a Snellen eye chart
4. Testing sensory function by asking the client to close eyes and then lightly touching the forehead, cheeks, and chin

283. The nurse is reinforcing instructions for a client in how to perform a testicular self-examination (TSE). The nurse explains that the best time to perform this exam is:
1. After a shower or bath
2. While standing to void
3. After having a bowel movement
4. While lying in bed before arising

284. The nurse notes that the physical assessment findings for a client with meningeal irritation indicate a positive Brudzinski sign. The nurse understands that which observation was made?
1. The client rigidly extends the arms with pronated forearms and plantar flexion of the feet.
2. The client flexes a leg at the hip and knee and reports pain in the vertebral column when the leg is extended.
3. The client passively flexes the hip and knee in response to neck flexion and reports pain in the vertebral column.
4. The client's upper arms are flexed and held tightly to the sides of the body and the legs are extended and internally rotated.

285. The clinic nurse is assisting to perform a focused data collection process on a client who is complaining of symptoms of a cold, a cough, and lung congestion. Which of the following would the nurse include for this type of data collection? **Select all that apply.**

❏ 1. Auscultating lung sounds
❏ 2. Obtaining the client's temperature
❏ 3. Checking the strength of peripheral pulses
❏ 4. Obtaining information about the client's respirations
❏ 5. Performing a musculoskeletal and neurological examination
❏ 6. Asking the client about a family history of any illness or disease

ANSWERS

276. 3
Rationale: The best action is to have a professional hospital-based interpreter translate for the client. English-speaking family members may not appropriately understand what is asked of them and may paraphrase what the client is actually saying. Also, client confidentiality as well as accurate information may be compromised when a family member or a non–health care provider acts as interpreter. Using a Spanish-English dictionary is not the best action; accurate interpretation is best done by a professional hospital-based interpreter.
Test-Taking Strategy: Note the strategic word "best." Initially focus on what the client needs. In this case the client needs and asks for an interpreter. Next keep in mind the issue of confidentiality and making sure that information is obtained in the most efficient and accurate way. This will assist in eliminating options 1, 2, and 4. Review the best nursing actions to take to obtain data from a non–English speaking client if you had difficulty with this question.
Level of Cognitive Ability: Applying
Client Needs: Psychosocial Integrity
Integrated Process: Communication and Documentation
Content Area: Adult Health: Health Assessment/Physical Exam
Reference: Jarvis, pp. 45–47. 2012.

277. 2
Rationale: Asthma is a respiratory disorder characterized by recurring episodes of dyspnea, constriction of the bronchi, and wheezing. Wheezes are described as high-pitched musical sounds heard when air passes through an obstructed or narrowed lumen of a respiratory passageway. Stridor is a harsh sound noted with an upper airway obstruction and often signals a life-threatening emergency. Diminished lung sounds are heard over lung tissue where poor oxygen exchange is occurring. A pleural friction rub is heard in individuals with pleurisy (inflammation of the pleural surfaces).
Test-Taking Strategy: Note the client's diagnosis and think about the pathophysiology that occurs in this disorder. Recalling that bronchial constriction occurs will assist in directing you to option 2. Also, thinking about the definition of each adventitious lung sound identified in the choices will direct you to option 2. Review the characteristics of adventitious breath sounds if you had difficulty with this question.
Level of Cognitive Ability: Analyzing
Client Needs: Physiological Integrity
Integrated Process: Nursing Process/Data Collection
Content Area: Adult Health: Health Assessment/Physical Exam
References: Christensen, Kockrow, pp. 426–427. 2011. *Adult health nursing.*
Jarvis, p. 430. 2012.

278. 3
Rationale: In the Romberg test, the client is asked to stand with the feet together and the arms at the sides and to close the eyes and hold the position. Normally the client can maintain posture and balance. A positive Romberg is a vestibular neurological sign that is found when a client elicits a loss of balance when closing the eyes. This may occur with cerebellar ataxia, loss of proprioception, and loss of vestibular function. A positive gaze nystagmus evaluation results in an involuntary rhythmic, rapid, twitching of the eyeballs. A positive Babinski test results with dorsiflexion of the ankle and great toe with fanning of the other toes. If this occurs in anyone older than 2 years it indicates the presence of central nervous system disease. A lack of normal sense of position coupled with an inability to return extended fingers to a point of reference is a finding in a past pointing test.
Test-Taking Strategy: Specific knowledge regarding the technique for performing the Romberg test is needed to answer this question. You can easily answer this question if you can recall that the client's balance is tested in this test. Review the procedure for performing Romberg's test and the purpose of the test if you had difficulty with this question.
Level of Cognitive Ability: Understanding
Client Needs: Physiological Integrity
Integrated Process: Nursing Process/Data Collection
Content Area: Adult Health: Health Assessment/Physical Exam
References: Jarvis, pp. 638–639. 2012.
Linton, p. 453. 2012.

279. 1
Rationale: Cheyne-Stokes respirations are rhythmic respirations with periods of apnea and can indicate a metabolic dysfunction in the cerebral hemisphere or basal ganglia. Neurogenic hyperventilation is a regular, rapid and deep, sustained respiration that can indicate a dysfunction in the low midbrain and middle pons. Ataxic respirations are totally irregular in rhythm and depth and indicate a dysfunction in the medulla. Apneustic respirations are irregular respirations with pauses at the end of inspiration and expiration and can indicate a dysfunction in the middle or caudal pons.
Test-Taking Strategy: Focus on the subject, the characteristics of Cheyne-Stokes respirations. If you can recall that periods of apnea occur with this type of respiration you will be able to answer this question correctly. Review the characteristics of Cheyne-Stokes respirations if you had difficulty with this question.
Level of Cognitive Ability: Understanding
Client Needs: Physiological Integrity
Integrated Process: Nursing Process/Data Collection
Content Area: Adult Health: Health Assessment/Physical Exam
Reference: Jarvis, p. 442. 2012.

280. 3

Rationale: A conductive hearing loss occurs as a result of a physical obstruction to the transmission of sound waves. A sensorineural hearing loss occurs as a result of a pathological process in the inner ear, a defect in the 8th cranial nerve, or a defect of the sensory fibers that lead to the cerebral cortex.

Test-Taking Strategy: Focus on the subject—a conductive hearing loss. Noting the relationship of the word "conductive" in the question and "transmission" in option 3 will direct you to this option. Review the causes of a conductive and a sensorineural hearing loss if you had difficulty with this question.

Level of Cognitive Ability: Understanding
Client Needs: Physiological Integrity
Integrated Process: Nursing Process/Data Collection
Content Area: Adult Health: Health Assessment/Physical Exam
Reference: Jarvis, p. 326. 2012.

281. 3

Rationale: A heart murmur is an abnormal heart sound and is described as a gentle, blowing, swooshing sound. Lubb-dubb sounds are normal and represent the S1 (first heart sound) and S2 (second heart sound), respectively. A pericardial friction rub is described as a scratchy, leathery heart sound. A click is described as an abrupt, high-pitched snapping sound.

Test-Taking Strategy: Focus on the subject, characteristics of a murmur. Eliminate option 1 because it describes normal heart sounds. Next use the process of elimination recalling that a murmur occurs as a result of the manner in which the blood is flowing through the cardiac chambers and valves. This will direct you to option 3. Review the characteristics of a murmur if you had difficulty with this question.

Level of Cognitive Ability: Understanding
Client Needs: Physiological Integrity
Integrated Process: Nursing Process/Data Collection
Content Area: Adult Health: Health Assessment/Physical Exam
Reference: Jarvis, p. 461. 2012.

282. 2

Rationale: Testing the six cardinal positions of gaze is done to check for muscle weakness in the eyes. The client is asked to hold the head steady, then to follow movement of an object through the positions of gaze. The client should follow the object in a parallel manner with the two eyes. A Snellen eye chart checks visual acuity and Cranial nerve II (optic). Testing sensory function by having the client close his or her eyes and then lightly touching areas of the face and testing the corneal reflexes check Cranial nerve V (trigeminal).

Test-Taking Strategy: Focus on the subject, checking for muscle weakness in the eyes. Note the relationship between the words extraocular movements in the question and positions of gaze in the correct option. Review the physical assessment technique for checking for muscle weakness in the eyes if you had difficulty with this question.

Level of Cognitive Ability: Understanding
Client Needs: Physiological Integrity
Integrated Process: Nursing Process/Planning
Content Area: Adult Health: Health Assessment/Physical Exam
Reference: Ignatavicius, Workman, p. 1078. 2010.

283. 1

Rationale: The nurse needs to teach the client how to perform a testicular self-examination (TSE). The nurse should instruct the client to select a day of the month and perform the exam on the same day each month. The nurse should also instruct the client that the best time to perform a TSE is after a shower or bath when the hands are warm and soapy and the scrotum is warm. This will provide ease in palpating and the client will be better able to identify any abnormalities. The client would stand to perform the exam, but it would be difficult to perform the exam while voiding. Having a bowel movement is unrelated to performing the TSE.

Test-Taking Strategy: Think about the purpose of the TSE and visualize this data collection technique. Review the instructions for performing a TSE. Eliminate option 3 because having a bowel movement is unrelated to performing the TSE. Next eliminate options 2 and 4 because it would be difficult to perform this self-exam lying down or during voiding.

Level of Cognitive Ability: Applying
Client Needs: Health Promotion and Maintenance
Integrated Process: Teaching and Learning
Content Area: Adult Health: Health Assessment/Physical Exam
Reference: Christensen, Kockrow, pp. 585-586. 2011. *Adult health nursing.*

284. 3

Rationale: Brudzinski's sign is tested with the client in the supine position. The examiner flexes the client's head and there should be no reports of pain or resistance to the neck flexion. A positive Brudzinski's sign is observed if the client passively flexes the hip and knee in response to neck flexion and reports pain in the vertebral column. Kernig's sign also tests for meningeal irritation and is positive when the client flexes the legs at the hip and knee and complains of pain along the vertebral column when the leg is extended. Decerebrate posturing is abnormal extension and occurs when the arms are fully extended, forearms pronated, wrists and fingers flexed, jaws clenched, neck extended, and feet plantar-flexed. Decorticate posturing is abnormal flexion and is noted when the client's upper arms are flexed and held tightly to the sides of the body and the legs are extended and internally rotated.

Test-Taking Strategy: Focus on the subject—a positive Brudzinski's sign. Recalling that a positive sign is elicited if the client reports pain will assist in eliminating options 1 and 4. Next it is necessary to know that a positive Brudzinski's sign is observed if the client passively flexes the hip and knee in response to neck flexion and reports pain in the vertebral column. Review the findings in a positive Brudzinski's sign if you had difficulty with this question.

Level of Cognitive Ability: Analyzing
Client Needs: Physiological Integrity
Integrated Process: Nursing Process/Data Collection
Content Area: Adult Health: Health Assessment/Physical Exam
Reference: Jarvis, p. 677. 2012.

285. 1, 2, 4

Rationale: A focused data collection process focuses on a limited or short-term problem, such as the client's complaint. Because the client is complaining of symptoms of a cold, a cough, and lung congestion the nurse would focus on the respiratory system and the presence of an infection. A complete data collection includes a complete health history and physical examination and forms a baseline database. Checking the strength of peripheral pulses relates to a vascular assessment, which is not related to this client's complaints. A musculoskeletal and neurological examination also is not related to this client's complaints. However, strength of peripheral pulses and a musculoskeletal and neurological examination would be included in a complete data collection. Likewise, asking the client about a family history of any illness or disease would be included in a complete assessment.

Test-Taking Strategy: Focus on the data in the question. Noting that the client's symptoms relate to the respiratory system and the presence of an infection will direct you to options 1, 2, and 4. Review the types of health and physical assessments and the components of a focused data collection process if you had difficulty with this question.

Level of Cognitive Ability: Applying

Client Needs: Health Promotion and Maintenance

Integrated Process: Nursing Process/Data Collection

Content Area: Adult Health: Health Assessment/Physical Exam

References: Christensen, Kockrow, p. 100. 2011. *Foundations of nursing.*

Jarvis, pp. 115-118. 2012.

Care of the Older Client

I. AGING AND GERONTOLOGY

A. Aging is the biopsychosocial process of change that occurs in a person between birth and death.

B. Gerontology is the study of the aging process.

II. PHYSIOLOGICAL CHANGES

A. Integumentary system
1. Loss of pigment in hair and skin
2. Wrinkling of the skin
3. Thinning of the epidermis; easy bruising and tearing of the skin
4. Decreased skin turgor, elasticity, and subcutaneous fat
5. Increased nail thickness and decreased nail growth
6. Decreased perspiration
7. Dry, itchy, and scaly skin
8. Seborrheic dermatitis and keratosis formation (overgrowth and thickening of the skin)

B. Neurological system
1. Slowed reflexes
2. Slight tremors and difficulty with fine motor movement
3. Loss of balance
4. An increased incidence of awakening after sleep onset
5. Increased susceptibility to hypothermia and hyperthermia
6. Short-term memory may decline
7. Long-term memory usually maintained

C. Musculoskeletal system
1. Muscle mass and strength decrease; muscles atrophy
2. Decreased mobility, range of motion, flexibility, coordination, and stability
3. Change of gait, with a shortened step and a wider base
4. Posture and stature changes that cause a decrease in height (Figure 30-1)
5. Increased brittleness of the bones
6. Deterioration of joint capsule components
7. Kyphosis of the dorsal spine (increased convexity in the curvature of the spine)

⚠ The older client is at risk for falls because of the changes that occur in the neurological and musculoskeletal systems.

D. Cardiovascular system
1. Diminished energy and endurance, with lowered tolerance to exercise
2. Decreased compliance of the heart muscle; heart valves become thicker and more rigid
3. Decreased cardiac output; decreased efficiency of blood return to the heart
4. Decreased compensatory response, so less able to respond to increased demands on the cardiovascular system
5. Decreased resting heart rate
6. Weak peripheral pulses
7. Increased blood pressure but susceptible to postural hypotension

E. Respiratory system
1. Decreased stretch and compliance of the chest wall
2. Decreased strength and function of the respiratory muscles
3. Decreased size and number of alveoli
4. The respiratory rate usually remains unchanged
5. Decreased depth of respirations and oxygen intake
6. Decreased ability to cough and expectorate sputum

F. Hematological system
1. Hemoglobin and hematocrit levels average toward the low end of normal
2. Prone to increased blood clotting
3. Decreased protein available for protein-bound medications

G. Immune system
1. Tendency for lymphocyte counts to be low with altered immunoglobulin production
2. Decreased resistance to infection and disease

H. Gastrointestinal system
1. Decreased need for calories because of lowered basal metabolic rate
2. Decreased appetite, thirst, and oral intake
3. Decreased lean body mass
4. Decreased stomach-emptying time

Height
— 5'6"
— 5'3"
— 5'
— 4'9"
— 4'6"
— 4'3"

Age   40   60   70

▲ **FIGURE 30-1** A normal spine at 40 years of age and osteoporotic changes at 60 and 70 years of age. These changes can cause a loss of as much as 6 inches in height and can result in a malformation called dowager's hump *(far right)* in the upper thoracic vertebrae. (From Ignatavicius, D., & Workman, M. [2010]. *Medical surgical nursing: Patient-centered collaborative care* [6th ed.]. St. Louis: Saunders).

5. Increased tendency toward constipation
6. Increased susceptibility to dehydration
7. Tooth loss
8. Difficulty with chewing and swallowing food
I. Endocrine system
    1. Decreased secretion of hormones, with specific changes related to each hormone function
    2. Decreased metabolic rate
    3. Decreased glucose tolerance, with resistance to insulin in the peripheral tissues
J. Renal system
    1. Decreased kidney size, function, and ability to concentrate urine
    2. Decreased glomerular filtration rate
    3. Decreased capacity of the bladder
    4. Increased residual urine; increased incidence of infection and possibly resultant incontinence
    5. Impaired medication excretion
K. Reproductive system
    1. Decreased testosterone production and size of testes
    2. Changes in the prostate gland, leading to urinary problems
    3. Decreased secretion of hormones, with the cessation of menses
    4. Vaginal changes, including decreased muscle tone and lubrication
    5. Impotence or sexual dysfunction for both genders; sexual function varies and depends on

general physical condition, mental health status, and medications
L. Special senses
    1. Decreased visual acuity
    2. Decreased accommodation in eyes, which requires increased time for adjustment to changes in light
    3. Decreased peripheral vision and increased sensitivity to glare
    4. Presbyopia and cataract formation
    5. Possible loss of hearing ability; low-pitched tones are more easily heard
    6. Inability to discern taste of food
    7. Decreased sense of smell
    8. Changes in touch sensation
    9. Decreased pain awareness

III.   PSYCHOSOCIAL CONCERNS

A. Adjustment to deterioration in physical and mental health and well-being
B. Threat to independent functioning; fear of becoming a burden to loved ones
C. Adjustment to retirement and loss of income
D. Loss of skills and competencies developed early in life
E. Coping with changes in role function and social life
F. Diminished quantity and quality of relationships and coping with loss
G. Dependence on governmental and social systems
H. Access to social support systems
I. Costs of health care and medications

IV.   MENTAL HEALTH CONCERNS (Box 30-1)

A. **Depression**: The increased dependency that older adults may experience can lead to hopelessness, helplessness, a lowered sense of self-control, and decreased self-esteem and self-worth. These changes can interfere with daily functioning and lead to **depression**.
B. Grief: Client reacts to the perception of loss, including physical, psychological, social, and spiritual aspects
C. Isolation: Client is alone and desires contact with others but is unable to make that contact
D. Suicide: **Depression** can lead to thoughts of self-harm.

Box 30-1 Mental Health Concerns

- Depression
- Grief
- Isolation
- Suicide

⚠ Any suicide threat from an older client should be taken seriously.

V. PAIN

A. Description
1. Pain can come about from numerous causes and most often occurs from degenerative changes in the musculoskeletal system.
2. The failure to alleviate pain in the older client can lead to functional limitations that affect the client's ability to function independently.

B. Data collection
1. Restlessness
2. Verbal reporting of pain
3. Agitation
4. Moaning
5. Crying

C. Interventions
1. Monitor the client for signs of pain.
2. Identify the pattern of pain.
3. Identify the precipitating factor(s) for the pain.
4. Monitor the impact of the pain on the client's activities of daily living.
5. Provide pain relief through measures such as distraction, relaxation, massage, and biofeedback.
6. Administer pain medications, as prescribed. Instruct the client in their use.
7. Evaluate the effects of pain-reducing measures.

VI. INFECTION

A. Confusion is a common sign of infection in the older adult, especially infection of the urinary tract.
B. Carefully monitor the older adult with an infection because of their diminished and altered immune response.
C. Nonspecific symptoms may indicate illness or infection (Box 30-2).

Box 30-2 Nonspecific Symptoms That May Indicate Illness or Infection

- Apathy
- Anorexia
- Changes in functional status
- Confusion
- Dyspnea
- Falling
- Fatigue
- Incontinence
- Self-neglect
- Shortness of breath
- Tachypnea
- Vital sign changes

VII. MEDICATIONS

A. Major problems with prescription medications include adverse effects, interactions, errors, noncompliance, and cost.
B. Determine the use of over-the-counter medications.
C. **Polypharmacy**
1. Routinely monitor the number of prescription and nonprescription medications used and determine if any can be eliminated or combined.
2. Keep the use of medications to a minimum.
3. Overprescribing medications leads to increased problems with more side effects, increased interaction among medications, replication of medication treatment, diminished quality of life, and increased costs.

D. Medication dosages normally are prescribed at one third to one half of the normal adult doses.
E. Closely monitor the client for side effects and adverse effects and response to therapy because of the increased risk for medication toxicity.
F. Assess for medication interactions in the client who is taking multiple medications.
G. Advise the client to use one pharmacy and notify the consulting health care providers of the medications taken.

⚠ A common sign of an adverse reaction to a medication in the older client is an acute change in mental status.

H. Administration of medications
1. Place the client in a sitting position when administering medication.
2. Check for mouth dryness, because medication may stick and dissolve in the mouth.
3. Administer liquid preparations if the client has difficulty swallowing tablets.
4. Crush tablets, if necessary, and give with textured food (e.g., nectar, applesauce) if not contraindicated.
5. Enteric-coated tablets are not crushed and capsules are not opened.
6. If administering a suppository, avoid inserting the suppository immediately after removing it from the refrigerator. A suppository may take a while to dissolve because of a decreased body core temperature.
7. When administering parenteral medication, monitor the site, because it may ooze medication or bleed as a result of decreased tissue elasticity. An immobile limb is not used for administering parenteral medication.
8. Monitor client compliance with the taking of prescribed medications.

9. Monitor the client for **safety** with regard to correctly taking medications, including an assessment of the client's ability to read the instructions and discriminate among the pills and their colorations.

10. Use a medication cassette to facilitate the proper administration of medication.

VIII. ABUSE OF THE OLDER ADULT

A. **Abuse** involves physical, emotional, or sexual **abuse** and also can involve **neglect** or economic exploitation.

B. Categories of mistreatment of the older client

1. Domestic mistreatment takes place in the home of the older adult and is usually carried out by a family member or significant other. This can include physical maltreatment, **neglect**, or abandonment.

2. Institutional mistreatment takes place when an older adult experiences **abuse** when hospitalized or living in another type of facility other than the home.

3. **Self-neglect** is the choice by a mentally competent individual to avoid medical care or other services that could improve optimal function; lack caring for oneself; and engage in actions that negatively affect his or her personal **safety**; unless declared legally incompetent, an individual has the right to refuse care.

! Individuals at most risk for abuse include those who are dependent because of their immobility or altered mental status.

C. Factors that contribute to **abuse** and **neglect** include longstanding family violence, caregiver stress, and the individual's increasing dependence on others.

D. Abusers tend to be male, engage in substance **abuse**, and have a mental illness or **dementia**; in addition, they tend to depend on the older client for financial assistance or other resources.

E. Victims may attempt to dismiss injuries as accidental, and abusers may prevent victims from receiving proper medical care to avoid discovery.

F. Victims often are isolated socially by their abusers.

G. For additional information about **abuse** of the older client, see Chapter 66

MORE QUESTIONS ON EVOLVE!

Practice Questions

286. An older client has been prescribed digoxin (Lanoxin). The nurse understands that which age-related change would place the client at risk for digoxin toxicity?

1. Decreased cough efficiency and vital capacity
2. Decreased salivation and gastrointestinal motility
3. Decreased muscle strength and loss of bone density
4. Decreased lean body mass and glomerular filtration rate

287. The nurse should plan which of the following to encourage autonomy in the client who is a resident in a long-term care facility?
1. Choosing his meals
2. Decorating his room
3. Scheduling his barber appointments
4. Allowing him to choose his social activities

288. Which data indicates to the nurse that a client may be experiencing ineffective coping?
1. Constantly neglects personal grooming
2. Visits her husband's grave once a month
3. Visits the senior citizens' center once a month
4. Frequently looks at snapshots of her husband and family

289. The nurse is preparing to communicate with an older client who is hearing impaired. Which intervention should be implemented initially?
1. Stand in front of the client.
2. Exaggerate the lip movements.
3. Obtain a sign-language interpreter.
4. Pantomime and write the client notes.

290. Which intervention should be implemented for the older client with presbycusis who has a hearing loss?
1. Speak louder
2. Speak slower
3. Use low-pitched tones
4. Use high-pitched tones

291. Which client is most likely at risk to become a victim of elder abuse?
1. A 75-year-old man with moderate hypertension
2. A 68-year-old man with newly diagnosed cataracts
3. A 90-year-old woman with advanced Parkinson's disease
4. A 70-year-old woman with early diagnosed Lyme disease

292. The nurse is planning to feed an older client who is at risk for aspiration of food. During the meal, how should the nurse position the client?
1. Upright in a chair
2. On the left side in bed
3. On the right side in bed
4. In a low-Fowler's position, with the legs elevated

293. The nurse is providing an education class to healthy older adults. Which exercise will best promote health maintenance?
1. Gardening every day for an hour
2. Sculpting once a week for 40 minutes
3. Cycling three times a week for 20 minutes
4. Walking three to five times a week for 30 minutes

294. The nurse should implement which activity to promote reminiscence among older clients?
1. Having storytelling hours
2. Setting up pet therapy sessions
3. Displaying calendars and clocks
4. Encouraging client participation in a pottery class

295. When the nurse is collecting data from the older adult, which of the following findings would be considered normal physiological changes? **Select all that apply.**
☐ 1. Increased heart rate
☐ 2. Decline in visual acuity
☐ 3. Decreased respiratory rate
☐ 4. Decline in long-term memory
☐ 5. Increased susceptibility to urinary tract infections
☐ 6. Increased incidence of awakening after sleep onset

ANSWERS

286. 4
Rationale: The older client is at risk for medication toxicity because of decreased lean body mass and an age-associated decreased glomerular filtration rate. Although options 1, 2, and 3 identify age-related changes that occur in the older client, they are not specifically associated with this risk.
Test-Taking Strategy: Use the process of elimination, and focus on the subject—age-related body change that could place the client at risk for medication toxicity. Note that option 4 is the only choice that addresses renal excretion. Review the physiological changes associated with aging if you had difficulty with this question.
Level of Cognitive Ability: Understanding
Client Needs: Physiological Integrity
Integrated Process: Nursing Process/Data Collection
Content Area: Fundamental Skills: Developmental Stages
References: Christensen, Kockrow, p. 732. 2011. *Foundations of nursing.*
deWit, p. 148. 2009.

287. 4
Rationale: Autonomy is the personal freedom to direct one's own life as long as it does not impinge on the rights of others. An autonomous person is capable of rational thought. This individual can identify problems, search for alternatives, and choose solutions that allow for continued personal freedom as long as the rights and property of others are not harmed. The loss of autonomy—and, therefore, independence—is a very real fear among older clients. Option 4 is the only choice that allows the client to be a decision maker.
Test-Taking Strategy: Use the process of elimination, and focus on the subject of encouraging autonomy. Recalling the definition of autonomy will direct you to the correct option. Remember that to promote independence in clients, it is essential to give the client choices. Review the concept of autonomy if you had difficulty with this question.
Level of Cognitive Ability: Applying
Client Needs: Safe and Effective Care Environment
Integrated Process: Caring

Content Area: Fundamental Skills: Developmental Stages
Reference: Linton, p. 28. 2012.

288. 1
Rationale: Coping mechanisms are behaviors that are used to decreased stress and anxiety. In response to a death, ineffective coping is manifested by an extreme behavior that in some instances may be harmful to the individual, physically, psychologically, or both. Option 1 is indicative of a behavior that identifies an ineffective coping behavior as part of the grieving process. The remaining options identify effective coping behaviors.
Test-Taking Strategy: Use the process of elimination, and note the subject—ineffective coping behavior. Eliminate options 2, 3, and 4, because they are comparable or alike and are positive activities that the individual is engaging in to get on with her life. Review the coping mechanisms for dealing with grief and loss if you had difficulty with this question.
Level of Cognitive Ability: Analyzing
Client Needs: Psychosocial Integrity
Integrated Process: Nursing Process/Data Collection
Content Area: Mental Health
References: Christensen, Kockrow, p. 227. 2011. *Foundations of nursing.*
Morrison-Valfre, pp. 192-194. 2009.

289. 1
Rationale: The nurse would ensure that the hearing-impaired client can see the nurse when the nurse is speaking by providing adequate lighting and standing in front of the client. The nurse should enunciate words clearly but not exaggerate lip movements. If the client is profoundly hearing impaired and uses signing, a sign-language interpreter should be obtained. If a client cannot understand by reading lips, the nurse would try using gestures, pantomiming, or writing notes.
Test-Taking Strategy: Note the strategic word "initially." To communicate effectively with a hearing-impaired client, the nurse first makes sure that the client can see him or her. Review the nursing interventions for the hearing-impaired client if you had difficulty with this question.
Level of Cognitive Ability: Applying

Client Needs: Physiological Integrity
Integrated Process: Nursing Process/Implementation
Content Area: Adult Health/Ear
Reference: Touhy, Jett, p. 32. 2010.

290. 3

Rationale: Presbycusis refers to the age-related, irreversible, degenerative changes of the inner ear that lead to decreased hearing acuity. As a result of these changes, the older client has a decreased response to high-frequency sounds. Low-pitched tones of voice are more easily heard and interpreted by the older client. Options 1, 2, and 4 are not accurate.
Test-Taking Strategy: Use the process of elimination. Recalling that the client with a hearing loss responds better to low-pitched tones will direct you to option 3. Review the characteristics associated with presbycusis and hearing loss if you had difficulty with this question.
Level of Cognitive Ability: Applying
Client Needs: Physiological Integrity
Integrated Process: Nursing Process/Implementation
Content Area: Adult Health/Ear
Reference: Touhy, Jett, pp. 79-80. 2010.

291. 3

Rationale: Elder abuse is widespread and occurs among all subgroups of the population. It includes physical and psychological abuse, the misuse of property, and the violation of rights. The typical abuse victim is a woman of advanced age with few social contacts and at least one physical or mental impairment that limits her ability to perform activities of daily living. In addition, the client usually lives alone or with the abuser and depends on the abuser for care.
Test-Taking Strategy: Use the process of elimination. Read each option carefully, and identify the client who is most defenseless as a result of the disease process. Review the characteristics of elder abuse if you had difficulty with this question.
Level of Cognitive Ability: Analyzing
Client Needs: Psychosocial Integrity
Integrated Process: Nursing Process/Data Collection
Content Area: Mental Health
Reference: Morrison-Valfre, p. 288. 2009.

292. 1

Rationale: It is preferable to get clients out of bed and sitting in a chair for meals. This position facilitates chewing and swallowing and prevents the reflux of stomach contents and aspiration. Options 2, 3, and 4 do not identify positions that will reduce the risk of aspiration.
Test-Taking Strategy: Use the process of elimination. Focus on the subject of the question—reducing the risk of aspiration. This should direct you to option 1. Review the measures that will prevent aspiration if you had difficulty with this question.
Level of Cognitive Ability: Applying
Client Needs: Safe and Effective Care Environment
Integrated Process: Nursing Process/Implementation
Content Area: Fundamental Skills: Safety/Infection Control
Reference: Touhy, Jett, p. 116. 2010.

293. 4

Rationale: Exercise and activity are essential for health promotion and maintenance in the older adult and for achieving an optimal level of functioning. Approximately half of the physical deterioration of the older client is caused by disuse rather than by the aging process or disease. One of the best exercises for an older adult is walking, with the goal of progressing to 30-minute sessions three to five times each week. Swimming and dancing are also beneficial.
Test-Taking Strategy: Use the process of elimination, and note the strategic word "best." Options 1, 2, and 3, although possible, are not the best activities. Remember that walking is one of the best forms of exercise. Review health promotion activities for the older client if you had difficulty with this question.
Level of Cognitive Ability: Applying
Client Needs: Health Promotion and Maintenance
Integrated Process: Nursing Process/Planning
Content Area: Fundamental Skills: Developmental Stages
Reference: Christensen, Kockrow, pp. 214, 1083. 2011. *Foundations of nursing.*

294. 1

Rationale: Clients who like to retell stories or to describe past events need to be provided with the opportunity to do so. This phenomenon is called life review or reminiscence. In a sense, it is a way for the older client to relive and restructure life experiences, and it is a part of achieving ego identity. Option 3 indicates reality orientation techniques. Options 2 and 4 indicate socialization and physical activity.
Test-Taking Strategy: Use the process of elimination. Focusing on the strategic word "reminiscence" and recalling its definition will direct you to option 1. Review this form of activity if you had difficulty with this question.
Level of Cognitive Ability: Applying
Client Needs: Psychosocial Integrity
Integrated Process: Caring
Content Area: Fundamental Skills: Developmental Stages
Reference: Touhy, Jett, pp. 40–41. 2010.

295. 2, 5, 6

Rationale: Anatomical changes to the eye affect the individual's visual ability, which leads to potential problems with activities of daily living. Light adaptation and visual fields are reduced. Respiratory rates are usually unchanged. The heart rate decreases, and the heart valves thicken. Age-related changes that affect the urinary tract increase an older client's susceptibility to urinary tract infections. Short-term memory may decline with age, but long-term memory is usually maintained. Changes in sleep patterns are consistent, age-related changes. Older persons experience an increased incidence of awakening after sleep onset.
Test-Taking Strategy: Knowledge regarding normal age-related changes is needed to answer this question. Read each characteristic carefully, and think about the physiological changes that occur with aging to select the correct items. Review normal age-related changes if you had difficulty with this question.
Level of Cognitive Ability: Analyzing
Client Needs: Health Promotion and Maintenance
Integrated Process: Nursing Process/Data Collection
Content Area: Fundamental Skills: Developmental Stages
Reference: Linton, pp. 145–150. 2012.

Pediatric Nursing

PYRAMID TERMS

atresia The congenital absence or closure of a body orifice.

child abuse The nonaccidental physical injury or nonaccidental act of omission of care by a parent or person responsible for a child; includes neglect as well as physical, sexual, and emotional maltreatment.

crackles Audible high-pitched crackling or popping sounds heard during lung auscultation; result from fluid in the airways, and are not cleared by coughing (formerly referred to as rales).

cyanosis The bluish color that is seen in tissues, nail beds, and mucous membranes when tissues are deprived of adequate amounts of oxygen.

developmental age The age based on a child's maturational progress. It is determined by standardized resources such as body size, physical and psychological functioning, motor skills, and aptitude tests. Developmental age does not necessarily correspond with chronological age (age in years).

functional age The age equivalent at which a child actually is able to perform specific self-care or related tasks.

growth Measurable physical and physiological body changes that occur over time.

grunting The sound made by forced expiration, which is the body's attempt to improve oxygenation when hypoxemia is present.

hereditary The transmission of genetic characteristics from parent to offspring.

nasal flaring A widening of the nares to enable an infant or child to take in more oxygen; a serious indicator of air hunger.

prodromal Pertaining to early symptoms that mark the onset of a disease.

puberty The period of time during which the adolescent experiences a growth spurt, develops secondary sex characteristics, and achieves reproductive maturity.

regurgitation An abnormal backward flow of body fluid.

retraction An abnormal movement of the chest wall during inspiration in which the skin appears to be drawn in between the ribs and above and/or below the clavicle and scapula; this condition indicates respiratory difficulty.

shunt The movement of blood or body fluid through an abnormal anatomical or surgically created opening.

stenosis The narrowing or constriction of an opening.

stridor A shrill harsh sound heard during inspiration, expiration, or both, that is produced by the flow of air through a narrowed segment of the respiratory tract.

vaccine A suspension of attenuated or killed microorganisms administered to induce active immunity to an infectious disease.

wheezing A high-pitched musical whistling sound that is heard with or without a stethoscope as air is compressed through narrowed or obstructed airways because of swelling, secretions, or tumors.

PYRAMID TO SUCCESS

The pyramid points focus on growth and development; safety and the age-appropriate measures to ensure a safe and hazard-free environment for the child, protection of the child, prevention of accidents, and acute disorders that occur in children. The focus is on nutrition, specific feeding techniques, positioning techniques, and interventions that will provide and maintain adequate airway, breathing, and circulation patterns in the child. Additionally, neglect and abuse of a child is a focus. On the NCLEX-PN examination, be alert to the age of the child if the age is presented in the question. If an age is presented in the question, think about the specific growth and development characteristics of the age group to answer the question correctly.

CLIENT NEEDS

Safe and Effective Care Environment

- Considering issues related to informed consent for minors
- Ensuring environmental and personal safety, including home safety, related to the developmental age of the child
- Establishing priorities
- Instituting measures related to the spread and control of infectious agents, particularly communicable diseases
- Maintaining confidentiality
- Preventing accidents
- Providing continuity of care
- Providing protective measures
- Protecting the child and other contacts to prevent illness
- Upholding parents' and child's rights

Health Promotion and Maintenance

- Ensuring that immunization schedules are up to date
- Focusing on developmental stages when planning care
- Performing data collection techniques specific to the pediatric client
- Preventing disease in the pediatric population
- Providing health-promotion programs for the pediatric client
- Providing instructions to the child and parents regarding care at home

Psychosocial Integrity

- Assessing for child abuse and neglect
- Communicating with the pediatric client
- Considering concepts of family dynamics when planning care
- Considering cultural, religious, and spiritual beliefs when planning care
- Considering end-of-life issues, grief, and loss in the pediatric population
- Identifying family and support systems for the child
- Providing play therapies

Physiological Integrity

- Following medication administration procedures
- Following nutritional guidelines for the pediatric population
- Identifying comfort measures that are appropriate for the child
- Maintaining sensitivity during intrusive procedures that are required for the pediatric client
- Managing childhood illnesses
- Monitoring elimination patterns
- Monitoring for age-appropriate normal body structure and function
- Monitoring for infectious diseases of the pediatric client
- Monitoring for potential alterations in body systems as a result of disease
- Monitoring for responses to treatments
- Providing for consistent rest and sleep patterns
- Responding to medical emergencies

Neurological, Cognitive, and Psychosocial Disorders

I. ATTENTION DEFICIT HYPERACTIVITY DISORDER

A. Description
   1. A behavior disorder that is characterized by inappropriate degrees of inattention, overactivity, and impulsivity
   2. Childhood problems include lowered intellectual development, some minor physical abnormalities, sleep disturbances, behavioral or emotional disorders, and difficulty with social relationships.
   3. Early diagnosis is important to prevent impaired emotional and psychological development.
   4. Diagnosis is established on the basis of self-reports, parent and teacher reports, and the use of assessment tools.

B. Data collection
   1. Fidgets with hands or feet or squirms in a seat
   2. Easily distracted by external or internal stimuli
   3. Difficulty with following through on instructions
   4. Poor attention span
   5. Shifts from one uncompleted activity to another
   6. Talks excessively
   7. Interrupts or intrudes on others
   8. Engages in physically dangerous activities without considering the possible consequences

C. Interventions
   1. Provide parents with information about the disorder and treatment plan; encourage support groups for the parents.
   2. Treatment included behavioral therapy, medication, maintaining a consistent environment, and appropriate classroom placement.
   3. Behavioral therapy focuses on preventing undesirable behavior.
   4. Maintain a consistent home and classroom environment, and provide environmental and physical safety measures.
   5. Promote self-esteem.
   6. Stimulant medications may be prescribed; possible side effects include appetite suppression and weight loss, nervousness, tics, insomnia, and increased blood pressure.
   7. Instruct the child and parents regarding medication administration and the need for regular follow-up.

II. AUTISM

A. Description
   1. Autism is a severe form of an autism spectrum disorder (pervasive developmental disorder).
   2. Symptoms are usually noted by the parents by 3 years of age.
   3. The cause of the disorder is not specifically known; however, it has been linked to a wide range of antepartum, intrapartum, and postpartum conditions and exposure to hazardous chemicals. Genetic predisposition is also linked to the disorder.
   4. The disorder is accompanied by intellectual and social behavioral deficits, and the child exhibits peculiar and bizarre characteristics with social interactions, communication, and behaviors.
   5. Diagnosis is established on the basis of symptoms and with the use of several screening tools.

B. Data collection
   1. Social
      a. Abnormal lack of comfort-seeking behaviors
      b. Abnormal or lack of social play
      c. Impairment in peer relationships
      d. Lack of awareness of the existence or feelings of others
      e. Abnormal or lack of imitation of others
   2. Communication
      a. Lack of, impaired, or abnormal speech such as producing a monotone voice or echolalia
      b. Abnormal nonverbal communication (does not use gestures to communicate)
      c. Lack of imaginative play
   3. Behavior
      a. Persistent preoccupation or attachment to objects; range of interests restricted
      b. Self-injurious behaviors
      c. Must maintain routine; any environmental change produces marked distress

d. Produces repetitive body movements such as rocking or head banging

C. Interventions
1. Determine the child's routines, habits, and preferences, and maintain consistency as much as possible.
2. Determine the specific ways in which the child communicates and use these methods.
3. Avoid placing demands on the child.
4. Evaluate the child for safety.
5. Implement safety precautions, as necessary, for self-injurious behaviors such as head banging.
6. Initiate referrals to special programs, as required.
7. Provide support to the parents.

⚠ Ensuring a safe environment for a child with autism is a priority.

III. CEREBRAL PALSY

A. Description
1. A disorder characterized by impaired movement and posture resulting from an abnormality in the extrapyramidal or pyramidal motor system
2. The most common clinical type is spastic cerebral palsy, which represents an upper motor neuron type of muscle weakness.
3. Less common types of cerebral palsy are athetoid, ataxic, and mixed.

B. Data collection
1. Extreme irritability and crying
2. Feeding difficulties
3. Abnormal motor performance
4. Alterations of muscle tone; stiff and rigid arms or legs
5. Delayed developmental milestones
6. Persistence of primitive infantile reflexes (e.g., Moro, tonic neck) after 6 months (most primitive reflexes disappear by 3 to 4 months of age)
7. Abnormal posturing (e.g., opisthotonic [exaggerated arching of the back]) (Figure 31-1)
8. Seizures may occur

C. Interventions
1. The goals of management are early recognition and intervention to maximize the child's abilities.
2. A multidisciplinary team approach is implemented to meet the many needs of the child.
3. Therapeutic management includes physical therapy, occupational therapy, speech therapy, education, and recreation.
4. Assess the child's developmental level and intelligence.
5. Encourage early intervention and participation in school programs.
6. Prepare for the use of mobilizing devices to help prevent or reduce deformities.

▲ **FIGURE 31-1** Abnormal posturing: Opisthotonos. (From Farrar, W.E. [1993]. *Atlas of infections of the nervous system.* London: Mosby-Wolfe).

7. Encourage communication and interaction with the child on his or her **developmental age** rather than his or her chronological age level.
8. Provide a safe environment by removing sharp objects, using a protective helmet if the child falls frequently, and implementing seizure precautions, if necessary.
9. Provide safe, appropriate toys for the child's age and developmental level.
10. Position the child upright after meals.
11. Medications may be prescribed to relieve muscle spasms, which cause intense pain; antiseizure medications may also be prescribed.
12. Provide the parents with information about the disorder and treatment plan; encourage support groups for parents.

IV. CHILD ABDUCTION

A. Description
1. Child abduction is the kidnapping of a child (or infant) by an older person.
2. Occurrences
   a. A stranger may kidnap a child for criminal or mischievous purposes.
   b. A stranger may kidnap a child (or infant) to bring up him or her as that person's own child.
   c. A parent removes or retains a child from the other parent's care (often during the course of or after divorce proceedings).
3. During the preschool years, the child becomes more independent and parents are less able to provide the constant protection provided in earlier years; interventions (including teaching the child) that ensure protection are necessary.

B. Interventions
1. Instruct the parents to teach the child basic guidelines about personal safety that include the following:
   a. Do not go anywhere alone.

b. Always tell an adult where he or she is going and when he or she will return.

c. Say "no" if he or she feels uncomfortable with a situation.

d. Do not talk with strangers or get into their cars.

e. Do not help anyone look for a lost dog or cat and do not accept candy from a stranger.

f. If lost in a store, do not wander around looking for the parent. Go at once to a clerk or guard.

2. Children need to learn their full name, address, and parents' names.

3. Watch for posttraumatic stress disorder in any child who has experienced abduction.

V. CHILD ABUSE

A. Description

1. **Child abuse** is the nonaccidental physical injury or the nonaccidental act of omission of care by a parent or person responsible for a child; includes neglect, physical, sexual, or emotional maltreatment.

2. Neglect can be in the form of physical or emotional neglect and involves the deprivation of basic needs, supervision, medical care, or education; and failure to meet the child's needs for attention and affection.

3. Sexual abuse can involve incest, molestation, exhibitionism, pornography, prostitution, or pediphilia; findings associated with sexual abuse may not be easily apparent in the child.

4. Shaken baby syndrome is caused by the violent shaking of a child younger than 1 year and results in intracranial (usually subdural hemorrhage) trauma; can lead to cerebral edema and death.

B. Data collection (Box 31-1)

C. Interventions

1. Support the child during a thorough physical assessment.

2. Check injuries.

3. If shaken baby syndrome is suspected, monitor the infant for a decrease in level of consciousness, which can indicate increased intracranial pressure (ICP).

4. Report a case of suspected **child abuse**.

5. Place the child in an environment that is safe, thereby preventing further injury.

6. Document information related to the suspected abuse in an objective manner.

7. Assess the parents' strengths and weaknesses, normal coping mechanisms, and the presence or absence of support systems.

8. Assist the family in identifying stressors, support systems, and resources.

9. Refer the family to appropriate support groups.

Box 31-1 Child Neglect and Abuse: Data Collection Findings

Neglect
Inadequate weight gain
Poor hygiene
Consistent hunger
Inconsistent school attendance
Constant fatigue
Reports of lack of child supervision
Delinquency

Physical Abuse
Unexplained bruises, burns, or fractures
Bald spots on the scalp
Apprehensive child
Extreme aggressiveness or withdrawal
Fear of parents
Lack of crying (older infant, toddler, or young preschool child) when approached by a stranger

Emotional Abuse
Speech disorders
Habit disorders such as sucking, biting, and rocking
Psychoneurotic reactions
Learning disorders
Suicide attempts

Sexual Abuse
Difficulty walking or sitting
Torn, stained, or bloody underclothing
Pain, swelling, or itching of the genitals
Bruises, bleeding, or lacerations in the genital or anal area
Unwillingness to change clothes or unwillingness to participate in gym activities
Poor peer relations

Shaken Baby Syndrome
External signs of trauma are usually absent
Ophthalmoscopic exam reveals retinal hemorrhages
Full bulging fontanels and head circumference greater than expected

⚠ Nurses are legally required to report all cases of suspected child abuse to the appropriate local or state agency.

VI. HEAD INJURY

A. Description

1. Head injury is the pathological result of any mechanical force to the skull, scalp, meninges, or brain.

a. Open head injury occurs when there is a fracture of the skull or a penetration of the skull by an object.

b. Closed head injury is the result of blunt trauma. It is more serious because of the chance of increased intracranial pressure

(ICP) in a "closed" vault. This type of injury can also be caused by shaken baby syndrome.
   2. Manifestations depend on the type of injury and the subsequent amount of increased ICP.
B. Data collection: Increased ICP
   1. Early signs
      a. Slight change in vital signs
      b. Slight change in level of consciousness
      c. Infant: Irritability, high-pitched cry, bulging fontanel, increased head circumference, dilated scalp veins, Macewen sign (cracked-pot sound on percussion of the head), setting-sun sign (sclera visible above the iris)
      d. Child: Headache, nausea, vomiting, visual disturbances (diplopia), seizures
   2. Late signs
      a. Decrease in level of consciousness
      b. Bradycardia
      c. Decreased motor and sensory responses
      d. Alteration in pupil size and reactivity
      e. Decorticate posturing: Adduction of the arms at the shoulders; arms are flexed on the chest with the wrists flexed and the hands fisted, and the lower extremities are extended and adducted; seen with severe dysfunction of the cerebral cortex (Figure 31-2)
      f. Decerebrate posturing: Rigid extension and pronation of the arms and the legs; a sign of dysfunction at the level of the midbrain (see Figure 31-2)
      g. Cheyne-Stokes respirations
      h. Coma

⚠ The child's level of consciousness provides the earliest indication of an improvement or deterioration of the neurological condition.

A

B

▲ **FIGURE 31-2 A,** Decorticate (flexion) posturing. **B,** Decerebrate (extension) posturing. (From Hockenberry, M., & Wilson, D. [2009]. *Wong's essentials of pediatric nursing* [8th ed.]. St. Louis: Mosby).

C. Interventions

⚠ Immobilize the neck and spine after a head injury if a cervical or other spinal injury is suspected. When a spinal cord injury is ruled out, elevate the head of the bed 15 to 30 degrees, if not contraindicated and as prescribed, to facilitate venous drainage.

   1. Monitor the airway and administer oxygen as prescribed.
   2. Check injuries. (Refer to Chapter 57 for information on spinal cord injuries).
   3. Position the client so that the head is maintained midline to avoid jugular vein compression, which can increase ICP.
   4. Monitor vital signs and neurological function. (Monitor level of consciousness closely.)
   5. Keep stimuli to a minimum; attempt to minimize crying in the infant.
   6. Plan to withhold sedating medications during the acute phase of the injury so that changes in levels of consciousness can be assessed.
   7. Initiate seizure precautions (Box 31-2).
   8. Monitor for decreased responsiveness to pain (a significant sign of altered level of consciousness).
   9. Maintain an NPO status or provide clear liquids, if prescribed, until it is determined that vomiting will not occur.
   10. Monitor prescribed intravenous fluids carefully to avoid aggravating any cerebral edema and to minimize the possibility of overhydration.
   11. Monitor for a fluid or electrolyte alteration (could indicate injury to the hypothalamus or posterior pituitary)
   12. Check wounds and dressings for the presence of drainage and monitor for nose or ear drainage, which could indicate leakage of cerebrospinal fluid (CSF).
   13. Administer tepid sponge baths or place on a hypothermia blanket as prescribed if hyperthermia occurs.

Box 31-2 Seizure Precautions

Raise the side rails when the child is sleeping or resting.
Pad the side rails and other hard objects.
Place a waterproof mattress or pad on the bed or crib.
Instruct the child to wear or carry medical identification.
Instruct the child regarding precautions to take during potentially hazardous activities.
Instruct the child to swim with a companion.
Instruct the child to use a protective helmet and padding during bicycle riding, skateboarding, and inline skating.
Alert caregivers to the need for any special precautions.

14. Avoid suctioning through the nares because of the possibility of the catheter entering the brain through a fracture, which places the child at high risk for a secondary infection.
15. As prescribed, administer acetaminophen (Tylenol) for headache, anticonvulsants for seizures, and antibiotics if a laceration is present; prepare to administer prophylactic tetanus toxoid.
16. A corticosteroid or osmotic diuretic may be prescribed to reduce cerebral edema.
17. Monitor for signs of brainstem involvement (Box 31-3).
18. Monitor for signs of epidural hematoma: Asymmetrical pupils (one dilated, nonreactive pupil) may indicate a neurosurgical emergency that requires evacuation of the hematoma.

⚠ Drainage from the nose or ear needs to be tested for the presence of glucose. Drainage that is positive for glucose (as tested with reagent strips) indicates leakage of CSF. The registered nurse and health care provider (HCP) must be notified immediately if the drainage tests positive for glucose.

VII. HYDROCEPHALUS

A. Description
  1. An imbalance of CSF absorption and production caused by malformations, tumors, hemorrhage, infections, or trauma
  2. Results in head enlargement and increased ICP
B. Types (Box 31-4)
C. Data collection
  1. Infant

Box 31-3 Signs of Brainstem Involvement

- Deep, rapid, or intermittent and gasping respirations
- Wide fluctuations or noticeable slowing of the pulse
- Widening pulse pressure or extreme fluctuations in blood pressure
- Sluggish, dilated, or unequal pupils

Notify the registered nurse or HCP immediately if these signs develop!

Box 31-4 Types of Hydrocephalus

Communicating
Hydrocephalus occurs as a result of impaired absorption within the subarachnoid space.
Interference of the cerebrospinal fluid in the ventricular system does not occur.

Noncommunicating
The obstruction of cerebrospinal fluid flow in the ventricular system occurs.

---

   a. Increased head circumference
   b. Thin, widely separated bones of the head that produce a cracked-pot sound (Macewen's sign) on percussion
   c. Anterior fontanel that is tense, bulging, and nonpulsating
   d. Dilated scalp veins
   e. Frontal bossing
   f. Setting sun eyes
  2. Child
   a. Behavior changes (e.g., irritability, lethargy)
   b. Headache on awakening
   c. Nausea and vomiting
   d. Ataxia
   e. Nystagmus
  3. Late signs: A high, shrill cry and seizures
D. Surgical interventions
  1. The goal of surgical treatment is to prevent further CSF accumulation by bypassing the blockage and draining the fluid from the ventricles to a location where it may be reabsorbed.
  2. In a ventriculoperitoneal **shunt**, the CSF drains into the peritoneal cavity from the lateral ventricle (Figure 31-3).
  3. In a ventriculoatrial **shunt**, the CSF drains into the right atrium of the heart from the lateral ventricle, bypassing the obstruction. This is used for older children and those with pathological conditions of the abdomen.
  4. **Shunt** revision may be necessary as the child grows.
  5. An alternative to **shunt** placement is endoscopic third ventriculostomy, in which a small opening in the floor of the third ventricle is made that allows CSF to bypass the fourth ventricle and return to the circulation to be absorbed. This treatment may not be appropriate for some types of hydrocephalus.
E. Preoperative interventions
  1. Monitor intake and output (I&O). Administer small frequent feedings as tolerated until a preoperative nothing-by-mouth status is prescribed.
  2. Reposition the head frequently and use special devices such as an eggcrate mattress under the head to prevent pressure sores.
  3. Prepare the child and family for diagnostic procedures and surgery.
F. Postoperative interventions
  1. Monitor the vital signs and the neurological signs.
  2. Position the child on the unoperated side to prevent pressure on the **shunt** valve.
  3. Keep the child flat, as prescribed, to avoid the rapid reduction of intracranial fluid.
  4. Observe for increased ICP. If increased ICP occurs, elevate the head of the bed to 15 to 30 degrees to enhance gravity flow through the **shunt**

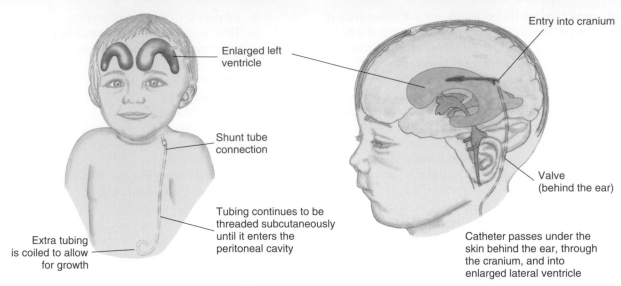

▲ FIGURE 31-3 Ventriculoperitoneal shunt. (From McKinney, E., James, S., Murray, S., & Ashwill, J. [2009]. *Maternal-child nursing* [3rd ed.]. Philadelphia: Saunders).

and report the observations to the registered nurse.
5. Monitor for signs of infection. Check dressings for drainage.
6. Measure the head circumference.
7. Monitor I&O.
8. Provide comfort measures. Administer medications, as prescribed.
9. Instruct the parents regarding how to recognize **shunt** infection or malfunction.
10. In an infant, irritability, lethargy, and feeding poorly may indicate **shunt** malfunction or infection.
11. In a toddler, headache and a lack of appetite are the earliest common signs of **shunt** malfunction.
12. In older children, the most valuable indicator of **shunt** malfunction is an alteration in the child's level of consciousness.

⚠ A high shrill cry in an infant can be a sign of increased ICP.

VIII. LATCHKEY CHILDREN

A. Description
1. Children who do not have adult supervision before or after school hours; they are left to care for themselves during these times
2. Occurs when the child or children are member(s) of a single-parent family, or the parent(s) work and need to leave the home before the child is brought to school.
3. This situation induces a stress-provoking environment for the child and places the child at risk for injury and delinquent behavior.

B. Interventions
1. Identify the latchkey child
2. Encourage the parent(s) to teach the child about self-care and self-help skills.
3. Inform the parent(s) about available community resources such as after-school programs for the children.

IX. MENINGITIS

A. Description
1. Meningitis is an infectious process of the central nervous system that is caused by bacteria and viruses that may be acquired as a primary disease or as a result of complications of neurosurgery, trauma, infection of the sinuses or ears, or systemic infections.
2. The diagnosis of bacterial meningitis is made by testing CSF obtained by lumbar puncture. The fluid of a child with meningitis is cloudy with increased pressure, increased white blood cell count, elevated protein, and decreased glucose levels.
3. Bacterial meningitis can be caused by a variety of organisms, most commonly *Haemophilus influenza* type B, *Streptococcus pneumoniae*, or *Neisseria meningitides*; meningococcal meningitis occurs in epidemic form and can be transmitted by droplets from nasopharyngeal secretions.
4. Viral meningitis is associated with viruses such as mumps, paramyxovirus, herpesvirus, and enterovirus.

B. Data collection
1. Signs and symptoms vary, depending on the type, the age of the child, and the duration of the preceding illness
2. Fever, chills, and headache
3. Vomiting and diarrhea

4. Poor feeding or anorexia
5. Nuchal rigidity
6. Poor or high-shrill cry
7. Altered level of consciousness (e.g., lethargy, irritability)
8. Bulging anterior fontanel in the infant
9. Positive Kernig's sign (the inability to extend the leg when the thigh is flexed anteriorly at the hip) and Brudzinski's sign (neck flexion causes adduction and flexion movements of the lower extremities) in children and adolescents
10. Muscle or joint pain (meningococcal infection and *Haemophilus influenzae* infection)
11. Petechial or purpuric rashes (meningococcal infection)
12. Ear that chronically drains (pneumococcal meningitis)

C. Interventions
1. Provide respiratory isolation precautions and maintain them for at least 24 hours after antibiotics are initiated.
2. Administer antibiotics and antipyretics as prescribed. (Administer antibiotics as soon as they are prescribed after lumbar puncture.) Antiseizure medications may also be prescribed.
3. Assist with performing a neurological assessment and monitor for seizures. Monitor for the complication of inappropriate antidiuretic hormone secretion, which causes fluid retention (cerebral edema) and dilutional hyponatremia.
4. Monitor for changes in the level of consciousness and irritability.
5. Monitor for a purpuric or petechial rash and for signs of thromboemboli.
6. Monitor nutritional status; monitor intake & output.
7. Monitor for hearing loss.
8. Determine close contacts of the child with meningitis because the contacts will need prophylactic treatment.
9. Pneumococcal conjugate **vaccine** is recommended for all children beginning at age 2 months to protect against meningitis; streptococcal pneumococci can cause many bacterial infections including meningitis (see Chapter 39 for information on **vaccines**).

X. MENTAL RETARDATION

A. Description
1. In mental retardation, the child manifests subaverage intellectual functioning along with deficits in adaptive skills.
2. Down syndrome is a congenital condition that results in moderate to severe retardation and has been linked to an extra group G chromosome (chromosome 21/trisomy 21).

B. Data collection
1. Deficits in cognitive skills and level of adaptive functioning
2. Delays in fine and gross motor skills
3. Speech delays
4. Decreased spontaneous activity
5. Nonresponsiveness
6. Irritability
7. Poor eye contact during feeding

C. Interventions
1. Medical strategies are focused at correcting structural deformities and treating associated behaviors.
2. Implement community and educational services with the use of a multidisciplinary approach.
3. Promote care skills as much as possible.
4. Assist with communication and socialization skills.
5. Facilitate appropriate playtime.
6. Initiate safety precautions, as necessary.
7. Assist the family with decisions regarding care.
8. Provide information regarding support services and community agencies.

XI. NEAR DROWNING

A. Description
1. Survival of at least 24 hours after submersion in a fluid medium
2. Hypoxia and asphyxiation is the primary problem because it results in extensive cell damage. Cerebral cells sustain irreversible damage after 4 to 6 minutes of submersion.
3. Additional problems include aspiration and hypothermia.
4. The outcome is predicted based on the length of submersion in non-icy water. The outcome may be good if submersion was for less than 5 minutes and the child exhibits neurological responsiveness, reactive pupils, and a normal cardiac rhythm.
5. A child who was submerged for more than 10 minutes and does not respond to cardiopulmonary life support measures within 25 minutes has an extremely poor prognosis (severe neurological impairment or death).

B. Interventions
1. Provide ventilatory and circulatory support; if child has had a severe cerebral insult, endotracheal intubation and mechanical ventilation may be required.
2. Monitor respiratory status because respiratory compromise and cerebral edema may occur 24 hours after the incident.
3. Monitor for aspiration pneumonia.
4. Monitor neurological status closely; if spontaneous purposeful movement and normal brainstem function is not apparent 24 hours after the event,

the child most likely suffered severe neurological deficits.

5. Teach the parents to provide adequate supervision of infants and small children around water to prevent accidents.

XII. REYE'S SYNDROME

A. Description
1. An acute encephalopathy that follows a viral illness. It is characterized pathologically by cerebral edema and fatty changes in the liver; a definitive diagnosis is made by liver biopsy.
2. The exact cause is not clear; most commonly follows a viral illness such as influenza or varicella.
3. Administration of aspirin and aspirin-containing salicylates is not recommended for children with a febrile illness or children with varicella or influenza because of its association with Reye's syndrome.
4. Acetaminophen (Tylenol) is usually prescribed for pediatric clients.
5. Early diagnosis and aggressive treatment is important; the goal of treatment is to maintain effective cerebral perfusion and control increasing ICP.

B. Data collection
1. History of systemic viral illness 4 to 7 days before the onset of symptoms
2. Malaise
3. Nausea and vomiting
4. Progressive neurological deterioration

C. Interventions
1. Provide rest and decrease stimulation in the environment.
2. Assess neurological status.
3. Monitor for altered level of consciousness and signs of increased ICP.
4. Monitor for signs of altered hepatic function and the results of liver function studies.
5. Monitor intake and output.
6. Monitor for signs of bleeding and signs of impaired coagulation, such as a prolonged bleeding time.

XIII. SEIZURE DISORDERS

A. Description (see Chapter 57 for additional information on seizures)
1. Excessive and unorganized neuronal discharges in the brain that activate associated motor and sensory organs.
2. Classified as generalized, partial, or unclassified, depending on the area of the brain involved.
3. Types of generalized seizures include tonic-clonic, absence, myoclonic, and atonic.

4. Partial seizures arise from a specific area in the brain and cause limited symptoms; types include simple partial and complex partial.

B. Data collection
1. Obtain information from the parents about the time of onset, precipitating events, and behavior before and after the seizure.
2. Determine the child's history related to seizures.
3. Ask the child about the presence of an aura (a warning sign of impending seizure).
4. Monitor for apnea and **cyanosis**.
5. Postseizure: The child is disoriented and sleepy.

C. Seizure precautions (see Box 31-2)

D. Interventions (Box 31-5)

E. Anticonvulsant medications (see Chapter 58 for information about medications)

 Never place anything, including an airway device or padded tongue blade, into the mouth of a child experiencing a seizure.

XIV. SPINA BIFIDA

A. Description
1. A central nervous system defect that results from the failure of the neural tube to close during embryonic development
2. Associated deficits may include sensorimotor disturbance, dislocated hips, talipes equinovarus (clubfoot), and hydrocephalus
3. Defect closure is performed immediately after birth.

B. Types
1. Spina bifida occulta

Box 31-5 Emergency Treatment for Seizures

Ensure airway patency.

Have suction equipment and oxygen available.

Time the seizure episode.

If the child is standing or sitting, ease the child down to the floor and place him or her in a side-lying position.

Place a pillow or folded blanket under the child's head. If no bedding is available, place your own hands under the child's head, or place the child's head in your own lap.

Loosen restrictive clothing.

Remove eyeglasses from the child, if present.

Clear the area of any hazards or hard objects.

Allow the seizure to proceed and end without interference.

If vomiting occurs, turn the child to one side as a unit.

Do not restrain the child, place anything in the child's mouth, or give any food or liquids to the child.

Prepare to administer medications, as prescribed.

Remain with the child until he or she fully recovers.

Observe for incontinence, which may have occurred during the seizure.

Document the occurrence.

    a. Posterior vertebral arches fail to close in the lumbosacral area.

    b. The spinal cord remains intact and usually is not visible.

    c. Meninges are not exposed on the skin surface.

    d. Neurological deficits are not usually present.

  2. Spina bifida cystica

    a. Protrusion of the spinal cord or its meninges or both occurs.

    b. The defect results in the incomplete closure of the vertebral and neural tubes, which results in a saclike protrusion in the lumbar or sacral area with varying degrees of nervous tissue involvement.

    c. The defect can include meningocele, myelomeningocele, lipomeningocele, and lipomeningomyelocele.

  3. Meningocele

    a. The protrusion involves meninges and a saclike cyst that contains CSF in the midline of the back, usually in the lumbosacral area.

    b. The spinal cord is not involved.

    c. Neurological deficits are usually not present.

  4. Myelomeningocele

    a. Protrusion of the meninges, CSF, nerve roots, and a portion of the spinal cord occurs.

    b. The sac (defect) is covered by a thin membrane that is prone to leakage or rupture.

    c. Neurological deficits are evident.

C. Data collection

  1. Depends on the spinal cord involvement

  2. Visible spinal defect

  3. Flaccid paralysis of the legs

  4. Altered bladder and bowel function

  5. Hip and joint deformities

  6. Hydrocephalus

D. Interventions

  1. Evaluate the sac and measure the lesion.

  2. Assist with performing a neurological assessment.

  3. Monitor for increased ICP, which may indicate developing hydrocephalus.

  4. Measure the head circumference. Check the anterior fontanel for fullness.

  5. Protect the sac. Cover with a sterile, moist (normal saline), nonadherent dressing to maintain the moisture of the sac and its contents.

  6. Change the dressing that covers the sac on a regular schedule, as prescribed, or whenever it becomes soiled to reduce the risk of infection. Diapering may be contraindicated until the defect has been repaired.

  7. Use aseptic technique to prevent infection.

  8. Place the child in a prone position to minimize tension on the sac and the risk of trauma; the head is turned to one side for feeding.

  9. Check the sac for redness, clear or purulent drainage, abrasions, irritation, and signs of infection.

  10. Early signs of infection include elevated axillary temperature, irritability, lethargy, and nuchal rigidity.

  11. Check for physical impairments such as hip and joint deformities.

  12. Prepare the child and family for surgery.

  13. Administer antibiotics preoperatively and postoperatively, as prescribed, to prevent infection.

  14. Teach the parents and eventually the child about long-term home care

    a. Positioning, feeding, skin care, and range-of-motion exercises.

    b. Instituting a bladder elimination program and performing clean intermittent catheterization technique.

    c. Administering antispasmodics (that act on the smooth muscle of the bladder) as prescribed to increase bladder capacity and improve continence.

    d. Implementing a bowel program including a high-fiber diet, increased fluids, suppositories, as needed.

    e. The child is at high risk for allergy to latex and rubber products because of the frequent exposure to latex during implementation of care measures.

MORE QUESTIONS ON EVOLVE!

Practice Questions

296. A nurse is collecting data about a child who has been admitted to the hospital with a diagnosis of seizures. The nurse checks for causes of the seizure activity by:

  1. Testing the child's urine for specific gravity

  2. Asking the child what happens during a seizure

  3. Obtaining a family history of psychiatric illness

  4. Obtaining a history regarding factors that may occur before the seizure activity

297. A child has a basilar skull fracture. Which of the following health care provider's prescriptions should the nurse question?

  1. Restrict fluid intake.

  2. Insert an indwelling urinary catheter.

  3. Keep an intravenous (IV) line patent.

  4. Suction via the nasotracheal route as needed.

298. Which of the following laboratory results would verify the diagnosis of bacterial meningitis?

  1. Clear cerebrospinal fluid with high protein and low glucose levels

2. Cloudy cerebrospinal fluid with low protein and low glucose levels
3. Cloudy cerebrospinal fluid with high protein and low glucose levels
4. Decreased pressure and cloudy cerebrospinal fluid with a high protein level

299. A child has been diagnosed with meningococcal meningitis. Which of the following isolation techniques is appropriate?
1. Enteric precautions
2. Neutropenic precautions
3. No precautions are required as long as antibiotics have been started.
4. Isolation precautions for at least 24 hours after the initiation of antibiotics

300. Which of the following represents a primary characteristic of autism?
1. Normal social play
2. Consistent imitation of others' actions
3. Lack of social interaction and awareness
4. Normal verbal and nonverbal communication

301. Which data collection finding would indicate the possibility of the sexual abuse of a child?
1. Poor hygiene
2. Consistent hunger
3. Bald spots on the scalp
4. Swelling of the genitals

302. A nurse is assisting with data collection from an infant who has been diagnosed with hydrocephalus. If the infant's level of consciousness diminishes, a priority intervention is:

1. Taking the apical pulse
2. Taking the blood pressure
3. Testing the urine for protein
4. Palpating the anterior fontanel

303. A mother arrives at the emergency department with her 5-year-old child and states that the child fell off a bunk bed. A head injury is suspected, and a nurse is monitoring the child continuously for signs of increased intracranial pressure (ICP). Which of the following is a late sign of increased ICP in this child?
1. Nausea
2. Bradycardia
3. Bulging fontanel
4. Dilated scalp veins

304. A child has been diagnosed with Reye's syndrome. The nurse understands that a major symptom associated with Reye's syndrome is:
1. Persistent vomiting
2. Protein in the urine
3. Symptoms of hyperglycemia
4. A history of a *Staphylococcus* infection

305. A nurse is developing a plan of care for a child who is at risk for seizures. Which interventions apply if the child has a seizure? **Select all that apply.**
❑ 1. Time the seizure.
❑ 2. Restrain the child.
❑ 3. Stay with the child.
❑ 4. Place the child in a prone position.
❑ 5. Move furniture away from the child.
❑ 6. Insert a padded tongue blade into the child's mouth.

ANSWERS

296. 4
Rationale: Fever and infections increase the body's metabolic rate. This can cause seizure activity among children who are less than 5 years old. Dehydration and electrolyte imbalance can also contribute to the occurrence of a seizure. Falls can cause head injuries, which would increase intracranial pressure or cerebral edema. Some medications could cause seizures. Specific gravity would not be a reliable test, because it varies, depending on the existing condition. Psychiatric illness has no impact on seizure occurrence or cause. Children do not remember what happened during the seizure itself.
Test-Taking Strategy: Use the process of elimination, and focus on the subject—cause of the seizure activity. Note the relationship between the subject and option 4. Review the precipitating factors associated with seizures if you had difficulty with this question.
Level of Cognitive Ability: Analyzing
Client Needs: Physiological Integrity
Integrated Process: Nursing Process/Data Collection

Content Area: Child Health: Neurological/Musculoskeletal
Reference: Christensen, Kockrow, pp. 1046–1047. 2011. *Foundations of nursing.*

297. 4
Rationale: Nasotracheal suctioning is contraindicated in a child with a basilar skull fracture. Because of the location of the injury, the suction catheter may be introduced into the brain. Fluids are restricted to prevent fluid overload. The child may require a urinary catheter for the accurate monitoring of intake and output. An IV line is maintained to administer fluids or medications, if necessary.
Test-Taking Strategy: Use the process of elimination, and note the strategic words "should the nurse question." Note that options 1, 2, and 3 are comparable or alike in that they all address the subject of fluid intake or output. Review the care of the child with a basilar skull fracture if you had difficulty with this question.
Level of Cognitive Ability: Analyzing
Client Needs: Safe and Effective Care Environment

Integrated Process: Nursing Process/Implementation
Content Area: Child Health: Neurological/Musculoskeletal
Reference: Hockenberry, Wilson, p. 992. 2009.

298. 3

Rationale: A diagnosis of meningitis is made by testing the cerebrospinal fluid (CSF) obtained by lumbar puncture. In the case of bacterial meningitis, findings usually include increased pressure, cloudy cerebrospinal fluid, a high protein level, and a low glucose level.

Test-Taking Strategy: Use the process of elimination and your knowledge regarding the diagnostic findings in clients with meningitis. Eliminate options 1 and 4 first, because clear CSF and decreased pressure are not likely to be found if an infectious process such as meningitis is suspected. From this point, recalling that a high protein level indicates a possible diagnosis of meningitis will direct you to option 3. Review the findings in clients with meningitis if you had difficulty with this question.

Level of Cognitive Ability: Analyzing
Client Needs: Physiological Integrity
Integrated Process: Nursing Process/Data Collection
Content Area: Fundamental Skills/Laboratory Values
Reference: Leifer, p. 541. 2011.

299. 4

Rationale: Meningococcal meningitis is transmitted primarily by droplet infection. Isolation is begun and maintained for at least 24 hours after antibiotics are given. Options 1, 2, and 3 are incorrect.

Test-Taking Strategy: Use the process of elimination, and eliminate options 1 and 2 first. Both enteric and neutropenic precautions are unrelated to the mode of transmission of meningococcal meningitis. Recalling that it takes approximately 24 hours for antibiotics to reach a therapeutic blood level will assist with directing you to option 4 from the remaining options. Review the mode of transmission of meningococcal meningitis if you had difficulty with this question.

Level of Cognitive Ability: Applying
Client Needs: Safe and Effective Care Environment
Integrated Process: Nursing Process/Planning
Content Area: Fundamental Skills: Safety/Infection Control
Reference: Leifer, pp. 541-542. 2011.

300. 3

Rationale: Autism is a severe form of an autism spectrum disorder. A primary characteristic is a lack of social interaction and awareness. Social behaviors in autism include a lack of or an abnormal imitation of others' actions and a lack of or abnormal social play. Additional characteristics include a lack of or impaired verbal communication and markedly abnormal nonverbal communication.

Test-Taking Strategy: Use the process of elimination. Eliminate options 1 and 4 first, because they address normal behaviors. From the remaining options, recalling that the autistic child lacks social interaction and awareness will direct you to option 3. Review the characteristics associated with autism if you had difficulty with this question.

Level of Cognitive Ability: Understanding
Client Needs: Psychosocial Integrity
Integrated Process: Nursing Process/Data Collection

Content Area: Child Health: Neurological/Musculoskeletal
References: Christensen, Kockrow, pp. 1070–1071. 2011. *Foundations of nursing.*
Leifer, pp. 410, 749. 2011.

301. 4

Rationale: The most likely findings among children who have been sexually abused include difficulty walking or sitting; torn, stained, or bloody underclothing; pain, swelling, or itching of the genitals; and bruises, bleeding, or lacerations in the genital or anal area. Poor hygiene and consistent hunger may be indicative of physical neglect. Bald spots on the scalp are most likely associated with physical abuse.

Test-Taking Strategy: Use the process of elimination. Note the strategic words "sexual abuse." The only choice that specifically addresses a finding related to sexual abuse is option 4. Review the findings in a child who is suspected of being abused if you had difficulty with this question.

Level of Cognitive Ability: Understanding
Client Needs: Physiological Integrity
Integrated Process: Nursing Process/Data Collection
Content Area: Mental Health
Reference: Christensen, Kockrow, pp. 1072–1074. 2011. *Foundations of nursing.*

302. 4

Rationale: A full or bulging anterior fontanel indicates an increase in cerebrospinal fluid collection in the cerebral ventricle. Apical pulse and blood pressure changes and proteinuria are not specifically associated with increasing cerebrospinal fluid in the brain tissue in an infant.

Test-Taking Strategy: Use the principles associated with excessive fluid buildup in the cranial cavity, and note that the question addresses an infant. Additionally, correlate "hydrocephalus" in the question with "anterior fontanel" in option 4. Review the symptoms associated with hydrocephalus if you had difficulty with this question.

Level of Cognitive Ability: Analyzing
Client Needs: Physiological Integrity
Integrated Process: Nursing Process/Data Collection
Content Area: Child Health: Neurological/Musculoskeletal
References: Christensen, Kockrow, pp. 1042–1044. 2011. *Foundations of nursing.*
Leifer, pp. 322-323. 2011.

303. 2

Rationale: Late signs of increased ICP include a significant decrease in the level of consciousness, bradycardia, and fixed and dilated pupils. Nausea is an early sign of increased ICP. A bulging fontanel and dilated scalp veins are early signs of increased ICP and would be noted in an infant rather than in a 5-year-old child.

Test-Taking Strategy: Use the process of elimination, and note the age of the child and the strategic word "late." Options 3 and 4 can be eliminated first, because these signs would be noted in an infant rather than a 5-year-old child. Focusing on the strategic word "late" will direct you to option 2. Review the early and late signs of increased ICP in an infant and in a child if you had difficulty with this question.

Level of Cognitive Ability: Analyzing

Client Needs: Physiological Integrity
Integrated Process: Nursing Process/Data Collection
Content Area: Child Health: Neurological/Musculoskeletal
References: Hockenberry, Wilson, p. 976. 2009.
McKinney, James, Murray, Ashwill, p. 1468. 2009.

304. 1

Rationale: Persistent vomiting is a major symptom that is associated with increased intracranial pressure (ICP). Options 2, 3, and 4 are incorrect. Protein is not present in the urine. Reye's syndrome is related to a history of viral infections, and hypoglycemia is a symptom of this disease.
Test-Taking Strategy: Note the strategic words "major symptom." Recalling that increased ICP is an associated characteristic will direct you to the correct option. Review the symptoms of Reye's syndrome and the signs of increased ICP if you had difficulty with this question.
Level of Cognitive Ability: Understanding
Client Needs: Physiological Integrity
Integrated Process: Nursing Process/Data Collection
Content Area: Child Health: Neurological/Musculoskeletal
Reference: Leifer, p. 540. 2011.

305. 1, 3, 5

Rationale: During a seizure, the child is placed on his or her side in a lateral position. This type of positioning will prevent aspiration, because saliva will drain out of the corner of the child's mouth. The child is not restrained, because this could cause injury. The nurse would loosen clothing around the child's neck and ensure a patent airway. Nothing is placed into the child's mouth during a seizure, because this action may cause injury to the child's mouth, gums, or teeth. The nurse would stay with the child to reduce the risk of injury and allow for the observation and timing of the seizure.
Test-Taking Strategy: Visualize this clinical situation. Recalling that airway patency and safety are the priorities will assist you with determining the appropriate interventions. Review the care of the child who is experiencing a seizure if you had difficulty with this question.
Level of Cognitive Ability: Applying
Client Needs: Physiological Integrity
Integrated Process: Nursing Process/Implementation
Content Area: Child Health: Neurological/Musculoskeletal
Reference: Christensen, Kockrow, pp. 1046–4047. 2011. *Foundations of nursing.*

Eye, Ear, Throat, and Respiratory Disorders

I. STRABISMUS

A. Description
1. Called squint or lazy eye
2. A condition in which the eyes are not aligned as a result of a lack of coordination of the extraocular muscles
3. Most often results from a muscle imbalance or the paralysis of the extraocular muscles, but it may also result from infection congenital defect
4. Amblyopia (reduced visual acuity) may occur if not treated early because the brain receives two messages as a result of the unparallel visual axes.
5. Permanent loss of vision can occur if not treated early.
6. This condition may be normally found in the young infant but should not be present after about age 4 months
7. Treatment of the condition depends on the cause

B. Data collection
1. Crossed eyes
2. Squinting; tilts the head or closes one eye to see
3. Loss of binocular vision
4. Impairment of depth perception
5. Frequent headaches
6. Diplopia; photophobia

C. Interventions
1. Corrective lenses to improve eye alignment
2. Instruct the parents regarding patching (occlusion therapy) of the "good" eye to strengthen the weak eye
3. Prepare for surgery to realign the weak muscles as prescribed if nonsurgical interventions are unsuccessful; this is usually performed before the age of 2 years.
4. Instruct the parents about the need for follow-up visits.

II. CONJUNCTIVITIS

A. Description
1. Inflammation of the conjunctiva; frequently known as pinkeye

2. May be caused by allergy, infection, or trauma
3. Bacterial or viral conjunctivitis is extremely contagious

B. Data collection
1. Itching, burning, or scratchy eyelids
2. Redness of the conjunctiva and sclera
3. Edema
4. Mucoid or purulent discharge; may vary in coloration from white to yellowish or greenish; may cause morning crusting and difficulty with opening the eyes first thing in the morning

⚠ Chlamydial conjunctivitis is rare among older children; if diagnosed in a child who is not sexually active, he or she should be assessed for possible sexual abuse.

C. Interventions
1. Instruct in infection control measures such as good handwashing and not sharing towels and washcloths
2. Administer antibiotic or antiviral eyedrops or ointment, as prescribed, if infection is present (severe infection may require therapy with systemic antibiotics).
3. Administer antihistamines, as prescribed, if an allergy is present.
4. Instruct the child and parents in the administration of the prescribed medications.
5. Instruct the parents that the child should be kept home from school or day care until antibiotics and/or antibiotic eyedrops have been administered for 24 hours.
6. Instruct the child and parents in the use of cool compresses to lessen irritation and in the wearing of dark glasses for photophobia.
7. Instruct the child to avoid rubbing the eye to prevent injury.
8. Instruct the child who is wearing contact lenses to discontinue wearing them until treatment is complete. New lenses need to be obtained to eliminate the chance of reinfection that can occur from the use of the old lenses.

9. Instruct the adolescent that the eye makeup currently being used should be discarded and replaced with new makeup to prevent reinfection.

III. OTITIS MEDIA

A. Description
1. Otitis media is an inflammatory disorder usually caused by an infection of the middle ear occurring as a result of a blocked eustachian tube, which prevents normal drainage; can be acute or chronic.
2. Otitis media is a common complication of an acute respiratory infection (most commonly from respiratory syncytial virus or influenza).
3. Infants and children have eustachian tubes that are shorter, wider, and straighter, which makes them more prone to otitis media.

B. Prevention
1. Feed infants in upright position, to prevent reflux.
2. Maintain routine immunizations
3. Encourage breastfeeding for at least the first 6 months of age
4. Avoid exposure to tobacco smoke and allergens

C. Data collection
1. Fever
2. Acute onset of ear pain
3. Crying, irritability, lethargy
4. Loss of appetite
5. Rolling of head from side to side
6. Pulling on or rubbing the ear
7. Purulent ear drainage may be present
8. Red, opaque, bulging, immobile tympanic membrane on otoscopic exam
9. Signs of hearing loss (indicative of chronic otitis media)

D. Interventions
1. Encourage fluid intake (may be difficult if the child is in pain).
2. Instruct the child to avoid chewing as much as possible during the acute period because chewing increases pain.
3. Provide local heat or cold as prescribed to relieve discomfort and have the child lie with the affected ear down.
4. Instruct the parents in the appropriate procedure to clean drainage from the external ear canal with sterile swabs or gauze; frequent cleansing and the application of moisture barriers may be prescribed to prevent ear excoriation from the drainage.
5. Instruct the parents in the administration of analgesics or antipyretics such as acetaminophen (Tylenol) to decrease fever and pain.
6. Instruct the parents in the administration of antibiotics if prescribed, emphasizing that the prescribed period of administration is necessary to eliminate infective organisms.

7. Instruct the parents that screening for hearing loss may be necessary.
8. Instruct the parents about the procedure for administering ear medications such as topical pain relief drops if prescribed

⚠ To administer ear medications in a child younger than age 3, pull the ear lobe down and back. In a child older than 3 years, pull the pinna up and back.

E. Myringotomy
1. Description
   a. A surgical incision into the tympanic membrane to provide drainage of the purulent middle ear fluid; may be done by a laser-assisted procedure
   b. Insertion of tympanoplasty tubes into the middle ear may be done to allow continued drainage and to equalize pressure and allow ventilation of the middle ear
2. Postoperative interventions
   a. Instruct the parents and child to keep the ears dry.
   b. The child should wear earplugs while bathing, shampooing, and swimming (diving and submerging under water are not allowed)
   c. Parents can administer an analgesic such as acetaminophen (Tylenol) to relieve discomfort following insertion of tympanoplasty tubes.
   d. Parents should be taught that the child should not blow his or her nose for 7 to 10 days after surgery.
   e. Instruct the parents that if the tubes fall out, it is not an emergency, but the health care provider (HCP) should be notified; inform the parents of the appearance of the tubes (tiny, white, spool-shaped tubes).

IV. TONSILLECTOMY AND ADENOIDECTOMY

A. Description
1. *Tonsillitis* refers to inflammation and infection of the tonsils, which is lymphoid tissue located in the pharynx (Figure 32-1)
2. *Adenoiditis* refers to inflammation and infection of the adenoids (pharyngeal tonsils), located on the posterior wall of the nasopharynx.
3. Tonsillectomy (surgical removal of the tonsils) and adenoidectomy (surgical removal of the adenoids) may be necessary.

B. Data collection
1. Persistent or recurrent sore throat
2. Enlarged bright red tonsils that may be covered with white exudate
3. Difficulty swallowing
4. Mouth breathing and an unpleasant mouth odor

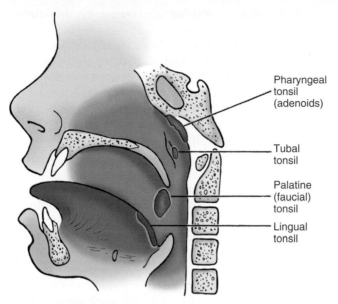

▲ FIGURE 32-1 Location of various tonsillar masses. (From Hockenberry, M., & Wilson, D. [2010]. *Wong's nursing care of infants and children* [9th ed.]. St. Louis: Mosby).

Labels on figure:
- Pharyngeal tonsil (adenoids)
- Tubal tonsil
- Palatine (faucial) tonsil
- Lingual tonsil

5. Fever
6. Cough
7. Enlarged adenoids may cause a nasal quality of speech, mouth breathing, hearing difficulty, snoring, or obstructive sleep apnea.
C. Interventions preoperatively
1. Monitor for signs of active infection.
2. Monitor bleeding and clotting studies, because the throat is very vascular.
3. Prepare the child for a sore throat postoperatively, and inform the child that he or she will need to drink liquids.
4. Check for any loose teeth to decrease the risk of aspiration during surgery.
D. Interventions postoperatively
1. Position the child prone or side-lying to facilitate drainage.
2. Have suction equipment available, but do not suction unless there is an airway obstruction.
3. Monitor for signs of bleeding (e.g., frequent swallowing). If bleeding occurs, turn the child to the side and notify the HCP.
4. Discourage coughing, clearing of the throat, or nose blowing to prevent bleeding.
5. Provide an ice collar or analgesics (rectally or intravenously) for discomfort, as prescribed.
6. Administer antiemetics, as prescribed, to prevent vomiting.
7. Provide clear, cool, non-citrus, and noncarbonated fluids (crushed ice, ice pops).
8. Avoid red, purple, or brown liquids, which will simulate the appearance of blood if the child vomits.

9. Avoid milk products such as milk, ice cream, and pudding initially, because they will coat the throat, causing the child to clear the throat.
10. Soft foods may be prescribed 1 to 2 days postoperatively.
11. Do not give the child any straws, forks, or sharp objects that can be put into the mouth.
12. Mouth odor, slight ear pain, and a low-grade fever may occur for a few days postoperatively, but the parents should be instructed to notify the HCP if bleeding, a persistent earache, or fever occurs.
13. Instruct the parents to keep the child away from crowds until healing has occurred; usually the child is able to resume normal activities after 1 to 2 weeks postoperatively.

V. EPISTAXIS (NOSEBLEEDS)

A. Description
1. The nose, especially the septum, is a highly vascular structure, and bleeding usually results from direct trauma, foreign bodies, nose picking, and mucosal inflammation.
2. Recurrent epistaxis and severe bleeding may indicate underlying disease.
B. Interventions
1. See Priority Nursing Actions.
2. If bleeding cannot be controlled, packing or cauterization of the bleeding vessel may be prescribed.

■■■■ PRIORITY NURSING ACTIONS! ■■■■

Actions to Take if a Child Has a Nosebleed
1. Remain calm and keep the child calm and quiet.
2. Have the child sit up and lean forward (not lying down).
3. Apply continuous pressure to the nose with the thumb and forefinger for at least 10 minutes.
4. Insert cotton or wadded tissue into each nostril, and apply ice or a cold cloth to the bridge of the nose if bleeding persists.

If a nosebleed occurs in a child, it is important for the nurse to remain calm; otherwise, the child becomes agitated and it is difficult to get the child to cooperate with the necessary interventions. The child should be assisted to a sitting up and leaning forward position to prevent aspiration of blood. The child should not be placed in a lying down position. Nosebleeds usually originate in the anterior part of the nasal septum and can be controlled by applying pressure to the soft lower portion of the nose with the thumb and forefinger for at least 10 minutes. If bleeding persists, cotton or wadded tissue should be placed into each nostril, and ice or a cold cloth should be applied to the bridge of the nose. If bleeding does persist, the HCP needs to be notified, and the nose may require packing by
Continued

the HCP. After the nosebleed has been stopped, petroleum or a water-soluble jelly may be inserted into each nostril to prevent crusting of old blood and to lessen the likelihood of the child picking at the crusted lesions and restarting the bleeding. Repeated bleeding episodes that last longer than 30 minutes may be an indication of the need for evaluation of a bleeding disorder.

Reference: Perry, S., Hockenberry, M., Lowdermilk, D., & Wilson, D. (2010). *Maternal child nursing care* (4th ed., p. 1507). St. Louis: Mosby.

VI. EPIGLOTTITIS

A. Description
1. A bacterial form of croup
2. An inflammation of the epiglottis occurs, which may be caused by *Haemophilus influenzae* type B or *Streptococcus pneumonia*; children immunized with *H influenza* type b (HIB **vaccine**) are at less risk for epiglottitis.
3. Occurs most frequently among children who are 2 to 8 years of age, but can occur from infancy to adulthood.
4. Onset is abrupt; occurs most often in the winter
5. Considered an emergency situation because it can progress rapidly to severe respiratory distress

B. Data collection
1. High fever
2. Sore, red, and inflamed throat (large, cherry red, edematous epiglottis) and pain on swallowing (Figure 32-2)
3. Absence of spontaneous cough
4. Drooling
5. Agitation
6. Muffled voice
7. **Retractions** and the child struggles to breathe (Figure 32-3)

8. Inspiratory **stridor** aggravated by the supine position
9. Tachycardia
10. Tachypnea progressing to more severe respiratory distress (hypoxia, hypercapnia, respiratory acidosis, decreased level of consciousness)
11. Tripod positioning: while supporting the body with the hands, the child leans forward, thrusts the chin forward and opens the mouth in an attempt to widen the airway.

C. Interventions
1. Maintain a patent airway.
2. Monitor respiratory status and breath sounds, noting **nasal flaring**, the use of accessory muscles, **retractions**, and the presence of **stridor**.
3. Check temperature by the axillary route, not the oral route.
4. Monitor pulse oximetry.
5. Prepare the child for lateral neck films to confirm the diagnosis (accompany the child to the radiology department).
6. Maintain an NPO status.
7. Do not leave the child unattended.
8. Avoid placing the child in a supine position because this position will further affect the respiratory status.
9. Do not restrain the child or take any other measure that may agitate the child.
10. Assist to administer intravenous (IV) fluids as prescribed; insertion of an IV may need to be delayed until an adequate airway is established because this procedure may agitate the child.
11. Intravenous antibiotics may be prescribed; these are usually followed by oral antibiotics.
12. Administer analgesics and antipyretics (acetaminophen [Tylenol] to reduce fever and throat pain as prescribed.

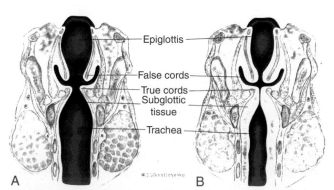

▲ **FIGURE 32-2 A,** Normal larynx. **B,** Obstruction and narrowing resulting from edema of croup. (From Hockenberry, M., & Wilson, D. [2010] *Wong's nursing care of infants and children* [9th ed.]. St. Louis: Mosby).

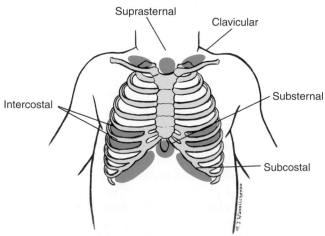

▲ **FIGURE 32-3** Location of retractions. (From Hockenberry, M., & Wilson, D. [2010]. *Wong's nursing care of infants and children* [9th ed.]. St. Louis: Mosby).

13. Administer corticosteroids to decrease inflammation and reduce throat edema as prescribed.
14. Nebulized epinephrine (racemic epinephrine) may be prescribed for severe cases (causes mucosal vasoconstriction and reduces edema); heliox (mixture of helium and oxygen) may be also prescribed to reduce mucosal edema.
15. Provide cool mist oxygen therapy as prescribed; high humidification cools the airway and decreases swelling.
16. Have resuscitation equipment available, and prepare for endotracheal intubation or tracheotomy for severe respiratory distress.
17. Ensure that the child is up to date with the immunization schedule, including *Haemophilus influenzae* type b (Hib) conjugate **vaccine**. (See Chapter 39 for information on immunizations.)

⚠ If epiglottitis is suspected, no attempts should be made to visualize the posterior pharynx, obtain a throat culture, or take an oral temperature. Otherwise, spasm of the epiglottis can occur, leading to complete airway occlusion.

VII. LARYNGOTRACHEOBRONCHITIS (CROUP)

A. Description (see Figure 32-2)
1. Inflammation of the larynx, trachea, and bronchi
2. Most common type of croup; may be viral or bacterial and most frequently occurs in children younger than 5 years
3. Common causative organisms include parainfluenzae virus types 1 and 2, respiratory syncytial virus (RSV), *Mycoplasma pneumoniae*, and influenza
4. Characterized by gradual onset that may be preceded by an upper respiratory infection

B. Data collection (Box 32-1)

C. Interventions
1. Maintain a patent airway.
2. Monitor the respiratory status, and check for **nasal flaring**, sternal **retraction**, and inspiratory **stridor**.
3. Monitor for adequate respiratory exchange; monitor for pallor or **cyanosis**.
4. Elevate the head of the bed and provide rest.
5. Provide humidified oxygen via a cool-mist tent for the hospitalized child.(Table 32-1).
6. Instruct the parents to use a cool-air vaporizer or humidifier at home. Other measures include having the child breathe in the cool night air or the air from an open freezer and taking the child to a cool basement or garage.
7. Provide and encourage fluid intake. IV fluids may be prescribed to maintain hydration status if the child is unable to take oral fluids.
8. Administer acetaminophen (Tylenol) as prescribed to reduce fever.

9. Teach the parents to avoid administering cough syrups and cold medicines, which may dry and thicken secretions.
10. Assist to administer corticosteroids, if prescribed, for their anti-inflammatory effects.
11. Assist to administer nebulized epinephrine (racemic epinephrine), as prescribed, for children with severe disease experiencing **stridor** at rest, **retractions**, or difficulty breathing.
12. Administer antibiotics, as prescribed, noting that they are not indicated unless a bacterial infection is present.
13. Heliox (mixture of helium and oxygen) may be prescribed; this medication reduces the work of breathing, reduces airway turbulence, and helps to relieve airway obstruction.
14. Have resuscitation equipment available.
15. Provide appropriate reassurance and education to the parents or caregivers.

⚠ Isolation precautions should be implemented for a hospitalized child with an upper respiratory infection until the cause of the infection is known.

Box 32-1 Progression of Symptoms in Laryngotracheobronchitis

Stage I
- Low-grade fever
- Hoarseness
- Seal bark and brassy cough (croup cough)
- Inspiratory stridor
- Fear
- Irritability and restlessness

Stage II
- Continuous respiratory stridor
- Retractions
- Use of accessory muscles
- Crackles and wheezing
- Labored respirations

Stage III
- Continued restlessness
- Anxiety
- Pallor
- Diaphoresis
- Tachypnea
- Signs of anoxia and hypercapnia

Stage IV
- Intermittent cyanosis that progresses to permanent cyanosis
- Apneic episodes that progress to cessation of breathing

Adapted from Perry, S., Hockenberry, M., Lowdermilk, D., & Wilson, D. (2010). *Maternal child nursing care* (4th ed., p. 1320). St. Louis: Mosby.

TABLE 32-1 Advantages and Disadvantages of Various Oxygen-Delivery Systems

Systems	Advantages	Disadvantages
Oxygen mask	Various sizes available Delivers higher O_2 concentration than cannula Able to provide a predictable concentration of oxygen (with Venturi mask) whether child breathes through nose or mouth	Skin irritation Fear of suffocation Accumulation of moisture on face Possibility of aspiration of vomitus Difficulty with controlling O_2 concentrations
Nasal cannula	Provides low to moderate O_2 concentration (22%-40%) Child able to eat and talk while receiving O_2 Possibility of more complete observation of child because nose and mouth remain unobstructed	Must have patent nasal passages May cause abdominal distention, discomfort, or vomiting Difficulty controlling O_2 concentration if child breathes through mouth Inability to provide mist, if desired
Oxygen tent	Provides lower O_2 concentrations (F_{IO_2} up to 0.3-0.5) Child able to receive desired inspired O_2 concentrations, even while eating	Necessity for proper fit around bed to prevent the leakage of gas Cool and wet tent environment Poor access to child; inspired O_2 levels fall when the tent is entered
Oxygen hood	Provides high O_2 concentrations (F_{IO_2} up to 1.00) Free access to child's chest for assessment	High-humidity environment Need to remove child for feeding and care

F_{IO_2}, Fraction of inspired oxygen; O_2, oxygen.
Adapted from Hockenberry, M., & Wilson, D. (2007). *Wong's nursing care of infants and children* (8th ed.). St. Louis: Mosby.

VIII. BRONCHITIS

A. Description: Inflammation of the trachea and bronchi; may be referred to as *tracheobronchitis*
B. Data collection
   1. Fever
   2. Dry, hacking, and nonproductive cough that is worse at night and becomes productive in 2 to 3 days
C. Interventions
   1. Treat the symptoms as necessary.
   2. Monitor for respiratory distress.
   3. Provide cool, humidified air to the child.
   4. Encourage increased fluid intake; child may drink beverages that he or she likes as long as the respiratory status is stable.
   5. Administer antipyretics for fever as prescribed.

6. Cough suppressants may be prescribed to promote rest.

IX. BRONCHIOLITIS AND RESPIRATORY SYNCYTIAL VIRUS

A. Description
   1. An inflammation of the bronchioles that causes a thick production of mucus, which occludes the bronchiole tubes and the small bronchi.
   2. Respiratory syncytial virus is an acute viral infection and a common cause of bronchiolitis (other organisms that cause bronchiolitis include adenoviruses, parainfluenza viruses, and human meta-pneumovirus).
   3. RSV, although not airborne, is highly communicable and is usually transferred by direct contact with respiratory secretions.
   4. Occurs primarily in the winter and spring
   5. Rarer in children older than 2 years, with a peak incidence at approximately 6 months of age
   6. At-risk children include those older than 1 year of age who have a chronic or disabling condition.
   7. Identification of the virus is done via testing of nasal or nasopharyngeal secretions.
   8. Prevention measures include encouraging breastfeeding, avoiding tobacco smoke exposure, using good handwashing techniques, and administering palivizumab (Synagis), a monoclonal antibody, to high-risk infants; palivizumab is administered via intramuscular injection monthly for a 5-month period (usually from November to March).
B. Data collection (Box 32-2)
C. Interventions
   1. For the child with bronchiolitis, interventions are aimed at treating symptoms and include airway maintenance, cool humidified air and oxygen, adequate fluid intake, and medications.
   2. For the hospitalized child with RSV, isolate the child in a single room or place in a room with another child with RSV.
   3. Ensure that nurses caring for the child with RSV do not care for other high-risk children.
   4. Use contact and standard precautions during care; using good handwashing techniques and wearing gloves and gowns are necessary.
   5. Monitor airway status and maintain a patent airway.
   6. For most effective airway maintenance, position the child at a 30- to 40-degree angle with the neck slightly extended to maintain an open airway and decrease pressure on the diaphragm.
   7. Provide cool, humidified oxygen as prescribed.
   8. Monitor pulse oximetry levels.
   9. Encourage fluids; fluids administered intravenously may be necessary until the acute stage has passed.

Box 32-2 Data Collection: Respiratory Syncytial Virus

Initial Manifestations
- Rhinorrhea
- Eye or ear drainage
- Pharyngitis
- Coughing
- Sneezing
- Wheezing
- Intermittent fever

Manifestations as the Disease Progresses
- Increased coughing and wheezing
- Signs of air hunger
- Tachypnea and retractions
- Periods of cyanosis

Manifestations in Severe Illness
- Tachypnea greater than 70 breaths per minute
- Decreased breath sounds and poor air exchange
- Listlessness
- Apneic episodes

Adapted from Perry, S., Hockenberry, M., Lowdermilk, D., & Wilson, D. (2010). *Maternal child nursing care* (4th ed., p. 1320). St. Louis: Mosby.

10. Periodic suctioning may be necessary if nasal secretions are copious; use of a bulb syringe for suctioning may be effective and should be done before feeding to promote comfort and adequate intake.
11. Assist to administer ribavirin (Virazole), an antiviral medication, if prescribed (administered via the inhalation route).

⚠ Cough suppressants are administered with caution because they can interfere with the clearance of respiratory secretions.

X. PNEUMONIA

A. Description
1. Inflammation of the pulmonary parenchyma and/or alveoli caused by a virus, mycoplasmal agents, bacteria, or aspiration of foreign substances
2. The causative agent usually is introduced into the lungs through inhalation or from the bloodstream.
3. Viral pneumonia occurs more frequently than bacterial pneumonia, is seen in children of all ages, and often is associated with a viral upper respiratory infection.
4. Primary atypical pneumonia, usually caused by *Mycoplasma pneumoniae or Chlamydia pneumoniae* occurs most often in the fall and winter months and is more common in crowded living conditions; most often seen in children between the ages of 5 and 12 years.

5. Bacterial pneumonia is often a serious infection requiring hospitalization when pleural effusion or empyema accompanies the disease; hospitalization is also necessary for children with staphylococcal pneumonia (*Streptococcus pneumoniae* is a common cause).
6. Aspiration pneumonia occurs when food, secretions, liquids, or other materials enter the lung and cause inflammation and a chemical pneumonitis. Classic symptoms include an increasing cough or fever with foul-smelling sputum, deteriorating results on chest x-rays, and other signs of airway involvement.
7. Prevention of viral and bacterial pneumonia includes immunization of infants and children with pneumococcal **vaccine**. (See Chapter 39 for information on immunizations).

B. Viral pneumonia
1. Data collection
   a. Mild fever, slight cough, and malaise to high fever, severe cough, and prostration
   b. Nonproductive or productive cough of small amounts of whitish sputum
   c. Wheezes or fine **crackles**
2. Interventions
   a. Treatment is symptomatic.
   b. Administer oxygen with cool humidified air as prescribed.
   c. Increase fluid intake.
   d. Administer antipyretics for fever as prescribed.
   e. Administer chest physiotherapy and postural drainage as prescribed.

C. Primary atypical pneumonia
1. Data collection
   a. Fever, chills, anorexia, headache, malaise, and muscle pain
   b. Rhinitis, sore throat, and dry, hacking cough
   c. Cough is nonproductive initially and then produces seromucoid sputum, which becomes mucopurulent or blood streaked
2. Interventions: Symptomatic

D. Bacterial pneumonia
1. Data collection
   a. Infant: Irritability, lethargy, poor feeding, abrupt fever (may be accompanied by seizures), and respiratory distress (air hunger, tachypnea, and circumoral **cyanosis**)
   b. Older child: Headache, chills, abdominal pain, chest pain, and meningeal symptoms (meningism)
   c. Hacking, nonproductive cough
   d. Diminished breath sounds or scattered **crackles**
   e. With consolidation, decreased breath sounds are more pronounced.
   f. As the infection resolves, the cough becomes productive and the child expectorates purulent sputum; coarse **crackles** and **wheezing** are noted.

2. Interventions
   a. Antibiotic therapy is initiated as soon as the diagnosis is suspected; in the hospitalized infant or child, intravenous antibiotics are usually prescribed.
   b. Administer oxygen for respiratory distress as prescribed and monitor oxygen saturation via pulse oximetry.
   c. Place the child in a cool mist tent as prescribed; cool humidification moistens the airways and assists in temperature reduction.
   d. Suction mucus from the infant using a bulb syringe to maintain a patent airway if the infant is unable to handle secretions.
   e. Administer chest physiotherapy and postural drainage every 4 hours as prescribed.
   f. Promote bed rest to conserve energy.
   g. Encourage the child to lie on the affected side (if pneumonia is unilateral) to splint the chest and reduce the discomfort caused by pleural rubbing.
   h. Encourage fluid intake (administer cautiously to prevent aspiration); intravenously administered fluids may be necessary.
   i. Administer antipyretics for fever and bronchodilators as prescribed.
   j. Monitor temperature frequently because of the risk for febrile seizures.
   k. Institute isolation precautions with pneumococcal or staphylococcal pneumonia (according to agency policy).
   l. Administer cough suppressant as prescribed before rest times and meals if the cough is disturbing.
   m. Continuous closed chest drainage may be instituted if purulent fluid is present (usually noted in *Staphylococcus* infections).
   n. Fluid accumulation in the pleural cavity may be removed by thoracentesis; thoracentesis also provides a means for obtaining fluid for culture and for instilling antibiotics directly into the pleural cavity.

⚠ Children with a respiratory disorder should be monitored for weight loss and for signs of dehydration. Signs of dehydration include a sunken fontanel, non-elastic skin turgor, decreased and concentrated urinary output, dry mucous membranes, and decreased tear production.

XI. ASTHMA

A. Description
   1. Asthma is a chronic inflammatory disease of the airways (see Chapter 49 for additional information about this disorder).

2. Asthma is classified based on disease severity; management includes medications, environmental control of allergens, and child/family education.
3. The allergic reaction in the airways caused by the precipitant can result in an immediate reaction with obstruction occurring, and it can result in a late bronchial obstructive reaction several hours after the initial exposure to the precipitant.
4. Mast cell release of histamine leads to a bronchoconstrictive process, bronchospasm, and obstruction.
5. Diagnosis is made based on the child's symptoms, history and physical exam, chest radiograph, and laboratory tests (Box 32-3)
6. Precipitants triggering an asthma attack (see Box 32-4)
7. Status asthmaticus is an acute asthma attack and the child displays respiratory distress despite vigorous treatment measures; this is a medical emergency that can result in respiratory failure and death if not treated.

B. Data collection
   1. Child has episodes of dyspnea, **wheezing**, breathlessness, chest tightness, and cough, particularly at night and/or in the early morning.
   2. Acute asthma attacks
      a. Episodes of progressively worsening shortness of breath, cough, **wheezing**, chest tightness, decreases in expiratory airflow secondary to bronchospasm, mucosal edema, and mucus

---

Box 32-3 Laboratory Tests to Assist in Diagnosing Asthma

Pulmonary function tests (PFTs): Spirometry testing assesses the presence and degree of disease and can determine the response to treatment.

Peak expiratory flow rate (PEFR) measurement: Measures the maximum flow of air that can be forcefully exhaled in 1 second; the child uses a peak expiratory flow meter (PEFM) to determine a "personal best value" that can be used for comparison at other times, such as during and after an asthma attack.

Bronchoprovocation testing: Testing done to identify inhaled allergens; the mucous membranes are directly exposed to the suspected allergen in increasing amounts.

Skin testing: Done to identify specific allergens.

Exercise challenges: Exercise is used to identify the occurrence of exercise-induced bronchospasm.

Radioallergosorbent test (RAST): A blood test used to identify a specific allergen.

Chest radiograph: May show hyperexpansion of the airways.

Note: Some tests place the child at risk for an asthma attack; therefore testing should be done under close supervision.

plugging; air is trapped behind occluded or narrow airways, and hypoxemia can occur.

b. The attack begins with irritability, restlessness, headache, feeling tired, and/or chest tightness; just before the attack, the child may present with itching localized at the front of the neck or over the upper part of the back.

c. Respiratory symptoms include a hacking, irritable, nonproductive cough caused by bronchial edema.

d. Accumulated secretions stimulate the cough; the cough becomes rattling and there is production of frothy, clear, gelatinous sputum.

e. The child experiences **retractions**.

f. Hyperresonance on percussion of the chest is noted.

g. Breath sounds are coarse and loud, with **crackles**, coarse rhonchi, and inspiratory and expiratory **wheezing**; expiration is prolonged.

h. Child may be pale or flushed, and the lips may have a deep, dark red color that may progress to **cyanosis** (also observed in the nail beds and skin, especially around the mouth).

i. Restlessness, apprehension, and diaphoresis occur.

j. Child speaks in short, broken phrases.

k. Younger children assume the tripod sitting position; older children sit upright, with the shoulders in a hunched-over position, the hands on the bed or a chair, and the arms braced to facilitate the use of the accessory muscles of breathing (child refuses to lie down).

l. Exercise-induced attack: A cough, shortness of breath, chest pain or tightness, **wheezing**, and endurance problems occur during exercise.

m. Severe spasm or obstruction: Breath sounds and **wheezing** cannot be heard (silent chest), and the cough is ineffective (represents a lack of air movement).

n. Ventilatory failure and asphyxia: Shortness of breath, with air movement in the chest restricted to the point of absent breath sounds is noted; this is accompanied by a sudden rise in the respiratory rate.

C. Interventions: Acute episode (see Priority Nursing Actions)

Box 32-4 Precipitants Triggering an Asthma Attack

- Outdoor allergens: trees, shrubs, weeds, grasses, molds, pollen, air pollution, spores
- Indoor allergens: dust, dust mites, mold, cockroach antigen
- Irritants: tobacco smoke, wood smoke, odors, sprays
- Exposure to occupational irritants
- Exercise
- Cold air
- Changes in weather or temperature
- Environmental change: moving to a new home, starting a new school, etc.
- Colds and infections
- Animals: cats, dogs, rodents, horses
- Medications: aspirin, nonsteroidal anti-inflammatory drugs (NSAIDs), antibiotics, beta-blockers
- Strong emotions: fear, anger, laughing, crying
- Conditions: gastroesophageal reflux disease, tracheoesophageal fistula
- Food additives: sulfite preservatives
- Foods: nuts, milk/dairy products
- Endocrine factors: menses, pregnancy, thyroid disease

Data from Perry, S., Hockenberry, M., Lowdermilk, D., & Wilson, D. (2010). *Maternal child nursing care* (4th ed., p. 1320). St. Louis: Mosby.

■■■■ PRIORITY NURSING ACTIONS! ■■■■

Actions to Take in the Event of an Acute Asthma Attack

1. Check airway patency and respiratory status.
2. Assist to administer humidified oxygen by nasal cannula or face mask.
3. Assist to administer quick-relief (rescue) medications.
4. Assist to initiate an intravenous (IV) line.
5. Prepare the child for a chest radiograph if prescribed.
6. Prepare to obtain a blood sample for determining arterial blood gas levels if prescribed.

In the event of an acute asthma attack, several interventions are necessary. First, the nurse checks airway status to ensure airway patency. If the airway is not patent, emergency interventions such as endotracheal intubation may be necessary. The nurse also quickly assesses the child's respiratory status. If the airway is patent, the nurse administers oxygen by nasal cannula or mask as prescribed. Quick-relief (rescue) medications are administered as prescribed to treat the symptoms. An IV line is initiated so that IV medications can be administered if prescribed.

The nurse prepares the child for a chest x-ray to assess airway status and to assist in ruling out a respiratory infection. Blood samples are obtained, and an arterial blood gas may be obtained. When the laboratory results are obtained, the nurse assists to administer medications as prescribed to correct dehydration, acidosis, or electrolyte imbalances. During the episode and during treatment, the nurse stays with the child and continuously monitors respiratory status, pulse oximetry, and color. The nurse also needs to be alert to decreased wheezing or a silent chest, which may signal the inability to move air.

Reference: McKinney, E., James, S., Murray, S., & Ashwill, J. (2009). *Maternal-child nursing* (3rd ed., p. 1204). St. Louis: Saunders.

Box 32-5 Quick-Relief (Rescue) Medications

Short-acting β_2-agonists
Anticholinergics (for the relief of acute bronchospasm)
Systemic corticosteroids (for their anti-inflammatory action to treat reversible airflow obstruction)

Box 32-6 Long-Term Control (Preventer) Medications

Corticosteroids (for anti-inflammatory action)
Antiallergic medications (to prevent an adverse response on exposure to an allergen)
Nonsteroidal anti-inflammatory drugs (for anti-inflammatory action)
Long-acting β_2 agonists (for long-acting bronchodilation)
Leukotriene modifiers (to prevent bronchospasm and inflammatory cell infiltration)
Monoclonal antibody (blocks the binding of IgE to mast cells to inhibit inflammation)

D. Medications

1. Quick-relief (rescue medications): Used to treat symptoms and exacerbations (Box 32-5)
2. Long-term control (preventer medications): Used to achieve and maintain control of inflammation (Box 32-6)
3. Nebulizer, metered-dose inhaler (MDI): may be used to administer medications; if the child has difficulty using the MDI, medication can be administered by nebulization (medication is mixed with saline and then nebulized with compressed air by a machine).
4. If the MDI is used to administer a corticosteroid, a spacer should be used to prevent yeast infections in the child's mouth.
5. The child's **growth** patterns need to be monitored when corticosteroids are prescribed.

E. Chest physiotherapy

1. Chest physiotherapy includes clapping, vibration, postural drainage, suctioning, and breathing exercises.
2. Chest physiotherapy will strengthen the respiratory musculature and produce more efficient breathing patterns.
3. Chest physiotherapy is not recommended during an acute exacerbation.

F. Allergen control

1. Testing may be done to identify allergens.
2. Teach the child and parents about measures to prevent and reduce exposure to allergens (see Box 32-4)

G. Home-care measures

1. Instruct the family in measures to eliminate environmental allergens.

2. Avoid extremes of environmental temperature; in cold temperatures, instruct the child to breathe through the nose, not the mouth, and to cover the nose and mouth with a scarf.
3. Avoid exposure to individuals with a respiratory infection.
4. Instruct the child and family in how to recognize early symptoms of an asthma attack.
5. Instruct the child and family how to administer medications as prescribed.
6. Instruct the child and family how to use a nebulizer, MDI, or peak expiratory flowmeter.
7. Instruct the child and family about the importance of home monitoring of the peak expiratory flow rate; a decrease in the expiratory flow rate may indicate impending infection or exacerbation.
8. Instruct the child in the cleaning of devices used for inhaled medications (yeast infections can occur with the use of aerosolized corticosteroids).
9. Encourage adequate rest, sleep, and a well-balanced diet.
10. Instruct the child in the importance of adequate fluid intake to liquefy secretions.
11. Assist in developing an exercise program.
12. Instruct the child in the procedure for respiratory treatments and exercises as prescribed.
13. Encourage the child to cough effectively.
14. Encourage the parents to keep immunizations up to date; annual influenza vaccinations are recommended for children 6 months of age and older.
15. Inform other HCP, and school personnel of the asthma condition.
16. Allow the child to take control of self-care measures based on age appropriateness.

XII. CYSTIC FIBROSIS (Figure 32-4)

A. Description

1. A chronic multisystem disorder and autosomal-recessive trait disorder that is characterized by exocrine gland dysfunction
2. The mucus produced by the exocrine glands is abnormally thick and copious, which causes the obstruction of the small passageways of the affected organs, particularly in the respiratory, gastrointestinal, and reproductive systems.
3. Common symptoms are associated with pancreatic enzyme deficiency and pancreatic fibrosis caused by duct blockage, progressive chronic lung disease as a result of infection, and sweat gland dysfunction resulting in increased sodium and chloride sweat concentrations.
4. An increase in sodium and chloride in sweat and saliva forms the basis for one diagnostic test, the sweat chloride test (Box 32-7).

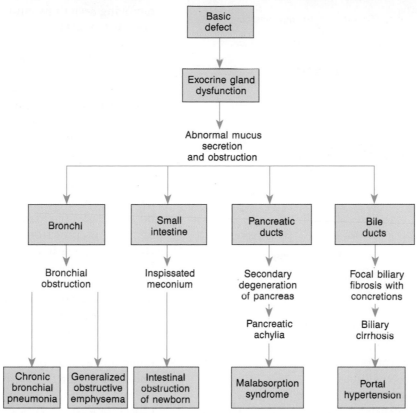

▲ **FIGURE 32-4** Various effects of exocrine gland dysfunction in cystic fibrosis. (From Hockenberry, M., & Wilson, D. [2010]. *Wong's nursing care of infants and children* [9th ed.]. St. Louis: Mosby).

Box 32-7 Quantitative Sweat Chloride Test

- The production of sweat is stimulated (pilocarpine iontophoresis), the sweat is collected, and the sweat electrolytes are measured (75 mg of sweat is needed).
- Normally, sweat chloride concentration is lower than 40 mEq/L.
- A chloride concentration higher than 60 mEq/L is a positive test result (higher than 40 mEq/L is diagnostic in infants younger than 3 months of age).
- Chloride concentrations between 40 to 60 mEq/L are highly suggestive of cystic fibrosis and require a repeat test.

5. CF is a progressive and incurable disorder and respiratory failure is a common cause of death; organ transplantations may be an option to increase survival rates.

B. Respiratory system
1. Symptoms are produced by the stagnation of mucus in the airway, which leads to bacterial colonization and the destruction of lung tissue.
2. Emphysema and atelectasis occur as the airways become increasingly obstructed.
3. Chronic hypoxemia causes the contraction and hypertrophy of the muscle fibers in the pulmonary arteries and arterioles, thus leading to pulmonary hypertension and eventual cor pulmonale.
4. Pneumothorax from ruptured bullae and hemoptysis from the erosion of the bronchial wall occur as the disease progresses.
5. Other respiratory symptoms
   a. **Wheezing** and cough
   b. Dyspnea
   c. **Cyanosis**
   d. Clubbing of the fingers and toes (Figure 32-5)
   e. Barrel chest
   f. Repeated episodes of bronchitis and pneumonia

C. Gastrointestinal system
1. Meconium ileus in the newborn is the earliest manifestation
2. Intestinal obstruction (distal intestinal obstructive syndrome) caused by thick intestinal secretions. Signs include pain, abdominal distention, nausea, and vomiting.
3. Steatorrhea (frothy, foul-smelling stools)
4. Deficiency of the fat-soluble vitamins A, D, E, and K, which causes easy bruising, bleeding, and anemia.
5. Malnutrition and failure to thrive. Demonstration of hypoalbuminemia from the diminished absorption of protein, which results in generalized edema

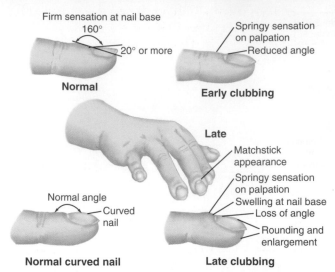

Firm sensation at nail base
160°
20° or more
Normal

Springy sensation
on palpation
Reduced angle
Early clubbing

Late
Matchstick
appearance
Springy sensation
on palpation
Swelling at nail base
Loss of angle
Rounding and
enlargement

Normal angle
Curved
nail
Normal curved nail

Late clubbing

▲ **FIGURE 32-5** Clubbing of fingers. (From Hockenberry, M., & Wilson, D. [2010]. *Wong's nursing care of infants and children* [9th ed.]. St. Louis: Mosby).

6. Rectal prolapse can result from the large, bulky stools and increased intraabdominal pressure.
7. Pancreatic fibrosis can occur and places the child at risk for diabetes mellitus.

D. Integumentary system
1. Abnormally high concentrations of sodium and chloride in the sweat
2. Parents report that the infant tastes "salty" when kissed.
3. Dehydration and electrolyte imbalances, especially during hyperthermic conditions

E. Reproductive system
1. Delayed **puberty** in females
2. Fertility can be inhibited by highly viscous cervical secretions, which act as a plug and block sperm entry.
3. Males are usually sterile as a result of the blockage of the vas deferens by abnormal secretions or the failure of the normal development of duct structures.

F. Diagnostic tests
1. Quantitative sweat chloride test is positive (see Box 32-7)
2. Newborn screening may be done in some states and may consist of immunoreactive trypsinogen analysis and direct DNA analysis for mutant genes.
3. Chest x-ray reveals atelectasis and obstructive emphysema.
4. Pulmonary function tests provide evidence of abnormal small airway function.
5. Stool fat and/or enzyme analysis: A 72-hour stool sample is collected to check the fat and/or enzyme (trypsin) content, or both (food intake is recorded during the collection).

G. Interventions: Respiratory system
1. Goals of treatment include preventing and treating pulmonary infection by improving aeration,

removing secretions, and administering antibiotic medications.
2. Monitor respiratory status, including lung sounds and the presence and characteristics of a cough.
3. Chest physiotherapy (percussion and postural drainage) on awakening and in the evening (more frequently during pulmonary infection) needs to be done every day to maintain pulmonary hygiene; it should not be performed before or immediately after a meal.
4. A Flutter Mucus Clearance Device (a small, hand-held plastic pipe with a stainless steel ball on the inside) facilitates the removal of mucus and may be prescribed; store away from small children because if the device separates, the steel ball poses a choking hazard.
5. Handheld percussors or a special vest device that provides high-frequency chest wall oscillation may be prescribed to help loosen secretions.
6. A positive expiratory pressure mask may be prescribed; use of this mask forces secretions to the upper airway for expectoration.
7. The child should be taught the forced expiratory technique (huffing) to mobilize secretions for expectoration.
8. Bronchodilator medication by aerosol may be prescribed and the medication opens the bronchi for easier expectoration (administered before the chest physiotherapy when the child has reactive airway disease or is **wheezing**); medications that decrease the viscosity of mucus may also be prescribed.
9. A physical exercise program with the aim of stimulating mucus expectoration and establishing an effective breathing pattern should be instituted.
10. Aerosolized antibiotics may be prescribed or intravenous antibiotics may be prescribed and administered at home through a central venous access device.
11. Oxygen may be prescribed during acute episodes; monitor closely for oxygen narcosis (signs include nausea and vomiting, malaise, fatigue, numbness and tingling of extremities, substernal distress) because the child with cystic fibrosis may have chronic carbon dioxide retention.
12. Monitor for hemoptysis; more than 250 mL in 24 hours for the older child (less for a younger child) needs to be reported to the HCP and treated immediately.
13. Hemoptysis may be controlled with measures such as bed rest, antibiotics if an infection is present, blood replacement therapy, and vitamin K; if hemoptysis persists, the site of bleeding may need to be cauterized.

H. Interventions: Gastrointestinal system

1. The child with cystic fibrosis requires a high-calorie, high-protein, and well-balanced diet to meet energy and **growth** needs; multivitamins and vitamins A, D, E, and K are also administered.
2. Monitor weight and for failure to thrive.
3. Monitor stool patterns and for signs of intestinal obstruction.
4. The goal of treatment for pancreatic insufficiency is to replace pancreatic enzymes; pancreatic enzymes are administered within 30 minutes of eating and administered with all meals and all snacks (not given if the child is NPO).
5. The amount of pancreatic enzymes administered depends on the HCP's preference and usually is adjusted to achieve normal **growth** and a decrease in the number of stools to two or three daily (additional enzymes are needed if the child is consuming high-fat foods).
6. Enteric-coated pancreatic enzymes should not be crushed or chewed; capsules can be taken apart and the contents can be sprinkled on a small amount of food for administration.
7. Monitor for constipation, intestinal obstruction, and rectal prolapse.
8. Monitor for signs of gastroesophageal reflux; place the infant in an upright position after eating and teach the child to sit upright after eating.

I. Additional interventions

1. Monitor blood glucose levels and for signs of diabetes mellitus.
2. Ensure adequate salt intake and fluids that provide an adequate supply of electrolytes during extremely hot weather and when the child has a fever.
3. Monitor bone **growth** in the child.
4. Monitor for signs of retinopathy or nephropathy.
5. Provide emotional support to the parents, particularly when the child is diagnosed; parents will be fearful and uncertain about the disorder and the care involved.
6. Provide support to the child as he or she transitions through the stages of **growth**.
7. Teach the child and parents about the care involved and encourage independence in the child to care for self, as it is age-appropriate.

J. Home care

1. Home care involves educating the parents and the child about all of the aspects of care for the disorder.
2. Informing the parents and child about the signs of complications and actions to take, and the importance of follow-up care is critical.
3. Instruct the parents to be sure that the child receives the recommended immunizations on schedule; additionally, the child should be immunized against influenza at age 6 months, followed by a yearly booster.
4. Inform the child and parents about the Cystic Fibrosis Foundation.

⚠ An alteration in respiratory status can create a frightening experience for both the child and parents. A calm and reassuring nursing approach will assist in reducing fear.

XIII. SUDDEN INFANT DEATH SYNDROME (SIDS)

A. Description

1. Unexpected death of an apparently healthy infant younger than 1 year for whom an investigation of the death and a thorough autopsy fails to demonstrate an adequate cause of death
2. Several theories are proposed as to the cause but the exact cause is unknown.
3. Most frequently occurs during winter months
4. Death usually occurs during sleep periods, but not necessarily at night.
5. Most frequently affects infants from 2 months to 3 months of age
6. Incidence is higher in males
7. Incidence is higher in Native Americans, African Americans, and Hispanics, and in lower socioeconomic groups
8. Incidence has been found to be lower in breastfed infants and infants sleeping with a pacifier
9. High-risk conditions for SIDS
   a. Prone position
   b. Use of soft bedding or sleeping in a noninfant bed such as a sofa
   c. Overheating (thermal stress)
   d. Co-sleeping
   e. Mother who is cigarette smoking or partakes in substance abuse during pregnancy.
   f. Exposure to tobacco smoke after birth.

B. Data collection

1. Child is apneic, blue, and lifeless.
2. Frothy blood-tinged fluid is in the nose and mouth
3. Child may be found in any position, but typically is found in a disheveled bed, with blankets over the head, and huddled in a corner.
4. Child may appear to have been clutching bedding.
5. Diaper may be wet and full of stool.

C. Prevention and interventions

1. Infants should be placed in the supine position for sleep.
2. Mother needs to be taught about the risk factors: cigarette smoking and substance abuse during pregnancy; use of soft bedding, sleeping in a non-infant bed such as a sofa, overheating (thermal stress), co-sleeping, exposure to tobacco smoke

FIRST-DEGREE
OBSTRUCTION

SECOND-DEGREE
OBSTRUCTION

COMPLETE
OBSTRUCTION

Obstruction
allows passage
of air in both
directions

Inhalation

Expiration

Air unable to
move in either
direction. FB and
edematous mucosa
obliterate
passage.

Air able to move past the obstruction
in one direction only. Air passages
enlarge during inspiration and diminish
during expiration.

▲ **FIGURE 32-6** Manifestations of airway obstruction by foreign body (FB). (From Hockenberry, M., & Wilson, D. [2010]. *Wong's nursing care of infants and children* [9th ed.]. St. Louis: Mosby).

after birth; stuffed animals or other toys should be removed from the crib while the infant is sleeping.
3. Teach the parents to monitor for positional plagiocephaly caused by the supine sleeping position; signs include flattened posterior occiput and development of a bald spot in the posterior occiput area.
4. To assist in preventing positional plagiocephaly, teach the parents to alter head position during sleep, avoid excessive time in infant seats and bouncers, and place the infant in a prone position while awake (monitor the infant when in the prone position).
5. If SIDS occurs, the parents need a great deal of support as they grieve and mourn, especially since the event was sudden, unexpected, and unexplained.

XIV. FOREIGN-BODY ASPIRATION

A. Description (Figure 32-6)
1. Swallowing and aspirating a foreign body (or bodies) into the air passages
2. Most inhaled foreign bodies lodge in the mainstem or lobar bronchus.
3. The most common offending foods are round in shape and include hot dogs, candy, peanuts, popcorn, and grapes.

B. Data collection
1. Initially, choking, gagging, coughing, and retractions are general findings.
2. If the condition worsens, **cyanosis** may occur.
3. Laryngotracheal obstruction leads to dyspnea, **stridor**, cough, and hoarseness.

4. Bronchial obstruction produces paroxysmal cough, **wheezing**, asymmetrical breath sounds, and dyspnea.
5. If any obstruction progresses, unconsciousness and asphyxiation may occur.
6. Partial obstructions may occur without symptoms.
7. The distressed child cannot speak, becomes cyanotic, and collapses.

C. Interventions
1. Emergency care (see Chapter 16)
2. Nonemergency management entails removal by endoscopy.
   a. Postprocedure, the child receives high-humidity air.
   b. Observe for signs and symptoms of airway edema.
3. Prevention
   a. Keep small objects including rubber balloons out of reach of small children.
   b. Avoid giving small children small, round, food items.
4. Parent, day care provider, babysitter education
   a. Teach about the hazards of aspiration.
   b. Discuss potential situations in which small items may be aspirated.
   c. Teach about the symptoms of aspiration.
   d. Teach how to perform emergency care measures.

XV. TUBERCULOSIS

A. Description
1. A contagious disease caused by *Mycobacterium tuberculosis*, which is an acid-fast bacillus

Box 32-8 Mantoux Test Results

Induration that measures 15 mm or more is considered to be a positive reaction in children 4 years old or older who do not have any risk factors.

Induration that measures 10 mm or more is considered to be a positive reaction in children younger than 4 years old and in those with chronic illness or who are at high risk for exposure to tuberculosis.

Induration that measures 5 mm or more is considered to be positive for those in the highest-risk groups, such as children with immunosuppressive conditions or human immunodeficiency virus infection.

2. Multidrug-resistant strains of M. tuberculosis occur as a result of client or family noncompliance with therapeutic regimens.
3. The route of transmission of M. tuberculosis is via the inhalation of droplets from an individual with active tuberculosis (TB).
4. There is an increased incidence in urban low-income areas, nonwhite racial or ethnic groups, and first-generation immigrants from endemic countries.
5. Most children are infected by a family member or another individual with whom they have frequent contact (e.g., a babysitter).

B. Data collection
1. May be asymptomatic or develop symptoms such as malaise, fever, cough, weight loss, anorexia, and lymphadenopathy
2. Specific symptoms are related to the site of infection (e.g., lungs, brain, bone) and may be present.
3. With increased time, asymmetrical expansion of the lungs, decreased breath sounds, **crackles**, and dullness to percussion develop.

C. Mantoux test (Box 32-8)
1. Will produce a positive reaction 2 to 10 weeks after the initial infection
2. Determines whether the child has been infected and has developed a sensitivity to the protein of the tubercle bacillus. A positive reaction does not confirm the presence of active disease (exposure versus presence).
3. After the child reacts positively, he or she will always react positively. A positive reaction in a previously negative child indicates that the child has been infected since the last test.
4. Tuberculosis testing should not be done at the same time as measles immunization (viral interference from the measles **vaccine** may cause a false-negative result).

D. Sputum culture
1. A definitive diagnosis is made by demonstrating the presence of mycobacteria in a culture.

2. Chest x-rays are supplemental to sputum cultures and are not definitive alone.
3. Because an infant or young child often swallows sputum rather than expectorates it, gastric washings (aspiration of lavaged contents from the fasting stomach) may be done to obtain a specimen; the specimen is obtained in the early morning before breakfast.

E. Interventions
1. Medications
    a. A 9-month course of isoniazid (INH) may be prescribed to prevent a latent infection from progressing to clinically active TB and to prevent initial infection in children in high-risk situations; a 12-month course may be prescribed for the child infected with human immunodeficiency virus.
    b. Recommendation for the child with clinically active tuberculosis may include combination administration of isoniazid (INH), rifampin (Rifadin), and pyrazinamide daily for 2 months, and then isoniazid and rifampin twice weekly for 4 months.
    c. Inform the parents and child that bodily fluids including urine may turn an orange-red color with some tuberculosis medications.
    d. Direct observed therapy may be necessary for some children.
2. Place children with active disease who are contagious on respiratory isolation until medications have been initiated, sputum cultures demonstrate a diminished number of organisms, and cough is improving; this includes use of a personally fitted air-purifying N95 or N100 respirator (mask) by the nurse caring for the child.
3. Stress the importance of adequate rest and adequate diet.
4. Instruct the child and family about measures to prevent the transmission of tuberculosis.
5. Case finding and follow-up with known contacts is critical to decrease the number of cases of individuals with active TB.

MORE QUESTIONS ON EVOLVE!

Practice Questions

306. The appropriate child position after a tonsillectomy is which of the following?
    1. Supine position
    2. Side-lying position
    3. High Fowler's position
    4. Trendelenburg's position

307. After a tonsillectomy, the child begins to vomit bright red blood. The initial nursing action would be to:

1. Turn the child to the side.
2. Notify the RN or health care provider (HCP).
3. Administer the prescribed antiemetic.
4. Maintain nothing-by-mouth (NPO) status.

308. After a tonsillectomy, which of the following fluid or food items would be appropriate to offer to the child?
1. Yellow Jell-O
2. Cold ginger ale
3. Vanilla pudding
4. Cherry Popsicle

309. A nurse reinforces instructions to the mother of a child with croup about the measures to take if an acute spasmodic episode occurs. Which statement by the mother indicates the need for further instruction?
1. "I will place a steam vaporizer in my child's room."
2. "I will take my child out into the cool, humid night air."
3. "I will place a cool-mist humidifier in my child's room."
4. "I will place my child in a closed bathroom and allow my child to inhale steam from the running water."

310. A nurse reinforces instructions to the mother of a child who has been hospitalized with croup. Which of the following statements, if made by the mother, would indicate the need for further instruction?
1. "I will give my child cough syrup if a cough develops."
2. "During an attack, I will take my child to a cool location."
3. "I will give acetaminophen (Tylenol) if my child develops a fever."
4. "I will be sure that my child drinks at least three to four glasses of fluids every day."

311. A nurse who is working in the emergency department is caring for a child who has been diagnosed with epiglottitis. Indications that the child may be experiencing airway obstruction include which of the following?
1. Nasal flaring and bradycardia
2. The child thrusts the chin forward and opens the mouth
3. A low-grade fever and complaints of a sore throat
4. The child leans backward, supporting himself or herself with the hands and arms

312. A nurse is caring for a hospitalized infant with bronchiolitis. Diagnostic tests have confirmed respiratory syncytial virus (RSV). On the basis of this

finding, which of the following would be the appropriate nursing action?
1. Initiate strict enteric precautions.
2. Wear a mask when caring for the child.
3. Plan to move the infant to a room with another child with RSV.
4. Leave the infant in the present room, because RSV is not contagious.

313. A nurse is instructing the mother of a child with cystic fibrosis (CF) about the appropriate dietary measures. Which of the following meals best illustrates the most appropriate diet for a client with cystic fibrosis?
1. A veggie salad and a caramel apple
2. A strawberry jelly sandwich and pretzels
3. A plate of nachos and cheese and a cupcake
4. A piece of fried chicken and a loaded baked potato

314. A nurse reviews the results of a Mantoux test performed on a 3-year-old child. The results indicate an area of induration that measures 10 mm. The nurse would interpret these results as:
1. Positive
2. Negative
3. Inconclusive
4. Definitive, requiring a repeat test

315. Isoniazid (INH) is prescribed for a 2-year-old child with a positive Mantoux test. The mother of the child asks the nurse how long the child will need to take the medication. The appropriate response is:
1. 6 months
2. 9 months
3. 15 months
4. 18 months

316. A day care nurse is observing a 2-year-old child and suspects that the child may have strabismus. Which of the following observations may be indicative of this condition?
1. The child has difficulty hearing.
2. The child does not respond when spoken to.
3. The child consistently tilts his or her head to see.
4. The child consistently turns his or her head to see.

317. A nurse has provided instructions to the mother of a child who has been diagnosed with bacterial conjunctivitis. Which of the following, if stated by the mother, would indicate the need for further instructions?
1. "I need to wash my hands frequently."
2. "I need to clean the eye, as prescribed."

3. "It is OK to share towels and washcloths."
4. "I need to give the eyedrops, as prescribed."

318. A nurse is assigned to care for a child after a myringotomy with the insertion of tympanostomy tubes. The nurse notes a small amount of reddish drainage from the child's ear after the surgery. On the basis of this finding, the nurse takes which action?
1. Documents the findings
2. Notifies the registered nurse immediately
3. Changes the ear tubes so that they do not become blocked
4. Checks the ear drainage for the presence of cerebrospinal fluid

319. A nurse prepares a teaching plan regarding the administration of eardrops for the parents of a 2-year-old child. Which of the following would be included in the plan?
1. Wear gloves when administering the eardrops.
2. Pull the ear up and back before instilling the eardrops.

3. Pull the earlobe down and back before instilling the eardrops.
4. Hold the child in a sitting position when administering the eardrops.

320. A nurse is preparing for the admission of an infant with a diagnosis of bronchiolitis caused by the respiratory syncytial virus (RSV). Choose the interventions that would be included in the plan of care. **Select all that apply.**
❏ 1. Place the infant in a private room.
❏ 2. Place the infant in a room near the nurses' station.
❏ 3. Ensure that the infant's head is in a flexed position.
❏ 4. Wear a mask at all times when in contact with the infant.
❏ 5. Place the child in a tent that delivers warm, humidified air.
❏ 6. Position the infant side-lying, with the head lower than the chest.

ANSWERS

306. 2
Rationale: The child should be placed in a semi-prone or side-lying position after tonsillectomy to facilitate drainage. Options 1, 3, and 4 will not achieve this goal.
Test-Taking Strategy: Visualize each of the positions described in the options. Keeping in mind that the goal is to facilitate drainage will direct you to option 2. Review positioning procedures after tonsillectomy if you had difficulty with this question.
Level of Cognitive Ability: Applying
Client Needs: Physiological Integrity
Integrated Process: Nursing Process/Implementation
Content Area: Child Health: Eye/Ear/Throat/Respiratory/Cardiovascular
References: Christensen, Kockrow, p. 1008. 2011. *Foundations of nursing.*
Leifer, p. 592. 2011.

307. 1
Rationale: After a tonsillectomy, if bleeding occurs, the child is turned to the side, and the RN or HCP is notified. An NPO status would be maintained, and an antiemetic may be prescribed; however, the initial nursing action would be to turn the child to the side.
Test-Taking Strategy: Note the strategic word "initial." Although all of the options may be appropriate, to maintain physiological integrity, the initial action is to turn the child to the side. Review the care to the child after tonsillectomy if you had difficulty with this question.
Level of Cognitive Ability: Applying
Client Needs: Physiological Integrity
Integrated Process: Nursing Process/Implementation
Content Area: Child Health: Eye/Ear/Throat/Respiratory/Cardiovascular

References: Hockenberry, Wilson, p. 764. 2009.
Perry, Hockenberry, Lowdermilk, Wilson, p. 1312. 2010.

308. 1
Rationale: After a tonsillectomy, clear, cool liquids should be administered. Citrus, carbonated, and extremely hot or cold liquids need to be avoided, because they may irritate the throat. Milk and milk products (pudding) are avoided, because they coat the throat and cause the child to clear the throat, thus increasing the risk of bleeding. Red liquids need to be avoided, because they give the appearance of blood if the child vomits.
Test-Taking Strategy: Use the process of elimination. Remember that avoiding foods and fluids that may irritate the throat or cause bleeding is the concern; this will assist you with eliminating options 2 and 3. The word "cherry" in option 4 should be the clue that this is not an appropriate food item. Review the dietary measures after tonsillectomy if you had difficulty with this question.
Level of Cognitive Ability: Applying
Client Needs: Physiological Integrity
Integrated Process: Nursing Process/Implementation
Content Area: Child Health: Eye/Ear/Throat/Respiratory/Cardiovascular
Reference: Leifer, pp. 592, 594. 2011.

309. 1
Rationale: Steam from warm running water in a closed bathroom and cool mist from a bedside humidifier are effective for reducing mucosal edema. Cool-mist humidifiers are recommended as compared with steam vaporizers, which present a danger of scalding burns. Taking the child out into the cool, humid night air may also relieve mucosal swelling. Remember, however, that a cold mist may precipitate bronchospasm.

Test-Taking Strategy: Note the strategic words "need for further instruction." Focus on the subjects of reducing mucosal edema and providing a safe environment. Option 1 is the option that would provide an unsafe environment for the child. Review the management of acute spasmodic croup if you had difficulty with this question.
Level of Cognitive Ability: Evaluating
Client Needs: Safe and Effective Care Environment
Integrated Process: Teaching and Learning
Content Area: Child Health: Eye/Ear/Throat/Respiratory/Cardiovascular
Reference: Leifer, p. 588. 2011.

310. 1
Rationale: Cough syrups and cold medicines are not to be given, because they may dry and thicken secretions. During a croup attack the child can be taken to a cool basement or garage. Acetaminophen is used if a fever develops. Adequate hydration of 500 to 1000 mL of fluids daily is important for thinning secretions.
Test-Taking Strategy: Note the strategic words "the need for further instruction." These words indicate a negative event query and ask you to select an option that is an incorrect statement. Knowledge of the pathophysiology related to croup will assist you with eliminating options 3 and 4 first. Recalling that taking the child to a cool location during an attack is appropriate will direct you to option 1 from the remaining options. Review the effects of cough medicines in a child with croup if you had difficulty with this question.
Level of Cognitive Ability: Evaluating
Client Needs: Physiological Integrity
Integrated Process: Teaching and Learning
Content Area: Child Health: Eye/Ear/Throat/Respiratory/Cardiovascular
Reference: McKinney, James, Murray, Ashwill, p. 1188. 2009.

311. 2
Rationale: Clinical manifestations that are suggestive of airway obstruction include tripod positioning (leaning forward supported by the hands and arms with the chin thrust out and the mouth open), nasal flaring, tachycardia, a high fever, and a sore throat.
Test-Taking Strategy: Use the process of elimination. Eliminate option 1 first, because tachycardia rather than bradycardia will occur in a child who is experiencing respiratory distress. Eliminate option 3 next, knowing that a high fever occurs with epiglottitis. From the remaining options, visualize the descriptions given in each, and determine which position would best assist a child who is experiencing respiratory distress. Review the tripod position if you had difficulty with this question.
Level of Cognitive Ability: Understanding
Client Needs: Physiological Integrity
Integrated Process: Nursing Process/Data Collection
Content Area: Child Health: Eye/Ear/Throat/Respiratory/Cardiovascular
Reference: Leifer, pp. 588–589. 2011.

312. 3
Rationale: RSV is a highly communicable disorder, but it is not transmitted via the airborne route. It is usually transferred by the hands, and meticulous handwashing is necessary to decrease the spread of organisms. The infant with RSV is isolated in a single room or placed in a room with another child with RSV. Enteric precautions are not necessary; however, the nurse should wear a gown when the soiling of clothing may occur.
Test-Taking Strategy: Knowledge regarding the transmission of RSV will direct you to option 3. Remember that RSV is usually transferred by the hands and that meticulous handwashing is necessary to decrease the spread of organisms. Review the care of the child with RSV if you had difficulty with this question.
Level of Cognitive Ability: Applying
Client Needs: Safe and Effective Care Environment
Integrated Process: Nursing Process/Implementation
Content Area: Child Health: Eye/Ear/Throat/Respiratory/Cardiovascular
Reference: Leifer, p. 590. 2011.

313. 4
Rationale: Children with CF are managed with a high-calorie, high-protein diet. Pancreatic enzyme replacement therapy is undertaken, and fat-soluble vitamin supplements are administered. Fats are not restricted unless steatorrhea cannot be controlled by increased levels of pancreatic enzymes. A piece of fried chicken and a loaded baked potato provides a high-calorie and high-protein meal that includes fat.
Test-Taking Strategy: Use the process of elimination. Eliminate options 1, 2, and 3 because they are not high in protein or calories. From the remaining options, recalling the appropriate diet for the child with CF will direct you to option 4. Review the treatment measures for CF if you had difficulty with this question.
Level of Cognitive Ability: Understanding
Client Needs: Physiological Integrity
Integrated Process: Teaching and Learning
Content Area: Child Health: Eye/Ear/Throat/Respiratory/Cardiovascular
Reference: Leifer, p. 605. 2011

314. 1
Rationale: An induration that measures 10 mm or more is considered to be a positive result for children who are younger than 4 years old and for those with chronic illness or with a high risk for environmental exposure to tuberculosis. A reaction of 5 mm or more is considered to be a positive result for those in the highest-risk groups.
Test-Taking Strategy: Use the process of elimination and your knowledge regarding a positive Mantoux test in children to answer this question. Option 4 can be easily eliminated first. Note the child's age in the question to determine the correct option from the remaining three options. Review the analysis of the Mantoux test for children if you had difficulty with this question.
Level of Cognitive Ability: Analyzing
Client Needs: Physiological Integrity
Integrated Process: Nursing Process/Data Collection
Content Area: Child Health: Eye/Ear/Throat/Respiratory/Cardiovascular
Reference: McKinney, James, Murray, Ashwill, pp. 1174, 1223. 2009.

315. 2

Rationale: Isoniazid is given to prevent tuberculosis (TB) infection from progressing to active disease. A chest x-ray film is obtained before the initiation of preventive therapy. In infants and children, the recommended duration of INH therapy is 9 months. For children with human immunodeficiency virus infection, a minimum of 12 months is recommended.

Test-Taking Strategy: Knowledge regarding treatment with INH in a 2-year-old child is required to answer this question. Remember that in infants and children, the recommended duration of INH therapy is 9 months. Review the recommended treatment plans for a child with TB if you had difficulty with this question.

Level of Cognitive Ability: Applying
Client Needs: Physiological Integrity
Integrated Process: Nursing Process/Implementation
Content Area: Child Health: Eye/Ear/Throat/Respiratory/Cardiovascular
Reference: McKinney, James, Murray, Ashwill, p. 1223. 2009.

316. 3

Rationale: The nurse may suspect strabismus in a child when the child complains of frequent headaches, squints, or tilts the head to see. Options 1, 2, and 4 are not indicative of this condition.

Test-Taking Strategy: Use the process of elimination. Begin by eliminating options 1 and 2, because they are comparable or alike and refer to hearing. From the remaining options, recalling the signs of strabismus will direct you to option 3. Review the signs of strabismus if you had difficulty with this question.

Level of Cognitive Ability: Understanding
Client Needs: Physiological Integrity
Integrated Process: Nursing Process/Data Collection
Content Area: Child Health: Eye/Ear/Throat/Respiratory/Cardiovascular
Reference: Leifer, p. 536. 2011.

317. 3

Rationale: Bacterial conjunctivitis is highly contagious, and infection control measures should be taught; these include frequent handwashing and not sharing towels and washcloths. Options 1, 2, and 4 are correct measures.

Test-Taking Strategy: Note the strategic words "indicate the need for further instructions." These words indicate a negative event query and ask you to select an option that is an incorrect statement. Recalling that bacterial conjunctivitis is highly contagious will direct you to option 3. Review the infection control measures for bacterial conjunctivitis if you had difficulty with this question.

Level of Cognitive Ability: Evaluating
Client Needs: Safe and Effective Care Environment
Integrated Process: Teaching and Learning
Content Area: Child Health: Eye/Ear/Throat/Respiratory/Cardiovascular
Reference: Christensen, Kockrow, p. 1008. 2011. *Foundations of nursing.*
Leifer, p. 537. 2011.

318. 1

Rationale: After a myringotomy with the insertion of tympanostomy tubes, the child is monitored for ear drainage. A small amount of reddish drainage is normal during the first few days after surgery. However, any heavy bleeding or bleeding that occurs after 3 days should be reported. The nurse would document the findings. Options 2, 3, and 4 are not necessary.

Test-Taking Strategy: Use the process of elimination. Note the strategic words "small amount." Considering both the anatomical location of the surgery and these strategic words will direct you to the correct option. Review postoperative findings after a myringotomy with the insertion of tympanostomy tubes if you had difficulty with this question.

Level of Cognitive Ability: Applying
Client Needs: Physiological Integrity
Integrated Process: Nursing Process/Implementation
Content Area: Child Health: Eye/Ear/Throat/Respiratory/Cardiovascular
Reference: McKinney, James, Murray, Ashwill, p. 1181. 2009.

319. 3

Rationale: When administering eardrops to a child who is less than 3 years old, the ear should be pulled down and back. For children who are more than 3 years old, the ear is pulled up and back. Gloves do not need to be worn by the parents, but handwashing needs to be performed before and after the procedure. The child should be in a side-lying position with the affected ear facing upward to facilitate the flow of medication down the ear canal by gravity.

Test-Taking Strategy: Use the process of elimination. Visualizing this procedure will assist you with eliminating options 1 and 4 first. From the remaining options, recalling the anatomy of the 2 year-old's ear canal will direct you to option 3. Review the administration of eardrops if you had difficulty with this question.

Level of Cognitive Ability: Applying
Client Needs: Physiological Integrity
Integrated Process: Teaching and Learning
Content Area: Child Health: Eye/Ear/Throat/Respiratory/Cardiovascular
Reference: Leifer, p. 504. 2011.

320. 1, 2

Rationale: The infant with RSV should be isolated in a private room or in a room with another child with RSV. The infant should be placed in a room near the nurses' station for close observation. The infant should be positioned with the head and chest at a 30- to 40-degree angle and the neck slightly extended to maintain an open airway and to decrease pressure on the diaphragm. Cool, humidified oxygen is delivered to relieve dyspnea, hypoxemia, and insensible water loss from tachypnea. Contact precautions (wearing gloves and a gown) reduce the nosocomial transmission of RSV.

Test-Taking Strategy: Recalling the mode of transmission of RSV will assist you with determining that the infant needs to be placed in a private room or in a room with another child with RSV and that contact precautions need to be maintained. Recalling the reasons to maintain a patent airway (edema and the accumulation of mucus obstruct the bronchioles) will assist you with determining that the infant needs to be observed closely, that the infant's head should be elevated, and that the infant should receive cool, humidified oxygen. Review the care of the child with bronchiolitis and RSV if you had difficulty with this question.

Level of Cognitive Ability: Analyzing

Client Needs: Physiological Integrity

Integrated Process: Nursing Process/Planning

Content Area: Child Health: Eye/Ear/Throat/Respiratory/Cardiovascular

Reference: Leifer, p. 590. 2011.

Cardiovascular Disorders

 I. CONGESTIVE HEART FAILURE

A. Description
1. The inability of the heart to pump sufficiently to meet the metabolic needs of the body
2. In infants and children, inadequate cardiac output is most commonly caused by congenital heart defects (**shunt**, obstruction, or a combination of both) that produce an excessive volume or pressure load on the myocardium
3. In infants and children, a combination of both left- and right-sided heart failure is usually present (Box 33-1).
4. The goals of treatment are to improve cardiac function, remove accumulated fluid and sodium, decrease cardiac demands, improve tissue oxygenation, and decrease oxygen consumption.

B. Data collection of early signs
1. Tachycardia, especially during rest and slight exertion
2. Tachypnea and **wheezing**
3. Profuse scalp diaphoresis (especially in infants) and on exertion such as with feeding
4. Fatigue and irritability
5. Sudden weight gain related to excess fluid retention
6. Respiratory distress

C. Interventions
1. Monitor for early signs of CHF.
2. Monitor for respiratory distress (count respirations for 1 minute).
3. Monitor apical pulse (count apical pulse for 1 minute) and monitor for abnormal rhythms.
4. Monitor temperature for hyperthermia and for other signs of infection, particularly respiratory infection.
5. Monitor strict intake and output; weigh diapers as appropriate for most accurate output.
6. Monitor daily weight to check for fluid retention; a weight gain of 0.5 kg (1 lb) in 1 day is caused by the accumulation of fluid.
7. Monitor for facial or peripheral dependent edema, listen to lung sounds, and report abnormal findings indicating excessive fluid in the body.
8. Elevate the head of the bed in a semi-Fowler's position.
9. Maintain a neutral thermal environment to prevent cold stress in infants.
10. Provide rest and decrease environmental stimuli.
11. Administer cool humidified oxygen as prescribed, using an oxygen hood for young infants and a nasal cannula or face mask for older infants and children.
12. Organize nursing activities to allow for uninterrupted sleep.
13. Maintain adequate nutritional status.
14. Feed when hungry and soon after awakening, conserving energy and oxygen supply.
15. Provide small, frequent feedings, conserving energy and oxygen supply.
16. Administer sedation as prescribed during the acute stage to promote rest.
17. Administer digoxin (Lanoxin) as prescribed
    a. Check apical heart rate for 1 minute before administration.
    b. Hold digoxin if the apical pulse is less than 90 to 110 beats/min in infants and young children and less than 70 beats/min in older children, as prescribed.
    c. Be aware that infants rarely receive more than 1 mL (50 mcg or 0.05 mg) of digoxin in one dose.
18. Monitor digoxin levels and for signs of digoxin toxicity, including anorexia, poor feeding, nausea, vomiting, bradycardia, dysrhythmias (report signs to the registered nurse immediately).
    a. Normal digoxin level is 0.5 to 2.0 mg/dL.
    b. Digoxin toxicity occurs when level is above 2.0 mg/dL.
19. Administer angiotensin-converting enzyme inhibitors as prescribed.
    a. Monitor for hypotension, renal dysfunction, and cough when angiotensin-converting enzyme inhibitors are administered.
    b. The blood pressure, serum protein, albumin, blood urea nitrogen, and creatinine levels, white blood cell count, urine output, urinary

Box 33-1 Signs and Symptoms of Congestive Heart Failure

Left-Sided Failure
- Crackles and wheezes
- Cough
- Dyspnea
- Grunting (infants)
- Head bobbing (infants)
- Nasal flaring
- Orthopnea
- Periods of cyanosis
- Retractions
- Tachypnea

Right-Sided Failure
- Ascites
- Hepatosplenomegaly
- Jugular vein distention
- Oliguria
- Peripheral edema, especially dependent edema and periorbital edema
- Weight gain

Box 33-2 Home Care Instructions for Administering Digoxin (Lanoxin)

Administer the medication as prescribed.

Administer the medication 1 hour before or 2 hours after feedings.

Use a calendar to mark off the dose that has been administered.

Do not mix the medication with food or fluid.

If a dose is missed and more than 4 hours have elapsed, withhold the dose, and give the next dose at the scheduled time. If less than 4 hours have elapsed, administer the missed dose.

If the child vomits, do not administer a second dose.

If more than two consecutive doses have been missed, notify the health care provider (HCP). Do not increase or double the dose to make up for missed doses.

If the child has teeth, give him or her water after the medication. If possible, brush the child's teeth to prevent tooth decay from the sweetened liquid.

Monitor for signs of toxicity such as poor feeding or vomiting.

If the child becomes ill, notify the HCP.

Keep the medication in a locked cabinet.

Call the poison control center immediately if accidental overdose occurs.

---

specific gravity, and urinary protein level is monitored.

20. Administer diuretics such as furosemide (Lasix) as prescribed.
    a. Monitor for signs and symptoms of hypokalemia (serum potassium level less than 3.5 mEq/L), including muscle weakness and cramping and confusion (child), irritability, restlessness, and inverted T wave on the electrocardiogram (ECG).
    b. If signs and symptoms of hypokalemia are present and the child is also being administered digoxin, then monitor closely for digoxin toxicity because hypokalemia potentiates digoxin toxicity.
21. Administer potassium supplements and provide dietary sources of potassium as prescribed.
    a. Supplemental potassium is prescribed if the need is indicated by low serum potassium levels and if adequate renal function is evident; supplemental potassium is usually necessary when administering a non–potassium-sparing diuretic such as furosemide (Lasix).
    b. Encourage foods that the child will eat that are high in potassium, as appropriate, such as bananas, baked potato skins, and peanut butter.
22. Monitor serum electrolyte levels, particularly the potassium level (normal level is 3.5 to 5.1 mEq/L).
23. Limit fluid intake as prescribed in the acute stage.

24. Monitor for signs and symptoms of dehydration, including sunken fontanel (infant), nonelastic skin turgor, dry mucous membranes, decreased tear production, decreased urine output, and concentrated urine.
25. Monitor sodium levels as prescribed.
    a. Normal level is 135 to 145 mEq/L.
    b. Many infant formulas have slightly more sodium than breast milk.
26. Instruct the parents regarding the description of the diagnosis and administration of medications (Box 33-2).
27. Instruct the parents in cardiopulmonary resuscitation (CPR); see Chapter 16 for information on CPR.

⚠ The parents should be provided with a medication guide for any medication prescribed for the infant or child. Additionally, the nurse needs to review the instructions in the guide and provide an opportunity for the parents to demonstrate medication administration procedures.

II. DEFECTS WITH INCREASED PULMONARY BLOOD FLOW (Box 33-3)

A. Description

1. Intracardiac communication along the septum or an abnormal connection between the great arteries allows blood to flow from the high-pressure

Box 33-3 Defects with Increased Pulmonary Blood Flow

- Atrial septal defect
- Atrioventricular canal defect
- Patent ductus arteriosus
- Ventricular septal defect

Box 33-4 Signs and Symptoms of Decreased Cardiac Output

- Decreased peripheral pulses
- Exercise intolerance
- Feeding difficulties
- Hypotension
- Irritability, restlessness, and lethargy
- Oliguria
- Pale, cool extremities
- Tachycardia

left side of the heart to the low-pressure right side of the heart (left-to-right **shunt**).
2. The infant typically demonstrates signs and symptoms of CHF.
B. Atrial septal defect (ASD)
   1. An abnormal opening between the atria that causes an increased flow of oxygenated blood into the right side of the heart
   2. Right atrial and ventricular enlargement occurs.
   3. Infant may be asymptomatic or may develop CHF.
   4. Signs and symptoms of decreased cardiac output may be present (Box 33-4).
   5. Nonsurgical treatment: May be closed with the use of devices during a cardiac catheterization.
   6. Management: Open repair with cardiopulmonary bypass is usually performed before the child reaches school age.
C. Atrioventricular canal defect
   1. Results from incomplete fusion of the endocardial cushions
   2. Most common cardiac defect in children with Down syndrome
   3. A characteristic murmur is present.
   4. The infant usually has mild to moderate CHF. **Cyanosis** increases with crying.
   5. Signs and symptoms of decreased cardiac output may be present.
   6. Management: Can include either pulmonary artery banding for infants with severe symptoms (palliative) or complete repair via cardiopulmonary bypass
D. Patent ductus arteriosus (PDA)
   1. Failure of the fetal ductus arteriosus (i.e., the artery that connects the aorta and the pulmonary artery) to close within the first weeks of life

Box 33-5 Obstructive Defects

- Aortic stenosis
- Coarctation of the aorta
- Pulmonary stenosis

2. A characteristic machine-like murmur is present. The infant may be asymptomatic or he or she may show signs of CHF.
3. A widened pulse pressure and bounding pulses are present.
4. Signs and symptoms of decreased cardiac output may be present.
5. Management
   a. Indomethacin (prostaglandin inhibitor) may be administered to close a patent ductus in premature infants and some newborns.
   b. The defect may be closed during cardiac catheterization or may require surgical management.
E. Ventricular septal defect (VSD)
   1. An abnormal opening between the right and left ventricles.
   2. Many VSDs close spontaneously during the first year of life in children who have small or moderate defects.
   3. A characteristic murmur is present; CHF is common.
   4. Signs and symptoms of CHF and of decreased cardiac output may be present.
   5. Management
      a. Device closure during cardiac catheterization may be possible.
      b. Open repair with cardiopulmonary bypass

III. **OBSTRUCTIVE DEFECTS** (Box 33-5)

A. Description
   1. Blood exiting the heart meets an area of anatomic narrowing (**stenosis**), thus causing obstruction of the blood flow.
   2. The location of narrowing is usually near the valve of the obstructive defect.
   3. Infants and children exhibit signs of CHF.
   4. Children with mild obstruction may be asymptomatic.
B. Aortic **stenosis**
   1. Aortic **stenosis** is a narrowing or stricture of the aortic valve, causing resistance to blood flow in the left ventricle, decreased cardiac output, left ventricular hypertrophy, and pulmonary vascular congestion.
   2. Valvular **stenosis** is the most common type and usually is caused by malformed cusps, resulting in a bicuspid rather than a tricuspid valve, or fusion of the cusps.

3. A characteristic murmur is present.
4. Infants with severe defects demonstrate signs of decreased cardiac output.
5. Children show signs of exercise intolerance, chest pain, and dizziness when standing for long periods of time.
6. Management
   a. Dilation of the narrowed valve may be done during cardiac catheterization.
   b. Surgical aortic valvotomy (palliative) may be done; a valve replacement may be required at a second procedure.
C. Coarctation of the aorta
1. Localized narrowing of the aortic arch or descending aorta, frequently near the insertion of the ductus arteriosus
2. Signs of CHF may occur in infants.
3. Signs and symptoms of decreased cardiac output may be present.
4. Children may experience headaches, dizziness, fainting, and epistaxis resulting from hypertension.
5. Management of the defect may be done via balloon angioplasty in children; restenosis can occur. Surgical intervention may be necessary.

⚠ With coarctation of the aorta, the blood pressure is higher in the upper extremities than the lower extremities. Additionally, bounding pulses in the arms, weak or absent femoral pulses, and cool lower extremities may be present.

D. Pulmonary **stenosis**
1. Narrowing at the entrance to the pulmonary artery
2. Resistance to blood flow causes right ventricular hypertrophy and decreased pulmonary blood flow. The right ventricle may be hypoplastic.
3. Pulmonary **atresia** is the extreme form of pulmonary **stenosis** (i.e., total fusion of the commissures and no blood flows to the lungs).
4. A characteristic murmur is present.
5. May be asymptomatic.
6. Newborns with severe narrowing will be cyanotic.
7. If pulmonary **stenosis** is severe, CHF occurs.
8. Signs and symptoms of decreased cardiac output may occur.
9. Management: Dilation of the narrowed valve may be done during cardiac catheterization. Surgical intervention may be necessary.

IV. DEFECTS WITH DECREASED PULMONARY BLOOD FLOW (Box 33-6)

A. Description
1. Obstructed pulmonary blood flow and an anatomic defect (ASD or VSD) between the right and left sides of the heart

---

Box 33-6 Defects with Decreased Pulmonary Blood Flow

- Tetralogy of Fallot
- Tricuspid atresia

---

2. Pressure on the right side of the heart increases, exceeding left-sided pressure, which allows desaturated blood to **shunt** right to left. This causes desaturation in the left side of the heart and the systemic circulation.
3. Typically, hypoxemia and **cyanosis** appear.
B. Tetralogy of Fallot
1. Includes four defects: ventricular septal defect, pulmonary **stenosis**, overriding aorta, and right ventricular hypertrophy
2. If pulmonary vascular resistance is higher than systemic resistance, the **shunt** is from right to left. If systemic resistance is higher than pulmonary resistance, the **shunt** is from left to right.
3. Infants
   a. May be acutely cyanotic at birth or may have mild **cyanosis** that progresses over the first year of life as the pulmonic **stenosis** worsens
   b. A characteristic murmur is present.
   c. Acute episodes of **cyanosis** and hypoxia (hypercyanotic spells), called blue spells or tet spells, occur when the infant's oxygen requirements exceed the blood supply (usually during crying, feeding, or defecating).
4. Children: With increasing **cyanosis**, squatting, clubbing of the fingers, and poor **growth** may occur.
   a. Squatting is a compensatory mechanism to facilitate increased return of blood flow to the heart for oxygenation.
   b. Clubbing (an abnormal enlargement in the distal phalanges seen in the fingers).
5. Surgical management: Palliative **shunt**
   a. The **shunt** increases pulmonary blood flow and increases oxygen saturation in infants who cannot undergo primary repair.
   b. The **shunt** provides blood flow to the pulmonary arteries from the left or right subclavian artery.
6. Surgical management: Complete repair
   a. Complete repair usually is performed in the first year of life.
   b. The repair requires a median sternotomy and cardiopulmonary bypass.
C. Tricuspid **atresia**
1. Failure of the tricuspid valve to develop
2. There is no communication from the right atrium to the right ventricle.
3. Blood flows through an ASD or a patent foramen ovale to the left side of the heart and through a VSD to the right ventricle and out to the lungs.

Box 33-7 Mixed Defects

- Hypoplastic left heart syndrome
- Total anomalous pulmonary venous connection
- Transposition of the great arteries or transposition of the great vessels
- Truncus arteriosus

4. Often associated with pulmonic **stenosis** and the transposition of the great arteries.
5. A complete mixing of unoxygenated and oxygenated blood in the left side of the heart occurs, which results in systemic desaturation, pulmonary obstruction, and decreased pulmonary blood flow.
6. **Cyanosis,** tachycardia, fatigability with feeding, and dyspnea are seen in the newborn.
7. Older children exhibit signs of chronic hypoxemia and clubbing.
8. Management: If the ASD is small, the defect may be closed during cardiac catheterization; otherwise, surgery is needed.

⚠ Clubbing is symptomatic of chronic hypoxia. Peripheral circulation is diminished and oxygenation of vital organs and tissues is compromised.

V. MIXED DEFECTS (Box 33-7)

A. Description
1. Fully saturated systemic blood flow mixes with the desaturated blood flow, which causes a desaturation of the systemic blood flow.
2. Pulmonary congestion occurs and cardiac output decreases.
3. Signs of CHF; symptoms depend on the degree of desaturation
B. Hypoplastic left heart syndrome
1. The underdevelopment of the left side of the heart that results in a hypoplastic left ventricle and aortic **atresia**
2. Mild **cyanosis** and signs of CHF occur until the ductus arteriosus closes. Progressive deterioration with **cyanosis** and decreased cardiac output then occurs, which lead to cardiovascular collapse.
3. This is fatal during the first few months of life without intervention.
4. Surgical treatment is necessary.
C. Transposition of the great arteries or transposition of the great vessels
1. The pulmonary artery leaves the left ventricle, and the aorta exits from the right ventricle.
2. No communication exists between the systemic and pulmonary circulations.
3. Infants with minimal communication are severely cyanotic and depressed at birth.

4. Infants with large septal defects or a patent ductus arteriosus may be less severely cyanotic but may have symptoms of CHF.
5. Cardiomegaly is evident a few weeks after birth.
6. Surgery is usually required
D. Total anomalous pulmonary venous connection
1. Failure of the pulmonary veins to join the left atrium
2. Results in mixed blood being returned to the right atrium and shunted from the right to the left through an ASD
3. The right side of the heart hypertrophies, whereas the left side of the heart may remain small.
4. Signs and symptoms of CHF develop.
5. **Cyanosis** worsens with pulmonary vein obstruction. After obstruction occurs, the infant's condition deteriorates rapidly.
6. Surgical treatment is necessary.
E. Truncus arteriosus
1. The failure of normal septation and the division of the embryonic bulbar trunk into the pulmonary artery and the aorta, which results in a single vessel that overrides both ventricles
2. Blood from both ventricles mixes in the common great artery, thus causing desaturation and hypoxemia.
3. A characteristic murmur is present.
4. The infant exhibits moderate to severe CHF, variable **cyanosis**, poor **growth**, and activity intolerance.
5. Surgical treatment is necessary.

VI. INTERVENTIONS: CARDIOVASCULAR DEFECTS

A. Monitor for signs of a defect in the infant or child.
B. Monitor the vital signs closely.
C. Monitor the respiratory status for the presence of **nasal flaring** and the use of accessory muscles. The HCP is notified if any changes occur.
D. Breath sounds are auscultated for **crackles**, wheezes, or rhonchi.
E. If respiratory effort is increased, place the child in reverse Trendelenburg's position (elevate the head and upper body) to decrease the work of breathing.
F. Administer humidified oxygen, as prescribed.
G. Endotracheal tube and ventilator care may be necessary.
H. Monitor for hypercyanotic spells and intervene immediately if they occur (see Priority Nursing Actions).

▬▬▬ PRIORITY NURSING ACTIONS! ▬▬▬

Actions to Take if a Hypercyanotic Spell Occurs in an Infant
1. Place the infant in a knee-chest position.
2. Prepare to administer 100% oxygen.
3. Assist to administer morphine sulfate. *Continued*

4. Assist to administer fluids intravenously.
5. Document occurrence, actions taken, and the infant's response.

Hypercyanotic spells are also known as tet spells or blue spells and occur in infants or children with certain types of heart defects. The infant or child becomes acutely cyanotic and hyperpneic because of the sudden infundibular spasm. These spells may occur as a result of stressful procedures or from feeding, crying, or defecation. If a spell occurs, the nurse needs to provide a calm and comforting approach while immediately placing the infant in the knee-chest position. This assists breathing and increases oxygenation to body tissues. Oxygen is administered by face mask or blow-by. Morphine sulfate is administered as prescribed subcutaneously or through an existing intravenous line (morphine sulfate helps reduce the infundibular spasm). Intravenous fluids are administered to replace fluids and to keep the infant well hydrated and the hematocrit and blood viscosity within acceptable limits. Depending on the infant's response, a repeated dose of morphine sulfate may be prescribed. Finally, the nurse documents the occurrence, actions taken, and the infant's response.

Reference: Perry, S., Hockenberry, M., Lowdermilk, D., & Wilson, D. (2010). *Maternal child nursing care* (4th ed., pp. 1465–1466). St. Louis: Mosby.

I. Monitor for signs of CHF, such as fluid retention in the hands, feet, chest, and around the eyes.
J. Monitor the peripheral pulses.
K. Monitor the I&O and notify the HCP if a decrease in urine output occurs.
L. Monitor the urine output, weighing diapers as necessary.
M. Obtain a daily weight.
N. Maintain fluid restriction, if prescribed.
O. Provide adequate nutrition (high-calorie requirements), as prescribed.
P. Administer medications, as prescribed.
Q. Keep the child as stress free as possible. Plan interventions to allow for maximal rest for the child.
R. Prepare the parents and child, if appropriate, for surgery.
S. Allow the parents and child to verbalize their feelings and concerns regarding the disorder.
T. Familiarize the parents and child with hospital procedures and equipment.

VII. CARDIAC CATHETERIZATION

A. Description
  1. An invasive diagnostic procedure used to determine cardiac defects
  2. Provides information about the oxygenation saturation of the blood in the great vessels and heart chambers
  3. May be diagnostic, interventional, or electrophysiological in purpose

  4. Risks include hemorrhage from the entry site, clot formation and subsequent blockage distally, and transient dysrhythmias
B. Preprocedure nursing interventions
  1. Check the accurate height and weight, because this assists with the selection of the correct catheter size.
  2. Obtain a history of the presence of allergic reactions to iodine.
  3. Check for symptoms of infection, including diaper rash.
  4. Check and mark bilateral pulses (e.g., dorsalis pedis, posterior tibial).
  5. Check the baseline oxygen saturation.
  6. Familiarize the parents and child with hospital procedures and equipment.
  7. Educate the parents and child, if he or she is of an appropriate age, about the procedure.
  8. Allow the parents and child to verbalize their feelings and concerns regarding the procedure and the disorder.
C. Postprocedure nursing interventions
  1. Monitor findings on the cardiac monitor and the oxygen saturation for up to 4 hours after the procedure.
  2. Check the pulses below the catheter site for equality and symmetry.
  3. Check the temperature and color of the affected extremity, and report coolness, which may indicate arterial obstruction.
  4. Monitor the vital signs frequently, per the HCP's prescriptions.
  5. Check the pressure dressing for intactness and signs of hemorrhage.
  6. Check for signs of bleeding under the extremity on the bedsheets, which may indicate bleeding from the entry site.
  7. If bleeding is present, apply continuous direct pressure above the entry site, and report it immediately.
  8. Immobilize the affected extremity for at least 4 to 6 hours for a venous entry site and for 6 to 8 hours for an arterial entry site, as prescribed.
  9. Hydrate the child via the oral route, the intravenous route, or both, as prescribed.
  10. Administer acetaminophen (Tylenol) or ibuprofen (Motrin) for pain or discomfort, as prescribed.
  11. Prepare the parents and child, if appropriate, for surgery.
D. Discharge teaching for the child and parents
  1. Remove the dressing on the day after the procedure and cover it with a Band-Aid for 2 to 3 days.
  2. Keep the site clean and dry.
  3. Have the child avoid tub baths for 2 to 3 days.
  4. Observe for redness, edema, drainage, bleeding, and fever, and report any of these signs immediately.

5. Avoid strenuous activity, if applicable (the child may return to school, if appropriate).
6. Provide a diet as tolerated.
7. Administer acetaminophen (Tylenol) or ibuprofen (Motrin) for pain, discomfort, or fever.
8. Stress the importance of keeping follow-up appointments with the primary care provider.

VIII. CARDIAC SURGERY

A. Postoperative interventions
1. Monitor the vital signs, per protocol.
2. Monitor the temperature. Notify the HCP if a fever occurs.
3. Monitor for signs of sepsis, such as fever, chills, diaphoresis, lethargy, and altered levels of consciousness.
4. Monitor for increased oxygen requirements and poor perfusion.
5. Maintain aseptic technique.
6. Assist with monitoring lines, tubes, or catheters that are in place. Remove them promptly, as prescribed, when they are no longer needed to prevent infection.
7. Monitor for signs of discomfort, such as irritability or restlessness; changes in heart rate, respiratory rate, and blood pressure.
8. Administer pain medications, as prescribed, and note their effectiveness.
9. Administer antibiotics and antipyretics, as prescribed.
10. Encourage rest periods.
11. Facilitate parent–child contact as soon as possible.

B. Postoperative home care (Box 33-8)

IX. RHEUMATIC FEVER

A. Description
1. An inflammatory autoimmune disease that affects the connective tissues of the heart, joints, subcutaneous tissues, and/or blood vessels of the central nervous system
2. The most serious complication is rheumatic heart disease, which affects the cardiac valves
3. Presents 2 to 6 weeks after an untreated or partially treated group A β-hemolytic streptococcal infection of the upper respiratory tract
4. Jones criteria are used to determine the diagnosis

B. Data collection (Figure 33-1)
1. Low-grade fever that spikes in the late afternoon
2. Elevated antistreptolysin O titer
3. Elevated sedimentation rate
4. Elevated C-reactive protein
5. Aschoff's bodies (lesions) in the heart, blood vessels, brain, and serous surfaces of the joints and pleurae

Box 33-8 Home Care After Cardiac Surgery (Based upon Health Care Provider's Prescription)

- Omit play outside for several weeks.
- Avoid activities in which the child could fall and injure self, such as bike riding, for 2 to 4 weeks.
- Avoid crowds for 2 weeks after discharge.
- Follow a no-added-salt diet if prescribed.
- Do not add any new foods to the infant's diet (if an allergy exists to the new food, the manifestations may be interpreted as a postoperative complication).
- Do not place creams, lotions, or powders on the incision until completely healed.
- The child may return to school usually the third week after discharge, starting with half-days.
- The child should not participate in physical education for 2 months.
- Instruct the parents to discipline the child normally.
- Instruct the parents about the importance of the 2-week follow-up.
- Avoid immunizations, invasive procedures, and dental visits for 2 months; following this time period, the immunization schedule and dental visits need to be resumed.
- Advise the parents regarding the importance of a dental visit every 6 months after age 3 years and to inform the dentist of the cardiac problem so that antibiotics can be prescribed if necessary.
- Instruct the parents to call the physician if coughing, tachypnea, cyanosis, vomiting, diarrhea, anorexia, pain, or fever occur, or any swelling, redness, or drainage occurs at the site of the incision.

6. A macular erythematous rash, primarily on the trunk and extremities

▲ Data collection of a child with suspected rheumatic fever includes inquiring about a recent sore throat because rheumatic fever manifests 2 to 6 weeks after an untreated or partially treated group A beta-hemolytic streptococcal infection of the upper respiratory tract.

C. Interventions
1. Monitor the vital signs.
2. Control joint pain and inflammation with massage and alternating hot and cold applications, as prescribed.
3. Provide bedrest during the acute febrile phase.
4. Limit physical exercise in the child with carditis.
5. Administer antibiotics, as prescribed.
6. Administer salicylates and anti-inflammatory agents, as prescribed. (These medications should not be instituted before the diagnosis is confirmed, because they mask polyarthritis.)
7. Initiate seizure precautions if the child is experiencing chorea.
8. Instruct the parents about the importance of follow-up and the need for antibiotic prophylaxis

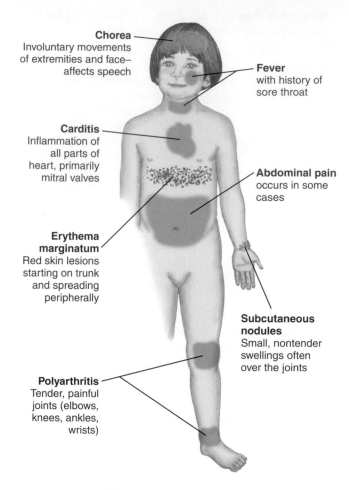

Chorea
Involuntary movements
of extremities and face–
affects speech

Fever
with history of
sore throat

Carditis
Inflammation of
all parts of
heart, primarily
mitral valves

Abdominal pain
occurs in some
cases

**Erythema
marginatum**
Red skin lesions
starting on trunk
and spreading
peripherally

**Subcutaneous
nodules**
Small, nontender
swellings often
over the joints

Polyarthritis
Tender, painful
joints (elbows,
knees, ankles,
wrists)

▲ **FIGURE 33-1** Clinical manifestations of rheumatic fever. (From
McKinney, E., James, S., Murray, S., & Ashwill, J. [2009]. *Maternal-child nursing* [3rd ed.]. Philadelphia: Saunders).

for dental work, infection, and invasive procedures.
9. Advise the child to tell the parents if anyone in school develops a streptococcal throat infection.

X. KAWASAKI DISEASE

A. Description
1. Also called mucocutaneous lymph node syndrome. It is an acute systemic inflammatory illness.
2. The cause is unknown but may be associated with an infection by an organism or toxin.
3. Cardiac involvement is the most serious complication. Aneurysms can develop.

B. Data collection
1. Acute stage
   a. Fever
   b. Conjunctival hyperemia
   c. Red throat
   d. Swollen hands, rash, and enlargement of the cervical lymph nodes
2. Subacute stage
   a. Cracking lips and fissures
   b. Desquamation of the skin on the tips of the fingers and toes
   c. Joint pain
   d. Cardiac manifestations
   e. Thrombocytosis
3. Convalescent stage: Child appears normal but signs of inflammation may be present.

C. Interventions
1. Monitor temperature frequently.
2. Check heart sounds, and the heart rate and rhythm.
3. Check extremities for edema, redness, and desquamation.

Box 33-9 Parent Education for Kawasaki Disease

- Follow-up care is essential to recovery.
- The signs and symptoms of Kawasaki disease include the following:
  - Irritability may last for up to 2 months after the onset of symptoms.
  - Peeling of the hands and feet may occur.
  - Pain in the joints may persist for several weeks.
  - Stiffness in the morning, after naps, and in cold temperatures may occur.
- Record the temperature (because fever is expected) until child has been afebrile for several days.
- Notify the physician if the temperature is 101° F or higher.
- Salicylates such as acetylsalicylic acid (aspirin) may be prescribed.
- Signs of aspirin toxicity include tinnitus, headache, vertigo, bruising; do not administer aspirin or aspirin-

containing products if child has been exposed to chickenpox or the flu.
- Signs and symptoms of bleeding include epistaxis (nose bleeds), hemoptysis (coughing up blood), hematemesis (vomiting up blood), hematuria (blood in urine), melena (blood in stool), and bruises on body.
- Signs and symptoms of cardiac complications include chest pain or tightness (older children), cool and pale extremities, abdominal pain, nausea and vomiting, irritability, restlessness, and uncontrollable crying.
- Child should avoid contact sports, if age appropriate, if taking aspirin or anticoagulants.
- Avoid administration of MMR or varicella vaccine to the child for 11 months post–intravenous immune globulin therapy, if appropriate.

4. Examine eyes for conjunctivitis.
5. Monitor mucous membranes for inflammation.
6. Monitor strict intake and output.
7. Administer soft foods and liquids that are neither too hot nor too cold.
8. Weigh the child daily.
9. Provide passive range-of-motion exercises to facilitate joint movement.
10. Administer acetylsalicylic acid (aspirin) as prescribed for its antipyretic and antiplatelet effects (additional anticoagulation may be necessary if aneurysms are present).
11. Intravenous immune globulin may be prescribed to reduce the duration of the fever and the incidence of coronary artery lesions and aneurysms; IV immune globulin (IVIG) is a blood product, so blood precautions when administering it are warranted.
12. Parent education (Box 33-9)

MORE QUESTIONS ON EVOLVE!

Practice Questions

321. A nurse reviews the record of a child who was just seen by a health care provider (HCP). The HCP has documented a diagnosis of suspected aortic stenosis. Which clinical manifestation that is specifically found in children with this disorder should the nurse anticipate?
1. Pallor
2. Hyperactivity
3. Exercise intolerance
4. Gastrointestinal disturbances

322. A nurse has reinforced home care instructions to the mother of a child who is being discharged after cardiac surgery. Which statement, if made by the mother, indicates the need for further instructions?
1. "A balance of rest and exercise is important."
2. "I can apply lotion or powder to the incision if it is itchy."
3. "Activities during which the child could fall need to be avoided for 2 to 4 weeks."
4. "Large crowds of people need to be avoided for at least 2 weeks after this surgery."

323. A nurse is told that a child with rheumatic fever (RF) will be arriving to the nursing unit for admission. Which question should the nurse ask the family to elicit information specific to the development of RF?
1. "Has the child complained of back pain?"
2. "Has the child complained of headaches?"
3. "Has the child had any nausea or vomiting?"
4. "Did the child have a sore throat or an unexplained fever within the past 2 months?"

324. Acetylsalicylic acid (aspirin) is prescribed for a child with rheumatic fever (RF). The nurse would question this prescription if the child had documented evidence of which condition?
1. Arthralgia
2. Joint pain
3. Facial edema
4. A viral infection

325. A nurse assists with admitting a child with a diagnosis of acute-stage Kawasaki disease. When obtaining the child's medical history, which clinical manifestation is likely to be reported?
1. Cracked lips
2. A normal appearance
3. Conjunctival hyperemia
4. Desquamation of the skin

326. A nurse caring for an infant with congenital heart disease is monitoring the infant closely for signs of congestive heart failure (CHF). The nurse looks for which early sign of CHF?
1. Pallor
2. Cough
3. Tachycardia
4. Slow and shallow breathing

327. A health care provider has prescribed oxygen as needed for a 10-year-old child with congestive heart failure (CHF). In which situation would the nurse administer the oxygen to the child?
1. When the child is sleeping
2. When changing the child's diapers
3. When the mother is holding the child
4. When drawing blood for the measurement of electrolyte levels

328. A nurse is monitoring the daily weight of an infant with congestive heart failure (CHF). Which of the following alerts the nurse to suspect fluid accumulation and thus to the need to notify the registered nurse?
1. Bradypnea
2. Diaphoresis
3. Decreased blood pressure (BP)
4. A weight gain of 1 lb in 1 day

329. A nurse provides home care instructions to the parents of a child with congestive heart failure regarding the procedure for the administration of digoxin (Lanoxin). Which statement, if made by a parent, indicates the need for further instruction?
1. "I will not mix the medication with food."
2. "If more than one dose is missed, I will call the health care provider."
3. "I will take my child's pulse before administering the medication."

4. "If my child vomits after medication administration, I will repeat the dose."

❖ **330.** A nurse is caring for an infant with a diagnosis of
tetralogy of Fallot. The infant suddenly becomes
cyanotic and the oxygen saturation reading drops
to 60%. Choose the interventions that the nurse
should perform. **Select all that apply.**

❏ 1. Call a code blue.
❏ 2. Notify the registered nurse.
❏ 3. Place the infant in a prone position.
❏ 4. Prepare to administer morphine sulfate.
❏ 5. Prepare to administer intravenous fluids.
❏ 6. Prepare to administer 100% oxygen by face
mask.

ANSWERS

321. 3
Rationale: The child with aortic stenosis shows signs of exercise intolerance, chest pain, and dizziness when standing for
long periods. Pallor may be noted, but it is not specific to this
type of disorder alone. Options 2 and 4 are not related to this
disorder.
Test-Taking Strategy: Use the process of elimination, and focus on the disorder. Options 2 and 4 can be eliminated first,
because they are not associated with a cardiac disorder. From
the remaining choices, noting the word "specifically" in the
question will direct you to option 3. Review the manifestations
associated with aortic stenosis if you had difficulty with this
question.
Level of Cognitive Ability: Analyzing
Client Needs: Physiological Integrity
Integrated Process: Nursing Process/Data Collection
Content Area: Child Health: Eye/Ear/Throat/Respiratory/
Cardiovascular
Reference: McKinney, James, Murray, Ashwill, p. 1250. 2009.

322. 2
Rationale: The mother should be instructed that lotions and
powders should not be applied to the incision site because
these items can affect the skin integrity and the healing process.
Options 1, 3, and 4 are accurate instructions regarding home
care after cardiac surgery.
Test-Taking Strategy: Note the strategic words "indicates the
need for further instructions." These words indicate a negative
event query and ask you to select an option that is an incorrect
statement. Using the general principles related to postoperative
incisional site care will direct you to option 2. Review the home
care instructions after cardiac surgery if you had difficulty with
this question.
Level of Cognitive Ability: Evaluating
Client Needs: Physiological Integrity
Integrated Process: Teaching and Learning
Content Area: Child Health: Eye/Ear/Throat/Respiratory/
Cardiovascular
Reference: McKinney, James, Murray, Ashwill, p. 1260. 2009.

323. 4
Rationale: Rheumatic fever (RF) characteristically presents 2 to
6 weeks after an untreated or partially treated group A β-
hemolytic streptococcal infection of the upper respiratory tract.
Initially, the nurse determines if the child has had a sore throat
or an unexplained fever within the past 2 months. Options 1,
2, and 3 are unrelated to RF.
Test-Taking Strategy: Use the process of elimination and think
about the etiology associated with RF. Note the similarity

between rheumatic "fever" in the question and the word "fe-
ver" in the correct option. Review the causes of RF if you had
difficulty with this question.
Level of Cognitive Ability: Analyzing
Client Needs: Physiological Integrity
Integrated Process: Nursing Process/Data Collection
Content Area: Child Health: Eye/Ear/Throat/Respiratory/
Cardiovascular
Reference: Leifer, p. 619. 2011.

324. 4
Rationale: Anti-inflammatory agents, including aspirin, may
be prescribed by the health care provider for the child with
RF. Aspirin should not be given to a child who has chickenpox
or other viral infections such as influenza because of the risk of
Reye's syndrome. Options 1 and 2 are clinical manifestations
of RF. Facial edema may be associated with the development
of a cardiac complication.
Test-Taking Strategy: Use the process of elimination and note
the strategic words "would question this prescription." Options 1 and 2 can be eliminated first, because they are compa-
rable or alike. Recalling that facial edema may indicate a
cardiac complication will assist you with eliminating this option. Review the contraindications related to the use of aspirin
if you had difficulty with this question.
Level of Cognitive Ability: Applying
Client Needs: Safe and Effective Care Environment
Integrated Process: Nursing Process/Implementation
Content Area: Child Health: Eye/Ear/Throat/Respiratory/
Cardiovascular
References: Leifer, pp. 539-540. 2011.
Perry, Hockenberry, Lowdermilk, Wilson, pp. 1473-1474.
2010.

325. 3
Rationale: During the acute stage of Kawasaki disease, the
child presents with fever, conjunctival hyperemia, a red throat,
swollen hands, a rash, and enlargement of the cervical lymph
nodes. During the subacute stage, cracking lips and fissures,
desquamation of the skin on the tips of the fingers and toes,
joint pain, cardiac manifestations, and thrombocytosis occur.
During the convalescent stage, the child appears normal, but
signs of inflammation may be present.
Test-Taking Strategy: Use the process of elimination. Noting
the strategic words "acute-stage" in the question will assist with
directing you to option 3. Review the clinical manifestations
associated with each stage of Kawasaki disease if you had difficulty with this question.
Level of Cognitive Ability: Analyzing
Client Needs: Physiological Integrity

Integrated Process: Nursing Process/Data Collection
Content Area: Child Health: Eye/Ear/Throat/Respiratory/Cardiovascular
Reference: Leifer, p. 623. 2011.

326. 3

Rationale: The early signs of CHF include tachycardia, tachypnea, profuse scalp sweating, fatigue, irritability, sudden weight gain, and respiratory distress. A cough may occur with CHF as a result of mucosal swelling and irritation, but it is not an early sign. Pallor may be noted in the infant with CHF, but it is also not an early sign.
Test-Taking Strategy: Use the process of elimination and note the strategic word "early." Think about the physiology and the effects on the heart when fluid overload occurs. These concepts will assist with directing you to option 3. Review the early signs of CHF in an infant if you had difficulty with this question.
Level of Cognitive Ability: Analyzing
Client Needs: Physiological Integrity
Integrated Process: Nursing Process/Data Collection
Content Area: Child Health: Eye/Ear/Throat/Respiratory/Cardiovascular
Reference: Leifer, p. 617. 2011.

327. 4

Rationale: Oxygen administration may be prescribed for the infant with CHF for stressful periods, especially during bouts of crying or invasive procedures. Drawing blood is an invasive procedure that would likely cause the child to cry.
Test-Taking Strategy: Use the process of elimination. Read the options and recall the situations that would place stress and an increased workload on the heart. This concept should direct you to option 4. Review care of the child with CHF if you had difficulty with this question.
Level of Cognitive Ability: Applying
Client Needs: Physiological Integrity
Integrated Process: Nursing Process/Implementation
Content Area: Child Health: Eye/Ear/Throat/Respiratory/Cardiovascular
Reference: Perry, Hockenberry, Lowdermilk, Wilson, pp. 1459-1460, 1463. 2010.

328. 4

Rationale: A weight gain of 0.5 kg (1 lb) in 1 day is a result of the accumulation of fluid. The nurse should monitor the urine output, monitor for evidence of facial or peripheral edema, check the lung sounds, and report the weight gain. Tachypnea and an increased BP would occur with fluid accumulation. Diaphoresis is a sign of CHF, but it is not specific to fluid accumulation, and it usually occurs with exertional activities.
Test-Taking Strategy: Use the process of elimination, and focus on the subject of fluid accumulation. Note the relationship between "fluid accumulation" in the question and "weight gain" in the correct option. Review the indications of fluid accumulation in the infant with CHF if you had difficulty with this question.
Level of Cognitive Ability: Analyzing
Client Needs: Physiological Integrity
Integrated Process: Nursing Process/Data Collection
Content Area: Child Health: Eye/Ear/Throat/Respiratory/Cardiovascular

Reference: Christensen, Kockrow, p. 988. 2011. *Foundations of nursing.* (p. 988).
Leifer, p. 617. 2011.

329. 4

Rationale: The parents need to be instructed that, if the child vomits after the digoxin is administered, they are not to repeat the dose. Options 1, 2, and 3 are accurate instructions regarding the administration of this medication. Additionally, the parents should be instructed that if a dose is missed and it is not noticed until 4 hours later, the dose should not be administered.
Test-Taking Strategy: Note the strategic words "need for further instruction." These words indicate a negative event query and ask you to select an option that is an incorrect statement. Principles related to the administration of medication to children will assist you with eliminating option 1. General knowledge regarding digoxin administration will assist you with eliminating option 3. From the remaining options, select option 4 over option 2, because, if the child vomits, it would be difficult to determine whether the medication was absorbed by the body. Review home care instructions regarding the administration of digoxin if you had difficulty with this question.
Level of Cognitive Ability: Evaluating
Client Needs: Physiological Integrity
Integrated Process: Teaching and Learning
Content Area: Child Health: Eye/Ear/Throat/Respiratory/Cardiovascular
Reference: Leifer, p. 618. 2011.

330. 2, 4, 5, 6 ❖

Rationale: The child who is cyanotic with oxygen saturations dropping to 60% is having a hypercyanotic episode. Hypercyanotic episodes often occur among infants with tetralogy of Fallot, and they may occur among infants whose heart defect includes the obstruction of pulmonary blood flow and communication between the ventricles. If a hypercyanotic episode occurs, the infant is placed in a knee-chest position immediately. The registered nurse is notified, who will then contact the health care provider. The knee-chest position improves systemic arterial oxygen saturation by decreasing venous return so that smaller amounts of highly saturated blood reach the heart. Toddlers and children squat to get into this position and relieve chronic hypoxia. There is no reason to call a code blue unless respirations cease. Additional interventions include administering 100% oxygen by face mask, morphine sulfate, and intravenous fluids, as prescribed.
Test-Taking Strategy: Focus on the infant's diagnosis and the data in the question. Noting that the infant is cyanotic and has an oxygen saturation of 60% will assist in selecting the correct interventions. Review the nursing interventions when a hypercyanotic episode occurs in an infant if you had difficulty with this question.
Level of Cognitive Ability: Analyzing
Client Needs: Physiological Integrity
Integrated Process: Nursing Process/Implementation
Content Area: Child Health: Eye/Ear/Throat/Respiratory/Cardiovascular
Reference: McKinney, James, Murray, Ashwill, p. 1244. 2009.

34

Metabolic, Endocrine, and Gastrointestinal Disorders

I. FEVER

A. Description

1. An abnormal body temperature elevation.
2. A child's temperature can vary depending on activity, emotional stress, the type of clothing that the child is wearing, and the temperature of the environment.
3. Data collection findings associated with the fever provides important indications of its seriousness.

B. Data collection

1. Temperature elevation: Normal temperature range for a child is 36.4° to 37° C (97.5° to 98.6° F)
2. Flushed skin; warm to touch
3. Diaphoresis
4. Chills
5. Restlessness or lethargy

C. Interventions

1. Monitor vital signs. Take the temperature via the tympanic or axillary route or per agency procedures.
2. Remove excess clothing and blankets, reduce the room temperature, and increase the air circulation. Use other cooling measures, such as the application of a cool compress to the forehead if appropriate.
3. Administer antipyretics such as acetaminophen (Tylenol) or ibuprofen (Motrin), as prescribed.
4. Do not administer aspirin (acetylsalicylic acid) unless specifically prescribed because of the risk of Reye's syndrome.
5. Retake the temperature 30 to 60 minutes after the antipyretic is administered.
6. Provide adequate fluid intake, as tolerated and prescribed.
7. Monitor for dehydration and fluid and electrolyte imbalance.
8. Instruct the parents regarding how to take the child's temperature, how to safely medicate the child, and when it is necessary to call the health care provider (HCP).

II. VOMITING

A. Description

1. The major concerns when a child is vomiting are the risk of dehydration, the loss of fluid and electrolytes, and the development of metabolic alkalosis.
2. Additional concerns include aspiration, atelectasis, and the development of pneumonia.
3. Causes of vomiting include acute infectious diseases, increased intracranial pressure, toxic ingestions, food intolerance, mechanical obstruction of the gastrointestinal tract, metabolic disorders, and psychogenic disorders.

B. Data collection

1. Signs of aspiration
2. Character of vomitus
3. Pain and abdominal cramping
4. Signs of dehydration
5. Signs of fluid and electrolyte imbalances
6. Signs of metabolic alkalosis

C. Interventions

1. Maintain a patent airway.
2. Position the child on his or her side to prevent aspiration.
3. Monitor the vital signs.
4. Monitor the character, amount, and frequency of vomiting.
5. Note the force of the vomiting, because projectile vomiting is indicative of pyloric **stenosis** or increased intracranial pressure.
6. Monitor the intake and output (I&O) and for signs of dehydration, such as a sunken fontanel (age-appropriate), nonelastic skin turgor, dry mucous membranes, decreased tear production, and oliguria.
7. Monitor the electrolyte levels.
8. Provide oral rehydration therapy, as tolerated and as prescribed. Start feeding slowly, with small amounts of fluid at frequent intervals (intravenous [IV] fluids may need to be prescribed).
9. Monitor for diarrhea or abdominal pain.

10. Tell the parents to contact the HCP when signs of dehydration, blood in the vomitus, forceful vomiting, or abdominal pain is present.

III. DIARRHEA

A. Description
1. Acute diarrhea is a cause of dehydration particularly in children younger than 5 years.
2. Some causes of acute diarrhea include acute infectious disorders of the gastrointestinal tract, antibiotic therapy, and parasitic infestation.
3. Some causes of chronic diarrhea include rotavirus, malabsorption syndromes, inflammatory bowel disease, immune deficiencies, food intolerances, and nonspecific factors.
4. Rotavirus is a cause of serious gastroenteritis and is a nosocomial (hospital-acquired) pathogen that is most severe in children ages 3 to 24 months; children younger than 3 months of age have some protection because of maternally acquired antibodies.

B. Data collection
1. Character of stools
2. Pain and abdominal cramping
3. Signs of dehydration
4. Signs of fluid and electrolyte imbalances
5. Signs of metabolic acidosis

C. Interventions
1. Monitor the vital signs.
2. Monitor the character, amount, and frequency of diarrhea.
3. Provide enteric isolation as required; instruct the parents in effective hand-washing technique (the child should be taught this technique also).
4. Monitor skin integrity.
5. Monitor strict intake and output.
6. Monitor electrolyte levels.
7. Monitor for signs and symptoms of dehydration
8. For mild to moderate dehydration, oral rehydration therapy with Pedialyte or a similar rehydration solution may be prescribed; avoid carbonated beverages because they are gas-producing, as well as fluids that contain high amounts of sugar, such as apple juice.
9. For severe dehydration, an NPO status may be prescribed to place the bowel at rest and fluid and electrolyte replacement by the intravenous (IV) route may be prescribed; if potassium is prescribed for IV administration, ensure that the child has voided before its administration and has adequate renal function.
10. Reintroduce a normal diet once rehydration is achieved.
11. Provide instructions to the parents about the types and amounts of fluid to encourage, signs of dehydration, and indications of the need to notify the HCP.

⚠ The major concerns when a child is having diarrhea are the risk of dehydration, the loss of fluid and electrolytes, and the development of metabolic acidosis.

IV. DEHYDRATION (Box 34-1)

A. Description
1. Dehydration is a common fluid and electrolyte imbalance in infants and children.
2. In infants and children, the organs that conserve water are immature, thus placing them at risk for fluid volume deficit.
3. The causes can include decreased fluid intake, diaphoresis, vomiting, diarrhea, diabetic ketoacidosis, and extensive burns or other serious injuries.

⚠ Infants and children are more vulnerable to fluid volume deficit because more of their body water is in the extracellular fluid compartment.

B. Data collection (findings depend on the extent of the dehydration)
1. Tachycardia
2. Dry skin and mucous membranes
3. Sunken periorbital areas and fontanels (age specific)
4. Decreased urine output and increased urine specific gravity
5. Changes in the level of consciousness and responses to stimuli
6. Loss of skin elasticity and turgor
7. Delayed capillary filling time
8. Weight loss
9. Thirst
10. Absence of tears
11. Decreased blood pressure. This is a late sign in infants and children. They can lose up to 25% of their circulating blood volume before their blood pressure is affected.

C. Interventions
1. The cause of the dehydration is treated. Monitor the vital signs.

Box 34-1 Types of Dehydration

Isotonic Dehydration
Electrolyte and water deficits occur in approximately balanced proportions.

Hypertonic Dehydration
Water loss exceeds electrolyte loss.

Hypotonic Dehydration
Electrolyte loss exceeds water loss

2. Monitor for signs of dehydration.
3. Monitor the weight and for weight changes, including fluid gains and losses.
4. Monitor the I&O and the urine for specific gravity.
5. Monitor the level of consciousness.
6. Monitor the skin turgor and mucous membranes for dryness.
7. For mild to moderate dehydration or severe dehydration, fluid replacement therapy is similar as for the child with vomiting or diarrhea.
8. Provide instructions to the parents about the types and amounts of fluid to encourage, the signs of dehydration, and indications of the need to notify the HCP.

V. PHENYLKETONURIA

A. Description
1. A genetic disorder (autosomal recessive disorder) that results in central nervous system damage from toxic levels of phenylalanine (an essential amino acid) in the blood.
2. Characterized by blood phenylalanine levels greater than 20 mg/dL. (A normal level is 1.2 to 3.4 mg/dL in newborns and 0.8 to 1.8 mg/dL thereafter.)
3. All 50 states require routine screening of all newborn infants for PKU.

B. Data collection
1. In all children:
   a. Digestive problems and vomiting
   b. Seizures
   c. Musty or mousy odor of the urine
   d. Mental retardation
2. In older children
   a. Eczema
   b. Hypertonia
   c. Hypopigmentation of the hair, skin, and irises
   d. Hyperactive behavior

C. Interventions
1. Screening of newborn infants for phenylketonuria: the infant should have begun formula or breast milk feeding before specimen collection.
2. If initial screening is positive, a repeat test is performed and further diagnostic evaluation is required to verify the diagnosis.
3. Rescreening of infants should be done by 14 days of age if the initial screening was done before 48 hours of age.
4. If phenylketonuria is diagnosed, prepare to implement the following:
   a. Restrict phenylalanine intake; high-protein foods (meats and dairy products) and aspartame are avoided because they contain large amounts of phenylalanine.
   b. Monitor physical, neurological, and intellectual development.

c. Stress the importance of follow-up treatment.
d. Encourage the parents to express feelings about the diagnosis and the risk of phenylketonuria in future children.
e. Educate the parents about use of special preparation formulas and about the foods that contain phenylalanine.
f. Consult with social care services to assist the parents with financial burdens of specially prepared formulas.

VI. DIABETES MELLITUS

A. Description (Figure 34-1)
1. Type 1 diabetes mellitus is characterized by the destruction of the pancreatic beta cells, which produce insulin. This results in absolute insulin deficiency.
2. Type 2 diabetes mellitus usually arises as a result of insulin resistance, in which the body fails to use insulin properly, in combination with relative (rather than absolute) insulin deficiency.
3. Complete insulin deficiency requires the use of exogenous insulin to promote appropriate glucose use and prevent complications related to elevated blood glucose levels, such as hyperglycemia, diabetic ketoacidosis, and death.

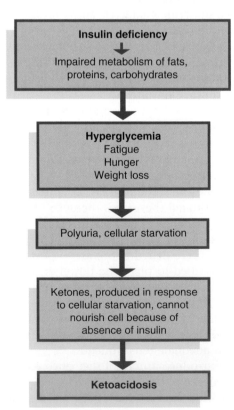

▲ **FIGURE 34-1** Insulin deficiency leading to ketoacidosis. (From McKinney, E., James, S., Murray, S., & Ashwill, J. [2009]. *Maternal-child nursing* [3rd ed.]. Philadelphia: Saunders.)

4. Diagnosis is based on the presence of classic symptoms and an elevated blood glucose level (a normal blood glucose level is between 70 and 110 mg/dL).
5. Children may be admitted directly to the pediatric intensive care unit because of the manifestations of diabetic ketoacidosis, which may be the initial occurrence when they are diagnosed with diabetes mellitus.

B. Data collection
1. Polyuria, polydipsia, and polyphagia
2. Hyperglycemia
3. Weight loss
4. Unexplained fatigue or lethargy
5. Headaches
6. Stomachaches
7. Occasional enuresis in a previously toilet-trained child
8. Vaginitis in adolescent girls (caused by *Candida vaginitis*, which thrives in hyperglycemic tissues)
9. Fruity odor to the breath
10. Dehydration
11. Blurred vision
12. Slow wound healing
13. Changes in the level of consciousness

C. Long-term effects
1. Failure to grow at a normal rate
2. Delayed maturation
3. Recurrent infections
4. Neuropathy
5. Cardiovascular disease
6. Retinal microvascular disease
7. Renal microvascular disease

D. Complications
1. Hypoglycemia
2. Hyperglycemia
3. Diabetic ketoacidosis
4. Coma
5. Hypokalemia
6. Hyperkalemia
7. Microvascular changes
8. Cardiovascular changes

⚠ For a child with diabetes mellitus, plan to initiate a consultation with the diabetic specialist to plan the child's care.

E. Diet
1. Normal, healthy nutrition is encouraged. The total number of calories is individualized on the basis of the child's age and **growth** expectations
2. As prescribed by the HCP, the child may be instructed to follow the food exchange from the American Diabetic Association diet or the dietary guidelines for Americans (MyPlate) issued by the U.S. Departments of Agriculture and Health and Human Services.
3. Dietary intake should include three meals per day, eaten at consistent intervals, plus a mid-afternoon carbohydrate snack and a bedtime snack that is high in protein. A consistent intake of carbohydrates at each meal and snack is needed.
4. Tell the child and the parents that the child should carry a source of glucose (e.g., glucose tablets) with him or her at all times to treat hypoglycemia if it occurs.
5. Incorporate the diet into the individual child's needs, likes, dislikes, lifestyle, and cultural and socioeconomic patterns.
6. Allow the child to participate in making food choices to provide a sense of control.

F. Exercise
1. Instruct the child regarding dietary adjustments to consider when exercising.
2. Extra food needs to be consumed for increased activity (usually 10 to 15 g of carbohydrates for every 30 to 45 minutes of activity).
3. Instruct the child to check the blood glucose level before exercising.
4. Plan an appropriate exercise regimen with the child, and incorporate the child's developmental stage.

G. Insulin
1. Diluted insulin may be required for some infants to provide small-enough doses to avoid hypoglycemia. Diluted insulin should be clearly labeled to avoid dosage errors.
2. A laboratory evaluation of the glycosylated hemoglobin level should be performed every 3 months.
3. Illness, infection, and stress increase the need for insulin. Insulin should not be withheld in these situations, because hyperglycemia and ketoacidosis can result.
4. When the child is NPO for a special procedure, verify with the HCP the need to withhold the morning insulin and when food, fluids, and insulin are to be given.
5. Instruct the child and parents regarding the administration of the insulin.
6. Instruct the child and parents regarding how to recognize the symptoms of hypoglycemia and hyperglycemia.
7. Instruct the parents in the administration of glucagon intramuscularly or subcutaneously if the child has a hypoglycemic reaction and is unable to consume items orally (if semi-conscious or unconscious).
8. Instruct the child and parents to always have a spare bottle of insulin available.
9. Advise the parents to obtain a Medic-Alert bracelet that indicates the type and daily insulin dosage that has been prescribed for the child.

10. See Chapter 46 for information on insulin types, administration sites, and administration procedure.
H. Blood glucose monitoring
1. Results provide information needed to maintain good glycemic control.
2. Blood glucose monitoring is more accurate than urine testing.
3. Requires that the child prick himself or herself several times a day, as prescribed (Box 34-2)
4. Instruct the child and parents in the proper procedure for obtaining the blood glucose level.
5. Inform the child and parents that the procedure must be performed precisely to obtain accurate results.
6. Stress the importance of handwashing before and after performing the procedure to prevent infection.
7. Stress the importance of following the manufacturer's instructions for the blood glucose monitoring device.
8. Instruct the child and parents to calibrate the monitor as instructed by the manufacturer.
9. Instruct the child and parents to check the expiration date on the test strips used for blood glucose monitoring.
10. Instruct the child and parents that, if the blood glucose results do not seem reasonable, to reread the instructions, reassess the technique, check the expiration date of the test strips, and perform the procedure again to verify the results.
I. Urine testing
1. Instruct the parents and child in the procedure for testing the urine for ketones and glucose.
2. Teach the child that the second voided urine specimen is the most accurate.

3. The presence of ketones may indicate impending ketoacidosis.

⚠ Urine glucose testing is an unreliable method of monitoring the glucose level; however, the urine should be tested for ketones when the child is ill or when the blood glucose level is greater than 240 mg/dL.

J. Hypoglycemia
1. Description
   a. A blood glucose level less than 70 mg/dL
   b. Occurs as a result of too much insulin, not enough food, or excessive activity
   c. Signs include headache, nausea, sweating, tremors, lethargy, hunger, confusion, slurred speech, tingling around the mouth, and anxiety.
2. Interventions (Boxes 34-3 and 34-4) (see Priority Nursing Actions)

Box 34-2 Lessening the Pain of Blood Glucose Monitoring

- Hold the finger under warm water for a few seconds before puncture (enhances blood flow to the finger).
- Use the ring finger or thumb to obtain a blood sample because blood flows more easily to these areas; puncture the finger just to the side of the finger pad because there are more blood vessels in this area and fewer nerve endings.
- Use lancet devices with adjustable-depth tips and begin using the shallowest setting.
- Press the lancet device lightly against the skin to prevent a deep puncture.
- Use glucose monitors that require very small blood samples for measurement.

Adapted from Perry, S., Hockenberry, M., Lowdermilk, D., & Wilson, D. (2010). *Maternal child nursing care* (4th ed., p. 1627). St. Louis: Elsevier.

Box 34-3 Interventions for Hypoglycemia

If possible, the nurse should confirm the hypoglycemia with a blood glucose reading.

Administer glucose immediately. The rapid-releasing glucose is followed by a complex carbohydrate and protein, such as a slice of bread or a peanut butter cracker.

Give the child an extra snack if the next meal is not planned for more than 30 minutes or if activity is planned.

If the child becomes unconscious, squeeze cake frosting or glucose paste onto the gums and retest the blood glucose level if the child does not improve within 15 to 20 minutes. If the reading remains low, administer additional glucose.

If the child remains unconscious, it may be necessary to administer glucagon.

In the hospital setting, prepare for the administration of intravenous dextrose if the child is unable to consume an oral glucose product.

Box 34-4 Food Items to Treat Hypoglycemia

- $1/2$ cup orange juice or a sugar-sweetened carbonated beverage
- 8 oz milk
- 1 small box of raisins
- 3 to 4 hard candies
- 4 sugar cubes (1 tbsp of sugar)
- 3 to 4 Life Savers
- 1 candy bar
- 1 tsp honey
- 2 or 3 glucose tablets

d. Develops over a period of several hours to days

e. The blood glucose level is more than 300 mg/dL, and urine and serum ketones are positive

⚠ Manifestations of diabetic ketoacidosis include signs of hyperglycemia, Kussmaul's respirations, acetone (fruity) breath odor, increasing lethargy, and decreasing level of consciousness.

2. Interventions
   a. Restore the circulating volume and protect against cerebral, coronary, or renal hypoperfusion.
   b. Dehydration is corrected with IV infusions of 0.9% or 0.45% saline, as prescribed.
   c. Hyperglycemia is corrected with IV regular insulin administration, as prescribed.
   d. Monitor the vital signs, urine output, and mental status closely.
   e. Correct acidosis and electrolyte imbalances as prescribed.
   f. Administer oxygen, as prescribed.
   g. Monitor the blood glucose level frequently.
   h. Monitor potassium level closely because when the child receives insulin to lower the blood glucose level, the serum potassium level will change; if the potassium level decreases, potassium replacement may be required.
   i. The child should be voiding adequately before administering potassium; if the child does not have an adequate output, hyperkalemia may result.
   j. Monitor the child closely for signs of fluid overload.

■■■ PRIORITY NURSING ACTIONS! ■■■

Actions to Take When a Hospitalized Child with Diabetes Mellitus Experiences Hypoglycemia

1. Check the child's blood glucose level.
2. Give the child ½ cup of fruit juice or other acceptable item.
3. Take the child's vital signs.
4. Retest the blood glucose level.
5. Give the child a small snack of carbohydrate and protein.
6. Document the child's complaints, actions taken, and outcome.

If a child with diabetes mellitus experiences hypoglycemia, the nurse first would check the child's blood glucose level to verify that the child is experiencing hypoglycemia. When this is verified, the nurse gives the child 10 to 15 g of carbohydrates. The nurse retests the blood glucose level in 15 minutes. In the meantime, the nurse checks the child's vital signs. If the child's symptoms of hypoglycemia do not resolve, the nurse gives the child another 10- to 15-g carbohydrate food item. Otherwise, the nurse provides a small snack of carbohydrates and protein if the child's next scheduled meal is more than 1 hour away from the time of the occurrence. After treatment and resolution of the hypoglycemic event, the nurse documents the occurrence, actions taken, and outcome.

References: Ignatavicius, D., & Workman, M. (2010). *Medical-surgical nursing: Patient-centered collaborative care* (6th ed., pp. 1507-1508). St. Louis: Saunders; and Perry, S., Hockenberry, M., Lowdermilk, D., & Wilson, D. (2010). *Maternal child nursing care* (4th ed., pp. 1621, 1624). St. Louis: Mosby.

K. Hyperglycemia
   1. Description: Elevated blood glucose level more than 250 mg/dL, or as specified by the HCP
   2. Interventions (Box 34-5)
   3. Sick-day rules (Box 34-6)

L. Diabetic ketoacidosis (see Figure 34-1)
   1. Description
      a. A complication of diabetes mellitus that develops when a severe insulin deficiency occurs
      b. A life-threatening condition
      c. Hyperglycemia that progresses to metabolic acidosis occurs

---

Box 34-5 Interventions for Hyperglycemia

Instruct the parents to notify the HCP when any of the following occur:
- Blood glucose results remain elevated (usually above 240 mg/dL).
- Moderate or high ketonuria is present.
- The child is unable to take food or fluids.
- The child vomits more than once.
- Illness persists.

Box 34-6 Sick-Day Rules for the Diabetic Child

- Always give insulin, even if the child does not have an appetite, or contact the health cae provider (HCP) for specific instructions.
- Test blood glucose levels at least every 4 hours.
- Test for urinary ketones with each voiding.
- Notify the HCP if moderate or large amounts of urinary ketones are present.
- Follow the child's usual meal plan.
- Encourage sugar-free liquids to aid in clearing ketones.
- Encourage rest, especially if urinary ketones are present.
- Notify the HCP if vomiting, fruity odor to the breath, deep rapid respirations, decreasing level of consciousness, or persistent hyperglycemia occurs.

Adapted from McKinney, E., James, S., Murray, S., & Ashwill, J. (2009). *Maternal-child nursing* (3rd ed., p. 1451). St. Louis: Elsevier.

k. Intravenously administered dextrose is added as prescribed when the blood glucose reaches an appropriate level.

l. The cause of the hyperglycemia is treated.

VII. CLEFT LIP AND CLEFT PALATE

A. Description
1. A congenital anomaly that occurs as a result of the failure of soft tissue or a bony structure to fuse during embryonic development.
2. Involves abnormal openings in the lip or palate that may occur unilaterally or bilaterally and that are readily apparent at birth
3. Causes include genetic, **hereditary**, and environmental factors, exposure to radiation or rubella virus, chromosome abnormalities, and teratogenic factors.
4. Closure of cleft lip defect precedes that of the cleft palate and is usually performed by age 3 to 6 months.
5. Cleft palate repair is performed sometime between 6 and 24 months of age to allow for the palatal changes that take place with normal **growth**; a cleft palate is closed as early as possible to facilitate speech development.
6. The child with cleft palate is at risk for developing frequent otitis media; this can result in hearing loss.
7. A multidisciplinary team approach is taken to address the many needs of the child; some of these professionals include audiologists, orthodontists, plastic surgeons, and occupational and speech therapists.

B. Data collection (Figure 34-2)
1. Cleft lip can range from a slight notch to a complete separation from the floor of the nose.
2. Cleft palate can include nasal distortion, midline or bilateral cleft, and variable extension from the uvula and the soft and hard palate.

C. Interventions
1. Check the ability to suck, swallow, handle normal secretions, and breathe without distress.
2. Monitor the fluid and calorie intake daily, and monitor the weight.
3. Modify feeding techniques; plan to use specialized feeding techniques, obturators, and special nipples and feeders.
4. Hold the child in an upright position and direct the formula to the side and back of the mouth to prevent aspiration.
5. Feed small amounts gradually and burp frequently.
6. Keep suction equipment and a bulb syringe at the bedside.
7. Teach the parents special feeding or suctioning techniques.
8. Teach the parents the *ESSR* method of feeding (*e*nlarge the nipple, *s*timulate the sucking reflex, *s*wallow, *r*est to allow the child to finish swallowing what has been placed in the mouth).

▲ **FIGURE 34-2** Variations in clefts of lip and palate at birth. **A,** Notch in vermilion border. **B,** Unilateral cleft lip and palate. **C,** Bilateral cleft lip and palate. **D,** Cleft palate. (From Hockenberry, M., & Wilson, D. [2010]. *Wong's nursing care of infants and children* [9th ed.]. St. Louis: Mosby.)

9. Encourage the parents to express their feelings about the disorder.
10. Encourage parental bonding with the child, including holding the child and calling the child by name.

D. Postoperative interventions
1. Cleft lip repair
   a. Provide lip protection; a metal appliance or adhesive strips may be taped securely to the cheeks to prevent trauma to the suture line.
   b. Avoid positioning the child on the side of the repair or in the prone position because these positions can cause rubbing of the surgical site on the mattress (position on the back upright and position to prevent airway obstruction by secretions, blood, or the tongue).
   c. Keep the surgical site clean and dry; after feeding, gently cleanse the suture line of formula or serosanguineous drainage with a solution such as normal saline or as designated by agency procedure.
   d. Apply antibiotic ointment to the site as prescribed.
   e. Elbow restraints should be used to prevent the infant from injuring or traumatizing the surgical site.
   f. Monitor for signs and symptoms of infection at the surgical site.
2. Cleft palate repair
   a. Feedings are resumed by bottle, breast, or cup per surgeon preference; some surgeons prescribe the use of an asepto syringe for feeding or a soft cup such as a Sipee cup.
   b. Oral packing may be secured to the palate (usually removed in 2 to 3 days).
   c. Do not allow the child to brush his or her teeth.
   d. Instruct the parents to avoid offering hard food items to the child, such as toast or cookies.
3. Soft elbow or jacket restraints may be used (check agency policies and procedures) to keep the child from touching the repair site; remove restraints at least every 2 hours (or per agency procedure) to check skin integrity and circulation and to allow for exercising the arms.
4. Avoid the use of oral suction or placing objects in the mouth such as a tongue depressor, thermometer, straws, spoons, forks, or pacifiers.
5. Provide analgesics for pain as prescribed.
6. Instruct the parents in feeding techniques and in the care of the surgical site.
7. Instruct the parents to monitor for signs of infection at the surgical site, such as redness, swelling, or drainage.
8. Encourage the parents to hold the child.
9. Initiate appropriate referrals such as a dental referral and speech therapist referral.

VIII. ESOPHAGEAL ATRESIA AND TRACHEOESOPHAGEAL FISTULA (Figure 34-3)

A. Description
1. The esophagus terminates before it reaches the stomach, ending in a blind pouch, and/or a fistula is present that forms an unnatural connection with the trachea.
2. The condition causes oral intake to enter the lungs or a large amount of air to enter the stomach. Choking, coughing, and severe abdominal distention can occur.
3. Aspiration pneumonia and severe respiratory distress will develop, and death will occur without surgical intervention.

▲ **FIGURE 34-3** Congenital atresia of esophagus and tracheoesophageal fistula. **A,** Upper and lower segments of esophagus end in blind sac (occurring in 5% to 8% of such infants). **B,** Upper segment of esophagus ends in atresia and connects to trachea by fistulous tract (occurring rarely). **C,** Upper segment of esophagus ends in blind pouch; lower segment connects with trachea by small fistulous tract (occurring in 80% to 95% of such infants). **D,** Both segments of esophagus connect by fistulous tracts to trachea (occurring in less than 1% of such infants). Infant may aspirate with first feeding. **E,** Esophagus is continuous but connects by fistulous tract to trachea; known as H-type. (From Hockenberry, M., & Wilson, D. [2010]. *Wong's nursing care of infants and children* [9th ed.]. St. Louis: Mosby).

4. Treatment includes maintenance of a patent airway, prevention of pneumonia, gastric or blind-pouch decompression, supportive therapy, and surgical repair.

B. Data collection

1. Frothy saliva in the mouth and nose; drooling
2. Coughing, choking during feedings, and unexplained **cyanosis** as a result of respiratory distress (also called "the 3 Cs")
3. **Regurgitation** and vomiting
4. Abdominal distention
5. Increased respiratory distress during and after feeding

C. Preoperative interventions

1. The infant may be placed in an incubator or radiant warmer in which humidified oxygen is administered (intubation and mechanical ventilation may be necessary if respiratory distress occurs).
2. Maintain NPO status.
3. Maintain IV fluids, as prescribed.
4. Suction accumulated secretions from the mouth and pharynx.
5. Maintain in a supine upright position (at least 30 degrees upright) to facilitate drainage and prevent aspiration of gastric secretions.
6. Keep the blind pouch empty of secretions by intermittent or continuous suction as prescribed; monitor its patency closely because clogging from mucus can easily occur.
7. If a gastrostomy tube is inserted, it may be left open so that air entering the stomach through the fistula can escape, minimizing the risk of **regurgitation** of gastric contents into the trachea.
8. Broad-spectrum antibiotics may be prescribed because of the high risk for aspiration pneumonia.

D. Postoperative interventions

1. Monitor vital signs and respiratory status.
2. Maintain IV fluids, antibiotics, and parenteral nutrition as prescribed.
3. Monitor strict intake and output.
4. Monitor daily weight; monitor for dehydration and possible fluid overload.
5. Monitor for signs of pain.
6. Maintain the chest tube if present.
7. Inspect the surgical site for signs and symptoms of infection.
8. Monitor for anastomotic leaks as evidenced by purulent drainage from the chest tube, increased temperature, and increased white blood cell count.
9. If a gastrostomy tube is present, it is usually attached to gravity drainage until the infant can tolerate feedings and the anastomosis is healed (usually the fifth to seventh day postoperatively); then feedings are prescribed.
10. Before oral feedings and removal of the chest tube, prepare for an esophagram as prescribed to check the integrity of the esophageal anastomosis.
11. Before feeding, elevate the gastrostomy tube and secure it above the level of the stomach to allow gastric secretions to pass to the duodenum and swallowed air to escape through the open gastrostomy tube.
12. Administer oral feedings with sterile water, followed by frequent small feedings of formula as prescribed.
13. Check the cervical esophagostomy site, if present, for redness, breakdown, or exudate; remove accumulated drainage frequently and apply protective ointment, barrier dressing, and/or a collection device as prescribed.
14. Provide non-nutritive sucking using a pacifier for infants who remain NPO for extended periods (a pacifier should not be used if the infant is unable to handle secretions).
15. Instruct the parents in the techniques of suctioning, gastrostomy tube care and feedings, and skin site care as appropriate.
16. Instruct the parents to identify behaviors that indicate the need for suctioning, signs of respiratory distress, and signs of a constricted esophagus (e.g., poor feeding, dysphagia, drooling, coughing during feedings, regurgitated undigested food).

IX. GASTROESOPHAGEAL REFLUX

A. Description

1. Gastroesophageal reflux is backflow of gastric contents into the esophagus as a result of relaxation or incompetence of the lower esophageal or cardiac sphincter.
2. Most infants with gastroesophageal reflux have a mild problem that improves in about 1 year and requires only medical therapy.
3. Gastroesophageal reflux disease (GERD) occurs when gastric contents reflux into the esophagus or oropharynx and produce symptoms.
4. Treatment (Box 34-7)

B. Data collection

1. Passive **regurgitation** or emesis
2. Poor weight gain
3. Irritability

Box 34-7 Treatment for Gastroesophageal Reflux

- Diet
- Positioning
- Medications
- Surgery (performed when severe complications occur)

4. Hematemesis
5. Melena
6. Heartburn (in older children)
7. Anemia from blood loss

C. Interventions
1. Monitor the amount and characteristics of the emesis.
2. Monitor the relationship of the vomiting to the times of feedings and infant activity.
3. Monitor the breath sounds before and after feedings.
4. Monitor for signs of aspiration, such as drooling, coughing, or dyspnea following feeding.
5. Place suction equipment at the bedside.
6. Monitor the I&O.
7. Monitor for signs and symptoms of dehydration.
8. Maintain the IV fluids, as prescribed.

⚠ Complications of gastroesophageal reflux disease include esophagitis, esophageal strictures, aspiration of gastric contents, and aspiration pneumonia.

D. Positioning
1. The infant is placed in the supine position during sleep (to reduce the incidence of sudden infant death syndrome) unless the risk of death from aspiration or other serious complications of GERD greatly outweigh the risks associated with the prone position (check the HCP's prescription); otherwise, the prone position is only acceptable while the infant is awake and can be monitored.
2. In children older than 1 year, position with the head of the bed elevated.

E. Diet
1. Provide small, frequent feedings with predigested formula to decrease the amount of **regurgitation**.
2. Nutrition via nasogastric tube feedings may be prescribed if severe **regurgitation** and poor **growth** are present.
3. For infants, formula may be thickened by adding rice cereal to the formula (follow agency procedure); then cross-cut the nipple.
4. Breast-feeding may continue, and the mother may provide more frequent feeding times or express milk for thickening with rice cereal.
5. Burp the infant frequently when feeding and handle the infant minimally after feedings; monitor for coughing during feeding and other signs of aspiration.
6. For toddlers, feed solids first, followed by liquids.
7. Instruct the parents to avoid feeding the child fatty foods, chocolate, tomato products, carbonated liquids, fruit juices, citrus products, and spicy foods.
8. Instruct the parents that the child should avoid vigorous play after feeding and avoid feeding just before bedtime.

F. Medications
1. Antacids for symptom relief
2. Proton pump inhibitors and histamine 2 (H_2) antagonists to decrease acid secretion
3. Prokinetics to accelerate gastric emptying.

G. Surgery
1. Fundoplication, in which a wrap to the stomach fundus is made around the distal esophagus (restores the competence of the lower esophageal sphincter)
2. A gastrostomy may be performed at the same time as the fundoplication for decompression of the stomach postoperatively.
3. Fundoplication may be combined with pyloroplasty in children with gastroesophageal reflux who also have delayed gastric emptying.
4. Postoperative care is similar to that for other types of abdominal surgery.
5. Instruct the parents about the potential postoperative problems, such as bloating symptoms or discomfort after consuming large, solid meals.

X. HYPERTROPHIC PYLORIC STENOSIS (Figure 34-4)

A. Description
1. Hypertrophy of the circular muscles of the pylorus causes the narrowing of the pyloric canal between the stomach and the duodenum.
2. Usually develops during the first few weeks of life and causes projectile vomiting, dehydration, metabolic alkalosis, and failure to thrive.

A

B

▲ **FIGURE 34-4** Hypertrophic pyloric stenosis. **A,** Enlarged muscular tumor nearly obliterates pyloric channel. **B,** Longitudinal surgical division of muscle down to submucosa establishes adequate passageway. (From Hockenberry, M., & Wilson, D. [2010]. *Wong's nursing care of infants and children* [9th ed.]. St. Louis: Mosby).

B. Data collection
1. Vomiting that progresses from mild **regurgitation** to forceful and projectile that usually occurs after a feeding.
2. Vomitus contains gastric contents, such as milk or formula. It may contain mucus, may be blood-tinged, and does not usually contain bile.
3. Hunger and irritability
4. Peristaltic waves visible from left to right across the epigastrium during or immediately after a feeding
5. Olive-shaped mass in the epigastrium just right of the umbilicus
6. Dehydration and malnutrition
7. Electrolyte imbalances
8. Metabolic alkalosis

C. Interventions
1. Monitor the vital signs.
2. Monitor the I&O and weight.
3. Monitor for signs of dehydration and electrolyte imbalances.
4. Prepare the child and parents for pyloromyotomy, if prescribed.

D. Pyloromyotomy
1. Description: An incision through the muscle fibers of the pylorus, which may be performed by laparoscopy.
2. Interventions preoperatively
   a. Monitor the hydration status by checking the daily weights, I&O, and urine for specific gravity.
   b. Correct fluid and electrolyte imbalances. IV fluids may be prescribed for rehydration.
   c. Maintain NPO status.
   d. Monitor the number and character of stools.
   e. Maintain the patency of the nasogastric (NG) tube that is placed for stomach decompression.
3. Postoperative interventions
   a. Monitor intake and output.
   b. Begin small, frequent feedings postoperatively as prescribed.
   c. Gradually increase amount and interval between feedings until a full feeding schedule has been reinstated.
   d. Feed the infant slowly, burping frequently and handle the infant minimally after feedings.
   e. Monitor for abdominal distention.
   f. Monitor the surgical wound and for signs of infection.
   g. Instruct the parents about wound care and feeding.

XI. LACTOSE INTOLERANCE

A. Description: The inability to tolerate lactose as a result of an absence or deficiency of lactase, which is an enzyme found in the secretions of the small intestine that is required for the digestion of lactose

B. Data collection (Box 34-8)
C. Interventions
1. Eliminate the offending dairy product or administer an enzyme replacement.
2. Provide information to the parents about enzyme tablets that predigest the lactose in milk or supplement the body's own lactase.
3. For infants, soy-based formula can be substituted for cow's milk formula or human milk.
4. Provide calcium and vitamin D supplements to prevent deficiency.
5. Limit milk consumption to one glass at a time.
6. If milk is consumed, it should be taken when other foods are consumed rather than by itself.
7. Encourage the consumption of hard cheese, cottage cheese, or yogurt (which contains inactive lactase enzyme) rather than milk.
8. Encourage the consumption of small amounts of dairy foods daily to help colonic bacteria adapt to ingested lactose.
9. Instruct the parents about the importance of calcium and vitamin D supplements.
10. Instruct the parents about the foods that contain lactose, including hidden sources.

⚠ A child with lactose intolerance can develop calcium and vitamin D deficiency. Instruct the parents about the importance of providing these supplements.

XII. CELIAC DISEASE

A. Description
1. Celiac disease also is known as gluten enteropathy or celiac sprue.
2. Intolerance to gluten, the protein component of wheat, barley, rye, and oats, is characteristic.
3. Celiac disease results in the accumulation of the amino acid glutamine, which is toxic to intestinal mucosal cells.
4. Intestinal villi atrophy occurs, which affects absorption of ingested nutrients.
5. Symptoms of the disorder occur most often between the ages of 1 and 5 years
6. There is usually an interval of 3 to 6 months between the introduction of gluten in the diet and the onset of symptoms.

Box 34-8 Data Collection Findings: Lactose Intolerance

- Symptoms occur after the ingestion of milk products
- Excessive flatus
- Diarrhea
- Abdominal distention
- Crampy abdominal pain; colic

7. Strict dietary avoidance of gluten minimizes the risk of developing malignant lymphoma of the small intestine and other gastrointestinal malignancies.

B. Data collection
1. Acute or insidious diarrhea. Stools are watery and pale with an offensive odor.
2. Anorexia
3. Abdominal pain and distention
4. Muscle wasting, particularly in the buttocks and extremities
5. Vomiting
6. Anemia
7. Irritability

C. Celiac crisis (Box 34-9)

D. Interventions
1. Gluten-free diet and the substitution of corn, rice, and millet as grain sources
2. Lifelong elimination of gluten sources such as wheat, rye, oats, and barley
3. Mineral and vitamin supplements, including iron, folic acid, and fat-soluble supplements A, D, E, and K
4. Teach the parents about a gluten-free diet and to read food labels carefully for hidden sources of gluten (Box 34-10).
5. Instruct the parents regarding measures to prevent celiac crisis.
6. Inform the parents about the Celiac Sprue Association

Box 34-9 Celiac Crisis

- Precipitated by infection, fasting, and the ingestion of gluten
- Can lead to electrolyte imbalance, rapid dehydration, and severe acidosis
- Causes profuse, watery diarrhea and vomiting

Box 34-10 Basics of a Gluten-Free Diet

Foods Allowed

Meat such as beef, pork, and poultry and fish, eggs, milk and dairy products, vegetables, fruits, rice, corn, gluten-free wheat flour, puffed rice, cornflakes, cornmeal, and pre-cooked gluten-free cereals

Foods Prohibited

Commercially prepared ice cream, malted milk, prepared puddings, and grains, including anything made from wheat, rye, oats, or barley, such as breads, rolls, cookies, cakes, crackers, cereal, spaghetti, macaroni noodles, beer, and ale

---

XIII. APPENDICITIS

A. Description
1. Inflammation of the appendix
2. When the appendix becomes inflamed or infected, perforation may occur within a matter of hours, leading to peritonitis, sepsis, septic shock, and potential death.
3. Treatment is the surgical removal of the appendix before perforation occurs.

B. Data collection
1. Pain in periumbilical area that descends to the right lower quadrant
2. Abdominal pain that is most intense at McBurney's point
3. Referred pain that indicates the presence of peritoneal irritation
4. Rebound tenderness and abdominal rigidity
5. Elevated white blood cell count
6. Side-lying position with abdominal guarding (legs flexed)
7. Difficulty walking and pain in the right hip
8. Low-grade fever
9. Anorexia, nausea, and vomiting after the pain develops
10. Diarrhea

C. Peritonitis
1. Data collection
   a. Results from a perforated appendix
   b. Increased fever
   c. Progressive abdominal distention
   d. Tachycardia and tachypnea
   e. Pallor
   f. Chills
   g. Restlessness and irritability

⚠ An indication of a perforated appendix is the sudden relief of pain and then a subsequent increase in pain accompanied by right guarding of the abdomen.

D. Appendectomy
1. Description: Surgical removal of the appendix
2. Preoperative interventions
   a. Maintain NPO status.
   b. IV fluids and electrolytes may be prescribed to prevent dehydration and correct electrolyte imbalances.
   c. Monitor for signs of a ruptured appendix and peritonitis.
   d. Antibiotics may be prescribed.
   e. Monitor for changes in the level of pain.
   f. Monitor the bowel sounds.
   g. Position the child in a right side-lying or low to semi-Fowler's position to promote comfort.
   h. Apply ice packs to the abdomen for 20 to 30 minutes every hour, if prescribed.

   i. Avoid the application of heat to the abdomen.
   j. Avoid the administration of laxatives or enemas.
3. Postoperative interventions
   a. Monitor the temperature for signs of infection.
   b. Maintain NPO status until bowel function has returned. Advance the diet gradually, as tolerated and as prescribed, when bowel sounds return.
   c. Monitor the incision for signs of infection, such as redness, swelling, drainage, and pain.
   d. Monitor Penrose drain drainage, which may be inserted if perforation occurred.
   e. Position in a right side-lying or low to semi-Fowler's position with the legs slightly flexed to facilitate drainage.
   f. Change the dressing, as prescribed, and record the type and amount of drainage.
   g. Perform wound irrigations, if prescribed.
   h. Maintain NG tube suction and the patency of the tube, if present.
   i. Administer antibiotics and analgesics, as prescribed.

XIV. HIRSCHSPRUNG'S DISEASE (Figure 34-5)

A. Description
   1. Congenital anomaly also known as congenital aganglionosis or aganglionic megacolon
   2. The disease occurs as the result of an absence of ganglion cells in the rectum and other areas of the affected intestine.
   3. The disease results in mechanical obstruction because of inadequate motility in an intestinal segment.
   4. The disease may be a familial congenital defect or may be associated with other anomalies, such as Down syndrome and genitourinary abnormalities.

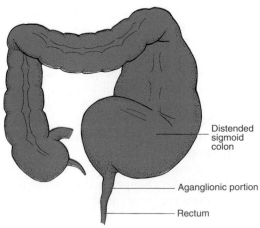

▲ **FIGURE 34-5** Hirschsprung's disease. (From Perry, S., Hockenberry, M., Lowdermilk, D., & Wilson, D. [2010]. *Maternal-child nursing care* [4th ed.]. St. Louis: Mosby).

5. A rectal biopsy demonstrates histological evidence of the absence of ganglionic cells.
6. The most serious complication is enterocolitis; signs include fever, severe prostration, gastrointestinal bleeding, and explosive watery diarrhea.
7. Treatment for mild or moderate disease is based on relieving the chronic constipation with stool softeners and rectal irrigations; however, many children require surgery.
8. Treatment for moderate to severe disease involves a two-step surgical procedure.
   a. Initially, in the neonatal period, a temporary colostomy is created to relieve obstruction and allow the normally innervated, dilated bowel to return to its normal size.
   b. A complete surgical repair is performed when the bowel returns to its normal size via a pull-through procedure to excise portions of the bowel; at this time, the colostomy is closed.

B. Data collection
   1. Newborn infants
      a. Failure to pass meconium stool
      b. Refusal to suck
      c. Abdominal distention
      d. Bile-stained vomitus
   2. Children
      a. Failure to gain weight and delayed **growth**
      b. Abdominal distention
      c. Vomiting
      d. Constipation alternating with diarrhea
      e. Ribbon-like and foul-smelling stools

C. Interventions: Medical management
   1. Maintain low-fiber, high-calorie, high-protein diet; parenteral nutrition may be necessary in extreme situations.
   2. Administer stool softeners as prescribed.
   3. Administer daily rectal irrigations with normal saline to promote adequate elimination and prevent obstruction as prescribed.

D. Surgical management: Preoperative interventions
   1. Monitor the bowel function and administer bowel preparations, as prescribed.
   2. Maintain NPO status.
   3. Monitor hydration and fluid and electrolyte status. IV fluids may be prescribed for hydration.
   4. Administer antibiotics or colonic irrigations with an antibiotic solution as prescribed to clear the bowel of bacteria.
   5. Monitor I&O and weight.
   6. Measure the abdominal girth.
   7. Avoid taking rectal temperatures.
   8. Monitor for respiratory distress associated with abdominal distention.

E. Postoperative interventions
   1. Monitor vital signs, avoiding taking the temperature rectally.
   2. Measure abdominal girth daily and PRN.

3. Check the surgical site for redness, swelling, and drainage.
4. Check the stoma if present for bleeding or skin breakdown (stoma should be red and moist).
5. Check the anal area for the presence of stool, redness, or discharge.
6. Maintain NPO status until bowel sounds return or flatus is passed and as prescribed, usually within 48 to 72 hours
7. Maintain the nasogastric tube to allow intermittent suction until peristalsis returns.
8. Maintain IV fluids until the child tolerates appropriate oral intake, advancing the diet from clear liquids to regular as tolerated and as prescribed.
9. Monitor for dehydration and fluid overload.
10. Monitor strict intake and output.
11. Obtain daily weight.
12. Monitor for pain and provide comfort measures as required.
13. Provide the parents with instructions regarding colostomy care and skin care.
14. Teach the parents about the appropriate diet and the need for adequate fluid intake.

XV. INTUSSUSCEPTION (Figure 34-6)

A. Description
1. The telescoping of one portion of the bowel into another
2. Results in an obstruction of the passage of intestinal contents
B. Data collection
1. Colicky abdominal pain that causes the child to scream and draw his or her knees to the abdomen

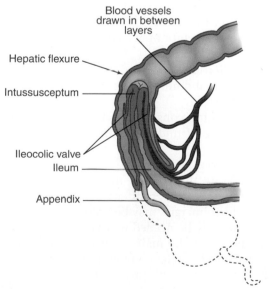

Blood vessels drawn in between layers

Hepatic flexure

Intussusceptum

Ileocolic valve

Ileum

Appendix

▲ **FIGURE 34-6** Ileocolic intussusception. (From Hockenberry, M., & Wilson, D. [2010]. *Wong's nursing care of infants and children* [9th ed.]. St. Louis: Mosby).

2. Vomiting of gastric contents
3. Bile-stained fecal emesis
4. Currant jelly–like stools that contain blood and mucus
5. Hypoactive or hyperactive bowel sounds
6. Tender and distended abdomen, possibly with a palpable sausage-shaped mass in the upper right quadrant
C. Interventions
1. Monitor for signs of perforation and shock as evidenced by fever, increased heart rate, changes in level of consciousness or blood pressure, and respiratory distress, and report immediately.
2. Antibiotics, IV fluids, and decompression via nasogastric tube may be prescribed.
3. Monitor for the passage of normal, brown stool, which indicates that the intussusception has reduced itself.
4. Prepare for hydrostatic reduction as prescribed, if no signs of perforation or shock occur (in hydrostatic reduction, air or fluid is used to exert pressure on area involved to lessen, diminish, or rid the intestine of prolapse).
5. Posthydrostatic reduction
   a. Monitor for the return of normal bowel sounds, for the passage of barium, and the characteristics of stool.
   b. Administer clear fluids and advance the diet gradually as prescribed.
6. If surgery is required, postoperative care is similar to that following any abdominal surgery.

XVI. ABDOMINAL WALL DEFECTS

A. Omphalocele
1. Occurs when there is a herniation of the abdominal contents through the umbilical ring (hernia of the umbilical cord), usually with an intact peritoneal sac
2. The protrusion is covered by a translucent sac that may contain bowel or other abdominal organs
3. Commonly associated with chromosomal abnormalities (trisomies 13, 18, and 21) and with cardiac, musculoskeletal, gastrointestinal, and genitourinary anomalies
4. Rupture of the sac results in the evisceration of the abdominal contents. Gastric decompression is essential to prevent visceral distention.
5. Immediately after birth, the sac is covered with sterile gauze soaked in normal saline to prevent the drying of the abdominal contents. A layer of plastic wrap is placed over the gauze to provide additional protection against heat and moisture loss.
6. Monitor the vital signs every 2 to 4 hours. Temperature is particularly important, because the infant can lose heat through the sac.

7. Preoperatively: Maintain NPO status. IV fluids will be prescribed to maintain hydration and electrolyte balance. Monitor for signs of infection, and handle the infant carefully to prevent the rupture of the sac.
8. Postoperatively: Control pain, prevent infection, maintain fluid and electrolyte balance, and ensure adequate nutrition.

B. Gastroschisis
1. Occurs when the herniation of the intestine is lateral (usually on the right) to the umbilical ring
2. There is no membrane covering the exposed bowel.
3. The exposed bowel is loosely covered in saline-soaked pads, and the abdomen is wrapped in a plastic drape. Wrapping around the exposed bowel is contraindicated, because if the exposed bowel expands, the wrapping could cause pressure and necrosis.
4. Gastric decompression is essential to prevent visceral distention.
5. Preoperatively: Care is similar to that for omphalocele. Surgery is performed within several hours after birth, because there is no membrane covering the sac.
6. Postoperatively: Most infants develop a prolonged ileus and require mechanical ventilation and parenteral nutrition. Otherwise, care is similar to that for omphalocele.

XVII.   UMBILICAL HERNIA

A. Description
1. A hernia is a protrusion of the bowel through an abnormal opening in the abdominal wall.
2. In children, a hernia most commonly occurs at the umbilicus and through the inguinal canal.
3. A hydrocele is the presence of abdominal fluid in the scrotal sac.

B. Data collection
1. Umbilical hernia: A soft swelling or protrusion around the umbilicus that is usually reducible with the finger
2. Inguinal hernia
   a. Painless inguinal swelling that is reducible
   b. Swelling may disappear during periods of rest and is most noticeable when the infant cries or coughs.
3. Incarcerated hernia
   a. Occurs when the descended portion of the bowel becomes tightly caught in the hernial sac, compromising blood supply
   b. Represents a medical emergency requiring surgical repair
   c. Data collection findings—irritability, tenderness at site, anorexia, abdominal distention, difficulty defecating

d. May lead to complete intestinal obstruction and gangrene
4. Noncommunicating hydrocele
   a. Occurs when residual peritoneal fluid is trapped with no communication with the peritoneal cavity
   b. Usually disappears by the age of 1 year
5. Communicating hydrocele
   a. Associated with a hernia that remains open from the scrotum to the abdominal cavity
   b. Data collection findings include a bulge in the inguinal area or the scrotum that increases with crying or straining and that decreases when the child is at rest.

C. Postoperative interventions (hernia)
1. Monitor the vital signs.
2. Monitor for wound infection (redness or drainage).
3. Monitor I&O and hydration status.
4. Advance the diet, as tolerated and as prescribed.
5. Administer analgesics, as prescribed.

D. Postoperative interventions (hydrocele)
1. Provide ice bags and a scrotal support to relieve pain and swelling.
2. Instruct the child and parents to avoid tub bathing until the incision heals.
3. Instruct the child and parents to avoid strenuous physical activities.

XVIII.   IRRITABLE BOWEL SYNDROME

A. Description
1. Occurs as a result of increased motility, which can lead to spasm and pain
2. Diagnosis is based on the elimination of pathology.
3. Self-limiting, intermittent problem with no definitive treatment
4. Stress and emotional factors may contribute to its occurrence

B. Data collection
1. Diffuse abdominal pain unrelated to meals or activity
2. Alternating constipation and diarrhea with the presence of undigested food and mucus in the stool

C. Interventions
1. Reassure the parents that the problem is self-limiting and intermittent and that it will resolve.
2. Anticholinergics may be prescribed. (Antidepressants may be needed in severe cases.)
3. Encourage the maintenance of a healthy, well-balanced, moderate-fiber and low-fat diet.
4. Encourage health-promotion activities, such as exercise and school activities.
5. Inform the parents about psychosocial resources, if required.

XIX. IMPERFORATE ANUS

A. Description: The incomplete development or absence of the anus in its normal position in the perineum

B. Data collection (Box 34-11)

C. Preoperative interventions
1. Determine the patency of the anus.
2. Monitor for the presence of stool in the urine and vagina. Report this immediately.
3. Administer IV fluids as prescribed
4. Prepare the child and parents for the surgical procedures, including the potential for colostomy.

D. Postoperative interventions
1. Monitor the skin for signs of infection.
2. The preferred position is a side-lying prone position with the hips elevated or a supine position with the legs suspended at a 90-degree angle to the trunk to reduce edema and pressure on the surgical site.
3. Keep the anal surgical incision clean and dry, and monitor for redness, swelling, or drainage.
4. Maintain NPO status and the NG tube, if one has been placed.
5. Maintain IV fluids until GI motility returns.
6. Provide colostomy care, if prescribed.
7. A fresh colostomy stoma will be red and edematous, but this should decrease with time.
8. Instruct the parents to perform anal dilation, if prescribed, to achieve and maintain bowel patency.
9. Instruct the parents to use only the dilators supplied by the HCP and a water-soluble lubricant and to insert the dilator no more than 1 to 2 cm into the anus to prevent damage to the mucosa.

XX. HEPATITIS

A. This section contains specific information regarding hepatitis as it relates to infants and children. Refer to Chapters 22 and 47 for additional information about hepatitis.

B. Description: An acute or chronic inflammation of the liver that may be caused by a virus, a medication reaction, or another disease process

C. Hepatitis A virus (HAV)
1. Highest incidence occurs among preschool or school-age children who are less than 15 years old

2. Many affected children are asymptomatic, but mild nausea, vomiting, and diarrhea may occur.
3. Infected children who are asymptomatic can still spread HAV to others.

D. Hepatitis B virus (HBV)
1. Most HBV in children is acquired perinatally.
2. Newborn infants are at risk if the mother is infected with HBV or was a carrier of HBV during pregnancy.
3. Possible routes of maternal-fetal (infant) transmission include the leakage of the virus across the placenta late in pregnancy or during labor, the ingestion of amniotic fluid or maternal blood, and breast-feeding, especially if the mother has cracked nipples.
4. The severity in the infant varies from no liver disease to fulminant (severe, acute course) or chronic, active disease.
5. In children and adolescents, HBV occurs in specific high-risk groups, including the following:
   a. Children with hemophilia or other disorders who have received multiple blood transfusions
   b. Children or adolescents who are involved in drug abuse
   c. Institutionalized children
   d. Preschool-age children in endemic areas
   e. Children who may be involved with heterosexual activity or sexual activity with homosexual males
6. HBV infection can cause a carrier state and lead to eventual cirrhosis or hepatocellular carcinoma during adulthood

E. Hepatitis C virus (HCV)
1. Transmission is primarily by the parenteral route.
2. Some children may be asymptomatic, but HCV often becomes a chronic condition, and it can cause cirrhosis and hepatocellular carcinoma.

F. Hepatitis D virus
1. Infection occurs in children already infected with HBV.
2. Acute and chronic forms tend to be more severe than HBV and can lead to cirrhosis.
3. Children with hemophilia are more likely to be infected, as are children who are IV drug users.

G. Hepatitis E virus
1. Uncommon among children
2. Is not a chronic condition, does not cause chronic liver disease, and has no carrier state

H. Hepatitis G virus
1. Blood-borne and similar to HCV
2. High-risk groups include transfusion recipients, IV drug users, and individuals infected with HCV.
3. Individuals are often asymptomatic, and most infections are chronic.

I. Data collection (Box 34-12)

J. Diagnostic evaluation: See Chapter 11 for the laboratory studies that are used to diagnose hepatitis

---

Box 34-11 Data Collection Findings: Imperforate Anus

- Failure to pass meconium stool
- Absence or stenosis of the anal rectal canal
- Presence of an anal membrane
- External fistula to the perineum

K. Prevention

1. Immune globulin (Ig) provides passive immunity and may be effective for preexposure prophylaxis to prevent HAV infection.
2. Hepatitis B immune globulin provides passive immunity and may be effective in preventing infection following a one-time exposure (should be given immediately after exposure), such as an accidental needle puncture or other contact of contaminated material with mucous membranes; should also be given to newborns whose mothers are HBsAg-positive.
3. Hepatitis A and hepatitis B **vaccines** (see Chapter 39 for information on immunizations)

⚠ Proper handwashing and standard precautions can prevent the spread of viral hepatitis.

L. Interventions

1. Strict handwashing
2. Hospitalization is required in the event of coagulopathy or fulminant hepatitis.
3. Standard precautions and enteric precautions are followed during hospitalization.
4. A hospitalized child is not usually isolated in a separate room unless he or she is fecally incontinent and items are likely to become contaminated with feces.
5. Children are discouraged from sharing toys.
6. Instruct the child and parents regarding good handwashing techniques.
7. Instruct the parents to thoroughly disinfect diaper-changing surfaces using ¼ cup of bleach in 1 gallon of water.
8. Maintain comfort and provide adequate rest and sleep.
9. Provide a low-fat, balanced diet.

Box 34-12 Data Collection Findings: Hepatitis

Prodromal or Anicteric Phase

- Lasts 5 to 7 days
- Absence of jaundice
- Anorexia, malaise, lethargy, and easy fatigability
- Fever (especially among adolescents)
- Nausea and vomiting
- Epigastric or right upper quadrant abdominal pain
- Arthralgia and skin rashes (more likely with hepatitis B virus)
- Hepatomegaly

Icteric Phase

- Jaundice, which is best assessed in the sclera, nail beds, and mucous membranes
- Dark urine and pale stools
- Pruritus

---

10. Provide enteric precautions for at least 1 week after the onset of jaundice with HAV.
11. Inform the parents that because HAV is not infectious 1 week after the onset of jaundice, the child may return to school at that time if he or she feels well enough.
12. Inform the parents that jaundice may get worse before it resolves.
13. Caution the parents about administering any medications to the child. (Remember that the liver is unable to detoxify and excrete medications.)
14. Instruct the parents regarding the signs that indicate the worsening of the child's condition, such as changes in the neurological status, bleeding, and fluid retention.

XXI. INGESTION OF POISONS (see Priority Nursing Actions)

▰▰▰ PRIORITY NURSING ACTIONS! ▰▰▰

Actions to Take in the Emergency Department in the Event of a Poisoning

1. Assess the child.
2. Terminate exposure to the poison.
3. Identify the poison.
4. Take measures to prevent absorption of the poison.
5. Document the occurrence, data collection findings, poison ingested, treatment measures, and the child's response.

In the event of a poisoning, the nurse treats the child first, not the poison. The ABCs, airway, breathing, and circulation and vital signs are assessed. Cardiopulmonary resuscitation is initiated immediately if necessary. Exposure to the poison is terminated next, such as emptying the mouth of pills or other materials or flushing the skin or other body area. The poison is identified next by questioning the parents or witnesses of the event to determine the appropriate treatment. The nurse assists to administer the antidote or takes other measures as prescribed by the HCP, such as administering activated charcoal. The nurse documents the occurrence, data collection findings, poison ingested, treatment measures, and the child's response.

Reference: Perry, S., Hockenberry, M., Lowdermilk, D., & Wilson, D. (2010). *Maternal child nursing care* (4th ed., pp. 1427–1430). St. Louis: Mosby.

A. Lead poisoning

1. Description: Excessive accumulation of lead in the blood
2. Causes
   a. The pathway for exposure may be food, air, or water.

b. Dust and soil contaminated with lead may be a source of exposure.

c. Lead enters the child's body through ingestion or inhalation or through placental transmission to an unborn child when the mother is exposed; the most common route is hand to mouth from contaminated objects, such as loose paint chips, pottery, or ceramic ware coupled with the inhalation of lead dust in the environment.

d. When lead enters the body, it affects the erythrocytes, bones, teeth, organs, and tissues, including the brain and nervous system. The most serious consequences are the effects on the central nervous system.

3. Universal screening
   a. Recommended in high-risk areas at the age of 1 to 2 years. Children at high risk should be screened earlier.
   b. Any child between the ages of 3 and 6 years who has not been screened should be tested.

4. Targeted screening
   a. Acceptable in low-risk areas
   b. At the age of 1 to 2 years (or a child between the ages of 3 and 6 years who has not been screened) may be targeted for screening if determined to be at risk.

5. Blood lead level test: Used for screening and diagnosis (Table 34-1)

6. Erythrocyte protoporphyrin test
   a. An indicator of anemia
   b. Normal value for a child is 35 mcg/100 mL of whole blood or less

7. Chelation therapy
   a. Removes lead from the circulating blood and from some organs and tissues
   b. Does not counteract any effects of the lead
   c. Medications include calcium disodium edetate (CaNa$_2$EDTA), and succimer (Chemet), an oral preparation; British anti-Lewisite (BAL, dimercaprol) is used in conjunction with EDTA.
   d. British anti-Lewisite (BAL, dimercaprol) is administered by the intravenous route or via deep intramuscular route and is contraindicated in children with an allergy to peanuts because the medication is prepared in a peanut oil solution; it is also contraindicated in children with a glucose 6-phosphate dehydrogenase (G6PD) deficiency and should not be given with iron.
   e. The function of the renal, hepatic, and hematological systems must be monitored closely.
   f. Ensure adequate urinary output before administering the medication and monitor the output and pH of the urine closely during and after therapy.

TABLE 34-1 Blood Lead Level Test Results and Intervention

Level	Intervention
Less than 10 mcg/dL	Reassess or rescreen in 1 year or sooner if exposure status changes.
10 to 14 mcg/dL	Provide family lead education, follow-up testing, and social service referral for home assessment if necessary.
15 to 19 mcg/dL	Provide family lead education, follow-up testing, and social service referral if necessary; on follow-up testing, initiate actions for blood lead level of 20 to 44 mcg/dL.
20 to 44 mcg/dL	Provide coordination of care, clinical management, including treatment, environmental investigation, and lead-hazard control
45 to 69 mcg/dL	Provide coordination of care and clinical management within 48 hours, including treatment, environmental investigation, and lead hazard control (the child must not remain in a lead-hazardous environment if resolution is necessary).
70 mcg/dL or greater	Medical treatment is provided immediately, including coordination of care, clinical management, environmental investigation, and lead-hazard control.

Adapted from Perry, S., Hockenberry, M., Lowdermilk, D., & Wilson, D. (2010). *Maternal child nursing care* (4th ed., p. 1436). St. Louis: Elsevier.

g. Provide adequate hydration and monitor kidney function for nephrotoxicity when the medication is given because the medication is excreted via the kidneys.

h. Follow-up of lead levels needs to be done to monitor progress.

i. Provide instructions to parents about safety from lead hazards, medication administration, and the need for follow-up.

j. Confirm that the child will be discharged to a home without lead hazards.

B. Acetaminophen (Tylenol) poisoning
   1. Description
      a. The seriousness of the ingestion is determined by the amount ingested and the length of time before intervention.
      b. A toxic dose is 150 mg/kg or higher in children.
   2. Data collection
      a. First 2 to 4 hours: Malaise, nausea, vomiting, sweating, pallor, and weakness
      b. Latent period: 24 to 36 hours; child improves
      c. Hepatic involvement: May last up to 7 days and be permanent; right upper quadrant pain, jaundice, confusion, stupor, elevated liver enzymes and bilirubin levels, and prolonged prothrombin time

3. Interventions
   a. Administer the antidote: *N*-Acetylcysteine (Mucomyst)
   b. Antidote is diluted in juice or soda because of its offensive odor.
   c. Loading dose is followed by maintenance doses.
   d. In the unconscious child, prepare to administer gastric lavage with activated charcoal to decrease the absorption of acetaminophen
   e. If using activated charcoal with lavage, do not also use *N*-acetylcysteine because activated charcoal will inactivate the antidote.

C. Acetylsalicylic acid (aspirin) poisoning
1. Description
   a. May be caused by acute or chronic ingestion
   b. Acute: Severe toxicity occurs with 300 to 500 mg/kg.
   c. Chronic: More than 100 mg/kg/day for 2 days or more; can be more serious than acute ingestion
2. Data collection
   a. GI effects: Nausea, vomiting, and thirst from dehydration
   b. Central nervous system effects: Hyperpnea, confusion, tinnitus, convulsions, coma, respiratory failure, and circulatory collapse
   c. Renal effects: Oliguria
   d. Hematopoietic effects: Bleeding tendencies
   e. Metabolic effects: Diaphoresis, fever, hyponatremia, hypokalemia, dehydration, and hypoglycemia
3. Interventions
   a. Prepare to administer activated charcoal to decrease the absorption of salicylate.
   b. Emesis or cathartic measures may be prescribed.
   c. Administer IV fluids; sodium bicarbonate may be prescribed to correct metabolic acidosis.
   d. Other interventions may include external cooling, anticonvulsants, vitamin K (if bleeding), and oxygen.
   e. Prepare the child for dialysis as prescribed if the child is unresponsive to the therapy.

D. Corrosives
1. Description
   a. Items that can cause poisoning include household cleaners, detergents, bleach, paint or paint thinners, or batteries.
   b. Liquid corrosives can cause more damage to the victim than other types of corrosives, such as granular.
2. Data collection
   a. Severe burning in the mouth, throat, or stomach
   b. Edema of the mucous membranes, lips, tongue, and pharynx

   c. Vomiting
   d. Drooling and inability to clear secretions
3. Interventions
   a. Dilute corrosive with water or milk as prescribed (usually no more than 4 oz).
   b. Inducing vomiting is contraindicated because vomiting re-damages the mucous membranes.
   c. Neutralization of the ingested corrosive is not done because it can cause a reaction producing heat and burns.

⚠ Educate parents to call the poison control center immediately in the event of poisoning. The parents need to be instructed to post the poison control center telephone number near each phone in the house.

XXII. INTESTINAL PARASITES

A. Description: Common infections in children are giardiasis and pinworms.
1. Giardiasis is caused by protozoa, and it is prevalent among children in crowded environments, such as classrooms and day-care centers.
2. Pinworms (enterobiasis) are universally present in temperate climate zones and easily transmitted in crowded environments.

B. Data collection
1. Giardiasis
   a. Diarrhea and vomiting
   b. Anorexia
   c. Failure to thrive
   d. Abdominal cramps with intermittent loose stools and constipation
   e. Steatorrhea
   f. Resolves in 4 to 6 weeks spontaneously
   g. Stool specimens from three or more collections are used for diagnosis
2. Pinworms
   a. Intense perianal itching
   b. Irritability and restlessness
   c. Poor sleeping
   d. Bed-wetting

C. Interventions
1. Giardiasis
   a. Medications that may be prescribed include metronidazole (Flagyl), tinidazole (Tindamax), nitazoxanide (Alinia), or albendazole (Albenza).
   b. Performance of meticulous handwashing by caregivers
   c. Provide education to the family and caregivers regarding sanitary practices.
2. Pinworms
   a. Perform a visual inspection of the anus with a flashlight 2 to 3 hours after sleep.
   b. The tape test is the most common diagnostic test.

c. Educate the family and caregivers regarding the tape test. A loop of transparent tape is placed firmly against the child's perianal area; it is removed in the morning and placed in a glass jar or plastic bag and transported to the primary care provider for analysis.

d. Medications that may be prescribed include ebendazole (Vermox), pyrantel pamoate (Pin-Rid, Antiminth) and albendazole (Albenza); these medications are not used in children under the age of 2 years.

e. The medication regimen may be repeated in 2 weeks to prevent reinfection

f. All members of the family are treated for the infection.

g. Teach the family and caregivers about the importance of meticulous hand washing and about washing all clothes and bed linens in hot water.

MORE QUESTIONS ON EVOLVE!

Practice Questions

331. A nurse reviews the record of a 3-week-old infant and notes that the health care provider has documented a diagnosis of suspected Hirschsprung's disease. The nurse understands that which of the following symptoms led the mother to seek health care for the infant?
1. Diarrhea
2. Projectile vomiting
3. The regurgitation of feedings
4. Foul-smelling, ribbon-like stools

332. A nurse is caring for a child with a diagnosis of intussusception. Which of the following symptoms would the nurse expect to note in this child?
1. Watery diarrhea
2. Ribbon-like stools
3. Profuse projectile vomiting
4. Blood and mucus in the stools

333. A child with a diagnosis of a hernia has been scheduled for a surgical repair in 2 weeks. The nurse reinforces instructions to the parents about the signs of possible hernial strangulation. The nurse tells the parents that which of the following signs would require health care provider (HCP) notification by the parents?
1. Fever
2. Diarrhea
3. Vomiting
4. Constipation

334. A nurse reinforces home-care instructions to the parents of a child with hepatitis regarding the care

of the child and the prevention of the transmission of the virus. Which statement by a parent indicates a need for further instruction?
1. "Frequent handwashing is important."
2. "I need to provide a well-balanced, high-fat diet to my child."
3. "I need to clean contaminated household surfaces with bleach."
4. "Diapers should not be changed near any surfaces that are used to prepare food."

335. A nursing instructor asks a nursing student about phenylketonuria (PKU). Which statement, if made by the student, indicates an understanding of this disorder?
1. "PKU is an autosomal-dominant disorder."
2. "PKU primarily affects the gastrointestinal system."
3. "Treatment of PKU includes the dietary restriction of tyramine."
4. "All 50 states require routine screening of all newborns for PKU."

336. A school-age child with type 1 diabetes mellitus has soccer practice three afternoons a week. The nurse reinforces instructions regarding how to prevent hypoglycemia during practice. The nurse tells the child to:
1. Drink a half a cup of orange juice before soccer practice.
2. Eat twice the amount that is normally eaten at lunchtime.
3. Take half of the amount of prescribed insulin on practice days.
4. Take the prescribed insulin at noontime rather than in the morning.

337. A mother of a 6-year-old child with type 1 diabetes mellitus calls the clinic nurse and tells the nurse that the child has been sick. The mother reports that she checked the child's urine and it showed positive ketones. Which of the following would the nurse instruct the mother to do?
1. Hold the next dose of insulin.
2. Come to the clinic immediately.
3. Encourage the child to drink liquids.
4. Administer an additional dose of regular insulin.

338. A nurse is caring for an 18-month-old child who has been vomiting. The appropriate position in which to place the child during naps and sleep time is:
1. A supine position
2. A side-lying position
3. Prone, with the head elevated
4. Prone, with the face turned to the side

339. A nurse is monitoring for signs of dehydration in a 1-year-old child who has been hospitalized for diarrhea and prepares to take the child's temperature. Which method of temperature measurement should be avoided?
1. Rectal
2. Axillary
3. Electronic
4. Tympanic

340. An infant returns to the nursing unit after the surgical repair of a cleft lip located on the right side of the lip. The best position in which to place this infant at this time is:
1. A flat position
2. A prone position
3. On his or her left side
4. On his or her right side

341. A nurse reviews the record of an infant who is seen in the clinic. The nurse notes that a diagnosis of esophageal atresia with tracheoesophageal fistula (TEF) is suspected. The nurse expects to note which most likely clinical manifestation of this condition in the medical record?
1. Incessant crying
2. Coughing at nighttime
3. Choking with feedings
4. Severe projectile vomiting

342. A nurse is reviewing the record of a child with a diagnosis of pyloric stenosis. Which data would the nurse expect to note as having been documented in the child's record?
1. Watery diarrhea
2. Projectile vomiting

3. Increased urine output
4. Vomiting large amounts of bile

343. A nurse reinforces instructions to the mother about dietary measures for a 5-year-old child with lactose intolerance. The nurse tells the mother that which of the following supplements will be required as a result of the need to avoid lactose in the diet?
1. Fats
2. Zinc
3. Calcium
4. Thiamine

344. A nurse reinforces home-care instructions to the parents of a child with celiac disease. Which of the following food items would the nurse advise the parents to include in the child's diet?
1. Rice
2. Oatmeal
3. Rye toast
4. Wheat bread

345. A nurse is assigned to care for a child who is scheduled for an appendectomy. Which prescriptions does the nurse anticipate will be prescribed? **Select all that apply.**
❒ 1. Administer a Fleet enema.
❒ 2. Initiate an intravenous line.
❒ 3. Maintain nothing-by-mouth status.
❒ 4. Administer intravenous antibiotics.
❒ 5. Administer preoperative medications.
❒ 6. Place a heating pad on the abdomen to decrease pain.

ANSWERS

331. 4
Rationale: Chronic constipation that begins during the first month of life and that results in foul-smelling, ribbon-like or pellet-like stools is a clinical manifestation of Hirschsprung's disease. The delayed passage or absence of meconium stool during the neonatal period is a characteristic sign. Bowel obstruction (especially during the neonatal period), abdominal pain and distention, and failure to thrive are also clinical manifestations. Options 1, 2, and 3 are incorrect.
Test-Taking Strategy: Knowledge regarding the clinical manifestations associated with Hirschsprung's disease is required to answer this question. Think about the pathophysiology associated with this disorder and recall that foul-smelling, ribbon-like or pellet-like stools are a clinical manifestation of this disorder. Review the manifestations of Hirschsprung's disease if you had difficulty with this question.
Level of Cognitive Ability: Understanding
Client Needs: Physiological Integrity
Integrated Process: Nursing Process/Data Collection

Content Area: Child Health: Gastrointestinal/Renal
Reference: Leifer, p. 653. 2011.

332. 4
Rationale: The child with intussusception classically presents with severe abdominal pain that is crampy and intermittent and that causes the child to draw in his or her knees to the chest. Vomiting may be present, but it is not projectile. Bright red blood and mucus are passed through the rectum and commonly described as currant jelly–like stools. Ribbon-like stools are not a manifestation of this disorder.
Test-Taking Strategy: Knowledge related to the clinical manifestations associated with intussusception is required to answer this question. Recalling that a classic manifestation is currant jelly–like stools will assist in directing you to the correct option. Review intussusception if you had difficulty with this question.
Level of Cognitive Ability: Understanding
Client Needs: Physiological Integrity
Integrated Process: Nursing Process/Data Collection

Content Area: Child Health: Gastrointestinal/Renal
Reference: Leifer, p. 654. 2011.

333. 3
Rationale: The parents of a child with a hernia need to be instructed about the signs of strangulation. These signs include vomiting, pain, and an irreducible mass. The parents should be instructed to contact the HCP immediately if strangulation is suspected. Fever, diarrhea, and constipation are not associated with strangulation of a hernia.
Test-Taking Strategy: Use the definition of the word "strangulation" to help answer this question; this will assist you with eliminating options 1 and 2. From the remaining options, thinking about the signs of strangulation will assist you with answering the question. Review the signs of strangulation if you had difficulty with this question.
Level of Cognitive Ability: Applying
Client Needs: Physiological Integrity
Integrated Process: Teaching and Learning
Content Area: Child Health: Gastrointestinal/Renal
Reference: Leifer, pp. 654-655. 2011.

334. 2
Rationale: The child with hepatitis should consume a well-balanced, low-fat diet to allow the liver to rest. Options 1, 3, and 4 are components of the home-care instructions to the family of a child with hepatitis.
Test-Taking Strategy: Note the strategic words "need for further instruction." These words indicate a negative event query and ask you to select an option that is an incorrect statement. Options 1, 3, and 4 can be eliminated by remembering the basic principles related to standard precautions. Review the home-care instructions for the parents of a child with hepatitis if you had difficulty with this question.
Level of Cognitive Ability: Evaluating
Client Needs: Safe and Effective Care Environment
Integrated Process: Teaching and Learning
Content Area: Child Health: Gastrointestinal/Renal
Reference: McKinney, James, Murray, Ashwill, p. 1134. 2009.

335. 4
Rationale: PKU is an autosomal-recessive disorder. Treatment includes the dietary restriction of phenylalanine intake (not tyramine intake). PKU is a genetic disorder that results in central nervous system (CNS) damage from toxic levels of phenylalanine in the blood.
Test-Taking Strategy: Use the process of elimination. Recalling that PKU is a recessive disorder will assist you with eliminating option 1. Reading option 3 carefully will direct you to eliminate it, because tyramine is restricted among clients taking monoamine oxidase inhibitors rather than among those with PKU. Recalling that PKU affects the CNS will direct you to option 4. Review the characteristics associated with PKU if you had difficulty with this question.
Level of Cognitive Ability: Understanding
Client Needs: Physiological Integrity
Integrated Process: Teaching and Learning
Content Area: Child Health: Metabolic/Endocrine
Reference: McKinney, James, Murray, Ashwill, p. 334. 2009

336. 1
Rationale: An extra snack of 10 g to 15 g of carbohydrates eaten before activities and for every 30 to 45 minutes of activity will prevent hypoglycemia. A half cup of orange juice will provide the needed carbohydrates. The child or parents should not be instructed to adjust the amount or time of insulin administration, and meal amounts should not be doubled.
Test-Taking Strategy: Use the process of elimination. Options 3 and 4 can be eliminated first using general medication guidelines, because insulin dosages and times should not be adjusted. From the remaining options, recalling the manifestations and treatment associated with hypoglycemia will direct you to option 1. Review the prevention of hypoglycemia if you had difficulty with this question.
Level of Cognitive Ability: Applying
Client Needs: Health Promotion and Maintenance
Integrated Process: Teaching and Learning
Content Area: Child Health: Metabolic/Endocrine
Reference: Swearingen, pp. 581-582. 2012.

337. 3
Rationale: When the child is sick, the mother should test for urinary ketones with each voiding. If ketones are present, liquids are essential to help with clearing them. The child should be encouraged to drink liquids. It is not necessary to bring the child to the clinic immediately, and insulin doses should not be adjusted or changed.
Test-Taking Strategy: Use the process of elimination. Eliminate options 1 and 4 first, because insulin doses should not be adjusted or changed. From the remaining options, note the words "positive ketones." This finding does not require immediate health care provider referral. Review the home-care instructions for the sick diabetic child if you had difficulty with this question.
Level of Cognitive Ability: Applying
Client Needs: Physiological Integrity
Integrated Process: Nursing Process/Implementation
Content Area: Child Health: Metabolic/Endocrine
Reference: McKinney, James, Murray, Ashwill, p. 1451. 2009.

338. 2
Rationale: The vomiting child should be placed in an upright or side-lying position to prevent aspiration. Options 1, 3, and 4 will place the child at risk for aspiration if vomiting occurs.
Test-Taking Strategy: Use the process of elimination. Eliminate options 3 and 4 first, because they are comparable or alike. In additional, these positions would place the child at risk for aspiration if vomiting occurred. Visualize the remaining two positions. Option 1 is also inappropriate and would cause aspiration. Review the appropriate positioning for the child who has been vomiting if you had difficulty with this question.
Level of Cognitive Ability: Applying
Client Needs: Safe and Effective Care Environment
Integrated Process: Nursing Process/Implementation
Content Area: Child Health: Gastrointestinal/Renal
References: Leifer, p. 656. 2011.
McKinney, James, Murray, Ashwill, p. 1083. 2009.

339. 1
Rationale: Rectal temperature measurements should be avoided if diarrhea is present. The use of a rectal thermometer can stimulate peristalsis and cause more diarrhea. Axillary or tympanic measurements of temperature would be acceptable. Most measurements are performed via electronic devices.
Test-Taking Strategy: Use the process of elimination, and note the strategic word "avoided." Eliminate option 3 first, because most methods of temperature measurement are performed with the use of an electronic device. Next, note the diagnosis stated in the question; this should direct you to option 1. Review the interventions for the child with diarrhea if you had difficulty with this question.
Level of Cognitive Ability: Applying
Client Needs: Physiological Integrity
Integrated Process: Nursing Process/Implementation
Content Area: Child Health: Gastrointestinal/Renal
Reference: Swearingen, p. 591. 2012.

340. 3
Rationale: After the repair of a cleft lip, the infant should be positioned on the side opposite to the repair to prevent contact of the suture lines with the bed linens. In this case, it is best to place the infant on his or her left side. Additionally, the flat or prone position can result in aspiration if the infant vomits.
Test-Taking Strategy: Use the process of elimination. Consider the anatomical location of the surgical site and the strategic words "right side." You should be easily directed to the correct option with the use of these concepts. Review postoperative positioning techniques following cleft lip repair if you had difficulty with this question.
Level of Cognitive Ability: Applying
Client Needs: Physiological Integrity
Integrated Process: Nursing Process/Implementation
Content Area: Child Health: Gastrointestinal/Renal
Reference: McKinney, James, Murray, Ashwill, p. 1095. 2009.

341. 3
Rationale: Any child who exhibits the "3 Cs"—coughing and choking during feedings and unexplained cyanosis—should be suspected of having TEF. Options 1, 2, and 4 are not specifically associated with TEF.
Test-Taking Strategy: Use the process of elimination, and focus on the diagnosis. Recalling the "3 Cs" associated with TEF will direct you to the correct option. Review the clinical manifestations associated with TEF if you had difficulty with this question
Level of Cognitive Ability: Analyzing
Client Needs: Physiological Integrity
Integrated Process: Nursing Process/Data Collection
Content Area: Child Health: Gastrointestinal/Renal
Reference: Leifer, p. 649. 2011.

342. 2
Rationale: Clinical manifestations of pyloric stenosis include projectile, nonbilious vomiting; irritability; hunger and crying; constipation; and signs of dehydration, including a decrease in urine output.

Test-Taking Strategy: Use the process of elimination. Considering the anatomical location of this disorder and the definition of the word *stenosis* will assist you with eliminating the incorrect options. Review the clinical manifestations of pyloric stenosis if you had difficulty with this question.
Level of Cognitive Ability: Analyzing
Client Needs: Physiological Integrity
Integrated Process: Nursing Process/Data Collection
Content Area: Child Health: Gastrointestinal/Renal
Reference: Leifer, p. 650. 2011.

343. 3
Rationale: Lactose intolerance is the inability to tolerate lactose, which is the sugar that is found in dairy products. Removing milk from the diet can provide relief from symptoms. Additional dietary changes may be required to provide adequate sources of calcium and, if the child is an infant, protein and calories.
Test-Taking Strategy: Knowledge that lactose is the sugar that is found in dairy products will easily direct you to option 3, because dairy products are major sources of calcium. Review the dietary management of lactose intolerance if you had difficulty with this question.
Level of Cognitive Ability: Applying
Client Needs: Physiological Integrity
Integrated Process: Nursing Process/Implementation
Content Area: Child Health: Gastrointestinal/Renal
Reference: McKinney, James, Murray, Ashwill, pp. 1127-1128. 2009.

344. 1
Rationale: Dietary management is the mainstay of treatment for celiac disease. All wheat, rye, barley, and oats should be eliminated from the diet and replaced with corn and rice. Vitamin supplements, especially fat-soluble vitamins and folate, may be required during the early period of treatment to correct deficiencies. These restrictions are likely to be lifelong, although small amounts of grains may be tolerated after the gastrointestinal ulcerations have healed.
Test-Taking Strategy: Use the process of elimination and your knowledge regarding the dietary management of celiac disease to answer this question. Recalling that corn and rice are substitute food replacements among clients with this disease will direct you to the correct option. Review the dietary management of celiac disease if you had difficulty with this question.
Level of Cognitive Ability: Applying
Client Needs: Health Promotion and Maintenance
Integrated Process: Teaching and Learning
Content Area: Child Health: Gastrointestinal/Renal
Reference: Leifer, p. 652. 2011.

345. 2, 3, 4, 5
Rationale: During the preoperative period, enemas or laxatives should not be administered. In addition, heat should not be applied to the abdomen. Any of these interventions can cause the rupture of the appendix and resultant peritonitis. Intravenous fluids would be started, and the child should receive nothing by mouth while awaiting surgery. Antibiotics are usually administered because of the risk of perforation. Preoperative medications are administered as prescribed.

Test-Taking Strategy: Consider the anatomical location of appendicitis, and think about the concern of rupture among clients with this disorder. This will assist you with determining the correct interventions. Review the preoperative care of the child with appendicitis if you had difficulty with this question.

Level of Cognitive Ability: Analyzing
Client Needs: Physiological Integrity
Integrated Process: Nursing Process/Planning
Content Area: Child Health: Gastrointestinal/Renal
Reference: Leifer, p. 666. 2011.

35

Renal and Urinary Disorders

I. GLOMERULONEPHRITIS

A. Description
1. Glomerulonephritis is a term that refers to a group of kidney disorders characterized by inflammatory injuries in the glomerulus, most of which are caused by an immunological reaction.
2. Results in proliferative and inflammatory changes within the glomerular structure
3. Destruction, inflammation, and sclerosis of the glomeruli of both kidneys occur.
4. Inflammation of the glomeruli results from an antigen–antibody reaction produced by an infection elsewhere in the body.
5. Loss of kidney function develops.

B. Causes
1. Immunological diseases
2. Autoimmune diseases
3. Antecedent group A β-hemolytic streptococcal infection of the pharynx or skin
4. History of pharyngitis or tonsillitis 2 to 3 weeks before the onset of symptoms

C. Types (Box 35-1)

D. Complications
1. Renal failure
2. Hypertensive encephalopathy
3. Pulmonary edema
4. Heart failure

E. Data collection
1. Periorbital and facial edema that is more prominent in the morning
2. Anorexia
3. Decreased urinary output
4. Cloudy, smoky, brown-colored urine (hematuria)
5. Pallor, irritability, and lethargy
6. In the older child, headaches, abdominal or flank pain, and dysuria
7. Hypertension
8. Proteinuria that produces a persistent and excessive foam in the urine
9. Azotemia
10. Increased blood urea nitrogen and creatinine levels

11. Increased antistreptolysin O titer (used to diagnose disorders caused by streptococcal infections)

F. Interventions
1. Monitor the vital signs, weight, intake and output (I&O), and characteristics of the urine.
2. Limit activity. Provide safety measures.
3. Provide high-quality nutrient foods.
   a. Restrictions depend on the stage and severity of the disease, especially the extent of the edema.
   b. In uncomplicated cases, a regular diet is permitted but sodium is restricted to a "no added salt to foods" diet.
   c. Moderate sodium and fluid restriction is prescribed for the child with hypertension or edema.
   d. Foods high in potassium are restricted during periods of oliguria.
   e. Protein is restricted if the child has severe azotemia resulting from prolonged oliguria.
4. Monitor for complications (i.e., renal failure, hypertensive encephalopathy, seizures, pulmonary edema, and heart failure).
5. Administer diuretics (if significant edema and fluid overload are present), antihypertensives (for hypertension), and antibiotics (to the child with evidence of persistent streptococcal infections), as prescribed.
6. Initiate seizure precautions and administer anticonvulsants, as prescribed, for seizures associated with hypertensive encephalopathy.
7. Instruct the parents to report signs of bloody urine, headache, or edema.
8. Instruct the parents that the child needs to obtain appropriate and adequate treatment for infections, specifically for sore throats, upper respiratory infections, and skin infections.

Box 35-1 Types of Glomerulonephritis

Acute: Occurs 2 to 3 weeks after a streptococcal infection
Chronic: Can occur after the acute phase or slowly over time

Measuring the daily weight and monitoring for weight changes is the most useful and effective method for determining fluid balance.

II. NEPHROTIC SYNDROME

A. Description
1. A kidney disorder characterized by massive proteinuria, hypoalbuminemia (hypoproteinemia), and edema (Figure 35-1)
2. The primary objectives of therapeutic management are to reduce the excretion of urinary protein and to maintain protein-free urine

B. Data collection (Box 35-2)

 The classic manifestations of nephrotic syndrome are massive proteinuria, hypoalbuminemia, and edema.

C. Interventions
1. Monitor the vital signs, I&O, and daily weights.
2. Monitor the urine for specific gravity, albumin, and protein.
3. Monitor for edema.
4. Nutrition: A regular diet without added salt is prescribed if the child is in remission. Sodium is restricted during periods of massive edema (fluids may also be restricted).

5. Corticosteroid therapy: Prescribed as soon as the diagnosis has been determined. Monitor the child closely for signs of infection (Box 35-3).
6. Immunosuppressant therapy may be prescribed to reduce the relapse rate and to induce long-term remission. This may be administered in conjunction with the corticosteroid.
7. Diuretics may be prescribed to reduce edema.
8. Plasma expanders such as salt-poor human albumin may be prescribed for the severely edematous child.
9. Instruct the parents about testing the urine for protein, medication administration, the side effects of the medications, and the general care of the child.

Box 35-2 Findings in Nephrotic Syndrome

The child gains weight.
Periorbital and facial edema are most prominent in the morning.
Leg, ankle, labial, or scrotal edema occurs.
Urine output decreases, and the urine is dark and frothy.
Ascites (fluid in the abdominal cavity) is present.
Blood pressure is normal or slightly decreased.
Lethargy, anorexia, and pallor occur.
Massive proteinuria is seen.
Decreased serum protein (hypoproteinemia) and elevated serum lipid levels occur.

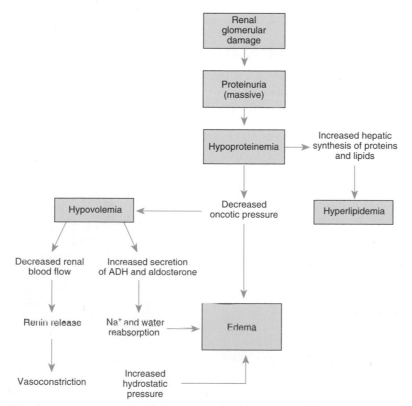

▲ **FIGURE 35-1** Sequence of events in the nephrotic syndrome. (From Perry, S., Hockenberry, M., Lowdermilk, D., & Wilson, D. [2010]. *Maternal child nursing care* [4th ed.]. St. Louis: Mosby.)

10. Instruct the parents regarding the signs of infection and the need to avoid contact with other children who may be infectious.

III. CRYPTORCHIDISM

A. Description: Occurs when one or both testes fail to descend through the inguinal canal and into the scrotal sac

B. Data collection: Testes not palpable or easily guided into the scrotum

C. Interventions
   1. Monitor during the first 12 months of life to determine whether spontaneous descent occurs.
   2. After the age of 1 year, medical or surgical treatment may be instituted.
   3. Human chorionic gonadotropin, a pituitary hormone that stimulates the production of testosterone, may be prescribed.
   4. Surgical correction, if needed, is performed by orchiopexy before the child's second birthday (preferably between 1 and 2 years of age) if the testes do not descend spontaneously.
   5. Monitor for bleeding and infection postoperatively.
   6. Instruct the parents regarding postoperative home care measures, including preventing infection, pain control, and activity restrictions.
   7. Provide an opportunity for parental counseling if the parents are concerned about the future fertility of the child.

IV. EPISPADIAS AND HYPOSPADIAS (Figure 35-2)

A. Description: Congenital defects that involve the abnormal placement of the urethral orifice of the penis; these anatomical defects can lead to the easy entry of bacteria into the urine.

B. Data collection
   1. Epispadias: Urethral orifice is located on the dorsal surface of the penis; often occurs with exstrophy of the bladder
   2. Hypospadias: Urethral orifice is located below the glans penis, along the ventral surface

---

Box 35-3 Adverse Effects of Corticosteroid Therapy

- Impaired wound healing
- Hyperglycemia
- Skin fragility
- Abnormal fat deposition
- Emotional lability
- Hirsutism
- Moon face
- Osteoporosis

C. Surgical interventions: Performed before the age of toilet training, preferably between 16 and 18 months of age.

⚠ Circumcision is not performed on a newborn with epispadias or hypospadias because the foreskin may be used in surgical reconstruction of the defect.

D. Postoperative interventions
   1. The child will have a pressure dressing and may have some type of urinary diversion or a urinary stent (used to maintain the patency of the urethral opening) while the healing of the meatus occurs.
   2. Monitor the vital signs.
   3. Encourage fluid intake to maintain adequate urine output and to maintain the patency of the stent.
   4. Monitor the I&O and the urine for cloudiness or a foul odor.
   5. Notify the registered nurse if there is no urinary drainage for 1 hour, because this may indicate kinks in the system or obstruction by sediment.
   6. Provide pain medication (acetaminophen [Tylenol]) or medication to relieve bladder spasms (anticholinergic), as prescribed.
   7. Administer antibiotics, as prescribed.

Epispadias

Dorsal placement of urethral opening

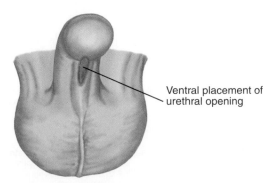

Hypospadias

Ventral placement of urethral opening

▲ **FIGURE 35-2** Epispadias and hypospadias are genital anomalies in which the urethral opening is above or below its normal location on the glans of the penis. (From James, S., Ashwill, J., & Droske, S. [2007]. *Nursing care of children: Principles and practice* [3rd ed.]. St. Louis: Saunders.)

8. Instruct the parents regarding the care of the urinary diversion or stent, if present.
9. Instruct the parents to avoid giving the child a tub bath until the stent, if present, is removed.
10. Instruct the parents about fluid intake, medication administration, the signs and symptoms of infection, and the need for health care provider follow-up for dressing removal approximately 4 days after surgery.

V. BLADDER EXSTROPHY

A. Description
1. A congenital anomaly characterized by the extrusion of the urinary bladder to the outside of the body through a defect in the lower abdominal wall
2. Cause is unknown
3. Treatment requires surgical management and occurs in a series of staged reconstructions
4. Initial surgery for the closure of the abdominal defect should occur within the first few days of life.
5. Goals of subsequent surgeries are to reconstruct the bladder and genitalia and enable the child to achieve urinary continence.

B. Data collection
1. Exposed bladder mucosa
2. Widened symphysis pubis
3. Defects of the external genitalia

C. Interventions
1. Monitor the urinary output.
2. Monitor for signs of urinary tract or wound infection.
3. Maintain the integrity of the exposed bladder mucosa.
4. Prevent the bladder tissue from drying while allowing for the drainage of urine until surgical closure is performed. The bladder is covered with sterile, nonadherent, clear plastic wrap or a sterile thin film dressing without adhesive.
5. Monitor the laboratory values and urinalysis to assess for renal function.
6. Administer antibiotics, as prescribed.
7. Provide emotional support to the parents, and encourage the verbalization of their fears and concerns.

⚠ Applying petroleum jelly to the bladder mucosa is avoided because it tends to dry out, adhere to the bladder mucosa, and damage the delicate tissues when the dressing is removed.

VI. HEMOLYTIC-UREMIC SYNDROME

A. Description
1. Thought to be associated with bacterial toxins, chemicals, and viruses that cause acute renal failure in children

---

Box 35-4 Manifestations of Hemolytic-Uremic Syndrome

- Vomiting
- Irritability
- Lethargy
- Marked pallor
- Hemorrhagic manifestations, such as bruising, petechiae, jaundice, and bloody diarrhea
- Oliguria or anuria
- Central nervous system involvement, including seizures, stupor, and coma

---

2. Occurs primarily among infants and small children between the ages of 6 months and 5 years
3. Clinical features include acquired hemolytic anemia, thrombocytopenia, renal injury, and central nervous system symptoms

B. Data collection
1. Triad of anemia, thrombocytopenia, and renal failure is diagnostic (Box 35-4)
2. Proteinuria, hematuria, and the presence of urinary casts
3. Blood urea nitrogen and serum creatinine levels are elevated. Hemoglobin and hematocrit levels are decreased.

C. Interventions
1. Hemodialysis or peritoneal dialysis may be prescribed if the child is anuric.
   a. Hemodialysis requires venous access (such as an arteriovenous [AV] fistula), and treatment is usually 3 to 8 hours in length (three times per week). Peritoneal dialysis requires the surgical placement of an abdominal catheter. (The correction of fluid and electrolyte imbalance is slower than hemodialysis.)
   b. Dialysate solution is prescribed to meet the child's electrolyte needs.
2. Strict monitoring of fluid balance is necessary. Fluid restrictions may be prescribed if the child is anuric.
3. Institute measures to prevent infection.
4. Provide adequate nutrition.
5. Other treatments may include medications to treat manifestations, or the administration of blood products to treat severe anemia (administered with caution to prevent fluid overload).

MORE QUESTIONS ON EVOLVE!

Practice Questions

346. A nurse is assigned to care for a child who is suspected of having glomerulonephritis. The nurse reviews the child's record and notes that which

finding is associated with the diagnosis of glomerulonephritis?
1. Hypotension
2. Red-brown urine
3. Low urinary specific gravity
4. A low blood urea nitrogen (BUN) level

347. A nurse is reviewing the health record of a child who has been recently diagnosed with glomerulonephritis. Which finding noted in the child's record is associated with the diagnosis of glomerulonephritis?
1. The child fell off a bike and onto the handlebars.
2. The child has had nausea and vomiting for the last 24 hours.
3. The child had urticaria and itching for 1 week before diagnosis.
4. The child had a streptococcal throat infection 2 weeks before diagnosis.

348. A nurse is planning care for a child with hemolytic-uremic syndrome (HUS). The child has been anuric and will be receiving peritoneal dialysis treatment. The nurse plans to:
1. Restrict fluids, as prescribed.
2. Administer analgesics, as prescribed.
3. Care for the arteriovenous (AV) fistula.
4. Encourage the intake of foods that are high in potassium.

349. A nurse is assisting with performing admission data collection on a 2-year-old child who has been diagnosed with nephrotic syndrome. The nurse collects data knowing that a common characteristic associated with nephrotic syndrome is:
1. Hypotension
2. Generalized edema
3. Increased urinary output
4. Frank, bright red blood in the urine

350. The child with cryptorchidism is being discharged after orchiopexy, which was performed on an outpatient basis. The nurse informs the parents about which priority care measure?
1. Measuring intake and output
2. Administering anticholinergics
3. Preventing infection at the surgical site
4. Applying cold, wet compresses to the surgical site

351. A nurse is reinforcing discharge instructions to the mother of a 2-year-old child who has had an orchiopexy to correct cryptorchidism. Which of the following statements, if made by the mother of the child, indicates that further teaching is necessary?

1. "I'll check his temperature."
2. "I'll give him medication so he'll be comfortable."
3. "I'll let him decide when to return to his play activities."
4. "I'll check his voiding to be sure there are no problems."

352. A nurse collects a urine specimen preoperatively from a child with epispadias who is scheduled for surgical repair. The nurse reviews the child's record for the laboratory results of the urine test and would most likely expect to note which of the following?
1. Hematuria
2. Bacteriuria
3. Glucosuria
4. Proteinuria

353. An 18-month-old child is being discharged after surgical repair of hypospadias. Which postoperative nursing care measure should the nurse stress to the parents as they prepare to take this child home?
1. Leave diapers off to allow the site to heal.
2. Avoid tub baths until the stent has been removed.
3. Encourage toilet training to ensure that the flow of urine is normal.
4. Restrict the fluid intake to reduce urinary output for the first few days.

354. The parents of a newborn have been told that their child was born with bladder exstrophy, and the parents ask the nurse about this condition. The nurse bases the response on knowledge that this condition is:
1. A hereditary disorder that occurs in every other generation
2. Caused by the use of medications taken by the mother during pregnancy
3. A condition in which the urinary bladder is abnormally located in the pelvic cavity
4. An extrusion of the urinary bladder to the outside of the body through a defect in the lower abdominal wall

355. A child is admitted to the hospital with a probable diagnosis of nephrotic syndrome. Which findings would the nurse expect to observe? **Select all that apply.**
☐ 1. Pallor
☐ 2. Edema
☐ 3. Anorexia
☐ 4. Proteinuria
☐ 5. Weight loss
☐ 6. Decreased serum lipids

ANSWERS

346. 2

Rationale: Gross hematuria resulting in dark, smoky, cola-colored or red-brown urine is a classic symptom of glomerulonephritis, and hypertension is also common. A mid to high urinary specific gravity is associated with glomerulonephritis. BUN levels may be elevated.

Test-Taking Strategy: Use the process of elimination. Eliminate options 1 and 3 first, because hypertension and a high specific gravity are likely to occur with this kidney disorder. Recalling that BUN levels elevate in clients with this condition will assist with directing you to option 2. Review the clinical manifestations associated with glomerulonephritis if you had difficulty with this question.

Level of Cognitive Ability: Understanding
Client Needs: Physiological Integrity
Integrated Process: Nursing Process/Data Collection
Content Area: Child Health: Gastrointestinal/Renal
Reference: Leifer, p. 683. 2011.

347. 4

Rationale: Group A β-hemolytic streptococcal infection is a cause of glomerulonephritis. The child often becomes ill with streptococcal infection of the upper respiratory tract and then develops symptoms of acute poststreptococcal glomerulonephritis after an interval of 1 to 2 weeks. The data presented in options 1, 2, and 3 are unrelated to a diagnosis of glomerulonephritis.

Test-Taking Strategy: Use your knowledge regarding the causes of glomerulonephritis and the process of elimination to answer the question. Option 1 relates to a kidney injury. Options 2 and 3 are not related to the diagnosis of glomerulonephritis. Review the causes of glomerulonephritis if you had difficulty with this question.

Level of Cognitive Ability: Understanding
Client Needs: Physiological Integrity
Integrated Process: Nursing Process/Data Collection
Content Area: Child Health: Gastrointestinal/Renal
Reference: Leifer, p. 683. 2011.

348. 1

Rationale: HUS is thought to be associated with bacterial toxins, chemicals, and viruses that cause acute renal failure in children. Clinical features of the disease include acquired hemolytic anemia, thrombocytopenia, renal injury, and central nervous system symptoms. A child with HUS who is undergoing peritoneal dialysis for the treatment of anuria will be on fluid restrictions. Pain is not associated with HUS, and potassium would be restricted rather than encouraged if the child was anuric. Peritoneal dialysis does not require an AV fistula (only hemodialysis does).

Test-Taking Strategy: Focus on the child's diagnosis, and recall your knowledge of the care of a client with acute renal failure. Also focus on the data in the question. Noting the word "peritoneal" will assist you with eliminating option 3. From the remaining options, remember that because the child is anuric, fluids will be restricted. Review the care of the child with HUS if you had difficulty with this question.

Level of Cognitive Ability: Analyzing

Client Needs: Physiological Integrity
Integrated Processes: Nursing Process/Planning
Content Area: Child Health: Gastrointestinal/Renal
Reference: McKinney, James, Murray, Ashwill, p. 1161. 2009.

349. 2

Rationale: Nephrotic syndrome is defined as massive proteinuria, hypoalbuminemia, and edema. The urine is dark, foamy, and frothy, but microscopic hematuria may be present. Frank, bright red blood in the urine does not occur. Urine output is decreased, and the blood pressure is normal or slightly decreased.

Test-Taking Strategy: Use the process of elimination. Eliminate option 3 first, because urine output is likely to be decreased in a client with a renal disorder. From the remaining options, associate edema with nephrotic syndrome, because this will be helpful to you if you encounter a similar question. Review the characteristics of nephrotic syndrome if you had difficulty with this question.

Level of Cognitive Ability: Understanding
Client Needs: Physiological Integrity
Integrated Process: Nursing Process/Data Collection
Content Area: Child Health: Gastrointestinal/Renal
Reference: Leifer, pp. 680–681. 2011.

350. 3

Rationale: The most common complications associated with orchiopexy are bleeding and infection. The parents are instructed in postoperative home care measures, including the prevention of infection, pain control, and activity restrictions. The measurement of intake and output is not required. Anticholinergics are prescribed for the relief of bladder spasms; they are not necessary after orchiopexy. Cold, wet compresses are not prescribed. The moisture from a wet compress presents a potential for infection.

Test-Taking Strategy: Note the strategic word "priority" in the question. Use Maslow's Hierarchy of Needs theory to answer the question. Of the options presented, the potential for infection is the physiological priority. Review the home care instructions after orchiopexy if you had difficulty with this question.

Level of Cognitive Ability: Applying
Client Needs: Physiological Integrity
Integrated Process: Teaching and Learning
Content Area: Child Health: Gastrointestinal/Renal
Reference: Leifer, p. 688. 2011.

351. 3

Rationale: All vigorous activities should be restricted for 2 weeks after surgery to promote healing and prevent injury. This will prevent dislodging of the suture, which is internal. Normally 2-year-old children will want to be very active. Therefore, allowing the child to decide when to return to his play activities may prevent healing and cause injury. The parents should be taught to monitor the child's temperature, provide analgesics, as needed, and monitor the urine output.

Test-Taking Strategy: Note the strategic words "further teaching is necessary." These words indicate a negative event query and ask you to select an option that is an incorrect statement. Option 1 is an important action for recognizing signs of infection. Option 2 is appropriate for keeping pain to a

minimum. Option 4 monitors the voiding pattern, which is also important after this type of surgery. Review the discharge instructions after the surgical correction of cryptorchidism if you had difficulty with this question.
Level of Cognitive Ability: Evaluating
Client Needs: Physiological Integrity
Integrated Process: Teaching and Learning
Content Area: Child Health: Gastrointestinal/Renal
References: McKinney, James, Murray, Ashwill, p. 1153. 2009. Perry, Hockenberry, Lowdermilk, Wilson, p. 1535. 2010.

352. 2
Rationale: Epispadias is a congenital defect that involves the abnormal placement of the urethral orifice of the penis. In clients with this condition, the urethral opening is located anywhere on the dorsum of the penis. This anatomical characteristic leads to the easy access of bacterial entry into the urine. Options 1, 3, and 4 are not characteristically noted with this condition.
Test-Taking Strategy: Use your knowledge regarding the anatomical characteristics of epispadias and the process of elimination to answer the question. Options 1, 3, and 4 do not relate to the potential for infection, which can be present with this condition. Review the diagnostic findings associated with epispadias if you had difficulty with this question.
Level of Cognitive Ability: Analyzing
Client Needs: Physiological Integrity
Integrated Process: Nursing Process/Data Collection
Content Area: Child Health: Gastrointestinal/Renal
Reference: Perry, Hockenberry, Lowdermilk, Wilson, p. 1531. 2010.

353. 2
Rationale: After hypospadias repair, the parents are instructed to avoid giving the child a tub bath until the stent has been removed to prevent infection. Diapers are placed on the child to prevent the contamination of the surgical site. Toilet training should not be an issue during this stressful period. Fluids should be encouraged to maintain hydration.
Test-Taking Strategy: Use the process of elimination. Option 3 is eliminated first, because toilet training should not be initiated during times of stress, such as after surgery. Eliminate option 1, because this action can cause the contamination of the surgical site. Option 4 is inappropriate, because fluids should be encouraged rather than restricted. Review the postoperative care after the surgical repair of hypospadias if you had difficulty with this question.

Level of Cognitive Ability: Applying
Client Needs: Physiological Integrity
Integrated Process: Teaching and Learning
Content Area: Child Health: Gastrointestinal/Renal
Reference: Hockenberry, Wilson, p. 958. 2009.

354. 4
Rationale: Bladder exstrophy is a congenital anomaly that is characterized by the extrusion of the urinary bladder to the outside of the body through a defect in the lower abdominal wall. The cause is unknown, and there is a higher incidence among males. Options 1, 2, and 3 are not characteristics of this disorder.
Test Taking Strategy: Use the process of elimination. If you are unfamiliar with this condition, note the relationship of the word "exstrophy" in the name of the disorder with the word "extrusion" in the correct option; this should remind you that this condition is located external to the body. Review the characteristics of bladder exstrophy if you had difficulty with this question.
Level of Cognitive Ability: Understanding
Client Needs: Physiological Integrity
Integrated Process: Nursing Process/Implementation
Content Area: Child Health: Gastrointestinal/Renal
Reference: Leifer, p. 678. 2011.

355. 1, 2, 3, 4
Rationale: Nephrotic syndrome is a kidney disorder that is characterized by massive proteinuria, hypoalbuminemia, edema, elevated serum lipids, anorexia, and pallor. The urine volume is decreased, and the urine is dark and frothy in appearance. The child with this condition gains weight.
Test-Taking Strategy: Note the child's diagnosis and think about the definition of nephrotic syndrome and its associated characteristics to answer the question. Remember it is characterized by massive proteinuria, hypoalbuminemia, edema, elevated serum lipids, anorexia, and pallor. Review the clinical manifestations associated with nephrotic syndrome if you had difficulty with this question.
Level of Cognitive Ability: Analyzing
Client Needs: Physiological Integrity
Integrated Process: Nursing Process/Data Collection
Content Area: Child Health: Gastrointestinal/Renal
References: Christensen, Kockrow, pp. 1026-1028. 2011. *Foundations of nursing.*
Leifer, pp. 680-681. 2011.

Integumentary Disorders

I. ATOPIC DERMATITIS (ECZEMA)

A. Description
1. A superficial inflammatory process that primarily involves the epidermis and that is characterized by pruritic lesions
2. Associated with family history of the disorder, allergies, asthma, or allergic rhinitis.
3. The major goals of management are to relieve pruritus, hydrate the skin, reduce inflammation, and prevent or control secondary infections

B. Forms of eczema (Box 36-1)

C. Data collection (Box 36-2)

D. Interventions
1. Avoid exposure to skin irritants such as soaps, detergents, fabric softeners, diaper wipes, and powder.
2. Avoid excessive bathing and washing of affected areas; bathing water should be tepid and the skin should be lubricated immediately after the bath.
3. Intermittently apply cool, wet compresses for short periods to soothe the skin and alleviate itching; pat the skin dry between cooling treatments.
4. Administer antihistamines and topical corticosteroids, as prescribed. Corticosteroids are applied in a thin layer and rubbed into the area thoroughly.
5. Immunomodulator medications may be prescribed.
6. Antibiotics may be prescribed if secondary infections occur.
7. Prevent or minimize scratching. Keep the nails short and clean, and place gloves or cotton socks over the hands.
8. Eliminate conditions that increase itching, such as wet diapers, excessive bathing, ambient heat, woolen clothes or blankets, and proximity to rough fabrics or furry stuffed animals; exposure to latex should also be avoided.
9. Instruct the parents to wash the child's clothing in a mild detergent and rinse it thoroughly. Putting the clothes through a second complete wash cycle without detergent will minimize the amount of residue remaining on the fabric.
10. Instruct the parents in the measures to prevent skin infections.
11. Instruct the parents to monitor the lesions for signs of infection (i.e., honey-colored crusts with surrounding erythema), and to seek immediate medical intervention if such signs are noted.

⚠ A child with an integumentary disorder needs to be monitored for signs of either a skin infection or a systemic infection.

II. IMPETIGO

A. Description
1. A highly contagious bacterial infection of the skin caused by β-hemolytic streptococci, *Staphylococcus aureus,* or both.
2. Impetigo can occur because of poor hygiene. It can be a primary infection or occur secondarily at a site that has been injured or at a site that was originally a rash, such as caused by exposure to poison ivy or poison oak.
3. The most common sites of infection are the face, around the mouth, the hands, the neck, and the extremities.
4. The lesions begin as vesicles or pustules surrounded by edema and redness (a pustule is similar to a vesicle except its fluid content is purulent).
5. After the crusting of the lesions, the initially serous vesicular fluid becomes cloudy, and the

---

Box 36-1 Forms of Eczema

Infantile
Usually begins at 2 to 6 months of age; generally undergoes spontaneous remission by 3 years of age

Childhood
May follow the infantile form; occurs at 2 to 3 years of age

Preadolescent and Adolescent
Begins at about 12 years of age; may continue into the early adult years or indefinitely

vesicle ruptures, leaving a honey-colored crust that covers an ulcerated base.

B. Data collection
1. Lesions
2. Erythema
3. Pruritus
4. Burning
5. Secondary lymph node involvement

C. Interventions
1. Contact isolation. Use standard precautions and implement agency-specific isolation procedures for the hospitalized child. Strict hygiene practices are important because it is a highly contagious condition.
2. Allow lesions to dry by air exposure.
3. Assist the child with daily bathing with antibacterial soap, as prescribed.
4. Apply warm compresses to lesions two or three times per day, as prescribed, to help with the removal of crusts and allow healing.
5. Apply topical antibiotic ointments and instruct the parents in their use; the infection is still communicable for 48 hours beyond initiation of antibiotic treatment.
6. Administer oral antibiotics, which may be prescribed if there is no response to topical antibiotic treatment. It is extremely important to comply with the prescribed antibiotic regimen because secondary infections such as glomerulonephritis may result if the infectious agent is of a streptococcal type that can affect the nephrons.
7. Apply and instruct the parents in the use of emollients, as prescribed, to prevent skin cracking.
8. Instruct the parents in the methods of preventing the spread of the infection, especially careful handwashing.
9. Inform the parents that the child needs to use separate towels, linens, and dishes.
10. Inform the parents that all linens and clothing should be washed separately with detergent in hot water.

III. PEDICULOSIS CAPITIS (LICE)

A. Description
1. An infestation of the hair and scalp with lice
2. The most common sites of involvement are the occipital area, behind the ears, at the nape of the neck, and, occasionally, the eyebrows and eyelashes.
3. The female louse lays her eggs (nits) on the hair shaft, close to the scalp. The incubation period is 7 to 10 days.
4. Head lice live and reproduce only on humans and are transmitted by direct and indirect contact, such as the sharing of brushes, hats, towels, and bedding.
5. All contacts of the infested child should be examined for lice infestation and referred for treatment as appropriate.

B. Data collection (Box 36-3)

C. Interventions
1. Use a pediculicide product (usually permethrin 1% cream rinse [Nix]) as prescribed; follow package instructions for timing the application and for contraindications for their use in children.
2. Daily removal of nits with an extra-fine-tooth metal nit comb should be done as a control measure after use of the pediculicide product. Gloves should be worn for removal of nits. Hairbrushes or combs should be discarded or soaked in boiling water for 10 minutes or in a commercially available lice-killing product for 1 hour.
3. Instruct the parents that siblings may also need treatment; grooming items are not to be shared and a single comb or brush should be used for each individual child.
4. Instruct the parents that bedding and clothing used by the child should be changed daily, laundered in hot water with detergent, and dried in a hot dryer for 20 minutes; this process should continue for 1 week.
5. Instruct the parents that nonessential bedding and clothing can be stored in a tightly sealed bag for 2 weeks and then washed.

Box 36-2 Data Collection Findings: Atopic Dermatitis (Eczema)

- Redness
- Scaliness
- Itching
- Minute papules (firm elevated circumscribed lesions smaller than 1 cm in diameter) and vesicles (similar to papules but fluid-filled)
- Weeping, oozing, and crusting of lesions
- Adolescent and early adult forms commonly occur in antecubital and popliteal areas.

Box 36-3 Data Collection Findings: Pediculosis Capitis

- Child scratches the scalp excessively.
- Pruritis is caused by the crawling insect and insect saliva on the skin
- Nits (white eggs) are observable on the hair shaft (it is important to differentiate nits from lint or dandruff, which flakes away easily)
- Adult lice are difficult to see and appear as small tan or grayish specks, which may crawl fast.

6. Instruct the parents to seal toys that cannot be washed or dry-cleaned in a plastic bag for 2 weeks.
7. Instruct the parents that furniture and carpets need to be vacuumed frequently, and that the dust bag from the vacuum should be discarded after vacuuming.
8. Teach the child not to share clothing, headwear, brushes, and combs.
9. Lice of the eyelashes or eyebrows may need to be removed manually.

IV. SCABIES

A. Description
1. A parasitic skin disorder caused by an infestation of *Sarcoptes scabiei* (itch mite)
2. Endemic among schoolchildren and institutionalized populations as a result of close personal contact
3. Incubation period
   a. Female mite burrows into the epidermis, lays eggs, and dies in the burrow after 4 to 5 weeks
   b. The eggs hatch in 3 to 5 days, and the larvae migrate to the skin to mature and complete their life cycle
4. Infectious period: During the course of the infestation

B. Data collection (Box 36-4)

⚠ Scabies is transmitted by close personal contact with an infected person. Household members and contacts of an infected child need to be treated simultaneously.

C. Interventions
1. Topical application of a scabicide such as permethrin (Elimite) kills the mites.
2. Lindane, an alternative product that may be prescribed, should not be used in children younger than 2 years because of the risk of neurotoxicity and seizures.
3. Instruct the parents in the application of the scabicide.
4. When permethrin is used, it is applied to cool dry skin at least 30 minutes after bathing, the cream is massaged thoroughly and gently into all skin surfaces (not just the areas that have the rash) from the head to the soles of the feet (avoid contact with the eyes), left on the skin for 8 to 14 hours,

and then removed by bathing. A repeat treatment may be necessary.
5. Household members and contacts of the infected child need to be treated at the same time.
6. Instruct the parents about the importance of frequent handwashing.
7. Instruct the parents that all clothing, bedding, and pillowcases used by the child need to be changed daily, washed in hot water with detergent, dried in a hot dryer, and ironed before reuse; this process should continue for one week.
8. Instruct the parents that nonwashable toys and other items should be sealed in plastic bags for 4 days.
9. Anti-itch topical treatment may be necessary and antibiotics may be prescribed if a secondary infection develops.

V. THE BURNED CHILD (see Priority Nursing Actions)

A. Pediatric differences (see Chapter 41 for additional information about burns)

■■■ PRIORITY NURSING ACTIONS! ■■■
Actions to Take in the Event of a Major Burn Injury
1. Stop the burning process.
2. Check circulation, airway, and breathing status.
3. Begin resuscitation if necessary.
4. Remove burned clothing and jewelry.
5. Cover the wound with a clean cloth.
6. Keep the child warm.
7. Transport the child to the emergency department.

The initial management of the burn injury begins at the scene of the injury. The first priority is to stop the burning process; this must be done before other interventions. To stop the burning process, flames should be smothered. The child should be placed in a horizontal position because a vertical position may cause the hair to ignite or the inhalation of flames, heat, or smoke. The child should be rolled in a blanket or other article taking care not to cover the face and head because of the danger of inhaling smoke and fumes. As soon as the flames are extinguished, the child's circulation, airway, and breathing status is checked. Measures are taken immediately if resuscitation is necessary. Burned clothing and jewelry are removed to prevent further burning of the skin and disruption of skin integrity, and then the burn is covered with a clean cloth, which prevents contamination of the wound, reduces pain by eliminating air contact, and prevents hypothermia. The child is also kept warm to prevent hypothermia and is immediately transported to the nearest emergency facility.

Reference: Perry, S., Hockenberry, M., Lowdermilk, D., & Wilson, D. (2010). *Maternal child nursing care* (4th ed., pp. 1664–1665). St. Louis: Mosby.

Box 36-4 Data Collection Findings: Scabies
- Pruritic papular rash
- Burrows on the skin (fine grayish-red lines that may be difficult to see)

1. Very young children who have been severely burned have a higher mortality rate than older children and adults with comparable burns.
2. Lower burn temperatures and shorter exposure to heat can cause a more severe burn in a child than an adult because a child's skin is thinner.
3. The degree of pain experienced by the child and the ability to communicate it will be different than in an adult with the same exposure.
4. Severely burned children are at increased risk for fluid and heat loss, dehydration, and metabolic acidosis than an adult.
5. The higher proportion of body fluid to mass in children increases the risk of cardiovascular problems.
6. Burns involving more than 10% of the total body surface area require some form of fluid resuscitation.
7. Infants and children are at increased risk for protein and calorie deficiency because they have smaller muscle mass and less body fat than adults.
8. Scarring is more severe in a child; disturbed body image will be a distinct issue for a child or adolescent, especially as **growth** continues.
9. An immature immune system presents an increased risk of infection for infants and young children.
10. A delay in **growth** may occur following a burn.

B. Extent of burn injury
1. The rule of nines, used for an adult with a burn injury, gives an inaccurate estimate in children because of the difference in body proportions between children and adults.
2. In the pediatric client, the extent of the burn is expressed as a percent of the total body surface area (TBSA) using age-related charts (Figure 36-1).

C. Fluid replacement therapy

⚠ To determine adequacy of fluid resuscitation, vital signs (especially heart rate), urine output, adequacy of capillary filling, and sensorium status are assessed.

1. Fluid replacement is necessary during the initial 24-hour period following the burn injury because of the fluid shifts that occur as a result of the injury.
2. Several formulas are available to calculate the child's fluid needs and the formula used depends on the health care provider's preference.
3. Crystalloid solutions are used during the initial phase of therapy; colloid solutions such as albumin, Plasma-Lyte (combined electrolyte solution), or fresh-frozen plasma are useful in maintaining plasma volume.
4. See Chapter 41 for additional information related to burns and their management.

A RELATIVE PERCENTAGES OF AREAS AFFECTED BY GROWTH

AREA	BIRTH	AGE 1 YR	AGE 5 YR
A = ½ of head	9½	8½	6½
B = ½ of one thigh	2¾	3¼	4
C = ½ of one leg	2½	2½	2¾

B RELATIVE PERCENTAGES OF AREAS AFFECTED BY GROWTH

AREA	AGE 10 YR	AGE 15 YR	ADULT
A = ½ of head	5½	4½	3½
B = ½ of one thigh	4½	4½	4¾
C = ½ of one leg	3	3¼	3½

▲ **FIGURE 36-1** Estimation of distribution of burns in children. **A,** Children from birth to age 5 years. **B,** Older children. (From Perry, S., Hockenberry, M., Lowdermilk, D., & Wilson, D. [2010]. *Maternal child nursing care* [4th ed.]. St. Louis: Mosby.)

MORE QUESTIONS ON EVOLVE!

Practice Questions

356. A school nurse prepares a list of home care instructions for the parents of school children who have been diagnosed with pediculosis capitis (head lice). Which is included in the list?
1. Use anti-lice sprays on all bedding and furniture.
2. Use a pediculicide shampoo and repeat treatment in 14 days.
3. Launder all the bedding and clothing in cold water and dry on low heat.
4. Vacuum floors, play areas, and furniture to remove any hairs that may carry live nits.

357. A mother of a 3-year-old child tells the nurse that the child has been continuously scratching the skin and has developed a rash. On data collection, which finding indicates that the child may have scabies?
1. Fine, grayish-red lines
2. Purple-colored lesions
3. Thick, honey-colored crusts
4. Clusters of fluid-filled vesicles

358. Permethrin 5% (Elimite) is prescribed for a 4-year-old child with a diagnosis of scabies. The nurse instructs the mother regarding the use of this treatment. Which instruction is appropriate?
1. Apply the lotion and leave it on for 4 hours.
2. Apply the lotion to the hair, the face, and the entire body.
3. The child should wear no clothing while the lotion is in place.
4. Apply the lotion to cool, dry skin at least half an hour after bathing.

359. A corticosteroid cream is prescribed by a health care provider for a child with atopic dermatitis (eczema). The nurse teaches the mother how to apply the cream. Which instruction is appropriate?
1. Apply the cream over the entire body.
2. Apply a thick layer of cream to affected areas only.
3. Avoid cleansing the area before applying the cream.
4. Apply a thin layer of cream, and rub it into the area thoroughly.

360. The nurse assists in planning care for a child who sustained a burn injury based on which of the following accurate statements?
1. Scarring is not as severe in a child as in an adult.
2. Children are at a lower risk of infection than adults because of their strong immune systems.
3. Lower burn temperatures and shorter exposure to heat can cause a more severe burn in a child than an adult because a child's skin is thinner.
4. Infants and children are at decreased risk for protein and calorie deficiency because they have smaller muscle mass and less body fat than adults.

ANSWERS

356. 4
Rationale: Thorough home cleaning is necessary to remove any remaining lice or nits. Anti-lice sprays are unnecessary. Additionally, they should never be used on bedding, furniture,or a child. The pediculicide product (usually permethrin 1% cream rinse [Nix]) needs to be used as prescribed and the parents are instructed to follow package instructions for timing the application and for contraindications for their use in children. Bedding and linens should be washed with hot water and dried on a hot setting.
Test-Taking Strategy: Use the process of elimination. Eliminate option 1, knowing that anti-lice sprays should not be used. The pediculicide product needs to be used based on the manufacturer's instructions. Knowing that bedding and linens should be washed in hot water and dried on a high heat setting will eliminate option 3. Review the home care instructions for the child with pediculosis capitis if you had difficulty with this question.
Level of Cognitive Ability: Applying
Client Needs: Safe and Effective Care Environment
Integrated Process: Teaching and Learning
Content Area: Fundamental Skills: Safety/Infection Control
Reference: McKinney, James, Murray, Ashwill, p. 1352. 2009.

357. 1
Rationale: Scabies appears as burrows or fine, grayish-red lines. They may be difficult to see if they are obscured by excoriation and inflammation. Purple-colored lesions may be indicative of various disorders, including systemic conditions. Thick, honey-colored crusts are characteristic of impetigo. Clusters of fluid-filled vesicles are seen in clients with herpesvirus.
Test-Taking Strategy: Use the process of elimination. Recalling that scabies infestation produces burrows will direct you to option 1. Review the characteristics of scabies if you had difficulty with this question.
Level of Cognitive Ability: Understanding
Client Needs: Physiological Integrity
Integrated Process: Nursing Process/Data Collection
Content Area: Child Health: Integumentary/AIDS/Infectious Diseases
Reference: McKinney, James, Murray, Ashwill, p. 1353. 2009.

358. 4
Rationale: Permethrin is applied from the neck downward, with care taken to ensure that the soles of the feet, the areas behind the ears, and the areas under the toenails and fingernails are covered. The lotion should be kept on for 8 to 14 hours, and

then the child should be given a bath. The lotion should be applied at least 30 minutes after bathing, and it should be applied only to cool, dry skin. The child should be clothed during treatment.

Test-Taking Strategy: Use the process of elimination. Reading options 2 and 3 carefully will assist you with eliminating these options. From the remaining options, recalling the treatment time for this medication will direct you to option 4. Review permethrin treatment if you had difficulty with this question.

Level of Cognitive Ability: Applying
Client Needs: Physiological Integrity
Integrated Process: Teaching and Learning
Content Area: Child Health: Integumentary/AIDS/Infectious Diseases
Reference: McKinney, James, Murray, Ashwill, p. 1353. 2009.

359. 4

Rationale: Corticosteroid cream should be applied sparingly and rubbed into the area thoroughly. The affected area should be cleansed gently before application. The cream should not be applied over extensive areas. Systemic absorption is more likely to occur with extensive application.

Test-Taking Strategy: Use the process of elimination. Eliminate option 1, because the cream should only be applied to the area that is affected. Eliminate option 2 because of the words "thick" and "only." Eliminate option 3, because it does not make sense to avoid cleansing an affected area. Review the procedure for the application of corticosteroid cream if you had difficulty with this question.

Level of Cognitive Ability: Applying
Client Needs: Physiological Integrity
Integrated Process: Teaching and Learning
Content Area: Child Health: Integumentary/AIDS/Infectious Diseases
Reference: McKinney, James, Murray, Ashwill, p. 1355. 2009.

360. 3

Rationale: Lower burn temperatures and shorter exposure to heat can cause a more severe burn in a child than an adult because a child's skin is thinner. Scarring is more severe in a child; additionally, disturbed body image will be a distinct issue for a child or adolescent, especially as growth continues. An immature immune system presents an increased risk of infection for infants and young children. Infants and children are at increased risk for protein and calorie deficiency because they have smaller muscle mass and less body fat than adults.

Test-Taking Strategy: Use the process of elimination. Read each option carefully. Thinking about the anatomy and physiology of an infant and child will assist in selecting the correct option. Review the care associated with an infant or child with a burn injury if you had difficulty with this question.

Level of Cognitive Ability: Understanding
Client Needs: Physiological Integrity
Integrated Process: Nursing Process/Planning
Content Area: Child Health: Integumentary/AIDS/Infectious Diseases
Reference: McKinney, James, Murray, Ashwill, p. 1365. 2009.

Musculoskeletal Disorders

I. **DEVELOPMENTAL DYSPLASIA OF THE HIP (DDH)**

A. Description
1. Refers to disorders related to abnormal development of the hip that may develop during fetal life, infancy, or childhood; in these disorders, the head of the femur is seated improperly in the acetabulum or hip socket of the pelvis.
2. Degrees of DDH (Box 37-1)

B. Data collection (Figure 37-1)
1. Neonates: Laxity of the ligaments around the hip.
2. Infants beyond the newborn period
   a. Shortening of the limb on the affected side (Galeazzi sign, Allis sign)
   b. Restricted abduction of the hip on the affected side when the child is placed supine with the knees and hips flexed
   c. Unequal gluteal folds when the infant is prone and the legs are extended against the examining table
   d. Positive Ortolani test: The Ortolani maneuver is a test to assess for hip instability. In the Ortolani maneuver, the examiner abducts the thigh and applies gentle pressure forward over the greater trochanter. A "clunking" sensation indicates a dislocated femoral head moving into the acetabulum.
   e. Positive Barlow test: The examiner adducts the hips and applies gentle pressure down and back with the thumbs. In hip dysplasia, the examiner can feel the femoral head move out of the acetabulum.
3. Older infant and child
   a. Affected leg is shorter than the other.
   b. The head of the femur can be felt to move up and down in the buttock when the extended thigh is pushed first toward the child's head and then pulled distally.
   c. Positive Trendelenburg's sign: The child stands on one foot and then the other foot, holding onto a support and bearing weight on the affected hip; the pelvis tilts downward on the normal side instead of upward, as it would with normal stability.

d. Greater trochanter is prominent.
e. Marked lordosis or waddling gait is noted in bilateral dislocations.

C. Interventions
1. Birth to 6 months of age, splinting of the hips with a Pavlik harness to maintain flexion, abduction and, external rotation; worn continuously until the hip is stable in about 3 to 6 months (Figure 37-2).
2. Age 6 to 18 months: Gradual reduction by traction followed by closed reduction or open reduction (if necessary) under general anesthesia. The child is then placed in a hip spica cast for 2 to 4 months until the hip is stable, and then a flexion-abduction brace is applied for approximately 3 months.
3. Operative reduction may be required in the older child.
4. Instruct the parents regarding the proper care of a Pavlik harness spica cast or abduction brace.

Box 37-1 Degrees of Developmental Dysplasia of the Hip (DDH)

Acetabular Dysplasia (Preluxation)
- Mildest form
- Neither subluxation nor dislocation
- Delay in acetabular development occurs
- Femoral head remains in the acetabulum

Subluxation
- Incomplete dislocation of the hip
- Femoral head remains in the acetabulum
- Stretched capsule and ligamentum teres causes head of the femur to be partially displaced

Dislocation
- Femoral head loses contact with acetabulum and is displaced posteriorly and superiorly over the fibrocartilaginous rim
- Ligamentum teres—elongated and taut

▲ **FIGURE 37-1** Signs of developmental dysplasia of the hip. **A,** Asymmetry of gluteal and thigh folds. **B,** Limited hip abduction, as seen in flexion. **C,** Apparent shortening of the femur, as indicated by the level of the knees in flexion. **D,** Ortolani click (if infant is under 4 weeks of age). **E,** Positive Trendelenburg's sign of gait (if child is weight bearing). (From Hockenberry, M. Wilson, D., & Wilkelstein, M. [2008]. *Wong's essentials of pediatric nursing* [8th ed.]. St. Louis: Mosby.)

Front   Back

▲ **FIGURE 37-2** Child in Pavlik harness. (From Hockenberry, M. Wilson, D., & Wilkelstein, M. [2008]. *Wong's essentials of pediatric nursing* [8th ed.]. St. Louis: Mosby.)

II. CONGENITAL CLUBFOOT

A. Description

1. Complex deformity of the ankle and foot that includes forefoot adduction, midfoot supination, hindfoot varus, and ankle equinus. The defect may be unilateral or bilateral.

2. The goal of treatment is to achieve a painless plantigrade (able to walk on the sole of the foot with the heel on the ground) and stable foot.

3. Long-term interval follow-up is required until the child reaches skeletal maturity.

B. Data collection: Deformities are described based on the position of the ankle and foot.

1. Talipes varus: An inversion or bending inward

2. Talipes valgus: An eversion or bending outward

3. Talipes equinus: Plantar flexion in which the toes are lower than the heel

4. Talipes calcaneus: Dorsiflexion in which the toes are higher than the heel

C. Interventions

1. Treatment begins as soon after birth as possible.

2. Manipulation and casting are performed weekly for about 8 to 12 weeks because of the rapid **growth** of early infancy; a splint is then applied if casting and manipulation are successful.

3. Surgical intervention may be necessary if normal alignment is not achieved by about 6 to 12 weeks of age.

4. Monitor for pain and monitor the neurovascular status of the toes.

⚠️ Contact the health care provider (HCP) immediately if signs of neurovascular impairment are noted in a child with a cast or brace.

III. IDIOPATHIC SCOLIOSIS

A. Description
1. A three-dimensional spinal deformity that usually involves lateral curvature, spinal rotation that results in rib asymmetry, and hypokyphosis of the thorax (Figure 37-3)
2. Usually diagnosed during the preadolescent **growth** spurt. Screenings are important at times when **growth** spurts occur.
3. Surgical (spinal fusion and placement of an instrumentation system) and nonsurgical (bracing) interventions are used. The type of treatment depends on the location and degree of the curvature, the age of the child, the amount of **growth** that is still anticipated, and any underlying disease processes.
4. Long-term monitoring is essential to detect any progression of the curve.

B. Data collection
1. Asymmetry of the ribs and flanks is noted when the child bends forward at the waist and hangs the arms down toward the feet (Adams' test).
2. Hip height, rib positioning, and shoulder height are asymmetrical. (This can be noted when standing behind the undressed child.) A leg-length discrepancy is also apparent.
3. Radiographs are performed to confirm the diagnosis.

C. Interventions
1. Monitor the progression of the curvatures.
2. Prepare the child and parents for the use of a brace, if prescribed.
3. Prepare the child and parents for surgery (spinal fusion and the placement of internal instrumentation systems), if prescribed.

⚠️ The potential for altered role performance, body image disturbance, fear, anger, and isolation exists for a child with a disabling condition and a condition that requires wearing a body brace.

D. Braces
1. Braces are not curative, but they may slow the progression of the curvature to allow for skeletal **growth** and maturity.
2. Braces usually are prescribed to be worn from 16 to 23 hours a day.
3. Inspect the skin for signs of redness or breakdown.
4. Keep the skin clean and dry, and avoid lotions and powders.

▲ **FIGURE 37-3** Scoliosis in a standing erect posture. (From Lemmi, F.O., & Lemmi, C.A.E. [2000]. *Physical assessment findings CD-ROM*. Philadelphia: Saunders.)

5. Advise the child to wear soft, nonirritating clothing under the brace.
6. Instruct the child and parents in the prescribed exercises, which help to maintain and strengthen the spinal and abdominal muscles during treatment.
7. Encourage verbalization about body image and other psychosocial issues.

E. Postoperative interventions
1. Maintain proper alignment. Avoid twisting movements.
2. Logroll the child when turning him or her to maintain alignment.
3. Assess the extremities for neurovascular status.
4. Encourage coughing, deep breathing, and the use of incentive spirometry.
5. Check for pain and administer analgesics, as prescribed.
6. Monitor for incontinence.
7. Monitor for signs and symptoms of infection.
8. Monitor for superior mesenteric artery syndrome, which is caused by mechanical changes in the position of the child's abdominal contents during surgery, and notify the HCP if it occurs. Symptoms include emesis and abdominal distention similar to that which occurs with intestinal obstruction or paralytic ileus.
9. Instruct the child and parents regarding activity restrictions.

10. Instruct the child how to logroll from a side-lying position to a sitting position, and assist with ambulation.
11. Prepare the child for the use of a molded plastic orthosis (brace) jacket to provide external stability of the spine when resuming activities.
12. Be alert to signs of a body image problem.

IV. JUVENILE IDIOPATHIC ARTHRITIS

A. Description
1. An autoimmune, inflammatory disease affecting the joints and other tissues, such as articular cartilage, that most often occurs in girls.
2. Treatment is supportive (there is no cure) and directed toward preserving joint function, controlling inflammation, minimizing deformity, and reducing the impact that the disease may have on the development of the child.
3. Treatment includes medications, physical and occupational therapies, and child and family education.
4. Surgical intervention may be implemented if the child has problems with joint contractures and unequal **growth** of extremities.

B. Data collection (Box 37-2)
1. There are no definitive tests to diagnose the condition.
2. Certain laboratory tests (e.g., an elevated erythrocyte sedimentation rate, the presence of leukocytosis) may support evidence of the disease.
3. Radiographs may show soft tissue swelling and joint space widening as a result of increased synovial fluid in the joint.

C. Interventions
1. Facilitate social and emotional development.
2. Instruct the parents and child in the administration of medications. Medications may be given alone or in combination and are prescribed in a steplike fashion that is dependent on the disease's response to each level (Box 37-3).

3. Assist the child with range-of-motion exercises. Instruct the child and parents with regard to prescribed exercises.
4. Encourage the normal performance of activities of daily living.
5. Instruct the parents and child in the use of hot and cold packs, splinting, and positioning the affected joint in a neutral position during painful episodes.
6. Encourage and support prescribed physical and occupational therapy.
7. Instruct the child and parents in the importance of preventive eye care and the reporting of visual disturbances.
8. Assess the child's and family's perceptions regarding the chronic illness. Plan to discuss the nature of a chronic illness and the grief associated with the new recognition of life alterations that result from the chronic progression of the disorder.

Box 37-3 Medications Used to Treat Juvenile Idiopathic Arthritis

Nonsteroidal Anti-inflammatory Drugs (NSAIDs)
- First medications used
- May cause gastrointestinal irritation and bruising

Methotrexate
- Used if NSAIDs are ineffective
- Complete blood cell counts and liver function studies are monitored closely

Corticosteroids
- Potent immunosuppressives that are used to treat life-threatening complications, incapacitating arthritis, and uveitis
- Administered at the lowest effective dose for the briefest period and discontinued on a tapering schedule
- Prolonged use can cause Cushing's syndrome, osteoporosis, increased infection risk, glucose intolerance, cataracts, and growth suppression

Tumor Necrosis Factor Receptor Inhibitors

Etanercept (Enbrel)

Infliximab (Remicade)
- Adverse effects include an allergic reaction at the injection site, increased risk for infection, demyelinating disease, and pancytopenia

Slower-Acting Antirheumatic Drugs (SAARDs)
- May require months to be effective
- Usually prescribed in combination with NSAIDs
- Category includes medications such as sulfasalazine (Azulfidine), hydroxychloroquine (Plaquenil), gold sodium thiomalate (Myochrysine), and D-penicillamine

---

Box 37-2 Data Collection: Juvenile Idiopathic Arthritis

Stiffness, swelling, and limited motion occur in the affected joints.

The affected joints are warm to the touch, tender, and painful.

Joint stiffness is present on arising in the morning and after inactivity.

Uveitis (the inflammation of structures in the uveal tract) can occur and cause blindness.

V. MARFAN SYNDROME

A. Description
1. A disorder of connective tissue that affects the skeletal system, cardiovascular system, eyes, and skin.
2. It is caused by defects in a gene called fibrillin-1, which serves as a building block for elastic tissue in the body; also, the disorder may be inherited.
3. There is no cure for the disorder.

B. Data collection
1. Tall and thin body structure; slender fingers, long arms and legs.
2. Curvature of the spine
3. Presence of cardiac problems

C. Interventions
1. Monitor for vision problems and obtain visual exams on a regular schedule.
2. Monitor for curvature of the spine, especially during adolescence.
3. Cardiac medications may be prescribed to slow the heart rate, which will decrease stress on the aorta.
4. Instruct the parents that the child should avoid participating in competitive athletics and contact sports to avoid injuring the heart.
5. Instruct the parents to inform the dentist of the condition; antibiotics should be taken before dental procedures to prevent endocarditis.
6. Surgical replacement of the aortic root and valve may be necessary.

VI. FRACTURES

A. Description
1. A break in the continuity of the bone as a result of trauma, twisting, or bone decalcification
2. Fractures in children usually occur as a result of increased mobility and inadequate or immature motor and cognitive skills; they may result from trauma or bone diseases such as congenital bone disease or bone tumors.

⚠ Fractures in infancy are generally rare and warrant further investigation to rule out the possibility of child abuse and recognize bone structure defects.

B. Data collection
1. Pain or tenderness over the involved area
2. Obvious deformity
3. Edema
4. Ecchymosis
5. Muscle spasm
6. Loss of function
7. Crepitation

C. Initial care of a fracture (see Priority Nursing Actions)

▰▰▰▰ PRIORITY NURSING ACTIONS! ▰▰▰▰

Actions to Take if a Child Sustains an Extremity Fracture

1. Check the extent of the injury and immobilize the affected extremity.
2. If a compound fracture exists, cover the wound with a sterile dressing. (Apply a clean dressing if a sterile dressing is unavailable.)
3. Elevate the injured extremity.
4. Apply cold packs to the injured area.
5. Continue to monitor neurovascular status.
6. Transport to the nearest emergency department.

If a child sustains a fracture, the extent of the injury is immediately assessed using the five "Ps"—pain and point of tenderness, pulses distal to fracture site, pallor, paresthesia (sensation) distal to the fracture site, and paralysis (movement distal to fracture site). The extremity is immobilized to prevent movement and further injury to soft tissues. If an open wound is present, it is covered to reduce the risk of infection. The extremity is elevated to reduce swelling, and cold packs are applied to assist in reducing the swelling and to reduce the pain. The neurovascular status is monitored closely, and the child is transported to the nearest emergency facility.

Reference: Perry, S., Hockenberry, M., Lowdermilk, D., & Wilson, D. (2010). *Maternal child nursing care* (4th ed., p. 1684). St. Louis: Mosby.

D. Interventions
1. Reduction
   a. Restoring the bone to proper alignment
   b. Closed reduction: Accomplished by the manual alignment of the fragments and followed by immobilization
   c. Open reduction: Requires the surgical insertion of internal fixation devices (e.g., rods, wires, pins) that help maintain alignment while healing occurs
2. Retention: The application of traction or a cast to maintain alignment until healing occurs

E. Traction
1. Russell's skin traction
   a. Used to stabilize a fractured femur before surgery
   b. Similar to Buck's traction but provides a double pull with the use of a knee sling
   c. Traction pulls at the knee and the foot
2. Balanced suspension
   a. Used with skin or skeletal traction to approximate fractures of the femur, tibia, or fibula
   b. Traction is produced by a counterforce other than the child
   c. Provide pin care if pins are used with the skeletal traction.

3. 90-degree–90-degree traction
   a. The lower leg is supported by a boot cast or a calf sling.
   b. A skeletal Steinmann pin or Kirschner wire is placed in the distal fragment of the femur, allowing 90-degree angle at both the hip and the knee.
4. Interventions
   a. Maintain the correct amount of weight, as prescribed.
   b. Ensure that the weights hang freely. They must not be resting on the floor or bed.
   c. Check the ropes for fraying, and be sure that they are placed appropriately on the pulleys.
   d. Monitor the neurovascular status of the involved extremity frequently.
   e. Protect the skin from breakdown.
   f. Monitor for signs and symptoms of complications of immobilization, such as constipation, skin breakdown, lung congestion, renal complications, and disuse syndrome of unaffected extremities.
   g. Monitor for sensory deprivation. Provide therapeutic and diversional play.

F. Casts
1. Description
   a. Made of plaster or fiberglass to provide for the immobilization of bones and joints after a fracture or injury
   b. Fractures of the hip or the knee may require a spica cast.
2. Interventions
   a. Examine the cast for pressure areas.
   b. Ensure that no rough casting material remains in contact with the skin; assist with petaling the cast edges as necessary.
   c. If a hip spica cast is placed, the cast edges around the perineum and buttocks may need to be taped with waterproof tape.
   d. Monitor the extremity for circulatory impairment, such as more pain than that expected for the type of injury, edema, rubor, pallor, numbness and tingling, coolness, decreased sensation or mobility, or diminished pulse.
   e. Notify the HCP if circulatory impairment occurs.
   f. Prepare for bivalving or cutting the cast if circulatory impairment occurs; prepare for emergency fasciotomy if cast removal does not improve the neurocirculatory compromise.
   g. Instruct the family and child not to stick objects down the cast.
   h. Teach the family and the child to keep the cast clean and dry.
   i. Instruct the family and the child in isometric exercises to prevent muscle atrophy.

Practice Questions

361. A nurse is providing instructions to the parents of a child with scoliosis regarding the use of a brace. Which statement by a parent indicates the need for further instruction?
1. "I need to have my child wear a soft fabric under the brace."
2. "I will apply lotion under the brace to prevent skin breakdown."
3. "I need to encourage my child to perform the prescribed exercises."
4. "I need to avoid applying powder under the brace, because it will cake."

362. The mother of a child with juvenile idiopathic arthritis calls the nurse because the child is experiencing a painful exacerbation of the disease. The mother asks the nurse if the child should perform range-of-motion (ROM) exercises at this time. The nurse makes which response to the mother?
1. "Avoid all exercise during painful periods."
2. "The ROM exercises must be performed every day."
3. "Have the child perform simple isometric exercises during this time."
4. "Administer additional pain medication before performing the ROM exercises."

363. A 4-year-old child sustains a fall at home and is brought to the emergency department by the mother. After an x-ray, it is determined that the child has a fractured arm, and a plaster cast is applied. The nurse provides instructions to the mother regarding cast care for the child. Which statement by the mother indicates the need for further instructions?
1. "The cast may feel warm as it dries."
2. "I can use lotion or powder around the cast edges to relieve itching."
3. "A small amount of white shoe polish can touch up a soiled white cast."
4. "If the cast becomes wet, a blow-dryer set on the cool setting may be used to dry it."

364. A nurse is preparing to perform a neurovascular check for tissue perfusion in the child with an arm cast. Which of the following is the priority when performing this procedure?
1. Taking the temperature
2. Taking the blood pressure
3. Checking the apical heart rate
4. Checking the peripheral pulse in the affected arm

365. A nurse is performing a neurovascular check on a child with a cast applied to the lower leg. The child complains of tingling in the toes distal to the fracture site. Which action should be taken by the nurse?
1. Elevate the extremity.
2. Document the findings.
3. Notify the health care provider (HCP).
4. Ambulate the child with crutches.

366. A nurse is assisting a health care provider (HCP) during the examination of an infant with hip dysplasia. The HCP performs the Ortolani maneuver. Which of the following best describes the action/purpose of the Ortolani maneuver?
1. Determining the extent of range of motion
2. Checking for asymmetry on the affected side
3. Pushing the unstable femoral head out of the acetabulum
4. Reducing the dislocated femoral head back into the acetabulum

367. A nurse provides information to the mother of a 2-week-old infant who was diagnosed with clubfoot at the time of birth. Which statement by the mother indicates the need for further instruction regarding this disorder?
1. "Treatment needs to be started as soon as possible."
2. "I realize my child will require follow-up care until full grown."
3. "I need to bring my child back to the clinic in 1 month for a new cast."
4. "I need to come to the clinic every week with my child for the casting."

368. A nurse is assigned to care for a child after a spinal fusion for the treatment of scoliosis. The child complains of abdominal discomfort and begins to have episodes of vomiting. On data collection, the nurse notes abdominal distention. Which action should the nurse take?
1. Administer an antiemetic.
2. Increase the intravenous fluids.
3. Notify the registered nurse (RN).
4. Place the child in a side-lying Sims' position.

369. A nurse is assigned to care for a child who is in skeletal traction. The nurse avoids which of the following when caring for the child?
1. Keeping the weights hanging freely
2. Ensuring that the ropes are in the pulleys
3. Placing the bed linens on the traction ropes
4. Ensuring that the weights are out of the child's reach

370. A nurse prepares a list of home care instructions for the parents of a child who has a plaster cast applied to the left forearm. Choose the instructions that would be included on the list. **Select all that apply.**
☐ 1. Use the fingertips to lift the cast while it is drying.
☐ 2. Keep small toys and sharp objects away from the cast.
☐ 3. Use a padded ruler or another padded object to scratch the skin under the cast if it itches.
☐ 4. Place a heating pad on the lower end of the cast and over the fingers if the fingers feel cold.
☐ 5. Contact the health care provider (HCP) if the child complains of numbness or tingling in the extremity.
☐ 6. Elevate the extremity on pillows for the first 24 to 48 hours after casting to prevent swelling.

ANSWERS

361. 2
Rationale: The use of either lotions or powders should be avoided, because they can become sticky or cake under the brace, thus causing irritation. Options 1, 3, and 4 are appropriate statements regarding the care of a child with a brace.
Test-Taking Strategy: Use the process of elimination, and note the strategic words "need for further instruction." These words indicate a negative event query and ask you to select an option that is an incorrect statement. Recalling that lotions and powders need to be avoided will direct you to option 2. Review the home care instructions for a child in a brace if you had difficulty with this question.
Level of Cognitive Ability: Evaluating
Client Needs: Physiological Integrity
Integrated Process: Teaching and Learning

Content Area: Child Health: Neurological/Musculoskeletal
Reference: McKinney, James, Murray, Ashwill, p. 1417. 2009.

362. 3
Rationale: During painful episodes, hot or cold packs, splinting, and positioning the affected joint in a neutral position help to reduce the pain. Although resting the extremity is appropriate, it is important to begin simple isometric or tensing exercises as soon as the child is able. These exercises do not involve joint movement.
Test-Taking Strategy: Use the process of elimination. Eliminate options 1, 2, and 4 because of the words "all," "must," and "additional," respectively, in each these options. Review pain management and care during exacerbations of juvenile idiopathic arthritis if you had difficulty with this question.
Level of Cognitive Ability: Applying

Client Needs: Physiological Integrity
Integrated Process: Nursing Process/Implementation
Content Area: Child Health: Neurological/Musculoskeletal
Reference: Christensen, Kockrow, p. 1003. 2011. *Foundations of nursing.*

363. 2

Rationale: The mother needs to be instructed to not use lotion or powders on the skin around the cast edges or inside the cast, because they can become sticky or caked and cause skin irritation. Options 1, 3, and 4 are appropriate instructions.
Test-Taking Strategy: Use the process of elimination, and note the strategic words "indicates the need for further instructions." These words indicate a negative event query and ask you to select an option that is an incorrect statement. Recalling the principles related to routine cast care should direct you to the correct option. Review home care instructions regarding cast care if you had difficulty with this question.
Level of Cognitive Ability: Evaluating
Client Needs: Physiological Integrity
Integrated Process: Teaching and Learning
Content Area: Child Health: Neurological/Musculoskeletal
Reference: Swearingen, p. 588. 2012.

364. 4

Rationale: The neurovascular check for tissue perfusion is performed on the toes or fingers distal to an injury or cast and includes checking peripheral pulse, color, capillary refill time, warmth, motion, and sensation. Options 1, 2, and 3 may be components of care, but they are not the priority in this situation.
Test-Taking Strategy: Use the process of elimination, and note the strategic word "priority." Option 4 is the only option that addresses a neurovascular check. Review the components of a neurovascular check if you had difficulty with this question.
Level of Cognitive Ability: Applying
Client Needs: Physiological Integrity
Integrated Process: Nursing Process/Data Collection
Content Area: Child Health: Neurological/Musculoskeletal
Reference: Swearingen, pp. 587–588. 2012.

365. 3

Rationale: Reduced sensation to touch or complaints of numbness or tingling at a site distal to the fracture may indicate poor tissue perfusion. This finding should be reported to the registered nurse or HCP. Options 1, 2, and 4 are inappropriate and would delay the required and immediate interventions.
Test-Taking Strategy: Use the process of elimination, and recall the signs of circulatory compromise. Noting the child's complaint will assist with directing you to the correct option. Review the complications associated with a cast if you had difficulty with this question.
Level of Cognitive Ability: Applying
Client Needs: Physiological Integrity
Integrated Process: Nursing Process/Implementation
Content Area: Child Health: Neurological/Musculoskeletal
Reference: Swearingen, pp. 587–588. 2012.

366. 4

Rationale: With the Ortolani maneuver, the examiner reduces the dislocated femoral head back into the acetabulum. A positive Ortolani maneuver is a palpable clunk as the femoral head

moves over the acetabular ring. Options 1 and 2 are data collection techniques for the identification of the clinical manifestations of hip dysplasia, but they do not describe the Ortolani maneuver. When performing the Barlow maneuver, the examiner pushes the unstable femoral head out of the acetabulum.
Test-Taking Strategy: Use the process of elimination. Eliminate options 1 and 2 first, because they are data collection techniques. From the remaining options, it is necessary to know the action/purpose of the Ortolani maneuver. Review the Ortolani maneuver if you had difficulty with this question.
Level of Cognitive Ability: Understanding
Client Needs: Physiological Integrity
Integrated Process: Nursing Process/Data Collection
Content Area: Child Health: Neurological/Musculoskeletal
Reference: Hockenberry, Wilson, pp. 1122–1123. 2009.

367. 3

Rationale: The treatment for clubfoot is started as soon as possible after birth. Serial manipulation and casting are performed at least weekly. If sufficient correction is not achieved within 3 to 6 months, surgery is usually indicated. Because clubfoot can recur, all children with the condition require long-term interval follow-up until they reach skeletal maturity to ensure an optimal outcome.
Test-Taking Strategy: Use the process of elimination, and focus on the subject, the treatment plan for clubfoot. Note the strategic words "indicates the need for further instruction." These words indicate a negative event query and the need to select the incorrect statement. This will assist you with eliminating options 1 and 2. Recalling that serial manipulations and casting are required weekly will direct you to option 3. Review the treatment procedures for clubfoot if you had difficulty with this question.
Level of Cognitive Ability: Evaluating
Client Needs: Physiological Integrity
Integrated Process: Teaching and Learning
Content Area: Child Health: Neurological/Musculoskeletal
References: Christensen, Kockrow, pp. 1038–1039. 2011. *Foundations of nursing.*
Leifer, pp. 329–330. 2011.

368. 3

Rationale: A complication after the surgical treatment of scoliosis is superior mesenteric artery syndrome. This disorder is caused by mechanical changes in the position of the child's abdominal contents that result from the lengthening of the child's body. It results in a syndrome of emesis and abdominal distention that is similar to that which occurs with intestinal obstruction or paralytic ileus. Postoperative vomiting among children with body casts or among those who have undergone spinal fusion warrants attention because of the possibility of superior mesenteric artery syndrome. Therefore, the remaining options are incorrect.
Test-Taking Strategy: Use the process of elimination. Eliminate option 2 first, because it should not be implemented without a prescription. Eliminate option 4 next, because this child requires logrolling, and the Sims' position may cause injury after surgery. From the remaining options, note the signs and symptoms in the question. These should alert you that the RN needs to be notified who will then contact the health care provider. Review superior mesenteric artery syndrome if you had difficulty with this question.

Level of Cognitive Ability: Analyzing
Client Needs: Physiological Integrity
Integrated Process: Nursing Process/Implementation
Content Area: Child Health: Neurological/Musculoskeletal
Reference: McKinney, James, Murray, Ashwill, p. 1418. 2009.

369. 3

Rationale: Bed linens should not be placed on the traction ropes because of the risk of disrupting the traction apparatus. Options 1, 2, and 4 are appropriate measures when caring for a child who is in skeletal traction.
Test-Taking Strategy: Note the strategic word "avoids." This word indicates a negative event query and asks you to select an option that is an incorrect intervention. Use the process of elimination and your knowledge regarding the care of the child in traction to direct you to option 3. Review the nursing measures for the child in traction if you had difficulty with this question.
Level of Cognitive Ability: Applying
Client Needs: Safe and Effective Care Environment
Integrated Process: Nursing Process/Implementation
Content Area: Child Health: Neurological/Musculoskeletal
References: Hockenberry, Wilson, p. 1120. 2009.
Leifer, p. 571. 2011.
McKinney, James, Murray, Ashwill, p. 1387. 2009.

370. 2, 5, 6

Rationale: While the cast is drying, the palms of the hands are used to lift the cast. If the fingertips are used, indentations in the cast could occur and cause constant pressure on the underlying skin. Small toys and sharp objects are kept away from the cast, and no objects (including padded objects) are placed inside of the cast because of the risk of altered skin integrity. A heating pad is not applied to the cast or fingers. Cold fingers could indicate neurovascular impairment, and the HCP should be notified. The extremity is elevated to prevent swelling, and the HCP is notified immediately if any signs of neurovascular impairment develop.
Test-Taking Strategy: Use of the ABCs—airway, breathing and circulation—and safety principles related to the care of a child with a cast will assist you with answering the question. Review these general cast care principles if you had difficulty with this question.
Level of Cognitive Ability: Applying
Client Needs: Physiological Integrity
Integrated Process: Teaching and Learning
Content Area: Child Health: Neurological/Musculoskeletal
References: Hockenberry, Wilson, p. 1116. 2009.
McKinney, James, Murray, Ashwill, p. 1388. 2009.
Swearingen, p. 588. 2012.

Hematological and Oncological Disorders

I. SICKLE CELL DISEASE

A. Description (Figure 38-1)
1. One of a group of diseases that are collectively called hemoglobinopathies in which hemoglobin (Hgb) A is partly or completely replaced by abnormal sickle hemoglobin (HgbS)
2. Caused by the inheritance of a gene for a structurally abnormal portion of the Hgb chain
3. Risk factors include having parents who are heterozygous for HgbS or being of African American descent.
4. HgbS is sensitive to changes in the oxygen content of the red blood cell (RBC).
5. Insufficient oxygen causes the cells to assume a sickle shape, and the cells become rigid and clumped together, thus obstructing capillary blood flow.
6. The clinical manifestations are primarily the result of obstruction caused by sickled RBCs and increased RBC destruction.
7. Situations that precipitate sickling include fever, dehydration, and emotional or physical stress; any condition that increases the body's need for oxygen or that alters the transport of oxygen can result in sickle cell crisis.
8. Sickle cell crises are acute exacerbations of the disease, which vary markedly in severity and frequency; these include vaso-occlusive crisis, splenic sequestration, and aplastic crisis.
9. The sickling response is reversible under conditions of adequate oxygenation and hydration; after repeated sickling, the cell becomes permanently sickled.
10. Care focuses on the prevention (preventing exposure to infection and maintaining normal hydration) and treatment (oxygen, hydration, pain management, and bedrest) of the crisis.

B. Sickle cell crisis: Data collection (Box 38-1)

C. Interventions
1. Maintain adequate hydration and blood flow with oral and intravenous (IV) administered fluids; electrolyte replacement is also provided as needed.
2. Administer oxygen, as prescribed, to increase tissue perfusion; blood transfusions may also be prescribed.
3. Assess pain; maintain effective pain management with the administration of analgesics (around the clock).
4. Assist the child with assuming a comfortable position so that the child keeps the extremities extended to promote venous return; elevate the head of the bed no more than 30 degrees, avoid putting strain on painful joints, and do not raise the knee gatch of the bed.
5. Encourage the consumption of a high-calorie, high-protein diet with folic acid supplementation.
6. Administer antibiotics, as prescribed, to prevent infection.
7. Monitor for signs of increasing anemia, decreased perfusion, and shock (i.e., mental status changes, pallor, and vital sign changes).
8. Instruct the child and parents about the early signs and symptoms of crisis and the measures to prevent and alleviate a painful vaso-occlusive crisis.
9. Emphasize the need to maintain strict adherence to immunization schedules; ensure that the child receives pneumococcal and meningococcal **vaccines** and an annual influenza **vaccine** because of the susceptibility to infection from functional asplenia.
10. A splenectomy may be necessary for those who experience recurrent splenic sequestration.
11. Inform the parents of the **hereditary** aspects of the disorder.

⚠ Administration of meperidine (Demerol) for pain is avoided because of the risk of normeperidine-induced seizures.

II. IRON DEFICIENCY ANEMIA

A. Description
1. Iron stores are depleted, which results in a decreased supply of iron for the manufacture of hemoglobin in RBCs.

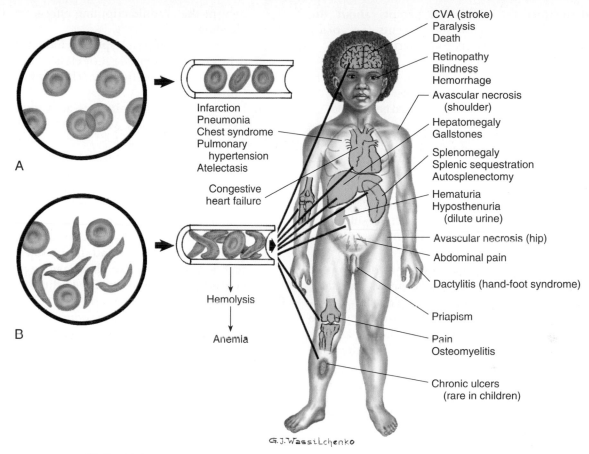

CVA (stroke)
Paralysis
Death

Retinopathy
Blindness
Hemorrhage

Avascular necrosis
(shoulder)

Hepatomegaly
Gallstones

Splenomegaly
Splenic sequestration
Autosplenectomy

Hematuria
Hyposthenuria
(dilute urine)

Avascular necrosis (hip)

Abdominal pain

Dactylitis (hand-foot syndrome)

Priapism

Pain
Osteomyelitis

Chronic ulcers
(rare in children)

Infarction
Pneumonia
Chest syndrome
Pulmonary
  hypertension
Atelectasis

Congestive
heart failure

Hemolysis

Anemia

A

B

G.J.Wassilchenko

▲ **FIGURE 38-1** Differences between **(A)** normal red blood cells and **(B)** sickled red blood cells in circulation with related complications. (From Hockenberry, M., & Wilson, D. [2010]. *Wong's nursing care of infants and children* [9th ed.]. St. Louis: Mosby.)

Box 38-1 Sickle Cell Crisis

Vaso-Occlusive Crisis

The crisis is caused by ischemia, infarction, and the stasis of blood with clumping of the cells in the microcirculation.

Manifestations include fever; painful swelling of the hands, feet, and joints; and abdominal pain.

Splenic Sequestration

This is caused by the pooling and clumping of blood in the spleen (hypersplenism).

Manifestations include profound anemia, hypovolemia, and shock.

Aplastic Crisis

This is caused by the diminished production and increased destruction of red blood cells, which is triggered by viral infection or the depletion of folic acid.

Manifestations include profound anemia and pallor.

2. Commonly results from blood loss, increased metabolic demands, syndromes of gastrointestinal (GI) malabsorption, and dietary inadequacy

3. Iron deficiency is associated with potentially irreversible developmental delays, behavioral disturbances, and learning impairments.

B. Data collection
1. Pallor
2. Weakness and fatigue
3. Irritability
4. Low hemoglobin and hematocrit levels
5. Red blood cells that are microcytic and hypochromic

C. Interventions
1. Increase oral intake of iron; iron-fortified formula will be needed for the infant.
2. Instruct the child and parents regarding food choices that are high in iron. (Refer to Chapter 12 for foods high in iron.)
3. Teach the parents how to administer the iron supplements.
   a. Give them between meals for maximum absorption.
   b. Give them with a multivitamin or fruit juice, because vitamin C increases absorption (fruit juice should be avoided among children who are less than 1 year old to prevent the introduction of allergens).
   c. Do not give them with milk or antacids, because these items decrease absorption.

d. Instruct the child and parents about the side effects of iron supplements (i.e., black stools, constipation, foul aftertaste).

⚠ Liquid iron preparation stains the teeth. Teach the parents and child that liquid iron should be taken through a straw and that the teeth should be brushed after administration.

III. APLASTIC ANEMIA

A. Description
1. A deficiency of circulating erythrocytes and all other formed elements of blood that results from the arrested development of RBCs within the bone marrow
2. There are several possible causes, including chronic exposure to myelotoxic agents, viruses, infection, autoimmune disorders, and allergic states.
3. The definitive diagnosis is determined by bone marrow aspiration, which demonstrates the conversion of red bone marrow to yellow fatty bone marrow.
4. Therapeutic management focuses on restoring function to the bone marrow and involves immunosuppressive therapy and bone marrow transplantation (BMT); BMT is the treatment of choice if a suitable donor exists, and the preferable donor is a matched sibling.

B. Data collection
1. Pancytopenia (a deficiency of erythrocytes, leukocytes, and thrombocytes)
2. Petechiae, purpura, bleeding, pallor, weakness, tachycardia, and fatigue

C. Interventions
1. Prepare the child for bone marrow transplantation, if planned.
2. Immunosuppressive medications: Antilymphocyte globulin or antithymocyte globulin may be prescribed to suppress the autoimmune response.
3. Colony-stimulating factors may be prescribed to enhance bone marrow production.
4. Corticosteroids and cyclosporine (Sandimmune) may be prescribed.
5. Blood or platelet transfusions may be prescribed.
6. Advise the parents to obtain a Medic-Alert bracelet for the child.

IV. HEMOPHILIA

A. Description
1. Refers to a group of bleeding disorders resulting from a deficiency of specific coagulation proteins
2. Identifying the specific coagulation deficiency is important so that definitive treatment with the specific replacement agent can be implemented; aggressive replacement therapy is initiated to

prevent the chronic crippling effects from joint bleeding.
3. The most common types include factor VIII deficiency (hemophilia A or classic hemophilia) and factor IX deficiency (hemophilia B or Christmas disease).
4. Hemophilia is transmitted as an X-linked recessive disorder (it may also occur as a result of a gene mutation).
5. Carrier females pass on the defect to affected males; female offspring are rarely born with the disorder, but may be if they inherit an affected gene from their mother and are offspring of a father with hemophilia.
6. The primary treatment is the replacement of the missing clotting factor; additional medications, such as those to relieve pain, may be prescribed depending on the source of bleeding.

B. Data collection
1. Abnormal bleeding in response to trauma or surgery; this condition is often diagnosed during the newborn period after circumcision or vitamin K injection.
2. Joint bleeding that causes pain, tenderness, swelling, and a limited range of motion
3. Tendency to bruise easily
4. Results of tests that measure platelet function are normal; results of tests that measure clotting factor function may be abnormal.

C. Interventions
1. Monitor for bleeding and maintain bleeding precautions.
2. Prepare to assist to administer replacement factors as prescribed.
3. DDAVP (1-deamino-8-D-arginine vasopressin), a synthetic form of vasopressin, increases plasma factor VIII and may be prescribed to treat mild hemophilia.
4. Monitor for joint pain; immobilize the affected extremity if joint pain occurs.
5. Monitor the neurological status; the child with this condition is at risk for intracranial hemorrhage.
6. Monitor the urine for hematuria.
7. Control bleeding by immobilization, elevation, and the application of ice; in addition, apply pressure (15 minutes) for superficial bleeding.
8. Instruct the child and parents about the signs of internal bleeding and how to control bleeding if it occurs.
9. Instruct the parents regarding activities for the child, emphasizing the avoidance of contact sports and the need for protective devices while learning to walk; assist in developing an appropriate exercise plan.
10. Instruct the child to wear protective devices such as helmets and knee and elbow pads when participating in sports such as bicycling and skating.

V.   VON WILLEBRAND'S DISEASE

A. Description
   1. A **hereditary** bleeding disorder characterized by a deficiency of or a defect in the protein called von Willebrand's factor (vWF)
   2. The disorder causes platelets to adhere to damaged endothelium; the vWF protein also serves as a carrier protein for factor VIII.
   3. It is characterized by an increased tendency to bleed from the mucous membranes.
B. Data collection
   1. Epistaxis
   2. Gum bleeding
   3. Easy bruising
   4. Excessive menstrual bleeding
C. Interventions
   1. Treatment and care are similar to those measures implemented for hemophilia, including the administration of clotting factors.
   2. Provide emotional support to the child and parents, especially if the child is experiencing an episode of bleeding.

⚠️ A child with a bleeding disorder needs to wear a Medic-Alert bracelet.

VI.   β-THALASSEMIA (Box 38-2)

A. Description
   1. An autosomal-recessive disorder characterized by the reduced production of a globin chain in the synthesis of hemoglobin (both parents must be carriers to produce a child with β-thalassemia major)
   2. The incidence is highest in individuals of Mediterranean descent, such as Italians, Greeks, Syrians, or their offspring.
   3. Treatment is supportive; the goal of therapy is to maintain normal hemoglobin levels by the administration of blood transfusions.
   4. Bone marrow transplantation may be offered as an alternative therapy.
   5. A splenectomy may be performed in a child with severe splenomegaly who requires repeated transfusions (assists in relieving abdominal pressure

and may increase the life span of supplemental red blood cells).
B. Data collection
   1. Frontal bossing
   2. Maxillary prominence
   3. Wide-set eyes with a flattened nose
   4. Greenish-yellow skin tone
   5. Hepatosplenomegaly
   6. Severe anemia
   7. Microcytic, hypochromic RBCs
C. Interventions
   1. Blood transfusions may be prescribed.
   2. Monitor for iron overload, and administer chelation therapy with deferasirox (Exjade) or deferoxamine (Desferal), as prescribed, to treat iron overload and to prevent organ damage from the elevated levels of iron caused by the multiple transfusion therapy.
   3. If the child has had a splenectomy, instruct the parents to report any signs of infection because of the risk of sepsis.
   4. Ensure that parents understand the importance of the child receiving pneumococcal and meningococcal **vaccines** in addition to the regularly scheduled **vaccines**.
   5. Provide resources for genetic counseling.

VII.   LEUKEMIA

A. Description (also refer to Chapter 43)
   1. Malignant exacerbation in the number of leukocytes, usually at an immature stage, in the bone marrow
   2. Affects the bone marrow, thus causing anemia from decreased erythrocytes, infection from neutropenia, and bleeding from decreased platelet production
   3. The cause is unknown and appears to involve the gene damage of cells, thus leading to the transformation of cells from a normal state to a malignant state.
   4. Risk factors include genetic, viral, immunological, and environmental factors and exposure to radiation, chemicals, and medications.
   5. Acute lymphocytic leukemia is the most frequent type of cancer in children; the peak onset is from the ages of 2 to 6 years.
   6. Leukemia is more common among boys than girls after 1 year of age
   7. Treatment involves the use of chemotherapeutic agents with or without radiation.
   8. The phases of treatment include the following: induction, which achieves a complete remission or disappearance of leukemic cells; intensification or consolidation therapy, which further decreases the tumor burden; central nervous system prophylactic therapy, which prevents leukemic cells from invading the central nervous

---

Box 38-2 Types of β-Thalassemia

Thalassemia minor: Asymptomatic silent carrier case
Thalassemia trait: Produces a mild microcytic anemia
Thalassemia intermedia: Manifested as splenomegaly and moderate to severe anemia
Thalassemia major: Results in severe anemia requiring transfusion support to sustain life (also known as Cooley's anemia)

system; and maintenance, which serves to maintain the remission phase.

9. Hematopoietic stem cell transplantation may also be performed to treat some children with leukemia.

B. Data collection

1. Infiltration of the bone marrow causes fever, pallor, fatigue, anorexia, hemorrhage (usually petechiae), and bone and joint pain; pathological fractures can occur as a result of bone marrow invasion with leukemic cells.
2. Signs of infection as a result of neutropenia
3. Hepatosplenomegaly and lymphadenopathy
4. Normal, elevated, or low white blood cell count, depending on the presence of infection or of immature versus mature white blood cells
5. Decreased hemoglobin and hematocrit levels
6. Decreased platelet count
7. Positive bone marrow biopsy identifying leukemic blast (immature) phase cells
8. Signs of increased intracranial pressure (see Box 38-5 later in this chapter)
9. Signs of cranial nerve (cranial nerve VII [the facial nerve] is most commonly affected) or spinal nerve involvement; clinical manifestations relate to the area involved
10. Clinical manifestations that indicate the invasion of leukemic cells in the kidneys, testes, prostate, ovaries, GI tract, and lungs

C. Infection (Box 38-3)

1. Infection can occur through self-contamination or cross-contamination.
2. Most common sites of infection are the skin (any break in the skin is a potential site of infection), respiratory tract, and gastrointestinal (GI) tract.

D. Bleeding (Box 38-4)

1. Children with platelet counts less than 20,000 cells/mm^3 may need a platelet transfusion.
2. For children with severe blood loss, packed red blood cells may be prescribed.

E. Fatigue and nutrition

1. Assist the child with selecting a well-balanced diet.
2. Provide small meals that require little chewing and will not be irritating to the oral mucosa
3. Assist the child with self-care and mobility activities.
4. Allow for adequate rest periods during care.
5. Do not perform nursing care activities unless they are essential.

F. Chemotherapy

1. Monitor for severe bone marrow suppression; during the period of greatest bone marrow suppression (the nadir), blood counts will be extremely low.
2. Monitor for infection and bleeding.
3. Protect the child from life-threatening infections.
4. Monitor for nausea, vomiting, and diarrhea.

Box 38-3 Protecting the Child from Infection

Initiate protective isolation procedures.

Maintain frequent and thorough handwashing.

Maintain the child in a private room with high-efficiency particulate air filtration or laminar airflow system, if possible.

Be sure that the child's room is cleaned daily.

Use strict aseptic technique for all nursing procedures.

Limit the number of caregivers entering the child's room, and ensure that anyone entering the child's room is wearing a mask.

Keep supplies for the child separate from supplies for other children.

Reduce exposure to environmental organisms by eliminating raw fruits and vegetables and fresh flowers and by not leaving standing water in the child's room.

Assist the child with daily bathing with the use of antimicrobial soap.

Assist the child with performing oral hygiene frequently.

Monitor for signs and symptoms of infection.

Monitor the temperature, pulse, and blood pressure.

Change wound dressings daily, and inspect wounds for redness, swelling, or drainage.

Monitor the urine for color and cloudiness.

Monitor the skin and oral mucous membranes for signs of infection.

Check the lung sounds.

Encourage the child to cough and deep breathe.

Monitor the white blood cell and the neutrophil count.

Notify the health care provider (HCP) if signs of infection are present; prepare to obtain specimens for the culture of open lesions, urine, and sputum.

Avoid invasive procedures, such as injections, rectal temperatures, and urinary catheterization.

Administer antibiotic, antifungal, and antiviral medication, as prescribed.

Administer granulocyte colony-stimulating factor, as prescribed.

Instruct the parents to keep the child away from crowds and those with infections.

Instruct the parents that the child should not receive immunization with a live virus (measles, mumps, rubella, polio) because if the immune system is depressed, the attenuated virus can result in a life-threatening infection; also, the child should not receive the varicella vaccine. The Salk (inactivated) vaccine for poliomyelitis may be administered.

Instruct the parents to inform the teacher that they should be notified immediately if a case of a communicable disease occurs in another child at school.

5. Administer antiemetics, as prescribed.
6. Monitor for signs of dehydration.
7. Monitor for signs of hemorrhagic cystitis.
8. Monitor for signs of peripheral neuropathy.
9. Check oral mucous membranes for mucositis; administer frequent mouth rinses per agency procedure and as prescribed; usually a mixture of normal saline with table salt or sodium bicarbonate will be prescribed to promote healing and/or prevent infection (local oral anesthetics may also be prescribed)
10. Instruct the parents regarding the signs and symptoms to monitor after chemotherapy and when to notify the HCP.
11. Inform the parents that hair loss may occur from chemotherapy; the hair will regrow in 3 to 6 months and may be a slightly different color or texture.
12. Instruct the parents about the care of a central venous access device, as necessary. (Refer to Chapter 13 for information on central venous access devices.)
13. Listen to the child and family, and encourage them to verbalize their feelings and express their concerns.
14. Introduce the family to other families of children with cancer.
15. Consult social services and chaplains, as necessary.

⚠ Monitor a child receiving chemotherapy closely for signs of infection. Infection is a major cause of death in the immunosuppressed child.

VIII. HODGKIN'S DISEASE

A. Description
1. A malignancy of the lymph nodes that originates in a single lymph node or a single chain of nodes

2. It predictably metastasizes to non-nodal or extra-lymphatic sites, especially the spleen, liver, bone marrow, lungs, and mediastinum (Figure 38-2).
3. Characterized by the presence of Reed-Sternberg cells in the lymph nodes
4. Peak incidence is in midadolescence.
5. Possible causes include viral infections and previous exposure to alkylating chemical agents.
6. The prognosis is excellent with long-term survival rates dependent on the stage of the disease.
7. The primary treatment modalities are radiation and chemotherapy; each may be used alone or in combination, depending on the clinical staging of the disease.

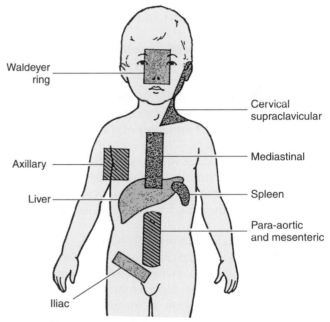

▲ **FIGURE 38-2** Main areas of lymphadenopathy and organ involvement in Hodgkin's disease. (From Hockenberry, M., Wilson, D., & Winklestein, M. [2009]. *Wong's essentials of pediatric nursing* [8th ed.]. St. Louis: Mosby.)

Box 38-4 Protecting the Child from Bleeding

Examine the child for signs and symptoms of bleeding.
Handle the child gently.
Measure the abdominal girth, which can indicate internal hemorrhage.
Instruct the child to use a soft toothbrush and to avoid dental floss.
Provide soft foods that are cool to warm in temperature.
Avoid injections, if possible, to prevent trauma to the skin and bleeding.
Apply firm and gentle pressure to a needle-stick site for at least 10 minutes.
Pad side rails and sharp corners of the bed and other furniture.
Discourage the child from engaging in activities that involve the use of sharp objects.
Instruct the child to avoid constrictive or tight clothing.

Use caution when taking the blood pressure to prevent skin injury.
Instruct the child to avoid blowing his or her nose.
Avoid rectal suppositories, enemas, and rectal thermometers; initiate a bowel program to prevent constipation and rectal trauma.
Examine all body fluids and excrement for the presence of blood.
Count the number of pads or tampons used if the female adolescent is menstruating.
Instruct the child regarding the signs and symptoms of bleeding.
Instruct the parents to avoid administering nonsteroidal anti-inflammatory drugs and products that contain aspirin to the child.

B. Data collection
1. Painless enlargement of the lymph nodes
2. Enlarged, firm, nontender, movable nodes in the supraclavicular area; in children, the sentinel node located near the left clavicle may be the first enlarged node
3. Nonproductive cough as a result of mediastinal lymphadenopathy
4. Abdominal pain as a result of enlarged retroperitoneal nodes
5. Advanced lymph node and extralymphatic involvement may cause systemic symptoms, such as low-grade and/or intermittent fever, anorexia, nausea, weight loss, night sweats, and pruritus.
6. Positive biopsy of a lymph node (presence of Reed-Sternberg cells) and positive bone marrow biopsy
7. Computed tomography scan of the liver, spleen, and bone marrow to detect metastasis

C. Interventions
1. For early stages without mediastinal node involvement, the treatment of choice is usually extensive external radiation of the involved lymph node regions.
2. With more extensive disease, radiation in combination with multiagent chemotherapy is used.
3. Monitor for drug-induced pancytopenia, which increases the risk for infection, bleeding, and anemia.
4. Protect the child from infection.
5. Provide a safe, hazard-free environment.
6. Monitor for side effects related to chemotherapy or radiation; the most common side effect of extensive irradiation is malaise, which can be difficult for older children and adolescents to tolerate both physically and psychologically (Table 38-1)
7. Monitor for nausea and vomiting; administer antiemetics, as prescribed.
8. Monitor for skin irritation and breakdown as a result of radiation therapy.

IX. NEPHROBLASTOMA (WILMS' TUMOR)

A. Description
1. Wilms' tumor is the most common intraabdominal and kidney tumor of childhood; it may present unilaterally and localized or bilaterally, sometimes with metastasis to other organs.
2. The peak incidence is at 3 years of age.
3. Associated with a genetic inheritance and with several congenital anomalies
4. Therapeutic management includes a combination treatment of surgery (partial to total nephrectomy) and chemotherapy with or without radiation, depending on the clinical stage and histologic pattern of the tumor.

TABLE 38-1 Side Effects of Radiation Therapy and Nursing Interventions

Body Area and Side Effects	Interventions
GASTROINTESTINAL TRACT	
Anorexia	Encourage fluids and foods as best tolerated. Provide small, frequent meals. Monitor for weight loss.
Nausea, vomiting	Administer antiemetics around the clock. Monitor for dehydration.
Mucosal ulceration	Provide soothing oral hygiene and prescribed mouth rinses. Topical anesthetic may be prescribed.
Diarrhea	Administer antispasmodics and antidiarrheal preparations as prescribed. Monitor for dehydration.
SKIN	
Alopecia (hair loss)	Introduce idea of a wig. Provide scalp hygiene. Stress the need for head covering in cold weather.
Dry or moist desquamation	Keep the skin clean. Wash the skin daily, using a mild soap sparingly. Do not remove skin markings for radiation. Avoid exposure to the sun and other extreme temperature changes. For dryness, apply lubricant as prescribed.
URINARY BLADDER	
Cystitis	Encourage fluid intake and frequent voiding. Monitor for hematuria.
BONE MARROW	
Myelosuppression	Monitor for fever. Administer antibiotics as prescribed. Avoid the use of suppositories and rectal temperatures. Institute bleeding precautions. Monitor for signs of anemia.

Adapted from Hockenberry, M., & Wilson, D. (2007). *Wong's nursing care of infants and children* (8th ed.). St. Louis: Mosby; and McKinney, E., James, S., Murray, S., & Ashwill, J. (2009). *Maternal-child nursing* (3rd ed.). St. Louis: Elsevier.

B. Data collection
1. A swelling or mass within the abdomen; the mass is characteristically firm, nontender, confined to one side, and deep within the flank
2. Abdominal pain
3. Urinary retention and/or hematuria
4. Anemia caused by hemorrhage within the tumor
5. Pallor, anorexia, and lethargy resulting from anemia
6. Hypertension, caused by the secretion of excess amounts of renin by the tumor
7. Weight loss and fever

8. Symptoms of lung involvement, such as dyspnea, shortness of breath, and pain in the chest, if metastasis has occurred

C. Preoperative interventions
1. Monitor the vital signs, particularly the blood pressure.
2. Avoid the palpation of the abdomen; Place a sign at the bedside that reads as follows: "Do not palpate abdomen."
3. Measure the abdominal girth at least once daily.

D. Postoperative interventions
1. Monitor the temperature and blood pressure closely.
2. Monitor for signs of hemorrhage and infection.
3. Monitor strict intake and output closely.
4. Monitor for abdominal distention, bowel sounds, and other signs of GI activity because of the risk for intestinal obstruction.

⚠ Avoid palpation of the abdomen in a child with Wilms' tumor and be cautious when bathing, moving, or handling the child. It is important to keep the encapsulated tumor intact. Rupture of the tumor can cause the cancer cells to spread throughout the abdomen, lymph system, and bloodstream.

X. NEUROBLASTOMA

A. Description
1. A tumor that originates from the embryonic neural crest cells that normally give rise to the adrenal medulla and the sympathetic ganglia.
2. Most tumors develop in the adrenal gland or the retroperitoneal sympathetic chain; other sites may be within the head, neck, chest, or pelvis.
3. Most children present with the tumor before 10 years of age. Most presenting signs are caused by the tumor compressing adjacent normal tissue and organs.
4. Diagnostic evaluation is aimed at locating the primary site of the tumor.
5. The prognosis is poor because of the frequency of invasiveness of the tumor and because, in most cases, the diagnosis is not made until after metastasis has occurred; the younger the child at diagnosis, the better the survival rate.
6. Surgery is performed to remove as much of the tumor as possible and to obtain samples for biopsy; in early stages, complete surgical removal of the tumor is the treatment of choice.
7. Surgery is usually limited to biopsy in the later stages because of the extensive metastasis.
8. Radiation is commonly used with late-stage disease and provides palliation for metastatic lesions in the bones, lungs, liver, or brain.
9. Chemotherapy is used for treatment for extensive local or disseminated disease.

B. Data collection: Signs and symptoms depend on the location of the primary tumor.
1. Firm, nontender, irregular mass in the abdomen that crosses the midline
2. Urinary frequency or retention from the compression of the kidney, ureter, or bladder
3. Lymphadenopathy, especially in the cervical and supraclavicular area
4. Bone pain if skeletal involvement occurs
5. Supraorbital ecchymosis (raccoon eyes), periorbital edema, and exophthalmos as a result of the invasion of retrobulbar soft tissue
6. Pallor, weakness, irritability, anorexia, weight loss
7. Signs of respiratory impairment (thoracic lesion)
8. Signs of neurological impairment (intracranial lesion)
9. Paralysis from the compression of the spinal cord

C. Preoperative interventions
1. Monitor for signs and symptoms related to the location of the tumor.
2. Provide emotional support to the child and parents.

D. Postoperative interventions
1. Monitor for postoperative complications related to the location (organ) of the surgery.
2. Monitor for complications related to chemotherapy or radiation, if prescribed.
3. Provide support for the parents, and encourage them to express their feelings; many parents suffer from guilt for not having recognized signs in the child earlier.
4. Refer the parents to appropriate community services.

XI. OSTEOGENIC SARCOMA

A. Description
1. The most common bone cancer in children; it is also known as osteosarcoma.
2. Usually found in the metaphysis of the long bones, especially in the lower extremities, with most tumors occurring in the femur.
3. Peak age of incidence is between 10 and 25 years.
4. Symptoms during the earliest stage are almost always attributed to extremity injury or normal growing pains.
5. Treatment may include surgical resection to save a limb or to remove affected tissue, or amputation.
6. Chemotherapy is used to treat the cancer and may be used before and after surgery.

B. Data collection
1. Localized pain at the affected site (may be severe or dull) that may be attributed to trauma or the vague complaint of "growing pains"; pain is often relieved by a flexed position.

2. Palpable mass
3. Limping if weight-bearing limb is affected
4. Progressively limited range of motion; child curtails physical activity
5. Child may be unable to hold heavy objects because of their weight and resultant pain in the affected extremity.
6. Pathological fractures at the tumor site

C. Interventions
1. Prepare the child and family for prescribed treatment modalities, which may include surgical resection to remove affected tissue, amputation, and chemotherapy.
2. Provide honesty and support to the child and family.
3. Prepare for prosthetic fitting, as necessary.
4. Assist the child with dealing with self-image problems.
5. Instruct the child and parents about the potential development of phantom limb pain that may occur after amputation, characterized by tingling, itching, and a painful sensation in the area where the limb was amputated.

XII. BRAIN TUMORS

A. Description
1. An infratentorial (below the tentorium cerebelli) tumor is located in the posterior third of the brain (primarily in the cerebellum or brainstem) and accounts for the frequency of symptoms that result from increased intracranial pressure (ICP).

2. A supratentorial tumor is located within the anterior two thirds of the brain, mainly the cerebrum.
3. The signs and symptoms of a brain tumor depend on its anatomical location and size and, to some extent, on the age of the child.
4. Therapeutic management includes surgery, radiation, and chemotherapy; the treatment of choice is the total removal of the tumor without residual neurological damage.

B. Data collection
1. Headache that is worse on awakening and that improves during the day
2. Vomiting that is unrelated to feeding or eating
3. Ataxia
4. Seizures
5. Behavioral changes
6. Clumsiness; awkward gait or difficulty walking
7. Diplopia
8. Facial weakness
9. Signs of increased intracranial pressure (Box 38-5)

⚠ Monitor for signs of increased ICP in a child with a brain tumor and after a craniotomy. If signs of increased ICP occur, notify the HCP immediately.

C. Preoperative interventions
1. Monitor the neurological status.
2. Institute seizure and safety measures.
3. Monitor the weight and nutritional status.
4. The child's head will be shaved (provide a favorite cap or hat for the child); shaving the head may also be done in the surgical suite

---

Box 38-5 Manifestations of Increased Intracranial Pressure in Infants and Children

Infants
Tense, bulging fontanel
Separated cranial sutures
Macewen's sign (cracked pot sound on percussion)
Irritability
High-pitched cry
Increased head circumference
Distended scalp veins
Poor feeding
Crying when disturbed
Setting sun sign (eyes appear to look only downward, with the sclera prominent over the iris)

Children
Headache
Nausea
Forceful vomiting
Diplopia; blurred vision
Seizures

Personality and Behavior Signs
Irritability, restlessness

Indifference, drowsiness
Decline in school performance
Diminished physical activity and motor performance
Increased sleeping
Inability to follow simple commands
Lethargy

Late Signs
Bradycardia
Decreased motor response to command
Decreased sensory response to painful stimuli
Alterations in pupil size and reaction
Decerebrate or decorticate posturing
Cheyne-Stokes respirations
Papilledema
Decreased consciousness
Coma

From Perry, S., Hockenberry, M., Lowdermilk, D., & Wilson, D. (2010). *Maternal child nursing care* (4th ed.). St. Louis: Elsevier.

5. Prepare the child as much as possible; tell the child that he or she will wake up with a large head dressing.

▲ **D.** Postoperative interventions
1. Monitor the neurological and motor function and the level of consciousness.
2. Monitor the temperature closely, because it may be elevated as a result of hypothalamus or brainstem involvement during surgery; maintain a cooling blanket by the bedside.
3. Monitor for signs of respiratory infection.
4. Monitor for signs of meningitis (opisthotonos, Kernig's and Brudzinski's signs).
5. Monitor for signs of increased ICP (see Box 38-5) or hemorrhage; check the back of the head dressing for the posterior pooling of blood.
6. Monitor the pupillary response; sluggish, dilated, or unequal pupils are reported immediately, because they may indicate increased ICP and potential brainstem herniation.
7. Monitor for colorless drainage on the dressing or from the ears or nose; this is indicative of cerebrospinal fluid and should be reported immediately. Assess for the presence of glucose in the drainage (dipstick).
8. Check the HCP's prescription for positioning, including the degree of neck flexion. (Refer to Chapter 57 for additional information on craniotomy.)
9. Monitor IV fluids closely to prevent volume overload.
10. Promote measures that prevent vomiting; vomiting increases ICP and the risk for incisional rupture.
11. Provide a quiet environment.
12. Administer analgesics, as prescribed.
13. Provide emotional support to the child and parents, and promote maximum functioning in the child.

MORE QUESTIONS ON EVOLVE!

Practice Questions

371. A nurse instructs the mother of a child with sickle cell disease regarding the precipitating factors related to pain crisis. Which of the following, if identified by the mother as a precipitating factor, indicates the need for further instructions?
1. Stress
2. Trauma
3. Infection
4. Fluid overload

372. Oral iron supplements are prescribed for a 6-year-old child with iron deficiency anemia. The nurse instructs the mother to administer the iron with which best food item?

1. Milk
2. Water
3. Apple juice
4. Orange juice

373. A nurse who is caring for a child with aplastic anemia reviews the laboratory results and notes a white blood cell (WBC) count of 6000 cells/mm^3 and a platelet count of 27,000 cells/mm^3. Which nursing intervention should be incorporated into the plan of care?
1. Encourage naps.
2. Encourage a diet high in iron.
3. Encourage quiet play activities.
4. Maintain strict isolation precautions.

374. A nurse reinforces home-care instructions to the parents of a 3-year-old child who has been hospitalized with hemophilia. Which statement by a parent indicates the need for further instructions?
1. "I will supervise my child closely."
2. "I will pad the corners of the furniture."
3. "I will remove household items that can easily fall over."
4. "I will avoid immunizations and dental hygiene treatments for my child."

375. A nurse provides instruction to the parents of a child with leukemia regarding measures related to monitoring for infection. Which statement by the parents indicates the need for further instructions?
1. "I need to use proper handwashing techniques."
2. "I need to take my child's rectal temperature daily."
3. "I need to inspect my child's skin daily for redness."
4. "I need to inspect my child's mouth daily for lesions."

376. A nurse is reviewing the health record of a 14-year-old child who is suspected of having Hodgkin's disease. Which of the following is the primary characteristic of this disease?
1. Fever and malaise
2. Anorexia and weight loss
3. Painful, enlarged inguinal lymph nodes
4. Painless, firm, and movable lymph nodes in the cervical area

377. A 4-year-old child is hospitalized with a suspected diagnosis of Wilms' tumor. The nurse assists with developing a plan of care. The nurse questions which intervention that is written in the plan of care?

1. Palpating the abdomen for a mass
2. Checking the urine for the presence of hematuria
3. Monitoring the blood pressure for the presence of hypertension
4. Monitoring the temperature for the presence of a kidney infection

378. A nursing instructor asks a student nurse to describe osteogenic sarcoma. Which statement by the student indicates the need to further research the disease?
1. "The femur is the most common site of this sarcoma."
2. "The child does not experience pain at the primary tumor site."
3. "If a weight-bearing limb is affected, then limping is a clinical manifestation."
4. "The symptoms of the disease during the early stage are almost always attributed to normal growing pains."

379. A nurse is monitoring for bleeding in a child after surgery for the removal of a brain tumor. The nurse checks the head dressing for the presence of blood and notes a colorless drainage on the back of the dressing. Which nursing action is appropriate?
1. Reinforce the dressing.
2. Notify the registered nurse (RN).
3. Document the findings and continue to monitor.
4. Circle the area of drainage and continue to monitor.

380. A nurse is reviewing a health care provider's prescription for a child with sickle cell anemia who was admitted to the hospital for the treatment of vaso-occlusive crisis. Which prescriptions documented in the child's record should the nurse question? **Select all that apply.**
☐ 1. Restrict fluid intake.
☐ 2. Position for comfort.
☐ 3. Avoid strain on painful joints.
☐ 4. Apply nasal oxygen at 2 L per minute.
☐ 5. Provide a high-calorie, high-protein diet.
☐ 6. Administer meperidine (Demerol) 25 mg for pain.

ANSWERS

371. 4
Rationale: Pain crisis may be precipitated by infection, dehydration, hypoxia, trauma, or general stress. The mother of a child with sickle cell disease should encourage a fluid intake of 1.5 to 2 times the daily requirement to prevent dehydration.
Test-Taking Strategy: Note the strategic words "need for further instructions." These words indicate a negative event query and ask you to select an option that is an incorrect statement. Recalling that fluid administration is a main component of the treatment of sickle cell disease to prevent dehydration and pain crisis will direct you to the correct option. Review the precipitating factors of pain crisis if you had difficulty with this question.
Level of Cognitive Ability: Evaluating
Client Needs: Physiological Integrity
Integrated Process: Teaching and Learning
Content Area: Child Health: Hematological/Oncological
Reference: Swearingen, pp. 606-607. 2012.

372. 4
Rationale: Vitamin C increases the absorption of iron by the body. The mother should be instructed to administer the medication with a citrus fruit or a juice that is high in vitamin C. Milk may affect absorption of the iron. Water will not assist in absorption. Orange juice contains a greater amount of vitamin C than apple juice.
Test-Taking Strategy: Use the process of elimination and note the strategic word "best." Recalling that vitamin C increases the absorption of iron will assist you with eliminating milk and water. From the remaining options, select orange juice, because this food item contains the highest amount of vitamin C. Review the procedure for administering oral iron if you had difficulty with this question.
Level of Cognitive Ability: Applying
Client Needs: Physiological Integrity
Integrated Process: Teaching and Learning
Content Area: Pharmacology
References: Christensen, Kockrow, p. 993. 2011. *Foundations of nursing.*
Leifer, p. 627. 2011.

373. 3
Rationale: Precautionary measures to prevent bleeding should be taken when a child has a low platelet count. These include no injections, no rectal temperatures, the use of a soft toothbrush, and abstinence from contact sports or activities that could cause an injury. Strict isolation would be required if the WBC count was low. Naps and a diet high in iron are unrelated to the risk of bleeding.
Test-Taking Strategy: Use the process of elimination. Note that the WBC count is normal and that the platelet count is low. Recall that a low platelet count places the client at risk for bleeding. This will assist you with eliminating the incorrect options. Review normal WBC and platelet counts if you had difficulty with this question.
Level of Cognitive Ability: Analyzing
Client Needs: Physiological Integrity
Integrated Process: Nursing Process/Planning
Content Area: Child Health: Hematological/Oncological
References: Leifer, p. 628. 2011.
McKinney, James, Murray, Ashwill, pp. 1300-1301. 2009.

374. 4

Rationale: The nurse needs to stress the importance of immunizations, dental hygiene, and routine well-child care. Options 1, 2, and 3 are appropriate statements. The parents are also provided instructions regarding measures to take in the event of blunt trauma (especially trauma that involves the joints), and they are instructed to apply prolonged pressure to superficial wounds until the bleeding has stopped.

Test-Taking Strategy: Use the process of elimination, and note the strategic words "need for further instructions." These words indicate a negative event query and ask you to select an option that is an incorrect statement. Recalling that bleeding is a concern among clients with this disorder will assist you with eliminating options 1, 2, and 3, because they include measures of protection and safety for the child. Review the home-care measures for the child with hemophilia if you had difficulty with this question.

Level of Cognitive Ability: Evaluating
Client Needs: Safe and Effective Care Environment
Integrated Process: Teaching and Learning
Content Area: Child Health: Hematological/Oncological
Reference: McKinney, James, Murray, Ashwill, p. 1295. 2009.

375. 2

Rationale: The risk of injury to the fragile mucous membranes is so great in the child with leukemia that only oral, axillary, or temporal or tympanic temperatures should be taken. Rectal abscesses can easily occur in damaged rectal tissue, so no rectal temperatures should be taken. In addition, oral temperatures should be avoided if the child has oral ulcers. Options 1, 3, and 4 are appropriate teaching measures.

Test-Taking Strategy: Use the process of elimination, and note the strategic words "need for further instructions." These words indicate a negative event query and ask you to select an option that is an incorrect statement. Options 1, 3, and 4 can be easily eliminated. Also, note the word "rectal" in option 2. Recalling that rectal temperatures should be avoided will direct you to this option. Review the home-care instructions for preventing infection in the leukemic child if you had difficulty with this question.

Level of Cognitive Ability: Evaluating
Client Needs: Safe and Effective Care Environment
Integrated Process: Teaching and Learning
Content Area: Child Health: Hematological/Oncological
Reference: Leifer, p. 639. 2011.

376. 4

Rationale: Clinical manifestations specifically associated with Hodgkin's disease include painless, firm, and movable adenopathy in the cervical and supraclavicular areas. Hepatosplenomegaly is also noted. Although anorexia, weight loss, fever, and malaise are associated with Hodgkin's disease, these manifestations are not the primary characteristics and are seen with many disorders.

Test-Taking Strategy: Note the strategic words "primary characteristic." Eliminate options 1 and 2 first, because these symptoms are general and vague. Recalling that painless adenopathy is associated with Hodgkin's disease will direct you to the correct option. Review the clinical manifestations of Hodgkin's disease if you had difficulty with this question.

Level of Cognitive Ability: Understanding
Client Needs: Physiological Integrity
Integrated Process: Nursing Process/Data Collection
Content Area: Child Health: Hematological/Oncological
References: Leifer, p. 638. 2011.
McKinney, James, Murray, Ashwill, pp. 1326-1327. 2009.

377. 1

Rationale: Wilms' tumor is an intra-abdominal and kidney tumor. If Wilms' tumor is suspected, the mass should not be palpated. Excessive manipulation can cause seeding of the tumor and thus cause the spread of the cancerous cells. Hematuria, hypertension, and fever are clinical manifestations that are associated with Wilms' tumor.

Test-Taking Strategy: Use the process of elimination, and note the strategic words, "questions which intervention." These words indicate a negative event query and ask you to select an option that is an incorrect intervention. Knowledge that Wilms' tumor is an intra-abdominal and kidney tumor will assist you with eliminating options 2, 3, and 4 because of the relationship of these options to renal function. Review the nursing interventions for the child with Wilms' tumor if you had difficulty with this question.

Level of Cognitive Ability: Analyzing
Client Needs: Safe and Effective Care Environment
Integrated Process: Nursing Process/Implementation
Content Area: Child Health: Hematological/Oncological
Reference: Leifer, p. 684. 2011.

378. 2

Rationale: Osteogenic sarcoma is the most common bone tumor in children. A clinical manifestation of osteogenic sarcoma is progressive, insidious, intermittent pain at the tumor site. By the time these children receive medical attention, they may be in considerable pain from the tumor. Options 1, 3, and 4 are accurate regarding osteogenic sarcoma.

Test-Taking Strategy: Note the strategic words "need to further research." These words indicate a negative event query and the need to select the incorrect student statement. Recalling that osteogenic sarcoma is a malignant tumor of the bone will direct you to the correct option. Review the clinical manifestations associated with osteogenic sarcoma if you had difficulty with this question.

Level of Cognitive Ability: Evaluating
Client Needs: Physiological Integrity
Integrated Process: Teaching and Learning
Content Area: Child Health: Hematological/Oncological
Reference: McKinney, James, Murray, Ashwill, p. 1329. 2009.

379. 2

Rationale: Colorless drainage on the dressing would indicate the presence of cerebrospinal fluid and should be reported to the RN immediately; the RN would then contact the health care provider. The colorless drainage should also be checked for evidence of cerebrospinal fluid; one method is to check for the presence of glucose using a dipstick. Options 1, 3, and 4 are incorrect and delay required immediate interventions.

Test-Taking Strategy: Use the process of elimination. Note the strategic words "colorless drainage." This should quickly alert you to the possibility of the presence of cerebrospinal fluid.

Therefore, eliminate options 1, 3, and 4. Review the care of the child with a brain tumor if you had difficulty with this question.

Level of Cognitive Ability: Applying
Client Needs: Physiological Integrity
Integrated Process: Nursing Process/Implementation
Content Area: Child Health: Hematological/Oncological
Reference: McKinney, James, Murray, Ashwill, p. 1324. 2009.

❖ **380. 1, 6**
Rationale: Sickle cell anemia is one of a group of diseases called hemoglobinopathies in which hemoglobin A is partly or completely replaced by abnormal sickle hemoglobin S. It is caused by the inheritance of a gene for a structurally abnormal portion of the hemoglobin chain. Hemoglobin S is sensitive to changes in the oxygen content of the red blood cell, and insufficient oxygen causes the cells to assume a sickle shape; the cells become rigid and clumped together, thus obstructing capillary blood flow. Oral and intravenous fluids are important parts of treatment. Meperidine (Demerol) is not recommended for the child with sickle cell disease because of the risk for normeperidine-induced seizures. Normeperidine, which is a metabolite of meperidine, is a central nervous system stimulant that produces anxiety, tremors, myoclonus, and generalized seizures when it accumulates with repetitive dosing. Therefore, the nurse would question the prescriptions for restricted fluids and meperidine for pain control. Positioning for comfort, avoiding strain in painful joints, oxygen, and a high-calorie, high-protein diet are important parts of the treatment plan.

Test-Taking Strategy: Focus on the pathophysiology that occurs with sickle cell disease to assist you with identifying the prescriptions that need to be questioned. Recalling that fluids are an important component of the treatment plan will help you to identify that a fluid-restriction prescription would need to be questioned. Recalling the effects of meperidine will assist you with identifying that this prescription needs to be questioned. Review the care of the child with sickle cell anemia who is experiencing a crisis if you had difficulty with this question.

Level of Cognitive Ability: Analyzing
Client Needs: Safe and Effective Care Environment
Integrated Process: Nursing Process/Implementation
Content Area: Child Health: Hematological/Oncological
References: Leifer, p. 631. 2011.
McKinney, James, Murray, Ashwill, pp. 1285, 1289. 2009.
Swearingen, pp. 607-609. 2012.

Communicable Diseases and Acquired Immunodeficiency Syndrome

I. RUBEOLA (MEASLES)

A. Description
1. Agent: Paramyxovirus virus
2. Incubation period: 10 to 20 days
3. Communicable period: From 4 days before to 5 days after the rash appears; mainly during the **prodromal** stage (this pertains to early symptoms that may mark the onset of disease)
4. Source: Respiratory tract secretions, blood, or urine of an infected person
5. Transmission: Airborne particles, direct contact with infectious droplets, or transplacental transmission

B. Data collection
1. Fever
2. Malaise
3. The "three Cs": Coryza, cough, and conjunctivitis
4. Rash appears as red, erythematous maculopapular eruption starting on the face and spreading downward to the feet; blanches easily with pressure and gradually turns a brownish color (lasts 6 to 7 days); may have desquamation.
5. Koplik spots: Small, red spots with a bluish-white center and a red base. They are located on the buccal mucosa and last for approximately 3 days.

C. Interventions
1. Use airborne droplet precautions if the child is hospitalized.
2. Restrict the child to quiet activities and bedrest.
3. Use a cool-mist vaporizer for cough and coryza.
4. Dim the lights if photophobia is present.
5. Administer antipyretics for fever, as prescribed.

II. ROSEOLA (*EXANTHEMA SUBITUM*)

A. Description
1. Agent: Human herpesvirus type 6 (HHV-6)
2. Incubation period: 5 to 15 days
3. Communicable period: Unknown, but thought to extend from the febrile stage to the time that the rash first appears
4. Source and transmission: Unknown

B. Data collection
1. Sudden high fever (greater than 102° F) of 3 to 5 days' duration in a child who appears well, followed by a rash (rose-pink macules that blanch with pressure)
2. The rash appears several hours to 2 days after the fever subsides and lasts 1 to 2 days

C. Interventions: Supportive

III. RUBELLA (GERMAN MEASLES)

A. Description
1. Agent: Rubella virus
2. Incubation period: 14 to 21 days
3. Communicable period: 7 days before to about 5 days after the rash appears
4. Source: Nasopharyngeal secretions. The virus is also present in the blood, stool, and urine.
5. Transmission
   a. Airborne or direct contact with infectious droplets
   b. Indirectly via articles that have been freshly contaminated with nasopharyngeal secretions, feces, or urine
   c. Transplacental

B. Data collection
1. Low-grade fever
2. Malaise
3. Pinkish-red maculopapular rash that begins on the face and spreads to the entire body within 1 to 3 days
4. Petechial red, pinpoint spots may occur on the soft palate.

C. Interventions
1. Provide supportive treatment.
2. Isolate the infected child from pregnant women.

IV. MUMPS

A. Description
1. Agent: Paramyxovirus
2. Incubation period: 14 to 21 days

3. Communicable period: Immediately before and after parotid gland swelling begins
4. Source: The saliva and possibly the urine of an infected person
5. Transmission: Direct contact or droplet spread from an infected person

B. Data collection
1. Fever
2. Headache and malaise
3. Anorexia
4. Jaw or ear pain aggravated by chewing, followed by parotid glandular swelling
5. Orchitis may occur.

C. Interventions
1. Institute droplet respiratory precautions.
2. Provide bedrest until the parotid gland swelling subsides.
3. Avoid foods that require chewing.
4. Apply hot or cold compresses to the neck, as prescribed.
5. Apply warmth and local support with tight-fitting underpants to relieve orchitis.
6. Monitor closely for signs of aseptic meningitis, a complication of mumps.

V. CHICKENPOX (VARICELLA)

A. Description
1. Agent: Varicella zoster virus (VZV)
2. Incubation period: 13 to 17 days
3. Communicable period: 1 to 2 days before the onset of the rash to 6 days after the first crop of vesicles, when crusts have formed
4. Source: Respiratory tract secretions of an infected person; skin lesions
5. Transmission: Direct contact, droplet (airborne) spread, and contaminated objects

B. Data collection
1. Slight fever, malaise, and anorexia are followed by a macular rash that first appears on the trunk and scalp and then moves to the face and extremities
2. Lesions become pustules, begin to dry, and develop a crust.
3. Lesions may appear on the mucous membranes of the mouth, the genital area, and the rectal area.

C. Interventions
1. In the hospital setting, ensure strict isolation (i.e., contact and droplet precautions).
2. In the home setting, isolate the infected child until the vesicles have dried.
3. Supportive care

⚠️ Isolate high-risk children, such as children who have immunosuppressive disorders, from a child with a communicable disease.

VI. PERTUSSIS (WHOOPING COUGH)

A. Description
1. Agent: *Bordetella pertussis*
2. Incubation period: 5 to 21 days (usually 10 days)
3. Communicable period: Greatest during the catarrhal stage (i.e., when discharge from respiratory secretions occurs)
4. Source: Discharge from the respiratory tract of the infected person
5. Transmission: Direct contact or droplet spread from the infected person; indirect contact with freshly contaminated articles

B. Data collection
1. Symptoms of respiratory infection followed by increased severity of cough with a loud whooping inspiration
2. May experience **cyanosis**, respiratory distress, and tongue protrusion
3. Listlessness, irritability, and anorexia

C. Interventions
1. Isolate the child during the catarrhal stage. If the child is hospitalized, institute droplet precautions.
2. Administer antimicrobial therapy, as prescribed.
3. Reduce environmental factors that cause coughing spasms, such as dust, smoke, and sudden changes in temperature.
4. Ensure adequate hydration and nutrition.
5. Provide suction and humidified oxygen, if needed.
6. Monitor the cardiopulmonary status (via a monitor as prescribed) and pulse oximetry.
7. Infants do not receive maternal immunity to pertussis.

VII. DIPHTHERIA

A. Description
1. Agent: *Corynebacterium diphtheriae*
2. Incubation period: 2 to 5 days
3. Communicable period: Variable; until virulent bacilli are no longer present (three negative cultures of discharge from the nose, nasopharynx, skin, and other lesions); usually 2 weeks but can be as long as 4 weeks
4. Source: Discharge from the mucous membrane of the nose, nasopharynx, skin, and other lesions of the infected person
5. Transmission: Direct contact with an infected person, carrier, or contaminated articles

B. Data collection
1. Low-grade fever, malaise, and sore throat
2. Foul-smelling and mucopurulent nasal discharge
3. Dense pseudomembrane formation of the throat that may interfere with eating, drinking, and breathing
4. Lymphadenitis, neck edema, and "bull neck"

C. Interventions
1. Ensure strict isolation for the hospitalized child
2. Assist to administer diphtheria antitoxin, as prescribed (after a skin or conjunctival test to rule out sensitivity to horse serum
3. Provide bedrest
4. Administer antibiotics, as prescribed
5. Provide suction and humidified oxygen, as needed
6. Provide tracheostomy care if a tracheostomy is necessary

VIII. POLIOMYELITIS

A. Description
1. Agent: Enteroviruses
2. Incubation period: 7 to 14 days
3. Communicable period: Not exactly known. The virus is present in the throat and feces shortly after infection and persists for about 1 week in the throat and 4 to 6 weeks in the feces.
4. Source: The oropharyngeal secretions and feces of an infected person
5. Transmission: Direct contact with an infected person; fecal-oral and oropharyngeal routes

B. Data collection
1. Fever, malaise, anorexia, nausea, headache, and sore throat
2. Abdominal pain followed by soreness and stiffness of the trunk, neck, and limbs that may progress to central nervous system paralysis

C. Interventions
1. Enteric precautions
2. Supportive treatment
3. Bedrest
4. Monitoring for signs of respiratory paralysis
5. Physical therapy

IX. SCARLET FEVER

A. Description
1. Agent: Group A β-hemolytic streptococci
2. Incubation period: 1 to 7 days
3. Communicable period: During the incubation period and clinical illness, which lasts about 10 days; during the first 2 weeks of the carrier stage, although this stage may persist for months
4. Source: Nasopharyngeal secretions of an infected person or carriers
5. Transmission: Direct contact with an infected person or droplet spread; indirectly by contact with contaminated articles or the ingestion of contaminated milk or other foods

B. Data collection
1. Abrupt high fever, flushed cheeks, vomiting, headache, enlarged lymph nodes in the neck, malaise, and abdominal pain

2. A red, fine, sandpaper-like rash develops in the axilla, groin, and neck and spreads to cover the entire body, except the face
3. The rash blanches with pressure (Schultz-Charlton reaction), except in areas of deep creases and folds of the joints (Pastia's sign).
4. Desquamation, a sheet-like sloughing of the skin of the palms and soles, appears by week 1 to week 3
5. The tongue is initially coated with a white, furry covering with red projecting papillae (white strawberry tongue). By the third to fifth day, the white coat sloughs off, leaving a red, swollen tongue (red strawberry tongue).
6. Tonsils are reddened, edematous, and covered with exudate.
7. Pharynx is edematous and beefy red

C. Interventions
1. Institute respiratory precautions until 24 hours after the initiation of antibiotic therapy
2. Provide supportive therapy.
3. Provide bedrest.
4. Encourage fluid intake.

X. ERYTHEMA INFECTIOSUM (FIFTH DISEASE)

A. Description
1. Agent: Human parvovirus B19
2. Incubation period: 4 to 14 days; may be as long as 20 days
3. Communicable period: Uncertain, but before the onset of symptoms in most children
4. Source: Infected person
5. Transmission: Unknown; possibly respiratory secretions and blood

B. Data collection
1. Before rash, asymptomatic or mild fever, malaise, headache, and runny nose
2. Stages of the rash
   a. Erythema of the face (slapped-cheek appearance) develops, chiefly on the cheeks, and disappears by 1 to 4 days
   b. About 1 day after the rash appears on the face, maculopapular red spots appear and are symmetrically distributed on the extremities. The rash progresses from the proximal to distal surfaces and may last a week or more.
   c. The rash subsides but may reappear if the skin is irritated or traumatized by factors such as the sun, heat, cold, exercise, or friction.

C. Interventions
1. The child is not usually hospitalized.
2. Pregnant women should avoid the infected individual.
3. Provide supportive care.
4. Administer antipyretics, analgesics, and anti-inflammatory medications, as prescribed.

XI. INFECTIOUS MONONUCLEOSIS

A. Description
1. Agent: Epstein-Barr virus
2. Incubation period: 4 to 6 weeks
3. Communicable period: Unknown
4. Source: Oral secretions
5. Transmission: Direct intimate contact

B. Data collection
1. Fever, sore throat, malaise, headache, fatigue, nausea, abdominal pain, and enlarged, red tonsils
2. Lymphadenopathy and hepatosplenomegaly
3. A discrete macular rash that is most prominent over the trunk may occur.

C. Interventions
1. Provide supportive care.
2. Monitor for signs of splenic rupture

⚠️ Teach the parents of a child with mononucleosis to monitor for signs of splenic rupture, which include abdominal pain, left upper quadrant pain, and left shoulder pain.

XII. ROCKY MOUNTAIN SPOTTED FEVER

A. Description
1. Agent: *Rickettsia rickettsii*
2. Incubation period: 2 to 14 days
3. Source: Tick from a mammal source, most often from wild rodents and dogs
4. Transmission: The bite of an infected tick

B. Data collection
1. Fever, malaise, anorexia, vomiting, headache, and myalgia
2. A maculopapular or petechial rash primarily on the extremities (ankles and wrists) but that may spread to other areas; characteristically on the palms and soles

C. Interventions
1. Provide vigorous supportive care.
2. Administer antibiotics, as prescribed.
3. Teach the child and parents about protection from tick bites (Box 39-1).

XIII. COMMUNITY-ASSOCIATED METHICILLIN-RESISTANT *STAPHYLOCOCCUS AUREUS* (CA-MRSA)

A. Description
1. *Staphylococcus aureus* is a bacterium that is normally located on the skin or in the nose of healthy people. When present without symptoms, it is called colonization, and when symptoms are present, it is called an infection.
2. MRSA is a strain of *S. aureus* that is resistant to methicillin and most often occurs in people who were hospitalized or treated at a health care facility (hospital-acquired MRSA).

Box 39-1 Protection from Tick Bites

Wear long-sleeved shirts, long pants tucked into long socks (socks should be pulled up over the pant legs), and a hat when walking in tick-infested areas.

Wear light-colored clothing to make ticks more visible if they get onto the child.

Check children for the presence of ticks after they have been in high-risk or tick-infested areas.

Follow paths rather than walking in tall grass and shrub areas because these are the places where most ticks are found.

Apply insect repellents containing diethyltoluamide (DEET) and permethrin before possible exposure to areas where ticks are found (use with caution in infants and small children).

Keep yards at home trimmed and free of accumulating leaves and other brush.

Apply tick repellent to dogs.

Save the tick for later identification if it is removed from the child's body.

3. CA-MRSA is a MRSA infection that occurs in a healthy person who has not been hospitalized or had a medical procedure done within the past year.
4. Community-associated MRSA is spread through person-to-person contact, contact with contaminated items, or infection of a preexisting cut or wound that is not protected by a dressing.
5. The bacteria can enter the bloodstream through the cut or wound and cause sepsis, cellulitis, endocarditis, osteomyelitis, septic arthritis, toxic shock syndrome, pneumonia, organ failure, and death.

B. Prevention measures
1. Handwashing and practicing good personal hygiene
2. Avoid sharing personal items.
3. Regular cleaning of shared equipment such as athletic equipment, whirlpools, or saunas
4. Cleaning a cut or wound thoroughly

C. Data collection
1. Appearance of a skin infection: Red, swollen area, warmth around the area, drainage of pus, pain at the site, fever
2. Symptoms of a more serious infection: Chest pain, cough, fatigue, chills, fever, malaise, headache, muscle aches, shortness of breath, rash

D. Interventions
1. Check skin lesions.
2. Prepare to drain an infected skin site and culture the wound and wound drainage.
3. Prepare to obtain blood cultures, sputum cultures, and urine cultures.

4. Prepare to administer antibiotics as prescribed.
5. Educate the parent and family about the causes and modes of transmission, signs and symptoms, and importance of treatment prescribed.

XIV. H1N1 INFLUENZA

A. Description
1. H1N1 is also known as swine flu and is a strain of influenza.
2. It is a viral infection that affects the respiratory system and is highly contagious.
3. It is caused by contact with an infected person or by touching something such as a toy or tissue that the infected person has touched.

B. Prevention
1. H1N1 flu **vaccine**
   a. Children age 6 months and older need to be vaccinated
   b. Children younger than 6 months are not old enough to receive the **vaccine**; therefore, family members and caregivers need to get vaccinated.
   c. Children 9 years and younger need two doses at least 3 weeks apart whereas children 10 years and older need one dose. (It takes about 2 weeks after receiving the second dose or the first dose in children needing only one dose before immunity develops.)
   d. The H1N1 **vaccine** and seasonal flu **vaccine** can be given at the same time.
   e. A nasal spray version of the H1N1 **vaccine** that contains a weakened live virus may be given to people 2 to 49 years of age who do not have a chronic health condition.
2. Wash the child's hands frequently and teach handwashing techniques.
3. Avoid children who are ill.
4. Keep the child home from school or away from others until the child has been fever-free (without the use of antipyretics) for at least 24 hours.

⚠ The signs and symptoms of H1N1 infection are similar to those of seasonal flu and usually last a week. If they last longer, the presence of complications should be suspected.

C. Data collection
1. Fever that occurs suddenly and is high
2. Headache, body aches, fatigue, chills, cough, congestion, sore throat, loss of appetite, vomiting, diarrhea

D. Interventions
1. Antiviral medications if prescribed, fluids, rest, pain relievers such as acetaminophen (Tylenol) or ibuprofen (Motrin)
2. Family and child teaching about prevention measures

■■■ PRIORITY NURSING ACTIONS! ■■■

Actions to Take When Administering a Parenteral Vaccine
1. Verify the prescription for the vaccine.
2. Obtain an immunization history from the parents and assess for allergies.
3. Provide information to the parents about the vaccine.
4. Obtain parental consent.
5. Check the lot number and expiration date and prepare the injection.
6. Select the appropriate site for administration.
7. Administer the vaccine.
8. Document the administration and site of administration and lot number and expiration date of the vaccine.
9. Provide a vaccination record to the parents.

The nurse should first verify the prescription and then obtain an immunization history from the parents to ensure that the immunizations are up to date. The nurse should also question the parents about the presence of any allergies in the child because some vaccines contain components to which the child may be allergic. The nurse next provides information to the parents about the vaccine and obtains consent. The expiration date and the lot number (located on the medication vial) of the vaccine should be checked before preparing the vaccine for administration. When the vaccine is prepared, the nurse prepares the child for the procedure, selects an appropriate site, and administers the vaccine. The nurse documents that the vaccination has been administered and provides an updated immunization record to the parents.

References: Hockenberry, M., & Wilson, D. (2009). *Wong's essentials of pediatric nursing* (8th ed., pp. 359, 363-364). St. Louis: Mosby; and McKinney, E., James, S., Murray, S., & Ashwill, J. (2009). *Maternal-child nursing* (3rd ed., pp. 68, 70). St. Louis: Saunders.

XV. IMMUNIZATIONS

A. Guidelines (see Priority Nursing Actions)
1. In the United States, the recommended age for beginning primary immunizations of infants is at birth.
2. Children who began primary immunizations at the recommended age but failed to receive all of the required doses do not need to begin the series again. Rather, they need to receive only the missed doses.
3. If there is a suspicion that the parent will not bring the child to the pediatrician or health care clinic for follow-up immunizations according to the optimal immunization schedule, any of the recommended **vaccines** can be administered simultaneously.

B. General contraindications and precautions
1. A **vaccine** is contraindicated if the child experienced an anaphylactic reaction to a previously administered **vaccine** or a component in the **vaccine**.

2. Live virus **vaccines** generally are not administered to individuals with severely deficient immune system, those with a severe sensitivity to gelatin, or pregnant women.

3. A **vaccine** is administered with caution to an individual with a moderate or severe acute illness, with or without fever.

C. Guidelines for administration (Box 39-2)

 Children born prematurely should receive the full dose of each vaccine at the appropriate chronological age.

D. Recommended immunization schedules: Refer to Centers for Disease Control and Prevention (CDC) for the 2012 immunization schedules for children, teens, and adults at http://www.immunize.org/CDC/schedules/.

XVI. REACTIONS TO A VACCINE

A. Local reactions
1. Tenderness, erythema, and swelling at the injection site
2. Low-grade fever
3. Behavioral changes, such as drowsiness, unusual crying, and eating less

B. Minimizing local reactions
1. Select a needle of adequate length to deposit the **vaccine** deep into the muscle or subcutaneous mass.
2. Inject the **vaccine** into the appropriate, recommended site.

C. Anaphylactic reactions
1. The goals of treatment are to secure and protect the airway, restore adequate circulation, and prevent further exposure to the antigen.
2. For a mild reaction with no evidence of respiratory distress or cardiovascular compromise, a subcutaneous injection of an antihistamine such as diphenhydramine (Benadryl) or epinephrine (Adrenalin) may be prescribed.
3. For moderate or severe distress, establish an airway; provide cardiopulmonary resuscitation if the child is not breathing; elevate the head; epinephrine, fluids, and vasopressors may be prescribed; monitor the vital signs and the urine output.

XVII. ACQUIRED IMMUNODEFICIENCY SYNDROME (AIDS)

A. Description
1. AIDS is a disorder caused by human immunodeficiency virus (HIV) and characterized by generalized dysfunction of the immune system (Figure 39-1)
2. HIV virus infects the $CD4^+$ T cells; a gradual decrease in the $CD4^+$ T cell count occurs and this results in a progressive immune deficiency; the risk for opportunistic infections is present.
3. HIV is transmitted through blood, semen, vaginal secretions, and breast milk; the incubation period is months to years.

Box 39-2 Guidelines for the Administration of Vaccines

Follow the manufacturer's recommendations for the route of administration, storage, and the reconstitution of the vaccine.

If refrigeration is necessary, store the vaccine on a center shelf and not on the door. Frequent temperature changes from opening the refrigerator door can alter the potency of the vaccine.

A vaccine information statement needs to be given to the parents or the individual, and informed consent for administration needs to be obtained.

Check the expiration date on the vaccine bottle.

Parenteral vaccines are given in separate syringes at different injection sites.

Vaccines that are administered intramuscularly are given in the vastus lateralis muscle (best site) or the ventrogluteal muscle. The deltoid can be used for children 36 months and older; the dorsogluteal site (the buttocks) is avoided.

Vaccines that are administered subcutaneously are given into the fatty areas in the lateral upper arms and the anterior thighs.

Adequate needle length and gauge are as follows: intramuscular, 1 inch, 23 to 25 gauge; subcutaneous, {5/8} inch, 25 gauge. (Needle length may vary depending on the child's size.)

Mild side effects may include fever, soreness, swelling, or redness at the injection site.

A topical anesthetic may be applied to the injection site before the injection.

For painful or red injection sites, advise the parent to apply cool compresses for the first 24 hours and to then use warm or cool compresses as long as needed.

An age-appropriate dose of acetaminophen (Tylenol) or ibuprofen (Motrin) may be administered every 4 to 6 hours for vaccine-associated discomfort.

Maintain an immunization record: document the day, month, and year of administration; the manufacturer and lot number of vaccine; the name, address, and title of the person who administered the vaccine; and the site and route of administration.

A Vaccine Adverse Event Report needs to be filed and the health department needs to be notified if an adverse reaction to an immunization occurs.

4. Horizontal transmission: occurs through intimate sexual contact or parenteral exposure to blood or body fluids that contain blood.
5. Vertical (perinatal) transmission: occurs through transmission from an HIV-infected pregnant woman to her fetus. (See Chapter 22 for additional information on HIV.)
6. The most common opportunistic infection that occurs in children infected with HIV is *Pneumocystis jiroveci* pneumonia (formerly known as *Pneumocystis carinii* pneumonia [PCP]); most frequently occurs between the ages of 3 and 6 months, when the HIV status may be indeterminate.

⚠ The infant or child infected with HIV is at risk for developing an opportunistic infection that can be life-threatening. Monitor the infant or child closely for signs of infection and report these signs immediately if they occur.

B. Data collection (Boxes 39-3 and Box 39-4)
C. Diagnostic tests: Before testing, counseling should be provided to parents; issues that should be addressed include the causes of HIV, reasons for testing, implications of positive test results, confidentiality issues, and beneficial effects of early intervention (Table 39-1).

Box 39-3 Common Data Collection Findings in Children with HIV Infection

Chronic cough
Chronic or recurrent diarrhea
Developmental delay or regression of developmental milestones
Failure to thrive
Hepatosplenomegaly
Lymphadenopathy
Malaise and fatigue
Night sweats
Oral candidiasis
Parotitis
Weight loss

Adapted from Perry, S., Hockenberry, M., Lowdermilk, D., & Wilson, D. (2010). *Maternal child nursing care* (4th ed.). St. Louis: Elsevier.

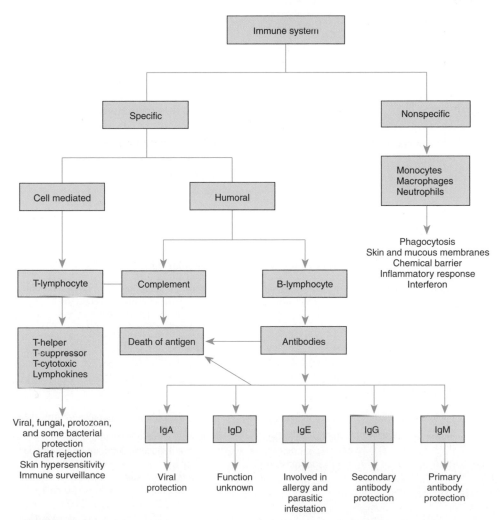

▲ **FIGURE 39-1** Components of the immune system. (From Hockenberry, M. [2007]. *Wong's nursing care of infants and children* [7th ed.]. St. Louis: Mosby.)

D. Prophylaxis (*P. jiroveci* pneumonia and other opportunistic infections)
  1. Provide prophylaxis as prescribed against *P. jiroveci* pneumonia and other opportunistic infections, particularly during the first year of life of the infant born to an HIV-infected mother.
  2. After 1 year of age, the need for prophylaxis is determined based on the presence and severity of immunosuppression or a history of *P. jiroveci* pneumonia.
  3. Continuing prophylaxis is based on the child's HIV status, history of opportunistic infections, and CD4$^+$ counts.
E. Antiretroviral medications (refer to Chapter 62)
  1. The goal of antiretroviral medications is to suppress viral replication to slow the decline in the number of CD4$^+$ cells, preserve immune function, reduce the incidence and severity of opportunistic infections, and delay disease progression.
  2. The medications affect different stages of the HIV life cycle to prevent reproduction of new virus particles.
  3. Combination therapy may be prescribed and includes the use of more than 1 antiretroviral medication.

⚠ Before administering an antiretroviral medication, ensure that the medication is safe for pediatric administration. Also check the contraindications for use and the adverse effects.

F. Immunizations: Symptomatic HIV or severe immunosuppression
  1. Only the inactivated influenza **vaccine** that is given intramuscularly should be used (influenza **vaccine** should be given yearly).
  2. Measles **vaccine** should not be given; immune globulin may be prescribed after measles exposure.
  3. Only the inactivated polio **vaccine** that is given intramuscularly should be used.
  4. Rotavirus should not be given
  5. Varicella zoster virus **vaccine** should not be given; varicella zoster immune globulin may be prescribed after chickenpox exposure.
  6. Tetanus immune globulin may be prescribed for tetanus-prone wounds.

⚠ Immunizations against common childhood illnesses are recommended for all children exposed to or infected with HIV.

Box 39-4 Common AIDS-Defining Conditions in Children

Candidal esophagitis
Cryptosporidiosis
Cytomegalovirus disease
Herpes simplex disease
HIV encephalopathy
Lymphoid interstitial pneumonitis
Mycobacterium avium-intracellulare infection
Pneumocystis jiroveci pneumonia
Pulmonary candidiasis
Recurrent bacterial infections
Wasting syndrome

From Perry, S., Hockenberry, M., Lowdermilk, D., & Wilson, D. (2010). *Maternal child nursing care* (4th ed.). St. Louis: Elsevier.

TABLE 39-1 Diagnostic Tests for HIV

Test	Age-Appropriate Use	Test Determines	Special Considerations
Enzyme-linked immunosorbent assay (ELISA)	18 mo or older	Response of antibodies to HIV virus	If used and found to be positive in infants younger than 18 mo, indicates only that the mother is infected, because maternal antibodies are transmitted transplacentally; use another diagnostic test.
Western blot	18 mo or older	Presence of HIV antibodies	Same as above
Polymerase chain reaction (PCR)	Younger than 18 mo	Presence of proviral DNA	Very accurate for diagnosing infants 1-4 mo of age
p24 antigen	Younger than 18 mo	HIV antigen specific	Very accurate for diagnosing infants 1-4 mo of age
CD4$^+$ lymphocyte count, T-lymphocyte count	Infant up to 13 yr	Immune system status related specifically to suppression	Age adjustment is essential, because normal counts are relatively high in infants and steadily decline until 6 yr of age. Severe suppression in all age groups is <15% total lymphocytes (less than 750 cells/L in an infant younger than 12 mo, less than 500 cells/L in a child 1-5 yr, less than 200 cells/L in a child 6-12 yr).

From http://www.cdc.gov/hiv/topics/testing/guideline.htm.

G. Caretaker instructions

1. Encourage routine good hygiene and frequent handwashing
2. Monitor for fever, malaise, fatigue, weight loss, vomiting, diarrhea, altered activity level, and oral lesions. Notify the health care provider if these occur.
3. Monitor for signs and symptoms of opportunistic infections, such as pneumonia.
4. Administer antiretroviral medications, as prescribed. Emphasize the importance of strict adherence to the treatment regimen.
5. The child needs to be restricted from having contact with persons who have infections or other contagious or potentially contagious illnesses.
6. Keep immunizations up to date.
7. Keep the child home when he or she is sick.
8. Avoid direct unprotected contact with the child's body fluids.
9. Monitor the child's weight.
10. Provide a high-calorie, high-protein diet.
11. Avoid fresh fruits, fresh vegetables, and raw fish (neutropenic diet if immunosuppressed).
12. Do not share eating utensils with the child.
13. Wash all eating utensils in the dishwasher.
14. Cover any of the child's unused food and formula and refrigerate (discard unused refrigerated formula and food after 24 hours).
15. Avoid sharing objects that may become contaminated with blood, such as toothbrushes.
16. Avoid sharing eating utensils; wash eating utensils in the dishwasher.
17. Cover unused food and formula, and refrigerate them.
18. Discard unused refrigerated formula and food after 24 hours.
19. Wear gloves for care, especially when in contact with body fluids and changing diapers.
20. Change diapers frequently and away from food areas.
21. Fold soiled disposable diapers inward, close with tabs, and dispose in a tightly covered plastic-lined container.
22. Dispose of trash daily.
23. Clean up any of the child's body fluid spills with bleach solution (10:1 ratio of water to bleach).

H. Education for an adolescent infected with HIV

1. High-risk behaviors and the importance of avoiding high-risk behaviors
2. Methods of transmission of HIV
3. The importance of abstinence from sexual contact, such as intercourse
4. The importance of using safe condoms if intercourse is planned
5. Resources available for support and other issues

MORE QUESTIONS ON EVOLVE!

Practice Questions

381. A child with rubeola (measles) is being admitted to the hospital. When preparing for the admission of the child, which precautions should be implemented?
1. Enteric
2. Contact
3. Protective
4. Respiratory

382. The nurse provides instructions regarding respiratory precautions to the mother of a child with mumps. The mother asks the nurse about the length of time required for the respiratory precautions. Which response by the nurse is accurate?
1. Respiratory isolation is not necessary.
2. Mumps is not transmitted by the respiratory system.
3. Respiratory precautions are indicated during the period of communicability.
4. Respiratory precautions are indicated for 18 days after the onset of parotid swelling.

383. A 6-month-old infant receives a diphtheria, tetanus, and acellular pertussis (DTap) immunization at the well-baby clinic. The mother returns home and calls the clinic to report that the infant has developed swelling and redness at the site of injection. Which instruction by the nurse is appropriate?
1. Monitor the infant for a fever.
2. Bring the infant back to the clinic.
3. Apply an ice pack to the injection site.
4. Leave the injection site alone, because this always occurs.

384. A child is diagnosed with scarlet fever. A nurse collects data regarding the child. Which of the following is a clinical manifestation of scarlet fever?
1. Pastia's sign
2. Abdominal pain and flaccid paralysis
3. Dense pseudoformation membrane in the throat
4. Foul-smelling and mucopurulent nasal drainage

385. A child is diagnosed with infectious mononucleosis. The nurse provides home-care instructions to the parents about the care of the child. Which information given by the nurse is accurate?
1. Maintain the child on bedrest for 2 weeks.
2. Maintain respiratory precautions for 1 week.
3. Notify the health care provider (HCP) if the child develops a fever.
4. Notify the HCP if the child develops abdominal or left shoulder pain.

386. The health care provider prescribes laboratory studies for an infant of a woman positive for human immunodeficiency virus (HIV) to determine the presence of HIV antigen in the infant. The nurse anticipates that which laboratory study will be prescribed for the infant?
1. Chest x-ray
2. Western blot
3. CD4$^+$ cell count
4. p24 antigen assay

387. A nursing student is assigned to help administer immunizations to children in a clinic. The nursing instructor asks the student about the contraindications to receiving an immunization. Immunization is contraindicated in the presence of which condition?
1. A cold
2. Otitis media
3. Mild diarrhea
4. A severe febrile illness

388. A mother with human immunodeficiency virus (HIV) infection brings her 10-month-old infant to the clinic for a routine checkup. A health care provider has documented that the infant is asymptomatic for HIV infection. After the checkup, the mother tells the nurse that she is so pleased that the infant will not get HIV. Which response by the nurse is appropriate?
1. "I am also so pleased that everything has turned out fine."
2. "Since symptoms have not developed, it is unlikely that the infant will develop HIV infection."
3. "Everything looks great, but be sure that you return with your infant next month for the scheduled visit."
4. "Most children infected with HIV develop symptoms within the first 9 months of life, and some become symptomatic at some point before the age of 3 years."

389. A child is scheduled to receive a measles, mumps, and rubella (MMR) vaccine. The nurse who is preparing to administer the vaccine reviews the child's record. Which finding should make the nurse question the health care provider's prescription?
1. Recent recovery from a cold
2. A history of frequent respiratory infections
3. A history of an anaphylactic reaction to neomycin
4. A local reaction at the site of a previous MMR vaccine injection

390. Choose the home care instructions that the nurse would provide to the mother of a child with acquired immunodeficiency syndrome (AIDS). **Select all that apply.**
- [ ] 1. Frequent handwashing is important.
- [ ] 2. The child should avoid exposure to other illnesses.
- [ ] 3. The child's immunization schedule will need revision.
- [ ] 4. Kissing the child on the mouth will never transmit the virus.
- [ ] 5. Clean up body fluid spills with bleach solution (10:1 ratio of water to bleach).
- [ ] 6. Fever, malaise, fatigue, weight loss, vomiting, and diarrhea are expected to occur and do not require special intervention.

ANSWERS

381. 4
Rationale: Rubeola is transmitted via airborne particles or direct contact with infectious droplets. Respiratory precautions are required, and a mask is worn by those who come in contact with the child. Gowns and gloves are not indicated. Articles that are contaminated should be bagged and labeled. Options 1, 2, and 3 are not indicated for rubeola.
Test-Taking Strategy: Use the process of elimination. Recalling that rubeola is transmitted via the airborne route will direct you to the correct option. Review the route of transmission and the therapeutic management of rubeola if you had difficulty with this question.
Level of Cognitive Ability: Applying
Client Needs: Safe and Effective Care Environment
Integrated Process: Nursing Process/Implementation
Content Area: Child Health: Integumentary/AIDS/Infectious Diseases
Reference: Christensen, Kockrow, p. 1059. 2011. *Foundations of nursing.*

382. 3
Rationale: Mumps is transmitted via direct contact or droplets spread from an infected person and possibly by contact with urine. Respiratory precautions are indicated during the period of communicability. Options 1, 2, and 4 are incorrect.
Test-Taking Strategy: Use the process of elimination. Options 1 and 2 can be eliminated first, because they are comparable or alike. From the remaining options, select option 3, because it is the umbrella option, and it addresses communicability. In addition, the time frame indicated in option 4 seems rather lengthy. Review the infectious period of mumps if you had difficulty with this question.
Level of Cognitive Ability: Applying
Client Needs: Safe and Effective Care Environment
Integrated Process: Teaching and Learning
Content Area: Child Health: Integumentary/AIDS/Infectious Diseases
Reference: Christensen, Kockrow, p. 1061. 2011. *Foundations of nursing.*

383. 3
Rationale: Occasionally tenderness, redness, or swelling may occur at the site of the injection. This can be relieved with cool packs for the first 24 hours and followed by warm or cool compresses if the inflammation persists. It is not necessary to bring the infant back to the clinic. Option 1 may be an appropriate intervention, but it is not specific to the subject of the question.
Test-Taking Strategy: Use the process of elimination. Option 4 can be eliminated first because of the closed-ended word "always." Eliminate option 1 next, because it does not relate specifically to the subject of the question. Next, eliminate option 2 as an unnecessary intervention. Review interventions after immunizations and injections if you had difficulty with this question.
Level of Cognitive Ability: Applying
Client Needs: Health Promotion and Maintenance
Integrated Process: Nursing Process/Implementation
Content Area: Child Health: Integumentary/AIDS/Infectious Diseases
Reference: McKinney, James, Murray, Ashwill, p. 70. 2009.

384. 1
Rationale: Pastia's sign is a rash seen among children with scarlet fever that will blanch with pressure, except in areas of deep creases and in the folds of joints. The tongue is initially coated with a white furry covering with red projecting papillae (white strawberry tongue). By the fourth to fifth day, the white strawberry tongue sloughs off and leaves a red, swollen tongue (strawberry tongue). The pharynx is edematous and beefy red in color. Option 2 is associated with poliomyelitis. Options 3 and 4 are characteristics of diphtheria.
Test-Taking Strategy: Focus on the subject, the clinical manifestations associated with scarlet fever. Remember that Pastia's sign describes the rash noted with scarlet fever. Review the clinical manifestations of scarlet fever if you had difficulty with this question.
Level of Cognitive Ability: Analyzing
Client Needs: Physiological Integrity
Integrated Process: Nursing Process/Data Collection
Content Area: Child Health: Integumentary/AIDS/Infectious Diseases
Reference: McKinney, James, Murray, Ashwill, p. 1029. 2009.

385. 4
Rationale: The parents need to be instructed to notify the HCP if abdominal pain (especially in the left upper quadrant) or it left shoulder pain occurs, because this may indicate splenic rupture. Children with enlarged spleens are also instructed to avoid contact sports until the splenomegaly resolves. Bedrest is not necessary, and children usually self-limit their activity. Respiratory precautions are not required, although transmission can occur via direct intimate contact or contact with infected blood. Fever is treated with acetaminophen (Tylenol).
Test-Taking Strategy: Use the process of elimination and your knowledge regarding the organs that are affected in clients with infectious mononucleosis. Options 1 and 2 can be eliminated first, because they are unnecessary interventions for this disease. From the remaining options, knowledge that splenic rupture is a concern will direct you to option 4. Review the complications associated with infectious mononucleosis if you had difficulty with this question.

Level of Cognitive Ability: Applying
Client Needs: Physiological Integrity
Integrated Process: Teaching and Learning
Content Area: Child Health: Integumentary/AIDS/Infectious Diseases
References: McKinney, James, Murray, Ashwill, p. 1025. 2009. Perry, Hockenberry, Lowdermilk, Wilson, p. 1318. 2010.

386. 4
Rationale: The detection of HIV in infants is confirmed by a p24 antigen assay, virus culture of HIV, or polymerase chain reaction. A chest x-ray evaluates the presence of other manifestations of HIV infection, such as pneumonia. A Western blot test confirms the presence of HIV antibodies. The CD4 cell count indicates how well the immune system is working.
Test-Taking Strategy: Note the strategic word *infant*. Recalling the laboratory tests used to determine the presence of HIV infection is needed to answer this question. If you are unfamiliar with the laboratory tests used to detect HIV in infants, review them. Specific laboratory tests to review include ELISA, Western blot, CD4$^+$ cell count, and p24 antigen assay.
Level of Cognitive Ability: Understanding
Client Needs: Physiological Integrity
Integrated Process: Nursing Process/Data Collection
Content Area:: Child Health: Integumentary/AIDS/Infectious Diseases
Reference: Pagana, Pagana, pp. 524-527. 2009.

387. 4
Rationale: A severe febrile illness is a reason to delay immunization, but only until the child has recovered from the acute stage of the illness. Minor illnesses such as a cold, otitis media, or mild diarrhea are not contraindications to immunization.
Test-Taking Strategy: Use the process of elimination, and focus on the subject of a contraindication to receiving an immunization. Noting the word "severe" in option 4 will direct you to this option. If you had difficulty with this question, review the contraindications associated with immunizations.
Level of Cognitive Ability: Understanding
Client Needs: Physiological Integrity
Integrated Process: Teaching and Learning
Content Area: Child Health: Integumentary/AIDS/Infectious Diseases
Reference: McKinney, James, Murray, Ashwill, p. 70. 2009.

388. 4
Rationale: Most children who are infected with HIV develop symptoms within the first 9 months of life. The remainder of these infected children become symptomatic sometime before the age of 3 years. Children, with their immature immune systems, have a much shorter incubation period than adults. Options 1, 2, and 3 are incorrect responses.
Test-Taking Strategy: Use the process of elimination. Eliminate options 1, 2, and 3, because they are comparable or alike in content. Option 4 is the only option that provides specific and accurate data regarding HIV infection in the infant. Review the data collection findings associated with HIV infection if you had difficulty with this question.
Level of Cognitive Ability: Applying

Client Needs: Psychosocial Integrity
Integrated Process: Nursing Process/Implementation
Content Area: Child Health: Integumentary/AIDS/Infectious Diseases
References: McKinney, James, Murray, Ashwill, p. 1054. 2009. Hockenberry, Wilson, p. 942. 2009.

389. 3

Rationale: The MMR vaccine contains minute amounts of neomycin. A history of an anaphylactic reaction to neomycin is considered a contraindication to the MMR vaccine. The general contraindication to all immunizations is a severe febrile illness. The presence of a minor illness such as the common cold is not a contraindication. In addition, a history of frequent respiratory infections is not a contraindication to receiving a vaccine. A local reaction to an immunization is treated with cool packs for the first 24 hours after injection, and this is followed by warm or cool compresses if the inflammation persists.

Test-Taking Strategy: Use the process of elimination. Recalling that a general contraindication to all immunizations is a severe febrile illness will assist you with eliminating options 1 and 2. From the remaining options, note that option 4 identifies a local reaction. This will direct you to option 3, which is a systemic reaction and a potentially life-threatening condition. Review the contraindications to receiving immunizations if you had difficulty with this question.

Level of Cognitive Ability: Analyzing
Client Needs: Physiological Integrity
Integrated Process: Nursing Process/Implementation
Content Area: Child Health: Integumentary/AIDS/Infectious Diseases
Reference: McKinney, James, Murray, Ashwill, p. 68. 2009.

❖ 390. 1, 2, 5

Rationale: AIDS is a disorder that is caused by the human immunodeficiency virus (HIV) and is characterized by a generalized dysfunction of the immune system. Both cellular and humoral immunity are compromised. The horizontal transmission of HIV occurs through intimate sexual contact or parenteral exposure to blood or body fluids that contain visible blood. Vertical (perinatal) transmission occurs when an HIV-infected pregnant woman passes the infection to her infant. Home care instructions include the following: frequent handwashing; monitoring for fever, malaise, fatigue, weight loss, vomiting, diarrhea, altered activity level, and oral lesions and notifying the health care provider if these occur; monitoring for signs and symptoms of opportunistic infections; administering antiretroviral medications, as prescribed; avoiding exposure to other illnesses; keeping immunizations up to date; avoiding kissing the child on the mouth; monitoring the weight and providing a high-calorie, high-protein diet; washing eating utensils in the dishwasher; and avoiding the sharing of eating utensils. Gloves are worn for care, especially when in contact with body fluids or changing diapers. Diapers are changed frequently and away from food areas, and soiled disposable diapers are folded inward, closed with their tabs, and disposed of in a tightly covered plastic-lined container. Any body fluid spills are cleaned with a bleach solution made up of a 10:1 ratio of water to bleach.

Test-Taking Strategy: Focus on the subject—the care of the child with AIDS. Recalling that this disorder is characterized by a generalized dysfunction of the immune system and recalling the modes of transmission will assist you with selecting the home care instructions. Review instructions regarding preventing the transmission of HIV/AIDS if you had difficulty with this question.

Level of Cognitive Ability: Applying
Client Needs: Safe and Effective Care Environment
Integrated Process: Teaching and Learning
Content Area: Child Health: Integumentary/AIDS/Infectious Diseases
Reference: McKinney, James, Murray, Ashwill, p. 1054. 2009.

Pediatric Medication Administration

I. MEDICATIONS AND THE PEDIATRIC CLIENT

A. Pediatric clients are smaller than adult clients, and their medications have to be adapted to their sizes and ages.

B. Neonates and premature infants have immature body systems.

C. The absorption, distribution, metabolism, and excretion of medications differ substantially, and the pediatric client will react more quickly to medication than will an adult client; also, their renal and hepatic function needs to be checked before medications are administered (Figure 40-1).

D. Medication reactions are not as predictable in pediatric clients as they are in adult clients.

II. ADMINISTERING ORAL MEDICATIONS

A. Most oral pediatric medications are in liquid or suspension form, because children usually cannot swallow a tablet.

B. Solutions may be measured by using an oral plastic syringe or other acceptable measurement or administration device; the device used depends on the developmental level of the child.

C. Medications in suspension settle to the bottom of the bottle between uses, so thorough mixing is required before the pouring of the medication.

D. Suspensions must be administered immediately after measurement to prevent settling and thus the administration of an incomplete dose.

E. Administer oral medications with the child sitting in an upright position with the head elevated to prevent aspiration if the child cries or resists.

F. Never pinch the infant or child's nostrils when administering medication.

G. If the medication is known to have an unpleasant taste, draw the required dose into a small syringe, and place the syringe into the side and toward the back of the infant's mouth; administer the medication slowly, allowing the infant to swallow.

H. Place the small child sideways on the adult's lap; the child's closest arm should be placed under the adult's arm and behind the adult's back; cradle the child's head, hold his or her hand, and administer the medication slowly with a plastic spoon, small plastic cup, or a syringe.

I. If a tablet or capsule has been administered, check the child's mouth to ensure that it has been swallowed; if swallowing is a problem, some tablets can be crushed and given in small amounts of puréed food or flavored syrup (enteric-coated tablets, timed-release tablets, and capsules should not be crushed).

J. Follow generally accepted medication administration guidelines for children (Box 40-1).

⚠ Newborns and infants have an immature liver and immature kidneys, so metabolism and elimination of medications is delayed.

III. ADMINISTERING PARENTERAL MEDICATIONS

A. Subcutaneous and intramuscularly administered medications

1. Medications usually given via the subcutaneous route are insulin and some immunizations.
2. Any site with sufficient subcutaneous tissue may be used for subcutaneous injections; common sites include the central third of the lateral aspect of the upper arm, the abdomen, and the center third of the anterior thigh.
3. The safe use of all injection sites is based on normal muscle development and the size of the child; the preferred site for intramuscular injections in infants is the vastus lateralis, but agency policies and procedures need to be followed (Table 40-1 and Figure 40-2).
4. The usual needle length and gauge for pediatric clients are $1/2$ to 1 inch and 22 to 25 gauge; needle length also can be estimated by grasping the muscle between the thumb and forefinger and half the resulting distance would be the needle length.
5. Pediatric dosages for subcutaneous and intramuscular administration are calculated to the nearest hundredth and measured with the use of a tuberculin syringe; always follow agency guidelines.

Immature blood-brain barrier

Increased permeability of skin and conjunctivae

Higher metabolic rate

Differences in protein binding

High total body water volume, low body fat

Immature cardiovascular system

Immature hepatic metabolism

Delayed gastric emptying, relative lack of gastric acid

Altered absorption patterns

Immature renal function

Rapidly growing tissues

Large body surface area

▲ **FIGURE 40-1** Some factors that affect drug disposition in children. (From Price, D., & Gwin, J. [2008]. *Pediatric nursing* [10th ed.]. Philadelphia: Saunders.)

Box 40-1 Medication Administration Guidelines for Children

- Two identifiers are required before medication administration, such as name, medical record number, birth date.
- Obtain information from the parents about successful methods for administering medications to their children.
- Ask the parents about any known allergies.
- To avoid aspiration, liquid forms of medication are safer to swallow than other forms.
- Straws often help older children swallow pills.
- Avoid putting medications in foods, such as milk, cereal, or baby food because it may cause an unpleasant taste to the food and the child may refuse to accept that same food in the future. Additionally, the child may not consume the entire serving and will not receive the required medication dosage.
- If the taste of the medication is unpleasant, have the child drink the medication through a straw.

- Offer juice, a soft drink, or a frozen juice bar after the child swallows a medication.
- Always read the pharmacological indications for administration. Some items such as fruit syrups can be acidic and should not be used with medications that react in an acid medium.
- Record the most successful method of administering medications and pertinent nursing prescriptions on the child's care plan for other nursing staff to follow; this notation also saves the child frustration, fear, and anxiety.

Adapted from Potter, P., & Perry, A. (2009). *Fundamentals of nursing* (7th ed.). St. Louis: Mosby; and Perry, S., Hockenberry, M., Lowdermilk, D., & Wilson, D. (2010). *Maternal-child nursing care* (4th ed.), St. Louis: Mosby.

TABLE 40-1 Intramuscular Injections: Amount of mL by Muscle Group

Muscle	Neonate	Infants 1 to 12 months	Toddlers 1 to 2 years	Preschool to child 3 to 12 years	Adolescent 12 to 18 years
Vastus lateralis	0.5	0.5 to 1	0.5 to 2	2	2
Rectus femoris	Not safe	Not safe	0.5 to 1	2	2
Ventrogluteal	Not safe	Not safe	Not safe	0.5 to 3	2 to 3
Dorsal gluteal	Not safe	Not safe	Not safe	0.5 to 2	2 to 3
Deltoid	Not safe	Not safe	0.5 to 1	0.5 to 1	1 to 1.5

Adapted from Kee, J., & Marshall, S. (2009). *Clinical calculations: With applications to general and specialty areas* (6th ed.). St. Louis: Saunders.

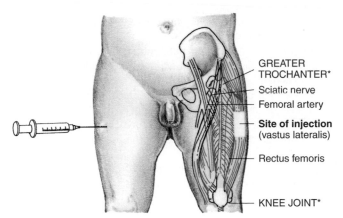

GREATER TROCHANTER*
Sciatic nerve
Femoral artery
Site of injection (vastus lateralis)
Rectus femoris
KNEE JOINT*

▲ **FIGURE 40-2** The appropriate site for intramuscular injections in children: the vastus lateralis. (From Hockenberry, M. [2009]. *Wong's essentials of pediatric nursing* [8th ed.]. St. Louis: Saunders.)

6. Place an adhesive bandage or decorated Band-Aid over the puncture site to help the child view the experience in a somewhat pleasant way.

B. Monitoring intravenous (IV) medications

1. When an infant or a child is receiving an IV medication, the IV site needs to be assessed for signs of infiltration and inflammation immediately before, during, and after the completion of the administration of each medication.
2. Signs of infiltration or inflammation need to be reported.

⚠ The 24-hour fluid intake must be monitored closely, and all IV fluid amounts including the amount of flush volume need to be documented accurately to prevent overhydration. For children, the maximum amount of IV fluid administered in a 24-hour period varies and is usually based on body weight and other factors. Check the health care provider's prescription and agency guidelines for the procedures for the administration of IV fluids and medications.

IV. CALCULATION OF MEDICATION DOSAGE BY BODY WEIGHT

A. Conversion of body weight (Box 40-2)
B. Calculating daily dosages
  1. Abbreviations (Box 40-3)

Box 40-2 Conversion of Body Weight

Measurements
1 lb = 16 oz
1 kg = 2.2 lb

Pounds to Kilograms
1 kg = 2.2 lbs
To convert pounds to kilograms, divide by 2.2. Kilograms are expressed to the nearest tenth.

Kilograms to Pounds
1 kg = 2.2 lbs
To convert kilograms to pounds, multiply by 2.2. Pounds are expressed to the nearest tenth.

Box 40-3 Abbreviations

BSA = body surface area
g = gram(s)
gr = grain(s)
kg = kilogram(s)
lb = pound(s)
m^2 = square meters
mcg = microgram(s)
mg = milligram(s)
mL = milliliter(s)
SA = surface area

2. Dosages are expressed in terms of mg/kg/day, mg/lb/day, or mg/kg/dose.
3. The total daily dosage is usually administered in divided doses (i.e., more than one) per day.
4. Express the child's body weight in kilograms or pounds to correlate with the dosage specifications.
5. Calculate the total daily dosage.
6. Divide the total daily dosage by the number of doses to be administered over the course of 1 day.

V. CALCULATION OF BODY SURFACE AREA

A. The body surface area (BSA) is determined by comparing body weight and height with averages or norms on a graph called a nomogram.

B. Not all children are the same size at the same age; therefore, the nomogram chart is used to determine the BSA of the child.

C. Look at the nomogram chart (Figure 40-3); the height is on the left-hand side of the chart, and the weight is on the right-hand side.

D. Place a ruler on the chart.

E. Line up the left side of the ruler on the height and the right side of the ruler on the weight; read the BSA at the point where the straight edge of the ruler intersects the surface area (SA) column.

F. The estimated SA is given in square meters (m^2).

G. See Box 40-4 for an example.

VI. CALCULATIONS BASED ON BODY SURFACE AREA

A. When dosage recommendations for children specify mg, mcg, or unit per m^2, calculating the dosage is simple multiplication (Box 40-5).

B. When dosages are specified only for adults, a formula is used to calculate the child's dosage from the adult dosage (Box 40-6).

VII. DEVELOPMENTAL CONSIDERATIONS FOR ADMINISTERING MEDICATIONS

A. When administering medications to children, **developmental age** must be taken into consideration to ensure safe and effective administration.

Box 40-4 How to Use the Nomogram

Example: Use the nomogram to estimate the body surface area (BSA) of a child whose height is 58 inches and whose weight is 12 kg.

Look at Figure 40-3 and note that the height is on the left-hand side of the chart and the weight is on the right-hand side of the chart.

Place a ruler on the chart, and line up the left side of the ruler on the height and the right side of the ruler on the weight. Read the BSA at the point where the straight edge of the ruler intersects the surface area (SA) column.

The estimated SA is given in square meters (m^2).
Answer: This child's BSA is 0.66 m^2

Box 40-5 Calculating Medication Dosage

When dosage recommendations for children specify milligrams, micrograms, or units per square meter, calculating the dosage is simple multiplication.

Example: The dosage recommendation is 4 mg/m^2. The child has a body surface area of 1.1 m^2. What is the dosage to be administered?

Answer: 1.1 × 4 mg = 4.4 mg

Box 40-6 Calculating a Child's Dosage From the Adult Dosage

When dosages are specified only for adults, a formula is used to calculate a child's dosage from the adult dosage. The adult dosage is based on a standardized body surface area of 1.73 m^2.

Example: A health care provider has prescribed an antibiotic for a child. The average adult dose is 250 mg. The child has a body surface area (BSA) of 0.41 m^2. What is the dose for the child?

Formula:

$$\frac{BSA\,of\,child\,(m^2)}{1.73\,m^2} \times Adult\,dose = Child's\,dose$$

$$\frac{0.41}{1.73} \times 250\,mg = 59.24\,mg$$

Answer: This child's dose is 59.24 mg.

▲ **FIGURE 40-3** Nomogram chart for estimating body surface area. (From Hockenberry, M. [2005]. *Wong's essentials of pediatric nursing* [7th ed.]. St. Louis: Saunders.)

Box 40-7 Developmental Considerations for Administering Medications

Infants
- Perform the procedure quickly; then offer comfort measures, such as holding, rocking, and cuddling.
- Allow self-comforting measures, such as the use of a pacifier.

Toddlers
- Offer a brief, concrete explanation of the procedure, and then perform it.
- Accept aggressive behavior, within reasonable limits, as a healthy response, and provide outlets for the toddler.
- Provide comfort measures immediately after the procedure, such as touch, holding, cuddling, and providing a favorite toy.

Preschoolers
- Offer a brief, concrete explanation of the procedure and then perform it.
- Provide comfort measures after the procedure, such as touch, holding, or providing a favorite toy.
- Accept aggressive behavior, within reasonable limits, as a healthy response, and provide outlets for the child.

School-Age Children
- Explain the procedure, allowing for some control over the body and situation.
- Explore feelings and concepts through therapeutic play, drawings of own body and self in the hospital, and the use of books and realistic hospital equipment.
- Set appropriate behavior limits, such as it is all right to cry or scream, but not to bite.
- Provide activities for releasing aggression and anger.
- Use the opportunity to teach about how medication helps the disorder.

Adolescents
- Explain the procedure, allowing for some control over body and situation.
- Explore concepts of self, hospitalization, and illness, and correct any misconceptions.
- Encourage self-expression, individuality, and self-care needs.
- Encourage participation in the procedure.

Adapted from McKenry, L., & Salerno, E. (2003). *Mosby's pharmacology in nursing.* St. Louis: Mosby.

B. General interventions
1. Always be prepared for the procedure with all necessary equipment and assistance.
2. For the hospitalized child, ask the parent and/or child if the parent should or should not remain for the procedure.
3. Determine appropriate preadministration and postadministration comfort measures.
4. Try to make the event as pleasant as is possible.
C. Box 40-7 lists developmental considerations when giving medications.

MORE QUESTIONS ON EVOLVE!

Practice Questions

391. Morphine sulfate, 2.5 mg, is prescribed for a child. The safe pediatric dose is 0.05 to 0.1 mg/kg/dose. The child weighs 50 kg. Which statement most accurately describes the prescribed dosage for this child?
1. The dose is too low.
2. The dose is too high.
3. The dose is within the safe dosage range.
4. There is not enough information to determine the safe dosage range.

392. A health care provider's prescription reads as follows: "Ampicillin, 125 mg intramuscular every 6 hours." The medication label reads "1 gram and reconstitute with 7.4 mL of bacteriostatic water." How many milliliters should the nurse draw up for one dose?
1. 0.54 mL
2. 0.92 mL
3. 1.1 mL
4. 7.4 mL

393. A health care provider has prescribed phenobarbital sodium (Luminal Sodium), 25 mg orally twice daily, for a child with febrile seizures. The medication label reads as follows: "Phenobarbital sodium, 20 mg/5 mL." The nurse has determined that the dose prescribed is a safe dose for the child. How many milliliters per dose should the nurse administer to the child?
1. 2 mL
2. 4.5 mL
3. 6.25 mL
4. 7 mL

394. Sulfisoxazole, 1 g orally four times daily, is prescribed for an adolescent with a urinary tract infection. The medication label reads "500-mg tablets." The nurse has determined that the prescribed dose is safe. How many tablets per dose should the nurse administer to the adolescent?
1. 0.5 tablet
2. 1 tablet
3. 2 tablets
4. 3 tablets

❖ **395.** Atropine sulfate, 0.2 mg given intramuscularly, is prescribed for a child. The medication label reads as follows: "0.4 mg/mL." The nurse has determined that the prescribed dose is safe.

How many milliliters should the nurse administer to the child? **Fill in the blank.**
Answer: _____ mL

ANSWERS

391. 3
Rationale: Use the formula for calculating a safe dosage range.
Dosage parameters:

0.05 mg/kg/dose × 50 kg = 2.5 mg/dose

0.1 mg/kg/dose × 50 kg = 5 mg/dose

The dose is within the safe dosage range.
Test-Taking Strategy: Identify the strategic components of the question and what the question is asking. In this case, the question asks for the safe dosage range of the medication. Calculate the dosage parameters with the use of the safe dosage range identified in the question and the child's weight in kilograms. Verify the answer with the use of a calculator. Review pediatric medication calculations if you had difficulty with this question.
Level of Cognitive Ability: Understanding
Client Needs: Physiological Integrity
Integrated Process: Nursing Process/Planning
Content Area: Fundamental Skills: Medications/Blood & IV Therapy
Reference: Kee, Marshall, pp. 126, 170. 2009.

392. 2
Rationale: Convert grams to milligrams. With the metric system, to convert larger to smaller, multiply by 1000 or move the decimal three places to the right. Then, use the medication calculation formula:

1 g = 1000 mg

Formula:

$$\frac{\text{Desired}}{\text{Available}} \times \text{Volume} = \frac{125 \text{ mg}}{1000 \text{ mg}} \times 7.4 \text{ mL} = 0.925 \text{ mL/dose}$$

Test-Taking Strategy: Identify the strategic components of the question and what the question is asking. In this case, the question asks for milliliters per dose. First, convert grams to milligrams. Next, use the formula to determine the correct dosage, knowing that 1000 mg = 7.4 mL. Verify the answer with the use of a calculator. Review pediatric medication calculations if you had difficulty with this question.
Level of Cognitive Ability: Applying
Client Needs: Physiological Integrity
Integrated Process: Nursing Process/Implementation
Content Area: Fundamental Skills: Medications/Blood & IV Therapy
Reference: Kee, Marshall, pp. 126, 170. 2009.

393. 3
Rationale: Use the medication calculation formula.
Formula:

$$\frac{\text{Desired}}{\text{Available}} \times \text{Volume} = \frac{25 \text{ mg}}{20 \text{ mg}} \times 5 \text{ mL} = 6.25 \text{ mL/dose}$$

Test-Taking Strategy: Identify the strategic components of the question and what the question is asking. In this case, the question asks for milliliters per dose. Use the formula to determine the correct dosage, and use a calculator to verify the answer. Review pediatric medication calculations if you had difficulty with this question.
Level of Cognitive Ability: Applying
Client Needs: Physiological Integrity
Integrated Process: Nursing Process/Implementation
Content Area: Fundamental Skills: Medications/Blood & IV Therapy
Reference: Kee, Marshall, pp. 126, 170. 2009.

394. 3
Rationale: Change grams to milligrams, knowing that 1000 mg = 1 g. When converting from grams to milligrams (larger to smaller), move the decimal point three places to the right; thus, 1.0 g = 1000 mg. Then, use the medication calculation formula.
Formula:

$$\frac{\text{Desired}}{\text{Available}} \times \text{Tablet} = \frac{1000 \text{ mg}}{500 \text{ mg}} \times 1 \text{ tablet} = 2 \text{ tablets}$$

Test-Taking Strategy: Identify the strategic components of the question and what the question is asking. In this case, the question asks for tablets per dose. Change grams to milligrams first. Then, use the formula to determine the correct dosage. Remember to verify the answer with the use of a calculator. Review pediatric medication calculations if you had difficulty with this question.
Level of Cognitive Ability: Applying
Client Needs: Physiological Integrity
Integrated Process: Nursing Process/Implementation
Content Area: Fundamental Skills: Medications/Blood & IV Therapy
Reference: Kee, Marshall, p. 126, 170. 2009.

395. 0.5

Rationale: Use the formula for calculating medication dosage.
Formula:

$$\frac{\text{Desired}}{\text{Available}} \times \text{Volume} = \frac{0.2 \text{ mg}}{0.4 \text{ mg}} \times 1 \text{ mL} = 0.5 \text{ mL}$$

Test-Taking Strategy: Identify what the question is asking. In this case, the question asks for the milliliters to be administered. Use the formula to determine the correct dose, and use a calculator to verify your answer. Review this formula if you had difficulty with this question.
Level of Cognitive Ability: Applying

Client Needs: Physiological Integrity
Integrated Process: Nursing Process/Implementation
Content Area: Fundamental Skills: Medications/Blood and IV Therapy
Reference: Kee, Marshall, p. 126. 2009.

The Adult Client with an Integumentary Disorder

PYRAMID TERMS

burns The cell destruction of the layers of the skin and the resultant depletion of fluid and electrolytes as a result of thermal or chemical injury.

carbon monoxide poisoning Carbon monoxide is a colorless, odorless, and tasteless gas that has an affinity for hemoglobin that is 200 times greater than that of oxygen. Oxygen molecules are displaced, and carbon monoxide reversibly binds to hemoglobin to form carboxyhemoglobin. Tissue hypoxia occurs.

chemical burn Tissue destruction caused by contact with strong acids, alkalis, or organic compounds. Systemic toxicity from cutaneous absorption can occur.

deep full-thickness burn A burn injury that involves damage of the muscle, bone, and tendons. The injured area appears black, and the eschar is hard and inelastic.

deep-partial thickness burn A burn injury that extends into the skin dermis. The wound is red and dry, with white areas in parts that are more deeply injured. The burn may also be painful and sensitive to cold air. Can convert to a full-thickness injury when tissue damage increases with infection, hypoxia, or ischemia.

electrical burn Tissue destruction caused by heat generated from electrical energy as it passes through the body and results in internal tissue damage.

full-thickness burn The injured area appears waxy white, deep red, yellow, brown, or black, and the injured surface appears dry. Edema is present under the eschar.

herpes zoster (shingles) An acute viral infection of the nerve structure caused by the varicella zoster virus. Herpes zoster is contagious to individuals who have not had chickenpox.

pressure ulcer A localized area of skin breakdown that occurs as a result of poor circulation to the area because of pressure between a surface and a bony prominence.

skin cancer A malignant lesion of the skin that may or may not metastasize. Causes include chronic friction and irritation to a skin area and exposure to ultraviolet rays. Diagnosis is confirmed by a skin biopsy that is positive for cancer cells.

smoke inhalation injury Injury that results when the victim is trapped in an enclosed, smoke-filled space.

superficial-thickness burn A burn injury that involves damage of the upper third of the dermis. Mild to severe erythema is noted, and the skin blanches with pressure. The burn is painful.

superficial partial-thickness burn A mottled red base and a broken epidermis and a wet, shiny, and weeping surface are present. Large blisters cover an extensive area. The skin is edematous and painful.

thermal burn Tissue injury caused by exposure to flames, hot liquids, steam, or hot objects.

PYRAMID TO SUCCESS

The Pyramid to Success focuses on the concept that the integumentary system provides the first line of defense against infections. Focus on the protective measures that are necessary to prevent infection. The pyramid points address the risk factors related to the development of integumentary disorders and the preventive measures related to skin cancer. Focus on the emergency measures related to a client with a burn, fluid resuscitation, monitoring for complications, and skin grafting. Psychosocial issues relate to the body-image disturbances that can occur as a result of an integumentary disorder.

CLIENT NEEDS

Safe and Effective Care Environment

- Consulting with members of the health care team regarding treatments
- Establishing priorities of care
- Handling hazardous and infectious materials
- Instituting standard and other precautions
- Maintaining confidentiality related to a disorder
- Making referrals to appropriate care providers
- Obtaining informed consent for treatments and procedures
- Practicing medical and surgical asepsis
- Preventing infection

Health Promotion and Maintenance

- Implementing disease prevention measures
- Performing data collection regarding the integumentary system
- Promoting health screening and health promotion programs to prevent skin disorders

- Providing instructions to the client regarding care for an integumentary disorder

Psychosocial Integrity

- Addressing end-of-life issues
- Discussing unexpected body-image changes
- Identifying coping mechanisms
- Identifying situational role changes
- Using support systems

Physiological Integrity

- Assessing for alterations in body systems
- Providing adequate nutrition for healing
- Providing basic care and comfort
- Providing emergency care
- Monitoring for the expected effects of treatments
- Monitoring for fluid and electrolyte imbalances and other complications
- Monitoring laboratory values

Integumentary System

I. ANATOMY AND PHYSIOLOGY

A. The skin is the largest sensory organ of the body, with a surface area of 15 to 20 square feet and a weight of about 9 lb.

B. Functions

   1. Provides the first line of defense against infections.
   2. Protects underlying tissues and organs from injury.
   3. Receives stimuli from the external environment; detects touch, pressure, pain, and temperature stimuli and relays that information to the nervous system.
   4. Maintains the normal body temperature.
   5. Excretes salts, water, and organic wastes.
   6. Protects the body from excessive water loss.
   7. Synthesizes vitamin D_3, which converts to calcitriol, for normal calcium metabolism.
   8. Stores nutrients.

C. Layers

   1. Epidermis
   2. Dermis
   3. Hypodermis (subcutaneous fat)

D. Epidermal appendages

   1. Nails
   2. Hair
   3. Glands
      a. Sebaceous
      b. Sweat

E. Normal bacterial flora

   1. Types of normal bacterial flora include the following:
      a. Gram-positive and gram-negative staphylococci
      b. Pseudomonas
      c. Streptococcus
   2. Organisms are shed with normal exfoliation.
   3. A pH of 4.2 to 5.6 halts the growth of bacteria.

II. RISK FACTORS FOR INTEGUMENTARY DISORDERS

A. Exposure to chemical and environmental pollutants

B. Exposure to radiation

C. Exposure to the sun

D. Lack of personal hygiene habits

E. Use of cosmetics and harsh soaps

F. Medications, such as long-term corticosteroid and anticoagulant therapy

G. Nutritional deficiencies

H. Moderate to severe emotional stress

I. Infection, with injured areas as the potential entry points for infection

J. Changes associated with developmental stages and aging

III. PSYCHOSOCIAL IMPACT

A. Changes in body image and decreased self-esteem

B. Social isolation and fear of rejection from embarrassment about changes in skin appearance

C. Restrictions in physical activity

D. Pain

E. Disruption or loss of employment

F. Cost of medications, hospitalizations, and follow-up care, including dressing supplies

IV. PHASES OF WOUND HEALING

A. Phases

   1. Inflammatory: Begins at the time of injury and lasts 3 to 5 days; manifestations include local edema, pain, redness, and warmth.
   2. Fibroblastic: Begins the fourth day after injury and lasts 2 to 4 weeks; scar tissue forms and granulation tissue forms in the tissue bed.
   3. Maturation: Begins as early as 3 weeks after the injury and may last for 1 year; scar tissue becomes thinner and is firm and inelastic on palpation.

B. Healing by intention

   1. First intention: Wound edges are approximated and held in place (i.e., with sutures) until healing occurs; wound is easily closed and dead space is eliminated.
   2. Second intention: This type of healing occurs with injuries or wounds that have tissue loss and require gradual filling in of the dead space with connective tissue.

3. Third intention: This type of healing involves delayed primary closure and occurs with wounds that are intentionally left open for several days for irrigation or removal of debris and exudates; once debris has been removed and inflammation resolves the wound may be closed by first intention.

V. SKIN ASSESSMENT

A. Skin assessment techniques: Refer to Chapter 29 for assessment of the integumentary system and Chapter 30 for skin changes that occur with the aging process.

B. Dark-skinned client
1. Cyanosis: Check lips and tongue for a gray color; nail beds, palms, and soles for a blue color; and conjunctiva for pallor.
2. Jaundice: Check oral mucous membranes for a yellow color; check the sclera nearest to the iris for a yellow color.
3. Bleeding: Look for skin swelling and darkening and compare the affected side with the unaffected side.
4. Inflammation: Check for warmth, a shiny or taut and pitting skin area, and compare with the unaffected side.

VI. DIAGNOSTIC TESTS

A. Skin biopsy
1. Description
   a. Skin biopsy is the collection of a small piece of skin tissue for histopathologic study.
   b. Methods include punch, excisional, incisional, and shave.
2. Preprocedure interventions
   a. Obtain informed consent.
   b. Cleanse site, as prescribed.
3. Postprocedure interventions
   a. Place specimen, when obtained by health care provider (HCP), in the appropriate container and send to pathology laboratory for analysis.
   b. Use surgically aseptic technique for biopsy site dressings.
   c. Assess the biopsy site for bleeding and infection.
   d. Instruct the client to keep the dressing dry and in place for at least 8 hours and to then clean the area daily and use antibiotic ointment, as prescribed.

B. Skin cultures
1. Description
   a. Noninvasive procedure
   b. A small skin culture sample is obtained with the use of a sterile applicator and the appropriate type of culture tube (bacterial versus viral).
   c. Viral culture is immediately placed on ice.

d. Sample is sent to the laboratory to identify an existing organism.
2. Preprocedure intervention: Obtain skin culture samples before instituting antibiotic therapy.

⚠ Obtain skin culture samples or any other type of culture specimens before instituting antibiotic therapy.

3. Postprocedure intervention: Send the skin culture sample to the laboratory.

C. Wood's light examination
1. Description: The skin is viewed under ultraviolet light through a special glass (Wood's glass) to identify superficial infections of the skin.
2. Preprocedure intervention: Darken the room before the examination.
3. Postprocedure intervention: Assist the client during adjusting to light after being in a darkened room.

D. Diascopy
1. Allows clearer inspection of lesions by eliminating the erythema caused by increased blood flow to the area.
2. A glass slide is pressed over the lesion, causing blanching and revealing the lesion more clearly.

VII. CANDIDA ALBICANS

A. Description
1. A superficial fungal infection of the skin and mucous membranes.
2. Is also known as a yeast infection and when it occurs in the mouth it is called thrush.
3. Risk factors include immunosuppression such as those clients with acquired immunodeficiency syndrome (AIDS); cancer clients receiving chemotherapy; use of long-term antibiotic therapy; clients with diabetes mellitus; and obesity.
4. Common areas of occurrence include the mucous membranes of the mouth, perineum, vagina, axilla, and under the breasts.

B. Data collection
1. Skin: red and irritated appearance that itches and burns.
2. Mucous membranes of the mouth: red and whitish patches.

C. Interventions
1. The client is instructed to keep skin-fold areas clean and dry.
2. For the hospitalized client, inspect skin fold areas frequently, turn and reposition the client frequently, and keep the skin and bed linens clean and dry.
3. Provide frequent mouth care as prescribed and avoid irritating products.
4. Provide food and fluids that are tepid in temperature and nonirritating to mucous membranes.
5. Antifungal medications may be prescribed.

VIII. HERPES ZOSTER (SHINGLES)

A. Description

1. With a history of chickenpox, **shingles** is caused by the reactivation of the varicella-zoster virus; **shingles** can occur during any immunocompromised state in a client with a history of chickenpox.

2. The dormant virus is located in the dorsal nerve root ganglion of the sensory cranial and spinal nerves.

3. **Herpes zoster** eruptions occur in a segmental distribution on the skin area along the infected nerve and show up after several days of discomfort in the area.

4. Diagnosis is determined by visual examination, and a Tzanck smear and viral culture that identify the organism.

5. Postherpetic neuralgia (severe pain) can remain after the lesions resolve.

6. It is contagious to individuals who never had chickenpox and have not been vaccinated against the disease.

7. Herpes simplex virus is another type of virus; Type 1 infection causes a cold sore (usually on the lip) and Type 2 causes a genital herpes (both types are contagious).

B. Data collection

1. Unilaterally clustered skin vesicles along peripheral sensory nerves on the trunk, thorax, or face

2. Fever; malaise

3. Burning and pain

4. Pruritus

5. Paresthesia

C. Interventions

1. Isolate the client because exudate from the lesions contains the virus (maintain standard and other precautions as appropriate, such as contact precautions).

2. Assess for signs and symptoms of infection including skin infections and eye infections; skin necrosis can also occur.

3. Assess neurovascular status and seventh cranial nerve function; Bell's palsy is a complication.

4. Use an air mattress and bed cradle on the client's bed if hospitalized and keep the environment cool; warmth and touch aggravate the pain.

5. Prevent the client from scratching and rubbing the affected area.

6. Instruct the client to wear lightweight, loose cotton clothing and to avoid wool and synthetic clothing.

7. Teach the client about the prescribed therapies; astringent compresses may be prescribed to relieve irritation and pain and to promote crust formation and healing.

8. Teach the client about measures to keep the skin clean to prevent infection.

9. Teach the client about topical treatment or antiviral medications if prescribed.

10. Vaccination for **shingles** is recommended for adults 60 years of age and older to reduce the risk of occurrence and the long-term pain associated with **shingles**.

11. Antiviral medications may include acyclovir (Zovirax), valacyclovir (Valtrex), or famiciclovir (Famvir); refer to Chapter 62 for information on antiviral medications.

IX. METHICILLIN-RESISTANT *STAPHYLOCOCCUS AUREUS* (MRSA)

A. Description

1. Skin or wound becomes infected with methicillin-resistant *Staphylococcus aureus*.

2. Infection can range from mild to severe and can present as folliculitis or furuncles.

3. Folliculitis is a superficial infection of the follicle caused by *Staphylococcus* and presents as a raised and red rash and pustules; furuncles are also caused by *Staphylococcus* and occur deep in the follicle and present as large raised bumps that may or may not have a pustule, and are very painful.

4. If MRSA gains access into the blood, sepsis, organ damage, and death can occur.

⚠ MRSA is contagious and is spread to others by direct contact with infected skin or infected articles; for the client with MRSA, the infection can also be spread to other parts of the body.

B. Data collection: A culture and sensitivity of the skin or wound will confirm the presence of MRSA and identify appropriate antibiotic therapy.

C. Interventions

1. Maintain standard precautions and isolation precautions as appropriate to prevent the spread to others.

2. Monitor the client closely for signs of further infection or worsening of the condition, which could indicate organ damage.

3. Administer antibiotic therapy as prescribed.

4. For additional information on MRSA, refer to Chapter 39.

X. ERYSIPELAS AND CELLULITIS

A. Description

1. Erysipelas is an acute, superficial, rapidly spreading inflammation of the dermis and lymphatics caused by *Streptococcus* group A, which enters the tissue via an abrasion, bite, trauma, or wound.

2. Cellulitis is a skin infection into the deeper dermis and subcutaneous fat, and the causative organism is usually *Streptococcus pyogenes*.

B. Data collection
  1. Pain
  2. Itching
  3. Swelling
  4. Redness and warmth
C. Interventions
  1. Promote rest of the affected area.
  2. Apply warm compresses as prescribed to promote circulation and to decrease discomfort, erythema, and edema.
  3. Clean the skin with an antibacterial type of soap as prescribed.
  4. Administer antibiotics as prescribed for an infection; obtain a culture of the area before initiating the antibiotics.

XI. POISON IVY, POISON OAK, AND POISON SUMAC

A. Description: A dermatitis that develops from contact with urushiol from poison ivy, oak, or sumac plants
B. Data collection
  1. Papulovesicular lesions
  2. Severe itching
C. Interventions
  1. Cleanse the skin of the plant oils immediately.
  2. Apply cool, wet compresses, as prescribed, to relieve the itching.
  3. Apply topical products to relieve the itching and discomfort.
  4. Topical or oral glucocorticoids may be prescribed for severe reactions.

XII. BITES AND STINGS

A. Spider bites
  1. Almost all types of spider bites are venomous and most are not harmful but bites or stings from brown recluse spiders, black widow spiders, tarantulas, scorpions, bees, and wasps can produce toxic reactions in humans.
  2. Brown recluse spider
    a. Can cause a skin lesion, a necrotic wound, or systemic effects from the toxin (loxoscelism).
    b. Application of ice to decrease enzyme activity of the venom and limit tissue necrosis should be done immediately and intermittently for up to 4 days after the bite.
    c. Topical antiseptics and antibiotics may be necessary if the site becomes infected.
  3. Black widow spider
    a. Causes a small red papule
    b. Venom cause neurotoxicity
    c. Ice is applied immediately to inhibit the action of the neurotoxin.
    d. Systemic toxicity can occur and the victim may require supportive therapy in the hospital.

  4. Tarantulas
    a. Cause swelling, redness, numbness, and lymph inflammation, and pain at the bite site.
    b. The tarantula launches its barbed hairs, which penetrate the skin and eyes of the victim producing a severe inflammatory reaction.
    c. Tarantula hairs are removed as soon as possible using sticky tape to pull hairs from the skin and the skin is thoroughly irrigated; saline irrigations are done for eye exposure.
    d. The involved extremity is elevated and immobilized to reduce the pain and swelling.
    e. Antihistamines and topical or systemic corticosteroids may be prescribed; tetanus prophylaxis is necessary.
B. Scorpion stings
  1. Scorpions inject venom into the victim through a stinging apparatus on their tail.
  2. Most stings cause local pain, inflammation, and mild systemic reactions that are treated with analgesics, wound care, and supportive treatment.
  3. The bark scorpion can inflict a severe and fatal systemic response and the venom is neurotoxic; the victim is taken to the emergency department immediately (an antivenom is administered for bark scorpion bites).
C. Bees and wasps
  1. Usually cause a wheal and flare reaction.
  2. Emergency care involves quick removal of the stinger and application of an ice pack.
  3. The stinger is removed by gently scraping or brushing it off with the edge of a needle or similar object; tweezers are not used because of the risk of pinching the venom sac.
  4. If the victim is allergic to the venom of a bee or wasp, a severe allergic response can occur (hives, pruritus, swelling of the lips and tongue) that can progress to life-threatening anaphylaxis; immediate emergency care is required.
  5. Individuals who are allergic should carry an EpiPen for the self-administration of intramuscular epinephrine if a bee or wasp sting occurs.
D. Snake bites
  1. Some snakes are venomous and can cause a serious systemic reaction in the victim.
  2. The victim should be immediately moved to a safe area away from the snake and should rest to decrease venom circulation; the extremity is immobilized and kept below the level of the heart.
  3. Constricting clothing and jewelry are removed before swelling occurs.
  4. The victim is kept warm and is not allowed to consume beverages such as alcohol or those that contain caffeine because they may speed absorption of the venom.
  5. If transport to the emergency room is not done immediately, a constricting band may be applied

proximal to the wound to slow the venom circulation; monitor the circulation frequently and loosen the band if edema occurs.

6. The wound is not incised or sucked to remove the venom; ice is not applied to the wound.

7. Emergency care in a hospital is required as soon as possible; an antivenom may be administered along with supportive care.

⚠ For spider bites, scorpion bites, or other stings or bites, the poison control center should be contacted as soon as possible to determine the best initial management.

XIII. FROSTBITE

A. Description
1. Frostbite is damage to tissues and blood vessels as a result of prolonged exposure to cold.
2. Fingers, toes, face, nose, and ears often are affected.

B. Data collection
1. First-degree: involves hyperemia and edema formation of the involved area.
2. Second-degree: large fluid-filled blisters with partial thickness skin necrosis occurs.
3. Third-degree: involves the formation of small blisters that contain dark fluid and an affected body part that is cool, numb, blue or red and does not blanch; full thickness and subcutaneous tissue necrosis occurs, requiring debridement.
4. Fourth-degree: no blisters or edema noted and the part is numb, cold, and bloodless; full thickness necrosis extends into muscle and bone and gangrene develops, which may require amputation of the affected part.

C. Interventions
1. Rewarm the affected part rapidly and continuously with a warm water bath to thaw the frozen part (hot towels can be used if a warming tub is not available).
2. Handle the part gently and immobilize and elevate the part above heart level.
3. Avoid the use of dry heat and never rub or massage the part (may result in further tissue damage).
4. Rewarming process may be painful; analgesics may be necessary.
5. Avoid compression of the injured tissues and apply only loose and nonadherent sterile dressings.
6. Monitor for signs of compartment syndrome.
7. Tetanus prophylaxis will be necessary and topical and systemic antibiotics may be precribed.
8. Debridement of necrotic tissue may be necessary; amputation may be necessary for those who develop gangrene.

XIV. ACTINIC KERATOSES

A. Actinic keratoses is caused by chronic exposure to the sun and appear as rough, scaly, red or brown lesions and are usually found on the face, scalp, arms, and back of the hands.

B. Lesions can progress to squamous cell carcinoma.

C. Treatment includes medications and therapies such as excision, cryotherapy, curettage, and laser therapy. (See Chapter 42 for information on medications.)

XV. SKIN CANCER

A. Description
1. **Skin cancer** is a malignant lesion of the skin, which may or may not metastasize.
2. Overexposure to the sun is a primary cause; other causes and conditions that place the individual at risk include chronic skin damage from repeated injury and irritation, an inherited genetic mutation, ionizing radiation, light-skinned races, age greater than 60 years, those who work outdoors, and exposure to chemical carcinogens.
3. Diagnosis is confirmed by a skin biopsy that is positive for cancer cells.

B. Types
1. Basal cell: Basal cell cancer arises from the basal cells contained in the epidermis; metastasis is rare but underlying tissue destruction can progress to organ tissue.
2. Squamous cell: Squamous cell cancer is a tumor of the epidermal keratinocytes and can infiltrate surrounding structures and metastasize to lymph nodes.
3. Melanoma: May occur any place on the body, especially where birthmarks or new moles are apparent; it is highly metastatic and can metastasize to the brain, lungs, bone, and liver, and survival depends on early diagnosis and treatment.

C. Data collection (Box 41-1)
1. Change in color, size, or shape of preexisting lesion
2. Pruritus
3. Local soreness

⚠ The client needs to be informed about the risks associated with overexposure to the sun and taught about the importance of performing monthly self-skin assessments.

D. Interventions
1. Instruct the client regarding the risk factors and preventive measures.
2. Instruct the client to perform monthly self-skin assessments and to monitor for lesions that do not heal or that change characteristics.

Box 41-1 Appearance of Skin Cancer Lesions

Basal Cell Carcinoma
- Waxy border
- Papule, with a red, central crater
- Rarely metastasizes

Squamous Cell Carcinoma
- Oozing, bleeding, crusting lesion
- Potentially metastatic
- Larger tumors associated with higher risk for metastasis

Melanoma
- Irregular, circular, bordered lesion with hues of tan, black, or blue
- Rapid infiltration into tissue
- Rapid metastasis
- Significant rates of morbidity and mortality

3. Instruct the client to have moles or lesions removed that are subject to chronic irritation.
4. Instruct the client to avoid contact with chemical irritants.
5. Instruct the client to wear layered clothing and use sunscreen lotions with an appropriate skin protection factor when outdoors.
6. Instruct the client to avoid sun exposure between 10 AM and 4 PM.
7. Management may include surgical or nonsurgical interventions; if medication is prescribed provide instructions about its use.
8. Assist with surgical management, which may include cryosurgery, curettage and electrodesication, or surgical excision of the lesion.

XVI. PSORIASIS

A. Description
   1. Psoriasis is a chronic, noninfectious skin inflammation involving keratin synthesis that results in psoriatic patches.
   2. Various forms exist, with psoriasis vulgaris being the most common.
   3. Possible causes of the disorder include stress, trauma, infection, hormonal changes, obesity, an autoimmune reaction, and climate changes; a genetic predisposition may also be a cause.
   4. The disorder also may be exacerbated by the use of certain medications.
   5. Koebner phenomenon is the development of psoriatic lesions at a site of injury, such as a scratched or sunburned area.
   6. Some individuals with psoriasis develop arthritis that leads to joint changes similar to those seen in rheumatoid arthritis.

7. The goal of therapy is to reduce cell proliferation and inflammation, and the type of therapy prescribed depends on the extent of the disease and the client's response to treatment.

B. Data collection
   1. Pruritus
   2. Shedding, silvery, white scales on a raised, reddened, round plaque that usually affects the scalp, knees, elbows, extensor surfaces of arms and legs, and sacral regions
   3. A yellow discoloration, pitting, and thickening of the nails is noted, if they are affected
   4. Joint inflammation with psoriatic arthritis

C. Pharmacological therapy: Refer to Chapter 42 for medications used to treat psoriasis.

D. Interventions and client education
   1. Provide emotional support to the client because of the risks associated with altered body image and decreased self-esteem.
   2. Instruct the client in the use of prescribed therapies and to avoid over-the-counter medications.
   3. Instruct the client not to scratch the affected areas and to keep the skin lubricated as prescribed to minimize itching.
   4. Monitor for and instruct the client to recognize the signs and symptoms of infection and to report these signs.
   5. Instruct the client to wear light cotton clothing over affected areas.
   6. Assist the client to identify ways to reduce stress if stress is a predisposing factor.

XVII. ACNE VULGARIS

A. Description
   1. Acne is a chronic skin disorder that usually begins in puberty and is more common in males; lesions develop on the face, neck, chest, shoulders, and back.
   2. Acne requires active treatment for control until it resolves.
   3. The types of lesions include comedones (open and closed), pustules, papules, and nodules.
   4. The exact cause is unknown but may include androgenic influence on sebaceous glands, increased sebum production, and proliferation of *Propionibacterium acnes* (the enzymes that reduce lipids to irritating fatty acids).
   5. Exacerbations coincide with the menstrual cycle because of hormonal activity; oily skin and a genetic predisposition may be contributing factors.

B. Data collection
   1. Closed comedones are whiteheads and noninflamed lesions that develop as follicles and enlarge, with the retention of horny cells.
   2. Open comedones are blackheads that result from continuing accumulation of horny cells and sebum, which dilates the follicles.

3. Pustules and papules result as the inflammatory process progresses.
4. Nodules result from total disintegration of a comedone and subsequent collapse of the follicle.
5. Deep scarring can result from nodules.

C. Interventions

1. Instruct the client in prescribed skin-cleansing methods, with emphasis on not scrubbing the face and using only the prescribed topical agents.
2. Instruct the client in the administration of topical or oral medications as prescribed.
3. Instruct the client not to squeeze, prick, or pick at lesions.
4. Instruct the client to use products labeled noncomedogenic and cosmetics that are water-based and to avoid contact with excessively oil-based products.
5. Instruct the client on the importance of follow-up treatment.
6. Refer to Chapter 42 for information on the medications used to treat acne.

XVIII. STEVENS-JOHNSON SYNDROME

A. A drug-induced skin reaction that occurs through an immunological response.
B. Is similar to toxic epidermal necrolysis, another drug-induced skin reaction that results in diffuse erythema and large blister formation.
C. The condition can be mild or severe and cause vesicles, erosions, and crusts on the skin; if severe, systemic reactions occur that involve the respiratory system, renal system, and eyes resulting in blindness.
D. Most commonly occurs in clients with cancer who are receiving chemotherapy or immunotherapy.
E. Treatment includes immediate discontinuation of the medication causing the syndrome; antibiotics, corticosteroids, and supportive therapy may be necessary.

XIX. PRESSURE ULCER

A. Description

1. A **pressure ulcer** causes impairment of skin integrity.
2. A **pressure ulcer** can occur anywhere on the body; tissue damage results when the skin and underlying tissue are compressed between a bony prominence and an external surface for an extended period of time.
3. The tissue compression restricts blood flow to the skin and this can result in tissue ischemia, inflammation, and necrosis; once a **pressure ulcer** forms, it is difficult to heal.
4. Prevention of skin breakdown in any part of the body is a major role of the nurse.

B. Risk factors

1. Skin pressure and skin shearing and friction
2. Immobility
3. Malnutrition
4. Excessive skin moisture such as that which occurs with incontinence
5. Decreased sensory perception

C. Data collection and staging (Box 41-2)
D. Interventions

⚠ Avoid direct massage to a reddened skin area because massage can damage the capillary beds and cause tissue necrosis.

1. Identify clients at risk for developing a **pressure ulcer**.
2. Institute measures to prevent **pressure ulcers** such as appropriate positioning, using pressure relief devices, ensuring adequate nutrition, and developing a plan for skin cleansing and care.
3. Perform frequent skin assessments and monitor for an alteration in skin integrity.
4. Keep the client's skin dry and the sheets wrinkle-free; if the client is incontinent, check the client frequently and change pads or any items placed under the client immediately.

Box 41-2 Stages of Pressure Ulcers

Stage I
The skin is intact.
The area is red and does not blanch with external pressure.
Area may be painful, firm, soft, warm, or cool compared with adjacent tissue.

Stage II
The skin is not intact.
Partial-thickness skin loss of the epidermis or dermis occurs.
Presents as a shallow open ulcer with a red-pink wound bed or as an intact or open/ruptured serum-filled blister.

Stage III
Full-thickness skin loss is present and extends into the dermis and subcutaneous tissues and slough may be present.
The subcutaneous tissue may be visible.
Purulent drainage is common.
Undermining and tunneling may or may not be present.

Stage IV
Full-thickness skin loss is present and extends into the muscle, bone, or other supporting structures.
Slough or eschar may be present.
Purulent, foul-smelling drainage is common.
Undermining and tunneling may develop.

5. Use creams and lotions to lubricate the skin and a barrier protection ointment for the incontinent client.
6. Turn and reposition the immobile client every 2 hours or more frequently if necessary; provide active and passive range of motion exercises at least every 8 hours.
7. If a **pressure ulcer** is present, record the location and size of the wound (length, width, depth), monitor and record the type and amount of exudates (a culture of the exudate may be prescribed), and assess for undermining and tunneling.
8. Serosanguineous exudate (blood-tinged amber fluid) is expected for the first 48 hours; purulent exudates indicate colonization of the wound with some type of bacteria.
9. Use agency protocols for skin assessment and management of a wound.
10. Treatment may include wound dressings, debridement procedures; skin grafting may be necessary
11. Other treatments may include electrical stimulation to the wound area (increases blood vessel growth and stimulates granulation), vacuum-assisted wound closure (removes infectious material from the wound and promotes granulation), hyperbaric oxygen therapy (administration of oxygen under high pressure raises tissue oxygen concentration), and the use of topical growth factors (biologically active substances that stimulate cell growth).

XX. BURN INJURIES

A. Description: Cell destruction of the layers of the skin and the resultant depletion of fluid and electrolytes
B. Burn size
1. Small **burns**: The response of the body to injury is localized to the injured area.
2. Large or extensive **burns**
   a. Large **burns** consist of 25% or more of the total body surface area for people less than 40 years of age and 20% or more of the total body surface area for people more than 40 years of age.
   b. The response of the body to the injury is systemic.
   c. The **burn** affects all the major systems of the body.
C. Estimating the extent of injury (Box 41-3 and Figure 41-1)
D. Burn depth
1. Superficial-thickness burn
   a. Involves injury to the upper third of the dermis; the blood supply to the dermis is still intact

b. Mild to severe erythema (pink to red) is present, but there are no blisters
c. The skin blanches with pressure
d. The **burn** is painful, with a tingling sensation and pain that is eased with cooling.
e. The discomfort lasts about 48 hours; healing occurs in about 3 to 5 days.
f. There is no scarring, and skin grafts are not required.
2. Superficial partial-thickness burn
   a. Involves injury deeper into the dermis; the blood supply is reduced
   b. Large blisters may cover an extensive area.

Box 41-3 Methods to Estimate the Extent of Burn Injury

Rule of Nines (Adult)
- Head: 9%
- Anterior trunk: 18%
- Posterior trunk: 18%
- Arms (9% each): 18%
- Legs (18% each): 36%
- Perineum: 1%

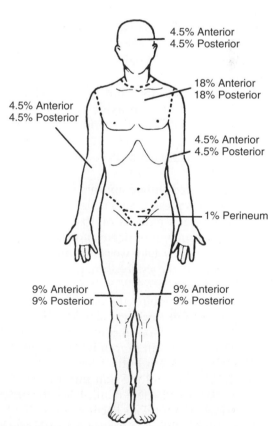

4.5% Anterior
4.5% Posterior

18% Anterior
18% Posterior

4.5% Anterior
4.5% Posterior

4.5% Anterior
4.5% Posterior

1% Perineum

9% Anterior
9% Posterior

9% Anterior
9% Posterior

▲ **FIGURE 41-1** The rule of nines for estimating burn percentage. (From Ignatavicius, D., & Workman, M. [2010]. *Medical surgical nursing: Patient-centered collaborative care* [6th ed.]. St. Louis: Saunders.)

c. Edema is present

d. The **burn** has a mottled pink to red base and a broken epidermis, with a wet, shiny, and weeping surface.

e. The **burn** is painful and sensitive to cold air.

f. Healing occurs in 10 to 21 days with no scarring, but some minor pigment changes may occur.

g. Grafts may be used if the healing process is prolonged.

3. Deep partial-thickness burn

a. Extends into the skin dermis

b. Blister formation usually does not occur, because the dead tissue layer is thick and sticks to the underlying viable dermis.

c. The wound surface is red and dry, with white areas in deeper parts.

d. The area may or may not blanch, and edema is moderate.

e. The **burn** may also be painful and sensitive to cold air.

f. Can convert to a **full-thickness burn** when tissue damage increases with infection, hypoxia, or ischemia

g. Generally heals in 3 to 6 weeks, but scar formation results, and skin grafting may be necessary

4. Full-thickness burn

a. Involves the injury and destruction of the epidermis and the dermis; the wound will not heal by re-epithelialization, and grafting may be required

b. Appears as a dry, hard, leathery eschar; this burn crust or dead tissue must slough off or be removed from the wound before healing can occur.

c. Appears waxy white, deep red, yellow, brown, or black

d. The injured surface appears dry

e. Edema is present under the eschar.

f. Sensation is reduced or absent as a result of the destruction of nerve endings.

g. Healing may take weeks to months and depends on the establishment of an adequate blood supply.

h. Treatment requires the removal of eschar and split- or **full-thickness** skin grafting.

i. Scarring and wound contractures are likely to develop without preventive measures.

5. Deep full-thickness burn

a. Extends beyond the skin into the underlying fascia and tissues; damage to the muscles, bones, and tendons occurs.

b. The injured area appears black, and sensation is completely absent.

c. The eschar is hard and inelastic.

d. Healing takes months, and grafts are required.

E. Age and general health

1. Mortality rates are higher for children less than 4 years old (particularly in the birth to 1-year-old age group) and for clients more than 65 years old.

2. Debilitating disorders (i.e., cardiac, respiratory, endocrine, and renal disorders) negatively influence the client's response to injury and treatment.

3. The mortality rate is higher when the client has a preexisting disorder at the time of the burn injury.

F. **Burn** location

1. **Burns** of the head, neck, and chest are associated with pulmonary complications.

2. **Burns** of the face are associated with corneal abrasion.

3. **Burns** of the ear are associated with auricular chondritis.

4. **Burns** of the hands and joints require intensive therapy to prevent disability.

5. **Burns** of the perineal area are prone to autocontamination by urine and feces.

6. Circumferential **burns** of the extremities can produce a tourniquet-like effect and lead to vascular compromise (compartment syndrome).

7. Circumferential thorax **burns** lead to inadequate chest wall expansion and pulmonary insufficiency.

XXI. TYPES OF BURNS

A. **Thermal burns** are caused by exposure to flames, hot liquids, steam, and hot objects.

B. **Chemical burns**

1. **Burns** are caused by tissue contact with strong acids, alkalis, and organic compounds.

2. Systemic toxicity from cutaneous absorption can occur.

C. Electrical burns

1. **Burns** are caused by heat generated by electrical energy as it passes through the body.

2. **Electrical burns** result in internal tissue damage.

3. Cutaneous **burns** cause muscle and soft tissue damage that may be extensive, particularly with high-voltage electrical injuries.

4. The voltage, type of current, contact site, and duration of contact are important to identify.

5. Alternating current is more dangerous than direct current, because it is associated with cardiopulmonary arrest, ventricular fibrillation, tetanic muscle contractions, and long-bone or vertebral fractures.

D. Radiation **burns** are caused by exposure to ultraviolet light, x-rays, and radioactive sources.

XXII. INHALATION INJURIES

A. Smoke inhalation injury

⚠️ Airway is a priority concern in an inhalation injury.

1. Description: Injury results when the victim is trapped in an enclosed, hot, smoke-filled space.
2. Data collection
   a. Facial burns
   b. Erythema
   c. Swelling of the oropharynx and nasopharynx
   d. Singed nasal hairs
   e. Flaring nostrils
   f. Stridor, wheezing, and dyspnea
   g. Hoarse voice
   h. Sooty (carbonaceous) sputum and cough
   i. Tachycardia
   j. Agitation and anxiety
   k. Risk factors

B. Carbon monoxide poisoning
1. Description
   a. Carbon monoxide is a colorless, odorless, and tasteless gas that has an affinity for hemoglobin 200 times greater than that of oxygen.
   b. Oxygen molecules are displaced, and carbon monoxide reversibly binds to hemoglobin to form carboxyhemoglobin.
   c. Tissue hypoxia occurs
2. Data collection (Table 41-1)

C. Smoke poisoning
1. Description
   a. Smoke poisoning is caused by the inhalation of the byproducts of combustion.
   b. A localized inflammatory reaction occurs and causes a decrease in bronchial ciliary action and in surfactant.
2. Data collection
   a. Mucosal edema occurs in the airways.
   b. Wheezing is evident on auscultation.
   c. After several hours, sloughing of the tracheobronchial epithelium may occur, and hemorrhagic bronchitis may develop.
   d. Adult respiratory distress syndrome can result.

D. Direct thermal heat injury
1. Description
   a. Thermal heat injury can occur to the lower airways as a result of the inhalation of steam or explosive gases or the aspiration of scalding liquids.
   b. Injury can occur to the upper airways, which appear erythematous and edematous, with mucosal blisters and ulcerations.
   c. Mucosal edema can lead to upper airway obstruction, especially during the first 24 to 48 hours.

TABLE 41-1 Carbon Monoxide Poisoning

Blood Level (%)	Clinical Manifestations
1-10	Normal level
11-20 (mild poisoning)	Headache Flushing Decreased visual acuity Decreased cerebral functioning Slight breathlessness
21-40 (moderate poisoning)	Headache Nausea and vomiting Drowsiness Tinnitus and vertigo Confusion and stupor Pale to reddish-purple skin Decreased blood pressure Increased and irregular heart rate
41-60 (severe poisoning)	Coma Seizures
61-80 (fatal poisoning)	Death

Adapted from Ignatavicius, D., & Workman, M. (2010). *Medical surgical nursing: Patient-centered collaborative care* (6th ed.). St. Louis: Saunders.

   d. All clients with head or neck burns should be monitored closely for the development of airway obstruction; these clients are considered immediately for endotracheal intubation if obstruction occurs.
2. Data collection
   a. Erythema and edema of the upper airways
   b. Mucosal blisters and ulcerations

XXIII. PATHOPHYSIOLOGY OF BURNS

A. After the burn, vasoactive substances are released from the injured tissue; these substances cause an increase in the capillary permeability, thus allowing plasma to seep into the surrounding tissues.

B. The direct injury to the vessels increases capillary permeability; capillary permeability decreases 18 to 26 hours after the **burn**, but it does not normalize until 2 to 3 weeks after the injury.

C. Extensive **burns** result in generalized body edema and a decrease in circulating intravascular blood volume.

D. The fluid losses result in a decrease in organ perfusion.

E. The heart rate increases, cardiac output decreases, and the blood pressure drops.

F. Initially hyponatremia and hyperkalemia occur.

G. The hematocrit level increases as a result of plasma loss; this initial increase falls to below normal on the third to fourth day after the burn as a result of red blood cell damage and loss at the time of injury.

H. Initially the body shunts blood from the kidneys, thereby causing oliguria; the body then begins to reabsorb fluid, and diuresis of the excess fluid occurs over the next days to weeks.

I. Blood flow to the gastrointestinal tract is diminished, which leads to intestinal ileus and gastrointestinal dysfunction.

J. Immune system function is depressed, which results in immunosuppression and thus increases the risk of infection and sepsis.

K. Pulmonary hypertension can develop, which results in decreases in the arterial oxygen tension level and lung compliance.

L. Evaporative fluid losses through the **burn** wound are greater than normal, and the losses continue until complete wound closure occurs.

M. If the intravascular space is not replenished with intravenous (IV) fluids, hypovolemic shock and ultimately death will occur.

XXIV. MANAGEMENT OF THE BURN INJURY (see Priority Nursing Actions)

■■■ PRIORITY NURSING ACTIONS! ■■■

Actions to Take in the Emergency Department for a Client with a Burn Injury

1. Check for airway patency.
2. Administer oxygen as prescribed.
3. Obtain vital signs.
4. Ensure initiation of an intravenous (IV) line and begin fluid replacement as prescribed.
5. Elevate the extremities if no fractures are obvious.
6. Keep the client warm and place the client on an NPO status.

The primary goal for a burn injury is to maintain a patent airway, administer IV fluids to prevent hypovolemic shock, and preserve vital organ functioning. Therefore the priority action is to assess for airway patency and to maintain a patent airway. The nurse then prepares to administer oxygen. The type of oxygen delivery system is prescribed by the HCP. Oxygen is necessary to perfuse tissues and organs. Vital signs should be assessed so that a baseline is obtained, which is needed for comparison of subsequent vital signs once fluid resuscitation is initiated. The nurse then initiates an IV line and begins fluid replacement as prescribed. The extremities are elevated (if no obvious fractures are present) to assist in preventing shock. The client is kept warm (using sterile linens) and is placed on NPO status because of the altered gastrointestinal function that occurs as a result of the burn injury. A Foley catheter may be inserted so that the response to the fluid resuscitation can be carefully monitored. Once these actions are taken the nurse performs a complete assessment, stays with the client, and monitors the client closely. Additionally, tetanus toxoid may be prescribed for prophylaxis.

Reference: Ignatavicius, D., & Workman, M. (2010). *Medical-surgical nursing: Patient-centered collaborative care* (6th ed., p. 528). St. Louis: Saunders.

A. Emergent phase

1. Description

a. The emergent phase begins at the time of injury and ends with the restoration of capillary permeability (fluid resuscitation), usually at 48 to 72 hours after the injury; the phase includes prehospital and emergency department care.

b. The primary goals are to prevent hypovolemic shock and to preserve vital organ functioning.

2. Prehospital care

a. Prehospital care begins at the scene of the accident and ends when emergency care is obtained.

b. Remove the victim from the source of the burn.

c. Remove the source of heat.

d. Assess airway, breathing, and circulation.

e. Assess for associated trauma.

f. Conserve body heat.

g. Cover **burns** with sterile or clean cloths.

h. Remove constrictive jewelry and clothing.

i. Assess the need for IV fluids.

j. Transport the client.

3. Emergency department care is a continuation of the care administered at the scene of the injury.

4. Major **burns**

a. Evaluate the degree and extent of the **burn**, and treat life-threatening conditions.

b. Ensure a patent airway, and administer 100% oxygen, as prescribed, if the **burn** occurred in an enclosed area.

c. Monitor for respiratory distress, and assess the need for intubation.

d. Assess the oropharynx for blisters and erythema.

e. Monitor the arterial blood gases and the carboxyhemoglobin level.

f. For an inhalation injury, administer 100% oxygen via a tight-fitting non-rebreather face mask, as prescribed, until the carboxyhemoglobin level falls below 15%.

g. Initiate peripheral IV access to nonburned skin proximal to any extremity **burn**, or prepare for the insertion of a central venous line, as prescribed.

h. Assess for hypovolemia, and prepare to administer IV fluids to maintain the fluid balance.

i. Monitor the vital signs closely.

j. Insert a Foley catheter, as prescribed, and maintain urine output at 30 to 50 mL per hour.

k. Maintain nothing-by-mouth (NPO) status.

l. Insert a nasogastric tube, as prescribed, to remove gastric secretions and to prevent aspiration.

m. Administer tetanus prophylaxis, as prescribed.
n. Administer pain medication, as prescribed, via the IV route.
o. Prepare the client for an escharotomy or fasciotomy, as prescribed.

5. Minor **burns**
   a. Administer pain medication with small doses of morphine sulfate or meperidine (Demerol), as prescribed.
   b. Instruct the client regarding the use of oral analgesics, as prescribed.
   c. Administer tetanus prophylaxis, as prescribed.
   d. Administer wound care, as prescribed; this may include cleansing, débriding loose tissue, removing any damaging agents, and applying topical antimicrobial cream and a sterile dressing.
   e. Instruct the client regarding follow-up care, including active range-of-motion exercises and wound care treatments.

B. Resuscitative phase
1. Description
   a. The resuscitative phase begins with the initiation of fluids and ends when capillary integrity returns to near-normal levels and the large fluid shifts have decreased.
   b. The amount of fluid administered is based on the client's weight and the extent of injury.
   c. Most fluid-replacement formulas are calculated from the time of injury rather than from the time of arrival at the hospital.
   d. The goal is to prevent shock by maintaining adequate circulating blood volume and vital organ perfusion.

2. Fluid resuscitation (Table 41-2)
   a. The amount of fluid administered depends on how much IV fluid is required to maintain a urinary output of 30 to 50 mL per hour.
   b. Successful fluid resuscitation is evaluated by stable vital signs, an adequate urine output, palpable peripheral pulses, and a clear sensorium.

c. Urinary output is the most common and most sensitive noninvasive assessment parameter for cardiac output and tissue perfusion.
d. IV fluid replacement may be titrated (adjusted) on the basis of urinary output plus serum electrolyte levels to meet the perfusion needs of the client with **burns**.
e. If the hemoglobin and hematocrit levels decrease or if the urinary output exceeds 50 mL/hour, the rate of IV fluid administration may be decreased.

3. Interventions

⚠ Urinary output is the most reliable and most sensitive noninvasive assessment parameter for cardiac output and tissue perfusion.

a. Monitor for tracheal or laryngeal edema, and administer respiratory treatments, as prescribed.
b. Monitor the pulse oximetry, and prepare to obtain arterial blood gas and carboxyhemoglobin levels if inhalation injury is suspected.
c. Elevate the head of the bed to 30 degrees or more for clients with **burns** of the face and head.
d. Initiate electrocardiogram monitoring.
e. Monitor the temperature, and assess for infection.
f. Initiate protective isolation techniques; maintain strict handwashing; use sterile sheets and linens when caring for the client; and wear gloves, cap, masks, shoe covers, scrub clothes, and plastic aprons.
g. Shave or cut the body hair around wound margins.
h. Monitor the client's daily weights; expect a weight gain of 15 to 20 lbs during the first 72 hours.
i. Monitor the gastric output and pH levels and for gastric discomfort and bleeding, which indicate a stress ulcer.

TABLE 41-2 Common Fluid Resuscitation Formulas for First 24 Hours After a Burn Injury

Formula	Solution	Rate of Administration
MODIFIED BROOKE		
0.5 mL to 15mL/kg/% TBSA burn	Protenate or 5% albumin in isotonic saline Lactated Ringer's without dextrose	Half given in first 8 hr Half given in next 16 hr
PARKLAND (BAXTER)		
4 mL/kg/% TBSA burn	Crystalloid only (lactated Ringer's)	Half given in first 8 hr, half given in next 16 hr
MODIFIED PARKLAND		
4 mL/kg/% TBSA burn + 15 mL/m^2 of TBSA	Crystalloid only (lactated Ringer's)	Half given in first 8 hr, half given in next 16 hr

TBSA, Total body surface area.
Adapted from Ignatavicius, D., & Workman, M. (2010). *Medical-surgical nursing: Patient-centered collaborative care* (6th ed.). St. Louis: Saunders.

j. Administer antacids, H$_2$-receptor antagonists, and antiulcer medications such as sucralfate (Carafate), as prescribed.

k. Auscultate the bowel sounds for ileus, and monitor for abdominal distention and gastrointestinal dysfunction.

l. Monitor the stools for occult blood.

m. Obtain a urine specimen for myoglobin and hemoglobin levels.

n. Monitor IV fluids and hourly intake and output to determine the adequacy of fluid replacement therapy; notify the HCP if urine output is less than 30 mL/hour or greater than 50 mL/hour.

o. Elevate circumferential **burns** of the extremities on pillows above the level of the heart to reduce dependent edema if no obvious fractures are present; diuretics increase the risk of hypovolemia and are generally avoided as a means of decreasing edema.

p. Monitor the pulses and capillary refill of the affected extremities, and assess the perfusion of the distal extremity with a circumferential **burn**.

q. Prepare for chest and other radiographs to rule out fractures or associated trauma.

r. Keep the room temperature warm.

s. Place the client on an air-fluidized bed, and use a bed cradle to keep the sheets off the client's skin.

4. Pain management

⚠ Avoid the intramuscular or subcutaneous medication routes for medication administration because absorption through the soft tissue is unreliable when hypovolemia and large fluid shifts occur.

a. Morphine sulfate or meperidine (Demerol) is administered as prescribed via the IV route.

b. Avoid intramuscular or subcutaneous medication routes, because absorption through the soft tissue is unreliable when hypovolemia and large fluid shifts are occurring.

c. Avoid administering medication by the oral route because of the possibility of gastrointestinal dysfunction.

d. Medicate the client before painful procedures.

5. Nutrition

a. Proper nutrition is essential to promote wound healing and prevent infection.

b. The basal metabolic rate is 40 to 100 times higher than normal in a client with a **burn** injury.

c. Maintain NPO status until bowel sounds are heard and then advance to clear liquids, as prescribed.

d. Nutrition may be provided via enteral tube feedings or parenteral nutrition.

e. Provide a diet that is high in protein, carbohydrates, fats, and vitamins.

f. Monitor the calorie intake.

6. Escharotomy

a. A lengthwise incision is made through the **burn** eschar to relieve constriction and pressure and to improve circulation.

b. Escharotomy is performed for circulatory compromise caused by circumferential **burns**.

c. Escharotomy is performed at the bedside without anesthesia, because nerve endings have been destroyed by the **burn** injury.

d. Escharotomy can be performed on the thorax to improve ventilation.

e. After the escharotomy, assess the pulses, color, movement, and sensation of the affected extremity, and control any bleeding with pressure.

f. Pack the incision gently with fine-mesh gauze for 24 hours after escharotomy, as prescribed.

g. Apply topical antimicrobial agents to the area, as prescribed, after the procedure.

7. Fasciotomy

a. An incision is made that extends through the subcutaneous tissue and fascia.

b. The procedure is performed if adequate tissue perfusion does not return after an escharotomy.

c. Fasciotomy is performed in the operating room with the client under general anesthesia.

d. After the procedure, assess the pulses, color, movement, and sensation of the affected extremity, and control any bleeding with pressure.

e. Apply topical antimicrobial agents and dressings to the area, as prescribed, after the procedure.

C. Acute phase

1. Description

a. The acute phase begins when the client is hemodynamically stable, capillary permeability is restored, and diuresis has begun.

b. The acute phase usually begins 48 to 72 hours after the time of injury.

c. Emphasis during this phase is placed on restorative therapy, and the phase continues until wound closure is achieved.

d. The focus is on infection control, wound care, wound closure, nutritional support, pain management, and physical therapy.

2. Interventions

a. Continue with protective isolation techniques.

b. Provide wound care, as prescribed, and prepare for wound closure.

c. Provide pain management.

d. Provide adequate nutrition, as prescribed.

e. Prepare the client for rehabilitation.

D. Wound care (Table 41-3)

1. Description: The cleansing, débridement, and dressing of the **burn** wounds

2. Hydrotherapy

   a. Wounds are cleansed by immersion, showering, or spraying.

   b. Hydrotherapy occurs for 30 minutes or less to prevent increased sodium loss through the **burn** wound, heat loss, pain, and stress.

   c. The client should be medicated before the procedure.

   d. Hydrotherapy is generally not used for clients who are hemodynamically unstable or for those with new skin grafts.

   e. Care is taken to minimize bleeding and to maintain body temperature during the procedure.

   f. If hydrotherapy is not used, wounds are washed and rinsed while the client is in bed before the application of antimicrobial agents.

3. Débridement

   a. Débridement is the removal of eschar or necrotic tissue to prevent bacterial proliferation under the eschar and to promote wound healing.

   b. Débridement may be mechanical, enzymatic, or surgical.

   c. **Deep partial-** or **full-thickness burns**: The wound is cleansed and débrided, and topical antimicrobial agents are applied once or twice daily.

E. Wound closure

1. Description

   a. Wound closure prevents infection and the loss of fluid.

   b. Closure promotes healing.

   c. Closure prevents contractures.

   d. Wound closure is performed on day 5 to 21 after the injury, depending on the extent of the **burn**.

2. Wound coverings (Box 41-4)

3. Autografting (see Box 41-4)

   a. Autografting provides permanent wound coverage.

   b. Autografting is the surgical removal of a thin layer of the client's own unburned skin, which is then applied to the excised burn wound.

   c. Autografting is performed in the operating room with the client under anesthesia.

   d. Monitor for bleeding after the graft, because bleeding beneath an autograft can prevent adherence.

   e. If prescribed, small amounts of blood or serum can be removed by gently rolling the fluid from the center of the graft to the periphery with a sterile gauze pad, where it can be absorbed.

   f. For large accumulations of blood, the HCP will aspirate the blood with the use of a small-gauge needle and syringe.

   g. Autografts are immobilized after surgery for 3 to 7 days to allow time for the graft to adhere and attach to the wound bed.

   h. Position the client for the immobilization and elevation of the graft site to prevent the movement and shearing of the graft.

4. Care of the graft site

   a. Elevate and immobilize the graft site.

   b. Keep the site free from pressure.

   c. Avoid weight bearing.

   d. When the graft takes, roll a cotton-tipped applicator over the graft to remove exudate, because exudate can lead to infection and prevent graft adherence.

TABLE 41-3 Open Versus Closed Method of Wound Care

Method	Advantages	Disadvantages
OPEN		
Antimicrobial cream is applied, and the wound is left open to the air without a dressing; antimicrobial cream may be prescribed every 12 hours.	Visualization of the wound; easier mobility and joint range of motion; simplicity of wound care	Increased chance of hypothermia from exposure
CLOSED		
Gauze dressings are carefully wrapped from the distal to the proximal area of the extremity to ensure that circulation is not compromised; no two burn surfaces should be allowed to touch; touching can promote the webbing of digits, contractures, and a poor cosmetic outcome; dressings are usually changed every 8 to 12 hours.	Decreases evaporative fluid and heat loss; aids in debridement	Mobility limitations; prevents effective range-of-motion exercises; wound assessment is limited

Box 41-4 Wound Coverings

Biological

Amniotic Membranes

Amniotic membranes from human placentas are used to adhere to the wound.

This is effective as a dressing until epithelial cell regrowth occurs.

Frequent changes are required, because amnion does not develop a blood supply, and it disintegrates in about 48 hours.

Allograft or Homograft (Human Tissue)

Donated human cadaver skin is provided through a skin bank.

Monitor for wound exudate and signs of infection.

Rejection can occur within 24 hours.

The risk of transmitting a blood-borne infection exists with the use of this covering.

Xenograft or Heterograft (Animal Tissue)

Pigskin is harvested after slaughter and preserved for storage.

Monitor for infection and wound adherence.

Rejection can occur within 24 to 72 hours.

This tissue is placed over granulation tissue and replaced every 2 to 5 days until the wound heals naturally or until closure with an autograft is complete.

Cultured Skin

Cultured skin is grown in a laboratory from a small specimen of epidermal cells from an unburned portion of the client's body.

Cell sheets are grafted onto the client to generate a permanent skin surface.

Cell sheets are not durable; care must be taken when applying them to ensure adherence and prevent sloughing.

Non-Biological

Artificial Skin

Artificial skin consists of two layers: a Silastic epidermis and a porous dermis made from bovine hide collagen and shark cartilage.

After application, fibroblasts move into the collagen part of the artificial skin and create a structure that is similar to that of normal dermis.

The artificial dermis then dissolves and is replaced with normal blood vessels and connective tissue called neodermis.

The neodermis supports a standard autograft that is placed over it when the Silastic layer is removed.

Biosynthetic

This type of covering is made of a combination of biosynthetic and synthetic materials.

It is placed in contact with the wound surface, and it forms an adherent bond until epithelialization has occurred.

Its porous substance allows exudate to pass through it.

Monitor for wound exudate and signs of infection.

Synthetic

Synthetic coverings are applied directly to the surface of a clean or surgically prepared wound, and they remain in place until they fall off or are removed.

The covering is transparent or translucent; therefore, the wound can be inspected without removing the dressing.

Pain at the wound site is reduced, because the covering prevents the contact of the wound with air.

Autograft

Skin is taken from a remote, unburned area of the client's own body and transplanted to cover the burn wound.

The graft is placed either on a clean granulated bed or over a surgically excised area of the burn.

Autograft provides for permanent skin coverage.

---

    e. Monitor for foul-smelling drainage, increased temperature, increased white blood cell count, hematoma, and fluid accumulation.

    f. Instruct the client to avoid using fabric softeners and harsh detergents in his or her laundry.

    g. Instruct the client to lubricate the healing skin with prescribed agents.

    h. Instruct the client to protect the affected area from sunlight.

    i. Instruct the client to use splints and support garments, as prescribed.

  5. Care of the donor site

    a. The method of care varies, depending on the HCP's preference.

    b. A moist gauze dressing is applied at the time of surgery to maintain pressure and to stop any oozing.

    c. The HCP may prescribe site treatment with single-layer gauze impregnated with petrolatum or with a biosynthetic dressing (e.g., Biobrane).

    d. Keep the donor site clean, dry, and free from pressure.

    e. Prevent the client from scratching the donor site.

    f. Apply lubricating lotions to soften the area and to reduce the itching after the donor site is healed.

    g. The donor site can be reused after healing has occurred; it should heal spontaneously within 7 to 14 days with proper care.

F. Physical therapy

  1. An individualized program of splinting, positioning, exercises, ambulation, and activities of daily living is implemented early during the acute phase of recovery to maximize the functional and cosmetic outcomes.

  2. Perform range-of-motion exercises, as prescribed, to reduce edema and to maintain strength and joint function.

  3. Ambulate the client, as prescribed, to maintain the strength of the lower extremities.

4. Apply splints, as prescribed, to maintain proper joint position and to prevent contractures.
   a. Static splints immobilize the joint and are applied for periods of immobilization, during sleeping, and for clients who cannot maintain proper positioning.
   b. Dynamic splints exercise the affected joint.
   c. Avoid pressure to skin areas when applying splints, which could lead to further tissue and nerve damage.
5. Scarring is controlled by elastic wraps and bandages that apply continuous pressure to the healing skin during the period of time when the skin is vulnerable to shearing.
6. Anti–burn scar support garments are usually worn 23 hours a day until the **burn** scar tissue has matured, which takes 18 months to 2 years.

G. Rehabilitative phase
1. Description
   a. Rehabilitation is the final phase of **burn** care.
   b. Rehabilitation overlaps with the acute care phase and goes well beyond hospitalization.
   c. The goals of this phase are designed so that the client can gain independence and achieve maximal function.
2. Goals
   a. Promote wound healing.
   b. Minimize deformities.
   c. Increase strength and function.
   d. Provide emotional support.

MORE QUESTIONS ON EVOLVE!

Practice Questions

396. A nurse is assigned to care for a client with herpes zoster. Which of the following characteristics would the nurse expect to note when assessing the lesions of this infection?
1. Clustered skin vesicles
2. A generalized body rash
3. Small blue-white spots with red bases
4. A fiery red edematous rash on the cheeks

397. A nurse who is employed in a long-term care facility is planning the clinical assignments for the day. The nurse knows not to assign which staff member to the client with a diagnosis of herpes zoster?
1. A staff member who has never had roseola
2. A staff member who has never had mumps
3. A nursing assistant who has never had German measles
4. An experienced nursing assistant who has never had chickenpox

398. A client returns to the clinic for follow-up treatment after a skin biopsy of a suspicious lesion that was performed 1 week ago. The biopsy report indicates that the lesion is a melanoma. The nurse understands that which of the following describes a characteristic of this type of a lesion?
1. Metastasis is rare.
2. It is encapsulated.
3. It is highly metastatic.
4. It is characterized by local invasion.

399. A nurse is reviewing the health care record of a client with a lesion that has been diagnosed as malignant melanoma. The nurse would expect which characteristic of this type of lesion to be documented in the client's record?
1. An irregularly shaped lesion
2. A small papule with a dry, rough scale
3. A firm nodular lesion topped with a crust
4. A pearly papule with a central crater and a waxy border

400. A nurse reinforces instructions to a group of clients regarding measures that will assist with the prevention of skin cancer. Which statement by a client indicates the need for further instruction?
1. "I need to wear sunscreen when participating in outdoor activities."
2. "I need to avoid sun exposure before 10:00 AM and after 4:00 PM."
3. "I need to wear a hat, opaque clothing, and sunglasses when in the sun."
4. "I need to examine my body monthly for any lesions that may be suspicious."

401. A client arrives at the emergency department and has experienced frostbite to the right hand. Which of the following would the nurse note when performing data collection regarding the client's hand?
1. A pink, edematous hand
2. Fiery red skin with edema in the nail beds
3. Black fingertips surrounded by an erythematous rash
4. A white color of the skin, which is insensitive to touch

402. An evening nurse reviews the nursing documentation in the client's chart and notes that the day nurse has documented that the client has a stage 2 pressure ulcer in the sacral area. Which of the following would the nurse expect to note when checking the client's sacral area?
1. Intact skin
2. The presence of tunneling
3. A deep, crater-like appearance
4. Partial-thickness skin loss of the epidermis

403. A nurse inspects the skin of a client who is suspected of having scabies. Which of the following

findings would the nurse note if this disorder was present?
1. Patchy hair loss and round, red macules with scales
2. The presence of wheal patches scattered about the trunk
3. Multiple straight or wavy threadlike lines beneath the skin
4. The appearance of vesicles or pustules with a thick, honey-colored crust

404. A nurse is told that an assigned client is suspected of having scabies. Which of the following precautions will the nurse institute during the care of the client?
1. Wear gloves only.
2. Wear a mask and gloves.
3. Wear a gown and gloves.
4. Avoid touching the client's clothes.

405. The client arrives at the emergency department after a burn injury that occurred in the basement at home, and an inhalation injury is suspected. Which of the following should the nurse anticipate as being prescribed for the client?
1. Oxygen via nasal cannula at 10 L
2. Oxygen via nasal cannula at 15 L
3. 100% oxygen via an aerosol mask
4. 100% oxygen via a tight-fitting, nonrebreather face mask

406. A nurse is caring for a client who has just been admitted to the nursing unit after receiving flame burns to the face and chest. The nurse notes a hoarse cough and that the client is expectorating sputum with black flecks. The client's eyelashes and eyebrows are singed, and the eyelids are swollen. The client suddenly becomes restless, and his color becomes dusky. The nurse interprets this data as indicating which of the following?
1. The client is hypotensive.
2. Pain is present from the burn injury.

3. The burn has probably caused laryngeal edema, which has occluded the airway.
4. The client is afraid and is having a panic attack as a result of the unfamiliar surroundings.

407. Which of the following would be the anticipated therapeutic outcome of an escharotomy procedure performed for a circumferential arm burn?
1. The return of distal pulses
2. Decreasing edema formation
3. Brisk bleeding from the injury site
4. The formation of granulation tissue

408. A nurse is caring for a client with circumferential burns of both legs. Which of the following leg positions is appropriate for this type of a burn?
1. A dependent position
2. Elevation of the knees
3. Flat, without elevation
4. Elevation above the level of the heart

409. A nurse is assisting with caring for a client who is receiving intravenous fluids and who has sustained full-thickness burn injuries of the back and legs. The nurse understands that which of the following would provide the most reliable indicator for determining the adequacy of the fluid resuscitation?
1. Vital signs
2. Urine output
3. Mental status
4. Peripheral pulses

410. An adult client was burned as a result of an explosion. The burn initially affected the client's entire face (the anterior half of the head) and the upper half of the anterior torso, and there were circumferential burns to the lower half of both of the arms. The client's clothes caught on fire, and the client ran, which caused subsequent burn injuries of the posterior surface of the head and the upper half of the posterior torso. According to the rule of nines, what is the extent of this client's burn injury? **Fill in the blank**.
Answer: _____%

ANSWERS

396. 1
Rationale: The primary lesion of herpes zoster is a vesicle. The classic presentation is grouped vesicles on a erythematous base along a dermatome. Because they follow nerve pathways, the lesions do not cross the body's midline. Options 2, 3, and 4 are incorrect descriptions.
Test-Taking Strategy: Use the process of elimination. Remembering that these lesions occur as grouped vesicles along a nerve pathway will assist you with answering the question. Review the characteristics of herpes zoster lesions if you had difficulty with this question.

Level of Cognitive Ability: Understanding
Client Needs: Physiological Integrity
Integrated Process: Nursing Process/Data Collection
Content Area: Adult Health/Integumentary
References: deWit, pp. 1027–1028. 2009.
Linton, pp. 1192-1193. 2012.

397. 4
Rationale: Herpes zoster is caused by a reactivation of the varicella zoster virus, which is the causative virus of chickenpox. Individuals who have not been exposed to the varicella zoster virus are susceptible to chickenpox. Options 1, 2, and 3 are not associated with the herpes zoster virus.

Test-Taking Strategy: Use the process of elimination, and note the strategic words "knows not to assign." Recalling that herpes zoster is caused by a reactivation of the varicella zoster virus will assist you with answering the question. Review the relationship between herpes zoster and chickenpox if you had difficulty with this question.
Level of Cognitive Ability: Applying
Client Needs: Safe and Effective Care Environment
Integrated Process: Nursing Process/Planning
Content Area: Fundamental Skills: Safety/Infection Control
Reference: Linton, p. 1193. 2012.

398. 3
Rationale: Melanomas are pigmented malignant lesions that originate in the melanin-producing cells of the epidermis. This skin cancer is highly metastatic, and a person's survival depends on early diagnosis and treatment. Basal cell carcinomas arise in the basal cell layer of the epidermis. Early malignant basal cell lesions often go unnoticed, and, although metastasis is rare, underlying tissue destruction can progress to include vital structures. Squamous cell carcinomas are malignant neoplasms of the epidermis. They are characterized by local invasion and the potential for metastasis.
Test-Taking Strategy: Knowledge regarding the various types of skin cancers and recalling that melanomas are highly metastatic will direct you to the correct option. Review the characteristics of skin cancers if you had difficulty with this question.
Level of Cognitive Ability: Understanding
Client Needs: Physiological Integrity
Integrated Process: Nursing Process/Data Collection
Content Area: Adult Health/Integumentary
Reference: Linton, p. 1196. 2012.

399. 1
Rationale: A melanoma is an irregularly shaped pigmented papule or plaque with a red, white, or blue color. Basal cell carcinoma appears as a pearly papule with a central crater and a rolled, waxy border. Squamous cell carcinoma is a firm nodular lesion that is topped with a crust or a central area of ulceration. Actinic keratosis, which is a premalignant lesion, appears as a small macule or papule with a dry, rough, adherent yellow or brown scale.
Test-Taking Strategy: Use the process of elimination. Remembering that irregularly shaped lesions are a cause for concern will assist you with answering the question. Review the characteristics of malignant skin lesions if you had difficulty with this question.
Level of Cognitive Ability: Understanding
Client Needs: Physiological Integrity
Integrated Process: Nursing Process/Data Collection
Content Area: Adult Health/Integumentary
Reference: Linton, p. 1196. 2012.

400. 2
Rationale: The client should be instructed to avoid sun exposure between the hours of approximately 10:00 AM and 4:00 PM. Sunscreen, a hat, opaque clothing, and sunglasses should be worn for outdoor activities. The client should be instructed to examine the body monthly for the appearance of any possible cancerous or precancerous lesions.
Test-Taking Strategy: Use the process of elimination. Note the strategic words "need for further instruction." These words

indicate a negative event query and ask you to select an option that is an incorrect statement. A careful reading of the question will direct you to option 2. Review client teaching for the prevention of skin cancer if you had difficulty with this question.
Level of Cognitive Ability: Understanding
Client Needs: Health Promotion and Maintenance
Integrated Process: Teaching and Learning
Content Area: Adult Health/Integumentary
Reference: Christensen, Kockrow, p. 92. 2011. *Adult health nursing.*

401. 4
Rationale: The findings related to frostbite include a white or blue skin color and skin that is hard, cold, and insensitive to touch. As thawing occurs, so does flushing of the skin, the development of blisters or blebs, or tissue edema. Gangrene can develop in 9 to 15 days.
Test-Taking Strategy: Use the process of elimination, and focus on the diagnosis of frostbite. The words "insensitive to touch" should assist with directing you to the correct option. Review the characteristics associated with frostbite if you had difficulty with this question.
Level of Cognitive Ability: Understanding
Client Needs: Physiological Integrity
Integrated Process: Nursing Process/Data Collection
Content Area: Adult Health/Integumentary
References: Christensen, Kockrow, pp. 757–758. 2011. *Foundations of nursing.*
Linton, p. 250. 2012.

402. 4
Rationale: With a stage 2 pressure ulcer, the skin is not intact. There is partial-thickness skin loss of the epidermis or dermis. The ulcer is superficial, and it may look like an abrasion, blister, or shallow crater. The skin is intact with a stage 1 pressure ulcer. A deep, crater-like appearance occurs during stage 3, and tunneling develops during stage 4.
Test-Taking Strategy: Use the process of elimination and your knowledge of the characteristics associated with each stage of pressure ulcers. Remember, with a stage 2 pressure ulcer, the skin is not intact. Review the characteristics associated with each stage of pressure ulcers if you had difficulty with this question.
Level of Cognitive Ability: Understanding
Client Needs: Physiological Integrity
Integrated Process: Nursing Process/Data Collection
Content Area: Adult Health/Integumentary
Reference: Linton, pp. 339–340. 2012.

403. 3
Rationale: Scabies can be identified by the multiple straight or wavy threadlike lines noted beneath the skin. The skin lesions are caused by the female, which burrows beneath the skin and lays its eggs. The eggs hatch in a few days, and the baby mites find their way to the skin surface, where they mate and complete the life cycle. Options 1, 2, and 4 are not characteristics of scabies.
Test-Taking Strategy: Recalling that scabies mites burrow beneath the skin surface will assist you with the process of elimination and provide direction for selecting the correct option. Review the characteristics associated with scabies if you had difficulty with this question.
Level of Cognitive Ability: Understanding

Client Needs: Physiological Integrity
Integrated Process: Nursing Process/Data Collection
Content Area: Adult Health/Integumentary
Reference: Christensen, Kockrow, pp. 89–90. 2011. *Adult health nursing.*

404. 3

Rationale: The Centers for Disease Control and Prevention recommend the wearing of gowns and gloves when in close contact with a person who is infested with scabies. Masks are not necessary. Transmission via clothing and other inanimate objects is uncommon. Scabies is usually transmitted from person to person by direct skin contact. All contacts that the client has had should be treated at the same time.
Test-Taking Strategy: Consider the mode of transmission of scabies, and use the process of elimination. Because scabies is transmitted by direct skin contact, eliminate options 1, 2, and 4. Review standard precautions and the transmission mode of scabies if you had difficulty with question.
Level of Cognitive Ability: Applying
Client Needs: Safe and Effective Care Environment
Integrated Process: Nursing Process/Implementation
Content Area: Adult Health/Integumentary
Reference: deWit, p. 1030. 2009.

405. 4

Rationale: If an inhalation injury is suspected, the administration of 100% oxygen via a tight-fitting, nonrebreather face mask is prescribed until the carboxyhemoglobin level falls below 15%. With inhalation injuries, the oropharynx is inspected for evidence of erythema, blisters, or ulcerations. The need for endotracheal intubation is also assessed. Options 1, 2, and 3 are incorrect.
Test-Taking Strategy: Use the process of elimination. Recalling that 100% oxygen is required after an inhalation injury will assist you with eliminating options 1 and 2. From the remaining options, recall that a tight-fitting nonrebreather mask is preferred so that the client will not rebreathe exhaled air. Review the care of the client after an inhalation injury if you had difficulty with this question.
Level of Cognitive Ability: Analyzing
Client Needs: Physiological Integrity
Integrated Process: Nursing Process/Planning
Content Area: Adult Health/Integumentary
References: Christensen, Kockrow, p. 97. 2011. *Adult health nursing.*
deWit, p. 1040. 2009.

406. 3

Rationale: The client exhibits several warning signs of an inhalation injury: a history of a flame burn to the face, hoarseness, cough, carbonaceous sputum, singed facial hair, facial edema, and color change. Additionally, one of the cardinal signs of hypoxia is restlessness.
Test-Taking Strategy: Use the ABCs—airway, breathing, and circulation—to answer the question. The only option that addresses the airway is option 3. Review the clinical manifestations associated with burns of the face if you had difficulty with this question.
Level of Cognitive Ability: Analyzing

Client Needs: Physiological Integrity
Integrated Process: Nursing Process/Data Collection
Content Area: Adult Health/Integumentary
References: Christensen, Kockrow, pp. 97-98. 2011. *Adult health nursing.*
Lewis, Dirksen, Heitkemper, Bucher, Camera, p. 478. 2011.

407. 1

Rationale: Escharotomies are performed to alleviate the compartment syndrome that can occur when edema forms under nondistensible eschar in a circumferential burn. Escharotomies are performed through avascular eschar to subcutaneous fat. Although bleeding may occur from the site, it is considered a complication rather than an anticipated therapeutic outcome. The formation of granulation tissue is not the intent of an escharotomy, and escharotomy will not affect the formation of edema.
Test-Taking Strategy: Note the subject of the question, a therapeutic outcome. Use the ABCs—airway, breathing, and circulation—to answer the question. The only option that addresses circulation is option 1. Review the purpose of an escharotomy if you had difficulty with this question.
Level of Cognitive Ability: Evaluating
Client Needs: Physiological Integrity
Integrated Process: Nursing Process/Evaluation
Content Area: Adult Health/Integumentary
Reference: deWit, pp. 1038, 1042. 2009.

408. 4

Rationale: Circumferential burns of the extremities may compromise circulation. Elevating injured extremities above the level of the heart and performing active exercise help to reduce dependent edema formation. Options 1, 2, and 3 are incorrect.
Test-Taking Strategy: Use the process of elimination. Remember that when an injury such as a burn occurs, edema occurs. Option 4 addresses a position that will reduce edema. Review the care of the client with a circumferential burn injury if you had difficulty with this question.
Level of Cognitive Ability: Applying
Client Needs: Physiological Integrity
Integrated Process: Nursing Process/Implementation
Content Area: Adult Health/Integumentary
Reference: Lewis, Dirksen, Heitkemper, Bucher, Camera, p. 477. 2011.

409. 2

Rationale: Successful or adequate fluid resuscitation in the adult is signaled by stable vital signs, adequate urine output, palpable peripheral pulses, and a clear sensorium. The most reliable indicator for determining the adequacy of fluid resuscitation is the urine output. For an adult, the hourly urine volume should be 30 to 50 mL.
Test-Taking Strategy: Use the process of elimination. Note the strategic word "reliable" and the subject of fluid resuscitation. Urine output is comparable or alike to the subject of administering fluids. Review the care of the burn client during fluid resuscitation if you had difficulty with this question.
Level of Cognitive Ability: Evaluating
Client Needs: Physiological Integrity
Integrated Process: Nursing Process/Evaluation
Content Area: Adult Health/Integumentary
Reference: deWit, p. 1040. 2009.

❖ **410. 36**

Rationale: According to the rule of nines, with the initial burn, the anterior half of the head equals 4.5%, the upper half of the anterior torso equals 9%, and the lower halves of both arms equal 9%. The subsequent burn included the posterior half of the head, which equals 4.5%, and the upper half of the posterior torso, which equals 9%. This totals 36%.

Test-Taking Strategy: Knowledge regarding the rule of nines is required to answer this question. According to the rule, the entire head equals 9%, each arm equals 9% (both arms, 18%), the anterior and posterior torso each equal 18% (entire torso, 36%), each leg equals 18% (both legs, 36%), and the perineum equals 1%. Remember the following. 9% (head) + 18% (arms) + 36% (torso) + 36% (legs) + 1% (perineum) = 100%. Review the rule of nines if you had difficulty with this question.

Level of Cognitive Ability: Analyzing

Client Needs: Physiological Integrity

Integrated Process: Nursing Process/Data Collection

Content Area: Adult Health/Integumentary

Reference: deWit, pp. 1037–1038. 2009.

42

Integumentary Medications

I. POISON IVY TREATMENT (Box 42-1 and Figure 42-1)

A. Treatment of lesions includes calamine lotion and other products that soothe lesions, Burow's solution compresses, and/or Aveeno baths to relieve discomfort.

B. Topical corticosteroids are effective to prevent or relieve inflammation, especially when used before blisters form.

C. Oral corticosteroids may be prescribed for severe reactions and a sedative such as diphenhydramine (Benadryl) may be prescribed.

II. MEDICATIONS TO TREAT ATOPIC DERMATITIS (Box 42-2)

A. Description
   1. A chronic inflammatory skin disease that is also known as eczema and is characterized by dry and scaly skin.
   2. May be treated with moisturizer and topical glucocorticoids. Systemic immunosuppressants may also be prescribed if topical treatment is ineffective.
   3. Systemic immunosuppressants may include methotrexate, cyclosporine (Sandimmune), or azathioprine (Imuran), and oral glucocorticoids.

B. Topical immunosuppressants
   1. Includes tacrolimus (Protopic) and Pimecrolimus 1% cream (Elidel)
   2. Side effects include redness, burning, and itching; causes sensitization of the skin to sunlight.
   3. Tacrolimus (Protopic) increases the risk of varicella zoster infection in children.
   4. Tacrolimus (Protopic) may cause **skin cancer** and lymphoma.

III. TOPICAL GLUCOCORTICOIDS

A. Description
   1. Have anti-inflammatory, antipruritic, and vasoconstrictive actions
   2. Preparations vary in potency and depend on the concentration and type of preparation, and method of application. (Occlusive dressings enhance absorption, increasing the effects.)
   3. Systemic effects are more likely to occur with prolonged therapy and when extensive skin surfaces are treated.

⚠ Topical glucocorticoids can be absorbed into the systemic circulation, and absorption is greater in permeable skin areas (scalp, axilla, face and neck, eyelids, perineum) and less in areas where permeability is poor (palms, soles, back).

B. Contraindications
   1. Clients demonstrating previous sensitivity to corticosteroids
   2. Clients with current systemic fungal, viral, or bacterial infections
   3. Clients with current complications related to glucocorticoid therapy

C. Local adverse effects
   1. Burning, dryness, irritation, itching
   2. Skin atrophy
   3. Thinning of the skin, striae, purpura, telangiectasia
   4. Acneiform eruptions
   5. Hypopigmentation
   6. Overgrowth of bacteria, fungi, and viruses

D. Systemic adverse effects
   1. Growth retardation in children
   2. Adrenal suppression
   3. Cushing's syndrome
   4. Striae, skin atrophy
   5. Ocular effects (glaucoma and cataracts)

E. Interventions
   1. Monitoring plasma cortisol levels may be prescribed if prolonged therapy is necessary.
   2. Wash the area just before application to increase medication penetration.
   3. Apply sparingly in a thin film, rubbing gently.
   4. Avoid the use of a dry occlusive dressing unless specifically prescribed by the health care provider (HCP).
   5. Instruct the client to report signs of adverse effects to the HCP.

⚠ In the adult, intact skin is generally impermeable to most topical medications. However, medications should not be applied to denuded areas unless prescribed because undesired absorption can occur.

Box 42-1 Poison Ivy Treatment Products

Bentoquatam—for preventive use (Ivy Block)
Calamine lotion (Caladryl lotion)
Hydrocortisone (Ivy Soothe, Ivy Stat)
Isopropanol; cetyl alcohol (Ivy Cleanse)
Zinc acetate; isopropanol (Ivy Dry)
Zinc acetate; isopropanol; benzyl alcohol (Ivy Super Dry)

Box 42-3 Medications to Treat Actinic Keratoses

Fluorouracil (Carac, Efudex, Fluoroplex)
Diclofenac sodium (Solaraze)
Imiquimod 5% cream (Aldara)
Aminolevulinic acid (Levulan Kerastick)

▲ **FIGURE 42-1** Poison ivy. Note "streaked" blisters surrounding one large blister. (From Habif, T. P. [2004]. *Clinical dermatology: A color guide to diagnosis and therapy* [4th ed.]. St. Louis, Mosby.)

Box 42-2 Medications to Treat Atopic Dermatitis

Systemic Immunosuppressants
Methotrexate
Cyclosporine (Sandimmune)
Azathioprine (Imuran)
Oral glucocorticoids

Topical Immunosuppressants
Tacrolimus (Protopic)
Pimecrolimus 1% cream (Elidel)

IV. MEDICATIONS TO TREAT ACTINIC KERATOSES (Box 42-3)

A. Description
1. Actinic keratoses are caused by chronic exposure to the sun and appear as rough, scaly, red or brown lesions and are usually found on the face, scalp, arms, and back of the hands.
2. Lesions can progress to squamous cell carcinoma.
3. Treatment includes medications and therapies such as excision, cryotherapy, curettage, and laser therapy.
4. Medications include fluorouracil (Carac, Efudex, Fluoroplex), diclofenac sodium (Solaraze), imiquimod 5% cream (Aldara), and aminolevulinic acid (Levulan Kerastick).

B. Fluorouracil (Carac, Efudex, Fluoroplex)
1. A topical medication that affects DNA and RNA synthesis and causes a sequence of response that results in healing. Results are usually seen in 2 to 6 weeks, but it may take 1 to 2 months longer for complete healing.
2. Side effects include itching, burning, inflammation, rash, and increased sensitivity to sunlight.

C. Diclofenac sodium (Solaraze)
1. A nonsteroidal anti-inflammatory topical drug, which may take 3 months to be effective.
2. Side effects include dry skin, itching, redness, and rash.

D. Imiquimod 5% cream (Aldara)
1. In addition to treating actinic keratoses, this topical medication has been used to treat venereal warts. It may take up to 4 months to be effective.
2. Side effects include redness, skin swelling, itching, burning, sores, blisters, scabbing, and crusting of the skin.

E. Aminolevulinic acid (Levulan Kerastick)
1. A topical medication used in conjunction with blue light photoactivation. The medication is applied, and 14 to 18 hours later the medication is activated by exposing the lesions to the blue light.
2. Can cause burning, stinging, redness, and swelling of the skin. Treated areas need to be protected from sunlight and bright indoor lights.

V. SUNCREENS

A. Ultraviolet (UV) light can damage the skin and can cause premalignant actinic keratoses and some types of **skin cancer**.

B. Sunscreens prevent the penetration of UV light and protect the skin.

C. Organic (chemical) sunscreen absorb UV light. Inorganic (physical) reflect and scatter UV light.

D. A sunscreen that protects against both UVB and UVA rays and one that has a sun protection factor (SPF) of at least 15 should be used.

E. Sunscreens are most effective when applied at least 30 minutes before exposure to the sun (sunscreens containing para-aminobenzoic acid [PABA] or padimate O require application 2 hours before sun exposure).

F. Sunscreen should be reapplied every 2 to 3 hours and after swimming or sweating; otherwise, the duration of protection is reduced.

G. Products containing PABA need to be avoided by individuals allergic to benzocaine, sulfonamides, or thiazides.

H. Sunscreens can cause contact dermatitis and photosensitivity reactions.

⚠ The client should be informed that UV light is greatest between the hours of 10:00 AM and 4:00 PM, and sunglasses, protective clothing, and a hat should be worn to reduce the risk of skin damage from the sun.

VI. MEDICATIONS TO TREAT PSORIASIS (Box 42-4)

A. Description
1. Psoriasis is a chronic inflammatory disorder that has varying degrees of severity.
2. Treatment is based on the severity of symptoms and aims to suppress the proliferation of keratinocytes or the activity of inflammatory cells.
3. There are numerous medications that can be used to treat psoriasis; some of these are presented in this section.

B. Topical medications
1. Glucocorticoids
   a. Used for mild psoriasis
   b. Should not be applied to the face, groin, axilla, or genitalia because the medication is readily absorbable, making the skin vulnerable to glucocorticoid-induced atrophy
2. Anthralin (Dritho-Scalp, Psoriatec)
   a. Can cause local irritation and skin redness
   b. Is applied to lesions at bedtime and allowed to remain on the skin overnight
   c. Client should be informed that the medication can stain clothing, skin, and hair
3. Tazarotene (Tazorac)
   a. Is a vitamin A derivative
   b. Can cause local reactions such as itching, burning, stinging, dry skin, and redness. Other less common effects include rash, desquamation, contact dermatitis, inflammation, fissuring, and bleeding.
   c. Sensitization to sunlight can occur, and the client should be instructed to use sunscreen and wear protective clothing.
   d. Medication is usually applied once daily in the evening to dry skin
4. Calcipotriene (Dovonex)
   a. Is an analog of vitamin D
   b. May take up to 1 to 3 weeks to produce a desired effect
   c. Can cause local irritation. High-dose applications may cause hypercalcemia.

Box 42-4 Medications and Treatments for Psoriasis

Topical Medications
Glucocorticoids
Keratolytics
Anthralin (Dritho-Scalp, Psoriatec)
Tazarotene (Tazorac)
Calcipotriene (Dovonex)
Coal tar
Others

Systemic Medications
Methotrexate
Acitretin (Soriatane)
Cyclosporine (Neoral)

Systemic Biologic Medications
Alefacept (Amevive)
Ustekinumab (Stelara)

Phototherapy
Coal tar and ultraviolet B irradiation
Photochemotherapy (PUVA [psoralen and ultraviolet A] therapy)

---

5. Coal tar
   a. Suppresses DNA synthesis, miotic activity, and cell proliferation
   b. Has an unpleasant odor and may cause irritation, burning, and stinging; can also stain the skin and hair
6. Keratolytics
   a. Soften scales and loosen the horny layer of the skin, resulting in minimal peeling to extensive desquamation
   b. Salicylic acid: Can be absorbed systemically and can cause salicylism, which is characterized by dizziness and tinnitus, hyperpnea, and psychologic disturbances. Salicylic acid is not applied to large surface areas or open wounds because of the risk of systemic effects.
   c. Sulfur: promotes peeling and drying and is used to treat acne, dandruff, seborrheic dermatitis, and psoriasis

C. Systemic medications
1. Methotrexate
   a. Reduces proliferation of epidermal cells
   b. Can be toxic; causes gastrointestinal effects such as diarrhea and ulcerative stomatitis and bone marrow depression leading to blood dyscrasias
   c. Can be hepatotoxic and hepatic function should be monitored during therapy
2. Acitretin (Soriatane)
   a. Inhibits keratinization, proliferation, and differentiation of cells; has anti-inflammatory and immunomodulatory actions; used for severe psoriasis and is reserved for use in those who have not responded to safer medications

b. Is embryotoxic and teratogenic and is contraindicated during pregnancy. Pregnancy needs to be ruled out, and two reliable forms of contraception need to be implemented before the medication is started. (Contraception needs to be implemented at least 1 month before treatment starts and continued for at least 3 years after treatment is discontinued.)

c. If pregnancy occurs during treatment with the medication, the medication is discontinued immediately and possible termination of the pregnancy is discussed.

d. Dermatological effects include hair loss, skin peeling, dry skin, rash, pruritus, and nail disorders. Other effects include rhinitis from mucous membrane irritation, inflammation of the lips, dry mouth, dry eyes, nosebleed, gingivitis, stomatitis, bone and joint pain, and spinal disorders.

e. Can be hepatotoxic; can elevate triglyceride levels and reduce levels of high-density lipoprotein cholesterol

f. Should be taken with meals to facilitate absorption; alcohol must be avoided

g. Is a derivative of vitamin A and can cause vitamin A toxicity if taken concurrently with vitamin A supplements

h. Should not be taken concurrently with tetracycline because it can cause increased intracranial pressure

3. Cyclosporine (Neoral)
   a. An immunosuppressant that inhibits proliferation of B and T cells
   b. Can be toxic and can cause kidney damage
   c. Is used for severe psoriasis and is reserved for use in those who have not responded to safer medications

D. Systemic biologic medications
   1. Alefacept (Amevive)
      a. Reduces the number and activity of memory CD4+T lymphocytes; therefore the medication is contraindicated in clients with HIV infection
      b. CD4+T cell counts should be monitored before each dose and discontinued if the count falls below 250 cells/mL.
      c. Increase the risk of cancer and should not be administered to a client with a history of malignancy and should be discontinued if cancer develops
      d. Can cause chills, cough, pruritus, myalgia, inflammation and pain at the intramuscular injection site
   2. Ustekinumab (Stelara)
      a. A human monoclonal antibody
      b. Can decrease the activity of the immune system and increase the risk for certain types of cancer

c. Side effects of the medication include upper respiratory infections, headache, and tiredness.

d. Contraindicated in clients who have a history of cancer; also contraindicated in clients with infection or posterior leukoencephalopathy syndrome. (This is a rare condition that affects the brain and can cause death.)

e. The client should not receive any live virus vaccines, because the viruses used in some types of vaccines can cause infection in those with a weakened immune system. Additionally the HCP needs to be informed if anyone in the household needs a vaccine.

f. The client should not receive the BCG vaccine during the one year before or after taking the medication.

g. The client should inform the HCP if he or she is receiving phototherapy, has any other medical condition, is pregnant or plans to become pregnant, or is breast-feeding or plans to breast-feed.

E. Phototherapy
   1. Coal tar and ultraviolet B irradiation: Treatment involves the application of coal tar for 8 to 10 hours. The coal tar is washed off and the area is exposed to short-wave UV radiation (ultraviolet B, UVB).
   2. Photochemotherapy (PUVA [psoralen and ultraviolet A] therapy)
      a. Combines the use of long-wave radiation (ultraviolet A, UVA) with oral methoxsalen (photosensitive medication).
      b. Can cause pruritus, nausea, erythema; may accelerate the aging process of the skin and may increase the risk of **skin cancer**.

VII. ACNE PRODUCTS (Box 42-5 and Figure 42-2)

A. Description
   1. Acne lesions that are mild may be treated with nonpharmacological measures such as gentle cleansing two or three times daily (oil-based moisturizing products need to be avoided), dermabrasion, or comedo extraction.
   2. Mild acne is usually treated pharmacologically with topical agents (antimicrobials and retinoids).
   3. Moderate acne is usually treated with oral antibiotics and comedolytics.
   4. Severe acne is usually treated with isotretinoin.
   5. Hormonal medications such as oral contraceptives may be prescribed to treat acne in females.
   6. Combination therapy may be prescribed to treat the acne.

Box 42-5 Acne Products

Topical Antibiotics
Benzoyl peroxide
Clindamycin (Cleocin) and erythromycin (Erythroderma)
Fixed dose combinations: clindamycin/benzoyl peroxide (BenzaClin) and erythromycin/benzoyl peroxide (Benzamycin)
Dapsone (Aczone)

Topical Retinoids
Tretinoin
Adapalene (Differin)
Tazarotene (Tazorac)
Azelaic acid (Azelex)

Oral Medications
Doxycycline (Vibramycin)
Minocycline (Dynacin, Minocin, Solodyn)
Tetracycline (Sumycin)
Erythromycin (Ery-Tab)
Isotretinoin (Accutane)

Hormonal Medications
Oral contraceptives

▲ **FIGURE 42-2** Acne vulgaris. **A,** Comedones with a few inflammatory pustules. **B,** Papulopustular acne. (From Weston, W. L., & Lane, A. T. [2007]. *Color textbook of pediatric dermatology* [4th ed.]. St. Louis, Mosby.)

7. Actions of the medications may include suppressing the growth of *Propionibacterium acnes*, reducing inflammation, promoting keratolysis, unplugging existing comedones and preventing their development, normalizing hyperproliferation of epithelial cells within the hair follicles; some medications cause thinning of the skin, which facilitates penetration of other medications.
8. For topical applications: The site should be washed and allowed to completely dry before application. Hands should be washed after application.
9. All topical products are kept away from the eyes, inside the nose, lips, mucous membranes, hair, and inflamed or denuded skin.

B. Topical antibiotic products
  1. Benzoyl peroxide
    a. Can produce drying and peeling
    b. Severe local irritation (burning, blistering, scaling, swelling) may require reducing the frequency of applications.
    c. Some products may contain sulfites. Monitor for allergic reactions.
  2. Clindamycin (Cleocin) and erythromycin (Erythroderma)
    a. Both products may be prescribed for use to prevent emergence of resistance.
    b. Combination therapy with benzoyl peroxide can be prescribed to prevent emergence of resistance. Fixed-dose combinations include clindamycin/benzoyl peroxide (BenzaClin) and erythromycin/benzoyl peroxide (Benzamycin).
  3. Dapsone (Aczone): side effects include oiliness, peeling, dryness, and erythema of the skin.
C. Topical retinoids
  1. Tretinoin
    a. A derivative of vitamin A (Vitamin A supplements should be discontinued during therapy.)
    b. In addition to treating acne, it may be prescribed to reduce fine wrinkles, skin roughness, mottled hyperpigmentation such as those that occur with age spots (tretinoin [Renova]).
    c. Can cause localized side effects such as blistering, peeling, crusting, burning, and swelling of the skin
    d. The use of abrasive products and keratolytic products should be discontinued before using tretinoin because they can cause localized side effects.
    e. Sensitizes the skin to ultraviolet light (UVL). The client needs to be instructed to apply sunscreen with a sun protection factor (SPF) of 15 or greater and to wear protective clothing when outdoors because the medication increases susceptibility to sunburn.
  2. Adapalene (Differin): similar to tretinoin and sensitizes the skin to UVL. Side effects include burning and itching after application, redness, dryness, and scaling of the skin.
  3. Tazarotene (Tazorac)
    a. Is a derivative of vitamin A (Vitamin A supplements should be discontinued during therapy.)
    b. In addition to acne, it is used to treat wrinkles and psoriasis.
    c. Can cause itching, burning, and dry skin and sensitizes the skin to UVL
  4. Azelaic acid (Azelex): can cause burning, itching, stinging, and redness of the skin; can also cause hypopigmentation of the skin in clients with a dark complexion

D. Oral antibiotics
1. Includes doxycycline (Vibramycin); minocycline (Dynacin, Minocin, Solodyn); tetracycline (Sumycin); and erythromycin (Ery-Tab)
2. Improvement develops slowly with the use of oral antibiotics and may take 3 to 6 months for some improvement to be noted. Following control of symptoms the client is usually switched to a topical antibiotic.

E. Isotretinoin
1. Derivative of vitamin A (Vitamin A supplements should be discontinued during therapy.) Additionally, the use of tetracyclines can increase the risk of adverse effects and should be discontinued before use of isotretinoin.
2. Used to treat severe cystic acne. Its use is reserved for persons who have not responded to other therapies, including systemic antibiotics.
3. Side effects include nosebleeds; inflammation of the lips or eyes; dryness or itching of the skin, nose, or mouth; pain, tenderness, or stiffness in the joints, bones, or muscles; and back pain.
4. Less common side effects include skin rash, hair loss, peeling of the skin, headache, and reduction in night vision.
5. Causes sensitization of the skin to UVL
6. Causes elevated triglyceride levels. The triglyceride level should be checked before and during therapy. Alcohol consumption needs to be eliminated during therapy because alcohol could potentiate elevation of serum triglyceride levels.
7. May cause depression in some clients. If this occurs the medication should be discontinued.

⚠ Isotretinoin is highly teratogenic and can cause fetal abnormalities and must not be used if the client is pregnant. The client needs to follow strict rules of the iPLEDGE Program.

F. iPLEDGE Program
1. A risk management program that ensures that no woman starting isotretoin is pregnant or no woman taking this medication becomes pregnant.
2. Access to the medication is controlled through a central automated system.
3. Strict rules must be followed by the client, HCP prescribing the medication, pharmacist dispensing the medication, and wholesaler of the medication to ensure safety and that no woman is pregnant on initiation of therapy or becomes pregnant while taking the medication.

G. Hormonal medications
1. Hormonal medications such as oral contraceptives and spironolactone (Aldactone) may be prescribed to treat acne in females.

Box 42-6 Burn Products

Mafenide acetate (Sulfamylon)
Nitrofurazone (Furacin)
Silver sulfadiazine (Silvadene)

2. These medications decrease androgen activity, resulting in decreased production of sebum (substance that combines with keratin to create a plug within a pore).
3. Spironolactone is teratogenic; therefore contraception during its use is necessary.
4. The adverse effects of spironolactone include breast tenderness, menstrual irregularities, and hyperkalemia.

VIII. BURN PRODUCTS (Box 42-6)

A. Nitrofurazone (Furacin)
1. Applied topically to the **burn** as a solution, ointment, or cream
2. Has a broad spectrum of antibacterial activity
3. Used for **burns** when bacterial resistance to other agents is a problem
4. Topical: Apply $\frac{1}{16}$-inch film directly to **burn**.
5. Side effects: Contact dermatitis, rash
6. Less common side effects: Pruritus, local edema

B. Mafenide acetate (Sulfamylon)
1. Water-soluble cream that is bacteriostatic for gram-negative and gram-positive organisms
2. Used to treat **burns** to reduce the bacteria present in avascular tissues
3. Diffuses through the devascularized areas of the skin and may precipitate metabolic acidosis (usually compensated for by hyperventilation)
4. Apply $\frac{1}{16}$-inch film directly to the **burn**.
5. Side effects can include local pain and rash.
6. Systemic effects include bone marrow depression, hemolytic anemia, and metabolic acidosis.
7. Keep **burn** covered with mafenide acetate at all times.
8. Notify the registered nurse who will then notify the HCP if hyperventilation occurs. If acidosis develops, mafenide acetate is washed off the skin and is usually discontinued for 1 to 2 days.

C. Silver sulfadiazine (Silvadene, Thermazene, SSD Cream)
1. Has broad spectrum of activity against gram-negative bacteria, gram-positive bacteria, and yeast
2. Released slowly from the cream, which is selectively toxic to bacteria
3. Used primarily to prevent sepsis in clients with **burns**

4. Not a carbonic anhydrase inhibitor; therefore, does not cause acidosis
5. Apply 1/16-inch film (keep **burn** covered at all times with silver sulfadiazine).
6. Side effects include rash and itching.
7. Systemic effects include leukopenia and interstitial nephritis.
8. Complete blood cell count, particularly the white blood cells, is frequently monitored. If leukopenia develops, the registered nurse and HCP are notified (and the medication is usually discontinued).

MORE QUESTIONS ON EVOLVE!

Practice Questions

411. Salicylic acid is prescribed for a client with a diagnosis of psoriasis. The nurse monitors the client, knowing that which of the following would indicate the presence of systemic toxicity from this medication?
1. Tinnitus
2. Diarrhea
3. Constipation
4. Decreased respirations

412. The camp nurse asks the children preparing to swim in the lake if they have applied sunscreen. The nurse reminds the children that chemical sunscreens are most effective when applied:
1. Immediately before swimming
2. 15 minutes before exposure to the sun
3. Immediately before exposure to the sun
4. At least 30 minutes before exposure to the sun

413. Mafenide acetate (Sulfamylon) is prescribed for the client with a burn injury. When applying the medication, the client complains of local discomfort and burning. Which of the following is the most appropriate nursing action?
1. Notifying the registered nurse
2. Discontinuing the medication
3. Informing the client that this is normal
4. Applying a thinner film than prescribed to the burn site

414. The burn client is receiving treatments of topical mafenide acetate (Sulfamylon) to the site of injury. The nurse monitors the client, knowing that which of the following indicates that a systemic effect has occurred?
1. Hyperventilation
2. Elevated blood pressure

3. Local pain at the burn site
4. Local rash at the burn site

415. Isotretinoin is prescribed for a client with severe acne. Before the administration of this medication, the nurse anticipates that which laboratory test will be prescribed?
1. Platelet count
2. Triglyceride level
3. Complete blood count
4. White blood cell count

416. A client with severe acne is seen in the clinic and the health care provider (HCP) prescribes isotretinoin. The nurse reviews the client's medication record and would contact the HCP if the client is taking which medication?
1. Vitamin A
2. Digoxin (Lanoxin)
3. Furosemide (Lasix)
4. Phenytoin (Dilantin)

417. The nurse is applying a topical corticosteroid to a client with eczema. The nurse would monitor for the potential for increased systemic absorption of the medication if the medication were being applied to which of the following body areas?
1. Back
2. Axilla
3. Soles of the feet
4. Palms of the hands

418. The clinic nurse is performing an admission assessment on a client. The nurse notes that the client is taking azelaic acid (Azelex). Because of the medication prescription, the nurse would suspect that the client is being treated for:
1. Acne
2. Eczema
3. Hair loss
4. Herpes simplex

419. The health care provider has prescribed silver sulfadiazine (Silvadene) for the client with a partial-thickness burn, which has cultured positive for gram-negative bacteria. The nurse is reinforcing information to the client about the medication. Which statement made by the client indicates a lack of understanding about the treatments?
1. "The medication is an antibacterial."
2. "The medication will help heal the burn."
3. "The medication will permanently stain my skin."
4. "The medication should be applied directly to the wound."

❖ **420.** The health education nurse provides instructions to a group of clients regarding measures that will assist in preventing skin cancer. Which instruction(s) should the nurse reinforce to the client? **Select all that apply.**

☐ 1. Use sunscreen when participating in outdoor activities.
☐ 2. Wear a hat, opaque clothing, and sunglasses when in the sun.
☐ 3. Avoid sun exposure in the late afternoon and early evening hours.
☐ 4. Examine your body monthly for any lesions that may be suspicious.
☐ 5. Sunscreen should be applied every 8 hours.

ANSWERS

411. 1
Rationale: Salicylic acid is absorbed readily through the skin, and systemic toxicity (salicylism) can result. Symptoms include tinnitus, dizziness, hyperpnea, and psychological disturbances. Constipation and diarrhea are not associated with salicylism.
Test-Taking Strategy: Use the process of elimination. Noting the name of the medication will assist in directing you to the correct option if you can recall the toxic effects that occur with acetylsalicylic acid (aspirin). Review the toxic effects of salicylic acid if you are unfamiliar with them.
Level of Cognitive Ability: Analyzing
Client Needs: Physiological Integrity
Integrated Process: Nursing Process/Data Collection
Content Area: Pharmacology
Reference: Lehne, p. 1228. 2010.

412. 4
Rationale: Sunscreens are most effective when applied at least 30 minutes before exposure to the sun so that they can penetrate the skin. All sunscreens should be reapplied after swimming or sweating.
Test-Taking Strategy: Use the process of elimination. Knowledge that sunscreens need to penetrate the skin will assist in eliminating options 2 and 3. Noting the strategic words *most effective* will assist in directing you to option 4. Review protective skin measures if you had difficulty with this question.
Level of Cognitive Ability: Applying
Client Needs: Physiological Integrity
Integrated Process: Teaching and Learning
Content Area: Pharmacology
Reference: Kee, Hayes, McCuistion, p. 765. 2009.

413. 3
Rationale: Mafenide acetate is bacteriostatic for gram-negative and gram-positive organisms and is used to treat burns to reduce bacteria present in avascular tissues. The client should be informed that the medication will cause local discomfort and burning and that this is a normal reaction; therefore options 1, 2, and 4 are incorrect
Test-Taking Strategy: Use the process of elimination. Eliminate options 2 and 4 because it is not within the scope of nursing practice to alter or discontinue a medication therapy. Recalling that this is a normal expected occurrence will direct you to option 3. If you had difficulty with this question, review the effects of this medication.
Level of Cognitive Ability: Applying
Client Needs: Physiological Integrity

Integrated Process: Nursing Process/Implementation
Content Area: Pharmacology
Reference: Kee, Hayes, McCuistion, p. 765. 2009.

414. 1
Rationale: Mafenide acetate is a carbonic anhydrase inhibitor and can suppress renal excretion of acid, thereby causing acidosis. Clients receiving this treatment should be monitored for signs of an acid-base imbalance (hyperventilation). If this occurs, the medication should be discontinued for 1 to 2 days. Options 3 and 4 describe local rather than systemic effects. An elevated blood pressure may be expected from the pain that occurs with a burn injury.
Test-Taking Strategy: Use the process of elimination. Note the strategic words *systemic effect*. Options 3 and 4 can be eliminated because these are local rather than systemic effects. From the remaining options, recall that the client in pain would likely have an elevated blood pressure. This should direct you to option 1. Review the systemic effects of this medication if you had difficulty with this question.
Level of Cognitive Ability: Analyzing
Client Needs: Physiological Integrity
Integrated Process: Nursing Process/Data Collection
Content Area: Pharmacology
Reference: Kee, Hayes, McCuistion, p. 765. 2009.

415. 2
Rationale: Isotretinoin can elevate triglyceride levels. Blood triglyceride levels should be measured before treatment and periodically thereafter until the effect on the triglycerides has been evaluated. Options 1, 3, and 4 do not need to be monitored specifically during this treatment.
Test-Taking Strategy: Use the process of elimination. Eliminate options 3 and 4 first because a complete blood count also will measure the white blood cell count. From the remaining options, recall that the medication can affect triglyceride levels in the client. Review this medication if you had difficulty with this question
Level of Cognitive Ability: Analyzing
Client Needs: Physiological Integrity
Integrated Process: Nursing Process/Data Collection
Content Area: Pharmacology
Reference: Lehne, p. 1232. 2010.

416. 1
Rationale: Isotretinoin is a metabolite of vitamin A and can produce generalized intensification of isotretinoin toxicity. Because of the potential for increased toxicity, vitamin A supplements should be discontinued before isotretinoin therapy.

Options 2, 3, and 4 are not contraindicated with the use of isotretinoin.

Test-Taking Strategy: Use the process of elimination. Recalling that isotretinoin is a metabolite of vitamin A will direct you to the correct option. If you are unfamiliar with this medication, review the contraindications associated with its use.

Level of Cognitive Ability: Analyzing
Client Needs: Physiological Integrity
Integrated Process: Nursing Process/Implementation
Content Area: Pharmacology
Reference: Lehne, p. 1232. 2010.

417. 2

Rationale: Topical corticosteroids can be absorbed into the systemic circulation. Absorption is higher from regions where the skin is especially permeable (scalp, axilla, face, eyelids, neck, perineum, genitalia), and lower from regions in which permeability is poor (back, palms, soles).

Test-Taking Strategy: Use the process of elimination. Focus on the subject of the question, areas of high permeability and the potential for increased systemic absorption. Eliminate options 3 and 4 because these body areas are comparable or alike in terms of skin substance. From the remaining options, think about permeability of the skin area. This should direct you to option 2. Review the principles related to the administration of topical corticosteroids if you had difficulty with this question.

Level of Cognitive Ability: Understanding
Client Needs: Physiological Integrity
Integrated Process: Nursing Process/Data Collection
Content Area: Pharmacology
Reference: Black, Hawks, p. 1204. 2009.

418. 1

Rationale: Azelaic acid is a topical medication used to treat mild to moderate acne. The acid appears to work by suppressing the growth of *Propionibacterium acnes* and decreasing the proliferation of keratinocytes. Options 2, 3, and 4 are incorrect.

Test-Taking Strategy: Use the process of elimination. Focusing on the name of the medication, azelaic acid, will direct you to the correct option. Review this medication if you are unfamiliar with it.

Level of Cognitive Ability: Understanding
Client Needs: Physiological Integrity

Integrated Process: Nursing Process/Data Collection
Content Area: Pharmacology
Reference: Lehne, p. 1231. 2010.

419. 3

Rationale: Silver sulfadiazine (Silvadene) is an antibacterial that has a broad spectrum of activity against gram-negative bacteria, gram-positive bacteria, and yeast. It is applied directly to the wound to assist in healing. It does not stain the skin.

Test-Taking Strategy: Note the strategic words *lack of understanding*. These words indicate a negative event query and ask you to select an option that is an incorrect statement. Recall the characteristics of this medication. Noting the words *permanently stain* in option 3 will direct you to this option. Review this medication if you had difficulty with this question.

Level of Cognitive Ability: Evaluating
Client Needs: Physiological Integrity
Integrated Process: Teaching and Learning
Content Area: Pharmacology
Reference: Lehne, p. 1027. 2010.

420. 1, 2, 4 ❖

Rationale: The client should be instructed to avoid sun exposure between the hours of 10 AM and 4 PM. Sunscreen, a hat, opaque clothing, and sunglasses should be worn for outdoor activities. The client should be instructed to examine the body monthly for the appearance of any possible cancerous or any precancerous lesions. Sunscreen should be reapplied every 2 to 3 hours and after swimming or sweating; otherwise the duration of protection is reduced.

Test-Taking Strategy: Use the process of elimination and focus on the subject, measures to prevent skin cancer. Reading each option carefully and thinking about the causes of cancer will direct you to the correct options. Review client teaching points for the prevention of skin cancer if you had difficulty with this question.

Level of Cognitive Ability: Applying
Client Needs: Health Promotion and Maintenance
Integrated Process: Teaching and Learning
Content Area: Adult Health/Integumentary
Reference: Ignatavicius, Workman, p. 511. 2010.

The Adult Client with an Oncological Disorder

PYRAMID TERMS

adenocarcinoma Cancer that arises from glandular tissues.

benign Usually refers to growths that are encapsulated, remain localized, and are slow-growing.

cancer A neoplastic disorder that can involve all body organs. Cells lose their normal growth-controlling mechanism, and the growth of cells is uncontrolled.

carcinogen A physical, chemical, or biological stressor that causes neoplastic changes in normal cells.

carcinoma A new growth or malignant tumor that originates from the epithelial cells, the skin, the gastrointestinal tract, the lungs, the uterus, the breast, or other organs.

carcinoma in situ A premalignant lesion with all of the histological characteristics of a malignancy except invasion.

hospice A concept of care for terminally ill clients that includes the idea of intensive caring rather than intensive care. The client and the family are the focus of nursing care, and the goals are to relieve pain and to facilitate an optimal quality of life.

leukemia or myeloma Neoplasms that originate from blood-forming organs.

lymphomas Neoplasms that originate from lymphoid tissue.

malignant Refers to growths that are not encapsulated but that metastasize and grow. These growths are cancerous lesions that have the characteristics of disorderly, uncontrolled, and chaotic proliferations of cells.

metastasis The transfer of disease from one organ or part to another organ or part that is not directly connected with it. Secondary malignant lesions, which originate from the primary tumor, are located in anatomically distant places.

nadir The period of time during which an antineoplastic medication has its most profound effects on the bone marrow.

neoplasm A new growth that may be benign or malignant.

sarcoma Neoplasm that originates from muscle, bone, fat, the lymph system, or connective tissues.

staging A method of classifying malignancies on the basis of the presence and extent of the tumor within the body.

tumor marker A specific body substance that seems to indicate tumor progression or regression.

undifferentiated cell A cell that has lost the capacity for specialized function.

PYRAMID TO SUCCESS

The pyramid points focus on the treatment modalities related to an oncological disorder (e.g., pain management, internal and external radiation, chemotherapy) and on oncological disorders such as skin cancer, leukemia, breast cancer, and lung cancer. The specific foci relate to the nursing care related to these treatment modalities and disorders, to client adaptation, and to the impact of the treatment or the disorder. Specifically, the emphasis is on the complications related to chemotherapy, the nursing measures required to monitor for these complications, and the prevention of life-threatening conditions such as infection and bleeding. Specific laboratory values include the white blood cell (WBC) count and the platelet count.

CLIENT NEEDS

Safe and Effective Care Environment

- Discussing oncology-related consultations and referrals
- Ensuring that advance directives are in the client's medical record
- Ensuring advocacy related to the client's decisions

- Establishing priorities
- Ensuring ethical practices
- Handling hazardous and infectious materials related to radiation and chemotherapy safely
- Implementing protective, standard, and other precautions
- Maintaining medical and surgical asepsis
- Preventing disease related to infection
- Providing confidentiality regarding the client's diagnosis
- Providing informed consent for treatments and procedures
- Upholding client's rights

Health Promotion and Maintenance

- Discussing expected body-image changes related to chemotherapy and treatments
- Providing client and family instructions regarding home care
- Providing instructions regarding monthly breast or testicular self-examinations
- Respecting client lifestyle choices
- Teaching about health promotion programs regarding risks for cancer
- Teaching about health screening measures for cancer

Psychosocial Integrity

- Determining the client's ability to cope, adapt, and/or problem solve during illness or stressful events

- Assisting the client and family with coping with alterations in body image
- Discussing end-of-life and grief and loss issues related to death and the dying process
- Mobilizing the appropriate support and resource systems
- Promoting a positive environment to maintain an optimal quality of life
- Respecting religious and cultural preferences

Physiological Integrity

- Assisting with administering blood and blood products
- Assisting with caring for central venous access devices
- Assisting with caring for the client who is receiving chemotherapy
- Caring for the client who is receiving radiation therapy
- Managing pain
- Monitoring diagnostic tests and laboratory values, such as white blood cell and platelet counts
- Monitoring for expected and unexpected responses to radiation and chemotherapy
- Protecting the client from the life-threatening adverse effects of treatments
- Providing basic care and comfort
- Providing nutrition

Oncological Disorders

I. CANCER

A. Description
1. A neoplastic disorder that can involve any body organ
2. Cells lose their normal growth-controlling mechanism, and the growth of cells is uncontrolled.
3. **Cancer** produces serious health problems such as impaired immune and hematopoietic (blood-producing) function; altered gastrointestinal (GI) tract structure and function; motor and sensory deficits; and decreased respiratory function.

B. **Metastasis** (Box 43-1)
1. **Cancer** cells move from their original location to other sites.
2. Routes of **metastasis**
   a. Local seeding: Distribution of shed **cancer** cells occurs in the local area of the primary tumor.
   b. Blood-borne **metastasis**: Tumor cells enter the blood; this is the most common cause of **cancer** spread.
   c. Lymphatic spread: Primary sites rich in lymphatics are more susceptible to early metastatic spread.

C. **Cancer** classification
1. Solid tumors: Associated with the organs from which they develop, such as breast **cancer** or lung **cancer**
2. Hematologic **cancers**: Originate from blood cell–forming tissues, such as the **leukemias** and the **lymphomas**

D. Grading and **staging**
1. A method used to describe the tumor
2. Includes the extent of the tumor, the extent to which malignancy has increased in size, the involvement of regional nodes, and metastatic development
3. Grading classifies the cellular aspects of the **cancer**
4. **Staging** classifies the clinical aspects of the **cancer**

E. Factors that influence **cancer** development
1. Environmental factors
   a. Chemical **carcinogens**: Industrial chemicals, drugs, and tobacco
   b. Physical **carcinogens**: Ionizing radiation (diagnostic and therapeutic x-rays) and ultraviolet radiation (sun, tanning beds, and germicidal lights); chronic irritation and tissue trauma
   c. Viral **carcinogens**: Viruses capable of causing **cancer** are known as oncoviruses (e.g., Epstein-Barr virus, hepatitis B virus, human papillomavirus).
   d. *Helicobacter pylori* infection is associated with an increased risk of gastric **cancer**.
2. Obesity and dietary factors including preservatives, contaminants, additives, and nitrates.
3. Genetic predisposition: Factors include an inherited predisposition to specific **cancers**, inherited conditions associated with **cancer**, familial clustering, and chromosomal aberrations.
4. Age: Advancing age is a significant risk factor for the development of **cancer**.
5. Immune function: The incidence of **cancer** is higher in immunosuppressed individuals, such as those with acquired immunodeficiency syndrome and organ transplant recipients who are taking immunosuppressive medications.

F. Prevention: Avoidance of known or potential **carcinogens** and avoidance or modification of the factors associated with the development of **cancer** cells

G. Early detection
1. Mammography
2. Papanicolaou (Pap) test
3. Stools for occult blood
4. Sigmoidoscopy
5. Breast self-examination
6. Testicular self-examination
7. Skin inspection

II. BREAST SELF-EXAMINATION

A. Performing breast self-examination (BSE)
1. Perform 7 to 10 days after menses
2. Postmenopausal clients or clients who have had a hysterectomy should select a specific day of the month and perform a BSE monthly on that day.

B. Procedure (Figure 43-1)

513

Box 43-1 Common Sites of Metastasis

Bladder Cancer
Lung
Bone
Liver
Pelvic, retroperitoneal
    structures

Brain Tumors
Central nervous system

Breast Cancer
Bone
Lung
Brain
Liver

Colorectal Cancer
Liver

Lung Cancer
Brain
Liver

Prostate Cancer
Bone
Spine
Lung
Liver
Kidneys

Testicular Cancer
Lung
Bone
Liver
Adrenal glands
Retroperitoneal lymph
    nodes

▲ **FIGURE 43-1** Breast self-examination (BSE). **A,** While in the shower or bath, when the skin is slippery with soap and water, examine your breasts. Use the pads of your second, third, and fourth fingers to firmly press every part of the breast. Use your right hand to examine your left breast and your left hand to examine your right breast. Using the pads of the fingers on your left hand, examine the entire breast with the use of small circular motions in a spiral or in an up-and-down motion so that the entire breast area is examined. Repeat the procedure using your right hand to examine your left breast. Repeat the pattern of palpation under the arm. Check for any lump, hard knot, or thickening of the tissue. **B,** Look at your breasts in a mirror. Stand with your arms at your side. **C,** Raise your arms overhead and check for any changes in the shape of your breasts, any dimpling of the skin, or any changes in the nipple. **D,** Place your hands on your hips and press down firmly, tightening the pectoral muscles. Observe for asymmetry or changes, keeping in mind that your breasts probably do not match exactly. **E,** While lying down, feel your breasts as described in part A. When examining your right breast, place a folded towel under your right shoulder, and put your right hand behind your head. Repeat the procedure when examining your left breast. Mark on your calendar that you have completed your BSE; note any changes or unique characteristics that you want to discuss with your health care provider. (From Lewis, S., Heitkemper, M., Dirksen, S., & Bucher, L. [2010]. *Medical-surgical nursing: Assessment and management of clinical problems* [8th ed.]. St. Louis: Mosby.)

 III. TESTICULAR SELF-EXAMINATION

A. Performing testicular self-examination (TSE): Select a day of the month and perform the examination on the same day each month.

B. Procedure (Figure 43-2)

IV. DIAGNOSTIC TESTS

A. Diagnostic tests to be performed depend on the suspected primary or metastatic sites of the **cancer** (Box 43-2).

 B. Biopsy
1. Description
    a. Definitive means of diagnosing **cancer**; provides histologic proof of malignancy
    b. Involves the surgical incision of a small piece of tissue for microscopic examination
2. Types
    a. Needle: Aspiration of cells
    b. Incisional: Wedge of suspected tissue is removed from a larger mass
    c. Excisional: Complete removal of the entire lesion
    d. **Staging**: Multiple needle or incisional biopsies in tissues in which **metastasis** is suspected or likely (see Box 43-1)
3. Tissue examination
    a. After excision, a frozen section or a permanent paraffin section is obtained to examine the specimen.
    b. The advantage of the frozen section is the speed with which the section can be prepared and the diagnosis made; only minutes are required for this test.

c. A permanent paraffin section takes about 24 hours; however, it provides clearer details than the frozen section.
4. Interventions
    a. The procedure is usually performed in an outpatient surgical setting.
    b. Prepare the client for the diagnostic procedure in accordance with the health care provider's (HCP's) instructions.
    c. Obtain informed consent

▲ **FIGURE 43-2** Testicular self-examination. (1) The best time to perform this examination is right after a shower when your scrotal skin is moist and relaxed, thus making the testicles easy to feel. (2) Gently lift each testicle. Each one should feel like an egg; it should be firm but not hard and smooth with no lumps. (3) Using both hands, place your middle fingers on the underside of each testicle and your thumbs on top. (4) Gently roll each testicle between the thumb and fingers to feel for any lumps, swellings, or masses. (5) If you notice any changes from one month to the next, notify your health care provider. (From Harkreader, H., & Hogan, M. A. [2007]. *Fundamentals of nursing: Caring and clinical judgment* [3rd ed.]. Philadelphia: Saunders.)

Box 43-2 Diagnostic Tests

- Biopsy
- Bone marrow examination (particularly if a hematolymphoid malignancy is suspected)
- Chest x-ray
- Complete blood count (CBC)
- Computed tomography (CT) scan
- Cytology studies (Papanicolaou smear)
- Liver function studies
- Magnetic resonance imaging (MRI)
- Evaluation of serum tumor markers (e.g., carcinoembryonic antigen and alpha-fetoprotein)
- Proctoscopic examination (including guaiac for occult blood)
- Radiographic studies (mammography)
- Radioisotope scanning (liver, brain, bone, lung)

 V. PAIN CONTROL

⚠ Assess the client's pain; pain is what the client describes or says that it is. Do not undermedicate the cancer client who is in pain.

A. Causes of pain
1. Bone destruction
2. Obstruction of an organ
3. Compression of peripheral nerves
4. Infiltration and distention of tissue
5. Inflammation and necrosis
6. Psychological causes (e.g., fear, anxiety)

B. Interventions
1. Collaborate with other members of the health care team to develop a pain management program.
2. Administer oral preparations if possible and if they provide adequate relief of pain; the transdermal route may also be prescribed.
3. Mild or moderate pain may be treated with salicylates, acetaminophen (Tylenol), and nonsteroidal anti-inflammatory drugs (NSAIDs); drug-drug interactions may occur with NSAIDs and anticoagulants, oral hypoglycemics, and antihypertensives.
4. Severe pain is treated with opioids, such as codeine sulfate, morphine sulfate, methadone, and hydromorphone hydrochloride (Dilaudid). Neuropathic pain is treated with a variety of anticonvulsants and antidepressants, as well as opioids.
5. Subcutaneous injections and continuous intravenous (IV) infusions of opioids provide rapid pain control; equianalgesic comparison charts should be used when switching routes of administration of opioids.
6. Monitor vital signs and for side effects of medications.
7. Monitor for effectiveness of medications.
8. Provide nonpharmacological techniques of pain control, such as relaxation, guided imagery, biofeedback, massage, and heat-cold application.

VI. SURGERY

A. Description: Used to diagnose, stage, and treat **cancer**

B. Prophylactic surgery
1. Performed in clients with an existing premalignant condition or a known family history that strongly predisposes the person to the development of **cancer**
2. An attempt is made to remove the tissue or organ at risk and thus prevent the development of **cancer**.

C. Ablation therapy: tumor is destroyed (burned) via radio-frequency, microwave therapy, or other type of therapy.

D. Curative surgery: All gross and microscopic tumor is either removed or destroyed.

E. Control (cytoreductive) surgery
1. A debulking procedure that consists of removing part of the tumor
2. It decreases the number of **cancer** cells and increases the chance that other therapies will be successful.

F. Palliative surgery
1. Performed to improve the quality of life during the survival time
2. Performed to reduce pain, relieve airway obstruction, relieve obstructions in the GI and urinary tracts, relieve pressure on the brain or spinal cord, prevent hemorrhage, remove infected or ulcerated tumors, or drain abscesses

G. Reconstructive or rehabilitative surgery: Performed to improve the quality of life by restoring maximal function and appearance (e.g., breast reconstruction after mastectomy)

H. Side effects of surgery
1. Loss of a specific body part
2. Reduced function as a result of organ loss
3. Scarring or disfigurement
4. Grieving about an altered body image or an imposed change in lifestyle

VII. CHEMOTHERAPY

A. Description
1. Kills or inhibits the reproduction of neoplastic cells; also attacks and kills normal cells
2. Effects are systemic; affects both healthy cells and cancerous cells
3. Normal cells most profoundly affected include those of the skin, the hair, the lining of the GI tract, the spermatocytes, and the hematopoietic cells.
4. Cell cycle phase–specific medications affect cells only during a certain phase of the reproductive cycle, and cell cycle phase–nonspecific medications affect cells during any phase of the reproductive cycle.
5. Usually several medications are used in combination (combination therapy) to increase the therapeutic response.
6. Combination chemotherapy is planned to avoid prescribing medications with **nadirs** (the times during which bone marrow activity and white blood cell counts are at their lowest) at or near the same time to minimize immunosuppression.
7. Antineoplastic therapy may be combined with other treatments, such as surgery and radiation.
8. The preferred route of administration is the IV route.
9. Side effects include alopecia, nausea, vomiting, mucositis, skin changes, immunosuppression, anemia, and thrombocytopenia.
10. See Chapter 44 for information about the care of the client who is receiving chemotherapy.

VIII. RADIATION THERAPY (see Priority Nursing Actions)

A. Description
1. Radiation therapy destroys **cancer** cells with minimal exposure of normal cells to the damaging effects of radiation; the cells that are damaged die or become unable to divide.

■■■■ PRIORITY NURSING ACTIONS! ■■■■

Actions to Take If a Sealed Radiation Implant Becomes Dislodged
1. Encourage the client to lie still.
2. Use a long-handled forceps to retrieve the radioactive source.
3. Deposit the radioactive source in a lead container.
4. Contact the radiation oncologist.
5. Document the occurrence and the actions taken.

The client with a sealed radiation implant can emit radiation. Therefore the nurse and any other person who is in contact with the client needs to take special precautions to protect self from radiation exposure. In the event that a radiation source becomes dislodged, the nurse would first encourage the client to lie still until the radioactive source has been placed in a safe closed container. The nurse would never touch the dislodged radiation source with his or her hands and would use a long-handled forceps to place the source in the lead container that should be kept in the client's room. The nurse calls the radiation oncologist and then documents the occurrence and the actions taken. In the event that the radiation source cannot be located, the nurse ensures that no linens or other articles in the client's room are disposed of, prohibits visitors, and notifies the radiation oncologist.

Reference: Ignatavicius, D., & Workman, M. (2010). *Medical-surgical nursing: Patient-centered collaborative care* (6th ed., p. 420). St. Louis: Saunders.

---

2. Radiation therapy is effective on tissues directly within the path of the radiation beam.
3. Side effects include local skin changes and irritation, alopecia (hair loss), fatigue (most common side effect of radiation), duplicate and altered taste sensation; the effects vary according to the site of treatment.
4. External-beam radiation (also called teletherapy) and brachytherapy are the types of radiation therapy that are most commonly used to treat **cancer**.

B. External-beam radiation (the actual radiation source is external to the client)
1. Instruct the client regarding skin care (Box 43-3).
2. The client does not emit radiation and does not pose a hazard to anyone else.

C. Brachytherapy
1. The radiation source comes into direct, continuous contact with tumor tissues for a specific time.
2. The radiation source is within the client; for a period of time, the client emits radiation and can pose a hazard to others.
3. Brachytherapy includes a sealed or unsealed source of radiation.
4. Unsealed radiation source
   a. Administration is via the oral or IV route or by instillation into the body cavities.

Box 43-3 Client Education Guide: Radiation Therapy for Cancer

Wash the irradiated area gently each day with either water alone or with a mild soap and water.

Use the hand rather than a washcloth to wash the area.

Rinse the soap thoroughly from the skin.

Take care not to remove the markings that indicate exactly where the beam of radiation is to be focused.

Dry the irradiated area with patting motions rather than rubbing motions; use a clean, soft towel or cloth.

Use no powders, ointments, lotions, or creams on the skin at the radiation site unless they are prescribed by the radiologist.

Wear soft clothing over the skin at the radiation site.

Avoid wearing belts, buckles, straps, or any type of clothing that binds or rubs the skin at the radiation site.

Avoid exposure of the irradiated area to the sun.

Avoid heat exposure.

From Ignatavicius, D., & Workman, M. (2010) Medical-surgical nursing: Patient-centered collaborative care (6th ed.). St. Louis: Saunders.

Box 43-4 Care of the Client with a Sealed Radiation Source

Place the client in a private room with a private bath.

Place a caution sign on the client's door.

Organize nursing tasks to minimize exposure to the radiation source.

Nursing assignments to a client with a radiation implant should be rotated.

Limit exposure time to 30 minutes per care provider per 8-hour shift.

Wear a dosimeter film badge to measure radiation exposure.

Wear a lead shield to reduce the transmission of radiation.

A nurse should never care for more than one client with a radiation implant at one time.

Do not allow a pregnant nurse to care for the client.

Do not allow children who are younger than 16 years old or pregnant women to visit the client.

Limit visitors to 30 minutes per day; visitors should be at least 6 feet from the source.

Save the bed linens and dressings until the source is removed, and then dispose of them in the usual manner.

Other equipment can be removed from the room at any time.

---

b. The source is not confined completely to one body area; it enters body fluids and eventually is eliminated via various excreta, which are radioactive and harmful to others; most of the source is eliminated from the body within 48 hours, at which time neither the client nor the excreta are radioactive or harmful.

5. Sealed radiation source (Box 43-4)
   a. A sealed temporary or permanent radiation source (solid implant) is implanted within the tumor target tissues.
   b. The client emits radiation while the implant is in place, but the excreta are not radioactive.

6. Removal of sealed radiation sources
   a. The client is no longer radioactive.
   b. Inform the client that sexual partners cannot "catch" **cancer**.
   c. Inform the female client that she may resume sexual intercourse after 7 to 10 days if the implant was cervical or vaginal.
   d. Provide a povidone-iodine douche, if prescribed, if the implant was placed in the cervix.
   e. Administer a Fleet enema, as prescribed.
   f. Advise the client who had a cervical or vaginal implant to notify the HCP if nausea, vomiting, diarrhea, frequent urination, vaginal or rectal bleeding, hematuria, foul-smelling vaginal discharge, abdominal pain or distention, or a fever occurs.

IX. BONE MARROW TRANSPLANTATION

A. Description
   1. Used for the treatment of **leukemia** for clients who have closely matched donors and who are experiencing temporary remission with chemotherapy.

2. The goal of treatment is to rid the client of **malignant** cells through treatment with high doses of chemotherapy.
3. Because these treatments are lethal to the bone marrow, without the replacement of bone marrow function through transplantation, the client would die of infection or hemorrhage.

B. Transplantation: Bone marrow is administered through the client's central line in a manner similar to that of a blood transfusion.

C. Post-transplantation period

 During the post-transplantation period, the client remains without any natural immunity until the donor stem cells begin to proliferate and engraftment occurs.

1. The client remains without any natural immunity until the donor marrow begins to proliferate and engraftment occurs.
2. Infection and severe thrombocytopenia are major concerns until engraftment occurs.

D. Complications: Major complications include failure to engraft and graft-versus-host disease.

X. SKIN CANCER (see Chapter 41)

XI. LEUKEMIA (Box 43-5)

A. Description
   1. **Malignant** exacerbation in the number of leukocytes, usually at an immature stage, in the bone marrow

Box 43-5 Classification of Leukemia

Acute Lymphocytic Leukemia
- Mostly lymphoblasts present in the bone marrow
- Age of onset is usually younger than 15 years

Acute Myelogenous Leukemia
- Mostly myeloblasts present in the bone marrow
- Age of onset is usually between 15 and 39 years

Chronic Myelogenous Leukemia
- Mostly granulocytes present in the bone marrow
- Age of onset is usually in the fourth decade

Chronic Lymphocytic Leukemia
- Mostly lymphocytes present in the bone marrow
- Age of onset is usually older than 50 years

2. May be acute, with a sudden onset and short duration, or chronic, with a slow onset and persistent symptoms over a period of years
3. Affects the bone marrow, thereby causing anemia, leukopenia, the production of immature cells, thrombocytopenia, and a decline in immunity
4. The cause is unknown but appears to involve gene damage of the cells, thus leading to the transformation of cells from a normal state to a **malignant** state.
5. Risk factors include genetic, viral, immunological, and environmental factors as well as exposure to radiation, chemicals, and medications.

 B. Data collection
   1. Anorexia, fatigue, weakness, dyspnea on exertion, and weight loss
   2. Bleeding: Nosebleeds, gum bleeding, rectal bleeding, hematuria, and increased menstrual flow
   3. Petechiae
   4. Prolonged bleeding after minor abrasions or lacerations
   5. Elevated temperature and fever
   6. Lymphadenopathy and splenomegaly
   7. Normal, elevated, or reduced white blood cell (WBC) count
   8. Decreased hemoglobin and hematocrit levels
   9. Decreased platelet count
   10. Positive bone marrow biopsy identifying leukemic blast-phase cells

 C. Infection

   ⚠ Infection is a major cause of death in the immunosuppressed client.

   1. Can occur through autocontamination or cross-contamination
   2. Common sites of infection are the skin, the respiratory tract, and the GI tract.

3. Initiate protective isolation procedures.
4. Ensure frequent and thorough handwashing.
5. Ensure that anyone entering the client's room is wearing a mask.
6. Use strict aseptic technique for all procedures.
7. Keep supplies for the client separate from supplies for other clients; keep frequently used equipment in the room for the client's use only.
8. Limit the number of caregivers that enter the client's room.
9. Maintain the client in a private room.
10. Place the client in a room with a high-efficiency particulate air filtration system or a laminar airflow system, if possible.
11. Reduce exposure to environmental organisms by eliminating raw fruits and vegetables (low-bacteria diet) from the diet and fresh flowers from the client's room and by not leaving standing water in the client's room.
12. Be sure that the client's room is cleaned daily.
13. Assist the client with daily bathing with the use of an antimicrobial soap.
14. Assist the client with performing oral hygiene frequently.
15. Initiate a bowel program to prevent constipation and rectal trauma.
16. Avoid invasive procedures (e.g., injections, rectal temperatures, urinary catheterization).
17. Change wound dressings daily, and inspect the wounds for redness, swelling, or drainage.
18. Monitor the urine for color and cloudiness.
19. Monitor the skin and oral mucous membranes for signs of infection (Box 43-6).
20. Encourage the client to cough and deep breathe.
21. Monitor the vital signs.
22. Monitor the white blood cell, neutrophil, and absolute granulocyte counts as well as the differential results.
23. The health care provider is notified if signs of infection are present; prepare to obtain specimens for the culture of open lesions, urine, and sputum.
24. Antibiotic, antifungal, and antiviral medication may be prescribed.
25. Instruct the client to avoid crowds and those with infections.
26. Instruct the client regarding a low-bacteria diet and to avoid drinking water that has been standing for longer than 15 minutes.
27. Instruct the client to avoid activities that expose him or her to infection, such as changing a pet's litter box or working with houseplants or in the garden.
28. Instruct the client that neither they nor their household contacts should receive immunization with a live virus such as measles, mumps, rubella, polio, varicella, shingles, and some influenza (including H1N1 vaccine).

Box 43-6 Mouth Care for the Client with Mucositis

Inspect the mouth daily.

Offer complete mouth care before and after every meal and at bedtime.

Brush the teeth and tongue with a soft-bristled toothbrush or sponges.

Provide mouth rinses every 12 hours with the prescribed solution

Administer topical anesthetic agents to mouth sores, as prescribed.

Avoid the use of alcohol- or glycerin-based mouthwashes or swabs because they are irritating to the mucosa. Offer soft foods that are cool to warm in temperature rather than foods that are hard or spicy.

⚠ During the period of greatest bone marrow suppression (the nadir), the platelet count and the white blood cell count may be extremely low.

D. Bleeding

1. The client is at risk for bleeding when the platelet count falls below 50,000 cells/mm^3; spontaneous bleeding frequently occurs when the platelet count is less than 20,000 cells/mm^3.

2. Clients with platelet counts less than 20,000/mm^3 may need a platelet transfusion.

3. For clients with anemia and fatigue, packed red blood cells may be prescribed.

4. Monitor the laboratory values (e.g., partial thromboplastin time, international normalized ratio, fibrinogen, fibrin degradation/split products, and platelet counts, as appropriate).

5. Examine the client for signs and symptoms of bleeding; examine all body fluids and excrement for the presence of blood.

6. Handle the client gently; use caution when obtaining blood pressure measurements to prevent skin injury.

7. Measure the abdominal girth, which can provide an indication of internal hemorrhage.

8. Provide soft foods at moderate temperatures; avoid foods that are at extreme temperatures.

9. Avoid injections, if possible, to prevent trauma to the skin and bleeding; apply firm and gentle pressure to a needle-stick site for at least 10 minutes.

10. Pad the side rails and sharp corners of the bed and furniture.

11. Avoid rectal suppositories, enemas, and thermometers.

12. If the female client is menstruating, count the number of pads or tampons used.

13. Blood products may be prescribed.

14. Instruct the client to use a soft toothbrush and to avoid dental floss.

15. Instruct the client to use only an electric razor for shaving.

16. Instruct the client to avoid blowing the nose.

17. Instruct the client to avoid constrictive or tight clothing or shoes.

18. Discourage the client from engaging in activities that involve the use of sharp objects.

19. Instruct the client to avoid using nonsteroidal anti-inflammatory drugs and products that contain aspirin.

E. Fatigue and nutrition

1. Assist the client with selecting a well-balanced diet.

2. Provide small, frequent, high-calorie, high-protein, high-carbohydrate meals that require little chewing.

3. Assist the client with self-care and mobility activities.

4. Allow for adequate rest periods during care.

5. Do not perform activities unless they are essential.

6. Administer blood products for anemia, as prescribed.

F. Additional interventions

1. Chemotherapy

2. Administer antibiotic, antibacterial, antiviral, and antifungal medications as prescribed.

3. Administer colony-stimulating factors as prescribed.

4. Administer blood replacements as prescribed.

5. Maintain infection and bleeding precautions.

6. Prepare the client for transplantation if indicated.

7. Instruct the client in appropriate home care measures.

8. Provide psychosocial support and support services for home care.

XII. LYMPHOMA: HODGKIN'S DISEASE

A. Description

1. A malignancy of the lymph nodes that originates in a single lymph node or a single chain of nodes.

2. **Metastasis** occurs to other, adjacent lymph structures and eventually invades nonlymphoid tissue.

3. Usually involves the lymph nodes, tonsils, spleen, and bone marrow; it is characterized by the presence of Reed-Sternberg cells in the nodes.

4. Possible causes include viral infections and previous exposure to alkylating chemical agents.

5. Prognosis is dependent on the stage of the disease

B. Data collection

1. Fever

2. Malaise, fatigue, and weakness

3. Night sweats

4. Loss of appetite and significant weight loss
5. Anemia and thrombocytopenia
6. Enlarged lymph nodes, spleen, and liver
7. Positive biopsy of lymph nodes, with cervical nodes most often affected first
8. Presence of Reed-Sternberg cells in nodes
9. Positive computed tomography scan of the liver and spleen

C. Interventions
1. For stages 1 and 2 without mediastinal node involvement, the treatment of choice is extensive external radiation of the involved lymph node regions.
2. With more extensive disease, radiation along with multiagent chemotherapy is used.
3. Monitor for side effects related to chemotherapy (drug-induced pancytopenia) or radiation.
4. Monitor for signs of infection and bleeding.
5. Maintain infection and bleeding precautions.
6. Discuss the possibility of sterility with the client who is receiving radiation; inform the male client of options related to sperm banks.

XIII. MULTIPLE MYELOMA

A. Description
1. A **malignant** proliferation of plasma cells and tumors within the bone
2. An excessive number of abnormal plasma cells invade the bone marrow, develop into tumors, and ultimately destroy the bone; the invasion of the lymph nodes, spleen, and liver occurs.
3. The abnormal plasma cells produce an abnormal antibody (**myeloma** protein or the Bence Jones protein) that is found in the blood and urine.
4. Causes the decreased production of immunoglobulin and antibodies and increased levels of uric acid and calcium, which can lead to renal failure
5. Multiple **myeloma** cells also produce excess cytokines that increase the **cancer** cell growth rates and destroy bone.
6. The cause is unknown.

B. Data collection
1. Bone (skeletal) pain, especially in the pelvis, spine, and ribs
2. Weakness and fatigue
3. Recurrent infections
4. Anemia
5. Bence Jones proteinuria and elevated total serum protein level
6. Osteoporosis (bone loss and the development of pathological fractures)
7. Thrombocytopenia and granulocytopenia
8. Elevated calcium and uric acid levels
9. Renal failure
10. Spinal cord compression and paraplegia

⚠ The client with multiple myeloma is at risk for pathological fractures. Therefore provide skeletal support during moving, turning, and ambulating and provide a hazard-free environment.

C. Interventions
1. Administer chemotherapy, as prescribed; autologous bone marrow transplantation may also be an option.
2. Provide supportive care to control symptoms and prevent complications, especially bone fractures, renal failure, and infections.
3. Maintain neutropenic and bleeding precautions, as necessary.
4. Monitor for signs of bleeding, infection, and skeletal fractures.
5. Encourage at least 2 L of fluid per day to offset potential problems associated with hypercalcemia, hyperuricemia, and proteinuria.
6. Monitor for signs of renal failure.
7. Encourage ambulation to prevent renal problems and slow down bone resorption.
8. Provide skeletal support during moving, turning, and ambulating to prevent pathological fractures; provide a hazard-free environment.
9. IV fluids and diuretics may be prescribed to increase the renal excretion of calcium.
10. Blood transfusions may be prescribed for anemia.
11. Administer analgesics, as prescribed, to control pain.
12. Administer antibiotics, as prescribed, for infection.
13. Prepare the client for local radiation therapy, if prescribed.
14. Instruct the client regarding home-care measures and the signs and symptoms of infection.

XIV. TESTICULAR CANCER

A. Description
1. Arises from the germinal epithelium of the sperm-producing germ cells or from the nongerminal epithelium of other structures in the testicles.
2. Incidence is higher among males who have an undescended testis (cryptorchidism).
3. Most often occurs between the ages of 15 and 40 years
4. **Metastasis** to the lung, liver, bone, and adrenal glands occurs

B. Prevention: Routine TSE (Figure 43-2)

C. Data collection
1. Painless testicular swelling
2. Dragging sensation in the scrotum as well as discomfort such as heaviness in the lower abdomen

3. Palpable lymphadenopathy, abdominal masses, and gynecomastia may indicate **metastasis**.
4. Late signs include back or bone pain and respiratory symptoms.

D. Interventions
1. Chemotherapy will be prescribed.
2. Prepare the client for radiation therapy, as prescribed.
3. Prepare the client for unilateral orchiectomy, if prescribed, for diagnosis and primary surgical management.
4. Prepare the client for radical retroperitoneal lymph node dissection, if prescribed, to stage the disease and reduce the tumor volume so that chemotherapy and radiation therapy are more effective.
5. Discuss reproduction, sexuality, and fertility information and options with the client.
6. Identify reproductive options such as sperm storage, donor insemination, and adoption.

E. Postoperative interventions
1. Monitor for signs of bleeding and wound infection.
2. Monitor the intake and output (I&O).
3. The HCP is notified if chills, fever, increasing pain or tenderness at the incision site, or drainage of the incision occurs.
4. Instruct the client that he may resume normal activities within 1 week, except for lifting objects heavier than 20 pounds and climbing stairs.
5. Instruct the client to perform a monthly TSE on the remaining testicle (see Figure 43-2).
6. Inform the client that sutures will be removed, usually 7 to 10 days after surgery.

XV. CERVICAL CANCER

A. Description
1. Preinvasive **cancer** is limited to the cervix and often asymptomatic.
2. Invasive **cancer** is in the cervix and other pelvic structures.
3. **Metastasis** is usually confined to the pelvis, but distant **metastasis** occurs through lymphatic spread.
4. Premalignant changes are described on a continuum from **dysplasia**, which is the earliest premalignancy change, to **carcinoma in situ**, which is the most advanced premalignant change.

B. Risk factors
1. Human papillomavirus (HPV) infection (vaccination against HPV is effective to avoid HPV infection, and thus cervical **cancer**)
2. Cigarette smoking, both active and passive
3. Reproductive behavior including early first intercourse (before age 17), multiple sex partners, or male partners with multiple sex partners.

4. Screening via regular gynecological examinations and Papanicolaou smear (Pap test), with treatment of precancerous abnormalities, decreases the incidence and mortality of cervical **cancer**.

C. Data collection
1. Painless vaginal bleeding, postmenstrually and postcoitally
2. Watery, blood-tinged vaginal discharge that becomes dark and foul-smelling or serosanguineous vaginal discharge
3. Pelvic, lower back, leg, or groin pain
4. Anorexia and weight loss
5. Leakage of urine and feces from the vagina
6. Dysuria
7. Hematuria
8. Cytological changes on Pap test
9. Indication of recurrence or **metastasis** includes unexplained weight loss, dysuria (painful urination), hematuria, rectal bleeding, chest pain, and cough.

D. Interventions (Box 43-7)

E. Laser therapy
1. Used when all boundaries of the lesion are visible during colposcopic examination
2. Energy from the beam is absorbed by fluid in the tissues, which causes them to vaporize.
3. Minimal bleeding is associated with the procedure.
4. Slight vaginal discharge is expected after the procedure; healing occurs in 6 to 12 weeks.

F. Cryosurgery
1. Freezing of the tissues by a probe with subsequent necrosis
2. No anesthesia is required, although cramping may occur during the procedure.
3. A heavy, watery discharge will occur for several weeks after the procedure.
4. Instruct the client to avoid intercourse and the use of tampons while the discharge is present.
5. Explain to the client that she should expect a heavy watery discharge for several weeks after the procedure.

Box 43-7 Treatment for Cervical Cancer

Nonsurgical
- Chemotherapy
- Cryosurgery
- External radiation
- Internal radiation implants (intracavitary)
- Laser therapy

Surgical
- Conization
- Hysterectomy
- Pelvic exenteration

G. Conization
1. A cone-shaped area of the cervix is removed.
2. Performed for women who want to preserve their fertility
3. Long-term follow-up care is needed, because new lesions can develop.
4. The risks of the procedure include hemorrhage, uterine perforation, incompetent cervix, cervical stenosis, and preterm labor in future pregnancies.

H. Hysterectomy
1. Description
   a. For microinvasive **cancer** if childbearing is not desired
   b. A vaginal approach is most commonly performed.
   c. A radical hysterectomy and bilateral lymph node dissection may be performed for **cancer** that has spread beyond the cervix but not to the pelvic wall.
2. Postoperative interventions
   a. Monitor the vital signs.
   b. Assist with coughing and deep-breathing exercises and the use of an incentive spirometer.
   c. Assist with range-of-motion (ROM) exercises and provide early ambulation.
   d. Apply antiembolism stockings, as prescribed.
   e. Monitor the I&O, Foley catheter drainage, and hydration status.
   f. Monitor the bowel sounds.
   g. Monitor vaginal bleeding; more than one saturated pad per hour may indicate excessive bleeding.
   h. Monitor the incision site for signs of infection.
   i. Administer pain medication, as prescribed.
   j. Instruct the client to avoid tub baths, sitting for long periods, and stair climbing for 1 month.
   k. Avoid strenuous activity or lifting anything that weighs more than 10 to 20 pounds.
   l. Instruct the client to consume foods that aid in healing.
   m. Instruct the client to avoid sexual intercourse for 3 to 6 weeks, as prescribed.
   n. Instruct the client regarding the signs that are associated with complications.

⚠ Monitor vaginal bleeding following hysterectomy. More than one saturated pad per hour may indicate excessive bleeding.

I. Pelvic exenteration (Box 43-8)
1. Description
   a. A radical surgical procedure that involves removal of all pelvic contents and is performed for recurrent **cancer** if there is no evidence of tumor outside of the pelvis and no lymph node involvement

---

Box 43-8 Types of Pelvic Exenteration

Anterior
Removal of the uterus, ovaries, fallopian tubes, vagina, bladder, urethra, and pelvic lymph nodes

Posterior
Removal of the uterus, ovaries, fallopian tubes, descending colon, rectum, and anal canal

Total
Combination of anterior and posterior

---

   b. When the bladder is removed, an ileal conduit will be created and located on the right side of the abdomen to divert urine.
   c. A colostomy may need to be created and will be located of the left side of the abdomen for the passage of feces.
2. Postoperative interventions
   a. Nursing care measures are similar to postoperative care after hysterectomy.
   b. Monitor the incision site for infection.
   c. Administer perineal irrigations with half-normal saline and hydrogen peroxide, as prescribed.
   d. Provide sitz baths, as prescribed.
   e. Instruct the client that the perineal opening, if present, may drain for several months.
   f. Instruct the client regarding the care of the ileal conduit and colostomy, if created.
   g. Provide sexual counseling; vaginal intercourse is not possible after anterior and total pelvic exenteration.

XVI. OVARIAN CANCER

A. Description
1. Ovarian **cancer** grows rapidly, spreads fast, and is often bilateral.
2. **Metastasis** occurs by direct spread to the organs in the pelvis, by distal spread through lymphatic drainage, or by peritoneal seeding.
3. In its early stages, ovarian **cancer** is often asymptomatic; because most women are diagnosed in advanced stages, ovarian **cancer** has more deaths than any other **cancer** of the female reproductive system, particularly white women between 55 and 65 years of age of North American or European descent.
4. An exploratory laparotomy is performed to diagnose and stage the tumor.

B. Data collection
1. Abdominal discomfort or swelling
2. GI disturbances with dyspepsia, indigestion, flatus, and distention
3. Dysfunctional vaginal bleeding
4. Abdominal mass

C. Interventions
1. External radiation is used if the tumor has invaded other organs.
2. Chemotherapy is used postoperatively for all stages of ovarian **cancer**.
3. Intraperitoneal chemotherapy, which involves the instillation of chemotherapy into the abdominal cavity, may be prescribed.
4. Immunotherapy, which alters the immunological response of the ovary and promotes tumor resistance, may be prescribed.
5. Total abdominal hysterectomy and bilateral salpingo-oophorectomy may be necessary.

XVII. ENDOMETRIAL (UTERINE) CANCER

A. Description
1. A slow-growing tumor that is associated with the menopausal years
2. **Metastasis** occurs through the lymphatic system to the ovaries and pelvis and via the blood to the lungs, liver, and bone, or intra-abdominally to the peritoneal cavity.

B. Risk factors
1. Use of estrogen replacement therapy (ERT)
2. Nulliparity
3. Polycystic ovary disease
4. Increased age
5. Late menopause
6. Family history of uterine **cancer** or hereditary nonpolyposis colorectal **cancer**
7. Obesity
8. Hypertension
9. Diabetes mellitus

C. Data collection
1. Postmenopausal bleeding
2. Watery, serosanguineous discharge
3. Low back, pelvic, or abdominal pain
4. Enlarged uterus in advanced stages

D. Nonsurgical interventions
1. External radiation or internal radiation (intracavitary radiation) used alone or in combination with surgery, depending on the stage of **cancer**
2. Chemotherapy to treat advanced or recurrent disease
3. Progestational therapy with medication for estrogen-dependent tumors may be prescribed.
4. Antiestrogen medication may also be prescribed.

E. Surgical interventions: Total abdominal hysterectomy and bilateral salpingo-oophorectomy

XVIII. BREAST CANCER

A. Description
1. Classified as invasive when it penetrates the tissue that surrounds the mammary duct and grows in an irregular pattern

2. **Metastasis** occurs via lymph nodes.
3. Common sites of **metastasis** are the bones and lungs; can also metastasize to the brain and liver.
4. Diagnosis is made by breast biopsy through a needle aspiration or by the surgical removal of the tumor with a microscopic examination for **malignant** cells.

B. Risk factors
1. Age
2. Family history of breast **cancer**
3. Early menarche and late menopause
4. Previous **cancer** of the breast, uterus, or ovaries
5. Nulliparity or late first birth
6. Obesity
7. High-dose radiation exposure of the chest

C. Data collection
1. Mass felt during BSE
2. Mass usually felt in the upper outer quadrant or beneath the nipple
3. A fixed, irregular, nonencapsulated mass
4. A painless mass, except during the very late stages
5. Nipple retraction or elevation
6. Asymmetry, with the affected breast being higher
7. Bloody or clear nipple discharge
8. Skin dimpling, retraction, or ulceration
9. Skin edema or peau d'orange skin, which may indicate lymphatic involvement (blocked skin drainage causes skin edema and an "orange peel" appearance)
10. Axillary lymphadenopathy
11. Lymphedema of the affected arm
12. Symptoms of **metastasis**
13. Presence of the lesion on mammography

D. Prevention: Monthly BSE (see Figure 43-1)

E. Nonsurgical interventions
1. Chemotherapy
2. Radiation therapy
3. Hormonal manipulation via the use of medication in postmenopausal women or other medications (e.g., tamoxifen [Nolvadex]) for estrogen receptor–positive tumors

F. Surgical interventions: Surgical breast procedures with possible breast reconstruction (Box 43-9)

G. Postoperative interventions
1. Monitor the vital signs.
2. Position the client in a semi-Fowler's position; turn her from the back to the unaffected side, with the affected arm elevated above the level of the heart to promote drainage and prevent lymphedema.
3. Encourage coughing and deep breathing.
4. If a drain (usually a Jackson-Pratt) is in place, maintain suction, and record the amount of drainage and the drainage characteristics.
5. Monitor the operative site for infection, swelling, or the presence of fluid collection under the skin flaps.

Box 43-9 Surgical Breast Procedures

Lumpectomy
The tumor is excised and removed.
Lymph node dissection may also be performed.

Simple Mastectomy
Breast tissue and the nipple are removed.
The lymph nodes are left intact.

Modified Radical Mastectomy
Breast tissue, the nipple, and the lymph nodes are removed.
The muscles are left intact.

Box 43-10 Client Instructions After Mastectomy

- Avoid overuse of the arm during the first few months.
- To prevent lymphedema, keep the affected arm elevated; consultation with lymphedema specialist may be prescribed.
- Provide incision care with an emollient to soften and prevent wound contracture.
- Encourage use of Reach for Recovery volunteers.
- Encourage the client to perform breast self-examination on the remaining breast.
- Protect the affected hand and arm.
- Avoid strong sunlight on the affected arm.
- Do not let the affected arm hang dependent.
- Do not carry a pocketbook or anything heavy over the affected arm.
- Avoid trauma, cuts, bruises, or burns to the affected side.
- Avoid wearing constricting clothing or jewelry on the affected side.
- Wear gloves when gardening.
- Use thick oven mitts when cooking.
- Use a thimble when sewing.
- Apply hand cream several times daily.
- Use cream cuticle remover.
- Call the HCP if signs of inflammation occur in the affected arm.
- Wear a Medic-Alert bracelet stating which arm is lymphedematous.

6. Monitor the incision site for constriction from the dressings, impaired sensation, or color changes of the skin.
7. If breast reconstruction was performed, the client will return from surgery with a surgical brassiere and the temporary prosthesis in place.
8. Provide the use of a pressure sleeve, as prescribed, if edema is severe.
9. Administer diuretics and provide a low-salt diet, as prescribed, for severe lymphedema.
10. Consult with the HCP and the physical therapist regarding the appropriate exercise program.
11. Instruct the client regarding home-care measures (Box 43-10).

⚠ No IVs, no injections, no blood pressure measurements, and no veniupunctures should be done on the arm on the side of the mastectomy. The arm on the side of the mastectomy is protected, and any intervention that could traumatize the affected arm is avoided.

XIX. GASTRIC CANCER

A. Description
   1. A **malignant** growth in the stomach
   2. Risk factors include *Helicobacter pylori* infection; a diet of smoked, highly salted, processed, or spiced foods; smoking; alcohol and nitrate ingestion; and a history of gastric ulcers.
   3. Complications include hemorrhage, obstruction, **metastasis**, and dumping syndrome.
   4. The goals of treatment are to remove the tumor and to provide a nutritional program.
B. Data collection
   1. Early symptoms of gastric **cancer**
      a. Indigestion
      b. Abdominal discomfort
      c. Full feeling
      d. Epigastric, back, or retrosternal pain
   2. Late symptoms of gastric **cancer**
      a. Weakness and fatigue
      b. Anorexia and weight loss
      c. Nausea and vomiting
      d. A sensation of pressure in the stomach
      e. Dysphagia and obstructive symptoms
      f. Iron deficiency anemia
      g. Ascites
      h. Palpable epigastric mass
C. Interventions
   1. Monitor the vital signs.
   2. Monitor the hemoglobin and hematocrit levels; blood transfusions may be prescribed.
   3. Monitor the weight daily.
   4. Monitor the nutritional status; encourage small, bland, easily digestible meals with vitamin and mineral supplements.
   5. Administer pain medication, as prescribed.
   6. Prepare the client for chemotherapy or radiation therapy, as prescribed.
   7. Prepare the client for surgical resection of the tumor, as prescribed (Box 43-11).
D. Postoperative interventions (see Chapter 47 for information regarding postoperative care)

XX. PANCREATIC CANCER

A. Description
   1. Most pancreatic tumors are highly **malignant**, rapidly growing **adenocarcinomas** that originate from the epithelium of the ductal system.

Box 43-11 Surgical Interventions for Gastric Cancer

Subtotal Gastrectomy

Billroth I
- Also called gastroduodenostomy
- Partial gastrectomy; the remaining segment is anastomosed to the duodenum

Billroth II
- Also called gastrojejunostomy
- Partial gastrectomy; the remaining segment is anastomosed to the jejunum

Total Gastrectomy
- Also called esophagojejunostomy
- Removal of the stomach, with the attachment of the esophagus to the jejunum or the duodenum

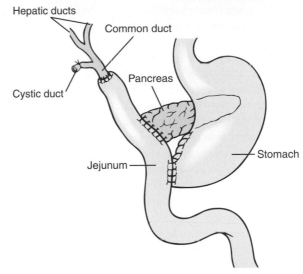

▲ **FIGURE 43-3** Whipple procedure or radical pancreaticoduodenectomy. (From Lewis, S., Heitkemper, M., Dirksen, S., & Bucher, L. [2010]. *Medical-surgical nursing: Assessment and management of clinical problems* [8th ed.]. St. Louis: Mosby.)

2. Pancreatic **cancer** is associated with increased age, a history of diabetes mellitus, alcohol use, a history of previous pancreatitis, smoking, the ingestion of a high-fat diet, and exposure to environmental chemicals.
3. Symptoms usually do not occur until the tumor is large; therefore, the prognosis is poor.

B. Data collection
1. Nausea and vomiting
2. Jaundice
3. Unexplained weight loss
4. Clay-colored stools
5. Glucose intolerance
6. Abdominal pain

C. Interventions
1. Radiation
2. Chemotherapy
3. Whipple procedure, which involves a pancreaticoduodenectomy with the removal of the distal third of the stomach, a pancreaticojejunostomy, a gastrojejunostomy, and a choledochojejunostomy (Figure 43-3)
4. Postoperative care measures are similar to those for the care of a client with pancreatitis and for a client after gastric surgery; monitor the blood glucose levels for transient hyperglycemia or hypoglycemia that results from the surgical manipulation of the pancreas.

XXI. INTESTINAL TUMORS

A. Description
1. **Malignant** lesions that develop in the cells lining the bowel wall or that develop as polyps in the colon or rectum
2. Complications include bowel perforation with peritonitis, abscess and/or fistula formation, hemorrhage, and complete intestinal obstruction.

3. **Metastasis** occurs via the circulatory or lymphatic system or by direct extension to other areas in the colon or other organs.

B. Risk factors for colorectal **cancer**
1. Age older than 50 years
2. Familial polyposis, family history of colorectal **cancer**
3. Previous colorectal polyps, history of colorectal **cancer**
4. History of chronic inflammatory bowel disease
5. History of ovarian or breast **cancer**

C. Data collection
1. Blood in the stool
2. Anorexia, vomiting, and weight loss
3. Malaise
4. Anemia
5. Abnormal stools
   a. Ascending colon tumor: Diarrhea
   b. Descending colon tumor: Constipation, some diarrhea, or flat, ribbon-like stool as a result of a partial obstruction
   c. Rectal tumor: Alternating constipation and diarrhea
6. Guarding or abdominal distention
7. Abdominal mass (late sign)
8. Cachexia (late sign)

D. Interventions
1. Monitor for signs of complications, which include bowel perforation with peritonitis, abscess and/or fistula formation, hemorrhage, and complete intestinal obstruction.
2. Monitor for signs of intestinal perforation, which include low blood pressure, rapid and weak pulse, distended abdomen, and elevated temperature.

3. Monitor for signs of intestinal obstruction, which include vomiting (may be fecal contents), pain, constipation, and abdominal distention.

4. Note that an early sign of intestinal obstruction is increased peristaltic activity, which produces an increase in bowel sounds; as the obstruction progresses, hypoactive sounds are heard.

5. Prepare for radiation preoperatively to facilitate surgical resection and postoperatively to decrease the risk of recurrence or to reduce pain, hemorrhage, bowel obstruction, or **metastasis**.

6. Chemotherapy is used postoperatively to assist with the control of symptoms and the spread of the disease.

E. Surgical interventions: Bowel resection and the creation of a colostomy or an ileostomy

F. Colostomy or ileostomy
   1. Preoperative interventions
      a. Consult with the enterostomal therapist to assist with identifying the optimal placement of the ostomy.
      b. Instruct the client to eat a low-residue diet for a day or two before surgery, as prescribed.
      c. Intestinal antiseptics and antibiotics may be prescribed to decrease the bacterial content of the colon and to reduce the risk of infection from the surgical procedure.
      d. Administer laxatives and enemas, as prescribed.
   2. Postoperative: Colostomy
      a. Place a petroleum jelly gauze over the stoma to keep it moist, and keep it covered by a dry sterile dressing if a pouch system is not in place.
      b. Place a pouch system on the stoma as soon as possible.
      c. Monitor the stoma for size, unusual bleeding, and necrotic tissue.
      d. Monitor for color changes in the stoma.
      e. Note that the normal stoma color is red or pink, which indicates high vascularity.
      f. Note that a pale pink stoma indicates low hemoglobin and hematocrit levels and that a purple-black stoma indicates compromised circulation that requires HCP notification.
      g. Monitor the pouch system for proper fit and signs of leakage.
      h. Assess the functioning of the colostomy.
      i. Expect that stool will be liquid postoperatively but that it will become more solid, depending on the area of the colostomy.
      j. Ascending colon colostomy: Expect liquid stool.
      k. Transverse colon colostomy: Expect loose to semiformed stool.
      l. Descending colon colostomy: Expect close-to-normal stool.

   m. Fecal matter should not be allowed to remain on the skin.
   n. Empty the pouch when it is one-third full.
   o. Administer analgesics and antibiotics, as prescribed.
   p. Irrigate the perineal wound, if present and if prescribed, and monitor for signs of infection.
   q. Instruct the client to avoid foods that cause excessive gas formation and odor.
   r. Instruct the client regarding stoma care and irrigations, as prescribed.
   s. Instruct the client that normal activities may be resumed when approved by the HCP.

3. Postoperative: Ileostomy
   a. A healthy stoma is red; a color change to dark blue or black should be reported to the HCP.
   b. Postoperative drainage will be dark green and progress to yellow as the client begins to eat.
   c. Stool is liquid.
   d. The risk for dehydration and electrolyte imbalance exists.
   e. Do not give suppositories through the ileostomy.

⚠ Monitor stoma color. A dark blue, purple, or black stoma indicates compromised circulation, requiring HCP notification.

XXII. LUNG CANCER

A. Description
   1. Lung **cancer**, **malignant** tumor of the bronchi and peripheral lung tissue, is one of the leading causes of **cancer**-related deaths in men and women in the United States.
   2. The lungs are a common target for **metastasis** from other organs.
   3. Bronchogenic **cancer** (tumors originate in the epithelium of the bronchus) spreads through direct extension and lymphatic dissemination.
   4. Classified according to histological cell type, there are two main types of lung **cancer**, small cell lung **cancer** (SCLC) and non–small cell lung **cancer** (NSCLC); epidermal (squamous cell), adenocarcinoma, and large cell anaplastic **carcinoma** are classified as NSCLC because of their similar responses to treatment.
   5. Diagnosis is made by a chest x-ray, CT scan, or magnetic resonance imaging (MRI), which will show a lesion or mass, and by bronchoscopy and sputum studies, which will demonstrate a positive cytological study for **cancer** cells.

B. Causes
   1. Cigarette smoking; also exposure to "passive" tobacco smoke

2. Exposure to environmental and occupational pollutants

C. Data collection
1. Cough
2. Dyspnea
3. Hoarseness
4. Hemoptysis
5. Chest pain
6. Anorexia and weight loss
7. Weakness

D. Interventions
1. Monitor the vital signs.
2. Monitor the breathing patterns and breath sounds and for signs of respiratory impairment.
3. Monitor for tracheal deviation.
4. Administer analgesics, as prescribed, for pain management.
5. Place the client in Fowler's position for ease of breathing.
6. Administer oxygen, as prescribed, and humidification to moisten and loosen secretions.
7. Monitor the pulse oximetry.
8. Provide respiratory treatments, as prescribed.
9. Administer bronchodilators and corticosteroids, as prescribed, to decrease bronchospasm, inflammation, and edema.
10. Provide a high-calorie, high-protein, high-vitamin diet.
11. Provide activity (as tolerated), rest periods, and active and passive range-of-motion (ROM) exercises.
12. Monitor for bleeding, infection, and electrolyte imbalances.

E. Nonsurgical interventions
1. Radiation therapy for localized intrathoracic lung **cancers** and for the palliation of hemoptysis, obstructions, dysphagia, and pain.
2. Chemotherapy may be prescribed for the treatment of nonresectable tumors or as adjuvant therapy.

F. Surgical interventions
1. Laser therapy: To relieve endobronchial obstruction
2. Ablation therapy to destroy the tumor
3. Thoracentesis and pleurodesis: To remove pleural fluid and relieve hypoxia
4. Thoracotomy (opening into the thoracic cavity) with pneumonectomy: Surgical removal of a lung
5. Thoracotomy with lobectomy: Surgical removal of one lobe of the lung for tumors that are confined to a single lobe
6. Thoracotomy with segmental resection: Surgical removal of a lobe segment

G. Preoperative interventions
1. Explain the potential postoperative need for chest tubes.
2. Note that closed-chest drainage is not usually used for a pneumonectomy and that the serum fluid that accumulates in the empty thoracic cavity eventually consolidates, thus preventing shifts of the mediastinum, heart, and remaining lung.

H. Postoperative interventions
1. Monitor the vital signs.
2. Monitor the cardiac and respiratory statuses; monitor for the absence or presence of lung sounds.
3. Monitor the chest tube drainage system, which will drain air and/or blood that accumulates in the pleural space.
4. Monitor the chest tube insertion site for crepitus (subcutaneous air) and drainage.
5. Administer oxygen, as prescribed.
6. Check the HCP's prescriptions regarding client positioning; complete lateral turning must be avoided.
7. Monitor the pulse oximetry.
8. Provide activity, as tolerated.
9. Encourage active ROM exercises of the operative shoulder, as prescribed.
10. See Chapter 19 for the care of the client with a chest tube.

⚠ Airway is the priority for a client with lung or laryngeal cancer.

XXIII. LARYNGEAL CANCER

A. Description
1. Laryngeal **cancer** is a **malignant** tumor of the larynx.
2. Laryngeal **cancer** presents as **malignant** ulcerations with underlying infiltration and is spread by local extension to adjacent structures in the throat and neck, and by the lymphatic system.
3. Diagnosis is made by laryngoscopy and biopsy showing a positive cytological study for **cancer** cells.
4. Laryngoscopy allows for evaluation of the throat and biopsy of tissues; chest radiography, CT, and MRI are used for **staging**.

B. Risk factors
1. Cigarette smoking
2. Heavy alcohol use and the combined use of tobacco and alcohol
3. Exposure to environmental pollutants (e.g., asbestos, wood dust)
4. Exposure to radiation

C. Data collection
1. Persistent hoarseness and sore throat
2. Painless neck mass
3. The feeling of a lump in the throat
4. Burning sensation in the throat
5. Dysphagia
6. Change in voice quality
7. Dyspnea

8. Weakness and weight loss
9. Hemoptysis
10. Foul breath odor

D. Interventions

1. Place the client in Fowler's position to promote optimal air exchange.
2. Monitor the respiratory status.
3. Monitor for signs of food and fluid aspiration.
4. Administer oxygen, as prescribed.
5. Provide respiratory treatments, as prescribed.
6. Provide activity, as tolerated.
7. Provide a high-calorie, high-protein, high-vitamin diet.
8. Prepare to provide nutritional support via parenteral nutrition or nasogastric, gastrostomy, or jejunostomy tube, as prescribed.
9. Administer analgesics for pain, as prescribed.

E. Nonsurgical interventions

1. Radiation therapy if the **cancer** is limited to a small area in one vocal cord
2. Chemotherapy, which may be performed in combination with radiation and surgery

F. Surgical interventions

1. Depend on the tumor size and the amount of tissue to be resected.
2. Types of resection include cordal stripping, cordectomy, partial laryngectomy, and total laryngectomy.
3. A tracheostomy is performed with a total laryngectomy; this airway opening is always permanent and is referred to as a laryngectomy stoma.

G. Preoperative interventions

1. Establish communication methods for the client.
2. Encourage the client to express feelings about changes in body image and the loss of the voice.
3. Describe the rehabilitation program and provide information about the tracheostomy and suctioning.

H. Postoperative interventions

1. Monitor the vital signs.
2. Monitor the respiratory status and airway patency, and provide frequent suctioning to remove bloody secretions.
3. Place the client in high Fowler's position.
4. Maintain mechanical ventilator support or a tracheostomy collar with humidification, as prescribed.
5. Monitor the pulse oximetry.
6. Maintain surgical drains in the neck area, if present.
7. Observe for hemorrhage and edema in the neck.
8. Monitor IV fluids or parenteral nutrition, if prescribed, until nutrition is administered via nasogastric, gastrostomy, or jejunostomy tube.
9. Provide oral hygiene.
10. Monitor the gag and cough reflexes and the ability to swallow.

11. Increase activity, as tolerated.
12. Monitor the color, amount, and consistency of the sputum.
13. Provide stoma and laryngectomy care (Box 43-12).
14. Provide consultation with a speech and language pathologist, as prescribed.
15. Reinforce the method of communication that is established preoperatively.
16. Prepare the client for rehabilitation and speech therapy (Box 43-13).

XXIV. PROSTATE CANCER

A. Description

1. Prostate **cancer**, a slow-growing malignancy of the prostate gland, is a common **cancer** in American men; most prostate tumors are adenocarcinomas arising from androgen-dependent epithelial cells.
2. The risk increases in men with each decade after the age of 50 years.
3. Prostate **cancer** can spread via direct invasion of surrounding tissues or by **metastasis**, through the bloodstream and lymphatics, to the bony pelvis and spine.
4. Bone **metastasis** is a concern, as is spread to the lungs, liver, and kidneys.
5. The cause of prostate **cancer** is unclear, but advancing age, heavy metal exposure, smoking, and history of sexually transmitted infection are contributing factors.

B. Data collection

1. Asymptomatic during the early stages
2. Hard, pea-sized nodule palpated on rectal examination

Box 43-12 Stoma Care After Laryngectomy

- Protect the neck from injury.
- Instruct the client in how to clean the incision and provide stoma care.
- Instruct the client to wear a stoma guard to shield the stoma.
- Demonstrate ways to prevent debris from entering the stoma.
- Advise the client to wear loose-fitting, high-collared clothing to cover the stoma.
- Avoid swimming, showering, and using aerosol sprays.
- Teach the client clean suctioning technique.
- Advise the client to increase humidity in the home.
- Increase fluid intake to 3000 mL/day as prescribed.
- Avoid exposure to persons with infections.
- Alternate rest periods with activity.
- Instruct the client in range-of-motion exercises for the arms, shoulders, and neck as prescribed.
- Advise the client to wear a Medic-Alert bracelet.

3. Hematuria (painless)
4. Late symptoms include weight loss, urinary obstruction, and pain radiating from the lumbosacral area down the leg.
5. Prostate-specific antigen level is elevated in various noncancerous conditions and therefore should not be used as a screening test without a digital rectal exam; it is routinely used to monitor response to therapy.
6. Diagnosis is made through biopsy of the prostate.

C. Nonsurgical interventions
1. Prepare the client for hormone manipulation therapy as prescribed.
2. Luteinizing hormone may be prescribed to slow the rate of growth of the tumor.
3. Pain medication, radiation therapy, corticosteroids, and bisphosphonates may be prescribed for palliation of advanced prostate **cancer**.
4. Prepare the client for external beam radiation or brachytherapy, which may be prescribed alone or with surgery, preoperatively or postoperatively, to reduce the lesion and limit **metastasis**.
5. Prepare the client for the administration of chemotherapy in cases of hormone-resistant tumors.

D. Surgical interventions
1. Prepare the client for orchiectomy (palliative), if prescribed, which will limit the production of testosterone.
2. Prepare the client for prostatectomy, if prescribed.
3. The radical prostatectomy can be performed via a retropubic, perineal, or suprapubic approach.

Box 43-13 Speech Rehabilitation After Laryngectomy

Esophageal Speech
- Client produces esophageal speech by "burping" the air that is swallowed
- Voice produced is monotone; it cannot be raised or lowered, and it carries no pitch
- Client must have adequate hearing, because he or she uses the mouth to shape words as they are heard

Mechanical Devices
- The devices are known as electrolarynges
- Placed against the side of the neck; air inside the neck and pharynx is vibrated, and the client articulates
- Other devices consist of a plastic tube that is placed inside the client's mouth and that vibrates on articulation

Tracheoesophageal Fistula
- Surgical creation of a fistula between the trachea and the esophagus, with the eventual placement of a prosthesis that is used to produce speech
- Prosthesis provides the client with a means to divert the air from the lungs through the trachea, into the esophagus, and out of the mouth
- Speech is produced by lip and tongue movement

---

4. Cryosurgical ablation is a minimally invasive procedure that may be an alternative to radical prostatectomy; liquid nitrogen freezes the gland, and the dead cells are absorbed by the body.

E. Transurethral resection of the prostate (TURP) may be performed for palliation in prostate **cancer** clients.
1. The procedure involves insertion of a scope into the urethra to excise prostatic tissue.
2. Monitor for hemorrhage; bleeding is common following TURP.
3. Postoperative continuous bladder irrigation (CBI) may be prescribed, which prevents catheter obstruction. (Box 43-14).
4. Assess for signs of transurethral resection syndrome, which include signs of cerebral edema and increased intracranial pressure, such as increased blood pressure, bradycardia, confusion, disorientation, muscle twitching, visual disturbances, and nausea and vomiting.
5. Antispasmodics may be prescribed for bladder spasm.
6. Instruct the client to monitor and report dribbling or incontinence postoperatively and teach perineal exercises.
7. Sterility is possible following the surgical procedure.

F. Suprapubic prostatectomy
1. Suprapubic prostatectomy is removal of the prostate gland by an abdominal incision with a bladder incision.
2. The client will have an abdominal dressing that may drain copious amounts of urine, and the abdominal dressing will need to be changed frequently.
3. Severe hemorrhage is possible, and monitoring for blood loss is an important nursing intervention.
4. Antispasmodics may be prescribed for bladder spasms.
5. Continuous bladder irrigation (CBI) is prescribed and carried out to keep the urine pink.
6. Sterility occurs with this procedure.

G. Retropubic prostatectomy
1. Retropubic prostatectomy is removal of the prostate gland by a low abdominal incision without opening the bladder.
2. Less bleeding occurs with this procedure compared with the suprapubic procedure, and the client experiences fewer bladder spasms.
3. Abdominal drainage is minimal.
4. CBI may be used.
5. Sterility occurs with this procedure.

H. Perineal prostatectomy
1. The prostate gland is removed through an incision made between the scrotum and anus.
2. Minimal bleeding occurs with this procedure.

Box 43-14 Continuous Bladder Irrigation

Description

Three-way (lumen) irrigation to decrease bleeding and to keep the bladder free from clots:

- One lumen for inflating the balloon (30 mL)
- One lumen for instillation (inflow)
- One lumen for outflow

Interventions

Maintain traction on the catheter, if applied to prevent bleeding, by pulling the catheter taut and taping it to the abdomen or thigh.

Instruct the client to keep the leg straight if traction is applied to the catheter and it is taped to the thigh.

Catheter traction is not released without a HCP's prescription; it is usually released after any bright-red drainage has diminished.

Use only normal saline or a prescribed solution to prevent water intoxication. Run the solution at a rate, as prescribed, to keep the urine pink. Run the solution rapidly if bright red drainage or clots are present; monitor output closely. Run the solution at about 40 gtt/min when the bright red drainage clears.

If the urinary catheter becomes obstructed, turn off the continuous bladder irrigation and irrigate the catheter with 30 to 50 mL of normal saline, if prescribed; notify the HCP if the obstruction does not resolve.

Monitor for transurethral resection syndrome or severe hyponatremia (water intoxication) caused by the excessive absorption of bladder irrigation (i.e., altered mental status, bradycardia, increased blood pressure, and confusion).

Discontinue continuous bladder irrigation and Foley catheterization as prescribed, usually 24 to 48 hours after surgery.

Monitor for continence and urinary retention when the catheter is removed.

Inform the client that some burning, frequency, and dribbling may occur after catheter removal.

Inform the client that he should be voiding 150 to 200 mL of clear yellow urine every 3 to 4 hours by 3 days after surgery.

Inform the client that he may pass small clots and tissue debris for several days.

Teach the client to avoid heavy lifting, stressful exercise, driving, Valsalva's maneuver, and sexual intercourse for 2 to 6 weeks to prevent strain.

Instruct the client to call the HCP if bleeding occurs or if there is a decrease in the urinary stream.

Instruct the client to drink 2400 to 3000 mL of fluid each day, preferably before 8:00 PM to prevent nocturia.

Instruct the client to avoid alcohol, caffeinated beverages, and spicy foods to prevent the overstimulation of the bladder.

Instruct the client that, if the urine becomes bloody, he should rest and increase the fluid intake; if the bleeding does not subside, he should notify the HCP.

---

3. The client needs to be monitored closely for infection, because the risk of infection is increased with this type of prostatectomy.
4. Urinary incontinence is common.
5. The procedure causes sterility.
6. Teach the client how to perform perineal exercises.

I. Postoperative interventions
   1. Monitor vital signs.
   2. Monitor urinary output and urine for hemorrhage or clots.
   3. Increase fluids to 2400 to 3000 mL/day, unless contraindicated.
   4. Monitor for arterial bleeding as evidenced by bright red urine with numerous clots; if it occurs, increase CBI and notify the surgeon immediately.
   5. Monitor for venous bleeding as evidenced by burgundy-colored urine output; if it occurs, inform the surgeon, who may apply traction on the catheter.
   6. Monitor hemoglobin and hematocrit levels.
   7. Expect red to light pink urine for 24 hours, turning to amber in 3 days.
   8. Ambulate the client as early as possible and as soon as urine begins to clear in color.

9. Inform the client that a continuous feeling of an urge to void is normal.
10. Instruct the client to avoid attempts to void around the catheter because this will cause bladder spasms.
11. Administer antibiotics, analgesics, stool softeners, and antispasmodics as prescribed.
12. Monitor the three-way Foley catheter, which usually has a 30- to 45-mL retention balloon.
13. Maintain CBI with sterile bladder irrigation solution as prescribed to keep the catheter free of obstruction and maintain the urine pink in color (see Box 43-14).

⚠ Following TURP, monitor for transurethral resection syndrome or severe hyponatremia (water intoxication) caused by the excessive absorption of bladder irrigation during surgery (altered mental status, bradycardia, increased blood pressure, and confusion).

J. Postoperative interventions: Suprapubic prostatectomy
   1. Monitor suprapubic and Foley catheter drainage.
   2. Monitor CBI if prescribed.
   3. Note that the Foley catheter will be removed 2 to 4 days postoperatively if the client has a suprapubic catheter.

4. If prescribed, clamp the suprapubic catheter after the Foley catheter is removed, and instruct the client to attempt to void; after the client has voided, assess the residual urine in the bladder by unclamping the suprapubic catheter and measuring the output.

5. Prepare for removal of the suprapubic catheter when the client consistently empties the bladder and residual urine is 75 mL or less.

6. Monitor the suprapubic incision dressing, which may become saturated with urine, until the incision heals; dressing may need to be changed frequently.

K. Postoperative interventions: Retropubic prostatectomy
1. Note that because the bladder is not entered, there is no urinary drainage on the abdominal dressing.
2. Assess for urinary or purulent drainage on the dressing; if this occurs, notify the surgeon.
3. Monitor for fever and increased pain, which may indicate an infection.

L. Postoperative interventions: Perineal prostatectomy
1. Note that the client will have an incision, which may or may not have a drain.
2. Avoid the use of rectal thermometers, rectal tubes, and enemas because they may cause trauma and bleeding.

XXV. BLADDER CANCER

A. Description
1. Papillomatous growths in the bladder urothelium that undergo **malignant** changes and that may infiltrate the bladder wall.
2. Predisposing factors include cigarette smoking, exposure to industrial chemicals, and exposure to radiation.
3. Common sites of **metastasis** include the liver, bones, and lungs.
4. As the tumor progresses, it can extend into the rectum, vagina, other pelvic soft tissues, and retroperitoneal structures.

B. Data collection
1. Gross, painless hematuria
2. Frequency, urgency, and dysuria
3. Clot-induced obstruction
4. Bladder biopsy confirms the diagnosis

C. Radiation
1. Most bladder **cancers** are poorly radiosensitive and require high doses of radiation.
2. Radiation therapy is more acceptable for advanced disease that cannot be eradicated by surgery.
3. Palliative radiation may be used to relieve pain and bowel obstruction and to control potential hemorrhage and leg edema secondary to venous or lymphatic obstruction.

4. Intracavitary radiation may be prescribed, which protects adjacent tissue.
5. External radiation combined with chemotherapy or surgery may be prescribed, because the external radiation alone may not be effective.
6. Complications of radiation
   a. Abacterial cystitis
   b. Proctitis
   c. Fistula formation
   d. Ileitis or colitis
   e. Bladder ulceration and hemorrhage

D. Chemotherapy
1. Intravesical instillation
   a. An alkylating chemotherapeutic agent is instilled into the bladder.
   b. This method provides a concentrated topical treatment with little systemic absorption.
   c. The medication is injected into a urethral catheter and retained for 2 hours.
   d. After instillation, the client's position is rotated every 15 to 30 minutes, starting in the supine position, to avoid lying on a full bladder.
   e. After 2 hours, the client voids in a sitting position and is instructed to increase fluids to flush the bladder.
   f. Treat the urine as a biohazard, and send it to the radioisotope laboratory for monitoring.
   g. For 6 hours after intravesical chemotherapy, disinfect the toilet with household bleach after the client has voided.
2. Systemic chemotherapy: Used to treat inoperable or late tumors
3. Complications of chemotherapy
   a. Bladder irritation
   b. Hemorrhagic cystitis

E. Surgical interventions
1. Transurethral resection of the bladder tumor
   a. Local resection and fulguration (destruction of tissue by electrical current through electrodes placed in direct contact with the tissue)
   b. Performed for very early tumors for cure or for inoperable tumors for palliation
2. Partial cystectomy
   a. The removal of up to half of the bladder
   b. Performed for early tumors and for clients who cannot tolerate a radical cystectomy
   c. During the initial postoperative period, the bladder capacity is markedly reduced to about 60 mL; however, as the bladder tissue expands, the capacity increases to 200 to 400 mL.
   d. Maintenance of a continuous output of urine after surgery is critical to prevent bladder distention and stress on the suture line.

e. A urethral catheter and a suprapubic catheter may be in place, and the suprapubic catheter may be left in place for 2 weeks until healing occurs.

3. Cystectomy and urinary diversion (Figure 43-4)
   a. Various surgical procedures performed to create alternate pathways for urine collection and excretion

b. Urinary diversion may be performed with or without cystectomy (bladder removal).

c. The surgery may be performed in two stages if the tumor is extensive, with the creation of the urinary diversion first and the cystectomy several weeks later.

d. If a radical cystectomy is performed, lower-extremity lymphedema may occur as a result of lymph node dissection, and male impotence may occur.

Ureterostomies divert urine directly to the skin surface through a ureteral skin opening (stoma). After ureterostomy, the patient must wear a pouch.

Cutaneous ureterostomy

Cutaneous ureteroureterostomy

Bilateral cutaneous ureterostomy

Conduits collect urine in a portion of the intestine, which is then opened onto the skin surface as a stoma. After the creation of a conduit, the patient must wear a pouch.

Ileal (Bricker's) conduit

Colon conduit

Ileal reservoirs divert urine into a surgically created pouch, or pocket, that functions as a bladder. The stoma is continent, and the patient removes urine by regular self-catheterization.

Catheter

Continent internal ileal reservoir (Kock's pouch)

Sigmoidostomies divert urine to the large intestine, so no stoma is required. The patient excretes urine with bowel movements, and bowel incontinence may result.

Ureterosigmoidostomy

Ureteroiliosigmoidostomy

▲ **FIGURE 43-4** Urinary diversion procedures used for the treatment of bladder cancer. (From Ignatavicius, D., & Workman, M. [2010]. *Medical-surgical nursing: Patient-centered collaborative care* [6th ed.]. St. Louis: Saunders.)

4. Ileal conduit
   a. Also called ureteroileostomy or Bricker's procedure
   b. Ureters are implanted into a segment of the ileum, with the formation of an abdominal stoma.
   c. The urine flows into the conduit and is continually propelled out through the stoma by peristalsis.
   d. The client is required to wear an appliance over the stoma to collect the urine.
   e. Complications include obstruction, pyelonephritis, leakage at the anastomosis site, stenosis, hydronephrosis, calculi, skin irritation and ulceration, and stomal defects.
5. Kock pouch
   a. A continent internal ileal reservoir created from a segment of the ileum and the ascending colon
   b. The ureters are implanted into the side of the reservoir, and a special nipple valve is constructed to attach the reservoir to the skin.
   c. Postoperatively, the client will have a size 24 to 26 Foley catheter in place to drain urine continuously until the pouch has healed.
   d. The catheter is irrigated gently with normal saline to prevent obstruction caused by mucus or clots.
   e. After the removal of the catheter, the client is instructed in how to self-catheterize and to drain the reservoir at 4- to 6-hour intervals.
6. Indiana pouch
   a. A continent reservoir is created from the ascending colon and the terminal ileum, thus making a pouch larger than the Kock pouch (additional continent reservoirs include the Mainz and Florida pouch systems).
   b. Postoperatively, the client will have a size 24 to 26 Foley catheter in place to drain urine continuously until the pouch has healed.
   c. The Foley catheter is irrigated gently with normal saline to prevent obstruction caused by mucus or clots.
   d. After the removal of the Foley catheter, the client is instructed in how to self-catheterize and to drain the reservoir at 4- to 6-hour intervals.
7. Creation of a neobladder
   a. Similar to the creation of an internal reservoir but different because, instead of emptying through an abdominal stoma, it empties through a pelvic outlet into the urethra.
   b. The client empties the neobladder by relaxing the external sphincter and creating abdominal pressure or by intermittent self-catheterization.
8. Percutaneous nephrostomy or pyelostomy
   a. Used when the **cancer** is inoperable, to prevent obstruction.

   b. Involves a percutaneous or surgical insertion of a nephrostomy tube into the kidney for drainage.
   c. Nursing interventions involve stabilizing the tube to prevent dislodgment and monitoring output.
9. Ureterostomy
   a. May be performed as a palliative procedure if the ureters are obstructed by the tumor
   b. The ureters are attached to the surface of the abdomen, where the urine flows directly into a drainage appliance without a conduit.
   c. Potential problems include infection, skin irritation, and the obstruction of urinary flow as a result of strictures at the opening.
10. Vesicostomy
    a. The bladder is sutured to the abdomen, and a stoma is created in the bladder wall.
    b. The bladder empties through the stoma.

F. Preoperative interventions
1. Administer bowel preparation, as prescribed, which may include a clear liquid diet 12 to 24 hours before the surgical procedure, laxatives and enemas, and antibiotics to lower the bacterial count in the bowel.
2. Assist the surgeon and the enterostomal nurse with selecting an appropriate skin site for the creation of the abdominal stoma.
3. Encourage the client to talk about his or her feelings related to the stoma creation.

G. Postoperative interventions

⚠ Monitor urinary output closely following bladder surgery. Irrigate the ureteral catheter (if present and if prescribed) gently to prevent obstruction. Follow the HCP's prescriptions and agency policy regarding irrigation.

1. Monitor the vital signs.
2. Monitor the incision site.
3. Assess the stoma (it should be red and moist) every hour for the first 24 hours.
4. Monitor for edema in the stoma, which may be present during the immediate postoperative period.
5. If the stoma appears dark and dusky, notify the HCP immediately, because this indicates necrosis.
6. Monitor for the prolapse or retraction of the stoma.
7. Monitor for the return of bowel function; monitor for peristalsis, which will return in 3 to 4 days.
8. Maintain nothing-by-mouth status, as prescribed, until bowel sounds return.
9. Monitor the urine flow, which is continuous (30 to 60 mL/hour) after surgery.
10. The HCP is notified if the urine output is less than 30 mL/hour or if there is no urine output for more than 15 minutes.

11. Ureteral stents or catheters may be in place for 2 to 3 weeks or until healing occurs; maintain stability of catheters to prevent dislodgment.
12. Monitor the urinary output closely and irrigate the catheter gently to prevent obstruction, as prescribed.
13. Monitor for hematuria.
14. Monitor for signs of peritonitis.
15. Monitor for bladder distention after a partial cystectomy.
16. Monitor for shock, hemorrhage, thrombophlebitis, and lower-extremity lymphedema after a radical cystectomy.
17. Monitor the urinary drainage pouch for leaks, and check the skin integrity.
18. Monitor the pH of the urine (do not place the dipstick into the stoma), because strong alkaline urine can cause skin irritation and facilitate crystal formation.
19. Instruct the client regarding the potential for urinary tract infection or the development of calculi.
20. Instruct the client to check the skin for irritation and to monitor the urinary drainage pouch for any leakage.
21. Encourage the client to express feelings about changes in body image and sexual function as well as embarrassment.

XXVI. ONCOLOGICAL EMERGENCIES

A. Sepsis and disseminated intravascular coagulation (DIC)
1. Description: The client with an oncological disorder is at increased risk for infection; DIC is caused by sepsis.
2. Interventions
   a. Maintain strict aseptic technique with the immunocompromised client, and monitor closely for infection.
   b. IV antibiotics may be prescribed.
   c. Anticoagulants may be prescribed during the early phase of DIC.
   d. Cryoprecipitated clotting factors may be prescribed when DIC progresses and hemorrhage is the primary problem.

⚠ Notify the HCP immediately if signs of an oncological emergency occur.

B. Syndrome of inappropriate antidiuretic hormone
1. Description
   a. Tumors can produce, secrete, or stimulate the brain to synthesize antidiuretic hormone.
   b. Mild symptoms include weakness, muscle cramps, loss of appetite, and fatigue; serum sodium levels range from 115 to 120 mEq/L.

c. More serious signs and symptoms relate to water intoxication and include weight gain, personality changes, confusion, and extreme muscle weakness.
   d. As the serum sodium level approaches 110 mEq/L, seizures, coma, and eventually death will occur unless the condition is rapidly treated.
2. Interventions
   a. Initiate fluid restriction and increased sodium intake, as prescribed.
   b. As prescribed, assist with the administration of an antagonist to antidiuretic hormone.
   c. Monitor the serum sodium levels.

C. Spinal cord compression
1. Description
   a. Occurs when a tumor directly enters the spinal cord or when the vertebral column collapses as a result of tumor entry
   b. Causes back pain, usually before neurological deficits occur
   c. Neurological deficits relate to the spinal level of compression and include numbness and tingling; the loss of urethral, vaginal, and rectal sensation; and muscle weakness.
2. Interventions
   a. Monitor for back pain and neurological deficits.
   b. Prepare the client for radiation and/or chemotherapy to reduce the size of the tumor and relieve compression.
   c. Surgery may need to be performed to remove the tumor and relieve the pressure on the spinal cord.
   d. Instruct the client regarding the use of neck or back braces, if prescribed.
   e. High doses of corticosteroids may be given to reduce the edema around the spinal cord.

D. Hypercalcemia
1. Description
   a. A late manifestation of extensive malignancy that occurs most often in clients with bone **metastasis**.
   b. Decreased physical mobility contributes to or worsens hypercalcemia.
   c. Early signs include fatigue, anorexia, nausea, vomiting, constipation, confusion, and polyuria.
   d. More serious signs and symptoms include severe muscle weakness, diminished deep tendon reflexes, paralytic ileus, dehydration, and electrocardiography changes.
2. Interventions
   a. Monitor the serum calcium level.
   b. Oral or parenteral (normal saline) fluids may be prescribed.
   c. Medications to lower the calcium level may be prescribed.

d. Prepare the client for dialysis if the condition becomes life threatening or is accompanied by renal impairment.

E. Superior vena cava (SVC) syndrome

1. Description

a. Occurs when the SVC is compressed or obstructed by tumor growth

b. Signs and symptoms result from the blockage of blood flow in the venous system of the head, neck, and upper trunk.

c. Early signs and symptoms generally occur in the morning and include edema of the face (especially around the eyes) and tightness of the shirt or blouse collar (Stokes' sign).

d. As the condition worsens, edema in the arms and hands, dyspnea, erythema of the upper body, and epistaxis (nosebleed) occur.

e. Life-threatening signs and symptoms include hemorrhage, cyanosis, mental status changes, decreased cardiac output, and hypotension.

2. Interventions

a. Monitor for signs and symptoms of SVC syndrome.

b. Prepare the client for radiation therapy to the mediastinal area.

F. Tumor lysis syndrome (TLS)

1. Description

a. Occurs when large quantities of tumor cells are destroyed rapidly and released into the bloodstream faster than the body's homeostatic mechanisms can handle them

b. TLS is a positive sign that **cancer** treatment is effective; however, if left untreated, it can cause severe tissue damage and death.

c. Hyperkalemia and hyperuricemia occur; hyperuricemia can lead to acute renal failure.

2. Interventions

a. Encourage oral hydration (at least 3 L for 3 days after treatment); IV hydration may be prescribed for the client who is experiencing nausea.

b. Instruct the client regarding the importance of fluid intake during chemotherapy.

c. Diuretics may be prescribed to increase the urine flow through the kidneys.

d. Medications that increase the excretion of purines (e.g., allopurinol [Zyloprim]) may be prescribed.

e. The IV infusion of glucose and insulin may be prescribed to treat hyperkalemia.

f. Prepare the client for dialysis if hyperkalemia and hyperuricemia persist despite treatment.

g. Provide antiemetics, as prescribed, to prevent dehydration as a result of nausea and vomiting.

MORE QUESTIONS ON EVOLVE!

Practice Questions

421. A nurse is assisting with developing a plan of care for the client with multiple myeloma. Which of the following is a priority nursing intervention for this client?
1. Encouraging fluids
2. Providing frequent oral care
3. Coughing and deep breathing
4. Monitoring the red blood cell count

422. A nurse is assisting with conducting a health-promotion program to community members regarding testicular cancer. The nurse determines that further teaching is needed if a community member states that which of the following is a sign of testicular cancer?
1. Alopecia
2. Back pain
3. Painless testicular swelling
4. A heavy sensation in the scrotum

423. A nurse is reviewing the laboratory results of a client with leukemia who has received a regimen of chemotherapy. Which laboratory value would the nurse specifically note as a result of the massive cell destruction that occurs with the chemotherapy?
1. Anemia
2. Decreased platelets
3. Increased uric acid level
4. Decreased leukocyte count

424. A client is receiving external radiation to the neck for cancer of the larynx. The nurse plans the client's care knowing that the most likely side effect to be expected is:
1. Dyspnea
2. Diarrhea
3. Sore throat
4. Constipation

425. A nurse is providing instructions to a client receiving external radiation therapy. The nurse determines that the client needs further instructions if the client states an intention to:
1. Eat a high-protein diet.
2. Avoid exposure to sunlight.
3. Wash the skin with a mild soap and pat it dry.
4. Apply pressure on the radiated area to prevent bleeding.

426. A nurse is caring for a client with an internal radiation implant. When caring for the client, the nurse should observe which principle?

1. Pregnant women are not allowed into the client's room.
2. Limit the time with the client to 1 hour per 8-hour shift.
3. Remove the dosimeter badge when entering the client's room.
4. Individuals less than 16 years old may be allowed to go in the room as long as they are 6 feet away from the client.

427. A nurse teaches skin care to the client who is receiving external radiation therapy. Which of the following statements, if made by the client, would indicate the need for further instruction?
1. "I will handle the area gently."
2. "I will wear loose-fitting clothing."
3. "I will avoid the use of deodorants."
4. "I will limit sun exposure to 1 hour daily."

428. A client is hospitalized for the insertion of an internal cervical radiation implant. While giving care, the nurse finds the radiation implant in the bed. The nurse would immediately:
1. Call the health care provider (HCP).
2. Reinsert the implant into the vagina immediately.
3. Pick up the implant with gloved hands and flush it down the toilet.
4. Pick up the implant with long-handled forceps and place into a lead container.

429. A nurse is assisting with developing a plan of care for a client who is experiencing hematological toxicity as a result of chemotherapy. The nurse suggests including which of the following in the plan of care?
1. Restricting all visitors
2. Restricting fluid intake
3. Restricting fresh fruits and vegetables in the diet
4. Inserting an indwelling urinary catheter to prevent skin breakdown

430. A nurse is reviewing the laboratory results of a client who is receiving chemotherapy and notes that the platelet count is 10,000 cells/mm^3. On the basis of this laboratory value, the priority action is to monitor which of the following?
1. Skin turgor
2. Temperature
3. Lung sounds
4. Level of consciousness

431. A client is admitted to the hospital with a diagnosis of suspected Hodgkin's disease. Which of the following findings would the nurse most likely expect to find documented in the client's record?
1. Fatigue
2. Weakness
3. Weight gain
4. Enlarged lymph nodes

432. When reviewing the health care record of a client with ovarian cancer, the nurse recognizes which symptom as being typical of the disease?
1. Diarrhea
2. Hypermenorrhea
3. Abnormal bleeding
4. Abdominal distention

433. A nurse is caring for a client after a modified radical mastectomy. Which of the following findings would indicate that the client is experiencing a complication related to the surgery?
1. Mild pain at the incisional site
2. Arm edema on the operative side
3. Sanguineous drainage in the drainage tube
4. Complaints of decreased sensation near the operative site

434. A nurse is caring for a client with cancer of the prostate after a prostatectomy. The nurse provides discharge instructions and plans to include which of the following?
1. Avoid driving the car for 1 week.
2. Restrict fluid intake to prevent incontinence.
3. Avoid lifting objects heavier than 20 pounds for at least 6 weeks.
4. Notify the health care provider if small blood clots are noticed during urination.

435. A client with carcinoma of the lung develops the syndrome of inappropriate antidiuretic hormone (SIADH) as a complication of the cancer. The nurse anticipates that which of the following may be prescribed? **Select all that apply.**
☐ 1. Radiation
☐ 2. Chemotherapy
☐ 3. Increased fluid intake
☐ 4. Serum sodium blood levels
☐ 5. Decreased oral sodium intake
☐ 6. Medication that is antagonistic to antidiuretic hormone (ADH)

ANSWERS

421. 1
Rationale: Hypercalcemia secondary to bone destruction is a priority concern in the client with multiple myeloma. The nurse should encourage fluids in adequate amounts to maintain an output of 1.5 to 2 L/day. Clients require about 3 L of fluid per day. The fluid is needed not only to dilute the calcium but also to prevent protein from precipitating in the renal tubules. Options 2, 3, and 4 may be components of the plan of care, but they are not the priorities for this client.

Test-Taking Strategy: Knowledge regarding the clinical manifestations that occur in clients with multiple myeloma is required to answer the question. Recalling that encouraging fluids is specific to the care of a client with this disorder will direct you to the correct option. Review the specific manifestations of this disorder if you had difficulty with this question.
Level of Cognitive Ability: Applying
Client Needs: Physiological Integrity
Integrated Process: Nursing Process/Planning
Content Area: Adult Health/Oncology
Reference: Christensen, Kockrow, pp. 291–292. 2011. *Adult health nursing.*

422. 1
Rationale: Alopecia is not a finding in clients with testicular cancer. However, it may occur as a result of radiation or chemotherapy. Options 2, 3, and 4 are findings in clients with testicular cancer. Back pain may indicate metastasis to the retroperitoneal lymph nodes.
Test-Taking Strategy: Note the strategic words "further teaching is needed." These words indicate a negative event query and ask you to select an option that is an incorrect sign. Use the process of elimination, and remember that alopecia occurs as a result of chemotherapy rather than of the disease. Review the manifestations associated with testicular cancer if you had difficulty with this question.
Level of Cognitive Ability: Evaluating
Client Needs: Health Promotion and Maintenance
Integrated Process: Teaching and Learning
Content Area: Adult Health/Oncology
Reference: Christensen, Kockrow, pp. 585–586. 2011. *Adult health nursing.*

423. 3
Rationale: Hyperuricemia is especially common after treatment for leukemias and lymphomas, because the therapy results in massive cell destruction. Although options 1, 2, and 4 may also be noted, an increased uric acid level is specifically related to cell destruction.
Test-Taking Strategy: Note the strategic words "specifically note" and "massive cell destruction." Recalling the cell response to destruction will assist with directing you to the correct option. Review this concept and the result of cell destruction if you had difficulty with this question.
Level of Cognitive Ability: Understanding
Client Needs: Physiological Integrity
Integrated Process: Nursing Process/Data Collection
Content Area: Adult Health/Oncology
References: Christensen, Kockrow, p. 117. *Adult health nursing.*
deWit, p. 182. 2009.
Lehne, p. 1177. 2010.

424. 3
Rationale: In general, only the area in the treatment field is affected by the radiation. Skin reactions, fatigue, nausea, and anorexia may occur with radiation to any site, whereas other side effects occur only when specific areas are involved in treatment. A client who is receiving radiation to the larynx is most likely to experience a sore throat. Options 2 and 4 may occur with radiation to the gastrointestinal (GI) tract. Dyspnea may occur with lung involvement.

Test-Taking Strategy: Use the process of elimination, and note the strategic words "most likely." Eliminate options 2 and 4 first, because they are comparable or alike, and both are GI related. Consider the anatomical location of the radiation therapy to direct you to option 3. Review the effects of radiation therapy if you had difficulty with this question.
Level of Cognitive Ability: Applying
Client Needs: Physiological Integrity
Integrated Process: Nursing Process/Planning
Content Area: Adult Health/Oncology
References: deWit, p. 304. 2009.
Lewis, Dirksen, Heitkemper, Bucher, Camera, p. 538. 2011.

425. 4
Rationale: The client should avoid pressure on the radiated area and should wear loose-fitting clothing to prevent a disruption in the skin integrity. Options 1, 2, and 3 are accurate instructions regarding radiation therapy.
Test-Taking Strategy: Use the process of elimination and note the strategic words "needs further instructions." These words indicate a negative event query and ask you to select an option that is an incorrect statement. The word "pressure" in option 4 should be an indication that this is an inappropriate measure. Review the client teaching points related to skin care and radiation therapy if you had difficulty with this question.
Level of Cognitive Ability: Evaluating
Client Needs: Physiological Integrity
Integrated Process: Teaching and Learning
Content Area: Adult Health/Oncology
Reference: Ignatavicius, Workman, p. 420. 2010.

426. 1
Rationale: The time that the nurse spends in the room of a client with an internal radiation implant is 30 minutes per 8-hour shift. The dosimeter badge must be worn when in the client's room. Children less than 16 years old and pregnant women are not allowed in the client's room.
Test-Taking Strategy: Use the process of elimination. Option 3 can be eliminated first. Knowledge of the time frame related to exposure to the client will assist you with eliminating option 2. From the remaining options, select option 1 because of the possible risks associated with exposure to the mother and fetus. Review the principles of radiation exposure if you had difficulty with this question.
Level of Cognitive Ability: Applying
Client Needs: Safe and Effective Care Environment
Integrated Process: Nursing Process/Implementation
Content Area: Adult Health/Oncology
References: Christensen, Kockrow, p. 792. 2011. *Adult health nursing.*
deWit, pp. 174–175. 2009.

427. 4
Rationale: The client needs to be instructed to avoid exposure to the sun. Options 1, 2, and 3 are accurate measures for the care of a client who is receiving external radiation therapy.
Test-Taking Strategy: Note the strategic words "need for further instruction." These words indicate a negative event query and ask you to select an option that is an incorrect statement. Eliminate option 1 because of the word "gently" and option 2 because of the word "loose." From the remaining options,

recalling that sun exposure is to be avoided will assist you with answering the question. Review skin care measures for the client who is receiving external radiation if you had difficulty with this question.
Level of Cognitive Ability: Evaluating
Client Needs: Physiological Integrity
Integrated Process: Teaching and Learning
Content Area: Adult Health/Oncology
Reference: Ignatavicius, Workman, p. 420. 2010.

428. 4
Rationale: A lead container and long-handled forceps should be kept in the client's room at all times during internal radiation therapy. If the implant becomes dislodged, the nurse should pick up the implant with long-handled forceps and place it into the lead container. Options 1, 2, and 3 are inaccurate interventions.
Test-Taking Strategy: Use the process of elimination. Note the strategic word "immediately." Option 2 is not an appropriate action. Eliminate option 3 next, because the implant would not be discarded. Although the HCP would be notified, the immediate action is option 4. Review the measures related to a dislodged implant if you had difficulty with this question.
Level of Cognitive Ability: Applying
Client Needs: Safe and Effective Care Environment
Integrated Process: Nursing Process/Implementation
Content Area: Adult Health/Oncology
Reference: deWit, p. 175. 2009.

429. 3
Rationale: In a client who is experiencing hematological toxicity, a low-bacteria diet is implemented. This includes avoiding fresh fruits and vegetables and performing a thorough cooking of all foods. Not all visitors are restricted, but the client is protected from people with known infections. Fluids should be encouraged. Invasive measures such as an indwelling urinary catheter should be avoided to prevent infections.
Test-Taking Strategy: Use the process of elimination. Eliminate option 1 because of the word "all." Next, eliminate option 2; it is not reasonable to restrict fluids for a client who is receiving chemotherapy because he or she is already at risk for fluid and electrolyte imbalances. Eliminate option 4 because of the risk of infection that exists with this measure. Review the interventions for the client with hematological toxicity if you had difficulty with this question.
Level of Cognitive Ability: Applying
Client Needs: Safe and Effective Care Environment
Integrated Process: Nursing Process/Planning
Content Area: Adult Health/Oncology
Reference: deWit, p. 181. 2009.

430. 4
Rationale: A high risk of hemorrhage exists when the platelet count is less than 20,000/mm³. Fatal central nervous system hemorrhage or massive gastrointestinal hemorrhage can occur when the platelet count is less than 10,000 cells/mm³. The client should be monitored for changes in the level of consciousness, which may be an early indication of an intracranial hemorrhage. Option 2 is a priority when the white blood cell count is low and the client is at risk for an infection. Although options 1 and 3 are important, they are not the priority in this situation.

Test-Taking Strategy: Use the process of elimination, and note the strategic word "priority." Recalling the normal platelet count and determining that a low count places the client at risk for bleeding will assist you with eliminating options 1, 2, and 3. Review the normal platelet count and the nursing interventions for a client with a low count if you had difficulty with this question.
Level of Cognitive Ability: Analyzing
Client Needs: Physiological Integrity
Integrated Process: Nursing Process/Implementation
Content Area: Adult Health/Oncology
Reference: Christensen, Kockrow, pp. 291–292. 2011. *Adult health nursing.*
deWit, pp. 181–182. 2009.

431. 4
Rationale: Hodgkin's disease is a chronic progressive neoplastic disorder of the lymphoid tissue that is characterized by the painless enlargement of the lymph nodes with progression to extralymphatic sites, such as the spleen and liver. Weight loss is most likely to be noted. Fatigue and weakness may occur, but they are not significantly related to the disease.
Test-Taking Strategy: Use the process of elimination, and note the strategic words "most likely." Option 3 can be eliminated first, because, in clients with such a disorder, weight loss is most likely to occur. Options 1 and 2 are comparable or alike and rather vague symptoms that can occur with many disorders. In addition, recalling that Hodgkin's disease affects the lymph nodes will direct you to option 4. Review the manifestations associated with Hodgkin's disease if you had difficulty with this question.
Level of Cognitive Ability: Understanding
Client Needs: Physiological Integrity
Integrated Process: Nursing Process/Data Collection
Content Area: Adult Health/Oncology
Reference: Christensen, Kockrow, pp. 293–294. 2011. *Adult health nursing.*

432. 4
Rationale: Clinical manifestations of ovarian cancer include abdominal distention, urinary frequency and urgency, pain from pressure caused by the growing tumor and the effects of urinary or bowel obstruction, and constipation. Abnormal bleeding is associated with uterine cancer and often results in hypermenorrhea.
Test-Taking Strategy: Use the process of elimination. Eliminate options 2 and 3 first, because they are comparable or alike. From the remaining options, consider the anatomical location of the diagnosis. This will assist with directing you to option 4. Review the manifestations associated with ovarian cancer if you had difficulty with this question.
Level of Cognitive Ability: Understanding
Client Needs: Physiological Integrity
Integrated Process: Nursing Process/Data Collection
Content Area: Adult Health/Oncology
Reference: Christensen, Kockrow, p. 568. 2011. *Adult health nursing.*

433. 2
Rationale: Arm edema on the operative side (lymphedema) is a complication after mastectomy that can occur immediately, months, or even years after surgery. Options 1, 3, and 4 are

expected occurrences after mastectomy and are not indicative of a complication.

Test-Taking Strategy: Use the process of elimination, and consider the normal and expected occurrences after a mastectomy. This will direct you to the correct option. Review the complications after mastectomy if you had difficulty with this question.

Level of Cognitive Ability: Analyzing
Client Needs: Physiological Integrity
Integrated Process: Nursing Process/Data Collection
Content Area: Adult Health/Oncology
Reference: Christensen, Kockrow, p. 579. 2011. *Adult health nursing.*

434. 3

Rationale: Small pieces of tissue or blood clots can be passed during urination for up to 2 weeks after surgery. Driving a car and sitting for long periods of time are restricted for at least 3 weeks. A daily fluid intake of 2 to 2.5 L/day should be maintained to limit clot formation and prevent infection. Option 3 is an accurate discharge instruction after prostatectomy.

Test-Taking Strategy: Use the process of elimination. Option 2 can easily be eliminated first. Eliminate option 1 next, because 1 week is a rather short time period. Recalling that small blood clots are expected after this type of surgery will direct you to option 3. Review the client teaching points after prostatectomy if you had difficulty with this question.

Level of Cognitive Ability: Applying
Client Needs: Physiological Integrity
Integrated Process: Teaching and Learning

Content Area: Adult Health/Oncology
Reference: deWit, p. 984. 2009.

435. 1, 2, 4, 6 ❖

Rationale: Cancer is a common cause of SIADH. In clients with SIADH, excessive amounts of water are reabsorbed by the kidney and put into the systemic circulation. The increased water causes hyponatremia (decreased serum sodium levels) and some degree of fluid retention. SIADH is managed by treating the condition and its cause, and treatment usually includes fluid restriction, increased sodium intake, and a medication with a mechanism of action that is antagonistic to ADH. Sodium levels are monitored closely, because hypernatremia can suddenly develop as a result of treatment. The immediate institution of appropriate cancer therapy (usually either radiation or chemotherapy) can cause tumor regression so that ADH synthesis and release processes return to normal.

Test-Taking Strategy: Focus on the client's diagnosis, and recall that in clients with SIADH, excessive amounts of water are reabsorbed by the kidney and put into the systemic circulation. Review the treatment for SIADH if you had difficulty with this question.

Level of Cognitive Ability: Analyzing
Client Needs: Physiological Integrity
Integrated Process: Nursing Process/Planning
Content Area: Adult Health/Oncology
References: Christensen, Kockrow, pp. 493–495. 2011. *Adult health nursing.*
deWit, pp. 338–339, 891–892. 2009.

Antineoplastic Medications

I. ANTINEOPLASTIC MEDICATIONS

A. Description
1. Antineoplastic medications kill or inhibit the reproduction of neoplastic cells.
2. Antineoplastic medications are used to cure, increase survival time, and decrease life-threatening complications.
3. The effect of antineoplastic medications may not be limited to neoplastic cells; normal cells also are affected by the medication.
4. Cell cycle phase-specific medications affect cells only during a certain phase of the reproductive cycle (Figure 44-1).
5. Cell cycle phase-nonspecific medications affect cells in any phase of the reproductive cycle (see Figure 44-1).
6. Usually, several medications are used in combination to increase the therapeutic response.
7. Antineoplastic medications may be combined with other treatments, such as surgery and radiation.
8. Although the intravenous (IV) route is most common for administration, antineoplastic medication may be given by the oral, intra-arterial, isolated limb perfusion, or intracavitary route; dosing is usually based on the client's body surface area and type of **cancer**.
9. Chemotherapy dosing is usually based on total body surface area (BSA), which requires a current, accurate height and weight for BSA calculation (before each medication administration) to ensure that the client receives optimal doses of chemotherapy medications.

⚠ Side effects from chemotherapy result from the effects of the antineoplastic medication on normal cells.

B. Side effects
1. Mucositis
2. Alopecia
3. Anorexia, nausea, and vomiting
4. Diarrhea
5. Anemia
6. Low white blood cell count (neutropenia)
7. Thrombocytopenia
8. Infertility, sexual alterations

C. General interventions
1. Physiological integrity
   a. Complete blood count (CBC), white blood cell count, platelet count, uric acid level, and electrolytes are monitored.
   b. Bleeding precautions are initiated if thrombocytopenia occurs.
   c. When the platelet count is less than 50,000 cells/mm^3, minor trauma can lead to episodes of prolonged bleeding; when less than 20,000 cells/mm^3, spontaneous and uncontrollable bleeding can occur.
   d. Monitor for petechiae, ecchymosis, bleeding of the gums, and nosebleeds because the decreased platelet count can precipitate bleeding tendencies.
   e. Intramuscular injections and venipunctures are avoided as much as possible to prevent bleeding.
   f. Neutropenic precautions are initiated if the white blood cell count decreases.
   g. Monitor for fever, sore throat, unusual bleeding, or signs and symptoms of infection.
   h. The client is informed that loss of appetite also may be the result of taste changes or a bitter taste in the mouth from the medications.
   i. Monitor for nausea and vomiting and provide a high-calorie diet with protein supplements.
   j. Antiemetics are administered several hours before chemotherapy and for 12 to 48 hours after as prescribed, because antineoplastic medications stimulate the vomiting center in the brain.
   k. Encourage hydration; IV fluids will be administered before and during therapy.
   l. Promote a fluid intake of at least 2000 mL/day to maintain adequate renal function.

⚠ Antineoplastic medication causes the rapid destruction of cells resulting in the release of uric acid. Allopurinol (Zyloprim) may be prescribed to lower the serum uric acid level.

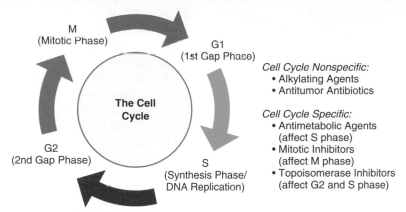

▲ **FIGURE 44-1** The cell cycle. G1, The cell is preparing for division; *S* (synthesis phase, DNA replication), the cell doubles its DNA content through DNA synthesis; *G2*, the cell produces proteins to be used in cell division and in normal physiological function after cell division is complete; and *M* (mitotic phase), the single cell splits apart into two cells.

2. Safe and effective care environment
   a. IV chemotherapy is prepared in an air-vented space (biohazard cabinet area).
   b. Gloves, gown, eye protectors, and mask are worn when handling IV medications.
   c. Nurses who are pregnant should consider avoiding chemotherapy preparation or the administration of chemotherapy.
   d. IV equipment is discarded in designated (biohazard) containers.
   e. Antineoplastic medication is administered precisely as prescribed to maximize antineoplastic effects while allowing normal cells to recover.
   f. IV administration can cause phlebitis because these medications may irritate the veins; the site needs to be monitored closely.
   g. Monitor for extravasation (leakage of medication into surrounding skin and subcutaneous tissue, which causes tissue necrosis) and notify the registered nurse if this occurs; heat or ice is applied depending on the medication, and an antidote may be injected into the site.
3. Psychosocial integrity
   a. The client is instructed about the possibility of hair loss and that varying degrees of hair loss may occur after the first or second treatment.
   b. Discuss the purchase of a wig before treatment starts.
   c. The client is informed that new hair growth will occur several months after the final treatment.
   d. The client is instructed about the need for contraception because these medications have teratogenic effects.
   e. The potential effect of infertility is discussed, which may be irreversible.
   f. Encourage pretreatment counseling.

4. Health promotion and maintenance
   a. The client is instructed that if diarrhea is a problem to avoid hot foods and high-fiber foods, which increase peristalsis.
   b. The client is instructed to inspect the oral mucosa frequently for erythema and ulcers, rinse the mouth after meals, and carry out good oral hygiene.
   c. The client is instructed to use mouth rinses as prescribed for mouth sores if necessary.
   d. The client is instructed in the use of antifungal agents for mouth sores, if prescribed, for the development of a fungal infection.
   e. The client is instructed to avoid crowds and persons with infections and to report signs of infection such as a low-grade fever, chills, or sore throat.
   f. Individuals with colds or infections are instructed to wear a mask when visiting or to avoid visiting the client.
   g. The client is instructed to use a soft toothbrush and electric razor to minimize the risk of bleeding.
   h. The client is instructed to avoid aspirin-containing products to minimize the risk of bleeding.
   i. The client is instructed to consult the health care provider (HCP) before receiving vaccinations (live vaccines should not be administered).
D. Anaphylactic reactions
   1. Precautions
      a. Obtain an allergy history.
      b. A test dose is administered when prescribed by the HCP.
      c. Stay with the client during the administration of medication.
      d. Monitor vital signs.
      e. Have emergency equipment and medications readily available.

f. An IV line is initiated for the administration of emergency medications if needed.

2. Signs of an anaphylactic reaction
   a. Dyspnea
   b. Chest tightness or pain
   c. Pruritis or urticaria
   d. Tachycardia
   e. Dizziness
   f. Anxiety or agitation
   g. Flushed appearance
   h. Hypotension
   i. Decreased sensorium
   j. Cyanosis
3. Interventions for an anaphylactic reaction (see Priority Nursing Actions)

■■■■■PRIORITY NURSING ACTIONS!■■■■■

Actions Taken if an Anaphylactic Reaction Occurs from Medication

1. Respiratory status is assessed.
2. The medication is stopped.
3. The HCP is contacted; the Rapid Response Team is also contacted if necessary.
4. Oxygen is administered.
5. The IV access is maintained with normal saline.
6. The client's feet and legs are raised, if not contraindicated.
7. Prescribed emergency medications are administered.
8. Vital signs are monitored.
9. The event, actions taken, and the client's response are documented.

If anaphylaxis occurs from a medication, the nurse immediately assesses the client's respiratory status. The medication is also immediately stopped. If the client's airway needs to be established or stabilized, the Rapid Response Team is called. Additionally, the HCP is contacted. The IV line is not removed because IV access is needed to administer emergency medications such as diphenhydramine (Benadryl) or epinephrine. The client is positioned appropriately. The legs and feet are elevated. The head of the bed is elevated to improve ventilation; elevate the head of the bed 10 degrees if hypotension is present and 45 degrees or higher if the blood pressure is normal. The nurse stays with the client and monitors the client's status, including the vital signs. The nurse documents the event, actions taken, and the client's response.

Reference: Ignatavicius, D., & Workman, M. (2010). *Medical-surgical nursing: Patient-centered collaborative care* (6th ed., p. 392). St. Louis: Saunders.

II. ALKYLATING MEDICATIONS (Box 44-1)

A. Description
1. Breaks DNA helix, thereby interfering with DNA replication
2. Cell cycle phase-nonspecific medications

B. Side effects
1. Anorexia, nausea, and vomiting may occur.
2. Stomatitis may occur.
3. Rash may occur.
4. Client may feel IV site pain during IV administration.
5. Busulfan (Myleran, Busulfex) may cause hyperuricemia.
6. Chlorambucil (Leukeran) and mechlorethamine (Mustargen) may cause gonadal suppression and hyperuricemia.
7. Cisplatin (Platinol-AQ), a platinum compound, may cause ototoxicity, tinnitus, hypokalemia, hypocalcemia, hypomagnesemia, and nephrotoxicity.
8. Cyclophosphamide (Neosar) may cause alopecia, gonadal suppression, hemorrhagic cystitis, and hematuria.

C. Interventions: Refer to General Interventions section under Antineoplastic Medications.
1. Medication is withheld if the platelet count is lower than 75,000 cells/mm^3 or the white blood cell count is lower than 2000 cells/mm^3, and the HCP is notified. (This may vary depending on the medication and agency policy.)
2. Monitor results of pulmonary function tests.
3. Monitor results of chest radiography and renal and liver function studies.
4. The client is hydrated with IV and/or oral fluids before administering the antineoplastic medication as prescribed.
5. As prescribed, IV site pain is reduced by altering IV rates or warming the injection site to distend vein and increase blood flow.

Box 44-1 Alkylating Medications

Nitrogen Mustards
Bendamustine (Treanda)
Chlorambucil (Leukeran)
Cyclophosphamide (Neosar)
Ifosfamide (Ifex)
Mechlorethamine (Mustargen)
Melphalan (Alkeran)

Nitrosoureas
Carmustine (BiCNU, Gliadel)
Lomustine (CeeNu)
Streptozocin (Zanosar)

Alkylating-Like Medications
Altretamine (Hexalen)
Busulfan (Myleran, Busulfex)
Carboplatin (Paraplatin)
Cisplatin (Platinol-AQ)
Dacarbazine (DTIC-Dome)
Oxaliplatin (Eloxatin)
Temozolomide (Temodar)
Thiotepa (Thioplex)

6. When administering cisplatin the client is monitored for dizziness, tinnitus, hearing loss, incoordination, and numbness or tingling of extremities.
7. Mesna (Mesnex) may be administered with ifosfamide to reduce the potential of ifosfamide-induced cystitis.
8. The client is instructed that cyclophosphamide, when prescribed orally, is administered without food.
9. The client is instructed to follow a diet low in purines to alkalinize the urine and lower uric acid blood levels.
10. The client is instructed in how to avoid infection.
11. The client is instructed to report signs of infection or bleeding.
12. The client is instructed about good oral hygiene and use of a soft toothbrush.

 Cyclophosphamide (Neosar) and ifosfamide (Ifex) are medications that can cause hemorrhagic cystitis. The client is encouraged to drink increased fluids (2 to 3 L per day) during therapy, unless contraindicated.

III. ANTITUMOR ANTIBIOTIC MEDICATIONS (Box 44-2)

A. Description
1. Interfere with DNA and RNA synthesis
2. Cell cycle phase-nonspecific medications

B. Side effects
1. Nausea and vomiting
2. Fever
3. Bone marrow depression
4. Rash
5. Alopecia
6. Stomatitis
7. Gonadal suppression
8. Hyperuricemia
9. Vesication (blistering of tissue at IV site)
10. Daunorubicin (DaunoXome) may cause congestive heart failure and dysrhythmias.
11. Doxorubicin (Adriamycin, Doxil) and idarubicin (Idamycin) may cause cardiotoxicity, cardiomyopathy, and electrocardiographic changes

Box 44-2 Antitumor Antibiotic Medications

Bleomycin sulfate
Dactinomycin (Cosmegen)
Daunorubicin (DaunoXome)
Doxorubicin (Adriamycin, Doxil)
Epirubicin (Ellence)
Idarubicin (Idamycin)
Mitomycin (Mutamycin)
Mitoxantrone (Novantrone)

(Dexrazoxane [Zinecard] may be administered with doxorubicin to reduce cardiomyopathy).
12. Pulmonary toxicity can occur with bleomycin.

C. Interventions: Refer to General Interventions section under Antineoplastic Medications.
1. Medication is withheld if the platelets are lower than 75,000 cells/mm^3 or the white blood cell count is lower than 2000 cells/mm^3, and the health care provider is notified. (This may vary depending on the medication and agency policy.)
2. Monitor results of pulmonary function tests.
3. Monitor for electrocardiographic changes.
4. Monitor lung sounds for crackles.
5. Monitor for signs of congestive heart failure, including dyspnea, crackles, peripheral edema, and weight gain.
6. Monitor results of chest radiography and renal and liver function studies.
7. The client is hydrated with IV and/or oral fluids before administration of antineoplastic medication.
8. As prescribed, IV site pain is reduced by altering IV rates or warming injection site to distend vein and increase blood flow.
9. Monitor IV site for irritation, phlebitis, and vesication; site is changed as needed.
10. Monitor for myocardial toxicity, dyspnea, dysrhythmias, hypotension, and weight gain when daunorubicin, doxorubicin, or idarubicin are administered.
11. Monitor pulmonary status when bleomycin is administered.

IV. ANTIMETABOLITE MEDICATIONS (Box 44-3)

A. Description
1. Antimetabolite medications halt the synthesis of cell protein; their presence impairs cell division.
2. Antimetabolite medications are cell cycle phase-specific and affect the S phase.

Box 44-3 Antimetabolite Medications

Capecitabine (Xeloda)
Cladribine (Leustatin)
Clofarabine (Clolar)
Cytarabine (Cytosar-U, DepoCyt, Tarabine PFS)
Floxuridine (FUDR)
Fludarabine (Fludara)
Fluorouracil (Adrucil)
Gemcitabine (Gemzar)
Hydroxyurea (Hydrea, Mylocel)
Mercaptopurine (Purinethol)
Methotrexate (Rheumatrex, Trexall)
Pemetrexed (Alimta)
Pentostatin (Nipent)
Thioguanine (Tabloid)

B. Side effects
1. Anorexia, nausea, and vomiting
2. Diarrhea
3. Alopecia
4. Stomatitis
5. Depression of bone marrow
6. Cytarabine (Cytosar-U, DepoCyt, Tarabine PFS) may cause alopecia, stomatitis, hyperuricemia, and hepatotoxicity.
7. Fluorouracil (Adrucil) may cause alopecia, stomatitis, diarrhea, phototoxicity reactions, and cerebellar dysfunction.
8. Mercaptopurine (Purinethol) may cause hyperuricemia and hepatotoxicity.
9. Methotrexate (Rheumatrex, Trexall) may cause alopecia, stomatitis, hyperuricemia, photosensitivity, hepatotoxicity, and hematological, gastrointestinal, and skin toxicity.

C. Interventions: Refer to General Interventions section under Antineoplastic Medications
1. Medication is withheld if the white blood cell count is lower than 2000 cells/mm^3 or the platelet count is lower than 75,000 cells/mm^3, and the HCP is notified. (This may vary depending on the medication and agency policy.)
2. Monitor renal function studies.
3. Monitor for cerebellar dysfunction.
4. Monitor for photosensitivity.
5. Monitor IV site for extravasation.
6. Fluid intake of 2 to 3 L/day is encouraged.
7. Good oral hygiene is encouraged.
8. The client is instructed in how to avoid infections and bleeding.
9. When fluorouracil is administered, monitor for signs of cerebellar dysfunction, such as dizziness, weakness, and ataxia, and monitor for stomatitis and diarrhea, which may necessitate medication discontinuation.
10. When fluorouracil or methotrexate are administered, the client is instructed to use sunscreen and wear protective clothing to prevent photosensitivity reactions.

⚠ When methotrexate is administered in large doses, leucovorin (folinic acid or citrovorum factor) may be administered as prescribed to prevent toxicity. This is known as leucovorin rescue.

V. ANTIMITOTIC MEDICATIONS (VINCA ALKALOIDS) (Box 44-4)

A. Description
1. Mitotic inhibitors prevent mitosis, causing cell death; mitotic inhibitors prevent cell division.
2. Mitotic inhibitors are cell cycle phase-specific and act on the M phase.

B. Side effects
1. Leukopenia
2. Neurotoxicity with vincristine (Oncovin, Vincasar) manifested as numbness and tingling in the fingers and toes, constipation, paralytic ileus.
3. Ptosis
4. Hoarseness
5. Motor instability
6. Anorexia, nausea, and vomiting
7. Peripheral neuropathy
8. Alopecia
9. Stomatitis
10. Hyperuricemia
11. Phlebitis at IV site

C. Interventions: Refer to the General Interventions section under Antineoplastic Medications.
1. Monitor for hoarseness.
2. Monitor eyes for ptosis.
3. Monitor motor stability and initiate safety precautions as necessary.
4. Monitor for neurotoxicity with vincristine sulfate manifested as numbness and tingling in the fingers and toes.
5. Monitor for constipation and paralytic ileus.

VI. TOPOISOMERASE INHIBITORS (Box 44-5)

A. Description
1. Block the enzyme needed for DNA synthesis and cell division.
2. Cell cycle phase-specific; act on the G2 and S phases

B. Side effects
1. Leukopenia, thrombocytopenia, anemia
2. Anorexia, nausea, and vomiting
3. Diarrhea
4. Alopecia

Box 44-4 Mitotic Inhibitors

Vinca Alkaloids
Vinblastine sulfate (Velban)
Vincristine sulfate (Oncovin, Vincasar)
Vinorelbine (Navelbine)

Taxanes
Docetaxel (Taxotere)
Paclitaxel (Abraxane, Taxol, Onxol)

Box 44-5 Topoisomerase Inhibitors

Etoposide (VePesid, Toposar, Etopophos)
Irinotecan (Camptosar)
Teniposide (Vumon)
Topotecan (Hycamtin)

5. Orthostatic hypotension
6. Hypersensitivity reaction

C. Interventions: Refer to General Interventions section under Antineoplastic Medications.

VII. HORMONAL MEDICATIONS AND ENZYMES
(Box 44-6)

A. Description
1. Suppress the immune system and block normal hormones in hormone-sensitive tumors.
2. Change the hormonal balance and slow the growth rates of certain tumors.

B. Side effects
1. Anorexia, nausea, and vomiting
2. Leukopenia
3. Impaired pancreatic function with asparaginase (Elspar)
4. Sex characteristic alterations
   a. Masculinizing effect in women: Chest and facial hair, menses stops (androgens, antiestrogen receptor drugs)
   b. Feminine manifestations in men: Gynecomastia (estrogens, progestins, antiestrogen receptors)
5. Breast swelling
6. Hot flashes
7. Weight gain

Box 44-6 Hormonal Medications and Enzymes

Estrogens
Diethylstilbestrol
Estramustine (Emcyt)
Ethinyl estradiol (Estinyl)

Antiestrogens
Anastrozole (Arimidex)
Exemestane (Aromasin)
Fulvestrant (Faslodex)
Letrozole (Femara)
Raloxifene (Evista)
Tamoxifen citrate
Toremifene (Fareston)

Antiandrogens
Bicalutamide (Casodex)
Flutamide (Eulexin)
Goserelin acetate (Zoladex)
Nilutamide (Nilandron)
Triptorelin (Trelstar)

Progestins
Medroxyprogesterone (Depo-Provera)
Megestrol acetate (Megace)

Other Hormonal Antagonists and Enzymes
Asparaginase (Elspar)
Leuprolide acetate (Lupron)
Mitotane (Lysodren)

---

8. Hemorrhagic cystitis, hypouricemia, and hyperlipidemia, with mitotane (Lysodren)
9. Hypertension
10. Thromboembolic disorders
11. Edema
12. Electrolyte imbalances
13. Tamoxifen citrate may cause edema, hypercalcemia, and elevated cholesterol and triglyceride levels.
14. Tamoxifen citrate decreases the effects of estrogen.
15. Diethylstilbestrol may cause impotence and gynecomastia in men.
16. Diethylstilbestrol may alter effects of insulin, orally administered anticoagulants, and orally administered hypoglycemic agents.

C. Interventions
1. Monitor vital signs.
2. Assess medications that the client is currently taking.
3. Monitor serum calcium levels with androgens.
4. Monitor for signs of alterations in sexual characteristics.
5. Monitor pancreatic function with asparaginase.
6. Encourage oral intake of 2 to 3 L of fluids per day.
7. Monitor uric acid and cholesterol levels.
8. Monitor for signs of hemorrhagic cystitis.

VIII. IMMUNOMODULATOR AGENTS: BIOLOGICAL RESPONSE MODIFIERS (Box 44-7)

A. Description
1. Immunomodulators stimulate the immune system to recognize **cancer** cells and take action to eliminate or destroy them.
2. Interleukins help different immune system cells recognize and destroy abnormal body cells.
3. Interferons slow down tumor cell division, stimulate proliferation, and cause **cancer** cells to differentiate into nonproliferative forms.

B. Colony-stimulating factors induce more rapid bone marrow recovery after suppression by chemotherapy (Box 44-8).

Box 44-7 Immunomodulator Agents

Aldesleukin (Proleukin, interleukin-2)
Interferon alfa-2a
Interferon alfa-2b
Interferon alfa-n3 (Alferon N)
Recombinant interferon alfa 2a (Intron A)
Recombinant interferon alfa-2b (Roferon-A)

Common Monoclonal Antibodies
Alemtuzumab (Campath)
Gemtuzumab ozogamicin (Mylotarg)
Ibritumomab (Zevalin)
Rituximab (Rituxan)
Trastuzumab (Herceptin)

Box 44-8 Colony-Stimulating Factors

Granulocyte-Macrophage Colony-Stimulating Factor
Sargramostim (Leukine)

Granulocyte Colony-Stimulating Factor
Filgrastim (Neupogen)
Pegfilgrastim (Neulasta)

Erythropoietin
Epoetin alfa (Epogen)
Darbepoetin alfa (Aranesp)
Thrombopoietic Growth Factor
Oprelvekin (Interleukin-11)

Box 44-9 Other Antineoplastic Medications

Asparaginase (Elspar)
Arsenic trioxide (Trisenox)
Bexarotene (Targretin)
Bortezomib (Velcade)
Imatinib (Gleevec)
Temozolomide (Temodar)

MORE QUESTIONS ON EVOLVE!

Practice Questions

IX. TARGETED THERAPY

A. Description
1. Medications used as targeted therapies are monoclonal antibodies that target a cellular element of the **cancer** cell or antisense medications that work at the gene level.
2. Some examples of monoclonal antibodies are rituximab (Rituxan), tositumomab (Bexxar), trastuzumab (Herceptin), alemtuzumab (Campath), and cetuximab (Erbitux).
B. Side effects: Allergic reactions (monoclonal antibodies)

X. OTHER ANTINEOPLASTIC MEDICATIONS
(Box 44-9)

A. Altretamine (Hexalen): Cytotoxic agent used to treat ovarian **cancer**
B. Denileukin diftitox (Ontak): Recombinant DNA-derived medication used to treat cutaneous T-cell **lymphoma**
C. Gemcitabine (Gemzar): Used to treat non–small cell lung **cancer** and **adenocarcinoma** of the pancreas and metastatic breast **cancer**, and lung **cancer** (in combination with paclitaxel [Abraxane, Taxol, Onxol]).
D. Irinotecan (Camptosar): Used to treat colorectal or rectal **cancer**
E. Paclitaxel (Abraxane, Taxol, Onxol): Used to treat ovarian or metastatic breast **cancer**
F. Pegaspargase (Oncaspar): Used in combination chemotherapies for acute lymphoblastic **leukemia** in clients unable to take asparaginase (Elspar)
G. Topotecan (Hycamtin): Indicated for the treatment of relapsed or refractory metastatic ovarian **cancer** after other therapies have failed
H. Trastuzumab (Herceptin): Used in combination chemotherapy to treat breast **cancer**
I. Bexarotene (Targretin): Use to treat advanced stage cutaneous T-cell **lymphoma**

436. A nurse is caring for a client who is receiving an intravenous (IV) infusion of an antineoplastic medication. During the infusion, the client complains of pain at the insertion site. During an inspection of the site, the nurse notes redness and swelling and that the rate of infusion of the medication has slowed. The nurse should take which appropriate action?
1. Notify the registered nurse.
2. Administer pain medication to reduce the discomfort.
3. Apply ice and maintain the infusion rate, as prescribed.
4. Elevate the extremity of the IV site, and slow the infusion.

437. The client with squamous cell carcinoma of the larynx is receiving bleomycin intravenously. The nurse caring for the client anticipates that which diagnostic study will be prescribed?
1. Echocardiography
2. Electrocardiography
3. Cervical radiography
4. Pulmonary function studies

438. The client with acute myelocytic leukemia is being treated with busulfan (Myleran). Which laboratory value would the nurse specifically monitor during treatment with this medication?
1. Clotting time
2. Uric acid level
3. Potassium level
4. Blood glucose level

439. The client with small cell lung cancer is being treated with etoposide (VePesid). The nurse who is assisting in caring for the client during its administration understands that which side effect is specifically associated with this medication?
1. Alopecia
2. Chest pain
3. Pulmonary fibrosis
4. Orthostatic hypotension

440. The clinic nurse is reviewing a teaching plan for the client receiving an antineoplastic medication. When implementing the plan, the nurse tells the client:
1. To take aspirin (acetylsalicylic acid) as needed for headache
2. Drink beverages containing alcohol in moderate amounts each evening
3. Consult with health care providers (HCPs) before receiving immunizations
4. That it is not necessary to consult HCPs before receiving a flu vaccine at the local health fair

441. The client with ovarian cancer is being treated with vincristine (Oncovin). The nurse monitors the client, knowing that which of the following indicates a side effect specific to this medication?
1. Diarrhea
2. Hair loss
3. Chest pain
4. Numbness and tingling in the fingers and toes

442. The nurse is reviewing the history and physical examination of a client who will be receiving asparaginase (Elspar), an antineoplastic agent. The nurse consults with the registered nurse regarding the administration of the medication if which of the following is documented in the client's history?
1. Pancreatitis
2. Diabetes mellitus
3. Myocardial infarction
4. Chronic obstructive pulmonary disease

443. Tamoxifen is prescribed for the client with metastatic breast carcinoma. The nurse understands that the primary action of this medication is to:
1. Increase DNA and RNA synthesis.
2. Promote the biosynthesis of nucleic acids.
3. Increase estrogen concentration and estrogen response.
4. Compete with estradiol for binding to estrogen in tissues containing high concentrations of receptors.

444. The client with metastatic breast cancer is receiving tamoxifen. The nurse specifically monitors which laboratory value while the client is taking this medication?
1. Glucose level
2. Calcium level
3. Potassium level
4. Prothrombin time

445. A nurse is assisting with caring for a client with cancer who is receiving cisplatin. Select the adverse effects that the nurse monitors for that are associated with this medication. **Select all that apply**.
☐ 1. Tinnitus
☐ 2. Ototoxicity
☐ 3. Hyperkalemia
☐ 4. Hypercalcemia
☐ 5. Nephrotoxicity
☐ 6. Hypomagnesemia

ANSWERS

436. 1
Rationale: When antineoplastic medications are administered via IV, great care must be taken to prevent the medication from escaping into the tissues surrounding the injection site, because pain, tissue damage, and necrosis can result. The nurse monitors for signs of extravasation, such as redness or swelling at the insertion site and a decreased infusion rate. If extravasation occurs, the registered nurse needs to be notified; he or she will then contact the health care provider.
Test-Taking Strategy: Use the process of elimination, and focus on the data in the question. Eliminate options 3 and 4 first. The nurse would not slow the IV rate, and the nurse would not be able to maintain the prescribed rate in this situation. Administering pain medication to reduce discomfort at an IV site is not an appropriate action. Further investigation of the cause of the discomfort is required. This leaves option 1 as the correct nursing action. Review the care of the client who is receiving IV chemotherapy if you had difficulty with this question.
Level of Cognitive Ability: Applying
Client Needs: Physiological Integrity
Integrated Process: Nursing Process/Implementation

Content Area: Pharmacology
Reference: Lewis, Dirksen, Heitkemper, Bucher, Camera, pp. 275–276. 2011.

437. 4
Rationale: Bleomycin is an antineoplastic medication that can cause interstitial pneumonitis, which can progress to pulmonary fibrosis. Pulmonary function studies along with hematological, hepatic, and renal function tests need to be monitored. The nurse needs to monitor lung sounds for dyspnea and crackles, which indicate pulmonary toxicity. The medication needs to be discontinued immediately if pulmonary toxicity occurs. Options 1, 2, and 3 are unrelated to the specific use of this medication.
Test-Taking Strategy: Use the process of elimination. Eliminate options 1 and 2 first because they are cardiac-related and are therefore comparable or alike. From the remaining options, use the ABCs—airway, breathing, and circulation—to direct you to option 4. If you had difficulty with this question, review the toxic effects of this medication.
Level of Cognitive Ability: Analyzing
Client Needs: Physiological Integrity
Integrated Process: Nursing Process/Planning

Content Area: Pharmacology
References: Gahart, Nazareno, pp. 204–206. 2011.
Hodgson, Kizior, p. 139. 2011.

438. 2

Rationale: Busulfan (Myleran) can cause an increase in the uric acid level. Hyperuricemia can produce uric acid nephropathy, renal stones, and acute renal failure. Options 1, 3, and 4 are not specifically related to this medication.
Test-Taking Strategy: Focus on the medication addressed in the question. It is necessary to know the adverse effects associated with this medication. Recalling that busulfan increases the uric acid level will direct you to the correct option. If you had difficulty with this question, review the effects of busulfan.
Level of Cognitive Ability: Analyzing
Client Needs: Physiological Integrity
Integrated Process: Nursing Process/Data Collection
Content Area: Pharmacology
References: Edmunds, p. 390. 2010.
Hodgson, Kizior, p. 34. 2011.

439. 4

Rationale: A side effect specific to etoposide is orthostatic hypotension. The client's blood pressure is monitored during the infusion. Hair loss occurs with nearly all the antineoplastic medications. Chest pain and pulmonary fibrosis are unrelated to this medication.
Test-Taking Strategy: Use the process of elimination. Eliminate option 1 first because this side effect is associated with many of the antineoplastic agents. Eliminate options 2 and 3 next because they are unrelated to etoposide. Note that the question asks for the side effect *specific* to this medication. Correlate hypotension with etoposide. Review the side effects of this medication if you had difficulty with this question.
Level of Cognitive Ability: Analyzing
Client Needs: Physiological Integrity
Integrated Process: Nursing Process/Data Collection
Content Area: Pharmacology
Reference: Gahart, Nazareno, p. 566. 2010.

440. 3

Rationale: Because antineoplastic medications lower the resistance of the body, clients must be informed not to receive immunizations without a HCP's approval. Clients also need to avoid contact with individuals who have recently received a live virus vaccine. Clients need to avoid aspirin and aspirin-containing products to minimize the risk of bleeding, and they need to avoid alcohol to minimize the risk of toxicity and side effects.
Test-Taking Strategy: Think about the adverse effects of antineoplastic medications. Recalling that antineoplastic medications lower the resistance of the body will direct you to the correct option. Review the client teaching points regarding these medications if you had difficulty with this question.
Level of Cognitive Ability: Applying
Client Needs: Physiological Integrity
Integrated Process: Teaching and Learning
Content Area: Pharmacology
Reference: Kee, Hayes, McCuistion, p. 541. 2009.
Edmunds, p. 206. 2010.

441. 4

Rationale: A side effect specific to vincristine is peripheral neuropathy, which occurs in almost every client. Peripheral neuropathy can be manifested as numbness and tingling in the fingers and toes. Depression of the Achilles tendon reflex may be the first clinical sign indicating peripheral neuropathy. Constipation rather than diarrhea is most likely to occur with this medication, although diarrhea may occur occasionally. Hair loss occurs with nearly all the antineoplastic medications. Chest pain is unrelated to this medication.
Test-Taking Strategy: Use the process of elimination. Eliminate options 1 and 2 first because these side effects are associated with many of the antineoplastic agents. Note that the question asks for the side effect "specific" to this medication. Correlate peripheral neuropathy with vincristine. Review the side effects of this medication if you had difficulty with this question.
Level of Cognitive Ability: Analyzing
Client Needs: Physiological Integrity
Integrated Process: Nursing Process/Data Collection
Content Area: Pharmacology
Reference: Lehne, p. 1193. 2010.

442. 1

Rationale: Asparaginase (Elspar) is contraindicated if hypersensitivity exists, in pancreatitis, or if the client has a history of pancreatitis. The medication impairs pancreatic function and pancreatic function tests should be performed before therapy begins and when a week or more has elapsed between administration of the doses. The client needs to be monitored for signs of pancreatitis, which include nausea, vomiting, and abdominal pain. The conditions noted in options 2, 3, and 4 are not contraindicated with this medication.
Test-Taking Strategy: Focus on the medication addressed in the question. It is necessary to know the contraindications associated with this medication. Recalling that this medication affects pancreatic function will direct you to the correct option. Review this medication if you had difficulty answering this question.
Level of Cognitive Ability: Analyzing
Client Needs: Physiological Integrity
Integrated Process: Nursing Process/Data Collection
Content Area: Pharmacology
References: Hodgson, Kizior, pp. 85–87. 2011.
Lehne, p. 1195. 2010.

443. 4

Rationale: Tamoxifen is an antineoplastic medication that competes with estradiol for binding to estrogen in tissues containing high concentrations of receptors. Tamoxifen is used to treat metastatic breast carcinoma in women and men. Tamoxifen is also effective in delaying the recurrence of cancer following mastectomy. Tamoxifen reduces DNA synthesis and estrogen response.
Test-Taking Strategy: Use the process of elimination. Eliminate options 1 and 2 first because they are comparable or alike. Nucleic acids include DNA and RNA. From this point, select option 4, because it is unlikely that treatment of metastatic breast carcinoma would focus on increasing estrogen concentration and estrogen response. If you had difficulty with this question, review the action of this medication.

Level of Cognitive Ability: Understanding
Client Needs: Physiological Integrity
Integrated Process: Nursing Process/Implementation
Content Area: Pharmacology
Reference: Lehne, pp. 1201–1202. 2010.

444. 2

Rationale: Tamoxifen may increase calcium, cholesterol, and triglyceride levels. Before the initiation of therapy, a complete blood count, platelet count, and serum calcium levels should be assessed. These blood levels, along with cholesterol and triglyceride levels, should be monitored periodically during therapy. The nurse should assess for hypercalcemia while the client is taking this medication. Signs of hypercalcemia include increased urine volume, excessive thirst, nausea, vomiting, constipation, hypotonicity of muscles, and deep bone and flank pain.

Test-Taking Strategy: Focus on the medication addressed in the question. It is necessary to know the adverse effects associated with this medication. Recalling that this medication causes hypercalcemia will direct you to the correct option. Review this medication if you had difficulty answering this question.

Level of Cognitive Ability: Analyzing
Client Needs: Physiological Integrity

Integrated Process: Nursing Process/Data Collection
Content Area: Pharmacology
Reference: Lehne, pp. 1201–1202. 2010.

445. 1, 2, 5, 6

Rationale: Cisplatin is an alkylating medication. Alkylating medications are cell cycle phase–nonspecific medications that affect the synthesis of DNA by causing the cross-linking of DNA to inhibit cell reproduction. Cisplatin may cause ototoxicity, tinnitus, hypokalemia, hypocalcemia, hypomagnesemia, and nephrotoxicity. Amifostine (Ethyol) may be administered before cisplatin to reduce the potential for renal toxicity.

Test-Taking Strategy: Note that cisplatin is an antineoplastic medication. Recall that most antineoplastic medications affect the bone marrow and the hematological system. This concept will assist you with determining that "hypo-" rather than "hyper-" conditions would occur. In addition, recall that this medication affects the ears (ototoxicity and tinnitus) and the kidneys (nephrotoxicity). Review the toxic effects of cisplatin if you had difficulty with this question.

Level of Cognitive Ability: Analyzing
Client Needs: Physiological Integrity
Integrated Process: Nursing Process/Data Collection
Content Area: Pharmacology
Reference: Hodgson, Kizior, pp. 243–245. 2011.

The Adult Client with an Endocrine Disorder

PYRAMID TERMS

addisonian crisis A life-threatening disorder caused by adrenal hormone insufficiency. It is precipitated by infection, trauma, stress, or surgery. Death can occur from shock, vascular collapse, or hyperkalemia.

Addison's disease The hyposecretion of adrenal cortex hormones (glucocorticoids and mineralocorticoids) from the adrenal gland that results in a deficiency of the steroid hormones. The condition is fatal if left untreated.

adrenalectomy The surgical removal of an adrenal gland. The lifelong replacement of glucocorticoids and mineralocorticoids is necessary with a bilateral adrenalectomy. Temporary replacement may be necessary for up to 2 years for a unilateral adrenalectomy.

Chvostek's sign A spasm of the facial muscles elicited by tapping the facial nerve just anterior to the ear. It is noted in clients with hypocalcemia.

Cushing's syndrome and Cushing's disease A condition that results from the hypersecretion of glucocorticoids from the adrenal cortex.

dawn phenomenon A condition that results from a nocturnal release of growth hormone, which may cause blood glucose level elevations before breakfast. Treatment includes administering an evening dose of intermediate-acting insulin at 10:00 PM.

diabetes insipidus The hyposecretion of antidiuretic hormone from the posterior pituitary gland, which results in the failure of the tubular reabsorption of water in the kidneys and profuse, dilute urine loss.

diabetes mellitus A chronic disorder of glucose intolerance and impaired carbohydrate, protein, and lipid metabolism caused by a deficiency of insulin or resistance to the action of insulin. A deficiency of effective insulin results in hyperglycemia.

diabetic ketoacidosis A life-threatening complication of diabetes mellitus that develops when a severe insulin deficiency occurs. Hyperglycemia progresses to ketoacidosis over a period of several hours to several days. It occurs in clients with type 1 diabetes mellitus, individuals with undiagnosed diabetes, and persons who stop taking the prescribed treatment for diabetes.

hyperglycemia An elevated blood glucose level.

hyperglycemic hyperosmolar nonketotic syndrome Extreme hyperglycemia without acidosis. It is a complication of type 2 diabetes mellitus, which may result in dehydration or vascular collapse. The onset is usually slow, taking from hours to days.

hyperthyroidism A condition that occurs as a result of excessive thyroid hormone secretion.

hypoglycemia A low blood glucose level (<60 mg/dL) that results from too much insulin, not enough food, or excess activity.

hypophysectomy The removal of the pituitary gland.

myxedema (hypothyroidism) A hypothyroid state that results from the hyposecretion of thyroid hormone. The condition occurs during adulthood.

myxedema coma A rare but serious disorder that results from the persistently low production of thyroid hormones. It can be precipitated by acute illness, the rapid withdrawal of thyroid medication, anesthesia, surgery, hypothermia, and the use of sedatives and opioids.

Somogyi phenomenon A rebound phenomenon that occurs in clients with type 1 diabetes mellitus. Normal or elevated blood glucose levels are present at bedtime, and hypoglycemia occurs at about 2:00 AM to 3:00 AM. Counterregulatory hormones, which are produced to prevent further hypoglycemia, result in hyperglycemia; this is evident in the prebreakfast blood glucose level. Treatment includes decreasing the evening (predinner or bedtime) dose of intermediate-acting insulin or increasing the bedtime snack.

Syndrome of inappropriate antidiuretic hormone (SIADH) In this condition excess antidiuretic hormone is released, but not in response to a bodily need for it. The syndrome results in water intoxication and hyponatremia.

thyroid storm An acute, potentially fatal exacerbation of hyperthyroidism. It may result from the manipulation of the thyroid gland during surgery, severe infection, or stress.

thyroidectomy The surgical removal of the thyroid gland to treat persistent hyperthyroidism or thyroid tumors.

Trousseau's sign A sign of hypocalcemia. Carpal spasm can be elicited by compressing the brachial artery with a blood pressure cuff for 3 minutes.

 PYRAMID TO SUCCESS

The endocrine system is made up of organs or glands that secrete hormones and release them directly into the circulation. The endocrine system can be easily understood if you remember that basically one of two situations can occur: either the hypersecretion or the hyposecretion of hormones from the organ or gland. When an excess of the hormone occurs, treatment is aimed at blocking the hormone release through medication or surgery. When a deficit of the hormone exists, treatment is aimed at replacement therapy. The pyramid points focus on diabetes mellitus, including the prevention and treatment of complications, insulin therapy, hypoglycemic and hyperglycemic reactions, and diabetic ketoacidosis; Addison's disease and addisonian crisis; Cushing's syndrome; thyroid disorders and thyroid storm; and care of the client after thyroidectomy or adrenalectomy.

 CLIENT NEEDS

Safe and Effective Care Environment

- Acting as a client advocate
- Collaborating with a multidisciplinary team regarding treatment
- Consulting with appropriate care providers
- Delegating care activities to others
- Establishing priorities of care
- Handling hazardous and infectious materials
- Obtaining informed consent for treatments and procedures

- Maintaining confidentiality related to the disorder
- Preventing accidents and client injury
- Using medical and surgical asepsis to prevent infection

Health Promotion and Maintenance

- Discussing expected body-image changes
- Identifying lifestyle choices related to treatment
- Performing data collection techniques related to the endocrine system
- Preventing disease
- Providing health screening
- Teaching about self-care measures

Psychosocial Integrity

- Discussing grief and loss issues related to complications of the disorder
- Discussing situational role changes related to the disorder
- Discussing unexpected body-image changes
- Identifying coping mechanisms
- Monitoring for sensory/perceptual alterations as a result of the disorder
- Making use of support systems

Physiological Integrity

- Administering medications safely
- Monitoring for alterations in body systems as a result of the disorder
- Monitoring for expected outcomes/effects of pharmacological therapy
- Monitoring for fluid and electrolyte imbalances that can occur
- Monitoring the laboratory values
- Monitoring for potential complications of diagnostic tests, treatments, and procedures
- Monitoring for potential complications from surgical procedures and health alterations
- Monitoring for problems with elimination as a result of the disorder
- Monitoring for unexpected responses to therapies
- Performing dosage calculations related to medication administration
- Preparing the client for diagnostic tests
- Providing nonpharmacological comfort interventions
- Providing nutrition and oral hydration measures
- Providing emergency care to the client

45

Endocrine System

I. ANATOMY AND PHYSIOLOGY OF THE ENDO-CRINE GLANDS

A. Functions
1. Maintenance and regulation of vital functions
2. Response to stress and injury
3. Growth and development
4. Energy metabolism
5. Reproduction
6. Fluid, electrolyte, and acid-base balance

B. Risk factors: See Box 45-1.

C. Hypothalamus
1. A portion of the diencephalon of the brain that forms the floor and part of the lateral wall of the third ventricle
2. Activates, controls, and integrates the peripheral autonomic nervous system, the endocrine processes, and many somatic functions, such as body temperature, sleep, and appetite

D. Pituitary gland (Figure 45-1)
1. The master gland; located at the base of the brain
2. Influenced by the hypothalamus; directly affects the function of the other endocrine glands
3. Promotes the growth of body tissue, influences water absorption by the kidney, and controls sexual development and function

E. Adrenal gland
1. One adrenal gland is on top of each kidney
2. Regulates sodium and electrolyte balance; affects carbohydrate, fat, and protein metabolism; influences the development of sexual characteristics; and sustains the "fight-or-flight" response
3. Adrenal cortex
   a. The outer shell of the adrenal gland
   b. Synthesizes glucocorticoids and mineralocorticoids; secretes small amounts of sex hormones (i.e., androgens, estrogens)
4. Adrenal medulla
   a. The inner core of the adrenal gland
   b. Works as part of the sympathetic nervous system; produces epinephrine and norepinephrine

F. Thyroid gland
1. Located in the anterior part of the neck
2. Controls the rate of body metabolism and growth; produces thyroxine (T_4), triiodothyronine (T_3), and thyrocalcitonin

G. Parathyroid glands
1. Located on the thyroid gland
2. Control calcium and phosphorus metabolism; produce parathyroid hormone

H. Pancreas
1. Located posteriorly to the stomach
2. Influences carbohydrate metabolism; indirectly influences fat and protein metabolism; and produces insulin and glucagon

I. Ovaries and testes
1. The ovaries are located in the pelvic cavity and produce estrogen and progesterone.
2. The testes are located in the scrotum. They control the development of the secondary sex characteristics and produce testosterone.

J. Negative feedback loop
1. Regulates hormone secretion by the hypothalamus and the pituitary gland
2. Increased amounts of target gland hormones in the bloodstream decrease the secretion of the same hormones and other hormones that stimulate their release.

II. DIAGNOSTIC TESTS

A. Stimulation and suppression tests
1. Stimulation testing

Box 45-1 Risk Factors for Endocrine Disorders

- Age
- Heredity
- Congenital
- Trauma
- Environmental
- Surgery
- Consequence of other disorders

a. For the client with suspected underactivity of an endocrine gland, a stimulus may be provided to determine whether the gland is capable of normal hormone production.

b. Measured amounts of selected hormones or substances are administered to stimulate the target gland to produce its hormone.

c. Hormone levels produced by the target gland are measured.

d. The failure of the hormone level to increase with stimulation indicates hypofunction.

2. Suppression tests

a. Suppression tests are used when hormone levels are high or in the upper range of normal.

b. Agents that normally induce a suppressed response are administered to determine whether normal negative feedback is intact.

c. The failure of hormone production to be suppressed during standardized testing indicates hyperfunction.

B. Radioactive iodine uptake

1. This thyroid function test measures the absorption of the iodine isotope to determine how the thyroid gland is functioning.

2. A small dose of radioactive iodine is given by mouth or the intravenous (IV) route. The amount of radioactivity is measured in 2 to 4 hours and again at 24 hours.

3. Normal values are 3% to 10% at 2 to 4 hours and 5% to 30% at 24 hours.

4. Elevated values indicate **hyperthyroidism**, decreased iodine intake, or increased iodine excretion.

5. Decreased values indicate a low T_4 level, the use of antithyroid medications, thyroiditis, **myxedema**, or **hypothyroidism**.

6. The test is contraindicated during pregnancy.

C. T_3 and T_4 resin uptake test

1. Blood tests are used to diagnose thyroid disorders.

2. T_3 and T_4 regulate thyroid-stimulating hormone.

3. Normal values (normal findings vary among laboratory settings)

   a. T_3: 80 to 230 ng/dL

   b. T_4: 5 to 12 mcg/dL

   c. Thyroxine, free (FT_4): 0.8 to 2.4 ng/dL

4. The T_3 is elevated in **hyperthyroidism**. It decreases with the aging process and may be decreased in **hypothyroidism**.

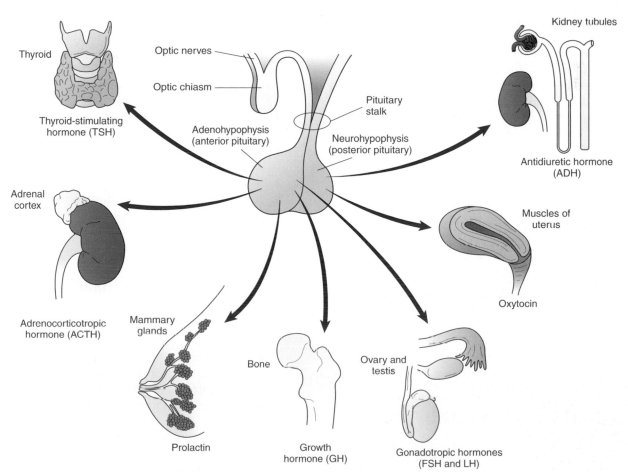

▲ **FIGURE 45-1** Pituitary hormones. (From Lilley, L., Harrington, S., & Snyder, J. [2010]. *Pharmacology and the nursing process* [6th ed.]. St. Louis: Mosby.)

5. The T_4 is elevated in **hyperthyroidism** and decreased in **hypothyroidism**.

 D. Thyroid-stimulating hormone
1. Blood test is used to differentiate the diagnosis of primary **hypothyroidism**.
2. Normal value is 0.2 to 5.4 microunits/mL; normal findings vary among laboratory settings.
3. Elevated values indicate primary **hypothyroidism**.
4. Decreased values indicate **hyperthyroidism** or secondary **hypothyroidism**.

E. Thyroid scan
1. A thyroid scan is performed to identify nodules or growths in the thyroid gland.
2. A radioisotope of iodine or technetium is administered before the scanning of the thyroid gland.
3. Reassure the client that the level of radioactive medication is not dangerous to self or others.
4. Determine whether the client has received radiographic contrast agents within the past 3 months, because these may invalidate the scan.
5. Check with the health care provider (HCP) regarding discontinuing medications that contain iodine for 14 days before the test and regarding the need to discontinue thyroid medication before the test.
6. Instruct the client to maintain nothing-by-mouth status after midnight on the day before the test. If iodine is used, the client will fast for an additional 45 minutes after the ingestion of the oral isotope, and the scan will be performed in 24 hours.
7. If technetium is used, it is administered by the IV route 30 minutes before the scan.
8. The test is contraindicated during pregnancy.

F. Needle aspiration of thyroid tissue
1. Aspiration of thyroid tissue is done for cytological examination.
2. No client preparation is necessary.
3. Light pressure is applied to the aspiration site after the procedure.

G. Glucose tolerance test
1. The glucose tolerance test aids in the diagnosis of **diabetes mellitus**.
2. A 2-hour post-load glucose level (2 hours after the injection or ingestion of glucose) greater than 200 mg/dL confirms the diagnosis of **diabetes mellitus**.
3. Client preparation (Box 45-2)
4. Many factors can alter the results; therefore this is not always a reliable test.

H. Glycosylated hemoglobin
1. Description
   a. Glycosylated hemoglobin is blood glucose that is bound to hemoglobin.
   b. Glycosylated hemoglobin A (HbA_{1c}) is a reflection of how well the blood glucose levels have been controlled for the prior 3 to 4 months.

Box 45-2 Client Preparation: Glucose Tolerance Test

Eat a diet that includes at least 200 to 300 g of carbohydrates for 3 days before the test.

Avoid alcohol, coffee, and smoking for 36 hours before the test.

Fast for 10 to 16 hours before the test.

Avoid strenuous exercise for 8 hours before and after the test.

If you have diabetes mellitus, withhold the morning insulin or oral hypoglycemic medication.

A fasting blood glucose is drawn, and you will be given a high-glucose drink.

Blood samples will be drawn at 30-minute intervals for a minimum of 2 hours. (Testing may take 3 to 5 hours.)

---

   c. Hyperglycemia in a client with diabetes mellitus is usually the cause of an increase in HbA_{1c}.

 Hyperglycemia in a client with diabetes mellitus is usually the cause of an increase in the HbA_{1c} value.

2. Values
   a. Values are expressed as a percentage of the total hemoglobin.
   b. The goal for clients with **diabetes mellitus** is 7% or less.
   c. For clients without **diabetes mellitus**, the normal range is 4% to 6%.
3. Nursing consideration: Fasting is not required.

I. Glycosylated serum albumin (fructosamine)
1. Reflects average serum glucose levels over a period of 2 to 3 weeks.
2. More sensitive to recent changes than the HbA_{1c}.
3. Normal ranges vary according to the method of testing used. For a nondiabetic client, the normal range is 1.5 to 2.7 mmol/L, and, for a diabetic client, it is 2.0 to 5.0 mmol/L.

III. DISORDERS OF THE PITUITARY GLAND

A. Hypopituitarism
1. Description: The hyposecretion of one or more of the pituitary hormones caused by tumors, trauma, encephalitis, autoimmunity, or stroke.
2. The hormones that are most often affected are growth hormone (GH) and the gonadotropins (luteinizing hormone and follicle-stimulating hormone), but thyroid-stimulating hormone (TSH), adrenocorticotropic hormone (ACTH), and antidiuretic hormone (ADH) may be involved.
3. Data collection
   a. Mild to moderate obesity (GH, TSH)
   b. Reduced cardiac output (GH, ADH)

c. Infertility and sexual dysfunction (gonadotropins, ACTH)

d. Fatigue and low blood pressure (TSH, ADH, ACTH, GH)

e. Tumors of the pituitary may also cause headaches and visual defects. (The pituitary is located near the optic nerve).

4. Interventions
   a. Provide emotional support to the client and family.
   b. Encourage the client and family to express feelings related to disturbed body image or sexual dysfunction.
   c. Client may need hormone replacement for specific deficient hormones.
   d. Client may require education regarding the signs and symptoms of both hypofunction and hyperfunction related to insufficient or excess hormone replacement.

B. Hyperpituitarism
1. Description
   a. The hypersecretion of growth hormone by the anterior pituitary gland in an adult and is caused primarily by pituitary tumors.
   b. Leads to conditions such as acromegaly and **Cushing's disease**
2. Data collection
   a. Large hands and feet
   b. Thickening and protrusion of the jaw
   c. Arthritic changes
   d. Visual disturbances
   e. Diaphoresis
   f. Oily, rough skin
   g. Organomegaly
   h. Hypertension
   i. Dysphagia
   j. Deepening of the voice
3. Interventions
   a. Provide emotional support to the client and family, and encourage the client and family to express feelings related to disturbed body image.
   b. Provide frequent skin care.
   c. Provide pharmacological and nonpharmacological interventions for joint pain as prescribed.
   d. Prepare the client for radiation of the pituitary gland, if prescribed.
   e. Prepare the client for **hypophysectomy**, if planned.

C. Hypophysectomy (pituitary adenectomy, transsphenoidal pituitary surgery)
1. Description
   a. The removal of the pituitary tumor via craniotomy or via transsphenoidal (endoscopic transnasal) approach. The latter approach is preferred, because it is associated with fewer complications.

b. Complications of craniotomy include increased intracranial pressure, bleeding, meningitis, and hypopituitarism.
   c. Complications of the transsphenoidal surgery include cerebrospinal fluid leak, infection, and hypopituitarism.

2. Postoperative interventions
   a. Initiate postoperative care similar to craniotomy care.
   b. Monitor the vital signs, neurological status, and level of consciousness.
   c. Elevate the head of the bed.
   d. Monitor for increased intracranial pressure.
   e. Monitor for bleeding.
   f. Instruct the client to avoid sneezing, coughing, and blowing the nose.
   g. Monitor electrolyte values for temporary **diabetes insipidus** or **syndrome of inappropriate ADH** as a result of ADH disturbances.
   h. Monitor the intake and output and avoid water intoxication.
   i. Administer glucocorticoids and other hormone replacements, as prescribed.
   j. Administer antibiotics, analgesics, and antipyretics, as prescribed.
   k. Instruct the client regarding the administration of prescribed medications, which may include vasopressin (synthetic ADH), levothyroxine (Synthroid), gonadotropic hormones, growth hormone (somatotropin), and glucocorticoids if the entire gland was removed.

⚠ Following transsphenoidal hypophysectomy, monitor for any postnasal drip or nasal drainage, which might indicate leakage of cerebrospinal fluid (check the nasal drainage for glucose).

D. Diabetes insipidus
1. Description
   a. The hyposecretion of ADH caused by strokes, trauma, or idiopathic causes
   b. The kidney tubules fail to reabsorb water
2. Data collection
   a. Polyuria of 4 to 24 L per day
   b. Polydipsia
   c. Dehydration (e.g., decreased skin turgor, dry mucous membranes)
   d. Inability to concentrate urine
   e. A low urinary specific gravity (1.006 or less)
   f. Fatigue
   g. Muscle pain and weakness
   h. Headache
   i. Postural hypotension that may progress to vascular collapse without rehydration
   j. Tachycardia

3. Interventions
    a. Monitor the vital signs and the neurological and cardiovascular statuses.
    b. Provide a safe environment, particularly for the client with postural hypotension.
    c. Monitor the electrolyte values and for signs of dehydration.
    d. Maintain the intake of adequate fluids.
    e. Monitor intake and output, weight, serum osmolality, and specific gravity of urine.
    f. Instruct the client to avoid foods or liquids that produce diuresis.
    g. Vasopressin tannate (Pitressin) or desmopressin acetate (DDAVP, Stimate) may be prescribed. These are used when the ADH deficiency is severe or chronic.
    h. Instruct the client regarding the administration of medications, as prescribed. DDAVP may be administered by injection, intranasally, or orally.
    i. Instruct the client to wear a Medic-Alert bracelet.

E. **Syndrome of inappropriate antidiuretic hormone (SIADH)**
    1. Description
        a. Excess ADH is released, but not in response to a bodily need for it.
        b. Causes include trauma, stroke, malignancies (often in the lungs or pancreas), medications, and stress.
        c. The syndrome results in water intoxication and hyponatremia.
    2. Data collection
        a. Signs of fluid volume overload
        b. Changes in the level of consciousness and mental status changes
        c. Weight gain
        d. Hypertension
        e. Tachycardia
        f. Anorexia, nausea, and vomiting
        g. Hyponatremia
    3. Interventions
        a. Monitor the vital signs and the cardiac and neurological status.
        b. Provide a safe environment, particularly for the client with changes in the level of consciousness or mental status.
        c. Monitor intake and output and obtain a daily weight.
        d. Monitor the fluid and electrolyte balance.
        e. Monitor the serum and urine osmolality.
        f. Restrict fluid intake, as prescribed.
        g. Administer diuretics and IV fluids (normal saline or hypertonic saline), as prescribed. Monitor IV fluids carefully because of the risk for fluid volume overload. (IV solutions containing water are contraindicated because of the risk of water intoxication.)

h. Medications that inhibit ADH-induced water reabsorption and produce water diuresis may be prescribed.

IV. DISORDERS OF THE ADRENAL GLANDS

A. Addison's disease
    1. Description
        a. Hyposecretion of adrenal cortex hormones (glucocorticoids and mineralocorticoids).
        b. Can be primary or secondary.
        c. The condition is fatal if left untreated.
    2. Data collection (Table 45-1)
    3. Interventions
        a. Monitor vital signs, particularly blood pressure, weight, and intake and output.
        b. Monitor white blood cell (WBC) count, blood glucose, potassium, sodium, and calcium levels.
        c. Administer glucocorticoid or mineralocorticoid medications, as prescribed.
        d. Observe for **addisonian crisis** caused by stress, infection, trauma, or surgery.
    4. Client education
        a. Avoid individuals with infections.
        b. Diet: High protein and carbohydrate intake; normal sodium intake
        c. Avoid strenuous exercise and stressful situations.
        d. Need for lifelong glucocorticoid therapy
        e. Avoid over-the-counter medications.
        f. Wear a Medic-Alert bracelet.
        g. Signs and symptoms related to the under- and over-replacement of hormones

TABLE 45-1 Data Collection: Addison's Disease and Cushing's Disease (Cushing's Syndrome)

Addison's Disease	Cushing's Disease and Syndrome
Lethargy, fatigue, and muscle weakness	Generalized muscle wasting and weakness
Gastrointestinal disturbances	Moonface and buffalo hump
Weight loss	Truncal obesity with thin extremities, supraclavicular fat pads, and weight gain
Menstrual changes in women; impotence in men	Hirsutism (masculine characteristics in females)
Hypoglycemia and hyponatremia	Hyperglycemia and hypernatremia
Hyperkalemia and hypercalcemia	Hypokalemia and hypocalcemia
Postural hypotension	Hypertension
Hyperpigmentation of the skin (bronzed) with primary disease	Fragile skin that easily bruises Reddish-purple striae on the abdomen and upper thighs

B. Addisonian crisis
1. Description (Box 45-3)
2. Data collection
   a. Severe headache
   b. Severe abdominal, leg, and lower back pain
   c. Generalized weakness
   d. Irritability and confusion
   e. Severe hypotension
   f. Shock
3. Interventions
   a. Prepare to administer IV glucocorticoids, as prescribed. Hydrocortisone sodium succinate (Solu-Cortef) is usually prescribed initially.
   b. After the resolution of the crisis, administer glucocorticoids and mineralocorticoids orally, as prescribed.
   c. Monitor the vital signs, particularly blood pressure.
   d. Monitor the neurological status, noting irritability and confusion.
   e. Monitor intake and output.
   f. Monitor the laboratory values, particularly sodium, potassium, and blood glucose levels.
   g. Administer IV fluids, as prescribed, to restore electrolyte balance.
   h. Protect the client from infection.
   i. Maintain the client on bedrest and provide a quiet environment.

⚠ Addison's disease is characterized by the hyposecretion of adrenal cortex hormones (glucocorticoids and mineralocorticoids), whereas Cushing's disease is characterized by a hypersecretion of glucocorticoids.

C. Cushing's disease and **Cushing's syndrome** (hypercortisolism)
1. Description
   a. Characterized by a hypersecretion of glucocorticoids from the adrenal cortex
   b. **Cushing's disease** is a metabolic disorder characterized by the abnormally increased secretion (endogenous) of adrenocortical steroids, particularly cortisol, caused by increased amounts of ACTH secreted by the pituitary gland.

Box 45-3 Addisonian Crisis

■ A life-threatening disorder caused by acute adrenal insufficiency
■ Precipitated by stress, infection, trauma, surgery, or the abrupt withdrawal of exogenous corticosteroid use
■ Can cause hyponatremia, hyperkalemia, hypoglycemia, and shock

---

   c. **Cushing's syndrome** is a metabolic disorder that results from the chronic and excessive production of cortisol by the adrenal cortex or from the administration of glucocorticoids in large doses for several weeks or longer (exogenous or iatrogenic).
2. Data collection (see Table 45-1)
3. Interventions
   a. Monitor the vital signs, particularly blood pressure.
   b. Monitor intake and output and weight.
   c. Monitor laboratory values, particularly the serum glucose level, the white blood cell count, and the sodium, potassium, and calcium levels.
   d. Provide meticulous skin care.
   e. Allow the client to discuss feelings related to body appearance.
   f. Administer chemotherapeutic agents, as prescribed, for inoperable adrenal tumors.
   g. Prepare the client for radiation, as prescribed, if the condition results from a pituitary tumor.
   h. Prepare the client for the removal of pituitary tumor (**hypophysectomy**, transsphenoidal adenectomy) if the condition results from the increased pituitary secretion of ACTH.
   i. Prepare the client for **adrenalectomy** if the condition results from an adrenal tumor. Glucocorticoid replacement may be required after **adrenalectomy**.
D. Primary hyperaldosteronism (Conn's syndrome)
1. Description
   a. A hypersecretion of mineralocorticoids (aldosterone) from the adrenal cortex of the adrenal gland
   b. Most commonly caused by a tumor
2. Data collection
   a. Symptoms related to hypokalemia, hypernatremia, and hypertension
   b. Headache, fatigue, muscle weakness, and nocturia
   c. Polydipsia and polyuria
   d. Paresthesias
   e. Visual changes
   f. Low urine specific gravity and increased urinary aldosterone
   g. Elevated serum aldosterone levels
   h. Metabolic alkalosis
3. Interventions
   a. Monitor the vital signs, particularly blood pressure.
   b. Monitor for signs of hypokalemia and hypernatremia.
   c. Monitor intake and output and the urine for specific gravity.
   d. Spironolactone (Aldactone) may be prescribed to promote fluid balance and to control

hypertension. The medication is a potassium-sparing diuretic and an aldosterone antagonist, and the client needs to be monitored for hyperkalemia, particularly in the presence of impaired renal function or excessive potassium intake.

   e. Administer potassium supplements, as prescribed.

   f. Prepare the client for **adrenalectomy**.

   g. Maintain sodium restriction preoperatively, if prescribed.

   h. Administer glucocorticoids preoperatively, as prescribed, to prevent adrenal hypofunction.

   i. Monitor the client for adrenal insufficiency postoperatively.

   j. Instruct the client regarding the need for glucocorticoid therapy after **adrenalectomy**.

   k. Instruct the client about the need to wear a Medic-Alert bracelet.

E. Pheochromocytoma

  1. Description

   a. A catecholamine-producing tumor that is usually found in the adrenal medulla. Extra-adrenal locations include the chest, bladder, abdomen, and brain. It is typically a benign tumor, but it can be malignant.

   b. Excessive amounts of epinephrine and norepinephrine are secreted.

   c. Diagnostic tests include a 24-hour urine collection for vanillylmandelic acid (VMA) (a product of catecholamine metabolism), metanephrine, and catecholamines, all of which are elevated in the presence of pheochromocytoma. The normal range of urinary catecholamines is up to 14 mcg/100 mL of urine, with higher levels occurring in pheochromocytoma.

   d. The surgical removal of the adrenal gland is the primary treatment.

   e. Symptomatic treatment is initiated if surgical removal is not possible.

   f. The complications associated with pheochromocytoma include hypertensive crisis, including hypertensive retinopathy and nephropathy; cardiac enlargement and dysrhythmias; congestive heart failure; myocardial infarction; increased platelet aggregation; and brain attack (stroke).

   g. Death can occur from shock, cerebrovascular stroke, renal failure, dysrhythmias, or dissecting aortic aneurysm.

  2. Data collection

   a. Paroxysmal or sustained hypertension

   b. Severe headaches

   c. Palpitations

   d. Flushing and profuse diaphoresis

   e. Pain in the chest or abdomen with nausea and vomiting

   f. Heat intolerance

   g. Weight loss

   h. Tremors

   i. **Hyperglycemia**

  3. Interventions

   a. Monitor the vital signs, particularly the blood pressure and heart rate.

   b. Monitor for hypertensive crisis and for complications that can occur with hypertensive crisis, such as stroke, cardiac dysrhythmias, and myocardial infarction.

   c. Instruct the client not to smoke, drink caffeine-containing beverages, or change position suddenly

   d. Prepare to administer an β-adrenergic blocking agent as prescribed, to control hypertension.

   e. Monitor the serum glucose level.

   f. Promote rest and a nonstressful environment.

   g. Provide a diet high in calories, vitamins, and minerals.

   h. Prepare the client for **adrenalectomy**.

⚠ For the client with pheochromocytoma, avoid stimuli that can precipitate a hypertensive crisis, such as increased abdominal pressure and vigorous abdominal palpation.

F. Adrenalectomy

  1. Description (Box 45-4)

  2. Preoperative interventions

   a. Monitor the electrolytes and correct electrolyte imbalances.

   b. Monitor for dysrhythmias.

   c. Monitor for hyperglycemia.

   d. Protect the client from infections.

   e. Administer glucocorticoids, as prescribed.

  3. Postoperative interventions

   a. Monitor the vital signs.

   b. Monitor intake and output. If the urinary output is less that 30 mL/hour, notify the HCP, because this may indicate renal failure and impending shock.

Box 45-4 Adrenalectomy

Surgical removal of an adrenal gland.

Lifelong glucocorticoid and mineralocorticoid replacement is necessary with a bilateral adrenalectomy.

Temporary glucocorticoid replacement for up to 2 years is necessary for a unilateral adrenalectomy.

Catecholamine levels drop as a result of surgery, which can result in cardiovascular collapse, hypotension, and shock. The client needs to be monitored closely.

Hemorrhage also can occur as a result of the high vascularity of the adrenal glands.

c. Monitor weight daily.

d. Monitor electrolyte and serum glucose levels.

e. Monitor for signs of shock and hemorrhage, particularly during the first 24 to 48 hours.

f. Monitor for manifestations of adrenal insufficiency (see Table 45-1).

g. Check the dressing for drainage.

h. Monitor for paralytic ileus, which is manifested by abdominal distention and pain, nausea, vomiting, and diminished or absent bowel sounds. This condition can develop from internal bleeding, anesthesia effects, and bowel manipulation.

i. Administer IV fluids, as prescribed, to maintain blood volume.

j. Administer glucocorticoids and mineralocorticoids, as prescribed.

k. Administer pain medication, as prescribed.

l. Provide pulmonary interventions to prevent atelectasis (e.g., coughing, deep breathing, incentive spirometry, splinting of the incision).

m. Instruct the client regarding the importance of hormone replacement therapy after surgery.

n. Instruct the client regarding the signs and symptoms of the under- and over-replacement of hormones.

o. Instruct the client regarding the need to wear a Medic-Alert bracelet.

V. DISORDERS OF THE THYROID GLAND

A. Hypothyroidism

1. Description

   a. A hypothyroid state that results from the hyposecretion of the thyroid hormones T_3 and T_4

   b. Characterized by a decreased rate of body metabolism

2. Data collection

   a. Lethargy and fatigue

   b. Weakness, muscle aches, and paresthesias

   c. Intolerance to cold

   d. Weight gain

   e. Dry skin and hair and loss of body hair

   f. Bradycardia

   g. Constipation

   h. Generalized puffiness and edema around the eyes and face (**myxedema**)

   i. Forgetfulness and loss of memory

   j. Menstrual disturbances

   k. Cardiac enlargement and the tendency to develop congestive heart failure

   l. Goiter may or may not be present

3. Interventions

   a. Monitor the vital signs, including heart rate and rhythm.

b. Administer thyroid replacement. Levothyroxine sodium (Synthroid) is most commonly prescribed.

c. Instruct the client about thyroid replacement therapy and about the clinical manifestations of both **hypothyroidism** and **hyperthyroidism** related to the under- or over-replacement of the hormone.

d. Instruct the client in a low-calorie, low-cholesterol, and low–saturated-fat diet

e. Monitor the client for constipation. Provide roughage and fluids to prevent constipation

f. Provide a warm environment for the client.

g. Avoid sedatives and opioid analgesics because of the client's increased sensitivity to these medications.

h. Monitor for the overdose of thyroid medications, which is characterized by tachycardia, chest pain, restlessness, nervousness, and insomnia.

i. Instruct the client to report episodes of chest pain or other signs of overdose immediately.

B. Myxedema coma

1. Description (Box 45-5)

2. Data collection

   a. Hypotension

   b. Bradycardia

   c. Hypothermia

   d. Hyponatremia

   e. **Hypoglycemia**

   f. Generalized edema

   g. Respiratory failure

   h. Coma

3. Interventions

   a. Maintain a patent airway.

   b. Administer IV fluids (normal or hypertonic saline), as prescribed.

   c. Administer IV levothyroxine sodium (Synthroid), as prescribed.

   d. Administer IV glucose, as prescribed.

   e. Administer corticosteroids, as prescribed.

   f. Monitor the client's temperature hourly.

   g. Monitor the blood pressure frequently.

   h. Keep the client warm.

   i. Monitor for changes in mental status.

   j. Monitor the electrolyte and glucose levels.

   k. Institute aspiration precautions.

Box 45-5 Myxedema Coma

This is a rare but serious disorder that results from persistently low thyroid production.

Coma can be precipitated by acute illness, the rapid withdrawal of thyroid medication, anesthesia, surgery, hypothermia, or the use of sedatives and opioid analgesics.

C. Hyperthyroidism
1. Description
   a. A hyperthyroid state that results from the hypersecretion of the thyroid hormones (T_3 and T_4).
   b. Characterized by an increased rate of body metabolism.
   c. A common cause is Graves' disease, which is also known as toxic diffuse goiter.
   d. Clinical manifestations are referred to as thyrotoxicosis.
2. Data collection for hyperthyroidism caused by Graves' disease
   a. Enlarged thyroid gland (goiter)
   b. Palpitations and cardiac dysrhythmias, such as tachycardia or atrial fibrillation
   c. Protruding eyeballs (exophthalmos) are possibly present.
   d. Hypertension
   e. Heat intolerance
   f. Diaphoresis
   g. Weight loss
   h. Diarrhea
   i. Smooth, soft skin and hair
   j. Nervousness and fine tremors of the hands
   k. Personality changes, such as irritability, agitation, and mood swings
3. Interventions
   a. Provide adequate rest.
   b. Administer sedatives, as prescribed.
   c. Provide a cool and quiet environment.
   d. Obtain the weight daily.
   e. Provide a high-calorie diet.
   f. Avoid the administration of stimulants.
   g. Administer antithyroid medications that block thyroid synthesis, as prescribed.
   h. Administer iodine preparations that inhibit the release of thyroid hormone, as prescribed.
   i. Administer propranolol (Inderal) for tachycardia, as prescribed.
   j. Prepare the client for radioactive iodine therapy, as prescribed, to destroy thyroid cells.
   k. Prepare the client for **thyroidectomy**, if prescribed.

D. Thyroid storm
1. Description (Box 45-6)
2. Data collection
   a. Elevated temperature
   b. Tachycardia
   c. Systolic hypertension
   d. Nausea, vomiting, and diarrhea
   e. Agitation, tremors, and anxiety
   f. Irritability, agitation, restlessness, confusion, and seizures as the condition progresses
   g. Delirium and coma

Box 45-6 Thyroid Storm

Thyroid storm is an acute and life-threatening condition that occurs in a client with uncontrollable hyperthyroidism.

It can occur as a result of the manipulation of the thyroid gland during surgery and the release of thyroid hormone into the bloodstream; it also can occur as a result of severe infection and stress.

Antithyroid medications, β-blockers, glucocorticoids, and iodides may be administered to the client before thyroid surgery to prevent its occurrence.

---

3. Interventions
   a. Maintain a patent airway and adequate ventilation.
   b. Administer antithyroid medications, sodium iodide solution, propranolol (Inderal), and glucocorticoids, as prescribed.
   c. Monitor the vital signs.
   d. Monitor continually for cardiac dysrhythmias.
   e. Administer nonsalicylate antipyretics, as prescribed. (Salicylates increase free thyroid hormone levels.)
   f. Use a cooling blanket to decrease the client's temperature, as prescribed.

E. Thyroidectomy
1. Description
   a. Removal of the thyroid gland
   b. Performed when persistent hyperthyroidism exists
2. Preoperative interventions
   a. Obtain the vital signs and weight.
   b. Monitor electrolyte levels.
   c. Monitor for **hyperglycemia**.
   d. Instruct the client regarding how to perform coughing and deep-breathing exercises and how to support the neck during the postoperative period when coughing and moving.
   e. Administer antithyroid medications, sodium iodide solution, propranolol (Inderal), and glucocorticoids, as prescribed, to prevent the occurrence of **thyroid storm**.
3. Postoperative interventions
   a. Monitor for respiratory distress.
   b. Have a tracheotomy set, oxygen, and suction at the bedside.
   c. Limit client talking, and determine the level of hoarseness.
   d. Monitor for laryngeal nerve damage as evidenced by respiratory obstruction, dysphonia, high-pitched voice, stridor, dysphagia, and restlessness.
   e. Monitor for signs of hypocalcemia and tetany, which can be the result of trauma to the parathyroid gland (Box 45-7).

Box 45-7 Signs of Tetany

- Cardiac dysrhythmias
- Carpopedal spasm
- Dysphagia
- Muscle and abdominal cramps
- Numbness and tingling of the face and extremities
- Positive Chvostek's sign
- Positive Trousseau's sign
- Visual disturbances (photophobia)
- Wheezing and dyspnea (bronchospasm, laryngospasm)
- Seizures

    f. Prepare to administer calcium gluconate, as prescribed, for tetany.

    g. Monitor for **thyroid storm**.

⚠ Following thyroidectomy, maintain the client in a semi-Fowler's position. Monitor the surgical site for edema and for signs of bleeding and check the dressing anteriorly and at the back of the neck.

VI. DISORDERS OF THE PARATHYROID GLAND

A. Hypoparathyroidism

1. Description
   a. A condition caused by the hyposecretion of parathyroid hormone by the parathyroid gland
   b. Can occur after **thyroidectomy** because of the removal of parathyroid tissue

2. Data collection
   a. Hypocalcemia and hyperphosphatemia
   b. Numbness and tingling in the face
   c. Muscle cramps and cramps in the abdomen or in the extremities
   d. Positive **Trousseau's sign** or **Chvostek's sign**
   e. Signs of overt tetany, such as bronchospasm, laryngospasm, carpopedal spasm, dysphagia, photophobia, cardiac dysrhythmias, and seizures
   f. Hypotension
   g. Anxiety, irritability, and depression

3. Interventions
   a. Monitor the vital signs.
   b. Monitor for signs of hypocalcemia and tetany.
   c. Initiate seizure precautions.
   d. Place a tracheotomy set, oxygen, and suctioning equipment at the bedside.
   e. Prepare to administer IV calcium gluconate for hypocalcemia.
   f. Provide a high-calcium, low-phosphorus diet.
   g. Instruct the client regarding the administration of calcium supplements, as prescribed.
   h. Instruct the client regarding the administration of vitamin D supplements, as prescribed.

Vitamin D enhances the absorption of calcium from the gastrointestinal tract.
   i. Instruct the client regarding the administration of phosphate binders, as prescribed, to promote the excretion of phosphate through the gastrointestinal tract.
   j. Instruct the client to wear a Medic-Alert bracelet.

B. Hyperparathyroidism

1. Description: A condition caused by the hypersecretion of parathyroid hormone by the parathyroid gland.

2. Data collection
   a. Hypercalcemia and hypophosphatemia
   b. Fatigue and muscle weakness
   c. Skeletal pain and tenderness
   d. Bone deformities that result in pathological fractures
   e. Anorexia, nausea, vomiting, and epigastric pain
   f. Weight loss
   g. Constipation
   h. Hypertension
   i. Cardiac dysrhythmias
   j. Renal stones

3. Interventions
   a. Monitor the vital signs, particularly the blood pressure.
   b. Monitor for cardiac dysrhythmias.
   c. Monitor intake and output and for signs of renal stones.
   d. Monitor for skeletal pain; move the client slowly and carefully.
   e. Encourage fluid intake.
   f. Administer furosemide (Lasix), as prescribed, to lower calcium levels.
   g. Administer IV normal saline, as prescribed, to maintain hydration.
   h. Administer phosphates, as prescribed. They interfere with calcium resorption.
   i. Administer calcitonin (Calcimar), as prescribed, to decrease skeletal calcium release and increase the renal clearance of calcium.
   j. Monitor the calcium and phosphorus levels.
   k. Prepare the client for parathyroidectomy, as prescribed.

⚠ For the client with a parathyroid gland disorder, notify the HCP immediately if hypocalcemia occurs. Monitor for tingling and numbness in the face and extremities and for other signs of hypocalcemia.

C. Parathyroidectomy

1. Description: The removal of one or more of the parathyroid glands

2. Preoperative interventions

a. Monitor the electrolyte, calcium, phosphate, and magnesium levels.

b. Ensure that calcium levels are decreased to near normal.

c. Inform the client that talking may be painful for the first day or two after surgery.

3. Postoperative interventions

a. Monitor for respiratory distress.

b. Place a tracheotomy set, oxygen, and suctioning equipment at the bedside.

c. Monitor the vital signs.

d. Position the client in a semi-Fowler's position.

e. Check the neck dressing for bleeding.

f. Monitor for hypocalcemic crisis as evidenced by tingling and twitching in the extremities and face.

g. Monitor for positive **Trousseau's** or **Chvostek's sign**. These signal the potential for tetany.

h. Monitor for changes in voice pattern and hoarseness.

i. Monitor for laryngeal nerve damage.

j. Instruct the client regarding the administration of calcium and vitamin D supplements, as prescribed.

VII. DISORDERS OF THE PANCREAS

A. Diabetes mellitus

1. Description

a. A chronic disorder of impaired carbohydrate, protein, and lipid metabolism that is caused by a deficiency of insulin.

b. An absolute or relative deficiency of insulin results in **hyperglycemia**.

c. Type 1 **diabetes mellitus** is a nearly absolute deficiency of insulin. If insulin is not given, fats are metabolized for energy, which results in ketonemia (acidosis).

d. Type 2 **diabetes mellitus** is a relative lack of insulin or resistance to the action of insulin; insulin is usually sufficient to stabilize fat and protein metabolism but not to deal with carbohydrate metabolism.

e. Metabolic syndrome is also known as syndrome X and the individual has coexisting risk factors for developing type 2 **diabetes mellitus**; these risk factors include abdominal obesity, **hyperglycemia**, hypertension, high triglyceride level, and a lowered HDL (high-density lipoprotein) cholesterol level.

f. **Diabetes mellitus** can lead to chronic health problems and early death as a result of complications that occur in the large and small blood vessels in tissues and organs.

g. Macrovascular complications include coronary artery disease, cardiomyopathy, hypertension, cerebrovascular disease, and peripheral vascular disease.

h. Microvascular complications include retinopathy, nephropathy, and neuropathy.

i. Infection is also a concern because of reduced healing ability.

j. Male erectile dysfunction can also occur as a result of the disease.

Obesity is a major risk factor for diabetes mellitus.

2. Data collection

a. Polyuria, polydipsia, and polyphagia (more common with type 1 **diabetes mellitus**)

b. **Hyperglycemia**

c. Weight loss (common with type 1 **diabetes mellitus**, rare with type 2 **diabetes mellitus**)

d. Blurred vision

e. Slow wound healing

f. Vaginal infections

g. Weakness and paresthesias

h. Signs of inadequate circulation to the feet

i. Signs of accelerated atherosclerosis (renal, cerebral, cardiac, and peripheral)

3. Diet

a. The total number of calories is individualized on the basis of the client's current or desired weight and the presence of other existing health problems.

b. Day-to-day consistency in timing and amount of food intake helps control the blood glucose level.

c. As prescribed by the health care provider, the client may be advised to follow the food exchange from the American Diabetic Association diet or the dietary guidelines for Americans (MyPlate) issued by the U.S. Departments of Agriculture and Health and Human Services.

d. Carbohydrate counting may be a simpler approach: It focuses on the total grams of carbohydrates eaten per meal. The client may be more compliant with carbohydrate counting, which results in better glycemic control and which is usually necessary for clients making use of intense insulin therapy.

e. Incorporate the diet into individual client needs, lifestyle, and cultural and socioeconomic patterns.

4. Exercise

a. Exercise lowers the blood glucose level, encourages weight loss, reduces cardiovascular risks, improves circulation and muscle tone, decreases total cholesterol and triglyceride levels, and decreases insulin resistance and glucose intolerance.

b. Instruct the client regarding dietary adjustments when exercising. Dietary adjustments are individualized.

c. If the client requires extra food during exercise to prevent **hypoglycemia**, it need not be deducted from the regular meal plan.

d. If the blood glucose level is greater than 250 mg/dL and urinary ketones are present in a client with type 1 **diabetes mellitus**, then the client is instructed not to exercise until the blood glucose is closer to normal and urinary ketones are absent.

⚠ Instruct the client with diabetes mellitus to monitor the blood glucose level before, during and after exercising.

5. Oral hypoglycemic medications
   a. Oral medications are prescribed for clients with type 2 **diabetes mellitus** when diet and weight control therapy have failed to maintain satisfactory blood glucose levels.
   b. Determine the client's knowledge of **diabetes mellitus** and the use of oral hypoglycemic agents.
   c. Monitor the vital signs and blood glucose levels.
   d. Determine the medications that the client is currently taking.
   e. Aspirin, alcohol, sulfonamides, oral contraceptives, and monoamine oxidase inhibitors increase the hypoglycemic effect, thereby causing a decrease in blood glucose levels.
   f. Glucocorticoids, thiazide diuretics, and estrogen increase blood glucose levels.
   g. Teach the client to recognize symptoms of **hypoglycemia** and **hyperglycemia**.
   h. Teach the client to avoid over-the-counter medications, unless prescribed by the HCP.
   i. Inform the client with type 2 **diabetes mellitus** that insulin may be needed during stress, surgery, or infection.
   j. Teach the client about the importance of compliance with the prescribed medication.
   k. Advise the client to wear a Medic-Alert bracelet.

⚠ To prevent a serious reaction, inform the client taking a sulfonylurea to avoid consuming alcohol.

6. Insulin
   a. Insulin is used to treat both type 1 and 2 **diabetes mellitus** when diet, weight-control therapy, and oral hypoglycemic agents have failed to maintain satisfactory blood glucose levels.
   b. Regular insulin is the only insulin that can be administered by IV for the emergency treatment of **diabetic ketoacidosis**.
   c. Aspirin, alcohol, oral anticoagulants, oral hypoglycemic medications, β-blockers, tricyclic antidepressants, tetracycline, and monoamine oxidase inhibitors increase the hypoglycemic effect of insulin, thus causing a further decrease in blood glucose levels.
   d. Glucocorticoids, thiazide diuretics, thyroid agents, oral contraceptives, and estrogen increase blood glucose levels.
   e. Illness, infection, and stress increase blood glucose levels and the need for insulin. Insulin should not be withheld during illness, infection, or stress, because **hyperglycemia** and **ketoacidosis** can result.
   f. Instruct the client to recognize symptoms of **hypoglycemia** and **hyperglycemia**.
   g. The peak action time of insulin is important because of the possibility of hypoglycemic reactions occurring during that time.

⚠ Regular insulin is the only insulin that can be administered intravenously. It is used in the emergency treatment of diabetic ketoacidosis.

B. Complications of insulin therapy
   1. Local allergic reactions
      a. Redness, swelling, tenderness, and an induration or wheal at the site of injection may occur 1 to 2 hours after administration.
      b. Reactions usually occur during the early stages of insulin therapy.
      c. Instruct the client to cleanse the skin with alcohol before injection.
   2. Insulin lipodystrophy
      a. Lipoatrophy is a loss of subcutaneous fat, and it appears as a slight dimpling or a more serious pitting of the subcutaneous fat. The use of human insulin helps to prevent this complication.
      b. Lipohypertrophy is the development of fibrous fatty masses at the injection site. It is caused by the repeated use of an injection site.
      c. Instruct the client to avoid injecting insulin into affected sites.
      d. Instruct the client about the importance of rotating insulin injections within one anatomical site.
   3. Insulin resistance
      a. The client who is receiving insulin develops immune antibodies that bind the insulin, thereby decreasing the insulin available for use in the body.
      b. Treatment consists of administering a purer insulin preparation.

c. Insulin resistance is also the term used for the lack of tissue sensitivity to the insulin from the body, which results in **hyperglycemia**.

4. **Dawn phenomenon**
   a. **Dawn phenomenon** results from reduced tissue sensitivity to insulin that develops between 5:00 AM and 8:00 AM (prebreakfast **hyperglycemia** occurs) and that may be caused by the nocturnal release of growth hormone.
   b. Treatment includes administering an evening dose (or increasing the amount of a current dose) of intermediate-acting insulin at 10:00 PM.

5. **Somogyi phenomenon**
   a. Normal or elevated blood glucose levels are present at bedtime; **hypoglycemia** occurs at 2:00 AM to 3:00 AM, which causes an increase in the production of counterregulatory hormones.
   b. By 7:00 AM, in response to the counterregulatory hormones, the blood glucose rebounds significantly to the hyperglycemic range.
   c. Treatment includes decreasing the evening (predinner or bedtime) dose of intermediate-acting insulin or increasing the bedtime snack.

C. Insulin administration
   1. See Chapter 46 for additional information about subcutaneous injections and mixing insulin.
   2. Insulin pens
      a. An insulin pen is a device that uses a small, prefilled insulin cartridge that is loaded into a pen-like holder. A disposable needle is attached to the device for injection, and the dosage is selected by dialing in the desired amount.
      b. The client inserts the needle for injection, and the insulin is delivered by pushing a button.
   3. Jet injectors
      a. A jet injector is a device that delivers insulin through the skin under pressure in an extremely fine stream.
      b. Insulin administered by this device is usually absorbed faster.
      c. The injector can cause bruising at the site of insulin delivery.
   4. Insulin pumps
      a. Continuous subcutaneous insulin infusion is administered by an externally worn device that contains a syringe attached to a long, thin, narrow-lumen tube with a needle or Teflon catheter attached to the end.
      b. The client inserts the needle or Teflon catheter into the subcutaneous tissue (usually on the abdomen) and secures it with tape or a transparent dressing. The pump is worn on a belt or

in a pocket. The needle or Teflon catheter is changed at least every 2 to 3 days.
      c. A continuous basal rate of insulin infuses; in addition, on the basis of the blood glucose level, the anticipated food intake, and the activity level, the client delivers a bolus of insulin before each meal.
      d. Both rapid-acting and regular insulin (buffered to prevent the precipitation of insulin crystals within the catheter) are appropriate for use in these pumps.
   5. Insulin pump and skin sensor
      a. A skin sensor device that monitors the client's blood continuously; the information is transmitted to the pump, determines the need for insulin, and then the insulin is injected.
      b. The pump holds up to a 3-day supply of insulin and can be easily disconnected for activities such as bathing.
   6. Pancreas transplants
      a. The goal of pancreatic transplantation is to halt or reverse the complications of **diabetes mellitus**.
      b. Transplants are performed on a limited number of clients, particularly clients who are receiving kidney transplantations simultaneously.
      c. Immunosuppressive therapy is prescribed to prevent and treat rejection.

D. Self-monitoring of blood glucose
   1. Self-monitoring provides the client with the current blood glucose level and with information to maintain good glycemic control.
   2. Monitoring requires a finger prick to obtain a drop of blood for testing.
   3. Alternative site testing (i.e., obtaining blood from the forearm, upper arm, abdomen, thigh, or calf) is now available with specific meters. These sites are not as reliable as the fingertip site when blood glucose levels are changing rapidly.
   4. Tests must be used with caution among clients with diabetic neuropathy.
   5. Client instructions (Box 45-8)

E. Urine testing
   1. Urine testing for glucose is not a reliable indicator of blood glucose and is therefore no longer used for monitoring purposes.
   2. Instruct the client regarding the procedure for testing urine ketones.
   3. The presence of ketones may indicate impending **ketoacidosis**.
   4. Urine ketone testing should be performed during illness and whenever the client with type 1 **diabetes mellitus** has persistently elevated blood glucose levels (greater than 240 mg/dL for two consecutive testing periods).

VIII. ACUTE COMPLICATIONS OF DIABETES MELLITUS (see Priority Nursing Actions)

■■■■ PRIORITY NURSING ACTIONS! ■■■■

Actions to Take if the Client Experiences a Hypoglycemic Reaction

1. Check the client's blood glucose level.
2. Give the client a 10- to 15-g carbohydrate item such as ½ cup of fruit juice to drink.
3. Take the client's vital signs.
4. Retest the blood glucose level.
5. Give the client a small snack of carbohydrate and protein.
6. Document the client's complaints, actions taken, and outcome.

If the client experiences symptoms of a hypoglycemic reaction such as hunger, irritability, shakiness, or weakness, the nurse first would check the client's blood glucose level to verify that he or she is experiencing hypoglycemia. Once this is verified, the nurse would give the client 10 to 15 g of carbohydrates. The nurse would retest the blood glucose level in 15 minutes. In the meantime, the nurse would check the client's vital signs. The nurse would give the client another 10- to 15-g carbohydrate food item if the client's symptoms do not resolve. Otherwise, the nurse would provide a small snack of carbohydrates and protein if the client's next scheduled meal is more than an hour away from the time of the occurrence. Following treatment and resolution of the hypoglycemic event, the nurse would document the occurrence, actions taken, and outcome.

Reference: Ignatavicius, D., & Workman, M. (2010). *Medical-surgical nursing: Patient-centered collaborative care* (6th ed., pp. 1507–1508). St. Louis: Saunders.

A. Hypoglycemia
1. Description
   a. **Hypoglycemia** occurs when the blood glucose level falls to less than 60 mg/dL or when the blood glucose drops rapidly from an elevated level.

Box 45-8 Client Instructions: Monitoring of Blood Glucose

Use the proper procedure for obtaining the blood glucose level.
Perform the procedure precisely to obtain accurate results.
Follow the manufacturer's instructions for the glucometer.
Wash your hands before and after performing the procedure to prevent infection.
Calibrate the monitor as instructed by the manufacturer.
Check the expiration date on the test strips.
If the blood glucose results do not seem reasonable, reread the instructions, reassess your technique, check the expiration date of the test strips, and perform the procedure again to verify your results.

---

b. **Hypoglycemia** is caused by too much insulin or oral hypoglycemic agents, too little food, or excessive activity.
c. The client needs to be instructed to always carry some form of fast-acting simple carbohydrate with them.
d. If the client has a hypoglycemic reaction and does not have any of the recommended emergency foods available, any available food should be eaten. High-fat foods slow the absorption of glucose, and the hypoglycemic symptoms may not resolve quickly.

2. Data collection (Box 45-9)
   a. Mild **hypoglycemia**: Client remains fully awake but displays adrenergic symptoms (e.g., sweating, nervousness, palpitations, tremors). The blood glucose level is usually less than 60 mg/dL.
   b. Moderate **hypoglycemia**: Client displays symptoms of worsening **hypoglycemia** (e.g., drowsiness, confusion, impaired coordination, inability to concentrate, slurred speech). The blood glucose level is usually less than 40 mg/dL.
   c. Severe **hypoglycemia**: Client displays severe neuroglycopenic symptoms (e.g., difficulty arousing, disoriented behavior, loss of consciousness, seizures). The blood glucose level is usually less than 20 mg/dL.

Box 45-9 Data Collection: Hypoglycemia

Mild
- Hunger
- Nervousness
- Palpitations
- Sweating
- Tachycardia
- Tremor

Moderate
- Confusion
- Double vision
- Drowsiness
- Emotional changes
- Headache
- Impaired coordination
- Inability to concentrate
- Irrational or combative behavior
- Lightheadedness
- Numbness of the lips and tongue
- Slurred speech

Severe
- Difficulty arousing
- Disoriented behavior
- Loss of consciousness
- Seizures

3. Interventions: Mild **hypoglycemia**
   a. Give 10 to 15 g of a fast-acting simple carbohydrate (Box 45-10).
   b. Retest the blood glucose level in 15 minutes, and repeat the treatment if symptoms do not resolve.
   c. After symptoms resolve, a snack that contains protein and carbohydrates (e.g., low-fat milk, cheese and crackers) is recommended unless the client plans to eat a regular meal within 60 minutes.
4. Interventions:
   a. Moderate **hypoglycemia**
   b. Administer 15 to 30 g of a fast-acting simple carbohydrate
   c. Administer additional food (e.g., low-fat milk or cheese) after 10 to 15 minutes
5. Interventions for severe **hypoglycemia**
   a. If the client is unconscious and cannot swallow, an injection of glucagon is administered subcutaneously or intramuscularly.
   b. Administer a second dose in 10 minutes if the client remains unconscious.
   c. A small meal is given to the client when he or she awakens as long as he or she is not nauseated.
   d. The HCP is notified if a severe hypoglycemic reaction occurs.
   e. In the hospital or emergency department, the client may be treated with an IV injection of 25 to 50 mL of 50% dextrose in water.
   f. Family members need to be instructed regarding the administration of glucagon.

⚠ Do not attempt to administer oral food or fluids to the client experiencing a severe hypoglycemic reaction that is semiconscious or unconscious and is unable to swallow. This client is at risk for aspiration. For this client, an injection of glucagon is administered subcutaneously or intramuscularly. In the hospital or emergency department, the client may be treated with an IV injection of 25 to 50 mL of 50% dextrose in water.

Box 45-10 Simple Carbohydrates to Treat Hypoglycemia

- Commercially prepared glucose tablets
- 6 to 10 Life Savers or hard candies
- 4 tsp of sugar
- 4 sugar cubes
- 1 Tbs of honey or syrup
- ½ cup of fruit juice or regular (nondiet) soft drink
- 8 oz low-fat milk
- 6 saltine crackers
- 3 graham crackers

B. Diabetic ketoacidosis (DKA)
1. Description (Figure 45-2)
   a. **Diabetic ketoacidosis** is a life-threatening complication of type 1 **diabetes mellitus** that develops when a severe insulin deficiency occurs
   b. The main clinical manifestations include **hyperglycemia**, dehydration, electrolyte imbalance, and acidosis
2. Data collection (Table 45-2)
3. Interventions
   a. Restore circulating blood volume and protect against cerebral, coronary, and renal hypoperfusion
   b. Treat dehydration with rapid IV infusions of 0.9% or 0.45% normal saline, as prescribed. Dextrose is added to IV fluids (D_5NS or 5% dextrose in 0.45% saline) when the blood glucose level reaches 250 to 300 mg/dL.
   c. Treat **hyperglycemia** with regular insulin administered intravenously, as prescribed.
   d. Correct electrolyte imbalances. (The potassium level may be elevated as a result of dehydration and acidosis.)
   e. Monitor the potassium level closely, because when the client receives treatment for the dehydration and acidosis, the serum potassium will decrease, and potassium replacement may be required.
4. Insulin IV administration
   a. Use regular insulin only.
   b. A dose of 5 to 10 units of regular insulin by IV bolus may be prescribed before a continuous infusion is begun.
   c. Mix the prescribed IV dose of regular insulin for continuous infusion in 0.9% or 0.45% normal saline, as prescribed.
   d. Flush the insulin solution through the entire IV infusion set, and discard the first 50 to 100 mL of solution before connecting and administering it to the client. Insulin molecules adhere to the plastic of IV infusion sets.
   e. Always place the insulin infusion on an IV infusion controller.
   f. Insulin is infused continuously until subcutaneous administration resumes.
   g. Monitor the vital signs.
   h. Monitor the urinary output and for signs of fluid overload.
   i. Monitor the potassium and glucose levels and for signs of increased intracranial pressure.
   j. The potassium level will fall rapidly within the first hour of treatment as the dehydration and the acidosis are treated.
   k. Potassium is administered by IV in a diluted solution, as prescribed, when the potassium reaches a normal level in order to prevent

▲ FIGURE 45-2 The pathophysiology of diabetic ketoacidosis. (From Black, J., & Hawks, J. [2008]. *Medical-surgical nursing: Clinical management for positive outcomes* [8th ed.]. Philadelphia: Saunders.)

TABLE 45-2 Differences Between Diabetic Ketoacidosis and Hyperglycemic-Hyperosmolar State

	Diabetic Ketoacidosis	Hyperglycemic-Hyperosmolar State
Onset	Sudden	Gradual
Precipitating factors	Infection	Infection
	Other stressors	Other stressors
	Inadequate insulin dose	Poor fluid intake
Manifestations	*Ketosis:* Kussmaul's respirations, fruity odor of the breath, nausea, and abdominal pain	Altered central nervous system function with neurologic symptoms
	Dehydration or electrolyte loss: polyuria, polydipsia, weight loss, dry skin, sunken eyes, soft eyeballs, lethargy, and coma	Dehydration or electrolyte loss; same as for DKA
LABORATORY FINDINGS		
Serum glucose	>300 mg/dL (16.7 mmol/L)	>800 mg/dL (44.5 mmol/L)
Osmolarity	Variable	>350 mOsm/L
Serum ketones	Positive at 1:2 dilutions	Negative
Serum pH	<7.35	>7.4
Serum HCO_3	<15 mEq/L	>20 mEq/L
Serum Na	Low, normal, or high	Normal or low
Serum K	Normal; elevated with acidosis, low following dehydration	Normal or low
BUN	>20 mg/dL; elevated because of dehydration	Elevated
Creatinine	>1.5 mg/dL; elevated because of dehydration	Elevated
Urine ketones	Positive	Negative

BUN, Blood urea nitrogen; *DKA*, diabetic ketoacidosis; *HCO_3*, bicarbonate; *K*, potassium; *Na*, sodium.
Adapted from Ignatavicius, D., & Workman, M. (2010). *Medical-surgical nursing: Patient-centered collaborative care* (6th ed.). St. Louis: Saunders.

hypokalemia. Ensure adequate renal function before administering potassium.

5. Client education (Box 45-11)

> ⚠ Monitor the client being treated for DKA closely for signs of increased intracranial pressure. If the blood glucose level falls too far or too fast before the brain has time to equilibrate, water is pulled from the blood to the cerebrospinal fluid and the brain, causing cerebral edema and increased intracranial pressure.

C. Hyperglycemic hyperosmolar state (HHS)
1. Description
   a. Extreme **hyperglycemia** occurs without ketosis and acidosis.
   b. The syndrome occurs most often among individuals with type 2 **diabetes mellitus**.
   c. The major difference between HHS and DKA is that ketosis and acidosis do not occur with HHS. Enough insulin is present with HHS to prevent the breakdown of fats for energy, thus preventing ketosis.
2. Data collection (see Table 45-2)
3. Interventions
   a. Treatment is similar to that for DKA.
   b. Treatment includes fluid replacement, the correction of electrolyte imbalances, and insulin administration.
   c. Fluid replacement in the older client must be done very carefully secondary to the potential for heart failure.
   d. Insulin plays a less critical role in the treatment of HHS than it does for the treatment of DKA, because ketosis and acidosis do not occur. Rehydration alone may decrease glucose levels.

Box 45-11 Client Education: Guidelines During Illness

Take insulin or oral antidiabetic medications, as prescribed.
Test the blood glucose level and the urine for ketones every 3 to 4 hours.
If the usual meal plan cannot be followed, substitute soft foods 6 to 8 times a day.
If vomiting, diarrhea, or fever occurs, consume liquids every 30 minutes to 1 hour to prevent dehydration and to provide calories.
Notify the HCP if vomiting, diarrhea, or fever persists; if blood glucose levels are greater than 250 to 300 mg/dL; when ketonuria is present for more than 24 hours; if unable to take food or fluids for a period of 4 hours; or if illness persists for more than 2 days.

IX. CHRONIC COMPLICATIONS OF DIABETES MELLITUS

A. Diabetic retinopathy
1. Description
   a. A chronic and progressive impairment of the retinal circulation that eventually causes hemorrhage
   b. Permanent vision changes and blindness can occur.
   c. The client has difficulty with carrying out the daily tasks of blood glucose testing and insulin injections.
2. Data collection
   a. A change in vision is caused by the rupture of small microaneurysms in the retinal blood vessels.
   b. Blurred vision results from macular edema.
   c. A sudden loss of vision results from retinal detachment.
   d. Cataracts result from lens opacity.
3. Interventions
   a. Maintain safety.
   b. Early prevention via the control of hypertension and blood glucose levels
   c. Photocoagulation (laser therapy) removes hemorrhagic tissue to decrease scarring and prevent the progression of the disease process.
   d. Vitrectomy removes vitreous hemorrhages and decreases tension on the retina, thus preventing detachment.
   e. Cataract removal with a lens implant improves vision.

B. Diabetic nephropathy
1. Description: A progressive decrease in kidney function
2. Data collection
   a. Microalbuminuria
   b. Thirst
   c. Fatigue
   d. Anemia
   e. Weight loss
   f. Signs of malnutrition
   g. Frequent urinary tract infections
   h. Signs of a neurogenic bladder
3. Interventions
   a. Early prevention measures include the control of hypertension and blood glucose levels.
   b. Monitor vital signs.
   c. Monitor intake and output.
   d. Monitor blood urea nitrogen and creatinine levels, as well as urine albumin levels.
   e. Restrict dietary protein, sodium, and potassium intake, as prescribed.
   f. Avoid nephrotoxic medications.
   g. Prepare the client for dialysis procedures, as prescribed.

h. Prepare the client for kidney transplant, as prescribed.

i. Prepare the client for pancreas transplant, as prescribed.

C. Diabetic neuropathy

1. Description
   a. A general deterioration of the nervous system throughout the body.
   b. Complications include the development of nonhealing ulcers of the feet, gastric paresis, and erectile dysfunction.

2. Classifications
   a. Focal or mononeuropathy: Involves a single nerve or a group of nerves, most frequently cranial nerves III (oculomotor) and VI (abducens), and results in diplopia. It usually resolves spontaneously.
   b. Sensory or peripheral neuropathy: Affects the distal portion of the nerves, most frequently in the lower extremities.
   c. Autonomic neuropathy: Symptoms vary according to the organ system involved.
   d. Cardiovascular: Cardiac denervation syndrome (i.e., the heart rate does not respond to changes in oxygenation needs) and orthostatic hypotension occur.
   e. Pupillary: Pupil does not dilate in response to decreased light
   f. Gastric: Decreased gastric emptying (gastroparesis)
   g. Urinary: Neurogenic bladder
   h. Sudomotor: Decreased sweating
   i. Adrenal: Hypoglycemic unawareness
   j. Reproductive: Impotence (male) and painful intercourse (female)

3. Data collection
   a. Paresthesias
   b. Decreased or absent reflexes
   c. Decreased sensation to vibration or light touch
   d. Pain, aching, and burning in the lower extremities
   e. Poor peripheral pulses
   f. Skin breakdown and signs of infection
   g. Weakness or loss of sensation in cranial nerves III (oculomotor), IV (trochlear), V (trigeminal), or VI (abducens)
   h. Dizziness and postural hypotension
   i. Nausea and vomiting
   j. Diarrhea or constipation
   k. Incontinence
   l. Dyspareunia
   m. Impotence
   n. Hypoglycemic unawareness

4. Interventions
   a. Early prevention measures include the control of hypertension and blood glucose levels.

b. Careful foot care is required to prevent trauma (Box 45-12).

c. Administer medications for pain relief, as prescribed.

d. Initiate bladder-training programs.

e. Instruct the client regarding the use of estrogen-containing lubricants for women with dyspareunia.

f. Prepare the male client with impotence for penile injections or implantable devices, as prescribed.

g. Prepare for surgical decompression of compression lesions related to the cranial nerves, as prescribed.

X. CARE OF THE DIABETIC CLIENT UNDERGOING SURGERY

A. Preoperative care

1. Check with the HCP regarding withholding oral hypoglycemic medications or insulin.
2. Some long-acting oral antidiabetic medications are discontinued 24 to 48 hours before surgery.

Box 45-12 Preventive Foot Care Instructions

Provide meticulous skin care and proper foot care.

Inspect the feet daily and monitor them for redness, swelling, or breaks in skin integrity.

Notify the HCP if redness or a break in the skin occurs.

Avoid thermal injuries from hot water, heating pads, and baths.

Wash the feet with warm (not hot) water, and dry them thoroughly (avoid foot soaks).

Consult a podiatrist for treating corns, blisters, or ingrown toenails.

Do not cross the legs or wear tight garments that may constrict blood flow.

Apply moisturizing lotion to the feet, but not between the toes.

Prevent moisture from accumulating between the toes.

Wear loose socks and well-fitting (not tight) shoes, and instruct the client not to go barefoot.

Wear clean cotton socks to keep the feet warm, and change the socks daily.

Do not wear the same pair of shoes 2 days in a row.

Do not wear open-toed shoes or shoes with a strap that goes between the toes.

Check the shoes for cracks or tears in the lining and for foreign objects before putting them on.

Break in new shoes gradually.

Cut the toenails straight across, and smooth the nails with an emery board.

Do not smoke.

3. Metformin (Glucophage) may need to be discontinued 48 hours before surgery, and it may not be restarted until renal function is normal postoperatively.
4. All other oral antidiabetic medications are stopped the day of surgery.
5. The insulin dose may be adjusted or withheld if IV insulin administration during surgery is planned.
6. Monitor the blood glucose level.
7. Administer IV fluids, as prescribed.

B. Intraoperative care
1. Monitor the blood glucose levels frequently.
2. Administer IV short- or rapid-acting insulin, as prescribed, to maintain blood glucose levels less than 200 mg/dL.

C. Postoperative care
1. Administer IV glucose and regular insulin infusions, as prescribed, until the client can tolerate oral feedings.
2. Administer supplemental short-acting insulin, as prescribed, on the basis of blood glucose results.
3. Monitor blood glucose levels frequently if the client is receiving parenteral nutrition.
4. When the client is tolerating food, ensure that he or she receives an adequate amount of carbohydrates daily to prevent **hypoglycemia** and ketosis.
5. The client is at higher risk for cardiovascular and renal complications postoperatively.
6. The client is also at risk for impaired wound healing.

MORE QUESTIONS ON EVOLVE!

Practice Questions

446. A nurse is caring for a client after thyroidectomy and notes that calcium gluconate is prescribed for the client. The nurse determines that this medication has been prescribed to:
1. Treat thyroid storm.
2. Prevent cardiac irritability.
3. Treat hypocalcemic tetany.
4. Stimulate the release of parathyroid hormone.

447. A nurse is collecting data regarding a client after a thyroidectomy and notes that the client has developed hoarseness and a weak voice. Which nursing action is appropriate?
1. Check for signs of bleeding.
2. Administer calcium gluconate.
3. Notify the registered nurse immediately.
4. Reassure the client that this is usually a temporary condition.

448. A client is admitted to the emergency department, and a diagnosis of myxedema coma is made. Which nursing action would the nurse prepare to carry out initially?
1. Warm the client.
2. Maintain a patent airway.
3. Infuse intravenous fluids.
4. Administer thyroid hormone.

449. A nurse is assisting with preparing a teaching plan for the client with diabetes mellitus regarding proper foot care. Which instruction should be included in the plan of care?
1. Soak the feet in hot water.
2. Avoid using soap to wash the feet.
3. Apply a moisturizing lotion to dry feet, but not between the toes.
4. Always have a podiatrist cut your toenails; never cut them yourself.

450. A nurse provides dietary instructions to a client with diabetes mellitus regarding the prescribed diabetic diet. Which statement, if made by the client, indicates the need for further teaching?
1. "I'll eat a balanced meal plan."
2. "I need to drink diet soft drinks."
3. "I need to buy special dietetic foods."
4. "I will snack on fruit instead of cake."

451. A client who has been newly diagnosed with diabetes mellitus has been stabilized with daily insulin injections. Which information should the nurse teach when carrying out plans for discharge?
1. Keep insulin vials refrigerated at all times.
2. Rotate the insulin injection sites systematically.
3. Increase the amount of insulin before unusual exercise.
4. Monitor the urine acetone level to determine the insulin dosage.

452. A nurse reinforces teaching with a client with diabetes mellitus regarding differentiating between hypoglycemia and ketoacidosis. The client demonstrates an understanding of the teaching by stating that glucose will be taken if which symptom develops?
1. Polyuria
2. Shakiness
3. Blurred vision
4. Fruity breath odor

453. When the nurse is teaching a client who has been newly diagnosed with type 1 diabetes mellitus, which statement by the client would indicate that teaching has been effective?

1. "I will stop taking my insulin if I'm too sick to eat."
2. "I will decrease my insulin dose during times of illness."
3. "I will adjust my insulin dose according to the level of glucose in my urine."
4. "I will notify my health care provider if my blood glucose level is greater than 250 mg/dL."

454. A nurse is monitoring a client who has been newly diagnosed with diabetes mellitus for signs of complications. Which of the following, if exhibited by the client, would indicate hyperglycemia and thus warrant health care provider notification?
1. Polyuria
2. Bradycardia
3. Diaphoresis
4. Hypertension

455. A nurse is reinforcing instructions with a client with diabetes mellitus who is recovering from diabetic ketoacidosis (DKA) regarding measures to prevent a recurrence. Which instruction is important for the nurse to emphasize?
1. Eat six small meals daily.
2. Test the urine ketone levels.
3. Monitor blood glucose levels frequently.
4. Receive appropriate follow-up health care.

456. A nurse is reviewing discharge teaching with a client who has Cushing's syndrome. Which statement by the client indicates that the instructions related to dietary management were understood?
1. "I can eat foods that contain potassium."
2. "I will need to limit the amount of protein in my diet."
3. "I am fortunate that I can eat all the salty foods I enjoy."
4. "I am fortunate that I do not need to follow any special diet."

457. A client with type 1 diabetes mellitus calls the nurse to report recurrent episodes of hypoglycemia. Which statement by the client indicates a correct understanding of NPH insulin and exercise?
1. "I should not exercise after lunch."
2. "I should not exercise after breakfast."
3. "I should not exercise in the late evening."
4. "I should not exercise in the late afternoon."

458. A nurse is caring for a postoperative parathyroidectomy client. Which of the following would require the nurse's immediate attention?
1. Incisional pain
2. Laryngeal stridor
3. Difficulty voiding
4. Abdominal cramps

459. When a nurse notes that a client with type 1 diabetes mellitus has lipodystrophy on both upper thighs, what information should the nurse obtain from the client?
1. Plan of injection rotation
2. Consistency of aspiration
3. Preparation of the injection site
4. Angle at which the medication is administered

460. A hospitalized client with type 1 diabetes mellitus received NPH and regular insulin 2 hours ago at 7:30 AM. The client calls the nurse and reports that he is feeling hungry, shaky, and weak. The client ate breakfast at 8:00 and is due to eat lunch at noon. List, in order of priority, the actions that the nurse would take. (Number 1 is the first action.)
___ Take the client's vital signs.
___ Retest the client's blood glucose level.
___ Check the client's blood glucose level.
___ Give the client half a cup of fruit juice to drink.
___ Give the client a small snack of carbohydrate and protein.
___ Document the client's complaints, the actions taken, and the outcome.

ANSWERS

446. 3
Rationale: Hypocalcemia can develop after thyroidectomy if the parathyroid glands are accidentally removed or injured during surgery. Manifestations develop 1 to 7 days after surgery. If the client develops numbness and tingling around the mouth, fingertips, or toes or muscle spasms or twitching, the health care provider is notified immediately. Calcium gluconate should be kept at the bedside.
Test-Taking Strategy: Noting the name of the medication (calcium gluconate) should easily direct you to the correct option. Calcium is given if hypocalcemic tetany occurs. Review calcium gluconate if you had difficulty with this question.

Level of Cognitive Ability: Analyzing
Client Needs: Physiological Integrity
Integrated Process: Nursing Process/Planning
Content Area: Pharmacology
References: deWit, p. 897. 2009.
Linton, pp. 1033, 1041. 2012.

447. 4
Rationale: Weakness and hoarseness of the voice can occur as a result of trauma of the laryngeal nerve. If this develops, the client should be reassured that the problem will subside in a few days. Unnecessary talking should be discouraged. It is not necessary to notify the registered nurse immediately. These signs

do not indicate bleeding or the need to administer calcium gluconate.

Test-Taking Strategy: Use the process of elimination. Options 1 and 2 can easily be eliminated, because they are unrelated to the signs presented in the question. From the remaining options, recall that these signs indicate a temporary condition. Review the expected findings after thyroidectomy if you had difficulty with this question.

Level of Cognitive Ability: Applying
Client Needs: Physiological Integrity
Integrated Process: Nursing Process/Implementation
Content Area: Adult Health/Endocrine
Reference: Ignatavicius, Workman, p. 1454. 2010.

448. 2

Rationale: The initial nursing action would be to maintain a patent airway. Oxygen would be administered, followed by fluid replacement. The nurse would also keep the client warm, monitor the vital signs, and administer thyroid hormones.

Test-Taking Strategy: Note the strategic words "carry out initially." All of the options are appropriate interventions, but the use of the ABCs—airway, breathing, and circulation—will direct you to the correct option. Review the care of the client with myxedema coma if you had difficulty with this question.

Level of Cognitive Ability: Applying
Client Needs: Physiological Integrity
Integrated Process: Nursing Process/Implementation
Content Area: Critical Care
Reference: Kunz Howard, Steinmann, p. 509. 2010.

449. 3

Rationale: The client should use a moisturizing lotion on his or her feet, but should avoid applying the lotion between the toes. The client should also be instructed to not soak the feet and to avoid hot water to prevent burns. The client may cut the toenails straight across and even with the toe itself, but he or she should consult a podiatrist if the toenails are thick or hard to cut or if his or her vision is poor. The client should be instructed to wash the feet daily with a mild soap.

Test-Taking Strategy: Use the process of elimination. Eliminate option 4 first because of the word "always," and eliminate option 1 because of the word "hot." From the remaining options, recalling the concern related to skin infection will assist you with eliminating option 2. Review diabetic foot care instructions if you had difficulty with this question.

Level of Cognitive Ability: Applying
Client Needs: Health Promotion and Maintenance
Integrated Process: Nursing Process/Planning
Content Area: Adult Health/Endocrine
Reference: Linton, p. 1052. 2012.

450. 3

Rationale: It is important to emphasize to the client and family that they are not eating a diabetic diet but rather following a balanced meal plan. Adherence to nutrition principles is an important component of diabetic management, and an individualized meal plan should be developed for the client. It is not necessary for the client to purchase special dietetic foods.

Test-Taking Strategy: Note the strategic words "indicates the need for further teaching." These words indicate a negative event query and ask you to select an option that is an incorrect statement. Basic principles related to the diabetic diet will direct you to the correct option. Review these principles if you had difficulty with this question.

Level of Cognitive Ability: Evaluating
Client Needs: Physiological Integrity
Integrated Process: Teaching and Learning
Content Area: Adult Health/Endocrine
References: deWit, pp. 912–913. 2009.
Linton, pp. 1056–1057. 2012.

451. 2

Rationale: Insulin dosages should not be adjusted or increased before unusual exercise. If acetone is found in the urine, it may possibly indicate the need for additional insulin. To minimize the discomfort associated with insulin injections, the insulin should be administered at room temperature. Injection sites should be systematically rotated from one area to another. The client should be instructed to give injections in one area, about 1 inch apart, until the whole area has been used and then to change to another site. This prevents dramatic changes in daily insulin absorption.

Test-Taking Strategy: Use the process of elimination. Eliminate option 1 first because of the words "at all times." Knowledge regarding insulin administration and the significance of acetone in the urine will assist you with eliminating options 3 and 4. Review insulin management if you had difficulty with this question.

Level of Cognitive Ability: Applying
Client Needs: Physiological Integrity
Integrated Process: Teaching and Learning
Content Area: Pharmacology
References: deWit, p. 917. 2009.
Linton, p. 1061. 2012.

452. 2

Rationale: Shakiness is a sign of hypoglycemia, and it would indicate the need for food or glucose. Fruity breath odor, blurred vision, and polyuria are signs of hyperglycemia.

Test-Taking Strategy: Knowledge regarding the signs and symptoms of hypoglycemia and hyperglycemia is required to answer this question. Remember that shakiness is a sign of hypoglycemia. Review the signs and symptoms of hypoglycemia and hyperglycemia if you had difficulty with this question.

Level of Cognitive Ability: Evaluating
Client Needs: Physiological Integrity
Integrated Process: Nursing Process/Evaluation
Content Area: Adult Health/Endocrine
Reference: deWit, p. 926. 2009.

453. 4

Rationale: During illness, the client should monitor the blood glucose level, and he or she should notify the health care provider (HCP) if the level is greater than 250 mg/dL. Insulin should never be stopped. In fact, insulin may need to be increased during times of illness. Doses should not be adjusted without the HCP's advice.

Test-Taking Strategy: Use the process of elimination. Note that options 1, 2, and 3 all relate to the adjustment of insulin

doses; therefore, eliminate these options. Review diabetic management during illness if you had difficulty with this question.
Level of Cognitive Ability: Evaluating
Client Needs: Physiological Integrity
Integrated Process: Nursing Process/Evaluation
Content Area: Adult Health/Endocrine
References: deWit, p. 927. 2009.
Linton, pp. 1064–1065. 2012.

454. 1
Rationale: The classic symptoms of hyperglycemia include polydipsia, polyuria, and polyphagia. Options 2, 3, and 4 are not signs of hyperglycemia.
Test-Taking Strategy: Focus on the subject, hyperglycemia. Remember the 3 Ps—polyuria, polydipsia, and polyphagia. Review the signs of hyperglycemia if you had difficulty with this question.
Level of Cognitive Ability: Understanding
Client Needs: Physiological Integrity
Integrated Process: Nursing Process/Data Collection
Content Area: Adult Health/Endocrine
References: deWit, p. 926. 2009.
Linton, p. 1048. 2012.

455. 3
Rationale: Client education after DKA should emphasize the need for home glucose monitoring four to five times per day. It is also important to instruct the client to notify the health care provider when illness occurs. The presence of urinary ketones indicates that DKA has already occurred. The client should eat well-balanced meals with snacks, as prescribed.
Test-Taking Strategy: Focus on the subject of preventing DKA. Recall that the treatment of DKA focuses on the maintenance of an appropriate blood glucose level. Option 1 is not an accurate component of diabetic care. Option 4 will not prevent DKA. Option 2 does not prevent DKA but helps to confirm the diagnosis. Review DKA if you had difficulty with this question.
Level of Cognitive Ability: Applying
Client Needs: Health Promotion and Maintenance
Integrated Process: Teaching and Learning
Content Area: Adult Health/Endocrine
References: Christensen, Kockrow, p. 525. 2011. *Adult health nursing.*
deWit, p. 929. 2009.
Swearingen, p. 365. 2012.

456. 1
Rationale: A diet that is low in calories, carbohydrates, and sodium but ample in protein and potassium content is encouraged for a client with Cushing's syndrome. Such a diet promotes weight loss, the reduction of edema and hypertension, the control of hypokalemia, and the rebuilding of wasted tissue.
Test-Taking Strategy: Note the strategic words "instructions related to dietary management were understood." Eliminate option 4, because it indicates that no dietary change is necessary. Eliminate option 2 next, because protein is usually only limited with renal disorders. Excess sodium is not healthy in general, so eliminate option 3. Review the dietary management of Cushing's syndrome if you had difficulty with this question.

Level of Cognitive Ability: Evaluating
Client Needs: Physiological Integrity
Integrated Process: Nursing Process/Evaluation
Content Area: Adult Health/Endocrine
References: Christensen, Kockrow, p. 505. 2011. *Adult health nursing.*
Ignatavicius, Workman, p. 1443. 2010.

457. 4
Rationale: A hypoglycemic reaction may occur in response to increased exercise. Clients should avoid exercise during the peak time of insulin. NPH insulin peaks at 12 to 14 hours; therefore, late afternoon exercise would occur during the peak of the medication.
Test-Taking Strategy: Use the process of elimination, and note the strategic words "a correct understanding." Recalling the peak time of insulin will direct you to option 4. Review the measures to prevent hypoglycemia if you had difficulty with this question.
Level of Cognitive Ability: Evaluating
Client Needs: Physiological Integrity
Integrated Process: Nursing Process/Evaluation
Content Area: Adult Health/Endocrine
Reference: deWit, pp. 913–914. 2009.

458. 2
Rationale: During the postoperative period, the nurse carefully observes the client for signs of hemorrhage, which cause swelling and the compression of adjacent tissue. Laryngeal stridor is a harsh, high-pitched sound heard on inspiration and expiration that is caused by the compression of the trachea and that leads to respiratory distress. It is an acute emergency situation that requires immediate attention to avoid the complete obstruction of the airway.
Test-Taking Strategy: Consider the anatomical location of the surgical procedure, and use the ABCs—airway, breathing, and circulation—to select the correct option. Options 1, 3, and 4 are usual postoperative problems that are not life threatening. Option 2 addresses the airway. Review the care of the client after parathyroidectomy if you had difficulty with this question.
Level of Cognitive Ability: Analyzing
Client Needs: Physiological Integrity
Integrated Process: Nursing Process/Data Collection
Content Area: Adult Health/Endocrine
Reference: deWit, pp. 895, 897–898. 2009.

459. 1
Rationale: Lipodystrophy (i.e., the hypertrophy of subcutaneous tissue at the injection site) occurs in some diabetic clients when the same injection sites are used for prolonged periods of time. Thus, clients are instructed to adhere to a rotating injection site plan to avoid tissue changes. Preparation of the site, aspiration, and the angle of insulin administration do not produce tissue damage.
Test-Taking Strategy: Recalling the definition of lipodystrophy will direct you to the correct option. Remember that lipodystrophy is the hypertrophy of subcutaneous tissue at the injection site. Review this potential complication of insulin therapy if you had difficulty with this question.
Level of Cognitive Ability: Understanding

Client Needs: Physiological Integrity
Integrated Process: Nursing Process/Data Collection
Content Area: Adult Health/Endocrine
Reference: Swearingen, p. 350. 2012.

❖ **460. 3, 4, 1, 2, 5, 6**
Rationale: The client is experiencing symptoms of mild hypoglycemia. If symptoms such as hunger, irritability, shakiness, or weakness occur, the nurse first would check the client's blood glucose level to verify that the client is experiencing hypoglycemia. After this is verified, the nurse would give the client 10 to 15 g of carbohydrates and then retest the blood glucose level in 15 minutes. In the meantime, the nurse would check the client's vital signs. The nurse would give the client another food item containing 10 to 15 g of carbohydrate if the client's symptoms do not resolve. Otherwise, the nurse would provide a small snack of carbohydrates and protein if the client's next scheduled meal is more than an hour away from the time of the occurrence. After treatment and the resolution of the hypoglycemic event, the nurse would document the occurrence, the actions taken, and the outcome.

Test-Taking Strategy: Focus on the client's symptoms. Noting that the client is hospitalized will assist you with determining that the first action would be to check the client's blood glucose level. After this has been done, treating the hypoglycemia is necessary. Recalling that an outcome cannot be determined until treatment has been instituted will assist you with selecting the documentation action as the last action. From the remaining three actions, select taking the vital signs as the third action. The nurse would not give the client a carbohydrate and protein item immediately after giving the client a 10- to 15-g carbohydrate item or before retesting the blood glucose level. Review the management of hypoglycemia if you had difficulty with this question.
Level of Cognitive Ability: Analyzing
Client Needs: Physiological Integrity
Integrated Process: Nursing Process/Implementation
Content Area: Leadership/Management/Delegating/Prioritizing
References: Christensen, Kockrow, p. 524. 2011. *Adult health nursing.*
Linton, p. 1053. 2012.

Endocrine Medications

I. PITUITARY MEDICATIONS

A. Description
  1. The anterior pituitary gland secretes growth hormone (GH), thyroid-stimulating hormone (TSH), adrenocorticotropic hormone (ACTH), prolactin, melanocyte-stimulating hormone (MSH), and gonadotropins (follicle-stimulating hormone [FSH] and luteinizing hormone [LH]).
  2. The posterior pituitary gland secretes antidiuretic hormone (vasopressin) and oxytocin.

B. Growth hormones and related medications (Box 46-1)
  1. Uses
     a. Growth hormones are used to treat pediatric or adult growth hormone deficiency.
     b. Growth hormone receptor antagonists are used to treat acromegaly.
     c. Growth hormone releasing factor is used to evaluate anterior pituitary function.
  2. Side effects
     a. May vary depending on the medication
     b. Development of antibodies to growth hormone
     c. Headache, muscle pain, weakness, vertigo
     d. Diarrhea, nausea, abdominal discomfort
     e. Mild **hyperglycemia**
     f. Hypertension
     g. Weight gain
     h. Allergic reaction (rash, swelling), pain at injection site
     i. Elevated aspartate aminotransferase (AST) and alanine aminotransferase (ALT)
  3. Interventions
     a. Check the child's physical growth and compare growth with standards.
     b. Recommend annual bone age determinations for children receiving growth hormones.
     c. Monitor vital signs, blood glucose levels, AST and ALT levels, and thyroid function tests.
     d. Reinforce teaching to the client and family about the clinical manifestations of **hyperglycemia** and about other side effects of therapy and the importance of follow-up regarding periodic blood tests.

II. ANTIDIURETIC HORMONES (Box 46-2)

A. Description
  1. Antidiuretic hormones enhance reabsorption of water in the kidneys, promoting an antidiuretic effect and regulating fluid balance.
  2. Antidiuretic hormones are used in **diabetes insipidus**.

B. Side effects
  1. Flushing
  2. Headache
  3. Nausea and abdominal cramps
  4. Water intoxication
  5. Hypertension with water intoxication
  6. Nasal congestion with nasal administration

C. Interventions
  1. Monitor weight.
  2. Monitor intake and output and urine osmolality.
  3. Monitor electrolyte levels.
  4. Monitor for signs of dehydration, indicating the need to increase the dosage.
  5. Monitor for signs of water intoxication (drowsiness, listlessness, shortness of breath, and headache), indicating need to decrease dosage.
  6. Monitor blood pressure.
  7. Instruct the client in how to use the intranasal medication.
  8. Instruct the client to weigh himself or herself daily to identify weight gain.
  9. Instruct the client to report signs of water intoxication or symptoms of headache or shortness of breath.

III. THYROID HORMONES (Box 46-3)

A. Description
  1. Thyroid hormones control the metabolic rate of tissues and accelerate heat production and oxygen consumption.
  2. Thyroid hormones are used to replace the thyroid hormone deficit in conditions such as **hypothyroidism** and **myxedema**.
  3. Thyroid hormones enhance the action of oral anticoagulants, sympathomimetics, and antidepressants

and decrease the action of insulin, oral hypoglycemics, and digitalis preparations. The action of thyroid hormones is decreased by phenytoin (Dilantin) and carbamazepine (Tegretol).

4. Thyroid hormones should be given at least 4 hours apart from multivitamins, aluminum hydroxide and magnesium hydroxide, simethicone, calcium carbonate, bile acid sequestrants, iron, and sucralfate (Carafate) because these medications decrease the absorption of thyroid replacements.

B. Side effects
1. Nausea and decreased appetite
2. Abdominal cramps and diarrhea
3. Weight loss
4. Nervousness and tremors
5. Insomnia
6. Sweating and heat intolerance
7. Tachycardia, dysrhythmias, palpitations, chest pain
8. Hypertension
9. Headache
10. Toxicity: **Hyperthyroidism**

C. Interventions
1. The client is assessed for a history of medications currently being taken.
2. Monitor vital signs.
3. Monitor weight.
4. Monitor triiodothyronine, thyroxine, and thyroid-stimulating hormone levels.
5. The client is instructed to take the medication at the same time each day, in the morning without food.
6. The client is instructed in how to monitor the pulse rate.
7. The client is instructed to avoid foods that can inhibit thyroid secretion, such as strawberries, peaches, pears, cabbage, turnips, spinach, kale, Brussels sprouts, cauliflower, radishes, and peas.
8. The client is advised to avoid over-the-counter medications.
9. The client is instructed to wear a Medic-Alert bracelet.

 The client taking a thyroid hormone is instructed to report symptoms of hyperthyroidism, such as tachycardia, chest pain, palpitations, and excessive sweating. These indicate signs of toxicity.

IV. ANTITHYROID MEDICATIONS (Box 46-4)

A. Description
1. Antithyroid medications inhibit the synthesis of thyroid hormone.
2. Antithyroid medications are used for **hyperthyroidism**, or Graves' disease.

B. Side effects
1. Nausea and vomiting
2. Diarrhea
3. Drowsiness, headache, fever
4. Hypersensitivity with skin rash
5. Agranulocytosis with leukopenia and thrombocytopenia
6. Alopecia and hyperpigmentation
7. Toxicity: **Hypothyroidism**
8. Iodism: Characterized by vomiting, abdominal pain, metallic or brassy taste in the mouth, rash, and sore gums and salivary glands

---

Box 46-1 Growth Hormones and Related Medications

Growth Hormones
Somatropin (Humatrope)
Mecasermin (Increlex)

Growth Hormone Receptor Antagonists
Octreotide acetate (Sandostatin)
Pegvisomant (Somavert)

Growth Hormone Releasing Factor
Sermorelin (Geref)

Box 46-2 Antidiuretic Hormones

Desmopressin acetate (DDAVP, Stimate, Minirin)
Vasopressin (Pitressin)

Box 46-3 Thyroid Hormones

Levothyroxine sodium (Synthroid, Levothroid, Levoxyl, Thyro-Tabs, Unithroid)
Liothyronine sodium (Cytomel, Triostat)
Liotrix (Thyrolar)
Thyroid (Armour Thyroid, Bio-Throid, Nature-Throid, Thyroid USP, Westhroid)

Box 46-4 Antithyroid Medications

Methimazole (Tapazole)
Propylthiouracil (PTU)
Strong iodine solution (Lugol's solution)
Potassium iodide
Iodide,[131] (Iodotope)

C. Interventions
1. Monitor vital signs.
2. Monitor triiodothyronine, thyroxine, and thyroid-stimulating hormone levels.
3. Monitor weight.
4. The client is instructed to take medication with meals to avoid gastrointestinal upset.
5. The client is instructed in how to monitor the pulse rate.
6. The client is informed of side effects and when to notify the health care provider (HCP).
7. The client is instructed in the signs of **hypothyroidism**.
8. The client is instructed regarding the importance of medication compliance and that abruptly stopping the medication could cause **thyroid storm**.
9. The client is instructed to monitor for signs and symptoms of **thyroid storm** (fever, flushed skin, confusion and behavioral changes, tachycardia, dysrhythmias, and signs of heart failure).
10. The client is instructed to monitor for signs of iodism.
11. The client is advised to consult the HCP before eating iodized salt and iodine-rich foods.
12. The client is instructed to avoid acetylsalicylic acid (aspirin) and medications containing iodine.

⚠ Propylthiouracil (PTU) causes agranulocytosis. Therefore, the client is advised to contact the HCP if a fever or sore throat develops.

V. PARATHYROID MEDICATIONS (Box 46-5)

A. Description
1. Parathyroid hormone regulates serum calcium levels.
2. Low serum levels of calcium stimulate parathyroid hormone release.
3. Hyperparathyroidism results in a high serum calcium level and bone demineralization. Medication is used to lower the serum calcium level.
4. Hypoparathyroidism results in a low serum calcium level, which increases neuromuscular excitability. Treatment includes calcium and vitamin D supplements.
5. Calcium salts administered with digoxin (Lanoxin) increases the risk of digoxin toxicity.
6. Oral calcium salts reduce the absorption of tetracycline hydrochloride.

B. Interventions
1. Monitor electrolyte and calcium levels.
2. Monitor for signs and symptoms of hypocalcemia and hypercalcemia.
3. Monitor for symptoms of tetany in the client with hypocalcemia.

4. Monitor for renal calculi in the client with hypercalcemia.
5. The client is instructed in the signs and symptoms of hypercalcemia and hypocalcemia.
6. The client is instructed to check over-the-counter medication labels for the possibility of calcium content.
7. The client receiving oral calcium supplements is instructed to maintain an adequate intake of vitamin D because vitamin D enhances absorption of calcium.
8. The client receiving calcium regulators such as alendronate sodium (Fosamax) is instructed to swallow the tablet whole with water at least 30 minutes before breakfast and not to lie down for at least 30 minutes.
9. The client using nasal spray of calcitonin (Calcimar) is instructed to alternate nares.
10. The client using antihypercalcemic agents is instructed to avoid foods rich in calcium such as green, leafy vegetables, dairy products, shellfish, and soy.
11. The client is instructed not to take other medications within 1 hour of taking a calcium salt.

Box 46-5 Medications to Treat Calcium Disorders

Oral Calcium Supplements
Calcium acetate (PhosLo)
Calcium carbonate (Rolaids, Tums, others)
Calcium chloride
Calcium citrate (Citracal)
Calcium glubionate (Calcionate, Calciquid)
Calcium gluconate
Calcium lactate (Cak-lac)
Tribasic calcium phosphate (Posture)

Vitamin D Supplements
Cholecalciferol (Vitamin D_3)
Ergocalciferol (Vitamin D_2)

Bisphosphonates and Calcium Regulators
Alendronate sodium (Fosamax)
Calcitonin salmon (Calcimar, Cibacalcin, Fortical)
Etidronate disodium (Didronel)
Ibandronate (Boniva)
Pamidronate disodium (Aredia)
Risedronate sodium (Actonel)
Tiludronate disodium (Skelid)
Zoledronate (Reclast)
Zoledronate (Zometa)

Medications to Treat Hypercalcemia
Cinacalcet hydrochloride (Sensipar)
Doxercalciferol (Hectorol)
Gallium nitrate (Ganite)
Paricalcitol (Zemplar)

12. The client is instructed to increase fluid and fiber in the diet to prevent constipation associated with calcium supplements.

VI. CORTICOSTEROIDS (MINERALOCORTICOIDS)
(Box 46-6)

A. Description
1. Mineralocorticoids are steroid hormones that enhance the reabsorption of sodium and chloride and promote the excretion of potassium and hydrogen from the renal tubules, thereby helping maintain fluid and electrolyte balance.
2. Mineralocorticoids are used for replacement - therapy in primary and secondary adrenal insufficiency in **Addison's disease**.

B. Side effects
1. Sodium and water retention (hypernatremia and edema), hypertension
2. Hypokalemia
3. Hypocalcemia
4. Osteoporosis, compression fractures
5. Weight gain
6. Heart failure

C. Interventions
1. Monitor vital signs.
2. Monitor intake and output and weight and for edema.
3. Monitor electrolyte and calcium levels.
4. The client is instructed to take medication with food or milk.
5. The client is instructed to consume a high-potassium diet.
6. The client is instructed to report illness, such as severe diarrhea, vomiting, and fever.
7. The client is instructed to notify the HCP if low blood pressure, weakness, cramping, palpitations, or changes in mental status occur.
8. The client is instructed to wear a Medic-Alert bracelet.

⚠ The client taking a corticosteroid is instructed not to stop the medication abruptly because this could result in adrenal insufficiency.

VII. CORTICOSTEROIDS (GLUCOCORTICOIDS)
(Box 46-7)

A. Description
1. Glucocorticoids affect glucose, protein, and bone metabolism, alter the normal immune response and suppress inflammation, and produce anti-inflammatory, antiallergic, and antistress effects.
2. Glucocorticoids may be used as a replacement for adrenocortical insufficiency.

B. Side effects
1. **Hyperglycemia**
2. Hypokalemia
3. Hypocalcemia, osteoporosis
4. Sodium and fluid retention
5. Weight gain
6. Mood swings
7. Moon face, buffalo hump, truncal obesity
8. Increased susceptibility to infection and masking of the signs and symptoms of infection
9. Cataracts
10. Hirsutism, acne, fragile skin, bruising
11. Growth retardation in children
12. Gastrointestinal (GI) irritation, peptic ulcer, pancreatitis
13. Seizures, psychosis

C. Contraindications and cautions
1. Contraindicated in clients with hypersensitivity, psychosis, and fungal infections
2. Should be used with caution in clients with **diabetes mellitus**
3. Used with extreme caution in clients with infections because they mask the signs and symptoms of an infection
4. Increase the potency of medications taken concurrently, such as aspirin, and nonsteroidal anti-inflammatory drugs, thus increasing the risk of gastrointestinal bleeding and ulceration.
5. Use of potassium-wasting diuretics increases potassium loss, resulting in hypokalemia.
6. Dexamethasone decreases the effects of orally administered anticoagulants and antidiabetic agents.
7. Barbiturates, phenytoin (Dilantin), and rifampin (Rifadin) decrease the effect of prednisone.

D. Interventions
1. Monitor vital signs.
2. Monitor serum electrolyte and blood glucose levels.
3. Monitor for hypokalemia and **hyperglycemia**.
4. Monitor intake and output and weight and for edema.
5. Monitor for hypertension.

Box 46-6 Corticosteroid: Mineralocorticoid

Fludrocortisone acetate

Box 46-7 Corticosteroids: Glucocorticoids

Betamethasone
Cortisone acetate
Dexamethasone
Hydrocortisone
Methylprednisolone
Prednisolone
Prednisone
Triamcinolone

6. Check medical history for glaucoma, cataracts, peptic ulcer, mental health disorders, or **diabetes mellitus**.
7. Monitor the older client for signs and symptoms of increased osteoporosis.
8. Check for changes in muscle strength.
9. Prepare a schedule for the client with information on short-term tapered doses.
10. The client is instructed that it is best to take medication in the early morning.
11. The client is advised to eat foods high in potassium.
12. The client is instructed to avoid individuals with respiratory infections.
13. The client is advised to inform all HCPs of the medication regimen.
14. The client is instructed to report signs and symptoms of a medication overdose or **Cushing's syndrome**, including a moon face, puffy eyelids, edema in the feet, increased bruising, dizziness, bleeding, and menstrual irregularities.
15. Note that the client may need additional doses during periods of stress, such as surgery.
16. The client is instructed not to stop the medication abruptly because abrupt withdrawal can result in severe adrenal insufficiency.
17. The client is advised to consult with the HCP before receiving vaccinations.
18. The client is advised to wear a Medic-Alert bracelet.

VIII. ANDROGENS (Box 46-8)

A. Description
1. Used to replace deficient hormones or to treat hormone-sensitive disorders
2. Can cause bleeding if the client is taking oral anticoagulants (increase the effect of anticoagulants)
3. Can cause decreased serum glucose concentration, thereby reducing insulin requirements in the client with **diabetes mellitus**
4. Hepatotoxic medications are avoided with the use of androgens because of the risk of additive damage to the liver.
5. Androgens usually are avoided in men with known prostate or breast carcinoma because androgens often stimulate growth of these tumors.

Box 46-8 Androgens

Fluoxymesterone
Methyltestosterone (Testred)
Testosterone preparations:
- Testosterone, pellets (Testopel)
- Testosterone, transdermal (Androderm)
- Testosterone cypionate (Depo-Testosterone)
- Testosterone enanthate (Delatestryl)
- Testosterone (Striant)

B. Side effects
1. Masculine secondary sexual characteristics (body hair growth, lowered voice, muscle growth)
2. Bladder irritation and urinary tract infections
3. Breast tenderness
4. Gynecomastia
5. Priapism
6. Menstrual irregularities
7. Virilism
8. Sodium and water retention with edema
9. Nausea, vomiting, or diarrhea
10. Acne
11. Changes in libido
12. Hepatotoxicity, jaundice
13. Hypercalcemia

C. Interventions
1. Monitor vital signs.
2. Monitor for edema, weight gain, and skin changes.
3. Check mental status and neurological function.
4. Check for signs of liver dysfunction, including right upper quadrant abdominal pain, malaise, fever, jaundice, and pruritus.
5. Check for the development of secondary sexual characteristics.
6. The client is instructed to take medication with meals or a snack.
7. The client is instructed to notify the HCP if priapism develops.
8. The client is instructed to notify the HCP if fluid retention occurs.
9. Women are instructed to use a nonhormonal contraceptive while on therapy.
10. For women, monitor for menstrual irregularities and decreased breast size.

IX. ESTROGENS AND PROGESTINS

A. Description
1. Estrogens are steroids that stimulate female reproductive tissue.
2. Progestins are steroids that specifically stimulate the uterine lining.
3. Estrogen and progestin preparations may be used to stimulate the endogenous hormones to restore hormonal balance or to treat hormone-sensitive tumors (suppress tumor growth) or for contraception (Boxes 46-9 and 46-10).

Box 46-9 Estrogens

Esterified estrogens (Menest)
Estradiol (Estrace, Femtrace)
Estrogens, conjugated (Premarin, Cenestin, Enjuvia)
Ethinyl estradiol (Estinyl)

B. Contraindications and cautions
1. Estrogens
   a. Estrogens are contraindicated in clients with breast cancer, endometrial hyperplasia, endometrial cancer, history of thromboembolism, known or suspected pregnancy, or lactation.
   b. Use estrogens with caution in clients with hypertension, gallbladder disease, or liver or kidney dysfunction.
   c. Estrogens increase the risk of toxicity when used with hepatotoxic medications.
   d. Barbiturates, phenytoin (Dilantin), and rifampin (Rifadin) decrease the effectiveness of estrogen.
2. Progestins are contraindicated in clients with thromboembolic disorders and should be avoided in clients with breast tumors or hepatic disease.

C. Side effects
1. Breast tenderness, menstrual changes
2. Nausea, vomiting, and diarrhea
3. Malaise, depression, excessive irritability
4. Weight gain
5. Edema and fluid retention
6. Atherosclerosis
7. Hypertension, stroke, myocardial infarction
8. Thromboembolism (estrogen)
9. Migraine headaches and vomiting (estrogen)

D. Interventions
1. Monitor vital signs.
2. Monitor for hypertension.
3. Check for edema and weight gain.
4. The client is advised not to smoke.
5. The client is advised to undergo routine breast and pelvic examinations.

X. CONTRACEPTIVES

A. Description
1. These medications contain a combination of estrogen and a progestin or a progestin alone.
2. Estrogen-progestin combinations suppress ovulation and change the cervical mucus, making it difficult for sperm to enter.

Box 46-10 Progestins

Estradiol/drospirenone (Angelic)
Estradiol/norgestimate (Prefest)
Estradiol/norethindrone (Femhrt)
Medroxyprogesterone acetate (Depo-Provera, Provera)
Medroxyprogesterone and conjugated estrogens (Premphase, Prempro)
Megestrol acetate (Megace)
Norethindrone acetate (Aygestin)
Norgestrel (Ovrette)
Progesterone (Prometrium)

---

3. Medications that contain only progestins are less effective than the combined medications.
4. Contraceptives usually are taken for 21 consecutive days and stopped for 7 days. The administration cycle is then repeated.
5. Contraceptives provide reversible prevention of pregnancy.
6. Contraceptives are useful in controlling irregular or excessive menstrual cycles.
7. Risk factors associated with the development of complications related to the use of contraceptives include smoking, obesity, and hypertension.
8. Contraceptives are contraindicated in women with hypertension, thromboembolic disease, cerebrovascular or coronary artery disease, estrogen-dependent cancers, and pregnancy.
9. Contraceptives should be avoided with the use of hepatotoxic medications.
10. Contraceptives interfere with the activity of bromocriptine mesylate (Parlodel) and anticoagulants and increase the toxicity of tricyclic antidepressants.
11. Contraceptives may alter blood glucose levels.
12. Antibiotics may decrease the absorption and effectiveness of oral contraceptives.

B. Side effects
1. Breakthrough bleeding
2. Excessive cervical mucus formation
3. Breast tenderness
4. Hypertension
5. Nausea, vomiting

C. Interventions
1. Monitor vital signs and weight.
2. The client is instructed in the administration of the medication. (It may take up to 1 week for full contraceptive effect to occur when the medication is begun.)
3. The client with **diabetes mellitus** is instructed to monitor blood glucose levels carefully.
4. The client is instructed to report signs of thromboembolic complications.
5. The client is instructed to notify the HCP if vaginal bleeding or menstrual irregularities occur or if pregnancy is suspected.
6. The client is advised to use an alternate method of birth control when taking antibiotics because these may decrease absorption of the oral contraceptive.
7. The client is instructed to perform breast self-examination monthly and about the importance of annual physical examinations.
8. Contraceptive patches
   a. Designed to be worn for 3 weeks and removed for a 1-week period
   b. Applied on clean, dry, intact skin on the buttocks, abdomen, upper outer arm, or upper torso

c. The client is instructed to peel away half of backing on patch, apply the sticky surface to the skin, remove the other half of the backing, and then press down on the patch with the palm for 10 seconds.

d. The client is instructed to change the patch weekly, using a new location for each patch.

e. If the patch falls off and remains off for less than 24 hours (such as when the client is sleeping or is unaware that it has fallen off), it can be reapplied if still sticky, or it can be replaced with a new patch.

f. If the patch is off for more than 24 hours, a new 4-week cycle must be started immediately.

9. Vaginal ring

a. Inserted into the vagina by the client, left in place for 3 weeks, and removed for 1 week

b. The medication is absorbed through mucous membranes of the vagina.

c. Removed rings should be wrapped in a foil pouch and discarded, not flushed down the toilet.

10. Implants and depot injections provide long-acting forms of birth control, from 3 months to 5 years in duration.

 If the client decides to discontinue the contraceptive to become pregnant, recommend that the client use an alternative form of birth control for 2 months after discontinuation to ensure more complete excretion of hormonal agents before conception.

XI. FERTILITY MEDICATIONS (Box 46-11)

A. Description

1. Fertility medications act to stimulate follicle development and ovulation in functioning ovaries and are combined with human chorionic gonadotropin to maintain the follicles once ovulation has occurred.

2. Fertility medications are contraindicated in the presence of primary ovarian dysfunction, thyroid or adrenal dysfunction, ovarian cysts, pregnancy, or idiopathic uterine bleeding.

Box 46-11 Fertility Medications

Chorionic gonadotropin (Profasi)
Clomiphene citrate (Clomid)
Follitropin alfa (Gonal-f)
Follitropin beta (Follistim AQ)
Menotropins (Pergonal, Repronex, Menopur)
Urotropin alfa (Bravelle, Fertinex, Metrodin)
Lutropin alfa (Luveris)

---

3. Fertility medications should be used with caution in clients with thromboembolic or respiratory disease.

B. Side effects

1. Risk of multiple births and birth defects
2. Ovarian overstimulation (abdominal pain, distention, ascites, pleural effusion)
3. Headache, irritability
4. Fluid retention and bloating
5. Nausea, vomiting
6. Uterine bleeding
7. Ovarian enlargement
8. Gynecomastia
9. Rash
10. Orthostatic hypotension
11. Febrile reactions

C. Interventions

1. The client is instructed regarding administration of the medication.
2. A calendar of treatment days is provided and instructions on when intercourse should occur to increase therapeutic effectiveness of the medication.
3. Information about the risks and hazards of multiple births is provided.
4. The client is instructed to notify the HCP if signs of ovarian overstimulation occur.
5. The client is informed about the need for regular follow-up for evaluation.

XII. MEDICATIONS FOR ERECTILE DYSFUNCTION

A. Description

1. Alprostadil (Caverject, Edex) is a prostaglandin that relaxes smooth muscle and promotes blood flow when injected directly into the corpus cavernosum.
2. Sildenafil (Viagra), tadalafil (Cialis), and vardenafil (Levitra) cause smooth muscle relaxation and allow blood flow into the corpus cavernosum.
3. Erectile dysfunction medications are contraindicated in the presence of any anatomical obstruction or condition that might predispose to priapism and in clients with penile implants.

4. Caution should be used in clients with bleeding disorders.
5. Sildenafil, tadalafil, and vardenafil are used cautiously in clients with coronary artery disease, active peptic ulcer disease, bleeding disorders, or retinitis pigmentosa.

6. Sildenafil, tadalafil, and vardenafil cannot be administered to clients taking nitrates, nitroprusside, or β-blockers (risk of severe hypotension).

B. Side effects

1. Alprostadil: Pain at the injection site, infection, priapism, fibrosis, rash, hypertension

2. Sildenafil, tadalafil, and vardenafil: Headache, flushing, dyspepsia, urinary tract infection, diarrhea, hypotension, dizziness, rash, neuralgia, insomnia
3. Blurred vision and changes in color vision

C. Interventions
1. A thorough assessment of health and medication history is performed.
2. The client is instructed regarding administration of the medication. Alprostadil is injected intracavernously. Sildenafil, tadalafil, and vardenafil are taken orally.
3. The client is informed of side effects necessitating the need to notify the HCP.

XIII. MEDICATIONS FOR DIABETES MELLITUS

A. Insulin and oral hypoglycemic medications
1. Description
   a. Insulin increases glucose transport into cells and promotes conversion of glucose to glycogen, decreasing serum glucose levels.
   b. Oral hypoglycemic agents stimulate the pancreas to produce more insulin, increase the sensitivity of peripheral receptors to insulin, decrease hepatic glucose output, or delay intestinal absorption of glucose, thus decreasing serum glucose levels.
2. Contraindications and concerns
   a. Insulin is contraindicated in clients with hypersensitivity.
   b. Oral hypoglycemic agents are contraindicated in type 1 **diabetes mellitus**.
   c. β-Adrenergic blocking agents may mask signs and symptoms of **hypoglycemia** associated with hypoglycemic medications.
   d. Anticoagulants, chloramphenicol (Chloromycetin), salicylates, propranolol (Inderal), monoamine oxidase inhibitors, pentamidine (Pentam 300), and sulfonamides may cause **hypoglycemia**.
   e. Corticosteroids, sympathomimetics, thiazide diuretics, phenytoin (Dilantin), thyroid preparations, oral contraceptives, and estrogen compounds may cause **hyperglycemia**.
   f. Side effects of the sulfonylureas include gastrointestinal symptoms and dermatological reactions. **Hypoglycemia** can occur when an excessive dose is administered or when meals are omitted or delayed, food intake is decreased, or activity is increased.

⚠ Sulfonylureas can cause a disulfiram (Antabuse) type of reaction when alcohol is ingested.

B. Oral hypoglycemic medications
1. Prescribed for clients with type 2 **diabetes mellitus**

2. Sulfonylureas (Box 46-12)
   a. Sulfonylureas may be classified as first- or second-generation sulfonylureas.
   b. Sulfonylureas stimulate the beta cells to produce more insulin.
3. Biguanides (see Box 46-12)
   a. May be used alone or in combination with a sulfonylurea
   b. Suppresses hepatic production of glucose and increases insulin sensitivity
   c. Side effects: Diarrhea (most common), lactic acidosis (most serious)
4. Alpha-glucosidase inhibitors (see Box 46-12)
   a. Delay absorption of ingested carbohydrates (sucrose and complex carbohydrates), resulting in smaller increase in blood glucose level after meals.
   b. Do not increase insulin production.
   c. Can be given alone or in combination with sulfonylureas
   d. Will not cause **hypoglycemia** when given alone
   e. Given with first bite of meal
5. Thiazolidinediones (see Box 46-12)
   a. Insulin-sensitizing agents that lower blood glucose by decreasing hepatic glucose production and improving target cell response to insulin
   b. May cause liver toxicity
6. Meglitinides (see Box 46-12)
   a. Stimulate pancreatic insulin secretion.

Box 46-12 Sulfonylureas and Nonsulfonylureas

Sulfonylureas
Acetohexamide (Dymelor)
Chlorpropamide (Diabinese)
Glimepiride (Amaryl)
Glipizide (Glucotrol)
Glyburide (DiaBeta, Micronase)
Tolazamide (Tolinase)
Tolbutamide (Orinase)

Biguanide
Metformin (Glucophage)

Alpha Glucosidase Inhibitors
Acarbose (Precose)
Miglitol (Glyset)

Thiazolidinediones
Pioglitazone (Actos)
Rosiglitazone (Avandia)

Meglitinides
Nateglinide (Starlix)
Repaglinide (Prandin)

Gliptins
Sitagliptin (Januvia)
Metformin and sitagliptin (Janumet)

b. Quicker and shorter duration of action; therefore, less chance of **hypoglycemia** because blood glucose–lowering effect wears off quickly

c. Very fast onset of action allows client to take the medication with meals and skip a dose when a meal is skipped

7. Interventions

a. The client's knowledge of **diabetes mellitus** and the use of oral antidiabetic agents is assessed.

b. A medication history regarding the medications that the client is taking currently is obtained.

c. Monitor vital signs and blood glucose levels.

d. The client is instructed to recognize the signs and symptoms of **hypoglycemia** and **hyperglycemia**.

e. The client is instructed to avoid over-the-counter medications unless prescribed by the HCP.

f. The client is instructed not to ingest alcohol with sulfonylureas.

g. The client is instructed that insulin may be needed during stress, surgery, or infection.

h. The client is instructed in the necessity of compliance with prescribed medication.

i. The client is instructed in how to take each specific medication, such as with the first bite of the meal for meglitinides and alpha-glucosidase inhibitors.

j. The client is advised to wear a Medic-Alert bracelet.

C. Insulin

1. Insulin primarily acts in the liver, muscle, and adipose tissue by attaching to receptors on cellular membranes and facilitating the passage of glucose, potassium, and magnesium.

2. Insulin is prescribed for clients with type 1 **diabetes mellitus** and type 2 **diabetes mellitus** in clients whose blood glucose level is not controlled with oral hypoglycemic agents.

3. The onset, peak, and duration of action depend on the insulin type (Table 46-1).

TABLE 46-1 Time Activity of Pharmacological Insulin*

Preparation	Brand	Onset (hr)	Peak (hr)	Duration (hr)
RAPID-ACTING INSULIN				
Insulin aspart	NovoLog	0.25	1-3	3-5
Insulin glulisine	Apidra	0.3	0.5-1.5	3-4
Human lispro injection	Humalog	0.25	0.5-1.5	5
SHORT-ACTING INSULIN				
Regular human insulin injection	Humulin R	0.5	2-4	5-7
	Novolin R	0.5	2.5-5	8
	ReliOn R			
Humulin R (concentrated U-500)	Humulin R (U 500)	1.5	4-12	24
INTERMEDIATE-ACTING INSULIN				
Isophane insulin NPH injection	Humulin N	1.5	4-12	16-24+
	Novolin N	1.5	4-12	16-24+
	ReliOn N			
Insulin detemir injection	Levemir	1	6-8	5.7-24
70% human insulin isophane suspension/30% human insulin injection	Humulin 70/30	0.5	2-12	24
	Novolin 70/30			
	ReliOn 70/30			
50% human insulin isophane suspension/50% human insulin injection	Humulin 50/50	0.5	3-5	24
70% insulin aspart protamine suspension/30% insulin aspart injection	NovoLog Mix 70/30	0.25	1-4	24
75% insulin lispro protamine suspension/25% insulin lispro injection	Humalog Mix 75/25	0.25	1-2	24
LONG-ACTING INSULIN				
Insulin glargine injection	Lantus	2-4	None	24

Time activity may be dose related.
From Ignatavicius, D., & Workman, M. (2010). *Medical surgical nursing: Patient-centered collaborative care* (6th ed.). St. Louis: Saunders.

4. Storing of insulin (Box 46-13)
5. Insulin injection sites
   a. The main areas for injections are the abdomen, arms (posterior surface), thighs (anterior surface), and hips (Figure 46-1).
   b. Insulin injected into the abdomen may absorb more evenly and rapidly than at other sites.
   c. Systematic rotation within one anatomical area is recommended to prevent lipodystrophy. The client should be instructed not to use the same site more than once in a 2- to 3-week period.
   d. Injections should be 1½ inches apart within the anatomical area.
   e. Heat, massage, and exercise of the injected area can increase absorption rates and may result in **hypoglycemia**.
   f. Injection into scar tissue may delay absorption of insulin.
6. Administering insulin

⚠️ Insulin glargine cannot be mixed with any other types of insulin.

Box 46-13 Storing Insulin

- Avoid exposing insulin to extremes in temperature.
- Insulin should not be frozen or kept in direct sunlight or a hot car.
- Before injection, insulin should be at room temperature.
- If a vial of insulin will be used up in 1 month, it may be kept at room temperature; otherwise, the vial should be refrigerated.

a. To prevent dosage errors, be certain that there is a match between the insulin concentration noted on the vial and the calibration of units on the insulin syringe. The usual concentration of insulin is U 100 (100 units/mL).
b. Most insulin syringes have a 27- to 29-gauge needle that is about ½-inch long.
c. Before use, the insulin vial is gently swirled or rotated between palms to ensure that the insulin and ingredients are mixed well. Otherwise, an inaccurate dose will be drawn. Vigorously shaking the bottle will cause bubbles to form.
d. Premixed insulins (NPH and regular insulin) are available as 70/30 (most commonly used) and 50/50. (Premixed insulin lispro protamine and insulin lispro 75/25 are also available.)
e. Air is injected into the insulin bottle. (A vacuum makes it difficult to draw up the insulin.)
f. When mixing insulins, the regular (shorter-acting) insulin is drawn up first (Figure 46-2).
g. Regular insulin may be mixed with NPH or Lente insulin.
h. Lispro insulin may be mixed with Humulin N or Humulin-U (Ultralente).

1 Wash hands.
2 Gently rotate NPH insulin bottle.
3 Wipe off tops of insulin vials with alcohol sponge.
4 Draw back amount of air into the syringe that equals total dose.
5 Inject air equal to NPH dose into NPH vial. Remove syringe from vial.   6 Inject air equal to regular dose into regular vial.

7 Invert regular insulin bottle and withdraw regular insulin dose.   8 Without adding more air to NPH vial, carefully withdraw NPH dose and add to regular insulin already in syringe.

Front   Back

▲ **FIGURE 46-1** Common insulin injection sites. (From Ignatavicius, D., & Workman, M. [2010]. *Medical surgical nursing: Patient-centered collaborative care* [6th ed.]. St. Louis: Saunders.)

▲ **FIGURE 46-2** Mixing insulins. (From Lewis, S., Heitkemper, M., & Dirksen, S. [2011]. *Medical-surgical nursing: Assessment and management of clinical problems* [8th ed.]. St. Louis: Mosby.)

i. Insulin aspart protamine may be mixed with NPH insulin only.

j. Insulin zinc suspensions may be mixed only with each other and regular insulin, not with other types of insulin.

k. A mixed dose of insulin is administered within 5 to 15 minutes of preparation. After this time, the regular insulin binds with the NPH insulin and its action is reduced.

l. Aspiration generally is not recommended with self-injection of insulin.

m. Insulin is administered at a 45- to 90-degree angle in clients with normal subcutaneous mass and at a 45- to 60-degree angle in thin persons or those with a decreased amount of subcutaneous mass.

⚠ Regular insulin is the only type of insulin that can be administered intravenously.

D. Exenatide (Byetta)

1. A synthetic hormone classified as an incretin mimetic that is administered subcutaneously.

2. Used for clients with type 2 **diabetes mellitus** (not recommended for clients taking insulin nor should clients be taken off of insulin and given exenatide)

3. Restores first-phase insulin response (first 10 minutes after food ingestion), lowers the production of glucagon after meals, slows gastric emptying (which limits the rise in the blood glucose level after a meal), reduces fasting and postprandial blood glucose levels, and reduces caloric intake, resulting in weight loss

4. Packaged in premeasured doses (pen) that require refrigeration (cannot be frozen)

5. Administered as a subcutaneous injection in the thigh, abdomen, or upper arm within 60 minutes before morning and evening meals; and is not taken after meals. If a dose is missed, the treatment regimen is resumed as prescribed with the next scheduled dose.

6. Can cause mild to moderate nausea that abates with use.

E. Pramlintide (Symlin)

1. Synthetic form of amylin, a naturally occurring hormone secreted by the pancreas

2. Used for clients with types 1 and 2 **diabetes mellitus** who use insulin; given before meals to lower blood glucose level after meals, leading to less fluctuation during the day and better long-term glucose control

3. Associated with an increased risk of insulin-induced severe **hypoglycemia**, particularly in clients with type 1 **diabetes mellitus**

4. Gastrointestinal side effects including nausea can occur.

5. Unopened vials are refrigerated. Opened vials can be refrigerated or kept at room temperature for up to 28 days.

F. Glucagon

1. Hormone secreted by the alpha cells of the islets of Langerhans in the pancreas

2. Increases blood glucose level by stimulating glycogenolysis in the liver

3. Can be administered subcutaneously, intramuscularly, or intravenously

4. Used to treat insulin-induced **hypoglycemia** when the client is semiconscious or unconscious and is unable to ingest liquids

5. The blood glucose level begins to increase within 5 to 20 minutes after administration.

6. Instruct the family in the procedure for administration.

7. See Chapter 45 for additional information regarding interventions for severe **hypoglycemia**.

MORE QUESTIONS ON EVOLVE!

Practice Questions

461. A nurse is reinforcing teaching for a client regarding how to mix regular insulin and NPH insulin in the same syringe. Which of the following actions, if performed by the client, indicates the need for further teaching?
1. Withdraws the NPH insulin first
2. Withdraws the regular insulin first
3. Injects air into NPH insulin vial first
4. Injects an amount of air equal to the desired dose of insulin into the vial

462. A home care nurse visits a client recently diagnosed with diabetes mellitus who is taking Humulin NPH insulin daily. The client asks the nurse how to store the unopened vials of insulin. The nurse tells the client to:
1. Freeze the insulin.
2. Refrigerate the insulin.
3. Store the insulin in a dark, dry place.
4. Keep the insulin at room temperature.

463. Glimepiride (Amaryl) is prescribed for a client with diabetes mellitus. A nurse reinforces instructions for the client and tells the client to avoid which of the following while taking this medication?
1. Alcohol
2. Organ meats
3. Whole-grain cereals
4. Carbonated beverages

464. Sildenafil (Viagra) is prescribed to treat a client with erectile dysfunction. A nurse reviews the

client's medical record and would question the prescription if which of the following is noted in the client's history?
1. Neuralgia
2. Insomnia
3. Use of nitroglycerin
4. Use of multivitamins

465. The health care provider (HCP) prescribes exenatide (Byetta) for a client with type 1 diabetes mellitus who takes insulin. The nurse knows that which of the following is the appropriate intervention?
1. The medication is administered within 60 minutes before the morning and evening meal.
2. The medication is withheld and the HCP is called to question the prescription for the client.
3. The client is monitored for gastrointestinal side effects after administration of the medication.
4. The insulin is withdrawn from the Penlet into an insulin syringe to prepare for administration.

466. A client is taking Humulin NPH insulin daily every morning. The nurse reinforces instructions for the client and tells the client that the most likely time for a hypoglycemic reaction to occur is:
1. 2 to 4 hours after administration
2. 4 to 12 hours after administration
3. 16 to 18 hours after administration
4. 18 to 24 hours after administration

467. A client with diabetes mellitus visits a health care clinic. The client's diabetes mellitus previously had been well controlled with glyburide (Dia-Beta) daily, but recently the fasting blood glucose level has been 180 to 200 mg/dL. Which medication, if added to the client's regimen, may have contributed to the hyperglycemia?
1. Prednisone
2. Phenelzine (Nardil)
3. Atenolol (Tenormin)
4. Allopurinol (Zyloprim)

468. A community health nurse visits a client at home. Prednisone 10 mg orally daily has been prescribed for the client and the nurse reinforces teaching for the client about the medication. Which statement, if made by the client, indicates that further teaching is necessary?
1. "I can take aspirin or my antihistamine if I need it."
2. "I need to take the medication every day at the same time."
3. "I need to avoid coffee, tea, cola, and chocolate in my diet."
4. "If I gain more than 5 pounds a week, I will call my doctor."

469. Desmopressin acetate (DDAVP) is prescribed for the treatment of diabetes insipidus. The nurse monitors the client after medication administration for which therapeutic response?
1. Decreased urinary output
2. Decreased blood pressure
3. Decreased peripheral edema
4. Decreased blood glucose level

470. The home health care nurse is visiting a client who was recently diagnosed with type 2 diabetes mellitus. The client is prescribed repaglinide (Prandin) and metformin (Glucophage) and asks the nurse to explain these medications. The nurse should reinforce which instructions to the client? **Select all that apply.**
☐ 1. Diarrhea can occur secondary to the metformin.
☐ 2. The repaglinide is not taken if a meal is skipped.
☐ 3. The repaglinide is taken 30 minutes before eating.
☐ 4. Candy or another simple sugar is carried and used to treat mild hypoglycemia episodes.
☐ 5. Metformin increases hepatic glucose production to prevent hypoglycemia associated with repaglinide.
☐ 6. Muscle pain is an expected side effect of metformin and may be treated with acetaminophen (Tylenol).

ANSWERS

461. 1

Rationale: When preparing a mixture of regular insulin with another insulin preparation, the regular insulin is drawn into the syringe first. This sequence will avoid contaminating the vial of regular insulin with insulin of another type. Options 2, 3, and 4 identify the correct actions for preparing NPH and regular insulin.
Test-Taking Strategy: Use the process of elimination, noting the strategic words "need for further teaching." These words

indicate a negative event query and ask you to select an option that is an incorrect action. Remember *RN*—draw up the *R*egular insulin before the *N*PH insulin. Review the procedure for preparing NPH and regular insulin if you had difficulty with this question.
Level of Cognitive Ability: Evaluating
Client Needs: Physiological Integrity
Integrated Process: Teaching and Learning
Content Area: Pharmacology
Reference: Kee, Hayes, McCuistion, p. 797. 2009.

462. 2

Rationale: Insulin in unopened vials should be stored under refrigeration until needed. Vials should not be frozen. When stored unopened under refrigeration, insulin can be used up to the expiration date on the vial. Options 1, 3, and 4 are incorrect.

Test-Taking Strategy: Use the process of elimination and note the strategic words "store the unopened vials" in the question. Remembering that insulin should not be frozen will assist in eliminating option 1. Options 3 and 4 are comparable or alike and should be eliminated. Review client teaching points related to insulin if you had difficulty with this question.

Level of Cognitive Ability: Applying
Client Needs: Physiological Integrity
Integrated Process: Teaching and Learning
Content Area: Pharmacology
Reference: Kee, Hayes, McCuistion, p. 793. 2009.

463. 1

Rationale: When alcohol is combined with glimepiride (Amaryl), a disulfiram-like reaction may occur. This syndrome includes flushing, palpitations, and nausea. Alcohol can also potentiate the hypoglycemic effects of the medication. Clients need to be instructed to avoid alcohol consumption while taking this medication. The items in options 2, 3, and 4 do not need to be avoided.

Test-Taking Strategy: Use the process of elimination. Eliminate options 2, 3, and 4 because these food items are allowed in a diabetic diet. Remembering that alcohol can affect the action of many medications will assist in directing you to option 1. Review this medication if you had difficulty with this question.

Level of Cognitive Ability: Applying
Client Needs: Physiological Integrity
Integrated Process: Teaching and Learning
Content Area: Pharmacology
References: Kee, Hayes, McCuistion, p. 802. 2009.
Lehne, p. 687. 2010.

464. 3

Rationale: Sildenafil (Viagra) enhances the vasodilating effect of nitric oxide in the corpus cavernosum of the penis, thus sustaining an erection. Because of the effect of the medication, it is contraindicated with concurrent use of organic nitrates and nitroglycerin. Sildenafil is not contraindicated with the use of vitamins. Neuralgia and insomnia are side effects of the medication.

Test-Taking Strategy: Use the process of elimination, noting the words "would question the prescription." Recalling the action of the medication will direct you to option 3. If you had difficulty with this question, review the contraindications associated with the use of this medication.

Level of Cognitive Ability: Analyzing
Client Needs: Physiological Integrity
Integrated Process: Nursing Process/Data Collection
Content Area: Pharmacology
Reference: Hodgson, Kizior, p. 1034. 2010.

465. 2

Rationale: Exenatide (Byetta) is an incretin mimetic used for type 2 diabetes mellitus only. It is not recommended for clients taking insulin. Hence, the nurse should hold the medication and question the HCP regarding this prescription. Although

options 1 and 3 are correct statements about the medication, in this situation the medication should not be administered. The medication is packaged in prefilled pens ready for injection without the need for drawing it up into another syringe.

Test-Taking Strategy: Use the process of elimination. Eliminate option 4 because the medication is packaged in prefilled pens ready for injection without the need for drawing it up into another syringe. From the remaining options, focus on the data in the question. Although options 1 and 3 are appropriate when administering this medication, this client should not receive the medication. Review this medication if you had difficulty with this question.

Level of Cognitive Ability: Applying
Client Needs: Physiological Integrity
Integrated Process: Nursing Process/Planning
Content Area: Pharmacology
Reference: http://www.diabetesmonitor.com/byetta.htm.
Lehne, p. 680. 2010.

466. 2

Rationale: Humulin NPH is an intermediate-acting insulin. The onset of action is 1.5 hours, it peaks in 4 to 12 hours, and its duration of action is 24 hours. Hypoglycemic reactions most likely occur during peak time.

Test-Taking Strategy: Use the process of elimination and knowledge regarding the onset, peak, and duration of action for NPH insulin. Remember that NPH peaks in 4 to 12 hours. If you had difficulty with this question, review the characteristics of NPH insulin.

Level of Cognitive Ability: Applying
Client Needs: Physiological Integrity
Integrated Process: Teaching and Learning
Content Area: Pharmacology
References: Edmunds, p. 335. 2010.
Kee, Hayes, McCuistion, p. 795. 2009.

467. 1

Rationale: Prednisone may decrease the effect of oral hypoglycemics, insulin, diuretics, and potassium supplements. Option 2, a monoamine oxidase inhibitor, and option 3, a β-blocker, have their own intrinsic hypoglycemic activity. Option 4 decreases urinary excretion of sulfonylurea agents, causing increased levels of the oral agents, which can lead to hypoglycemia.

Test-Taking Strategy: Use the process of elimination and focus on the subject, an increase in the blood glucose level. Recalling that prednisone decreases the effects of oral hypoglycemics will direct you to the correct option. Review medication interactions with hypoglycemics if you had difficulty with this question.

Level of Cognitive Ability: Analyzing
Client Needs: Physiological Integrity
Integrated Process: Nursing Process/Data Collection
Content Area: Pharmacology
Reference: Lehne, p. 855. 2010.

468. 1

Rationale: Aspirin and other over-the-counter medications should not be taken unless the client consults with the health care provider (HCP). The client needs to take the medication at the same time every day and should be instructed not to stop the medication. A slight weight gain as a result of an improved appetite is expected, but after the dosage is stabilized, a weight gain of 5 lb or more weekly should be reported to the HCP. Caffeine-containing foods and fluids need to be avoided because they may contribute to steroid-ulcer development.

Test-Taking Strategy: Use the process of elimination, noting the strategic words "further teaching is necessary." These words indicate a negative event query and ask you to select an option that is an incorrect statement. Remember that a client should not take other medications, especially over-the-counter medications, without first consulting with his or her HCP. Review teaching points for the client taking prednisone if you had difficulty with this question.

Level of Cognitive Ability: Evaluating
Client Needs: Physiological Integrity
Integrated Process: Teaching and Learning
Content Area: Pharmacology
Reference: Lehne, p. 855. 2010.

469. 1

Rationale: Desmopressin promotes renal conservation of water. The hormone carries out this action by acting on the collecting ducts of the kidney to increase their permeability to water, which results in increased water reabsorption. The therapeutic effect of this medication would be manifested by a decreased urine output. Options 2, 3, and 4 are unrelated to the effects of this medication.

Test-Taking Strategy: Use the process of elimination. Focus on the diagnosis in the question to assist in answering the question. Recalling the manifestations related to the loss of large volumes of urine in this disorder will help direct you to option 1. Review diabetes insipidus and the action of desmopressin if you had difficulty with this question.

Level of Cognitive Ability: Evaluating
Client Needs: Physiological Integrity
Integrated Process: Nursing Process/Evaluation
Content Area: Pharmacology
References: Hodgson, Kizior, p. 323. 2010. Lehne, p. 709. 2010.

470. 1, 2, 3, 4

Rationale: Repaglinide is a rapid-acting oral hypoglycemic agent that stimulates pancreatic insulin secretion that should be taken before meals, and that should be withheld if the client does not eat. Hypoglycemia is a side effect of repaglinide and the client should always be prepared by carrying a simple sugar with her or him at all times. Metformin is an oral hypoglycemic given in combination with repaglinide and works by decreasing hepatic glucose production. A common side effect of metformin is diarrhea. Muscle pain may occur as an adverse effect from metformin but it might signify a more serious condition that warrants health care provider notification, not the use of acetaminophen.

Test-Taking Strategy: Focus on the data in the question and the client's diagnosis to assist in answering the question. Also, recalling the actions and effects of these medications will assist in answering correctly. Review these medications if you are not familiar with them.

Level of Cognitive Ability: Applying
Client Needs: Physiological Integrity
Integrated Process: Nursing Process/Implementation
Content Area: Pharmacology
Reference: Lehne, pp. 674, 676. 2010.

The Adult Client with a Gastrointestinal Disorder

PYRAMID TERMS

ascites The accumulation of fluid within the peritoneal cavity

asterixis A coarse tremor characterized by rapid, nonrhythmic extensions and flexions in the wrist and fingers; also termed liver flap

Billroth I Also called gastroduodenostomy; partial gastrectomy and remaining segment are anastomosed to the duodenum

Billroth II Also called gastrojejunostomy; partial gastrectomy and remaining segment are anastomosed to the jejunum

cholecystectomy Removal of the gallbladder

cholecystitis An inflammation of the gallbladder that may occur as an acute or chronic process. Acute inflammation is associated with gallstones (cholelithiasis). Chronic cholecystitis results when inefficient bile emptying and gallbladder muscle wall disease result in a fibrotic and contracted gallbladder

choledocholithotomy Incision into the common bile duct to remove a gallstone

cirrhosis A chronic, progressive disease of the liver in which liver cells are replaced by scar tissue

Crohn's disease An inflammatory disease that can occur anywhere in the gastrointestinal (GI) tract, but most often affects the terminal ileum and leads to thickening and scarring, a narrowed lumen, fistulas, ulcerations, and abscesses. It is characterized by remissions and exacerbations

Cullen's sign Bluish discoloration of the abdomen and periumbilical area seen in acute hemorrhagic pancreatitis

diverticulitis Inflammation of one or more diverticuli in the lining of the intestinal wall, caused by intestinal contents becoming lodged in diverticula

diverticulosis Outpouchings or herniations of the intestinal mucosa; this condition can occur in any part of the intestine, but is most common in the sigmoid colon

dumping syndrome Rapid emptying of the gastric contents into the small intestine; occurs after gastric resection

esophageal varices Dilated veins in the submucosa of the esophagus; they are caused by portal hypertension, are often associated with liver cirrhosis, and are at high risk for rupture if portal circulation pressure rises

fetor hepaticus The fruity, musty breath odor associated with severe chronic liver disease

gastrectomy Also called esophagojejunostomy; involves removal of the stomach, with attachment of the esophagus to the jejunum or duodenum

gastric resection Also called antrectomy; involves removal of the lower half of the stomach and usually includes a vagotomy

hepatitis Inflammation of the liver that causes cell damage, often caused by a virus; viral types of hepatitis are classified as A, B, C, D, E, and G

hiatal hernia Also known as esophageal or diaphragmatic hernia; a portion of the stomach herniates through the diaphragm and into the thorax; hiatal hernia results from weakening of the muscles of the diaphragm and is aggravated by factors that increase abdominal pressure, such as pregnancy, ascites, obesity, tumors, and heavy lifting

Kock ileostomy (continent ileostomy) An intra-abdominal pouch is constructed from the terminal ileum; the pouch is connected to the stoma with a nipple-like valve constructed from a portion of the ileum; the stoma is flush with the skin

Murphy's sign A sign of gallbladder disease consisting of pain on taking a deep breath when the examiner's fingers are on the approximate location of the gallbladder

pancreatitis An acute or chronic inflammation of the pancreas, with associated escape of pancreatic enzymes into surrounding tissue; acute pancreatitis occurs suddenly as one attack or can be recurrent but resolves; chronic pancreatitis is a continual inflammation and destruction of the pancreas, with scar tissue replacing pancreatic tissue

peristalsis Wavelike rhythmic contractions that propel material through the GI tract

portal hypertension A persistent increase in pressure within the portal vein that develops as a result of obstruction to flow

pyloroplasty Enlarging the pylorus to prevent or decrease pyloric obstruction, thereby enhancing gastric emptying

Turner's sign A gray-blue discoloration of the flanks seen in acute hemorrhagic pancreatitis

ulcerative colitis Ulcerative and inflammatory disease of the bowel that results in poor absorption of nutrients; acute ulcerative colitis results in vascular congestion, hemorrhage, edema, and ulceration of the bowel mucosa; chronic ulcerative colitis causes muscular hypertrophy, fat deposits, and fibrous tissue with bowel thickening, shortening, and narrowing

vagotomy Surgical division of the vagus nerve to eliminate the vagal impulses that stimulate hydrochloric acid secretion in the stomach

 PYRAMID TO SUCCESS

Pyramid points focus on diagnostic tests, nursing care related to the various gastric or intestinal tubes, gastric surgery, cirrhosis, hepatitis, pancreatitis, and colostomy care. Focus on preprocedure and postprocedure care of the client undergoing a gastrointestinal diagnostic test. Remember that an informed consent is required for any invasive procedure. Focus on diet restrictions before and after the diagnostic test, and remember that the gag reflex or bowel sounds must return before allowing a client to consume food or fluids. Pyramid points include instructions to the client and family regarding the prevention of gastrointestinal disorders and the complications associated with the disorder. Focus on teaching the client and family about diet and nutrition specific to the disorder, tube and wound care, preventing the transmission of infection, and care of a colostomy or ileostomy.

 CLIENT NEEDS

Safe and Effective Care Environment

- Consulting with other health care professionals regarding the client's nutritional status
- Ensuring that confidentiality issues related to the gastrointestinal disorder are maintained
- Establishing priorities of care

- Handling infectious drainage and secretions safely
- Maintaining standard precautions and other precautions as appropriate
- Obtaining informed consent for treatments and surgical procedures
- Obtaining referrals for home care and community services
- Preventing disease transmission

Health Promotion and Maintenance

- Performing data collection techniques of the gastrointestinal system
- Preventing disease related to the gastrointestinal system
- Providing health screening and health promotion programs related to gastrointestinal disorders
- Teaching related to colostomy or ileostomy care
- Teaching related to preventing the transmission of disease
- Teaching related to prescribed dietary and other treatment measures

Psychosocial Integrity

- Assessing coping mechanisms
- Considering end-of-life and grief and loss issues
- Identifying available support systems
- Monitoring for expected body image changes related to colostomy or ileostomy

Physiological Integrity

- Administering medications as prescribed specific to the gastrointestinal disorder
- Assessing for signs and symptoms of infectious diseases of the gastrointestinal tract
- Assisting with personal hygiene
- Monitoring elimination patterns
- Monitoring for complications related to tests, procedures, and surgical interventions
- Monitoring for fluid and electrolyte imbalances
- Monitoring laboratory values related to gastrointestinal disorders
- Monitoring parenterally administered fluids, including parenteral nutrition
- Providing adequate nutrition and oral hydration
- Providing care for gastrointestinal tubes
- Providing nonpharmacological and pharmacological comfort measures
- Providing preprocedure and postprocedure care for diagnostic tests related to the gastrointestinal system

Gastrointestinal System

I. ANATOMY AND PHYSIOLOGY

A. Functions of the gastrointestinal system
1. Process food substances.
2. Absorb the products of digestion into the blood.
3. Excrete unabsorbed materials
4. Provide an environment for microorganisms to synthesize nutrients, such as vitamin K.
5. For risk factors associated with the gastrointestinal system, see Box 47-1.

B. Mouth
1. Contains the lips, cheeks, palate, tongue, teeth, salivary glands, muscles, and maxillary bones
2. Saliva contains the amylase enzyme (ptyalin) that aids in digestion

C. Esophagus
1. A collapsible muscular tube about 10 inches long
2. Carries food from the pharynx to the stomach

D. The stomach
1. Contains the cardia, fundus, body, and pylorus
2. Mucous glands are located in the mucosa and prevent autodigestion by providing an alkaline protective covering.
3. The lower esophageal (cardiac) sphincter prevents reflux of gastric contents into the esophagus.
4. The pyloric sphincter regulates the rate of stomach emptying into the small intestine.
5. Hydrochloric acid kills microorganisms, breaks food into small particles, and provides a chemical environment that facilitates gastric enzyme activation.
6. Pepsin is the chief coenzyme of gastric juice, which converts proteins into proteases and peptones.
7. Intrinsic factor is necessary for the absorption of vitamin B_{12}.
8. Gastrin controls gastric acidity.

E. Small intestine
1. The duodenum contains the openings of the bile and pancreatic ducts.
2. The jejunum is about 8 feet long.
3. The ileum is about 12 feet long.
4. The small intestine terminates into the cecum.

F. Pancreatic intestinal juice enzymes
1. Amylase digests starch to maltose.
2. Maltase reduces maltose to monosaccharide glucose.
3. Lactase splits lactose into galactose and glucose.
4. Sucrase reduces sucrose to fructose and glucose.
5. Nucleuses split nucleic acids to nucleotides.
6. Enterokinase activates trypsinogen to trypsin.

G. Large intestine
1. Is about 5 feet long
2. Absorbs water and eliminates wastes
3. Intestinal bacteria play a vital role in the synthesis of some B vitamins and vitamin K
4. Colon: includes the ascending, transverse, descending, sigmoid, and rectum
5. The ileocecal valve prevents contents of the large intestine from entering the ileum.
6. The anal sphincters control/guard the anal canal.

H. Peritoneum: lines the abdominal cavity and forms the mesentery that supports the intestines and blood supply

I. Liver
1. The largest gland in the body, weighing 3 to 4 lb
2. Contains Kupffer's cells, which remove bacteria in the portal venous blood
3. Removes excess glucose and amino acids from the portal blood
4. Synthesizes glucose, amino acids, and fats
5. Aids in the digestion of fats, carbohydrates, and proteins
6. Receives blood supply from the hepatic artery and portal vein (1500 mL of blood flows through the liver every minute)
7. Stores vitamins A, D, and B, as well as iron
8. Secretes bile to emulsify fats (500 to 1000 mL of bile a day)
9. Hepatic ducts
   a. Deliver bile to the gallbladder via the cystic duct and to the duodenum via the common bile duct
   b. The common bile duct opens into the duodenum with the pancreatic duct at the ampulla of Vater.

Box 47-1 Risk Factors Associated with the Gastrointestinal (GI) System

Allergic reactions to food or medications
Cardiac, respiratory, and endocrine disorders that may lead to constipation
Chronic alcohol use
Chronic high stress levels
Chronic laxative use
Chronic use of aspirin or nonsteroidal anti-inflammatory drugs
Diabetes mellitus, which may predispose to oral candidal infections or other GI disorders
Family history of GI disorders
Long-term GI conditions, such as ulcerative colitis, that may predispose to colorectal cancer
Neurological disorders that can impair movement, particularly with chewing and swallowing
Previous abdominal surgery or trauma, which may lead to adhesions
Tobacco use

   c. The sphincter prevents the reflux of intestinal contents into the common bile duct and pancreatic duct.

J. Gallbladder
  1. Stores and concentrates bile and contracts to force bile into the duodenum during the digestion of fats
  2. The cystic duct joins the hepatic duct to form the common bile duct.
  3. The sphincter of Oddi is located at the entrance into the duodenum.
  4. The presence of fatty materials in the duodenum stimulates the liberation of cholecystokinin, which causes contraction of the gallbladder and relaxation of the sphincter of Oddi.

K. Pancreas
  1. Exocrine gland
    a. Secretes sodium bicarbonate to neutralize the acidity of the stomach contents that enter the duodenum
    b. Pancreatic juices contain enzymes for digesting carbohydrates, fats, and proteins
  2. Endocrine gland
    a. Secretes glucagon to raise blood glucose levels and secretes somatostatin to exert a hypoglycemic effect
    b. The islets of Langerhans secrete insulin
    c. Insulin is secreted into the bloodstream and is important for carbohydrate metabolism.

II. DIAGNOSTIC PROCEDURES

A. Upper gastrointestinal tract study (barium swallow)
  1. Description: An examination of the upper gastrointestinal tract under fluoroscopy after the client drinks barium sulfate

  2. Preprocedure: NPO after midnight before the day of the test
  3. Postprocedure
    a. A laxative may be prescribed.
    b. Instruct the client to increase oral fluid intake to help pass the barium.
    c. Monitor stools for the passage of barium (stools will appear chalky white) because barium can cause a bowel obstruction.

B. Lower gastrointestinal tract study (barium enema)
  1. Description
    a. A fluoroscopic and radiographic examination of the large intestine is performed after rectal instillation of barium sulfate.
    b. The study may be done with or without air.
  2. Preprocedure
    a. A low-residue diet for 1 to 2 days before the test
    b. A clear liquid diet and a laxative the evening before the test
    c. NPO after midnight before the day of the test
    d. Cleansing enemas on the morning of the test
  3. Postprocedure
    a. Instruct the client to increase oral fluid intake to help pass the barium.
    b. Administer a mild laxative as prescribed to facilitate emptying of the barium.
    c. Monitor stools for the passage of barium.
    d. Notify the health care provider (HCP) if a bowel movement does not occur within 2 days.

C. Gastric analysis
  1. Description
    a. Gastric analysis requires the passage of a nasogastric tube into the stomach to aspirate gastric contents for the analysis of acidity (pH), appearance, and volume. The entire gastric contents are aspirated, and then specimens are collected every 15 minutes for 1 hour.
    b. Histamine or pentagastrin may be administered subcutaneously to stimulate gastric secretions. These medications may produce a flushed feeling.
    c. Esophageal reflux of gastric acid may be performed by ambulatory pH monitoring. A probe is placed just above the lower esophageal sphincter, is connected to an external recording device, and provides a computer analysis and graphic display of results.
  2. Preprocedure
    a. Fasting for 8 to 12 hours is required before the test.
    b. Tobacco and chewing gum are avoided for 6 hours before the test.
    c. Medications that stimulate gastric secretions are withheld for 24 to 48 hours
  3. Postprocedure
    a. Client may resume normal activities

b. Refrigerate gastric samples if not tested within 4 hours.

D. Upper gastrointestinal fiberoscopy
1. Description
   a. Is also known as esophagogastroduodenoscopy
   b. Following sedation, an endoscope is passed down the esophagus to view the gastric wall, sphincters, and duodenum. Tissue specimens can be obtained.
2. Preprocedure
   a. The client must be NPO for 6 to 12 hours before the test.
   b. A local anesthetic (spray or gargle) is administered along with medication that provides conscious sedation and relieves anxiety, such as midazolam (Versed), intravenously, just before the scope is inserted.
   c. Atropine sulfate may be administered to reduce secretions, and glucagon may be administered to relax smooth muscle.
   d. The client is positioned on the left side to facilitate saliva drainage and provide easy access of the endoscope.
   e. Airway patency is monitored during the test, and pulse oximetry is used to monitor oxygen saturation. Emergency equipment should be readily available.
3. Postprocedure
   a. The client must be NPO until the gag reflex returns (1 to 2 hours).
   b. Monitor for signs of perforation (pain, bleeding, unusual difficulty swallowing, elevated temperature).
   c. Maintain bedrest for the sedated client until he or she is alert.
   d. Lozenges, saline gargles, or oral analgesics can relieve a minor sore throat (not given to the client until the gag reflex returns).

E. Anoscopy, proctoscopy, and sigmoidoscopy
1. Description
   a. Anoscopy requires the use of a rigid scope to examine the anal canal. The client is placed in the knee-chest position with the back inclined at a 45-degree angle.
   b. Proctoscopy and sigmoidoscopy require the use of a flexible scope to examine the rectum and sigmoid colon. The client is placed on the left side with the right leg bent and placed anteriorly.
   c. Biopsies and polypectomies can be performed.
2. Preprocedure: Enemas are given until the returns are clear.
3. Postprocedure: Monitor for rectal bleeding and signs of perforation and peritonitis (Box 47-2).

Box 47-2 Signs of Bowel Perforation and Peritonitis

Guarding of the abdomen
Increased fever and chills
Pallor
Progressive abdominal distention and abdominal pain
Restlessness
Tachycardia and tachypnea

F. Fiberoptic colonoscopy
1. Description
   a. Colonoscopy is a fiberoptic endoscopy study in which the lining of the large intestine is visually examined. Biopsies and polypectomies can be performed.
   b. Cardiac and respiratory functions are monitored continuously during the test.
   c. Colonoscopy is performed with the client lying on the left side with the knees drawn up to the chest. The position may be changed during the test to facilitate passing of the scope.
2. Preprocedure
   a. Adequate cleansing of the colon is necessary, as prescribed by the HCP.
   b. A clear liquid diet is started on the day before the test.
   c. Consult with the HCP regarding medications that must be withheld before the test.
   d. The client is NPO after midnight on the day before the test.
   e. A sedative may be administered.
3. Postprocedure
   a. Provide bedrest until he or she is alert.
   b. Monitor for signs of bowel perforation and peritonitis (see Box 47-2).
   c. Instruct the client to report any bleeding to the HCP.

⚠ The client receiving laxatives and enemas is at risk for fluid and electrolyte balances.

G. Laparoscopy (peritoneoscopy) is performed with a fiberoptic laparoscope that allows direct visualization of organs and structures within the abdomen. Biopsies may be obtained.

H. Cholecystography
1. Description: Performed to detect gallstones and to assess the ability of the gallbladder to fill, concentrate its contents, contract, and empty.
2. Preprocedure
   a. Assess for allergies to iodine or seafood.
   b. Contrast agents may be administered 10 to 12 hours (evening before) before the test.

    c. Client is NPO after the contrast agent is administered.

    d. Instruct the client to report to the emergency department if a rash, itching, hives, or difficulty in breathing occurs after taking the contrast agent.

  3. Postprocedure

    a. Inform the client that dysuria is common because the contrast agent is excreted in the urine.

    b. A normal diet may be resumed. (A fatty meal may enhance excretion of the contrast agent.)

I. Endoscopic retrograde cholangiopancreatography (ERCP)

  1. Description

    a. Examination of the hepatobiliary system is performed via a flexible endoscope inserted into the esophagus to the descending duodenum. Multiple positions are required during the procedure to pass the endoscope.

    b. If medication is administered before the procedure, the client is monitored closely for signs of respiratory and central nervous system depression, hypotension, oversedation, and vomiting (risk for aspiration).

  2. Preprocedure

    a. The client is NPO for several hours before the procedure.

    b. Sedation is administered before the procedure.

  3. Postprocedure

    a. Monitor the vital signs.

    b. Monitor for the return of the gag reflex.

    c. Monitor for signs of perforation or peritonitis (see Box 47-2).

⚠ Following endoscopic procedures, monitor for the return of a gag reflex before giving the client any oral substance. If the gag reflex has not returned, the client could aspirate.

J. Percutaneous transhepatic cholangiography

  1. Description

    a. The examination involves the injection of dye directly into the biliary tree.

    b. The hepatic ducts within the liver, the entire length of the common bile duct, the cystic duct, and the gallbladder are outlined clearly.

  2. Preprocedure

    a. The client is NPO.

    b. Sedating medication is administered.

  3. Postprocedure

    a. Monitor the vital signs.

    b. Monitor for signs of bleeding, peritonitis (see Box 47-2), and septicemia. Report the presence of pain immediately.

    c. Administer antibiotics as prescribed to reduce the risk of sepsis.

K. Paracentesis

  1. Description: transabdominal removal of fluid from the peritoneal cavity for analysis

  2. Preprocedure

    a. Have the client void before the start of the procedure to empty the bladder and move the bladder out of the way of the paracentesis needle.

    b. Measure abdominal girth, weight, and baseline vital signs.

    c. Note that the client is positioned upright on the edge of the bed with the back supported and the feet resting on a stool. (Fowler's position is used for the client confined to bed.)

⚠ The rapid removal of fluid from the abdominal cavity during paracentesis leads to decreased abdominal pressure, which can cause vasodilation and resultant shock.

  3. Postprocedure

    a. Monitor vital signs.

    b. Measure fluid collected, describe, and record.

    c. Label fluid samples and send to the laboratory for analysis.

    d. Apply a dry sterile dressing to the insertion site. Monitor the site for bleeding.

    e. Measure abdominal girth and weight.

    f. Monitor for hypovolemia, electrolyte loss, mental status changes, or encephalopathy.

    g. Monitor for hematuria caused by bladder trauma.

    h. Instruct the client to notify the HCP if the urine becomes bloody, pink, or red (see Priority Nursing Actions).

L. Liver biopsy

  1. Description: A needle is inserted through the abdominal wall to the liver to obtain a tissue sample for biopsy and microscopic examination.

  2. Preprocedure

    a. Assess results of coagulation tests (prothrombin time, partial thromboplastin time, platelet count).

    b. Administer a sedative as prescribed.

    c. Note that the client is placed in the supine or left lateral position during the procedure to expose the right side of the upper abdomen.

  3. Postprocedure

    a. Assess vital signs.

    b. Assess biopsy site for bleeding.

    c. Monitor for peritonitis (see Box 47-2).

    d. Maintain bedrest as prescribed.

    e. Place the client on the right side with a pillow under the costal margin to decrease the risk of bleeding, and instruct the client to avoid coughing and straining.

═══ **PRIORITY NURSING ACTIONS!** ═══

Actions to Take in Caring for a Client with a Paracentesis

1. Ensure that the client understands the procedure and that informed consent has been obtained.
2. Obtain vital signs, including weight.
3. Have the client void.
4. Position the client upright.
5. Assist the HCP. Monitor the vital signs and provide comfort and support during the procedure.
6. Apply a dressing to the site of puncture.
7. Weigh the client, and maintain the client on bedrest.
8. Measure the amount of fluid removed.
9. Label and send the fluid for laboratory analysis.
10. Document the event, client's response, and appearance and amount of fluid removed.

Paracentesis is the transabdominal removal of fluid from the peritoneal cavity. The nurse first ensures that the client understands the procedure and that informed consent has been obtained because the procedure is invasive. The nurse next obtains preprocedure vital signs, including weight so that a baseline is obtained. Weight is taken before and after the procedure to provide an indication of the effectiveness of the procedure in fluid removal. The client is positioned upright on the edge of the bed with the back supported and the feet resting on a stool or in a Fowler's position in bed. The nurse assists the HCP, monitors vital signs per protocol, and provides comfort and support to the client during the procedure. Once the procedure is complete the nurse applies a dressing to the site of puncture and monitors for leakage or bleeding. The client is placed in a position of comfort, bedrest is maintained as prescribed, and vital signs are monitored to assess for complications. The fluid removed from the client is measured, labeled and sent to the laboratory for analysis. The nurse documents the event, the client's response, the appearance and amount of fluid removed, and any additional pertinent data.

Reference: Ignatavicius, D., & Workman, M. (2010). *Medical-surgical nursing: Patient-centered collaborative care* (6th ed., p. 1352). St. Louis: Saunders.

    f. Instruct the client to avoid heavy lifting and strenuous exercise for 1 week.

   ⚠ After a liver biopsy, place the client on the right side with a pillow under the costal margin at the anatomical location of the liver to decrease the risk of bleeding.

M. Stool specimens
  1. Testing of stool specimens includes inspecting the specimen for consistency and color and testing for occult blood.
  2. Tests for fecal urobilinogen, fat, nitrogen, parasites, pathogens, food substances, and other substances may be performed. These tests require that the specimen be sent to the laboratory.

  3. Random specimens are sent promptly to the laboratory.
  4. Quantitative 24- to 72-hour collections must be kept refrigerated until they are taken to the laboratory.
  5. Some specimens require that a certain diet be followed or that certain medications be withheld. Check agency guidelines regarding specific procedures.

N. Urea breath test
  1. The urea breath test detects the presence of *Helicobacter pylori,* the bacteria that causes peptic ulcer disease.
  2. The client consumes a capsule of carbon-labeled urea and provides a breath sample 10 to 20 minutes later.
  3. Certain medications may need to be avoided before testing and these may include the following: antibiotics or bismuth subsalicylate (Pepto-Bismol) for 1 month before the test; sucralfate (Carafate) and omeprazole (Prilosec) for 1 week before the test; and cimetidine (Tagamet), famotidine (Pepcid), ranitidine (Zantac), or nizatidine (Axid) for 24 hours before breath testing.
  4. *Helicobacter pylori* can also be detected by assessing serum antibody levels.

O. Liver and pancreas laboratory studies (refer to Chapter 11).
  1. Alkaline phosphatase is released during liver damage or biliary obstruction.
  2. Prothrombin time is prolonged with liver damage.
  3. Serum ammonia assesses the ability of the liver to deaminate protein by-products.
  4. Liver enzymes (transaminase studies) are elevated with liver damage.
  5. An increase in cholesterol indicates **pancreatitis** or biliary obstruction.
  6. An increase in bilirubin indicates liver damage or biliary obstruction.
  7. Increased values for amylase and lipase indicate **pancreatitis**.

III. DATA COLLECTION (see Chapter 29 for data collection technique)

IV. GASTROINTESTINAL TUBES (refer to Chapter 19 for information regarding care of the client with these tubes)

V. GASTROESOPHAGEAL REFLUX DISEASE

A. Description
  1. Gastroesophageal reflux is the backflow of gastric and duodenal contents into the esophagus.

2. The reflux is caused by an incompetent lower esophageal sphincter, pyloric stenosis, or a motility disorder.

B. Data collection
1. Heartburn
2. Epigastric pain
3. Dyspepsia
4. Regurgitation
5. Pain and difficulty with swallowing
6. Hypersalivation

C. Interventions
1. The client is instructed to avoid factors that decrease lower esophageal sphincter pressure or cause esophageal irritation.
2. The client is instructed to eat a low-fat, high-fiber diet; avoid caffeine, tobacco, and carbonated beverages; avoid eating and drinking 2 hours before bedtime; avoid wearing tight clothes; and elevate the head of the bed on 6- to 8-inch blocks.
3. Avoid the use of anticholinergics, which delay stomach emptying.
4. The client is instructed regarding prescribed medications, such as antacids, histamine 2 (H_2)-receptor antagonists, or proton pump inhibitors.
5. The client is instructed regarding the administration of prokinetic medications, if prescribed, which accelerate gastric emptying.
6. If medical management is unsuccessful, surgery may be required and involves a fundoplication (wrapping a portion of the gastric fundus around the sphincter area of the esophagus). Surgery may be performed by laparoscopy.

VI. GASTRITIS

A. Description
1. Inflammation of the stomach or gastric mucosa
2. Acute gastritis is caused by the ingestion of food contaminated with disease-causing microorganisms or food that is irritating or too highly seasoned, the overuse of aspirin or other nonsteroidal anti-inflammatory drugs (NSAIDs), excessive alcohol intake, bile reflux, or radiation therapy.
3. Chronic gastritis is caused by benign or malignant ulcers or by the bacteria *H. pylori*, and it may be caused by autoimmune diseases, dietary factors, medications, alcohol, smoking, or reflux.

B. Data collection (Box 47-3)

C. Interventions
1. Acute gastritis: Food and fluids may be withheld until symptoms subside. Afterward, ice chips, followed by clear liquids, and then solid food is introduced.
2. Monitor for signs of hemorrhagic gastritis such as hematemesis, tachycardia, and hypotension. Notify the HCP if these signs occur.

Box 47-3 Data Collection: Acute and Chronic Gastritis

Acute Gastritis
Abdominal discomfort
Anorexia, nausea, and vomiting
Headache
Hiccuping

Chronic Gastritis
Anorexia, nausea, and vomiting
Belching
Heartburn after eating
Sour taste in the mouth
Vitamin B_{12} deficiency

---

3. Instruct the client to avoid irritating foods, fluids, and other substances such as spicy and highly seasoned foods, caffeine, alcohol, and nicotine.
4. Instruct the client on the use of prescribed medications, such as antibiotics and antacids.
5. Provide the client with information about the importance of vitamin B_{12} injections, if a deficiency is present.

VII. PEPTIC ULCER DISEASE

A. Description
1. A peptic ulcer is ulceration in the mucosal wall of the stomach, pylorus, duodenum, or esophagus in portions that are accessible to gastric secretions. Erosion may extend through the muscle.
2. The ulcer may be referred to as gastric, duodenal, or esophageal, depending on its location.
3. The most common peptic ulcers are gastric ulcers and duodenal ulcers.

B. Gastric ulcers
1. Description
   a. A gastric ulcer involves ulceration of the mucosal lining that extends to the submucosal layer of the stomach.
   b. Predisposing factors include stress, smoking, the use of corticosteroids, NSAIDs, alcohol, a history of gastritis, a family history of gastric ulcers, or infection with *H. pylori*.
   c. Complications include bleeding, perforation, and pyloric obstruction.
2. Data collection (Box 47-4)
3. Interventions
   a. Monitor the vital signs and for signs of bleeding.
   b. Administer small, frequent bland feedings during the active phase.
   c. Administer H_2-receptor antagonists or proton pump inhibitors as prescribed to decrease the secretion of gastric acid.
   d. Administer antacids as prescribed to neutralize gastric secretions.

Box 47-4 Data Collection: Gastric and Duodenal Ulcers

Gastric Ulcers

Gnawing, sharp pain in or left of the midepigastric region occurs 30 to 60 minutes after a meal (food ingestion accentuates the pain)

Hematemesis is more common than melena

Duodenal Ulcers

Burning pain in the midepigastric area 1.5 to 3 hours after a meal and during the night (often awakens the client)

Melena is more common than hematemesis

Pain is often relieved by the ingestion of food

    e. Administer anticholinergics as prescribed to reduce gastric motility.

    f. Administer mucosal barrier protectants as prescribed 1 hour before each meal.

    g. Administer prostaglandins as prescribed for their protective and antisecretory actions.

  4. Client education

    a. Avoid consuming alcohol and substances that contain caffeine or chocolate.

    b. Avoid smoking.

    c. Avoid aspirin or NSAIDs.

    d. Obtain adequate rest and reduce stress.

  5. Interventions during active bleeding

    a. Monitor the vital signs closely.

    b. Monitor for signs of dehydration, hypovolemic shock, sepsis, and respiratory insufficiency.

    c. Maintain NPO status and administer intravenous (IV) fluid replacement as prescribed. Monitor intake and output (I&O).

    d. Monitor hemoglobin and hematocrit.

    e. Administer blood transfusions as prescribed.

    f. Prepare to assist with administering medications as prescribed to induce vasoconstriction and reduce bleeding.

  6. Surgical interventions

    a. Total **gastrectomy**: removal of the stomach with attachment of the esophagus to the jejunum or duodenum; also called esophagojejunostomy or esophagoduodenostomy

    b. **Vagotomy**: surgical division of the vagus nerve to eliminate the vagal impulses that stimulate hydrochloric acid secretion in the stomach

    c. **Gastric resection**: removal of the lower half of the stomach and usually includes a **vagotomy**; also called antrectomy

    d. **Billroth I**: partial **gastrectomy**, with the remaining segment anastomosed to the duodenum; also called gastroduodenostomy

    e. **Billroth II**: partial **gastrectomy**, with the remaining segment anastomosed to the jejunum; also called gastrojejunostomy

    f. **Pyloroplasty**: enlargement of the pylorus to prevent or decrease pyloric obstruction, thereby enhancing gastric emptying

  7. Postoperative interventions

    a. Monitor the vital signs.

    b. Position in Fowler's for comfort and to promote drainage

    c. Administer fluids and electrolyte replacements intravenously as prescribed. Monitor intake and output.

    d. Check bowel sounds.

    e. Monitor nasogastric suction as prescribed.

    f. Maintain NPO status as prescribed for 1 to 3 days until **peristalsis** returns.

    g. Progress the diet from NPO to sips of clear water to six small, bland meals a day as prescribed when the bowel sounds return.

    h. Monitor for postoperative complications of hemorrhage, **dumping syndrome**, diarrhea, hypoglycemia, and vitamin B_{12} deficiency.

⚠ After gastric surgery, do not irrigate or remove the nasogastric (NG) tube unless specifically prescribed because of the risk for disruption of the gastric sutures. Monitor closely to ensure proper functioning of the NG tube to prevent strain on the anastomosis site. Contact the HCP if the tube is not functioning properly.

C. Duodenal ulcers

  1. Description

    a. A duodenal ulcer is a break in the mucosa of the duodenum.

    b. Risk factors and causes include alcohol intake; smoking; stress; caffeine; the use of aspirin, corticosteroids, and NSAIDs; and infection with *H. pylori*.

    c. Complications include bleeding, perforation, gastric outlet obstruction, and intractable disease.

  2. Data collection (see Box 47-4)

  3. Interventions

    a. Monitor the vital signs.

    b. Instruct the client in a bland diet with small frequent meals.

    c. Provide for adequate rest.

    d. Encourage the cessation of smoking.

    e. Instruct the client to avoid alcohol intake, caffeine, and the use of aspirin, corticosteroids, and NSAIDs.

    f. Administer medications to treat *H. pylori* and antacids to neutralize acid secretions as prescribed.

    g. Administer H_2-receptor antagonists as prescribed to block the secretion of acid.

  4. Surgical interventions: Surgery is performed only if the ulcer is unresponsive to medications or if hemorrhage, obstruction, or perforation occurs.

D. Dumping syndrome
1. Description: the rapid emptying of the gastric contents into the small intestine that occurs following **gastric resection**
2. Data collection
   a. Symptoms occurring 30 minutes after eating
   b. Nausea and vomiting
   c. Feelings of abdominal fullness and abdominal cramping
   d. Diarrhea
   e. Palpitations and tachycardia
   f. Perspiration
   g. Weakness and dizziness
   h. Borborygmi (loud gurgles indicating hyperperistalsis, or stomach growling)
3. Client education (Box 47-5)

VIII. VITAMIN B$_{12}$ DEFICIENCY

A. Description
1. Vitamin B$_{12}$ deficiency results from an inadequate intake of vitamin B$_{12}$ or a lack of absorption of ingested vitamin B$_{12}$ from the intestinal tract.
2. Pernicious anemia results from a deficiency of intrinsic factor, which is necessary for intestinal absorption of vitamin B$_{12}$. Gastric disease or surgery can result in a lack of intrinsic factor.

B. Data collection
1. Severe pallor
2. Fatigue
3. Weight loss
4. Smooth, beefy red tongue
5. Slight jaundice
6. Paresthesias of the hands and feet
7. Disturbances with gait and balance

C. Interventions
1. Increase dietary intake of foods rich in vitamin B$_{12}$ if the anemia is the result of a dietary deficiency (refer to Chapter 12).
2. Administer vitamin B$_{12}$ injections initially as prescribed weekly and then monthly for maintenance (lifelong) if the anemia is the result of a deficiency of the intrinsic factor or disease or surgery of the ileum.

IX. BARIATRIC SURGERY

A. Description
1. Surgical reduction of gastric capacity that may be performed on a client with morbid obesity to produce permanent weight loss.
2. Surgery may be performed by laparoscope. The decision is based on the client's weight, body build, history of abdominal surgery, and current medical disorders.
3. Obese clients are at increased postoperative risk for pulmonary and thromboembolic complications and death.
4. Surgery can prevent the complications of obesity such as diabetes mellitus, hypertension and other cardiovascular disorders, depression, or sleep apnea.
5. The client needs to agree to modify his or her lifestyle, lose weight and keep the weight off, and obtain support from available community resources (Box 47-6).
6. Various procedures are available; the type preformed depends on the HCP and the client's choice (Figure 47-1).

B. Postoperative interventions
1. Care is similar to that for the client undergoing abdominal surgery
2. Clear liquids are introduced slowly once bowel sounds have returned and the client passes flatus (1-ounce cups are used for each serving).
3. Clear fluids are followed by pureed foods, juices, thin soups, and milk 24 to 48 hours after clear fluids are tolerated (the diet is limited to liquids or pureed foods for 6 weeks). Then the diet is progressed to nutrient-dense regular food.

C. Client teaching points about diet are provided (Box 47-7).

X. GASTRIC CANCER (see Chapter 43)

XI. HIATAL HERNIA

A. Description
1. A **hiatal hernia** is also known as esophageal or diaphragmatic hernia.
2. A portion of the stomach herniates through the diaphragm and into the thorax.

Box 47-5 Client Education: Preventing Dumping Syndrome

Avoid sugar, salt, and milk.
Eat a high-protein, high-fat, low-carbohydrate diet.
Eat small meals and avoid consuming fluids with meals.
Lie down after meals.
Take antispasmodic medications as prescribed to delay gastric emptying.

Box 47-6 Community Resources After Bariatric Surgery

American Obesity Association
American Society of Bariatric Surgery
Overeaters Anonymous

3. Herniation results from weakening of the muscles of the diaphragm and is aggravated by factors that increase abdominal pressure such as pregnancy, **ascites**, obesity, tumors, and heavy lifting.

4. Complications include ulceration, hemorrhage, regurgitation, and aspiration of stomach contents, strangulation, and incarceration of the stomach in the chest with possible necrosis, peritonitis, and mediastinitis.

B. Data collection
1. Heartburn
2. Regurgitation or vomiting
3. Dysphagia
4. Feeling of fullness

C. Interventions
1. Medical and surgical management is similar to that for gastroesophageal reflux disease.
2. Provide small frequent meals and limit the amount of liquids taken with meals.
3. Advise the client not to recline for 1 hour after eating.
4. Avoid anticholinergics, which delay stomach emptying.

XII. CHOLECYSTITIS

A. Description
1. An inflammation of the gallbladder that may occur as an acute or chronic process
2. Acute inflammation is associated with gallstones (cholelithiasis).
3. Chronic **cholecystitis** results when inefficient bile emptying and gallbladder muscle wall disease cause a fibrotic and contracted gallbladder.

Box 47-7 Dietary Measures for the Client After Bariatric Surgery

Avoid alcohol, high-protein foods, and foods high in sugar and fat.
Eat slowly and chew food well.
Progress food types and amounts as prescribed.
Take nutritional supplements as prescribed, which may include calcium, iron, multivitamins, and vitamin B_{12}.
Monitor and report signs and symptoms of complications such as dehydration.

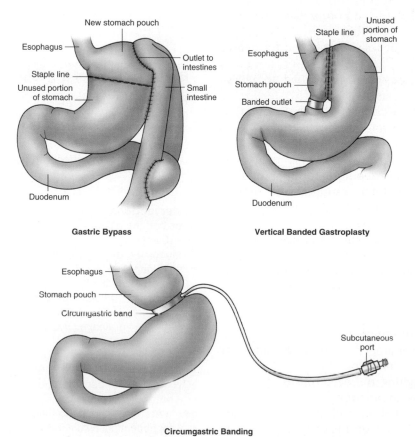

▲ FIGURE 47-1 Bariatric surgical procedures. (From Ignatavicius, D., & Workman, M. [2010]. *Medical-surgical nursing: Patient-centered collaborative care* [6th ed.]. St. Louis: Saunders.)

4. Acalculous **cholecystitis** occurs in the absence of gallstones and is caused by bacterial invasion via the lymphatic or vascular systems.

B. Data collection
1. Nausea and vomiting
2. Indigestion
3. Belching
4. Flatulence
5. Epigastric pain that radiates to the scapula 2 to 4 hours after eating fatty foods and may persist for 4 to 6 hours
6. Pain localized in right upper quadrant
7. Guarding, rigidity, and rebound tenderness
8. Mass palpated in the right upper quadrant
9. **Murphy's sign** (pain on taking a deep breath when the examiner's fingers are on the approximate location of the gallbladder)
10. Elevated temperature
11. Tachycardia
12. Signs of dehydration

C. Biliary obstruction
1. Jaundice
2. Dark orange and foamy urine
3. Steatorrhea and clay-colored feces
4. Pruritus

D. Interventions
1. Maintain NPO status during nausea and vomiting episodes.
2. Maintain nasogastric decompression as prescribed for severe vomiting.
3. Administer antiemetics as prescribed for nausea and vomiting.
4. Administer analgesics as prescribed to relieve pain and reduce spasm.
5. Administer antispasmodics (anticholinergics) as prescribed to relax smooth muscle.
6. Instruct the client with chronic **cholecystitis** to eat small, low-fat meals
7. Instruct the client to avoid gas-forming foods.
8. Prepare the client for nonsurgical and surgical procedures as prescribed.

E. Surgical interventions
1. **Cholecystectomy** is the removal of the gallbladder.
2. **Choledocholithotomy** requires incision into the common bile duct to remove the stone.
3. Surgical procedures may be performed by laparoscopy.

F. Postoperative interventions
1. Monitor for respiratory complications caused by pain at the incisional site.
2. Encourage coughing and deep breathing.
3. Encourage early ambulation.
4. Instruct the client about splinting the abdomen to prevent discomfort during coughing.
5. Administer antiemetics as prescribed for nausea and vomiting.

6. Administer analgesics as prescribed for pain relief.
7. Maintain NPO status and nasogastric tube suction as prescribed.
8. Advance diet from clear liquids to solids when prescribed and as tolerated by the client.
9. Maintain and monitor drainage from the T-tube, if present (Box 47-8).

XIII. CIRRHOSIS (Box 47-9)

A. Description
1. A chronic, progressive disease of the liver characterized by diffuse degeneration and destruction of hepatocytes
2. Repeated destruction of hepatic cells causes the formation of scar tissue.

B. Complications
1. **Portal hypertension**: A persistent increase in pressure within the portal vein that develops as a result of obstruction to flow
2. **Ascites**
   a. The accumulation of fluid within the peritoneal cavity that results from venous congestion of the hepatic capillaries
   b. Capillary congestion leads to plasma leaking directly from the liver surface and portal vein.

Box 47-8 Care of a T-Tube

Purpose and Description

A T-tube is placed after surgical exploration of the common bile duct. The tube preserves the patency of the duct and ensures drainage of bile until edema resolves and bile is effectively draining into the duodenum. A gravity drainage bag is attached to the T-tube to collect the drainage.

Interventions

Position the client in a semi-Fowler's position to facilitate drainage.

Monitor the amount, color, consistency, and odor of the drainage.

Report sudden increases in bile output to the HCP.

Monitor for inflammation and protect the skin from irritation.

Keep the drainage system below the level of the gallbladder.

Monitor for foul odor and purulent drainage and report its presence to the HCP.

Avoid irrigation, aspiration, or clamping of the T-tube without a HCP's prescription.

As prescribed, clamp the tube before a meal, and observe for abdominal discomfort and distention, nausea, chills, or fever; unclamp the tube if nausea or vomiting occurs.

3. Bleeding **esophageal varices**: fragile, thin-walled, distended esophageal veins that become irritated and rupture

4. Coagulation defects
   a. Decreased synthesis of bile fats in the liver prevents the absorption of fat-soluble vitamins.
   b. Without vitamin K and clotting factors II, VII, IX, and X, the client is prone to bleeding.

5. Jaundice: Occurs because the liver is unable to metabolize bilirubin and the edema, fibrosis, and scarring of the hepatic bile ducts interfere with normal bile and bilirubin secretion

6. Portal systemic encephalopathy: End-stage hepatic failure and **cirrhosis** characterized by altered level of consciousness, neurological symptoms, impaired thinking, and neuromuscular disturbances

7. Hepatorenal syndrome
   a. Progressive renal failure associated with hepatic failure
   b. Characterized by a sudden decrease in urinary output, elevated blood urea nitrogen and creatinine, decreased urine sodium excretion, and increased urine osmolarity

C. Data collection (Figure 47-2)

D. Interventions
   1. Elevate the head of the bed to minimize shortness of breath.
   2. If **ascites** and edema are absent and the client does not exhibit signs of impending coma, a high-protein diet supplemented with vitamins is prescribed.

Box 47-9 Types of Cirrhosis

Laënnec's Cirrhosis
Cirrhosis is alcohol induced, nutritional, or portal.
Cellular necrosis causes eventual widespread scar tissue, with fibrotic infiltration of the liver.

Postnecrotic Cirrhosis
Cirrhosis occurs after massive liver necrosis.
Cirrhosis results as a complication of acute viral hepatitis or exposure to hepatotoxins.
Scar tissue causes destruction of liver lobules and entire lobes.

Biliary Cirrhosis
Cirrhosis develops from chronic biliary obstruction, bile stasis, and inflammation resulting in severe obstructive jaundice.

Cardiac Cirrhosis
Cirrhosis is associated with severe, right-sided congestive heart failure and results in an enlarged, edematous, congested liver.
The liver becomes anoxic, resulting in liver cell necrosis and fibrosis.

---

3. Provide supplemental vitamins (B complex; vitamins A, C, and K; folic acid; and thiamine) as prescribed.
4. Restrict sodium intake and fluid intake as prescribed.
5. Initiate enteral feedings or parenteral nutrition as prescribed.
6. Administer diuretics as prescribed to treat **ascites**.
7. Monitor I&O and electrolyte balance.
8. Weigh client and measure abdominal girth daily.
9. Monitor level of consciousness; assess for precoma state (tremors, delirium).
10. Monitor for **asterixis**, a coarse tremor characterized by rapid, nonrhythmic extension and flexions in the wrist and fingers.
11. Monitor for **fetor hepaticus**—the fruity, musty breath odor of severe chronic liver disease.
12. Maintain gastric intubation to assess bleeding or esophagogastric balloon tamponade to control bleeding varices if prescribed.
13. Administer blood products as prescribed.
14. Monitor coagulation laboratory results. Administer vitamin K if prescribed.
15. Administer low-sodium antacids as prescribed.
16. Administer lactulose (Chronulac) as prescribed, which decreases the pH of the bowel, decreases production of ammonia by bacteria in the bowel, and facilitates the excretion of ammonia.
17. Administer antibiotics as prescribed to inhibit protein synthesis in bacteria and decrease the production of ammonia.
18. Avoid medications such as opioids, sedatives, and barbiturates and any hepatotoxic medications or substances.
19. Instruct the client about the importance of abstinence of alcohol intake.
20. Prepare the client for paracentesis to remove abdominal fluid.
21. Prepare the client for surgical shunting procedures if prescribed to divert fluid from **ascites** into the venous system.

XIV. ESOPHAGEAL VARICES

A. Description
   1. Dilated and tortuous veins in the submucosa of the esophagus
   2. Caused by **portal hypertension**, are often associated with liver **cirrhosis**, and are at high risk for rupture if portal circulation pressure rises
   3. Bleeding varices are an emergency.
   4. The goal of treatment is to control bleeding, prevent complications, and prevent the reoccurrence of bleeding.

B. Data collection
   1. Hematemesis
   2. Melena

3. Tarry stools
4. **Ascites**
5. Jaundice
6. Hepatomegaly and splenomegaly
7. Dilated abdominal veins
8. Signs of shock

⚠ Rupture and resultant hemorrhage of the esophageal varices is the primary concern because it is a life-threatening situation.

C. Interventions
1. Monitor the vital signs.
2. Elevate the head of the bed.
3. Monitor for orthostatic hypotension.

4. Monitor lung sounds and for the presence of respiratory distress.
5. Administer oxygen as prescribed to prevent tissue hypoxia.
6. Monitor the level of consciousness.
7. Maintain NPO status.
8. Administer fluids intravenously as prescribed to restore fluid volume and electrolyte imbalances. Monitor intake and output.
9. Monitor hemoglobin, hematocrit, and coagulation factors.
10. Administer blood transfusions or clotting factors as prescribed.
11. Assist in inserting a nasogastric tube or a balloon tamponade as prescribed; balloon tamponade is

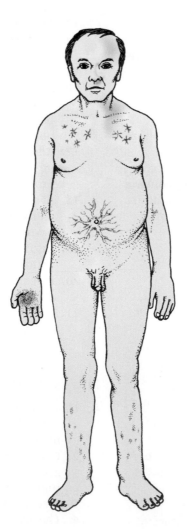

NEUROLOGIC FINDINGS
Asterixis
Paresthesias of feet
Peripheral nerve degeneration
Portal-systemic encephalopathy
Reversal of sleep-wake pattern
Sensory disturbances

GASTROINTESTINAL (GI) FINDINGS
Abdominal pain
Anorexia
Ascites
Clay-colored stools
Diarrhea
Esophageal varices
Fetor hepaticus
Gallstones
Gastritis
Gastrointestinal bleeding
Hemorrhoidal varices
Hepatomegaly
Hiatal hernia
Hypersplenism
Malnutrition
Nausea
Small nodular liver
Vomiting

RENAL FINDINGS
Hepatorenal syndrome
Increased urine bilirubin

ENDOCRINE FINDINGS
Increased aldosterone
Increased antidiuretic hormone
Increased circulating estrogens
Increased glucocorticoids
Gynecomastia

IMMUNE SYSTEM DISTURBANCES
Increased susceptibility to infection
Leukopenia

CARDIOVASCULAR FINDINGS
Cardiac dysrhythmias
Development of collateral circulation
Fatigue
Hyperkinetic circulation
Peripheral edema
Portal hypertension
Spider angiomas

PULMONARY FINDINGS
Dyspnea
Hydrothorax
Hyperventilation
Hypoxemia

HEMATOLOGIC FINDINGS
Anemia
Disseminated intravascular coagulation
Impaired coagulation
Splenomegaly
Thrombocytopenia

DERMATOLOGIC FINDINGS
Axillary and pubic hair changes
Caput medusae
Ecchymosis
Increased skin pigmentation
Jaundice
Palmar erythema
Pruritus
Spider angiomas

FLUID AND ELECTROLYTE DISTURBANCES
Ascites
Decreased effective blood volume
Dilutional hyponatremia or hypernatremia
Hypocalcemia
Hypokalemia
Peripheral edema
Water retention

▲ **FIGURE 47-2** The clinical picture of a client with liver dysfunction. Manifestations vary according to the progression of the disease. (From Ignatavicius, D., & Workman, M. [2010]. *Medical-surgical nursing: Patient-centered collaborative care* [6th ed.]. St. Louis: Saunders.)

not used frequently because it is very uncomfortable for the client and its use is associated with complications.

12. Prepare to assist with administering medications to induce vasoconstriction and reduce bleeding.
13. Instruct the client to avoid activities that will initiate vasovagal responses.
14. Prepare the client for endoscopic procedures or surgical procedures as prescribed.

D. Endoscopic injection (sclerotherapy)
1. The procedure involves the injection of a sclerosing agent into and around bleeding varices.
2. Complications include chest pain, pleural effusion, aspiration pneumonia, esophageal stricture, and perforation of the esophagus.

E. Endoscopic variceal ligation
1. The procedure involves ligation of the varices with an elastic rubber band.
2. Sloughing, followed by superficial ulceration, occurs in the area of ligation within 3 to 7 days.

F. Surgical shunting procedures
1. Description: shunt blood away from the **esophageal varices**
2. Portacaval shunting involves anastomosis of the portal vein to the inferior vena cava, diverting blood from the portal system to the systemic circulation.
3. Distal splenorenal shunt
   a. The shunt involves splenectomy, with anastomosis of the splenic vein to the left renal vein.
   b. The splenic vein conducts blood from the high-pressure varices to the low-pressure renal vein.
4. Mesocaval shunting involves a side anastomosis of the superior mesenteric vein to the proximal end of the inferior vena cava.
5. Transjugular intrahepatic portal/systemic shunt (TIPS)
   a. The nonsurgical procedure uses the normal vascular anatomy of the liver to create a shunt with the use of a metallic stent.

b. The shunt is between the portal and systemic venous system within the liver and is aimed at relieving **portal hypertension**.

XV. HEPATITIS

A. Description
1. An inflammation of the liver caused by a virus, bacteria, or exposure to medications or hepatotoxins
2. The goals of treatment include resting the inflamed liver to reduce metabolic demands and increasing the blood supply, thus promoting cellular regeneration and preventing complications.
3. General home care instructions (Box 47-10)

B. Types of viral **hepatitis**
1. **Hepatitis** A virus (HAV): infectious **hepatitis**
2. **Hepatitis** B virus (HBV): serum **hepatitis**
3. **Hepatitis** C virus (HCV): non-A, non-B **hepatitis** or post-transfusion **hepatitis**
4. **Hepatitis** D virus (HDV): delta agent **hepatitis**
5. **Hepatitis** E virus (HEV): enterically transmitted or epidemic non-A, non-B **hepatitis**
6. **Hepatitis** G virus: non-A, non-B, non-C **hepatitis**

C. Stages of viral **hepatitis** (Box 47-11)

D. Data collection
1. Preicteric stage
   a. Flulike symptoms: malaise, fatigue
   b. Anorexia, nausea, vomiting, or diarrhea
   c. Pain: headache, muscle aches, or polyarthritis
   d. Elevated serum bilirubin and enzyme levels
2. Icteric stage
   a. Jaundice
   b. Pruritus
   c. Brown urine
   d. Lighter-colored stools
   e. Decrease in preicteric-phase symptoms
3. Posticteric stage
   a. Increased energy levels
   b. Subsiding of pain

Box 47-10 Home Care Instructions About Hepatitis

Hand washing must be strict and frequent.
Bathrooms should not be shared unless the client strictly adheres to personal hygiene measures.
Individual washcloths, towels, drinking and eating utensils, toothbrushes, and razors must be labeled and identified.
The client must not prepare food for other family members.
The client should avoid alcohol and over-the-counter medications, particularly acetaminophen (Tylenol) and sedatives because these medications are hepatotoxic.
The client should increase activity gradually to prevent fatigue.
The client should consume small, frequent, high-carbohydrate, low-fat foods.
The client is not to donate blood.

The client may maintain normal contact with persons as long as proper personal hygiene is maintained.
Close personal contact such as kissing should be discouraged until hepatitis B surface antigen test results are negative.
The client is to avoid sexual activity until hepatitis B surface antigen results are negative.
The client needs to carry a Medic-Alert card noting the date of hepatitis onset.
The client needs to inform other health professionals, such as medical or dental personnel, of the onset of hepatitis.
The client needs to keep follow-up appointments with the HCP.

Box 47-11 Stages of Viral Hepatitis

Preicteric Stage

The first stage of hepatitis preceding the appearance of jaundice; includes flulike symptoms

Icteric Stage

The second stage of hepatitis, which includes the appearance of jaundice and associated symptoms such as elevated bilirubin levels, dark or brown-colored urine, and clay-colored stools

Posticteric Stage

The convalescent stage in which the jaundice decreases and the color of the urine and stool returns to normal

---

    c. Minimal to absent gastrointestinal symptoms

    d. Serum bilirubin and enzyme levels return to normal

E. Laboratory assessment

    1. Alanine aminotransferase: elevated into the thousands (normal is 4 to 36 international units/L)

    2. Aspartate aminotransferase: elevated into the thousands (normal is 8 to 33 units/L)

    3. Alkaline phosphatase levels: may be normal or mildly elevated (normal is 4.5 to 13 King-Armstrong units/dL)

    4. Total bilirubin levels: elevated in the serum and urine (normal is less than 1.5 mg/dL)

XVI. HEPATITIS A

A. Description

    1. Formerly known as infectious **hepatitis**

    2. Commonly seen during the fall and early winter

B. Individuals at increased risk

    1. Commonly seen in young children

    2. Individuals in institutionalized settings

    3. Health care personnel

C. Transmission

    1. Fecal-oral route

    2. Person-to-person contact

    3. Parenteral

    4. Contaminated fruits, vegetables, or uncooked shellfish

    5. Contaminated water or milk

    6. Poorly washed utensils

D. Incubation and infectious period

    1. Incubation period: 2 to 6 weeks

    2. Infectious period: 2 to 3 weeks before and 1 week after development of jaundice

E. Testing

    1. Infection is established by the presence of HAV antibodies (anti-HAV) in the blood.

    2. Immunoglobulin M (IgM) and G (IgG) are normally present in the blood, and increased levels indicate infection and inflammation.

    3. Ongoing inflammation of the liver is evidenced by the presence of elevated IgM antibodies, which persist in the blood for 4 to 6 weeks.

    4. Previous infection is indicated by the presence of elevated IgG antibodies.

F. Complication: fulminant (severe acute and often fatal) **hepatitis**

G. Prevention

    1. Strict hand washing

    2. Stool and needle precautions

    3. Treatment of municipal water supplies

    4. Serological screening of food handlers

    5. **Hepatitis** A vaccine (Havrix VAQTA)

    6. Immune globulin: For individuals exposed to HAV who have never received the **hepatitis** A vaccine, administer immune globulin during the period of incubation and within 2 weeks of exposure.

    7. Immune globulin and **hepatitis** A vaccine are recommended for household members and sexual contacts of individuals with **hepatitis** A.

    8. Pre-exposure prophylaxis with immunoglobulin is recommended for individuals traveling to countries with poor or uncertain sanitation conditions.

⚠ Strict and frequent handwashing is essential to preventing the spread of all types of hepatitis.

XVII. HEPATITIS B

A. Description

    1. **Hepatitis** B is nonseasonal.

    2. All age groups are affected.

B. Individuals at increased risk

    1. IV drug user

    2. Clients undergoing long-term hemodialysis

    3. Health care personnel

C. Transmission

    1. Blood or body fluid contact

    2. Infected blood products

    3. Infected saliva or semen

    4. Contaminated needles

    5. Sexual contact

    6. Parenteral

    7. Perinatal period

    8. Blood or body fluids contact at birth

D. Incubation period: 6 to 24 weeks

E. Testing

    1. Infection is established by the presence of **hepatitis** B antigen-antibody systems in the blood

    2. Presence of **hepatitis** B surface antigen (HBsAg) is the serological marker to establish the diagnosis of **hepatitis** B

    3. The client is considered infectious if these antigens are present in the blood.

4. If the serological marker (HBsAg) is present after 6 months, it indicates a carrier state or chronic **hepatitis**.
5. Normally the serological marker (HBsAg) level declines and disappears after the acute **hepatitis** B episode.
6. The presence of antibodies to HBsAg (anti-HBs) indicates recovery and immunity to **hepatitis** B.
7. **Hepatitis** B early antigen (HBeAg) is detected in the blood about 1 week after the appearance of HBsAg, and its presence determines the infective state of the client.

F. Complications
1. Fulminant **hepatitis**
2. Chronic liver disease
3. **Cirrhosis**
4. Primary hepatocellular carcinoma

G. Prevention
1. Strict hand washing
2. Screening blood donors
3. Testing of all pregnant women
4. Needle precautions
5. Avoiding intimate sexual contact if test for HBsAg is positive in a person
6. **Hepatitis** B vaccine: Engerix-B (adult), Recombivax HB (pediatric); there is also an adult vaccine that protects against **hepatitis** A and B known as Twinrix.
7. **Hepatitis** B immune globulin: for individuals exposed to HBV through sexual contact or through the percutaneous or transmucosal routes, who have never had **hepatitis** B, and who have never received **hepatitis** B vaccine

XVIII. HEPATITIS C

A. Description
1. **Hepatitis** C virus infection occurs year-round.
2. Infection can occur in any age group.
3. Infection with HCV is common among drug abusers and is the major cause of post-transfusion **hepatitis**.
4. Risk factors are similar to those for HBV because **hepatitis** C is also transmitted parenterally.

B. Individuals at increased risk
1. Parenteral drug users
2. Clients receiving frequent transfusions
3. Health care personnel

C. Transmission: Same as for HBV; primarily through blood

D. Incubation period: 5 to 10 weeks

E. Testing: Anti-HCV is the antibody to HCV and is most accurate in detecting chronic states of **hepatitis** C.

F. Complications
1. Chronic liver disease
2. **Cirrhosis**
3. Primary hepatocellular carcinoma

G. Prevention
1. Strict hand washing
2. Needle precautions
3. Screening of blood donors

XIX. HEPATITIS D

A. Description
1. **Hepatitis** D is common in the Mediterranean and Middle Eastern areas.
2. **Hepatitis** D occurs with **hepatitis** B and may cause infection only in the presence of active HBV infection.
3. Coinfection with the delta-agent (HDV) intensifies the acute symptoms of **hepatitis** B.
4. Transmission and risk of infection are the same as for HBV, via contact with blood and blood products.
5. Prevention of HBV infection with vaccine also prevents HDV infection because HDV depends on HBV for replication.

B. High-risk individuals
1. Drug users
2. Clients receiving hemodialysis
3. Clients receiving frequent blood transfusions

C. Transmission: Same as for HBV

D. Incubation period: 7 to 8 weeks

E. Testing: Serological HDV determination is made by detection of the **hepatitis** D antigen (HDAg) early in the course of the infection and by detection of anti-HDV antibody in the later disease stages.

F. Complications
1. Chronic liver disease
2. Fulminant **hepatitis**

G. Prevention: Because **hepatitis** D must coexist with **hepatitis** B, the precautions that help prevent **hepatitis** B are also useful in preventing delta **hepatitis**.

XX. HEPATITIS E

A. Description
1. **Hepatitis** E is a waterborne virus.
2. **Hepatitis** E is prevalent in areas where sewage disposal is inadequate or communal bathing in contaminated rivers is practiced.
3. The risk of infection is the same as for HAV.
4. Infection with HEV presents as a mild disease except in infected women in the third trimester of pregnancy, with whom the mortality rate is high.

B. Individuals with increased risk
1. Travelers to countries that have a high incidence of **hepatitis** E such as India, Burma (Myanmar), Afghanistan, Algeria, and Mexico
2. Eating or drinking of food or water contaminated with the virus

C. Transmission: Same as for HAV

D. Incubation period: 2 to 9 weeks

E. Testing: Specific serological tests for HEV include detection of IgM and IgG antibodies to **hepatitis** E (anti-HEV)

F. Complications
  1. High mortality rate in pregnant women
  2. Fetal demise

G. Prevention
  1. Strict hand washing
  2. Treatment of water supplies and sanitation measures

XXI. HEPATITIS G

A. **Hepatitis** G is non-A, non-B, non-C **hepatitis**.

B. Autoantibodies are absent.

C. Risk factors are similar to those for **hepatitis** C.

D. **Hepatitis** G virus has been found in some blood donors, IV drug users, hemodialysis clients, and clients with hemophilia; however, **hepatitis** G virus does not appear to cause significant liver disease.

XXII. PANCREATITIS

A. Description
  1. An acute or chronic inflammation of the pancreas with associated escape of pancreatic enzymes into surrounding tissue
  2. Acute **pancreatitis** occurs suddenly as one attack or can be recurrent with resolutions.
  3. Chronic **pancreatitis** is a continual inflammation and destruction of the pancreas, with scar tissue replacing pancreatic tissue.
  4. Precipitating factors include trauma, the use of alcohol, biliary tract disease, viral or bacterial disease, hyperlipidemia, cholelithiasis, hyperparathyroidism, ischemic vascular disease, and peptic ulcer disease.

B. Acute pancreatitis
  1. Data collection
    a. Abdominal pain, including a sudden onset at the midepigastric or left upper quadrant location with radiation to the back
    b. Pain that is aggravated by a fatty meal or alcohol or by lying in a supine and flat (recumbent) position
    c. Abdominal tenderness and guarding
    d. Nausea and vomiting
    e. Weight loss
    f. Absent or decreased bowel sounds
    g. Elevated white blood cell count, glucose, bilirubin, alkaline phosphatase, or urinary amylase
    h. Elevated serum lipase and amylase

  ⚠ Cullen's sign is the discoloration of the abdomen and periumbilical area. Turner's sign is the bluish discoloration of the flanks. Both signs are indicative of pancreatitis.

  2. Interventions
    a. Maintain NPO status and maintain hydration with IV fluids as prescribed.
    b. Administer parenteral nutrition for severe nutritional depletion.
    c. Administer supplemental preparations and vitamins and minerals to increase caloric intake if prescribed.
    d. Maintain nasogastric tube to decrease gastric distention and suppress pancreatic secretion.
    e. Administer medication as prescribed for pain.
    f. Administer antacids as prescribed to neutralize gastric secretions.
    g. Administer H_2-receptor antagonists as prescribed to decrease hydrochloric acid production and prevent activation of pancreatic enzymes.
    h. Administer anticholinergics as prescribed to decrease vagal stimulation, decrease gastrointestinal motility, and inhibit pancreatic enzyme secretion.
    i. The client is instructed on the importance of avoiding alcohol.
    j. The client is instructed on the importance of follow-up visits with the HCP.
    k. The client is instructed to notify the HCP if acute abdominal pain, jaundice, clay-colored stools, or dark urine develops.

C. Chronic **pancreatitis**
  1. Data collection
    a. Abdominal pain and tenderness
    b. Left upper quadrant mass
    c. Steatorrhea and foul-smelling stools that may increase in volume as pancreatic insufficiency increases
    d. Weight loss
    e. Muscle wasting
    f. Jaundice
    g. Signs and symptoms of diabetes mellitus
  2. Interventions
    a. The client is instructed on the prescribed dietary measures (fat and protein intake may be limited).
    b. The client is instructed to avoid heavy meals.
    c. The client is instructed about the importance of avoiding alcohol.
    d. Provide supplemental preparations and vitamins and minerals to increase caloric intake.
    e. Administer pancreatic enzymes as prescribed to aid in the digestion and absorption of fat and protein.
    f. Administer insulin or oral hypoglycemic medications as prescribed to control diabetes mellitus, if present.
    g. The client is instructed on the use of pancreatic enzyme medications.

h. The client is instructed on the treatment plan for glucose management.

i. The client is instructed to notify the HCP if increased steatorrhea occurs or if abdominal distention or cramping and skin breakdown develops.

j. The client is instructed in the importance of follow-up visits.

XXIII. PANCREATIC TUMORS, INTESTINAL TUMORS, AND BOWEL OBSTRUCTIONS (refer to Chapter 43)

XXIV. ULCERATIVE COLITIS

A. Description

1. An ulcerative and inflammatory disease of the bowel that results in poor absorption of nutrients.

2. Commonly begins in the rectum and spreads upward toward the cecum

3. The colon becomes edematous and may develop bleeding lesions and ulcers. The ulcers may lead to perforation.

4. Scar tissue develops and causes loss of elasticity and loss of the ability to absorb nutrients.

5. Colitis is characterized by various periods of remissions and exacerbations.

6. Acute **ulcerative colitis** results in vascular congestion, hemorrhage, edema, and ulceration of the bowel mucosa.

7. Chronic **ulcerative colitis** causes muscular hypertrophy, fat deposits, and fibrous tissue with bowel thickening, shortening, and narrowing.

B. Data collection

1. Anorexia

2. Weight loss

3. Malaise

4. Abdominal tenderness and cramping

5. Severe diarrhea that may contain blood and mucus

6. Dehydration and electrolyte imbalances

7. Anemia

8. Vitamin K deficiency

C. Interventions

1. Acute phase: Maintain NPO status and administer intravenous fluids and electrolytes or parenteral nutrition as prescribed.

2. Restrict the client's activity to reduce intestinal activity.

3. Monitor bowel sounds and for abdominal tenderness and cramping.

4. Monitor stools, noting color, consistency, and the presence or absence of blood.

5. Monitor for bowel perforation, peritonitis (see Box 47-3), and hemorrhage.

6. After the acute phase, the diet progresses from clear liquids to low fiber as tolerated.

7. Instruct the client to consume a low-fiber, high-protein diet. Vitamins and iron supplements may be prescribed.

8. Instruct the client to avoid gas-forming foods and milk products, and foods such as whole grains, nuts, raw fruits and vegetables, pepper, alcohol, and caffeine-containing products.

9. Instruct the client to avoid smoking.

10. Administer medications as prescribed, which may include a combination of medications such as salicylate compounds, corticosteroids, immunosuppressants, and antidiarrheals.

D. Surgical interventions

1. Total proctocolectomy with permanent ileostomy

a. The procedure is curative and involves the removal of the entire colon (colon, rectum, and anus with anal closure).

b. The end of the terminal ileum forms the stoma, which is located in the right lower quadrant.

2. **Kock ileostomy (continent ileostomy)** (Figure 47-3)

a. The **Kock ileostomy** is an intra-abdominal pouch that stores the feces and is constructed from the terminal ileum.

b. The pouch is connected to the stoma with a nipple-like valve constructed from a portion of the ileum. The stoma is flush with the skin.

c. A catheter is used to empty the pouch, and a small dressing or adhesive bandage is worn over the stoma between emptyings.

3. Ileoanal reservoir (Figure 47-4).

a. Creation of an ileoanal reservoir is a two-stage procedure that involves the excision of the rectal mucosa, an abdominal colectomy, construction of a reservoir to the anal canal, and a temporary loop ileostomy.

b. The ileostomy is closed 3 to 4 months after the capacity of the reservoir is increased and has had time to heal.

4. Ileoanal anastomosis (ileorectostomy)

a. Does not require an ileostomy

b. A 12- to 15-cm rectal stump is left after the colon is removed, and the small intestine is inserted into this rectal sleeve and anastomosed.

c. Ileorectostomy requires a large, compliant rectum.

5. Preoperative colostomy/ileostomy interventions

a. Consult with an enterostomal therapist to assist in identifying optimal placement of the ostomy.

b. The client is instructed to eat a low-fiber diet for 1 to 2 days before surgery as prescribed.

c. Administer intestinal antiseptics and antibiotics as prescribed to cleanse the bowel and decrease the bacterial content of the colon.

d. Administer laxatives and enemas as prescribed.

1. A reservoir, in which the patient will retain stool until draining it, is constructed from a loop of ileum folded and sutured together, then cut.

2. A portion of the ileum is intussuscepted to form a nipple valve, and the upper part of the stitched and cut ileum is pulled down and sutured to form a pouch.

3. The nipple valve, which shuts tight against pressure from a filled pouch, is pulled through the stoma and sutured flush with the abdomen.

▲ **FIGURE 47-3** The creation of a Kock's (continent) ileostomy. (From Ignatavicius, D., & Workman, M. [2010]. *Medical-surgical nursing: Patient-centered collaborative care* [6th ed.]. St. Louis: Saunders.)

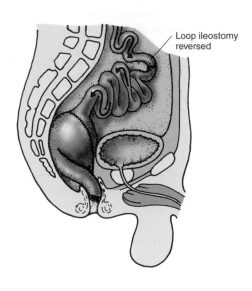

Stage 1.
After removal of the colon, a temporary loop ileostomy is created and an ileoanal reservoir is formed. The reservoir is created in an S-shaped reservoir (using three loops of ileum) or a J-shaped reservoir (suturing a portion of ileum to the rectal cuff, with an upward loop).

Stage 2.
After the reservoir has had time to heal—usually several months—the temporary loop ileostomy is reversed, and stool is allowed to drain into the reservoir.

▲ **FIGURE 47-4** The creation of an ileoanal reservoir. (From Ignatavicius, D., & Workman, M. [2010]. *Medical-surgical nursing: Patient-centered collaborative care* [6th ed.]. St. Louis: Saunders.)

6. Postoperative colostomy interventions
   a. Place petrolatum gauze over the stoma as prescribed to keep it moist, followed by a dry sterile dressing if a pouch (external) system is not in place.
   b. Place a pouch system on the stoma as soon as possible.
   c. Monitor the stoma for size, unusual bleeding, or necrotic tissue.
   d. Monitor for color changes in the stoma.
   e. Note that the normal stoma color is pink to bright red and shiny, indicating high vascularity.
   f. Note that a pale pink stoma indicates low hemoglobin and hematocrit levels, and a purple-black stoma indicates compromised circulation, requiring HCP notification.
   g. Monitor the functioning of the colostomy and check for bowel sounds.

h. Expect that stool is liquid in the immediate postoperative period but becomes more solid depending on the area of the colostomy: ascending colon—liquid; transverse colon—loose to semiformed; and descending colon—close to normal.

i. Monitor the pouch system for proper fit and signs of leakage.

j. Empty the pouch when it is one-third full.

k. Fecal matter should not be allowed to remain on the skin.

l. Administer analgesics and antibiotics as prescribed.

m. Irrigate the perineal wound (if present) as prescribed and monitor for signs of infection.

n. Instruct the client to avoid foods that cause excess gas formation and odor.

o. Instruct the client about stoma care and irrigations as prescribed. (Refer to Chapter 43 for information on colostomy irrigation.)

p. Instruct the client that normal activities may be resumed when approved by the HCP.

7. Postoperative ileostomy interventions
   a. Note that normal stool is liquid.
   b. Monitor for dehydration and electrolyte imbalance.

⚠ A stoma that is purple-black in color indicates compromised circulation, requiring immediate HCP notification.

XXV. CROHN'S DISEASE

A. Description
   1. An inflammatory disease that can occur anywhere in the gastrointestinal tract, but most often affects the terminal ileum and leads to thickening and scarring, a narrowed lumen, fistulas, ulcerations, and abscesses.
   2. Characterized by remissions and exacerbations
B. Data collection
   1. Fever
   2. Cramp-like and colicky pain after meals
   3. Diarrhea (semisolid), which may contain mucus and pus
   4. Abdominal distention
   5. Anorexia, nausea, and vomiting
   6. Weight loss
   7. Anemia
   8. Dehydration
   9. Electrolyte imbalances
   10. Malnutrition (may be worse than that seen in **ulcerative colitis**)
C. Interventions: Care is similar to the client with **ulcerative colitis**; however, surgery is avoided as much as possible because recurrence of the disease process in the same region is likely to occur.

XXVI. APPENDICITIS

A. Description
   1. Inflammation of the appendix
   2. When the appendix becomes inflamed or infected, rupture may occur within a matter of hours, leading to peritonitis and sepsis.
B. Data collection
   1. Pain in the periumbilical area that descends to the right lower quadrant
   2. Abdominal pain that is most intense at McBurney's point
   3. Rebound tenderness and abdominal rigidity
   4. Low-grade fever
   5. Elevated white blood cell count
   6. Anorexia, nausea, and vomiting
   7. Client in side-lying position, with abdominal guarding and legs flexed
   8. Constipation or diarrhea
C. Peritonitis: Inflammation of the peritoneum (see Box 47-2)
D. Appendectomy: surgical removal of the appendix
   1. Preoperative interventions
      a. Maintain NPO status.
      b. Administer fluids intravenously to prevent dehydration.
      c. Monitor for changes in level of pain.
      d. Monitor for signs of ruptured appendix and peritonitis (see Box 47-2).
      e. Position right side–lying or low to semi-Fowler's position to promote comfort.
      f. Monitor bowel sounds.
      g. Apply ice packs to the abdomen for 20 to 30 minutes every hour as prescribed.
      h. Administer antibiotics as prescribed.
      i. Avoid laxatives or enemas.

⚠ Avoid the application of heat to the abdomen of a client with appendicitis. Heat can cause rupture of the appendix, leading to peritonitis, a life-threatening condition.

   2. Postoperative interventions
      a. Monitor temperature for signs of infection.
      b. Assess incision for signs of infection such as redness, swelling, and pain.
      c. Maintain NPO status until bowel function has returned.
      d. Advance diet gradually as tolerated and as prescribed, when bowel sounds return.
      e. If rupture of the appendix occurred, expect insertion of a Penrose drain, or the incision may be left open to heal from the inside out.
      f. Expect that drainage from the Penrose drain may be profuse for the first 12 hours.
      g. Position the client in a right side–lying or low to semi-Fowler's position, with legs flexed, to facilitate drainage.

h. Change the dressing as prescribed and record the type and amount of drainage.

i. Perform wound irrigations if prescribed.

j. Maintain nasogastric suction and patency of the nasogastric tube if present.

k. Administer antibiotics and analgesics as prescribed.

XXVII. DIVERTICULOSIS AND DIVERTICULITIS

A. Description

1. **Diverticulosis**

   a. **Diverticulosis** is an outpouching or herniation of the intestinal mucosa.

   b. The disorder can occur in any part of the intestine, but is most common in the sigmoid colon.

2. **Diverticulitis**

   a. **Diverticulitis** is the inflammation of one or more diverticula that occurs from penetration of fecal matter through the thin-walled diverticula and can result in local abscess formation and perforation.

   b. A perforated diverticulum can progress to intra-abdominal perforation with generalized peritonitis.

B. Data collection

1. Left lower quadrant abdominal pain that increases with coughing, straining, or lifting

2. Elevated temperature

3. Nausea and vomiting

4. Flatulence

5. Cramp-like pain

6. Abdominal distention and tenderness

7. Palpable, tender rectal mass

8. Blood in the stools

C. Interventions

1. Provide bedrest during the acute phase.

2. Maintain NPO status or provide clear liquids during the acute phase as prescribed.

3. Introduce a fiber-containing diet gradually, when the inflammation has resolved.

4. Administer antibiotics, analgesics, and anticholinergics to reduce bowel spasms as prescribed.

5. Instruct the client to refrain from lifting, straining, coughing, or bending to avoid increased intra-abdominal pressure.

6. Monitor for perforation (see Box 47-2), hemorrhage, fistulas, and abscesses.

7. Instruct the client to increase fluid intake to 2500 to 3000 mL daily, unless contraindicated.

8. Instruct the client to eat soft high-fiber foods, such as whole grains; the client should avoid high-fiber foods when inflammation occurs because these foods will irritate the mucosa further.

9. Instruct the client to avoid gas-forming foods or foods containing indigestible roughage, seeds, or nuts because these food substances become trapped in diverticula and cause inflammation.

10. Instruct the client to consume a small amount of bran daily and to take bulk-forming laxatives as prescribed to increase stool mass.

D. Surgical interventions

1. Colon resection with primary anastomosis may be an option.

2. Temporary or permanent colostomy may be required for increased bowel inflammation.

XXVIII. HEMORRHOIDS

A. Description

1. Dilated varicose veins of the anal canal

2. May be internal, external, or prolapsed

3. Internal hemorrhoids lie above the anal sphincter and cannot be seen on inspection of the perianal area.

4. External hemorrhoids lie below the anal sphincter and can be seen on inspection.

5. Prolapsed hemorrhoids can become thrombosed or inflamed.

6. Hemorrhoids are caused by **portal hypertension**, straining, irritation, or increased venous or abdominal pressure.

B. Data collection

1. Bright red bleeding with defecation

2. Rectal pain

3. Rectal itching

C. Interventions

1. Apply cold packs to the anal/rectal area followed by sitz baths as prescribed.

2. Apply witch hazel soaks and topical anesthetics as prescribed.

3. Encourage a high-fiber diet and fluids to promote bowel movements without straining.

4. Administer stool softeners as prescribed.

D. Surgical interventions: May include ultrasound, sclerotherapy, circular stapling, or simple resection of the hemorrhoids (hemorrhoidectomy)

E. Postoperative interventions after hemorrhoidectomy

1. Assist the client to a prone or side-lying position to prevent bleeding.

2. Maintain ice packs over the dressing as prescribed until the packing is removed by the HCP.

3. Monitor for urinary retention.

4. Administer stool softeners as prescribed.

5. Instruct the client to increase fluids and high-fiber foods.

6. Instruct the client to limit sitting to short periods.

7. Instruct the client in the use of sitz baths three to four times a day as prescribed.

MORE QUESTIONS ON EVOLVE!

Practice Questions

471. A nurse is teaching the client about an upcoming colonoscopy procedure. The nurse would include in the instructions that the client will be placed in which of the following positions for the procedure?
1. Left Sims' position
2. Lithotomy position
3. Knee-chest position
4. Right Sims' position

472. A nurse is preparing to perform an abdominal examination. The initial step would be which of the following?
1. Palpation
2. Inspection
3. Percussion
4. Auscultation

473. A nurse provides instructions to a client after a liver biopsy. The nurse tells the client to:
1. Avoid alcohol for 8 hours.
2. Remain NPO for 24 hours.
3. Lie on the right side for 2 hours.
4. Save all stools to be checked for blood.

474. A nurse is caring for a client with a diagnosis of chronic gastritis. The nurse anticipates that this client is at risk for which vitamin deficiency?
1. Vitamin A
2. Vitamin C
3. Vitamin E
4. Vitamin B_{12}

475. A nurse is caring for a client after a Billroth II procedure. On review of the postoperative prescriptions, which of the following, if prescribed, would the nurse question and verify?
1. Leg exercises
2. Early ambulation
3. Irrigating the nasogastric (NG) tube
4. Coughing and deep breathing exercises

476. The nurse is providing discharge instructions to a client after gastrectomy. Which measure will the nurse instruct the client to follow to help prevent dumping syndrome?
1. Ambulate after a meal.
2. Eat high-carbohydrate foods.
3. Limit the fluids taken with meals.
4. Sit in a high-Fowler's position during meals.

477. A nurse is monitoring a client for the early signs and symptoms of dumping syndrome. Which of the following symptoms indicate this occurrence?

1. Sweating and pallor
2. Dry skin and stomach pain
3. Bradycardia and indigestion
4. Double vision and chest pain

478. A nurse is reviewing the record of a client with Crohn's disease. Which of the following stool characteristics would the nurse expect to see documented in the record?
1. Diarrhea
2. Constipation
3. Bloody stools
4. Stool constantly oozing from the rectum

479. A client with ascites is scheduled for a paracentesis. The nurse is assisting the health care provider in performing the procedure. Which of the following positions will the nurse assist the client to assume for this procedure?
1. Flat
2. Upright
3. Left side–lying
4. Right side–lying

480. An ultrasound of the gallbladder is scheduled for the client with a suspected diagnosis of cholecystitis. The nurse explains to the client that this test:
1. Is uncomfortable
2. Requires that the client be NPO
3. Requires the client to lie still for short intervals
4. Is preceded by the administration of oral tablets

481. It has been determined that a client with hepatitis has contracted the infection from contaminated food. What type of hepatitis is this client most likely experiencing?
1. Hepatitis A
2. Hepatitis B
3. Hepatitis C
4. Hepatitis D

482. A nurse is reviewing the health care provider's prescriptions written for a client admitted with acute pancreatitis. Which health care provider prescription would the nurse verify if noted on the client's chart?
1. NPO status
2. An anticholinergic medication
3. Position the client supine and flat
4. Prepare to insert a nasogastric tube.

483. A client with hiatal hernia chronically experiences heartburn after meals. The nurse would teach the client to avoid which of the following, which is contraindicated with hiatal hernia?
1. Lying recumbent after meals
2. Eating small, frequent, bland meals

3. Raising the head of the bed on 6-inch blocks
4. Taking histamine receptor antagonist medication, as prescribed

484. A nurse is monitoring for stoma prolapse in a client with a colostomy. The nurse would observe which of the following appearances in the stoma if prolapse occurred?
1. Dark and bluish
2. Sunken and hidden
3. Narrowed and flattened
4. Protruding and swollen

485. A nurse is reviewing the prescriptions of a client admitted to the hospital with a diagnosis of acute pancreatitis. Choose the interventions that the nurse would expect to be prescribed for the client. **Select all that apply.**
❏ 1. Administer antacids, as prescribed.
❏ 2. Small, frequent high-calorie feedings.
❏ 3. Encourage coughing and deep breathing.
❏ 4. Administer anticholinergics, as prescribed.
❏ 5. Maintain the client in a supine and flat position.

ANSWERS

471. 1
Rationale: The client is placed in the left Sims' position for the procedure. This position takes the best advantage of the client's anatomy for ease in introducing the colonoscope. The other options are incorrect.
Test-Taking Strategy: Use concepts related to gastrointestinal anatomy to answer this question. The position would be the same as that used for giving the client an enema while lying down. When answering factual questions such as these, remember the guiding principles and attempt to visualize the procedure to help you select the correct option. Review this procedure if you had difficulty with this question.
Level of Cognitive Ability: Applying
Client Needs: Physiological Integrity
Integrated Process: Nursing Process/Implementation
Content Area: Adult Health/Gastrointestinal
References: Ignatavicius, Workman, p. 1228. 2010. Pagana, Pagana, p. 273. 2009.

472. 2
Rationale: The appropriate technique for abdominal examination is inspection, auscultation, percussion, and palpation. Auscultation is performed after inspection and before percussion and palpation to ensure that the motility of the bowel and bowel sounds are not altered. The sequence of maneuvers is inspect, auscultate, percuss, and palpate.
Test-Taking Strategy: Use the process of elimination and think about the procedure. Remember that the sequence for abdominal examination is different than the usual systematic approach. Review this technique if you had difficulty with this question.
Level of Cognitive Ability: Applying
Client Needs: Health Promotion and Maintenance
Integrated Process: Nursing Process/Data Collection
Content Area: Adult Health: Health Assessment/Physical Exam
References: deWit, pp. 21, 23. 2009. Jarvis, pp. 115–116. 2012

473. 3
Rationale: To splint the puncture site, the client is kept on his or her right side for a minimum of 2 hours. It is not necessary to remain NPO for 24 hours. Permission regarding the consumption of alcohol should be obtained from the health care provider. It is not necessary to save all stools.
Test-Taking Strategy: Use the process of elimination and focus on the subject—a liver biopsy. Recalling the anatomical location of this procedure will direct you to the correct option. Review postprocedure instructions after a liver biopsy if you had difficulty with this question.
Level of Cognitive Ability: Applying
Client Needs: Physiological Integrity
Integrated Process: Nursing Process/Implementation
Content Area: Adult Health/Gastrointestinal
Reference: Pagana, Pagana, p. 604. 2009.

474. 4
Rationale: Deterioration and atrophy of the lining of the stomach lead to the loss of function of the parietal cells. When the acid secretion decreases, the source of the intrinsic factor is lost, which results in the inability to absorb vitamin B_{12}. This leads to the development of pernicious anemia. Options 1, 2, and 3 are incorrect.
Test-Taking Strategy: Use the process of elimination. Knowledge regarding the pathophysiology related to the lining of the stomach is required to answer this question. If you are unfamiliar with vitamin B_{12} deficiency and its relationship to gastric disorders, review this content.
Level of Cognitive Ability: Understanding
Client Needs: Physiological Integrity
Integrated Process: Nursing Process/Data Collection
Content Area: Adult Health/Gastrointestinal
Reference: Linton, p. 804. 2012.

475. 3
Rationale: In a Billroth II resection, the proximal remnant of the stomach is anastomosed to the proximal jejunum. Patency of the NG tube is critical for preventing the retention of gastric secretions. The nurse, however, should never irrigate or reposition the gastric tube after gastric surgery unless specifically prescribed by the health care provider. In this situation, the nurse should clarify the prescription. Options 1, 2, and 4 are appropriate postoperative interventions.
Test-Taking Strategy: Use the process of elimination. Eliminate the incorrect options because they are general postoperative measures. Also, consider the anatomical location of the surgical procedure to assist in directing you to the correct

option. Review these postoperative measures if you had difficulty with this question.
Level of Cognitive Ability: Analyzing
Client Needs: Safe and Effective Care Environment
Integrated Process: Nursing Process/Implementation
Content Area: Adult Health/Gastrointestinal
References: Christensen, Kockrow, pp. 196–197. 2011. *Adult health nursing.*
Linton, p. 809. 2012.

476. 3

Rationale: The client should be instructed to decrease the amount of fluid taken at meals. The client should also be instructed to avoid high-carbohydrate foods including fluids, such as fruit nectars; assume a low-Fowler's position during meals; lie down for 30 minutes after eating to delay gastric emptying; and take antispasmodics as prescribed.
Test-Taking Strategy: Use the process of elimination. Eliminate options 1 and 4 first because these measures will promote gastric emptying. From the remaining options, select option 3 because this measure will delay gastric emptying. If you are unfamiliar with this syndrome, review these client-teaching points.
Level of Cognitive Ability: Applying
Client Needs: Physiological Integrity
Integrated Process: Teaching and Learning
Content Area: Adult Health/Gastrointestinal
References: Christensen, Kockrow, p. 196. 2011. *Adult health nursing.*
deWit, p. 702. 2009.

477. 1

Rationale: Early manifestations occur 5 to 30 minutes after eating. Symptoms include vertigo, tachycardia, syncope, sweating, pallor, palpitations, and the desire to lie down.
Test-Taking Strategy: Knowledge regarding the early manifestations associated with dumping syndrome is required to answer this question. Remember, sweating and pallor occur and are early signs of dumping syndrome. If you are unfamiliar with these manifestations, review this content.
Level of Cognitive Ability: Understanding
Client Needs: Physiological Integrity
Integrated Process: Nursing Process/Data Collection
Content Area: Adult Health/Gastrointestinal
Reference: deWit, p. 702. 2009.
Christensen, Kockrow, p. 640. 2011. *Foundations of nursing.*

478. 1

Rationale: Crohn's disease is characterized by non-bloody diarrhea of usually not more than four or five stools daily. Over time, the diarrhea episodes increase in frequency, duration, and severity. Options 2, 3, and 4 are not characteristics of Crohn's disease.
Test-Taking Strategy: Use the process of elimination. Recalling the pathophysiology related to Crohn's disease will direct you to the correct option. If you are unfamiliar with this disorder, review this content.
Level of Cognitive Ability: Understanding
Client Needs: Physiological Integrity
Integrated Process: Nursing Process/Data Collection

Content Area: Adult Health/Gastrointestinal
Reference: Linton, pp. 827–828. 2012.

479. 2

Rationale: An upright position allows the intestine to float posteriorly and helps prevent intestinal laceration during catheter insertion. Options 1, 3, and 4 are incorrect positions.
Test-Taking Strategy: Use the process of elimination and visualize this procedure in selecting the correct option. Knowing that fluid will be aspirated from the abdominal cavity will assist in directing you to the correct option. If you had difficulty with this question, review this procedure.
Level of Cognitive Ability: Applying
Client Needs: Physiological Integrity
Integrated Process: Nursing Process/Implementation
Content Area: Adult Health/Gastrointestinal
References: Linton, p. 852. 2012.
Pagana, Pagana, p. 696. 2009.

480. 3

Rationale: Ultrasound of the gallbladder is a noninvasive procedure and is frequently used for emergency diagnosis of acute cholecystitis. The client does not need to be NPO, but may be instructed to avoid carbonated beverages for 48 hours before the test to help decrease intestinal gas. It is a painless test and does not require the administration of oral tablets as preparation.
Test-Taking Strategy: Focus on the subject—an ultrasound. Visualizing this procedure will direct you to the correct option. Review this procedure if you had difficulty with this question.
Level of Cognitive Ability: Applying
Client Needs: Physiological Integrity
Integrated Process: Nursing Process/Implementation
Content Area: Adult Health/Gastrointestinal
References: Linton, p. 844. 2012.
Pagana, Pagana, p. 3. 2009.

481. 1

Rationale: Hepatitis A is transmitted by the fecal-oral route via contaminated food or infected food handlers. Hepatitis B, C, and D are most commonly transmitted via infected blood or body fluids.
Test-Taking Strategy: Knowledge regarding the modes of transmission of the various types of hepatitis is required to answer this question. Remember, hepatitis A is transmitted by the fecal-oral route via contaminated food or infected food handlers. If you are unfamiliar with the modes of transmission of hepatitis, review this content.
Level of Cognitive Ability: Understanding
Client Needs: Physiological Integrity
Integrated Process: Nursing Process/Data Collection
Content Area: Adult Health/Gastrointestinal
Reference: Linton, p. 847. 2012.

482. 3

Rationale: The pain associated with acute pancreatitis is aggravated when the client lies in a supine and flat position. Therefore, the nurse would verify this prescription. Options 1, 2, and 4 are appropriate interventions for the client with acute pancreatitis.

Test-Taking Strategy: Use the process of elimination and note the strategic word "acute" in the question. Recalling the treatment measures for acute pancreatitis and the contraindications in the care of the client will direct you to the correct option. Review these measures if you had difficulty with this question.
Level of Cognitive Ability: Analyzing
Client Needs: Safe and Effective Care Environment
Integrated Process: Nursing Process/Implementation
Content Area: Adult Health/Gastrointestinal
Reference: Linton, p. 870. 2012.

483. 1
Rationale: Hiatal hernia is caused by a protrusion of a portion of the stomach above the diaphragm, where the esophagus usually is positioned. The client generally experiences pain caused by reflux resulting from ingestion of irritating foods, lying flat following meals or at night, and consuming large or fatty meals. Relief is obtained by eating small, frequent, and bland meals; histamine antagonists and antacids; and elevation of the thorax after meals and during sleep.
Test-Taking Strategy: Use the process of elimination. Note the strategic word "contraindicated." This tells you that the correct answer will be the option that represents an aggravating factor for hiatal hernia discomfort. Visualize each option and think about the anatomical location of a hiatal hernia to direct you to option 1. Review these teaching points if you had difficulty with this question.
Level of Cognitive Ability: Applying
Client Needs: Physiological Integrity
Integrated Process: Teaching and Learning
Content Area: Adult Health/Gastrointestinal
References: deWit, pp. 690–691. 2009.
Linton, p. 803. 2012.

484. 4
Rationale: A prolapsed stoma is one in which bowel protrudes through the stoma, with an elongated and swollen appearance. A stoma retraction is characterized by sinking of the stoma.

Ischemia of the stoma would be associated with dusky or bluish color. A stoma with a narrowed opening, either at the level of the skin or fascia, is said to be stenosed.
Test-Taking Strategy: Use the process of elimination. Focusing on the strategic word "prolapse" will direct you to option 4. Review the different complications that can occur with ostomy formation if you had difficulty with this question.
Level of Cognitive Ability: Analyzing
Client Needs: Physiological Integrity
Integrated Process: Nursing Process/Data Collection
Content Area: Adult Health/Gastrointestinal
Reference: Linton, p. 432. 2012.

485. 1, 3, 4
Rationale: The client with acute pancreatitis is normally placed on an NPO status to rest the pancreas and suppress gastrointestinal (GI) secretions. Because abdominal pain is a prominent symptom of pancreatitis, pain medication will be prescribed. Some clients experience lessened pain by assuming positions that flex the trunk and draw the knees up to the chest. A side-lying position with the head elevated 45 degrees decreases tension on the abdomen and may also help ease the pain. The client is susceptible to respiratory infections because the retroperitoneal fluid raises the diaphragm, which causes the client to take shallow, guarded abdominal breaths. Therefore measures such as turning, coughing, and deep breathing are instituted. Antacids and anticholinergics may be prescribed to suppress GI secretions.
Test-Taking Strategy: Focus on the pathophysiology associated with pancreatitis and note the word "acute" in the question. This will assist in selecting the correct interventions. Review treatment measures for acute pancreatitis if you had difficulty with this question.
Level of Cognitive Ability: Analyzing
Client Needs: Physiological Integrity
Integrated Process: Nursing Process/Planning
Content Area: Adult Health/Gastrointestinal
Reference: Swearingen, pp. 430–432, 436. 2012.

Gastrointestinal Medications

I. ANTACIDS (Table 48-1 and Figure 48-1)

A. React with gastric acid to produce neutral salts or salts of low acidity.

B. Inactivate pepsin and enhance mucosal protection but do not coat the ulcer crater to protect it from the acid and pepsin.

C. These medications are used for peptic ulcer disease and gastroesophageal reflux disease.

D. These medications should be taken on a regular schedule. Some are prescribed to be taken 1 and 3 hours after each meal and at bedtime.

E. To provide maximum benefit, treatment should elevate the gastric pH above 5.

F. Antacid tablets should be chewed thoroughly and followed with a glass of water or milk.

G. Liquid preparations should be shaken before dispensing.

⚠ To prevent interactions with other medications and the interference with the action of other medications, 1 hour should be allowed between antacid administration and the administration of other medications.

II. GASTRIC PROTECTANTS (Box 48-1)

A. Misoprostol (Cytotec)
1. An antisecretory medication that enhances mucosal defenses.
2. Suppresses secretion of gastric acid and maintains submucosal blood flow by promoting vasodilation
3. Used to prevent gastric ulcers caused by nonsteroidal anti-inflammatory drugs and aspirin
4. Administered with meals
5. Causes diarrhea and abdominal pain
6. Contraindicated for use in pregnancy

B. Sucralfate (Carafate)
1. Creates a protective barrier against acid and pepsin
2. Administered orally; should be taken on an empty stomach
3. May cause constipation

4. May impede absorption of warfarin sodium (Coumadin), phenytoin (Dilantin), theophylline, digoxin (Lanoxin), and some antibiotics. Should be administered at least 2 hours apart from these medications

III. MUSCARINIC ANTAGONIST

A. Description: Suppresses acid secretion by blocking muscarinic cholinergic receptors

B. Medication: Pirenzepine (Gastrozepine)

IV. HISTAMINE 2 (H_2)-RECEPTOR ANTAGONISTS (Box 48-2)

A. Description
1. Suppress secretion of gastric acid
2. Alleviate symptoms of heartburn and assist in preventing complications of peptic ulcer disease
3. Prevent stress ulcers and reduce the recurrence of all ulcers
4. Promote healing in gastroesophageal reflux disease
5. Are contraindicated in hypersensitive clients
6. Should be used with caution in clients with impaired renal or hepatic function

B. Cimetidine (Tagamet)
1. Can be administered orally, intramuscularly, or intravenously
2. Food reduces the rate of absorption. If taken with meals, absorption will be slowed.
3. Intravenous administration can cause hypotension and dysrhythmias.
4. Antacids can decrease the absorption of oral cimetidine.
5. Cimetidine and antacids should be administered at least 1 hour apart from each other.
6. Cimetidine passes the blood-brain barrier, and central nervous system side effects can occur. It may cause mental confusion, agitation, psychosis, depression, anxiety, and disorientation.
7. Dosage should be reduced in clients with renal impairment.

TABLE 48-1 Classification of Antacids and Considerations

Classification	Consideration
Aluminum compounds	Aluminum hydroxide is used to treat hyperphosphatemia; therefore it can cause hypophosphatemia. Aluminum hydroxide can reduce the effects of tetracyclines, warfarin sodium (Coumadin), and digoxin (Lanoxin) and can reduce phosphate absorption and thereby cause hypophosphatemia Contain significant amounts of sodium; should be used with caution in clients with hypertension and heart failure. The most common side effect is constipation.
Magnesium compounds	Magnesium hydroxide is also a saline laxative and the most prominent side effect is diarrhea. It is usually administered in combination with aluminum hydroxide, an antacid that assists in preventing diarrhea. Contraindicated in clients with intestinal obstruction, appendicitis, or undiagnosed abdominal pain. In clients with renal impairment, magnesium can accumulate to high levels, causing signs of toxicity.
Calcium compounds	Calcium carbonate can cause acid rebound. Rapid-acting; release carbon dioxide in the stomach, causing belching and flatulence A common side effect is constipation. Milk-alkali syndrome (headache, urinary frequency, anorexia, nausea/vomiting, fatigue) can occur (the client should avoid milk products and vitamin D supplements).
Sodium bicarbonate	Has a rapid onset and liberates carbon dioxide, increases intra-abdominal pressure, and promotes flatulence. Should be used with caution in clients with hypertension and heart failure. Can cause systemic alkalosis in clients with renal impairment. Useful for treating acidosis and elevating urinary pH to promote excretion of acidic medications after overdose

Gastric Ulcer

Duodenal Ulcer

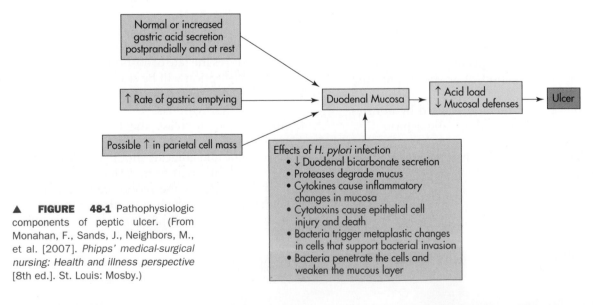

▲ **FIGURE 48-1** Pathophysiologic components of peptic ulcer. (From Monahan, F., Sands, J., Neighbors, M., et al. [2007]. *Phipps' medical-surgical nursing: Health and illness perspective* [8th ed.]. St. Louis: Mosby.)

Box 48-1 Gastric Protectants

Misoprostol (Cytotec)   Sucralfate (Carafate)

Box 48-2 Histamine 2 (H$_2$)-Receptor Antagonists

Cimetidine (Tagamet)   Nizatidine (Axid)
Famotidine (Pepcid)   Ranitidine (Zantac)

8. If cimetidine is administered with warfarin sodium (Coumadin), phenytoin (Dilantin), theophylline, or lidocaine, the dosages of these medications should be reduced.
C. Ranitidine (Zantac)
   1. Can be administered orally, intramuscularly, or intravenously
   2. Side effects are uncommon and do not penetrate the blood-brain barrier, as does cimetidine.
   3. Ranitidine is not affected by food.
D. Famotidine (Pepcid) and nizatidine (Axid)
   1. Famotidine and nizatidine are similar to ranitidine and cimetidine.
   2. These medications do not need to be administered with food.

V. **PROTON PUMP INHIBITORS** (Box 48-3)

A. Suppress gastric acid secretion
B. Used to treat active ulcer disease, erosive esophagitis, and pathological hypersecretory conditions
C. Contraindicated in hypersensitivity
D. Common side effects include headache, diarrhea, abdominal pain, and nausea

VI. **MEDICATION REGIMENS TO TREAT HELICO-BACTER PYLORI INFECTIONS** (Box 48-4)

A. An antibacterial agent alone is not effective for eradicating *Helicobacter pylori* because the bacterium readily becomes resistant to the agent.
B. Triple or quadruple therapy with a variety of medication combinations is used (if triple therapy fails, quadruple therapy is recommended).

VII. **PROKINETIC AGENT**

A. Medication: Metoclopramide (Reglan)
B. Stimulates motility of the upper gastrointestinal tract and increases the rate of gastric emptying without stimulating gastric, biliary, or pancreatic secretions
C. Used to treat gastroesophageal reflux and paralytic ileus

Box 48-3 Proton Pump Inhibitors

Esomeprazole (Nexium)   Pantoprazole (Protonix)
Lansoprazole (Prevacid)   Rabeprazole (AcIpHex)
Omeprazole (Prilosec)

Box 48-4 Medication Regimens for Treating *Helicobacter pylori* Infections

Triple Therapy
Esomeprazole (Nexium), amoxicillin (Amoxil), clarithromycin (Biaxin)

Quadruple Therapies
Esomeprazole (Nexium), metronidazole (Flagyl), tetracycline, bismuth subsalicylate
Ranitidine (Zantac), metronidazole (Flagyl), tetracycline, bismuth subsalicylate

Note: Additional medications may be prescribed for each level of therapy.

D. May cause restlessness, drowsiness, extrapyramidal reactions, dizziness, insomnia, and headache
E. Usually administered 30 minutes before meals and at bedtime
F. Contraindicated in clients with sensitivity and those with mechanical obstruction, perforation, or gastrointestinal hemorrhage
G. Can precipitate hypertensive crisis in clients with pheochromocytoma
H. Safety in pregnancy is not established
I. Metoclopramide (Reglan) can cause parkinsonian reactions. If this occurs, the medication will be discontinued by the health care provider.
J. Anticholinergics and opioid analgesics antagonize the effects of metoclopramide.
K. Alcohol, sedatives, cyclosporine (Sandimmune), and tranquilizers produce an additive effect.

VIII. **BILE ACID SEQUESTRANTS** (Box 48-5)

A. Act by absorbing and combining with intestinal bile salts, which then are secreted in the feces, preventing intestinal reabsorption
B. Used to treat hyperlipidemia in adults, biliary obstruction, and pruritis associated with biliary disease
C. With powdered forms, taste and palatability are often reasons for noncompliance and can be improved by the use of flavored products or mixing the medication with various juices.
D. Side effects include nausea, bloating, and constipation. Fecal impaction and intestinal obstruction can result.
E. Stool softeners and other sources of fiber can be used to abate the gastrointestinal side effects.

⚠ Bile acid sequestrants should be used cautiously in clients with suspected bowel obstruction or severe constipation because they can worsen these conditions.

IX. TREATING HEPATIC ENCEPHALOPATHY

A. Medication: Lactulose (Constulose, Enulose)
B. Used in the prevention and treatment of portal systemic encephalopathy, including hepatic precoma and coma; also used in the treatment of chronic constipation.
C. Promotes increased **peristalsis** and bowel evacuation, expelling ammonia from the colon and thus lowering the ammonia level.
D. Improves protein tolerance in clients with advanced hepatic **cirrhosis**
E. Administered orally in the form of a syrup or rectally

X. PANCREATIC ENZYME REPLACEMENTS (Box 48-6)

A. Used to supplement or replace pancreatic enzymes and thus improve nutritional status and reduce the amount of fatty stools. (A deficiency of pancreatic enzymes can compromise digestion, especially the digestion of fats.)
B. They should be taken with every meals and snack.
C. Side effects include abdominal cramps or pain, nausea, and diarrhea.
D. Products that contain calcium carbonate or magnesium hydroxide interfere with the action of the medication.

XI. TREATMENT FOR INFLAMMATORY BOWEL DISEASE (Box 48-7)

A. Inflammatory bowel disease has two forms, including **Crohn's disease** and **ulcerative colitis**.
B. Antimicrobials: May be prescribed to prevent or treat secondary infection (see Chapter 62 for information on antimicrobials)
C. 5-Aminosalicylates (5-ASA): Decrease gastrointestinal inflammation. Adverse effects include nausea, rash, arthralgia, and hematological disorders.
D. Corticosteroids: Act as an anti-inflammatory to decrease gastrointestinal inflammation (see Chapter 46 for information on glucocorticoids and corticosteroids).
E. Immunosuppressants: Suppress the immune system. Can cause **pancreatitis** and neutropenia secondary to bone marrow depression. Their use is reserved for those who have not responded to other traditional therapies (see Chapter 62 for information on immunosuppressants).
F. Immunomodulators: These medications are monoclonal antibodies that modulate the immune response to induce and maintain remission.

XII. TREATMENT FOR IRRITABLE BOWEL SYNDROME (IBS)

A. Irritable bowel syndrome is a gastrointestinal disorder that is characterized by crampy abdominal pain accompanied by diarrhea, constipation, or both.
B. Symptomatic relief is sometimes provided with the use of antispasmodics that relax the smooth muscle of the gastrointestinal tract, bulk-forming medications, antidiarrheals, and antidepressants.
C. Alosetron (Lotronex)
  1. Used for severe IBS
  2. Can cause severe adverse effects such as constipation, impaction, bowel obstruction, perforation of the bowel, and ischemic colitis

---

Box 48-6 Pancreatic Enzyme Replacements

Pancreatin
Pancrelipase (Pancrease MT, Viokase, Lipram, Pancrecarb MS)

Box 48-7 Medications to Treat Inflammatory Bowel Disease

Antimicrobial
Metronidazole (Flagyl)
Ciprofloxacin (Cipro)

5-Aminosalicylates
Sulfasalazine (Azulfidine)
Mesalamine (Rowasa, Asacol, Pentasa, Canasa)
Olsalazine (Dipentum)
Balsalazide (Colazal)

Corticosteroids
Prednisone
Budesonide (Entocort-EC)

Immunosuppressants
Azathioprine (Imuran)
Cyclosporine (Sandimmune, Neoral, Gengraf)
Mercaptopurine (Purinethol)

Immunomodulators
Adalimumab (Humira)
Certolizumab (Cimzia)
Infliximab (Remicade)
Natalizumab (Tysabri)

Box 48-5 Bile Acid Sequestrants

Colesevelam (WelChol)
Cholestyramine (Questran, Prevalite)
Colestipol (Colestid)

3. A strict risk management procedure must be followed by both the prescriber of the medication and the client, which includes several guidelines that must be followed including monitoring for serious adverse effects, reporting them, and immediate discontinuation of the medication if they arise.

D. Lubiprostone (Amitiza)
1. Increases intestinal motility and increases the passage of stool, thereby reducing abdominal pain
2. Side effects include nausea, headache, diarrhea, flatulence. Adverse effects include urinary tract infection and upper respiratory tract infection.

E. Tegaserod (Zelnorm)
1. Decreases visceral sensation and increase gastrointestinal motility and secretions
2. Most serious adverse effect is diarrhea and cardiovascular events such as myocardial infarction and stroke
3. Use of the medication is restricted. Only those who do not have cardiovascular disease and have not responded to an alternative treatment may be eligible for treatment with this medication.

XIII. ANTIEMETICS (Box 48-8)

A. Medications used to control vomiting and motion sickness

B. The choice of the antiemetic is determined by the cause of the nausea and vomiting.
C. Monitor for drowsiness and protect the client from injury.
D. Monitor vital signs and intake and output.
E. Limit odors in the client's room when the client is nauseated or vomiting.
F. Limit oral intake to clear liquids when the client is nauseated or vomiting.

 Antiemetics can cause drowsiness; therefore a priority intervention is to protect the client from injury.

XIV. LAXATIVES (Box 48-9)

A. Bulk-forming
1. Description
a. Absorb water into the feces and increase bulk to produce large and soft stools
b. Contraindicated in bowel obstruction
c. Dependency can occur with chronic use.
2. Side effects include gastrointestinal disturbances, dehydration, and electrolyte imbalances.

B. Stimulants: Stimulate motility of large intestine.
C. Surfactants
1. Inhibit absorption of water so fecal mass remains large and soft
2. Used to avoid straining
D. Osmotics: Attract water into the large intestine to produce bulk and stimulate **peristalsis**

Box 48-8 Commonly Administered Antiemetics

Serotonin Antagonists
Ondansetron (Zofran)
Granisetron (Kytril)
Dolasetron (Anzemet)
Palonosetron (Aloxi)

Glucocorticoids
Dexamethasone (Decadron)
Methylprednisolone (Solu-Medrol)

Substance P/Neurokinin1 Antagonists
Aprepitant (Emend)

Benzodiazepines
Lorazepam (Ativan)
Diazepam (Valium)

Dopamine Antagonists

Phenothiazines
Chlorpromazine (Thorazine)
Perphenazine (Trilafon)
Prochlorperazine (Compazine)
Promethazine (Phenergan)

Butyrophenones
Haloperidol (Haldol)
Droperidol (Inapsine)

Others
Metoclopramide (Reglan)
Domperidone (Motilium)

Cannabinoids
Dronabinol (Marinol)
Nabilone (Cesamet)

Anticholinergics

Antihistamines
Cyclizine (Marezine)
Dimenhydrinate (Dramamine)
Diphenhydramine (Benadryl)
Hydroxyzine (Vistaril, Atarax)
Meclizine hydrochloride (Bonine, Antivert)

Others
Scopolamine transdermal (Transderm Scop)

Adapted from Lehne, R. (2010). *Pharmacology for nursing care* (7th ed.). Philadelphia: Saunders.

E. Lubricants
1. Act to soften the feces, ease the strain of passing stool, and lessen irritation to hemorrhoids
2. Mineral oil: Interferes with absorption of the fat-soluble vitamins A, D, E, and K and can cause lipid pneumonia if accidentally aspirated

⚠ The client receiving a laxative needs to increase fluid intake to prevent dehydration.

XV. MEDICATIONS TO CONTROL DIARRHEA (Box 48-10)

A. The goals of treatment for diarrhea are to identify and treat the underlying cause, treat dehydration, replace fluids and electrolytes, relieve abdominal discomfort and cramping, and reduce the passage of stool.

Box 48-9 Laxatives

Bulk-Forming
Methylcellulose (Citrucel)
Polycarbophil (FiberCon)
Psyllium (Metamucil, others)

Stimulants
Bisacodyl (Correctol, Dulcolax, Feen-a-Mint, Fleet laxative, others)
Senna (Senokot Ex-Lax, others), Cascara sagrada

Surfactant
Docusate sodium (Colace, others)

Osmotics
Magnesium hydroxide (Milk of Magnesia)
Magnesium citrate (citrate of magnesia)
Sodium phosphates (Fleet enema, Fleet Phospho-Soda)
Polyethylene glycol and electrolytes (GoLYTELY)

Lubricant
Mineral oil

Box 48-10 Medications to Control Diarrhea

Opioids and Related Medications
Difenoxin with atropine sulfate (Motofen)
Diphenoxylate with atropine sulfate (Lomotil)
Loperamide (Imodium)
Paregoric (camphorated tincture of opium)
Tincture of opium

Other Antidiarrheals
Bismuth subsalicylate (Pepto-Bismol, Kaopectate, Kapectolin)

B. Opioids
1. Opioids are very effective antidiarrheal medications and decrease intestinal motility and **peristalsis**.
2. When poisons, infections, or bacterial toxins are the cause of the diarrhea, opioids worsen the condition by delaying the elimination of toxins.
3. Tincture of opium has an unpleasant taste and can be diluted with 15 to 30 mL of water for administration.

C. Other antidiarrheals: See Box 48-10.

MORE QUESTIONS ON EVOLVE!

Practice Questions

486. A client with Crohn's disease is scheduled to receive an infusion of infliximab (Remicade). The nurse assisting in caring for the client should take which action to monitor the effectiveness of treatment?
1. Monitoring the leukocyte count for 2 days after the infusion
2. Checking the frequency and consistency of bowel movements
3. Checking serum liver enzyme levels before and after the infusion
4. Carrying out a Hematest on gastric fluids after the infusion is completed

487. The client has a PRN prescription for loperamide hydrochloride (Imodium). The nurse understands that this medication is used for which condition?
1. Constipation
2. Abdominal pain
3. An episode of diarrhea
4. Hematest-positive nasogastric tube drainage

488. The client has a PRN prescription for ondansetron (Zofran). For which condition should this medication be administered to the postoperative client?
1. Paralytic ileus
2. Incisional pain
3. Urinary retention
4. Nausea and vomiting

489. The client has begun medication therapy with pancrelipase (Pancrease MT). The nurse evaluates that the medication is having the optimal intended benefit if which effect is observed?
1. Weight loss
2. Relief of heartburn
3. Reduction of steatorrhea
4. Absence of abdominal pain

490. An older client recently has been taking cimetidine (Tagamet). The nurse monitors the client for which most frequent central nervous system side effect of this medication?
1. Tremors
2. Dizziness
3. Confusion
4. Hallucinations

491. The client with a gastric ulcer has a prescription for sucralfate (Carafate), 1 g by mouth four times daily. The nurse schedules the medication for which times?
1. With meals and at bedtime
2. Every 6 hours around the clock
3. One hour after meals and at bedtime
4. One hour before meals and at bedtime

492. The client who chronically uses nonsteroidal anti-inflammatory drugs has been taking misoprostol (Cytotec). The nurse determines that the medication is having the intended therapeutic effect if which of the following is noted?
1. Resolved diarrhea
2. Relief of epigastric pain
3. Decreased platelet count
4. Decreased white blood cell count

493. The client has been taking omeprazole (Prilosec) for 4 weeks. The ambulatory care nurse evaluates that the client is receiving optimal intended effect of the medication if the client reports the absence of which symptom?

1. Diarrhea
2. Heartburn
3. Flatulence
4. Constipation

494. A client with a peptic ulcer is diagnosed with a *Helicobacter pylori* infection. The nurse is reinforcing teaching for the client about the medications prescribed, including clarithromycin (Biaxin), esomeprazole (Nexium), and amoxicillin (Amoxil). Which statement by the client indicates the best understanding of the medication regimen?
1. "My ulcer will heal because these medications will kill the bacteria."
2. "These medications are only taken when I have pain from my ulcer."
3. "The medications will kill the bacteria and stop the acid production."
4. "These medications will coat the ulcer and decrease the acid production in my stomach."

495. A histamine (H_2)-receptor antagonist will be prescribed for a client. The nurse understands that which medications are H_2-receptor antagonists? **Select all that apply**. ❖
☐ 1. Nizatidine (Axid)
☐ 2. Ranitidine (Zantac)
☐ 3. Famotidine (Pepcid)
☐ 4. Cimetidine (Tagamet)
☐ 5. Esomeprazole (Nexium)
☐ 6. Lansoprazole (Prevacid)

ANSWERS

486. 2
Rationale: The principal manifestations of Crohn's disease are diarrhea and abdominal pain. Infliximab (Remicade) is an immunomodulator that reduces the degree of inflammation in the colon, thereby reducing the diarrhea. Options 1, 3, and 4 are unrelated to this medication.
Test-Taking Strategy: Focus on the client's diagnosis, Crohn's disease. Eliminate option 1 because gastric bleeding is not a characteristic of Crohn's disease. Monitoring the leukocyte count and liver enzyme levels is appropriate when infliximab (Remicade) is given but not to evaluate the effectiveness of treatment, eliminating options 3 and 4. Review the manifestations of Crohn's disease and the actions of this medication if you had difficulty with this question.
Level of Cognitive Ability: Evaluating
Client Needs: Physiological Integrity
Integrated Process: Nursing Process/Evaluation
Content Area: Pharmacology
Reference: Gahart, Nazareno, pp. 761–762. 2011.

487. 3
Rationale: Loperamide is an antidiarrheal agent. It is used to manage acute and also chronic diarrhea in conditions such

as inflammatory bowel disease. Loperamide also can be used to reduce the volume of drainage from an ileostomy. It is not used for the conditions in options 1, 2, and 4.
Test-Taking Strategy: Focus on the name of the medication. Recalling that this medication is an antidiarrheal agent will direct you to option 3. Review the action of this medication if you had difficulty with this question.
Level of Cognitive Ability: Understanding
Client Needs: Physiological Integrity
Integrated Process: Nursing Process/Planning
Content Area: Pharmacology
Reference: Lehne, p. 941. 2010.

488. 4
Rationale: Ondansetron is an antiemetic used to treat postoperative nausea and vomiting, as well as nausea and vomiting associated with chemotherapy. The other options are incorrect.
Test-Taking Strategy: Use the process of elimination. Recalling that this medication is an antiemetic will direct you to the correct option. Review this medication if you had difficulty with this question.
Level of Cognitive Ability: Applying
Client Needs: Physiological Integrity
Integrated Process: Nursing Process/Implementation

Content Area: Pharmacology
Reference: Lehne, pp. 937–938. 2010.

489. 3
Rationale: Pancrelipase (Pancrease MT) is a pancreatic enzyme used in clients with pancreatitis as a digestive aid. The medication should reduce the amount of fatty stools (steatorrhea). Another intended effect could be improved nutritional status. It is not used to treat abdominal pain or heartburn. Its use could result in weight gain but should not result in weight loss if it is aiding in digestion.
Test-Taking Strategy: Use the process of elimination and focus on the name of the medication. Use knowledge of physiology of the pancreas to assist in directing you to the correct option. Review this medication if you had difficulty with this question.
Level of Cognitive Ability: Evaluating
Client Needs: Physiological Integrity
Integrated Process: Nursing Process/Evaluation
Content Area: Pharmacology
References: Hodgson, Kizior, p. 895. 2012.
Lehne, p. 949. 2010.

490. 3
Rationale: Cimetidine is a histamine 2 (H_2)-receptor antagonist. Older clients are especially susceptible to central nervous system side effects of cimetidine. The most frequent of these is confusion. Less common central nervous system side effects include headache, dizziness, drowsiness, and hallucinations.
Test-Taking Strategy: Use the process of elimination and note the strategic words *most frequent*. Use knowledge of the older client and medication effects to direct you to the correct option. Review the side effects of cimetidine if you had difficulty with this question.
Level of Cognitive Ability: Analyzing
Client Needs: Physiological Integrity
Integrated Process: Nursing Process/Data Collection
Content Area: Pharmacology
Reference: Hodgson, Kizior, p. 238. 2012.

491. 4
Rationale: Sucralfate is a gastric protectant. The medication should be scheduled for administration 1 hour before meals and at bedtime. The medication is timed to allow it to form a protective coating over the ulcer before food intake stimulates gastric acid production and mechanical irritation. The other options are incorrect.
Test-Taking Strategy: Use the process of elimination. Focusing on the client's diagnosis and thinking about the pathophysiology associated with a gastric ulcer will assist in directing you to the correct option. Review the administration of this medication if you had difficulty with this question.
Level of Cognitive Ability: Applying
Client Needs: Physiological Integrity
Integrated Process: Nursing Process/Implementation
Content Area: Pharmacology
Reference: Hodgson, Kizior, p. 1083. 2012.

492. 2
Rationale: The client who chronically uses nonsteroidal anti-inflammatory drugs (NSAIDs) is prone to gastric mucosal injury. Misoprostol is a gastric protectant and is given specifically to prevent this occurrence. Diarrhea can be a side effect of the medication, but is not an intended effect. Options 3 and 4 are incorrect.
Test-Taking Strategy: The strategic words in this question are *intended therapeutic effect*. This tells you that the medication is being given to prevent the occurrence of specific symptoms. Recalling that NSAIDs can cause gastric mucosal injury will direct you to the correct option. Review this medication and the side effects of NSAIDs if you had difficulty with this question.
Level of Cognitive Ability: Evaluating
Client Needs: Physiological Integrity
Integrated Process: Nursing Process/Evaluation
Content Area: Pharmacology
Reference: Hodgson, Kizior, pp. 780–781. 2012.

493. 2
Rationale: Omeprazole is a proton pump inhibitor classified as an antiulcer agent. The intended effect of the medication is relief of pain from gastric irritation, often called heartburn by clients. Omeprazole is not used to treat the conditions identified in options 1, 3, and 4.
Test-Taking Strategy: Use the process of elimination. Recalling that this medication is a proton pump inhibitor will direct you to the correct option. Review the action of this medication if you had difficulty with this question.
Level of Cognitive Ability: Evaluating
Client Needs: Physiological Integrity
Integrated Process: Nursing Process/Evaluation
Content Area: Pharmacology
Reference: Hodgson, Kizior, pp. 866–867. 2012.

494. 3
Rationale: Triple therapy for *Helicobacter pylori* infection usually includes two antibacterial drugs and a proton pump inhibitor. Clarithromycin and amoxicillin are antibacterials. Esomeprazole is a proton pump inhibitor. These medications will kill the bacteria and decrease acid production.
Test-Taking Strategy: Focus on the name of the medications and their actions. Eliminate option 1 because the medications do more than kill the bacteria. These medications are taken not only when there is pain but continually until gone, usually for 1 to 2 weeks. This will eliminate option 2. These medications do not coat the ulcer, eliminating option 4. Review the medication regimens for treatment of *H. pylori* and their actions if you had difficulty with this question.
Level of Cognitive Ability: Evaluating
Client Needs: Physiological Integrity
Integrated Process: Nursing Process/Evaluation
Content Area: Pharmacology
References: Ignatavicius, Workman, pp. 1274–1275. 2010.
Kee, Hayes, McCuistion, p. 724. 2009.

495. 1, 2, 3, 4
Rationale: H_2-receptor antagonists suppress secretion of gastric acid, alleviate symptoms of heartburn, and assist in preventing complications of peptic ulcer disease. These medications also suppress gastric acid secretions and are used in active ulcer disease, erosive esophagitis, and pathological hypersecretory conditions. The other medications listed are proton pump inhibitors.

Test-Taking Strategy: Focus on the subject, H_2 receptor antagonists. Recalling that these medication names end with -*dine* will assist in answering this question. Also, recall that proton pump inhibitors medication names end with -*zole*. Review the H_2-receptor antagonists if you had difficulty with this question.

Level of Cognitive Ability: Understanding
Client Needs: Physiological Integrity
Integrated Process: Nursing Process/Implementation
Content Area: Pharmacology
References: Kee, Hayes, McCuistion, p. 731. 2009. Lehne, pp. 919–920. 2010.

The Adult Client with a Respiratory Disorder

PYRAMID TERMS

asthma A chronic inflammatory disorder of the airways marked by airway hyperresponsiveness. Asthma causes recurrent episodes of wheezing, breathlessness, chest tightness, and coughing associated with airflow obstruction that is often reversible with treatment.

Bacille Calmette-Guérin vaccine A vaccine containing attenuated tubercle bacilli that may be given to persons in foreign countries or to those traveling to foreign countries to produce increased resistance to tuberculosis

chronic obstructive pulmonary disease A disease state characterized by pulmonary airflow obstruction that is usually progressive, not fully reversible, and sometimes accompanied by airway hyperreactivity; airflow obstruction may be caused by chronic bronchitis and/or emphysema; in chronic hypercapnia the stimulus to breathe is a low P_{O_2} instead of an increased P_{CO_2}

emphysema A chronic pulmonary disease marked by a narrowing of the small airways and the trapping of air, with destructive changes in their walls; also known as chronic obstructive pulmonary disease; also described as an abnormal permanent enlargement of airspaces distal to the terminal bronchioles with destruction of alveolar walls, without obvious fibrosis

Mantoux skin test A skin test that determines infection with tuberculosis; a small amount (0.1 mL) of intermediate-strength purified protein derivative containing 5 tuberculin units is given intradermally in the forearm; an area of induration measuring 10 mm or more in diameter, 48 to 72 hours after injection, indicates that the individual has been exposed to tuberculosis

mechanical ventilation The use of a ventilator to move room air or oxygen-enriched air into and out of the lungs mechanically if a client is unable to ventilate enough on his or her own to maintain proper levels of oxygen and carbon dioxide in the blood.

multidrug-resistant strain A multidrug-resistant strain of tuberculosis (MDR-TB) can occur as a result of improper or noncompliant use of prescribed treatment programs and the development of mutations in the tubercle bacilli

Mycobacterium tuberculosis The causative organism (bacillus) of tuberculosis; an aerobic bacterium that is a nonmotile, nonsporulating, acid-fast rod that secretes niacin

pneumothorax The accumulation of atmospheric air in the pleural space caused by a rupture in the visceral or parietal pleura, which results in a rise in intrathoracic pressure and reduced vital capacity; the loss of negative intrapleural pressure results in collapse of the lung; diagnosis of pneumothorax is made by chest radiography

suctioning A sterile procedure that involves the removal of respiratory secretions that accumulate in the tracheobronchial airway when the client is unable to expectorate secretions; performed to maintain a patent airway

tuberculosis A highly communicable disease caused by *Mycobacterium tuberculosis;* tuberculosis is transmitted by the airborne route via droplet infection

PYRAMID TO SUCCESS

The Pyramid to Success focuses on maintaining a patent airway. Pyramid points focus on infectious diseases, particularly tuberculosis, and on the client with pneumonia, respiratory failure, chronic obstructive pulmonary disease, or pneumothorax. The Pyramid to Success includes the care of the client with tuberculosis, especially with regard to the importance of the medication regimen, providing adequate nutrition and rest to promote the healing process, and preventing disease progression. Focus on assisting the client to cope with the social isolation issues that exist during the period of illness and on teaching the client and family the critical measures of screening and preventing respiratory disease and the transmission of disease.

 CLIENT NEEDS

Safe and Effective Care Environment

- Collaborating with multidisciplinary team in the management of the respiratory disorder
- Discussing consultations and referrals related to the respiratory disorder
- Establishing priorities
- Safely handling infectious materials such as sputum or body fluids
- Maintaining asepsis when caring for wounds or tracheostomy sites and during suctioning
- Maintaining confidentiality related to the respiratory disorder
- Maintaining respiratory precautions, standard precautions, and other precautions
- Obtaining informed consent related to diagnostic and surgical procedures
- Upholding client rights

Health Promotion and Maintenance

- Educating the client about adequate fluid and nutritional intake
- Educating the client about breathing exercises and respiratory therapy and care
- Educating the client about medication administration
- Educating the client about the need for follow-up care
- Educating the client about the prevention of transmission of infection

- Informing the client about health promotion programs
- Performing data collection techniques
- Preventing respiratory disorders and infectious diseases
- Providing health screening related to risks for respiratory disorders

Psychosocial Integrity

- Considering religious, cultural, and spiritual influences when providing care
- Discussing body image changes related to tracheostomy if performed
- Discussing end-of-life and grief and loss issues
- Discussing situational role changes
- Identifying coping mechanisms
- Identifying support systems
- Informing the client about community resources

Physiological Integrity

- Administering medications
- Caring for the client on mechanical ventilation
- Caring for the client receiving respiratory care and oxygen
- Managing illnesses
- Monitoring for acid-base imbalances
- Monitoring for alterations in body systems
- Monitoring for infectious diseases
- Providing comfort
- Providing nutrition and oral hygiene
- Providing personal hygiene and promoting rest and sleep

Respiratory System

I. ANATOMY AND PHYSIOLOGY

A. Primary functions of the respiratory system
1. Provides oxygen for metabolism in the tissues
2. Removes carbon dioxide, the waste product of metabolism

B. Secondary functions of the respiratory system
1. Facilitates sense of smell
2. Produces speech
3. Maintains acid-base balance
4. Maintains body water levels
5. Maintains heat balance

C. Upper respiratory tract
1. Nose: Humidifies, warms, and filters inspired air
2. Sinuses: Air-filled cavities within the hollow bones that surround the nasal passages and provide resonance during speech
3. Pharynx
   a. A passageway for the respiratory and digestive tracts that is located behind the oral and nasal cavities
   b. Is divided into the nasopharynx, oropharynx, and laryngopharynx
4. Larynx
   a. Located above the trachea, just below the pharynx at the root of the tongue and commonly called the voice box
   b. Contains two pairs of vocal cords: the false and true cords
   c. The opening between the true vocal cords is the glottis
   d. The glottis plays an important role in coughing, which is the most fundamental defense mechanism of the lungs.
5. Epiglottis
   a. A leaf-shaped elastic structure that is attached along one end to the top of the larynx
   b. Prevents food from entering the tracheobronchial tree by closing over the glottis during swallowing

D. Lower respiratory tract
1. Trachea: Located in front of the esophagus, branching into the right and left mainstem bronchi at the carina

2. Mainstem bronchi
   a. Begin at the carina
   b. The right bronchus is slightly wider, shorter, and more vertical than the left bronchus.
   c. The mainstem bronchi divide into secondary or lobar bronchi that enter each of the five lobes of the lung.
   d. The bronchi are lined with cilia, which propel mucus up and away from the lower airway to the trachea, where it can be expectorated or swallowed.
3. Bronchioles
   a. Branch from the secondary bronchi and subdivide into the small terminal and respiratory bronchioles
   b. The bronchioles contain no cartilage and depend on the elastic recoil of the lung for patency.
   c. The terminal bronchioles contain no cilia and do not participate in gas exchange.
4. Alveolar ducts and alveoli
   a. Acinus (plural acini) is a term used to indicate all structures distal to the terminal bronchiole.
   b. Alveolar ducts branch from the respiratory bronchioles.
   c. Alveolar sacs, which arise from the ducts, contain clusters of alveoli, which are the basic units of gas exchange.
   d. Type II alveolar cells in the walls of the alveoli secrete surfactant, a phospholipid protein that reduces the surface tension in the alveoli. Without surfactant, the alveoli would collapse.
5. Lungs
   a. Located in the pleural cavity in the thorax
   b. Extend from just above the clavicles to the diaphragm, the major muscle of inspiration
   c. The right lung, which is larger than the left, is divided into three lobes: upper, middle, and lower.
   d. The left lung, which is narrower than the right lung to accommodate the heart, is divided into two lobes.
   e. Innervation of the respiratory structures is accomplished by the phrenic nerve, the vagus nerve, and the thoracic nerves.

f. The parietal pleura line the inside of the thoracic cavity, including the upper surface of the diaphragm.

g. The visceral pleura cover the pulmonary surfaces.

h. A thin fluid layer, which is produced by the cells lining the pleura, lubricates the visceral pleura and the parietal pleura, allowing them to glide smoothly and painlessly during respiration.

i. Blood flow through the lungs occurs via the pulmonary system and bronchial systems.

6. Accessory muscles of respiration include the scalene muscles, which elevate the first two ribs; the sternocleidomastoid muscles, which raise the sternum; and the trapezius and pectoralis muscles, which fix the shoulders.

7. The respiratory process

a. The diaphragm descends into the abdominal cavity during inspiration, causing negative pressure in the lungs.

b. The negative pressure draws air from the area of greater pressure, the atmosphere, into the area of lesser pressure, the lungs.

c. In the lungs, air passes through the terminal bronchioles into the alveoli to oxygenate the body tissues.

d. At the end of inspiration, the diaphragm and intercostal muscles relax and the lungs recoil.

e. As the lungs recoil, pressure within the lungs becomes greater than atmospheric pressure, causing the air, which now contains the cellular waste products of carbon dioxide and water, to move from the alveoli in the lungs to the atmosphere.

f. Effective gas exchange depends on distribution of gas (ventilation) and blood (perfusion) in all portions of the lungs.

II. DIAGNOSTIC TESTS

A. Risk factors for respiratory disorders (Box 49-1)

B. Chest x-ray film (radiograph)

1. Description: Provides information regarding the anatomical location and appearance of the lungs

2. Preprocedure

a. Remove all jewelry and other metal objects from the chest area.

b. Assess the client's ability to inhale and hold breath.

3. Postprocedure: Assist the client to dress.

⚠ Question women regarding pregnancy or the possibility of pregnancy before performing radiography studies.

Box 49-1 Risk Factors for Respiratory Disorders

Allergies
Chest injury
Crowded living conditions
Exposure to chemicals and environmental pollutants
Family history of infectious disease
Frequent respiratory illnesses
Geographic residence and travel to foreign countries
Smoking
Surgery
Use of chewing tobacco
Viral syndromes

C. Sputum specimen

1. Description: A specimen obtained by expectoration or tracheal **suctioning** to assist in the identification of organisms or abnormal cells

2. Preprocedure

a. Determine the specific purpose of collection and check with institutional policy for the appropriate collection of the specimen.

b. Obtain an early morning sterile specimen from **suctioning** or expectoration after a respiratory treatment, if a treatment is prescribed.

c. Instruct the client to rinse the mouth with water before collection.

d. Obtain 15 mL of sputum.

e. Instruct the client to take several deep breaths and then cough deeply to obtain sputum.

f. Always collect the specimen before the client begins antibiotic therapy (see Priority Nursing Actions).

3. Postprocedure

a. If a culture of sputum is prescribed, transport the specimen to the laboratory immediately.

b. Assist the client with mouth care.

D. Laryngoscopy and bronchoscopy

1. Description: Direct visual examination of the larynx, trachea, and bronchi with a fiberoptic bronchoscope

2. Preprocedure

a. Obtain informed consent.

b. Maintain NPO status for the client from midnight before the procedure.

c. Obtain the vital signs.

d. Assess the results of coagulation studies.

e. Remove dentures or eyeglasses.

f. Prepare suction equipment.

g. Establish an intravenous (IV) access as necessary and administer medication for sedation as prescribed.

h. Have emergency resuscitation equipment readily available.

3. Postprocedure
   a. Monitor the vital signs.
   b. Maintain the client in the semi-Fowler's position.
   c. Assess for the return of the gag reflex.

PRIORITY NURSING ACTIONS!

Actions to Take to Perform Respiratory Suctioning
1. Explain the procedure to the client.
2. Assist the client to an upright position.
3. Perform hand hygiene and don protective garb.
4. Prepare suctioning equipment and turn on the suction.
5. Hyperoxygenate the client.
6. Insert the catheter without suction applied.
7. Once inserted, apply suction intermittently while rotating and withdrawing the catheter.
8. Hyperoxygenate the client.
9. Listen to breath sounds.
10. Document the procedure, client response, and effectiveness.

Once the nurse has assessed the client, the nurse would explain the procedure. The client is assisted to a sitting upright position such as semi-Fowler's with the head hyperextended (unless contraindicated). The nurse next performs hand hygiene and applies appropriate protective garb using aseptic technique. The nurse prepares the needed suctioning equipment, turns on the suction device, and sets it to the appropriate pressure. The nurse hyperoxygenates the client by a resuscitation bag, increasing the oxygen flow rate, or asking the client to take deep breaths. The nurse next lubricates the catheter with sterile water or water-soluble lubricant (per agency procedure), inserts the catheter without the application of suction, and then applies intermittent suction for up to 10 seconds while rotating and withdrawing the catheter. After suctioning, the nurse hyperoxygenates the client again and encourages the client to take deep breaths if possible. During the procedure the nurse monitors the client for toleration of the procedure and the presence of complications. Finally, the nurse listens to breath sounds to assist in determining effectiveness and documents the procedure, the client's response, and effectiveness.

Reference: Perry, A., & Potter, P. (2010). *Clinical nursing skills & techniques* (7th ed., pp. 676–680). St. Louis: Mosby.

---

d. Maintain NPO status until the gag reflex returns.
e. Have an emesis basin readily available for the client to expectorate sputum.
f. Monitor for bloody sputum.
g. Monitor respiratory status, particularly if sedation was administered.
h. Monitor for complications, such as bronchospasm, bronchial perforation indicated by facial or neck crepitus, dysrhythmias, fever, bacteremia, hemorrhage, hypoxemia, and **pneumothorax.**
i. Notify the health care provider (HCP) if fever, difficulty in breathing, or other signs of complications occur after the procedure.

E. Pulmonary angiography
   1. Description
      a. An invasive fluoroscopic procedure in which a catheter is inserted through the antecubital or femoral vein into the pulmonary artery or one of its branches
      b. Involves an injection of iodine or radiopaque or contrast material
   2. Preprocedure
      a. Obtain informed consent.
      b. Assess for allergies to iodine, seafood, or other radiopaque dyes.
      c. Maintain NPO status of the client for 8 hours before the procedure.
      d. Monitor the vital signs.
      e. Assess the results of coagulation studies.
      f. Establish an IV access.
      g. Administer sedation as prescribed.
      h. Instruct the client to lie still during the procedure.
      i. Instruct the client that he or she may feel an urge to cough, flushing, or nausea or experience a salty taste after injection of the dye.
      j. Have emergency resuscitation equipment available.
   3. Postprocedure
      a. Monitor the vital signs.
      b. Avoid taking blood pressures for 24 hours in the extremity used for the injection.
      c. Monitor peripheral neurovascular status of the affected extremity.
      d. Assess the insertion site for bleeding.
      e. Monitor for delayed reaction to the dye.

F. Thoracentesis
   1. Description: Removal of fluid or air from the pleural space via a transthoracic aspiration
   2. Preprocedure
      a. Obtain informed consent.
      b. Obtain vital signs.
      c. Prepare the client for ultrasound or chest radiograph, if prescribed, before the procedure.
      d. Assess the results of coagulation studies.
      e. Note that the client is positioned sitting upright, with the arms and shoulders supported by a table at the bedside during the procedure.
      f. If the client cannot sit up, he or she is placed lying in bed toward the unaffected side with the head of the bed elevated.
      g. Instruct the client not to cough, breathe deeply, or move during the procedure.
   3. Postprocedure
      a. Monitor the vital signs.
      b. Monitor the respiratory status.
      c. Apply a pressure dressing, and assess the puncture site for bleeding and crepitus.
      d. Monitor for signs of **pneumothorax**, air embolism, and pulmonary edema.

G. Pulmonary function test
 1. Description: A number of different tests used to evaluate lung mechanics, gas exchange, and acid-base disturbance through spirometric measurements, lung volumes, and arterial blood gases.
 2. Preprocedure
    a. Determine whether an analgesic that may depress the respiratory function is being administered.
    b. Consult with the HCP regarding holding bronchodilators before testing.
    c. Instruct the client to void before the procedure and to wear loose clothing.
    d. Remove dentures.
    e. Instruct the client to refrain from smoking; also, the client should avoid eating a heavy meal for 4 to 6 hours before the test.
 3. Postprocedure: The client may resume a normal diet and any bronchodilators and respiratory treatments that were held before the procedure.

H. Lung biopsy
 1. Description
    a. A transbronchial biopsy and a transbronchial needle aspiration are performed during biopsy and are performed to obtain tissue for analysis by culture or cytological examination.
    b. An open lung biopsy is performed in the operating room.
 2. Preprocedure
    a. Obtain informed consent.
    b. Maintain NPO status of the client before the procedure.
    c. Inform the client that a local anesthetic will be used, but that a sensation of pressure during needle insertion and aspiration may be felt.
    d. Administer analgesics and sedatives as prescribed.
 3. Postprocedure
    a. Monitor the vital signs.
    b. Apply a dressing to the biopsy site and monitor for drainage or bleeding.
    c. Monitor for signs of respiratory distress, and notify the HCP if they occur.
    d. Monitor for signs of **pneumothorax** and air emboli, and notify the HCP if they occur.
    e. Prepare the client for chest radiography if prescribed.

I. Ventilation-perfusion lung scan
 1. Description
    a. The perfusion scan evaluates blood flow to the lungs.
    b. The ventilation scan determines the patency of the pulmonary airways and detects abnormalities in ventilation.

 c. A radionuclide may be injected for the procedure.
 2. Preprocedure
    a. Obtain informed consent.
    b. Assess the client for allergies to dye, iodine, or seafood.
    c. Remove jewelry around the chest area.
    d. Review breathing methods that may be required during testing.
    e. Establish an IV access.
    f. Administer sedation if prescribed.
    g. Have emergency resuscitation equipment available.
 3. Postprocedure
    a. Monitor the client for reaction to the radionuclide.
    b. Instruct the client that the radionuclide clears from the body in about 8 hours.

J. Skin tests: A skin test is an intradermal injection used to assist in diagnosing various infectious diseases (Box 49-2).

K. Arterial blood gases (ABGs)
 1. Description: Measurement of the dissolved oxygen and carbon dioxide in the arterial blood to reveal the acid-base state and how well the oxygen is being carried to the body
 2. Preprocedure and postprocedure care (see Chapter 10)

⚠ Avoid suctioning the client before drawing an ABG sample because the suctioning procedure will deplete the client's oxygen, resulting in inaccurate ABG results.

L. Pulse oximetry
 1. Description
    a. Pulse oximetry is a noninvasive test that registers the oxygen saturation (Sa_{O_2}) of the client's hemoglobin.

Box 49-2 Skin Test Procedure

Determine hypersensitivity or previous reactions to skin tests.
Use a skin site that is free of excessive body hair, dermatitis, and blemishes.
Apply the injection at the upper one third of the inner surface of the left arm.
Circle and mark the injection test site.
Document the date, time, and test site.
Advise the client not to scratch the test site in order to prevent infection and possible abscess formation.
Instruct the client to avoid washing the test site.
Interpret the reaction at the injection site 24 to 72 hours after administration of the test antigen.
Assess the test site for the amount of induration (hard swelling) in millimeters and for the presence of erythema and vesiculation (small blister-like elevations).

b. The capillary Sao_2 is recorded as a percentage.

c. The normal value is 96% to 100%.

d. After a hypoxic client uses up the readily available oxygen (measured as the arterial oxygen pressure [Pao_2] on ABG testing), the reserve oxygen—that oxygen attached to the hemoglobin (Sao_2)—is drawn on to provide oxygen to the tissues.

e. A pulse oximeter reading can alert the nurse to hypoxemia before clinical signs occur.

2. Procedure

a. A sensor is placed on the client's finger, toe, nose, ear lobe, or forehead to measure Sao_2, which is then displayed on a monitor.

b. Maintain the transducer at heart level.

c. Do not select an extremity with an impediment to blood flow.

d. Results lower than 91% necessitate immediate treatment.

e. If the Sao_2 is less than 85%, oxygenation to body tissues is compromised. An Sao_2 of less than 70% is life threatening.

⚠ A pulse oximetry reading lower than 91% necessitates HCP notification; if the reading is lower than 85%, oxygenation to body tissues is compromised; and a reading lower than 70% is life threatening.

III. RESPIRATORY TREATMENTS

A. Breathing retraining (Box 49-3)

B. Chest physiotherapy (CPT)
1. Description: Percussion, vibration, and postural drainage techniques performed over the thorax to loosen secretions in the affected area of the lungs and move them into more central airways
2. Interventions (Box 49-4)
3. Contraindications
   a. Unstable vital signs
   b. Increased intracranial pressure
   c. Increase in bronchospasm from CPT
   d. History of pathological fractures
   e. Rib fractures
   f. Chest incisions

C. Incentive spirometry (Box 49-5)

Box 49-3 Client Education: Breathing Retraining and Huff Coughing

Breathing Retraining

Includes exercises to decrease the use of accessory muscles of breathing to decrease fatigue

The main types of exercises include pursed-lip breathing and diaphragmatic breathing.

The client should inhale slowly through the nose.

The client should place the hand over the abdomen while inhaling. The abdomen should expand with inhalation and contract during exhalation.

The client should exhale three times longer than inhalation by blowing through pursed lips.

Huff Coughing

An effective coughing technique that conserves energy, reduces fatigue, and facilitates mobilization of secretions.

The client should perform three to four deep breaths using pursed lip and diaphragmatic breathing. Leaning slightly forward, the client should cough three to four times during exhalation.

The client may need to splint the thorax or abdomen to achieve a maximum cough.

Box 49-4 Chest Physiotherapy (CPT) Procedure

Perform CPT in the morning on rising, 1 hour before meals, or 2 to 3 hours after meals.

Stop CPT if pain occurs.

If the client is receiving a tube feeding, stop the feeding and aspirate the residual before beginning CPT.

Administer the bronchodilator (if prescribed) 15 minutes before the procedure.

Place a layer of material (gown or pajamas) between the hands or percussion device and the client's skin.

Position the client for postural drainage based on assessment.

Percuss the area for 1 to 2 minutes.

Vibrate the same area while the client exhales four to five deep breaths.

Monitor for respiratory tolerance to the procedure.

Stop the procedure if cyanosis or exhaustion occurs.

Maintain the position for 5 to 20 minutes after the procedure.

Repeat in all necessary positions until the client no longer expectorates mucus.

Dispose of sputum properly.

Provide mouth care after the procedure.

Box 49-5 Client Instructions for Incentive Spirometry

Instruct the client to assume a sitting or upright position.

Instruct the client to place the mouth tightly around the mouthpiece of the device.

Instruct the client to inhale slowly to raise and maintain the flow rate indicator between the 600 and 900 marks.

Instruct the client to hold the breath for 5 seconds and then to exhale through pursed lips.

Instruct the client to repeat this process 10 times every hour.

IV. OXYGEN

A. Interventions
1. Assess color and vital signs before and during treatment.
2. Place an OXYGEN IN USE sign at the client's bedside.
3. Assess for chronic lung problems.
4. Humidify the oxygen if prescribed.

B. Nasal cannula (nasal prongs)
1. Description
   a. A nasal cannula is used at flow rates of 1 to 6 L/min, providing approximate oxygen concentrations of 24% (at 1 L/min) to 44% (at 6 L/min).
   b. Flow rates higher than 6 L/min do not significantly increase oxygenation because the anatomical reserve or dead space (oral and nasal cavities) is full.
   c. A nasal cannula is used for the client with chronic airflow limitation and for long-term oxygen use.
   d. Effective oxygen concentration can be delivered to nose breathers and mouth breathers with the use of a nasal cannula.

   ⚠️ A client who is hypoxemic and has chronic hypercapnia requires low levels of oxygen delivery at 1 to 2 L/min because a low arterial oxygen level is the client's primary drive for breathing.

2. Interventions
   a. Place the nasal prongs in the nostrils, with the openings facing the client.
   b. Add humidification if prescribed when a flow rate higher than 2 L/min is prescribed.
   c. Check the water level and change the humidifier as needed.
   d. Assess the client for changes in respiratory rate or depth.
   e. Assess the nasal mucosa because high flow rates have a drying effect and increase mucosal irritation.
   f. Assess skin integrity because the oxygen tubing can irritate the skin.

C. Simple face mask (Figure 49-1)
1. Description
   a. A face mask is used to deliver oxygen concentrations of 40% to 60% for short-term oxygen therapy or to deliver oxygen in an emergency.
   b. A minimal flow rate of 5 L/min is needed to prevent the rebreathing of exhaled air.
2. Interventions
   a. Be sure the mask fits securely over the nose and mouth because a poorly fitting mask reduces the fraction of inspired oxygen (FIO_2) delivered.

   b. Assess the skin and provide skin care to the area covered by the mask because pressure and moisture under the mask may cause skin breakdown. (Remove mucus and saliva from the mask.)
   c. Monitor the client closely for the risk of aspiration because the mask limits the client's ability to clear the mouth, especially if vomiting occurs.
   d. Provide emotional support to decrease anxiety in the client who feels claustrophobic.
   e. Consult with the HCP regarding switching the client from a mask to a nasal cannula during eating.

D. Partial rebreather mask (Figure 49-2)
1. Description
   a. A partial rebreather mask consists of a mask with a reservoir bag that provides an oxygen concentration of 70% to 90% with flow rates of 6 to 15 L/min.
   b. The client rebreathes one third of the exhaled tidal volume, which is high in oxygen, thus providing a high FIO_2.
2. Interventions
   a. Make sure that the reservoir does not twist, kink, or become deflated.
   b. Adjust the flow rate to keep the reservoir bag inflated two-thirds full during inspiration because deflation results in decreased oxygen delivered and rebreathing of exhaled air.

E. Non-rebreather mask (Figure 49-3)
1. Description
   a. A non-rebreather mask provides the highest concentration of the low-flow systems and can deliver an FIO_2 greater than 90%, depending on the client's ventilatory pattern.

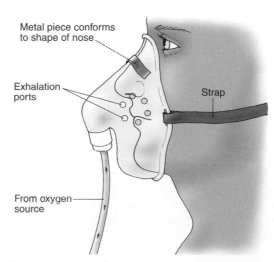

Metal piece conforms to shape of nose

Exhalation ports

Strap

From oxygen source

▲ **FIGURE 49-1** Simple face mask used to deliver oxygen. (From Ignatavicius, D., & Workman, M. [2010]. *Medical-surgical nursing: Patient-centered collaborative care* [6th ed.]. St. Louis: Saunders.)

b. A non-rebreather mask is used most frequently in the client with a deteriorating respiratory status who might require intubation.

▲ **FIGURE 49-2** Partial rebreather mask. (From Ignatavicius, D., & Workman, M. [2010]. *Medical-surgical nursing: Patient-centered collaborative care* [6th ed.]. St. Louis: Saunders.)

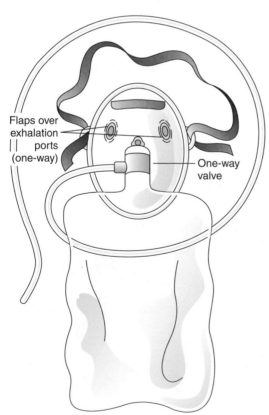

▲ **FIGURE 49-3** Non-rebreather mask. (From Ignatavicius, D., & Workman, M. [2010]. *Medical-surgical nursing: Patient-centered collaborative care* [6th ed.]. St. Louis: Saunders.)

c. The non-rebreather mask has a one-way valve between the mask and the reservoir and two flaps over the exhalation ports.
   d. The valve allows the client to draw the entire quantity of oxygen from the reservoir bag.
   e. The flaps prevent room air from entering through the exhalation ports.
   f. During exhalation, air leaves through these exhalation ports while the one-way valve prevents exhaled air from reentering the reservoir bag.
2. FiO_2 delivered: 60% to 100% FiO_2 at a liter flow that maintains the bag two-thirds full
3. Interventions
   a. Remove mucus or saliva from the mask.
   b. Assess the client closely.
   c. Ensure that the valve and flaps are intact and functional during each breath.
   d. Valves should open during expiration and close during inhalation.
   e. Suffocation can occur if the reservoir bag kinks or the oxygen source disconnects.

F. Face tent
   1. A face tent fits over the client's chin, with the top extending halfway across the face.
   2. The oxygen concentration varies, but the face tent is useful instead of a tight-fitting mask for the client who has facial trauma or burns.

G. Aerosol mask: Used for the client who requires high humidity after extubation or upper airway surgery or for the client who has thick secretions

H. Tracheostomy collar and T piece
   1. The tracheostomy collar can be used to deliver high humidity and the desired oxygen to the client with a tracheostomy.
   2. A special adapter, called the T piece, can be used to deliver any desired FiO_2 to the client with a tracheostomy, laryngectomy, or endotracheal tube.
   3. Refer to Chapter 19 for information on endotracheal and tracheostomy tubes.

I. Interventions for face tent, aerosol mask, tracheostomy collar, and T piece
   1. Change the delivery system to a nasal cannula during mealtimes if prescribed for the client with a face mask or aerosol mask.
   2. Ensure that the aerosol mist escapes from the vents of the delivery system during inspiration and expiration.
   3. Empty condensation from the tubing to prevent the client from being lavaged with water and to promote an adequate flow rate. Remove and clean the tubing at least every 4 hours.
   4. Ensure that sufficient water is in the aerosol water container, and change the container as needed.
   5. Keep the exhalation port on the T piece open and uncovered. (If the port is occluded, the client can suffocate.)

6. Position the T piece so that it does not pull on the tracheostomy or endotracheal tube and cause erosion of the skin at the tracheostomy insertion site.
7. Make sure the humidifier creates enough mist. A mist should be seen during inspiration and expiration.

J. Venturi mask (Figure 49-4)
1. Description
    a. Provides a high-flow oxygen delivery system
    b. Operation of the Venturi mask is based on a mechanism that pulls in a specific proportional amount of room air for each liter flow of oxygen.
    c. An adapter is located between the bottom of the mask and the oxygen source. The adapter contains holes of different sizes that allow only specific amounts of air to mix with the oxygen.
    d. The adapter allows selection of the amount of oxygen desired.
2. FIO_2 delivered: 24% to 55% FIO_2 with flow rates of 4 to 10 L/min
3. Interventions
    a. Monitor the client closely to ensure an accurate flow rate for specific FIO_2 .
    b. Keep the air entrapment port for the Venturi adapter open and uncovered to ensure adequate oxygen delivery.
    c. Ensure that the mask fits snugly and the tubing is free of kinks because the FIO_2 is altered if kinking occurs or if the mask fits poorly.
    d. Assess the client for dry mucous membranes. Humidity or aerosol can be added to the system.

▲ **FIGURE 49-4** Venturi mask for precise oxygen delivery. (From Ignatavicius, D., & Workman, M. [2010]. *Medical-surgical nursing: Patient-centered collaborative care* [6th ed.]. St. Louis: Saunders.)

V. MECHANICAL VENTILATION

A. Description: Used to overcome the client's inability to ventilate or oxygenate adequately
B. Interventions

⚠ For a client receiving mechanical ventilation, always assess the client first and then assess the ventilator.

1. Assess the client first and the ventilator second.
2. Assess vital signs, lung sounds, respiratory status, and breathing patterns. The client will never breathe at a rate less than the rate set on the ventilator.
3. Monitor skin color, particularly in the lips and nail beds.
4. Monitor the chest for bilateral expansion.
5. Obtain pulse oximetry readings.
6. Monitor ABG results.
7. Assess the need for **suctioning** and observe the type, color, and amount of secretions.
8. Assess ventilator settings.
9. Assess the level of water in the humidifier and the temperature of the humidification system because extremes in temperature can cause damage to the mucosa in the airway.
10. Ensure that the alarms are set. (Never shut alarms off.)
11. If a cause for an alarm cannot be determined, ventilate the client manually with a resuscitation bag until the problem is corrected.
12. Empty the ventilator tubing when moisture collects.
13. Turn the client at least every 2 hours or get the client out of bed, as prescribed, to prevent complications of immobility.
14. Have resuscitation equipment available at the bedside.

C. Causes of alarms (Box 49-6)

Box 49-6 Causes of Ventilator Alarms

High-Pressure Alarm
Increased secretions are in the airway.
Wheezing or bronchospasm causes decreased airway size.
The endotracheal tube is displaced.
The endotracheal tube is obstructed as a result of water or a kink in the tubing.
The client coughs, gags, or bites on the oral endotracheal tube.
The client is anxious or fights the ventilator.

Low-Pressure Alarm
Disconnection or leak in the ventilator or in the client's airway cuff occurs.
The client stops spontaneous breathing.

⚠ Never set ventilator alarm controls to the off position.

D. Complications
1. Hypotension caused by the application of positive pressure, which increases intrathoracic pressure and inhibits blood returning to the heart
2. Respiratory complications such as **pneumothorax** or subcutaneous **emphysema** as a result of positive pressure can occur.
3. Gastrointestinal alterations such as stress ulcers
4. Malnutrition, if nutrition is not maintained
5. Infections
6. Muscular deconditioning
7. Ventilator dependence or inability to wean

E. Weaning: The process of going from ventilator dependence to spontaneous breathing

VI. CHEST INJURIES

A. Rib fracture
1. Description
   a. Results from direct blunt chest trauma and causes a potential for intrathoracic injury, such as **pneumothorax** or pulmonary contusion
   b. Pain with movement and chest splinting result in impaired ventilation and inadequate clearance of secretions
2. Data collection
   a. Pain at the injury site that increases with inspiration
   b. Tenderness at the site
   c. Shallow respirations
   d. Client splints chest
   e. Fractures noted on chest x-ray film
3. Interventions
   a. Note that the ribs usually unite spontaneously.
   b. Place the client in the high Fowler's position.
   c. Administer pain medication as prescribed to maintain adequate ventilatory status.
   d. Monitor for increased respiratory distress.
   e. Instruct the client to self-splint with hands and arms.
   f. Prepare the client for an intercostal nerve block as prescribed if the pain is severe.

B. Flail chest
1. Description
   a. Occurs from blunt chest trauma associated with accidents, which may result in hemothorax and rib fractures
   b. The loose segment of the chest wall becomes paradoxical to the expansion and contraction of the rest of the chest wall.
2. Data collection
   a. Paradoxical respirations (inward movement of a segment of the thorax during inspiration with outward movement during expiration)

b. Severe pain in the chest
   c. Dyspnea
   d. Cyanosis
   e. Tachycardia
   f. Hypotension
   g. Tachypnea; shallow respirations
   h. Diminished breath sounds
3. Interventions
   a. Maintain the client in the high Fowler's position.
   b. Administer humidified oxygen as prescribed.
   c. Monitor for increased respiratory distress.
   d. Encourage coughing and deep breathing.
   e. Administer pain medication as prescribed.
   f. Maintain bedrest and limit activity to reduce oxygen demands.
   g. Prepare for intubation with **mechanical ventilation**. (Positive end expiratory pressure [PEEP] is used for flail chest associated with respiratory failure and shock.)

C. Pulmonary contusion
1. Description
   a. Is characterized by interstitial hemorrhage associated with intraalveolar hemorrhage, resulting in decreased pulmonary compliance
   b. The major complication is acute respiratory distress syndrome.
2. Data collection
   a. Dyspnea
   b. Hypoxemia
   c. Increased bronchial secretions
   d. Hemoptysis
   e. Restlessness
   f. Decreased breath sounds
   g. Crackles and wheezes
3. Interventions
   a. Maintain a patent airway and adequate ventilation.
   b. Place the client in the high Fowler's position.
   c. Administer oxygen as prescribed.
   d. Monitor for increased respiratory distress.
   e. Maintain bedrest and limit activity to reduce oxygen demands.
   f. Prepare for **mechanical ventilation** with PEEP if required.

D. **Pneumothorax** (Figure 49-5)
1. Description
   a. The accumulation of atmospheric air in the pleural space, which results in a rise in intrathoracic pressure and in a reduction in vital capacity
   b. The loss of negative intrapleural pressure results in collapse of the lung.
   c. A spontaneous **pneumothorax** occurs with the rupture of a pulmonary bleb.
   d. An open **pneumothorax** occurs when an opening through the chest wall allows the entrance of positive atmospheric air pressure into the pleural space.

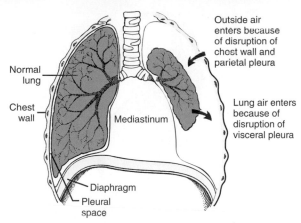

▲ FIGURE 49-5 Pneumothorax. Air in the pleural space causes the lung to collapse around the hilus and may push mediastinal contents (heart and great vessels) toward the other lung. (From McCance, K., & Huether, S. [2010]. *Pathophysiology: The biologic basis for disease in adults and children* [6th ed.]. St. Louis: Mosby.)

Labels in figure: Normal lung; Chest wall; Mediastinum; Outside air enters because of disruption of chest wall and parietal pleura; Lung air enters because of disruption of visceral pleura; Diaphragm; Pleural space

Box 49-7 Data Collection Findings: Pneumothorax

Absent breath sounds on affected side
Cyanosis
Decreased chest expansion unilaterally
Dyspnea
Hypotension
Sharp chest pain
Subcutaneous emphysema as evidenced by crepitus on palpation
Sucking sound with open chest wound
Tachycardia
Tachypnea
Tracheal deviation to the unaffected side with tension pneumothorax

e. A tension **pneumothorax** occurs from a blunt chest injury or **mechanical ventilation** with PEEP when a buildup of positive pressure occurs in the pleural space.

f. Diagnosis of **pneumothorax** is made by chest x-ray film.

2. Data collection (Box 49-7)
3. Interventions
   a. Apply a dressing over an open chest wound.
   b. Administer oxygen as prescribed.
   c. Place the client in the high Fowler's position.
   d. Prepare for chest tube placement until the lung has expanded fully.
   e. Monitor the chest tube drainage system.
   f. Monitor for subcutaneous **emphysema**.
   g. Refer to Chapter 19 for information on chest tubes.

⚠ Clients with a respiratory disorder should be positioned with the head of the bed elevated.

VII. ACUTE RESPIRATORY FAILURE

A. Description
1. Occurs when insufficient oxygen is transported to the blood or inadequate carbon dioxide is removed from the lungs and the client's compensatory mechanisms fail.
2. Causes include a mechanical abnormality of the lungs or chest wall, a defect in the respiratory control center in the brain, or an impairment in the function of the respiratory muscles.
3. In oxygenation failure, or hypoxemic respiratory failure, oxygen may reach the alveoli but cannot be absorbed or used properly, resulting in a PaO_2 less than 60 mm Hg, arterial SaO_2 lower than 90%, or partial pressure of arterial carbon dioxide ($PaCO_2$) greater than 50 mm Hg occurring with acidemia.
4. Many clients experience both hypoxemic and hypercapnic respiratory failure and retained carbon dioxide in the alveoli displaces oxygen contributing to the hypoxemia.
5. Manifestations of respiratory failure are related to the extent and rapidity of change in PaO_2 and $PaCO_2$.

B. Data collection
1. Dyspnea
2. Headache
3. Restlessness
4. Confusion
5. Tachycardia
6. Hypertension
7. Dysrhythmias
8. Decreased level of consciousness
9. Alterations in respirations and breath sounds

C. Interventions
1. Identify and treat the cause of the respiratory failure.
2. Administer oxygen to maintain the PaO_2 level greater than 60 to 70 mm Hg.
3. Place the client in the high Fowler's position.
4. Encourage deep breathing.
5. Administer bronchodilators as prescribed.
6. Prepare the client for **mechanical ventilation** if supplemental oxygen cannot maintain acceptable PaO_2 and $PaCO_2$ levels.

VIII. ACUTE RESPIRATORY DISTRESS SYNDROME

A. Description
1. A form of acute respiratory failure that occurs as a complication of some other condition. It is caused by a diffuse lung injury and leads to extravascular lung fluid.
2. The major site of injury is the alveolar capillary membrane.
3. The interstitial edema causes compression and obliteration of the terminal airways and leads to reduced lung volume and compliance.

4. The ABGs identify respiratory acidosis and hypoxemia that does not respond to an increased percentage of oxygen.
5. The chest x-ray film shows bilateral interstitial and alveolar infiltrates. Interstitial edema may not show until there is a 30% increase in fluid content.
6. Some of the causes include sepsis, fluid overload, shock, trauma, neurological injuries, burns, disseminated intravascular coagulation, drug ingestion, aspiration, and the inhalation of toxic substances.

B. Data collection
1. Tachypnea
2. Dyspnea
3. Decreased breath sounds
4. Deteriorating arterial blood gas levels
5. Hypoxemia despite high concentrations of delivered oxygen
6. Decreased pulmonary compliance
7. Pulmonary infiltrates

C. Interventions
1. Identify and treat the cause of the acute respiratory distress syndrome.
2. Administer oxygen as prescribed.
3. Place the client in the high Fowler's position.
4. Restrict fluid intake as prescribed.
5. Provide respiratory treatments as prescribed.
6. Administer diuretics, anticoagulants, or corticosteroids as prescribed.
7. Prepare the client for intubation and **mechanical ventilation** using PEEP.

IX. ASTHMA (refer to Chapter 32 for information on **asthma**)

X. CHRONIC OBSTRUCTIVE PULMONARY DISEASE

A. Description
1. Is also known as chronic obstructive lung disease and chronic airflow limitation.
2. **Chronic obstructive pulmonary disease** is a disease state characterized by airflow obstruction caused by **emphysema** or chronic bronchitis.
3. Progressive airflow limitation occurs, associated with abnormal inflammatory response of the lungs that is not completely reversible.
4. **Chronic obstructive pulmonary disease** leads to pulmonary insufficiency, pulmonary hypertension, and cor pulmonale.

B. Data collection
1. Cough
2. Exertional dyspnea
3. Wheezing and crackles
4. Sputum production
5. Weight loss

▲ **FIGURE 49-6** Typical barrel chest in the client with chronic obstructive pulmonary disease. (From Ignatavicius, D., & Workman, M. [2010]. *Medical-surgical nursing: Patient-centered collaborative care* [6th ed.]. St. Louis: Saunders.)

6. Barrel chest (**emphysema**) (Figure 49-6)
7. Use of accessory muscles for breathing
8. Prolonged expiration
9. Orthopnea
10. Cardiac dysrhythmias
11. Congestion and hyperinflation on chest x-ray film (Figure 49-7)
12. ABGs that indicate respiratory acidosis and hypoxemia
13. Pulmonary function tests that demonstrate decreased vital capacity

C. Interventions
1. Monitor the vital signs.
2. Administer a low concentration of oxygen (1 to 2 L/min) as prescribed. The stimulus to breathe is a low arterial P_{O_2} instead of an increased P_{CO_2}.
3. Monitor pulse oximetry.
4. Provide respiratory treatments and CPT.
5. Instruct the client in diaphragmatic or abdominal breathing techniques and pursed lip breathing techniques.
6. Record the color, amount, and consistency of sputum.
7. Suction fluids from the client's lungs, if necessary, to clear the airway and prevent infection.
8. Monitor weight.
9. Encourage small, frequent meals to maintain nutrition and prevent dyspnea.
10. Provide a high-calorie, high-protein diet with supplements.
11. Encourage fluid intake up to 3000 mL/day to keep secretions thin, unless contraindicated.

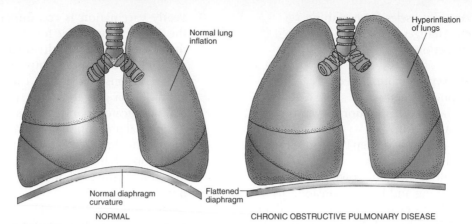

▲ **FIGURE 49-7** Diaphragm shape and lung inflation in the normal client and in the client with chronic obstructive pulmonary disease. (From Ignatavicius, D., & Workman, M. [2010]. *Medical-surgical nursing: Patient-centered collaborative care* [6th ed.]. St. Louis: Saunders.)

12. Place the client in the high Fowler's position and leaning forward to aid in breathing.
13. Allow activity as tolerated.
14. Administer bronchodilators as prescribed, and instruct the client in the use of oral and inhalant medications.
15. Administer corticosteroids as prescribed to treat exacerbation.
16. Administer mucolytics to thin secretions as prescribed.
17. Administer antibiotics for infection if prescribed.
D. Client education (Box 49-8).

XI. SEVERE ACUTE RESPIRATORY SYNDROME (SARS)

A. A respiratory illness caused by the coronavirus, called *SARS-associated coronavirus*
B. The syndrome begins with a fever, an overall feeling of discomfort, body aches, and mild respiratory symptoms.
C. After 2 to 7 days, the client may develop a dry cough and dyspnea.
D. Infection is spread by close person-to-person contact by direct contact with infectious material (respiratory secretions or by contact with persons or objects infected with infectious droplets).
E. Prevention includes avoiding contact with those suspected of having SARS, avoiding travel to countries with an outbreak of SARS, avoiding close contact with crowds in areas where SARS exists, and frequent handwashing if in an area where SARS exists.

XII. PNEUMONIA

A. Description
   1. An infection of the pulmonary tissue, including the interstitial spaces, the alveoli, and the bronchioles

Box 49-8 Client Education: Chronic Obstructive Pulmonary Disease

Adhere to activity limitations, alternating rest periods with activity.
Avoid gas-producing foods, spicy foods, and extremely hot or cold foods.
Avoid exposure to individuals with infections, and avoid crowds.
Avoid extremes in temperature.
Avoid fireplaces, pets, feather pillows, and other environmental allergens.
Avoid powerful odors.
Meet nutritional requirements.
Receive immunizations as recommended.
Recognize the signs and symptoms of respiratory infection and hypoxia.
Stop smoking.
Use medications and inhalers as prescribed.
Use oxygen therapy as prescribed.
Use pursed lip and diaphragmatic or abdominal breathing.
When dusting, use a wet cloth.

   2. The edema associated with inflammation stiffens the lung, decreases lung compliance and vital capacity, and causes hypoxemia.
   3. Pneumonia can be community acquired or hospital acquired.
   4. The chest x-ray film shows lobar or segmental consolidation, pulmonary infiltrates, or pleural effusions.
   5. A sputum culture identifies the organism.
   6. The white blood cell count and erythrocyte sedimentation rate are elevated.
B. Data collection
   1. Chills
   2. Elevated temperature
   3. Pleuritic pain
   4. Tachypnea
   5. Rhonchi and wheezes

6. Use of accessory muscles for breathing
7. Mental status changes
8. Sputum production

C. Interventions

1. Administer oxygen as prescribed.
2. Monitor respiratory status.
3. Monitor for labored respirations, cyanosis, and cold and clammy skin.
4. Encourage coughing and deep breathing and use of the incentive spirometer.
5. Place the client in the semi-Fowler's position to facilitate breathing and lung expansion.
6. Change the client's position frequently and ambulate as tolerated to mobilize secretions.
7. Provide CPT.
8. Perform nasotracheal **suctioning** if the client is unable to clear secretions.
9. Monitor pulse oximetry.
10. Monitor and record color, consistency, and amount of sputum.
11. Provide a high-calorie, high-protein diet with small frequent meals.
12. Encourage fluids up to 3 L a day to thin secretions unless contraindicated.
13. Provide a balance of rest and activity, gradually increasing activity.
14. Administer antibiotics as prescribed.
15. Administer antipyretics, bronchodilators, cough suppressants, mucolytic agents, and expectorants as prescribed.
16. Prevent the spread of infection by handwashing and the proper disposal of secretions.

D. Client education

1. Instruct the client about the importance of rest, proper nutrition, and adequate fluid intake.
2. Avoid chilling and exposure to individuals with respiratory infections or viruses.
3. Instruct the client regarding medications and the use of inhalants as prescribed.
4. Instruct the client to notify the HCP if chills, fever, dyspnea, hemoptysis, or increased fatigue occurs.
5. Instruct the client on the importance of receiving immunizations as recommended.

 Teach clients that using proper hand washing techniques, disposing respiratory secretions properly, and receiving vaccines as appropriate will assist in preventing the spread of infection.

XIII. INFLUENZA

A. Description

1. A highly contagious acute viral respiratory infection; also known as the flu
2. May be caused by several viruses usually known as A, B, and C

3. Yearly vaccination is recommended to prevent the disease, especially for those who are older than 50 years of age, individuals with chronic illness or who are immunocompromised, those living in institutions, and health care individuals providing direct care to clients. (The vaccination is contraindicated in individuals with egg allergies.)
4. Additional prevention measures include avoiding those who have developed influenza, frequent and proper handwashing, and cleaning and disinfecting surfaces that have become contaminated with secretions.
5. Avian influenza A (H5N1)
   a. Affects birds; does not usually affect humans; however, human cases have been reported in some countries.
   b. An H5N1 vaccine has been developed for use if a pandemic virus were to emerge.
   c. Reported symptoms are similar to those that are associated with influenza A, B, and C.
   d. Prevention measures include thoroughly cooking poultry products, avoiding contact with wild animals, frequent and proper handwashing, and cleaning and disinfecting surfaces that have become contaminated with secretions.
6. Swine (H1N1) influenza
   a. It is a new strain of flu that consists of genetic materials from swine, avian, and human influenza viruses.
   b. Signs and symptoms are similar to those that present with seasonal flu; additionally vomiting and diarrhea commonly occur.
   c. Prevention measures and treatment is the same as for the seasonal flu.
   d. Refer to Chapter 39 for additional information on swine flu and Chapter 50 for information on H1N1 vaccines.

B. Data collection

1. Acute onset of fever and muscle aches
2. Headache
3. Fatigue, weakness, and anorexia
4. Sore throat, cough, and rhinorrhea

C. Interventions

1. Encourage rest.
2. Encourage fluids to prevent pulmonary complications (unless contraindicated).
3. Monitor lung sounds.
4. Provide supportive therapy such as antipyretics or antitussives, as indicated.
5. Administer antiviral medications as prescribed for current strain of influenza (refer to Chapter 50).

XIV. LEGIONNAIRE'S DISEASE

A. Description

1. An acute bacterial infection caused by *Legionella pneumophila*

2. Sources of the organism include contaminated air conditioner cooling towers and warm stagnant water supplies, including water vaporizers, water sonicators, whirlpool spas, and showers.
3. Person-to-person contact does not occur and the risk for infection is increased by the presence of other conditions.

B. Data collection: Influenza-like symptoms with a high fever, chills, muscle aches, and headache that may progress to dry cough, pleurisy, and sometimes diarrhea

C. Interventions: Treatment is supportive and antibiotics may be prescribed.

XV. PLEURAL EFFUSION

A. Description
1. Pleural effusion is the collection of fluid in the pleural space.
2. Any condition that interferes with secretion or drainage of fluid in the pleural space will lead to pleural effusion.

B. Data collection
1. Pleuritic pain that is sharp and increases with inspiration
2. Progressive dyspnea with decreased movement of the chest wall on the affected side
3. Dry, nonproductive cough caused by bronchial irritation or mediastinal shift
4. Tachycardia
5. Elevated temperature
6. Decreased breath sounds over affected area
7. Chest x-ray film that shows pleural effusion and a mediastinal shift away from the fluid if the effusion is greater than 250 mL

C. Interventions
1. Identify and treat the underlying cause.
2. Monitor breath sounds.
3. Place the client in the high Fowler's position.
4. Encourage coughing and deep breathing.
5. Prepare the client for thoracentesis.
6. If pleural effusion is recurrent, prepare the client for pleurectomy or pleurodesis as prescribed.

D. Pleurectomy
1. Consists of surgically stripping the parietal pleura away from the visceral pleura
2. This produces an intense inflammatory reaction that promotes adhesion formation between the two layers during healing.

E. Pleurodesis
1. Involves the instillation of a sclerosing substance into the pleural space via a thoracotomy tube
2. The substance creates an inflammatory response that scleroses tissues together.

XVI. EMPYEMA

A. Description
1. The collection of pus within the pleural cavity
2. The fluid is thick, opaque, and foul smelling.
3. The most common cause is pulmonary infection and lung abscess caused by thoracic surgery or chest trauma, in which bacteria are introduced directly into the pleural space.
4. Treatment focuses on treating the infection, emptying the empyema cavity, re-expanding the lung, and controlling the infection.

B. Data collection
1. Recent febrile illness or trauma
2. Chest pain
3. Cough
4. Dyspnea
5. Anorexia and weight loss
6. Malaise
7. Elevated temperature and chills
8. Night sweats
9. Pleural exudate on chest x-ray film

C. Interventions
1. Monitor breath sounds.
2. Place the client in the semi-Fowler's or high Fowler's position.
3. Encourage coughing and deep breathing.
4. Administer antibiotics as prescribed.
5. Instruct the client to splint the chest as necessary.
6. Assist with thoracentesis or chest tube insertion to promote drainage and lung expansion.
7. If marked pleural thickening occurs, prepare the client for decortication, if prescribed. This is a surgical procedure that involves removal of the restrictive mass of fibrin and inflammatory cells.

XVII. PLEURISY

A. Description
1. The inflammation of the visceral and parietal membranes that may be caused by pulmonary infarction or pneumonia
2. The visceral and parietal membranes rub together during respiration and cause pain
3. Pleurisy usually occurs on one side of the chest, usually in the lower lateral portions in the chest wall.

B. Data collection
1. Knife-like pain that is aggravated on deep breathing and coughing
2. Dyspnea
3. Pleural friction rub heard on auscultation
4. Apprehension

C. Interventions
1. Identify and treat the cause.
2. Monitor lung sounds.
3. Administer analgesics as prescribed.
4. Apply hot or cold applications as prescribed.

5. Encourage coughing and deep breathing.
6. Instruct the client to lie on the affected side to splint the chest.

XVIII. PULMONARY EMBOLISM

A. . Description
  1. Occurs when a thrombus forms (most commonly in a deep vein), detaches, and travels to the right side of the heart and then lodges in a branch of the pulmonary artery
  2. Clients prone to pulmonary embolism are those at risk for deep vein thrombosis, including those who underwent surgery or those with prolonged immobilization, obesity, pregnancy, congestive heart failure, advanced age, or a history of thromboembolism.
  3. Fat emboli can occur as a complication after a fracture of a long bone and can cause pulmonary emboli.
  4. Treatment is aimed at prevention through risk factor recognition and elimination.

B. Data collection (Box 49-9)
C. Interventions (see Priority Nursing Actions)

■ PRIORITY NURSING ACTIONS! ■

Actions to Take if a Pulmonary Embolism Is Suspected

1. Notify the Rapid Response Team.
2. Reassure the client and elevate the head of the bed.
3. Prepare to administer oxygen.
4. Obtain vital signs and check lung sounds.
5. Prepare to obtain an arterial blood gas.
6. Prepare for the administration of heparin therapy or other therapies.
7. Document the event, interventions taken, and the client's response to treatment.

Signs and symptoms of a pulmonary embolism include the sudden onset of dyspnea, apprehension and restlessness, a feeling of impending doom, cough, hemoptysis, tachypnea, crackles, petechiae over the chest and axillae, and a decreased arterial oxygen saturation. If suspected, the nurse immediately notifies the Rapid Response Team. The nurse stays with the client, reassures the client, and elevates the head of the bed. The nurse prepares to administer oxygen and obtains the vital signs and checks lung sounds. The nurse continues to monitor the client closely, prepares the client for tests prescribed to confirm the diagnosis, and prepares to obtain an arterial blood gas. When prescribed, the client is prepared for the administration of heparin therapy or other therapies such as embolectomy or placement of a vena cava filter if necessary. Finally, the nurse documents the event, interventions taken, and the client's response to treatment.

Reference: Ignatavicius, D., & Workman, M. (2010). *Medical-surgical nursing: Patient-centered collaborative care* (6th ed., p. 680). St. Louis: Saunders.

XIX. LUNG CANCER AND LARYNGEAL CANCER
(see Chapter 43)

XX. CARBON MONOXIDE POISONING
(see Chapter 41)

XXI. HISTOPLASMOSIS

A. Description
  1. A pulmonary fungal infection caused by spores of *Histoplasma capsulatum*
  2. Transmission occurs by the inhalation of spores, which are commonly located in contaminated soil.
  3. Spores are also usually found in bird droppings.
B. Data collection
  1. Similar to pneumonia
  2. Positive skin test for histoplasmosis
  3. Positive agglutination test
  4. Splenomegaly and hepatomegaly
C. Interventions
  1. Administer oxygen as prescribed.
  2. Monitor breath sounds.
  3. Administer antiemetics, antihistamines, antipyretics, and corticosteroids as prescribed.
  4. Administer fungicidal medications as prescribed.
  5. Encourage coughing and deep breathing.
  6. Place the client in the semi-Fowler's position.
  7. Monitor the vital signs.
  8. Monitor for nephrotoxicity from fungicidal medications.
  9. As appropriate, educate about the importance of spraying the floor area with water before sweeping barn and chicken coops.

XXII. SARCOIDOSIS

A. Description
  1. The presence of epithelioid cell tubercles in the lung

Box 49-9 Data Collection Findings: Pulmonary Embolism

Apprehension and restlessness
Blood-tinged sputum
Chest pain
Cough
Crackles and wheezes on auscultation
Cyanosis
Distended neck veins
Dyspnea accompanied by anginal and pleuritic pain, exacerbated by inspiration
Feeling of impending doom
Hypotension
Petechiae over the chest and axilla
Shallow respirations
Tachypnea and tachycardia

2. The cause is unknown, but a high titer of Epstein-Barr virus may be identified.

3. Viral incidence is highest in blacks and young adults.

B. Data collection

1. Night sweats
2. Fever
3. Weight loss
4. Cough
5. Skin nodules
6. Polyarthritis
7. Kveim test: Sarcoid node antigen is injected intradermally and causes a local nodular lesion in about 1 month.

C. Interventions

1. Administer corticosteroids to control symptoms.
2. Monitor temperature.
3. Increase fluid intake.
4. Provide frequent periods of rest.
5. Encourage small, nutritious meals.

XXIII. OCCUPATIONAL LUNG DISEASE

A. Description

1. Caused by exposure to environmental or occupational fumes, dust, vapors, gases, bacterial or fungal antigens, and allergens; can result in acute reversible effects or chronic lung disease

2. Common disease classifications include occupational **asthmas**, pneumoconiosis (silicosis or coal miner's [black lung] disease), diffuse interstitial fibrosis (asbestosis, talcosis, berylliosis), or extrinsic allergic alveolitis (farmer's lung, bird fancier's lung, or machine operator's lung)

B. Data collection: Manifestations depend on the type of disease and are respiratory symptoms.

C. Interventions

1. Prevention through the use of respiratory protective devices
2. Treatment is based on the symptoms experienced by the client.

XXIV. TUBERCULOSIS

A. Description

1. A highly communicable disease caused by *Mycobacterium tuberculosis*

2. *Mycobacterium tuberculosis* is a nonmotile, nonsporulating, acid-fast rod that secretes niacin. When the bacillus reaches a susceptible site, it multiplies freely.

3. Because *Mycobacterium tuberculosis* is an aerobic bacterium, it primarily affects the pulmonary system, especially the upper lobes where the oxygen content is greatest, but it can also affect other areas of the body, such as the brain, intestines, peritoneum, kidney, joints, and liver.

4. An exudative response causes a nonspecific pneumonitis and the development of granulomas in the lung tissue.

5. **Tuberculosis** has an insidious onset, and many clients are not aware of symptoms until the disease is well advanced.

6. Improper or noncompliant use of treatment programs may cause the development of mutations in the tubercle bacilli, resulting in a **multidrug-resistant strain** of tuberculosis (MDR-TB).

7. The goal of treatment is to prevent transmission, control symptoms, and prevent progression of the disease.

B. Risk factors (Box 49-10)

C. Transmission

1. Transmission of **tuberculosis** is via the airborne route by droplet infection.

2. When an infected individual coughs, laughs, sneezes, or sings, droplet nuclei containing **tuberculosis** bacteria enter the air and may be inhaled by others.

3. Identification of those individuals in close contact with the infected individual is important so they can be tested and treated as necessary.

4. When contacts have been identified, these persons are assessed with a tuberculin skin test and chest x-ray films to determine infection with **tuberculosis**.

5. After the infected individual has received **tuberculosis** medication for 2 to 3 weeks, the risk of transmission is reduced greatly.

D. Disease progression

1. Droplets enter the lungs, and the bacteria form a tubercle lesion.

2. The defense systems of the body encapsulate the tubercle, leaving a scar.

Box 49-10 Risk Factors for Tuberculosis

Children younger than 5 years of age

Drinking of unpasteurized milk if the cow is infected with bovine tuberculosis

Homeless individuals or those from a lower socioeconomic group, minority groups, or immigrant group

Individuals in constant, frequent contact with an untreated or undiagnosed individual

Individuals living in crowded areas, such as long-term care facilities, prisons, and mental health facilities

Older clients

Individuals with malnutrition, an infection, or an immune dysfunction or human immunodeficiency virus infection, or individuals who are immunosuppressed as a result of medication therapy

Individuals who abuse alcohol or are intravenous drug users

3. If encapsulation does not occur, bacteria may enter the lymph system, travel to the lymph nodes, and cause an inflammatory response called granulomatous inflammation.

4. Primary lesions form. The primary lesions may become dormant but can be reactivated and become a secondary infection when re-exposed to the bacterium.

5. In an active phase, **tuberculosis** can cause necrosis and cavitation in the lesions, leading to rupture and the spread of necrotic tissue, as well as damage to various parts of the body.

E. Client history
1. Past exposure to **tuberculosis**
2. Client's country of origin and travel to foreign countries in which the incidence of **tuberculosis** is high
3. Recent history of influenza, pneumonia, febrile illness, cough, or foul-smelling sputum production
4. Previous positive tests for **tuberculosis**
5. Recent **Bacille Calmette-Guérin vaccine** (a vaccine containing attenuated tubercle bacilli that may be given to persons in foreign countries or to persons traveling to foreign countries, to produce increased resistance to **tuberculosis**)

⚠️ An individual who has received a bacilli Calmette-Guérin vaccine will have a positive tuberculin skin test result and should be evaluated for tuberculosis with a chest x-ray.

F. Clinical manifestations
1. May be asymptomatic in primary infection
2. Fatigue
3. Lethargy
4. Anorexia
5. Weight loss
6. Low-grade fever
7. Chills
8. Night sweats
9. Persistent cough and the production of mucoid and mucopurulent sputum, which is occasionally streaked with blood
10. Chest tightness and a dull, aching chest pain that may accompany the cough

G. Chest data collection
1. A physical examination of the chest does not provide conclusive evidence of **tuberculosis**.
2. A chest x-ray film is not definitive, but the presence of multinodular infiltrates with calcification in the upper lobes suggests **tuberculosis**.
3. If the disease is active, caseation and inflammation may be seen on the chest x-ray film.
4. Advanced disease
   a. Dullness with percussion over the involved parenchymal areas, bronchial breath sounds, rhonchi, and crackles indicate advanced disease.

b. Partial obstruction of a bronchus caused by endobronchial disease or compression by lymph nodes may produce localized wheezing and dyspnea.

H. QuantiFERON-TB Gold test
1. A blood analysis test by an enzyme-linked immunosorbent assay.
2. A sensitive and rapid test (results can be available in 24 hours) that assists in diagnosing the client.

I. Sputum cultures
1. Sputum specimens are obtained for an acid-fast smear.
2. A sputum culture identifying *Mycobacterium tuberculosis* confirms the diagnosis.
3. After medications are started, sputum samples are obtained again to determine the effectiveness of therapy.
4. Most clients have negative cultures after 3 months of treatment.

J. **Mantoux skin test**
1. A positive Mantoux reaction does not mean that active disease is present, but indicates exposure to **tuberculosis** or the presence of inactive (dormant) disease.
2. Once the test result is positive, it will be positive in any future tests.
3. Purified protein derivative containing 5 tuberculin units is administered intradermally in the forearm.
4. An area of induration measuring 10 mm or more in diameter, 48 to 72 hours after injection, indicates that the individual has been exposed to **tuberculosis**.
5. For individuals with human immunodeficiency virus infection or who are immunosuppressed, a reaction of 5 mm or greater is considered positive.
6. Once an individual's skin test is positive, a chest x-ray film is necessary to rule out active **tuberculosis** or to detect old, healed lesions.

K. The hospitalized client
1. The client with active **tuberculosis** is placed with respiratory isolation precautions in a negative-pressure room. To maintain negative pressure, the door of the room must be tightly closed.
2. The room should have at least six exchanges of fresh air per hour and should be ventilated to the outside environment if possible.
3. The nurse wears a particulate respirator (a special individually fitted mask) when caring for the client and a gown when a possibility exists of contamination of clothing.
4. Always thoroughly wash hands before and after caring for the client.
5. If the client needs to leave the room for a test or procedure, he or she must wear a mask.

Box 49-11 Client Education: Tuberculosis

Provide the client and family with information about tuberculosis and allay concerns about the contagious aspect of the infection.

Instruct the client to follow the medication regimen exactly as prescribed and always to have a supply of the medication on hand.

Advise the client of the side effects of the medication and ways of minimizing them to ensure compliance.

Reassure the client that after 2 to 3 weeks of medication therapy, it is unlikely that the client will infect anyone.

Inform the client to resume activities gradually.

Instruct the client about the need for adequate nutrition and a well-balanced diet to promote healing and prevent recurrence of the infection.

Instruct the client to increase intake of foods rich in iron, protein, and vitamin C.

Inform the client and family that respiratory isolation is not necessary because family members have already been exposed.

Instruct the client to cover the mouth and nose when coughing or sneezing and confine used tissues to plastic bags.

Instruct the client and family about thorough handwashing.

Inform the client that a sputum culture is needed every 2 to 4 weeks once medication therapy is initiated.

Inform the client that when the results of three sputum cultures are negative, the client is no longer considered infectious and usually can return to former employment.

Advise the client to avoid excessive exposure to silicone or dust because these substances can cause further lung damage.

Instruct the client regarding the importance of compliance with treatment, follow-up care, and sputum cultures, as prescribed.

---

6. Respiratory isolation is discontinued when the client is no longer considered infectious.
7. After the infected individual has received **tuberculosis** medication for 2 to 3 weeks, the risk of transmission is reduced greatly.

L. Client education (Box 49-11)
M. Medications (see Chapter 50)

MORE QUESTIONS ON EVOLVE!

Practice Questions

496. A nurse is providing instructions to a hospitalized client with a diagnosis of emphysema about positions that will enhance the effectiveness of breathing during dyspneic periods. Which position will the nurse instruct the client to assume?
1. Sitting up in bed
2. Side-lying in bed
3. Sitting in a recliner chair
4. Sitting on the side of the bed, leaning on an overbed table

497. A nurse is gathering data on a client with a diagnosis of tuberculosis (TB). The nurse reviews the results of which diagnostic test that will confirm this diagnosis?
1. Chest x-ray
2. Bronchoscopy
3. Sputum culture
4. Tuberculin skin test

498. Which of the following identifies the route of transmission of tuberculosis (TB)?
1. Hand to mouth
2. The enteric route
3. The airborne route
4. Blood and body fluids

499. A nurse is caring for a client with emphysema who is receiving oxygen. The nurse checks the oxygen flow rate to ensure that it does not exceed:
1. 1 L/min
2. 2 L/min
3. 6 L/min
4. 10 L/min

500. A nurse is instructing a client about pursed lip breathing, and the client asks the nurse about its purpose. The nurse tells the client that the primary purpose of pursed lip breathing is to:
1. Promote oxygen intake
2. Strengthen the diaphragm
3. Strengthen the intercostal muscles
4. Promote carbon dioxide elimination

501. The low-pressure alarm sounds on the ventilator. The nurse checks the client and then attempts to determine the cause of the alarm but is unsuccessful. Which initial action will the nurse take?
1. Administer oxygen.
2. Ventilate the client manually.
3. Check the client's vital signs.
4. Start cardiopulmonary resuscitation (CPR).

502. A nurse is assigned to care for a client after a left pneumonectomy. Which one of the follow positions would be contraindicated for this client?
1. On the side
2. In a low Fowler's position
3. In a semi-Fowler's position
4. With the head of the bed elevated 40 degrees

503. A nurse is caring for a client after pulmonary angiography via catheter insertion into the left

groin. The nurse monitors for an allergic reaction to the contrast medium by noting the presence of:
1. Hypothermia
2. Respiratory distress
3. Hematoma in the left groin
4. Discomfort in the left groin

504. A nurse is providing discharge instructions to the client with pulmonary sarcoidosis. The nurse knows that the client understands the information if the client verbalizes which early sign of exacerbation?
1. Fever
2. Fatigue
3. Weight loss
4. Shortness of breath

505. A nurse is caring for several clients with respiratory disorders. Which client is at least risk for developing a tuberculosis infection?
1. An uninsured man who is homeless
2. A woman newly immigrated from Korea
3. A man who is an inspector for the U.S. Postal Service
4. An older woman admitted from a long-term care facility

506. A nurse is reading the results of a Mantoux skin test on a client with no documented health problems. The site has no induration and a 1-mm area of ecchymosis. The nurse interprets that the result is:
1. Positive
2. Negative
3. Uncertain
4. Borderline

507. A nurse notes that a hospitalized client has experienced a positive reaction to the Mantoux skin test. Which action by the nurse is the priority?
1. Report the findings.
2. Document the finding in the client's record.
3. Call the employee health service department.
4. Call the radiology department for a chest x-ray.

508. A client being discharged from the hospital to home with a diagnosis of tuberculosis (TB) is worried about the possibility of infecting the family and others. The nurse determines that the client would get the most reassurance from the knowledge that:
1. The family does not need therapy, and the client will not be contagious after 1 month of medication therapy
2. The family does not need therapy, and the client will not be contagious after 6 consecutive weeks of medication therapy
3. The family will receive prophylactic therapy, and the client will not be contagious after 1 continuous week of medication therapy
4. The family will receive prophylactic therapy, and the client will not be contagious after 2 to 3 consecutive weeks of medication therapy

509. A nurse has reinforced discharge teaching with a client who was diagnosed with tuberculosis (TB) and has been on medication for 1½ weeks. The nurse knows that the client has understood the information if the client makes which statement?
1. "I can't shop at the mall for the next 6 months."
2. "I need to continue medication therapy for 2 months."
3. "I can return to work if a sputum culture comes back negative."
4. "I should not be contagious after 2 to 3 weeks of medication therapy."

510. The nurse is preparing a list of home care instructions for the client who has been hospitalized and treated for tuberculosis. Choose the instructions that the nurse will include on the list. **Select all that apply.**
☐ 1. Activities should be resumed gradually.
☐ 2. Avoid contact with other individuals, except family members, for at least 6 months.
☐ 3. A sputum culture is needed every 2 to 4 weeks once medication therapy is initiated.
☐ 4. Respiratory isolation is not necessary because family members have already been exposed.
☐ 5. Cover the mouth and nose when coughing or sneezing and confine used tissues to plastic bags.
☐ 6. When one sputum culture is negative, the client is no longer considered infectious and can usually return to his or her former employment.

ANSWERS

496. 4

Rationale: Positions that will assist the client with breathing include sitting up and leaning on an overbed table, sitting up and resting with the elbows on the knees, or standing or leaning against the wall. The positions in options 1, 2, and 3 will not enhance the effectiveness of breathing.

Test-Taking Strategy: Use the process of elimination. Eliminate option 2 because side-lying will not promote appropriate lung expansion. Next, eliminate options 1 and 3 because they are comparable or alike and will restrict lung expansion. If you had difficulty with this question, review the positions that will decrease the work of breathing in a client with emphysema.

Level of Cognitive Ability: Applying

Client Needs: Physiological Integrity
Integrated Process: Teaching and Learning
Content Area: Adult Health/Respiratory
Reference: Linton, pp. 587–588, 592. 2012.

497. 3

Rationale: A definitive diagnosis of TB is confirmed through culture and isolation of *Mycobacterium tuberculosis*. A presumptive diagnosis is made on the basis of a tuberculin skin test, a sputum smear that is positive for acid-fast bacteria, a chest x-ray, and histologic evidence of granulomatous disease on biopsy.
Test-Taking Strategy: Use the process of elimination and note the strategic word "confirm" in the question. Confirmation is made by identifying *Mycobacterium tuberculosis*. If you had difficulty with this question, review the diagnostic procedures related to TB.
Level of Cognitive Ability: Understanding
Client Needs: Physiological Integrity
Integrated Process: Nursing Process/Data Collection
Content Area: Adult Health/Respiratory
Reference: Linton, p. 596. 2012.

498. 3

Rationale: Tuberculosis is an infectious disease caused by the bacillus *Mycobacterium tuberculosis* and spread primarily by the airborne route. Options 1, 2, and 4 are incorrect.
Test-Taking Strategy: Use the process of elimination. Recalling that TB is a respiratory disease will direct you to option 3. If you had difficulty with this question, review the transmission of this disease.
Level of Cognitive Ability: Understanding
Client Needs: Safe and Effective Care Environment
Integrated Process: Nursing Process/Planning
Content Area: Adult Health/Respiratory
Reference: Linton, p. 598. 2012.

499. 2

Rationale: Between 1 and 3 L/min of oxygen by nasal cannula may be required to raise the Pao_2 level to 60 to 80 mm Hg. However, oxygen is used cautiously in the client with emphysema and should not exceed 2 L/min. Because of the long-standing hypercapnia that occurs in this disorder, the respiratory drive is triggered by low oxygen levels rather than by increased carbon dioxide levels, which is the case in a normal respiratory system.
Test-Taking Strategy: Recalling the physiology associated with emphysema is required to answer this question. Remember that oxygen is used cautiously in the client with emphysema and should not exceed 2 L/min. If you are unfamiliar with this disorder, review this content.
Level of Cognitive Ability: Applying
Client Needs: Physiological Integrity
Integrated Process: Nursing Process/Data Collection
Content Area: Adult Health/Respiratory
References: Christensen, Kockrow, p. 423. 2011. *Adult health nursing.*
Linton, pp. 589, 592. 2012.

500. 4

Rationale: Pursed lip breathing facilitates maximal expiration for clients with obstructive lung disease and promotes carbon dioxide elimination. This type of breathing allows better expiration by increasing airway pressure, which keeps air passages open during exhalation. Options 1, 2, and 3 are not the purposes of this type of breathing.
Test-Taking Strategy: Use the process of elimination. Visualize the use of this breathing technique to assist in answering correctly. Recalling the respiratory conditions in which this type of breathing is helpful will also assist in directing you to the correct option. Review the purpose of this breathing technique if you had difficulty with this question.
Level of Cognitive Ability: Applying
Client Needs: Physiological Integrity
Integrated Process: Teaching and Learning
Content Area: Adult Health/Respiratory
References: deWit, p. 336. 2009.
Linton, pp. 553–554. 2012.

501. 2

Rationale: If an alarm is sounding at any time and the nurse cannot quickly ascertain the problem, the client is disconnected from the ventilator and a manual resuscitation device is used to support respirations until the problem can be corrected. Although oxygen is helpful, it will not provide ventilation to the client. Checking vital signs is not the initial action. There is no reason to begin CPR.
Test-Taking Strategy: Use the process of elimination. Read the question carefully and note that the subject relates to adequate ventilation of the client. Focusing on this subject will direct you to option 2. If you are unfamiliar with the management of a client on a ventilator, review this content.
Level of Cognitive Ability: Applying
Client Needs: Physiological Integrity
Integrated Process: Nursing Process/Implementation
Content Area: Adult Health/Respiratory
Reference: Ignatavicius, Workman, p. 695. 2010.

502. 1

Rationale: Complete lateral positioning is contraindicated for a client following pneumonectomy. Because the mediastinum is no longer held in place on both sides by lung tissue, lateral positioning may cause mediastinal shift and compression of the remaining lung. The head of the bed should be elevated.
Test-Taking Strategy: Use the process of elimination and note the strategic word "contraindicated." This word indicates a negative event query and the need to select the incorrect position. Eliminate options 2, 3, and 4 because they are comparable or alike. If you had difficulty with this question, review care of the client after pneumonectomy.
Level of Cognitive Ability: Applying
Client Needs: Physiological Integrity
Integrated Process: Nursing Process/Implementation
Content Area: Adult Health/Respiratory
Reference: Linton, pp. 561–562. 2012.

503. 2

Rationale: Signs of allergic reaction to the contrast medium include localized itching and edema, respiratory distress, stridor, and decreased blood pressure. Hypothermia is an unrelated event. Hematoma formation is a complication of the procedure but does not indicate an allergic reaction. Discomfort is expected.
Test-Taking Strategy: Use ABCs—airway, breathing, and circulation—and focus on the subject, an allergic reaction. This will

direct you to the correct option. Review the signs of an allergic reaction to the contrast medium if you had difficulty with this question.
Level of Cognitive Ability: Applying
Client Needs: Physiological Integrity
Integrated Process: Nursing Process/Data Collection
Content Area: Adult Health/Respiratory
Reference: Christensen, Kockrow, p. 478. 2011. *Foundations of nursing.*

504. 4
Rationale: Shortness of breath is an early sign of exacerbation of pulmonary sarcoidosis. Others include chest pain, hemoptysis, and pneumothorax. Systemic signs and symptoms that occur later include weakness and fatigue, malaise, fever, and weight loss.
Test-Taking Strategy: Note the strategic word "early" in the question. Because sarcoidosis is a pulmonary problem, eliminate options 1 and 3 first. Choose option 4 over option 2, because the shortness of breath (and impaired ventilation) appears first and would cause the fatigue as a secondary symptom. Review this disorder if you had difficulty with this question.
Level of Cognitive Ability: Evaluating
Client Needs: Physiological Integrity
Integrated Process: Nursing Process: Evaluation
Content Area: Adult Health/Respiratory
References: Linton, p. 601. 2012.

505. 3
Rationale: People at high risk for acquiring tuberculosis include children younger than 5 years of age; homeless individuals or those from a lower socioeconomic group, minority groups, or immigrant group; individuals in constant, frequent contact with an untreated or undiagnosed individual; individuals living in crowded areas, such as long-term care facilities, prisons, and mental health facilities; older clients; individuals with malnutrition, an infection, or an immune dysfunction or human immunodeficiency virus infection, or individuals who are immunosuppressed as a result of medication therapy; and individuals who abuse alcohol or are intravenous drug users.
Test-Taking Strategy: Use the process of elimination and note the strategic words "least risk." Begin to answer this question by eliminating options 1 and 2, because immigrants and the medically underserved are more frequently affected by this infection. From the remaining options, note that the postal inspector may or may not come in contact with many people, depending on job description. The client from the long-term care facility, however, lives in a group setting, where a large number of people share a common environment 24 hours a day. Review the risks associated with tuberculosis if you had difficulty with this question.
Level of Cognitive Ability: Analyzing
Client Needs: Health Promotion and Maintenance
Integrated Process: Nursing Process/Data Collection
Content Area: Adult Health/Respiratory
Reference: deWit, pp. 324–325. 2009.

506. 2
Rationale: A positive Mantoux reading has an induration measuring 10 mm or more in diameter and indicates exposure to tuberculosis. A small area of ecchymosis is insignificant and is probably related to injection technique.

Test-Taking Strategy: To answer this question accurately, it is necessary to know that induration is necessary for a positive response. Because the client in this question has no induration, the result is negative. Review Mantoux skin test results if you had difficulty with this question.
Level of Cognitive Ability: Understanding
Client Needs: Physiological Integrity
Integrated Process: Nursing Process/Data Collection
Content Area: Adult Health/Respiratory
Reference: Linton, pp. 548, 596. 2012.

507. 1
Rationale: The nurse who interprets a Mantoux skin test as positive notifies the health care provider (HCP) immediately. The HCP would prescribe a chest x-ray to determine whether the client has clinically active tuberculosis (TB) or old, healed lesions. A sputum culture would be done to confirm the diagnosis of active TB. The client is placed on TB precautions prophylactically until a final diagnosis is made. The findings are documented in the client's record, but this action is not the highest priority. Calling the employee health service would be of no benefit to the client.
Test-Taking Strategy: Use the process of elimination and note the strategic word "priority." Because the nurse may not prescribe diagnostic tests, eliminate option 4 first. Option 3 can be eliminated, because calling the employee health service is of no benefit to the client. From the remaining options, notifying the HCP should have a higher priority than the documentation, even though both may be done in the same narrow time period. Review nursing interventions related to Mantoux skin testing if you had difficulty with this question.
Level of Cognitive Ability: Applying
Client Needs: Safe and Effective Care Environment
Integrated Process: Nursing Process/Implementation
Content Area: Adult Health/Respiratory
References: Linton, pp. 587–588, 592. 2012.
deWit, p. 325. 2009.
Linton, pp. 596–597. 2012.

508. 4
Rationale: Family members or others who have been in close contact with a client diagnosed with TB are placed on prophylactic therapy with isoniazid (INH) for 6 to 12 months. The client is usually not contagious after taking medication for 2 to 3 consecutive weeks. However, the client must take the full course of therapy (for 6 months or longer) to prevent reinfection or drug-resistant TB.
Test-Taking Strategy: Use the process of elimination. Recalling that the family requires prophylactic therapy allows you to eliminate options 1 and 2. From the remaining options, it is necessary to know that the client is not contagious after 2 to 3 weeks of therapy. Review the concepts related to the prevention of the spread of TB if you had difficulty with this question.
Level of Cognitive Ability: Understanding
Client Needs: Psychosocial Integrity
Integrated Process: Nursing Process/Planning
Content Area: Adult Health/Respiratory
References: Ignatavicius, Workman, pp. 670, 672. 2010.
Linton, p. 598. 2012.

509. 4

Rationale: The client is continued on medication therapy for 6 to 12 months, depending on the situation. The client is generally considered to be not contagious after 2 to 3 weeks of medication therapy. The client is instructed to wear a mask if there will be exposure to crowds, until the medication is effective in preventing transmission. The client is allowed to return to employment when the results of three sputum cultures are negative.

Test-Taking Strategy: Use the process of elimination. Knowing that the medication therapy lasts for at least 6 months helps you eliminate option 2 first. Knowing that three sputum cultures must be negative helps you eliminate option 3 next. From the remaining options, recalling that the client is not contagious after 2 to 3 weeks of therapy helps you choose option 4. If you had difficulty with this question, review the infectious period of TB.

Level of Cognitive Ability: Evaluating
Client Needs: Physiological Integrity
Integrated Process: Nursing Process/Evaluation
Content Area: Adult Health/Respiratory
Reference: Ignatavicius, Workman, pp. 670, 672. 2010.

❖ **510. 1, 3, 4, 5**

Rationale: The nurse should provide the client and family with information about tuberculosis and allay concerns about the contagious aspect of the infection. The client is to follow the medication regimen exactly as prescribed and always to have a supply of the medication on hand. The client is advised of the side effects of the medication and ways of minimizing them to ensure compliance. The client is reassured that, after 2 to 3 weeks of medication therapy, it is unlikely that the client will infect anyone. The client is also informed that activities should be resumed gradually and about the need for adequate nutrition and a well-balanced diet that is rich in iron, protein, and vitamin C to promote healing and prevent recurrence of infection. The client and family are informed that respiratory isolation is not necessary, because family members have already been exposed. The client is instructed about thorough handwashing and to cover the mouth and nose when coughing or sneezing and confine used tissues to plastic bags. The client is informed that a sputum culture is needed every 2 to 4 weeks once medication therapy is initiated and, when the results of three sputum cultures are negative, the client is no longer considered infectious and can usually return to his or her former employment.

Test-Taking Strategy: Knowledge regarding the pathophysiology, transmission, and treatment of tuberculosis is needed to answer this question. Using this knowledge will assist in directing you to the correct options. Review home care instructions for the client with tuberculosis if you had difficulty with this question.

Level of Cognitive Ability: Applying
Client Needs: Safe and Effective Care Environment
Integrated Process: Teaching and Learning
Content Area: Adult Health/Respiratory
Reference: deWit, p. 328. 2009.

Respiratory Medications

I. USE OF AN INHALER

A. Client instructions for use of a metered-dose inhaler (MDI; see Figures 50-1 and 50-2)

B. If two different inhaled medications are prescribed and one of the medications contains a glucocorticoid (corticosteroid), administer the bronchodilator first and the corticosteroid second.

⚠ If two different inhaled medications are prescribed, instruct the client to wait 5 minutes after administration of the first before inhaling the second.

II. BRONCHODILATORS (Box 50-1)

A. Description

1. Sympathomimetic bronchodilators dilate the airways of the respiratory tree, making air exchange and respiration easier for the client, and relax the smooth muscle of the bronchi.
2. Methylxanthine bronchodilators stimulate the central nervous system and respiration, dilate coronary and pulmonary vessels, cause diuresis, and relax smooth muscle.
3. Bronchodilators are used to treat allergic rhinitis and sinusitis, acute bronchospasm, acute and chronic asthma, bronchitis, **chronic obstructive pulmonary disease**, **emphysema**, and other restrictive airway diseases.
4. Bronchodilators are contraindicated in individuals with hypersensitivity, peptic ulcer disease, severe cardiac disease and cardiac dysrhythmias, hyperthyroidism, or uncontrolled seizure disorders.
5. Bronchodilators should be used with caution in clients with hypertension, diabetes mellitus, or narrow-angle glaucoma.
6. Theophylline increases the risk of digoxin toxicity and decreases the effects of lithium and phenytoin (Dilantin).
7. If theophylline and a β_2-adrenergic agonist are administered together, cardiac dysrhythmias may result.

8. β-Blockers, cimetidine (Tagamet), and erythromycin increase the effects of theophylline.
9. Barbiturates and carbamazepine (Tegretol) decrease the effects of theophylline.

B. Side effects
1. Palpitations and tachycardia
2. Dysrhythmias
3. Restlessness, nervousness, tremors
4. Anorexia, nausea, and vomiting
5. Headaches and dizziness
6. Hyperglycemia
7. Decreased clotting time
8. Mouth dryness and throat irritation with inhalers
9. Tolerance and paradoxical bronchoconstriction with inhalers

C. Interventions
1. Monitor vital signs and lung sounds.
2. Monitor for cardiac dysrhythmias.
3. Check for cough, wheezing, decreased breath sounds, and sputum production.
4. Monitor for restlessness and confusion.
5. Provide adequate hydration.
6. The medication is administered at regular intervals around the clock to maintain a sustained therapeutic level.
7. Oral medications are administered with or after meals to decrease gastrointestinal irritation.
8. The client is instructed not to crush enteric-coated or sustained-release tablets or capsules.
9. The client is instructed to avoid caffeine-containing products such as coffee, tea, cola, and chocolate.
10. The client is instructed in the side effects of bronchodilators.
11. The client is instructed in how to monitor the pulse and to report any abnormalities to the health care provider (HCP).
12. The client is instructed in how to use an inhaler or nebulizer and how to monitor the amount of medication remaining in an inhaler canister. How to use a spacer (a device that enhances the delivery of medication) is also taught (see Figures 50-1 and 50-2).

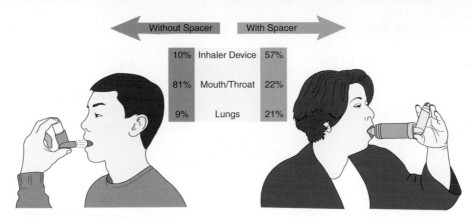

▲ **FIGURE 50-1** Distribution of medication with and without a spacer. (From Kee, J., & Marshall, S. [2009]. *Clinical calculations: With applications to general and specialty areas* [6th ed.]. Philadelphia: Saunders.)

▲ **FIGURE 50-2** Inhaled drugs commonly used in asthma treatment include β-adrenergic bronchodilators, cromolyn sodium, and aerosol glucocorticoids. **A,** The metered-dose inhaler should not be put in the mouth but held about two finger widths (1½ inches) in front of the mouth. **B,** Alternatively, an inhaler with a spacer device can be used. Patients should breathe deeply once before activating the inhaler, and then continue breathing in for about 5 seconds. Patients then should hold their breath for 10 to 15 seconds before breathing out slowly. If a second dose is needed, patients should wait 1 to 2 minutes before taking another dose. (From Clark, J., Queener, S., & Karb, V. [2000]. *Pharmacologic basis of nursing practice* [6th ed.]. St. Louis: Mosby.)

13. The client is instructed to avoid over-the-counter medications.
14. The client is instructed to stop smoking and is provided information regarding support resources.
15. The client with diabetes mellitus is instructed to monitor blood glucose levels.
16. The client with asthma is instructed to wear a Medic-Alert bracelet.
17. Monitor for a therapeutic serum theophylline level of 10 to 20 mcg/mL.
18. Intravenously administered theophylline preparations should be administered slowly and always via an infusion pump.

⚠ Theophylline toxicity is likely to occur when the serum level is higher than 20 mcg/mL. Early signs of toxicity include restlessness, nervousness, tremors, palpitations, and tachycardia.

III. ANTICHOLINERGICS (see Box 50-1)

A. Inhaled medications improve lung function by blocking muscarinic receptors in the bronchi, which results in bronchodilation.
B. Effective for treating **chronic obstructive pulmonary disease**, allergy-induced asthma, and exercise-induced bronchospasm.
C. Side effects include dry mouth and irritation of the pharynx. Sucking on sugarless candy will help to relieve symptoms.
D. Systemic anticholinergic effects rarely occur but can include increased intraocular pressure, blurred vision, tachycardia, cardiovascular events, urinary retention, and constipation.

⚠ The client with a peanut allergy should not take ipratropium (Atrovent) HFA and ipratropium/albuterol (Combivent) because both products contain soy lecithin, which is in the same plant family as peanuts.

Box 50-1 Medications to Treat Restrictive Airway Disorders

Bronchodilators

β_2-**Adrenergic Agonists**

Inhaled
Albuterol (Proventil HFA, AccuNeb, ProAir HFA, Ventolin, HFA)
Arformoterol (Brovana)
Formoterol (Foradil Aerolizer, Perforomist)
Levalbuterol (Xopenex, Xopenex HFA)
Pirbuterol (Maxair Autohaler)
Salmeterol (Serevent Diskus)

Oral
Albuterol (VoSpire)
Terbutaline (Brethine)

Methylxanthines
Theophylline, oral (Theo-24, Theochron, Uniphyl, Elixophyllin)

Anticholinergics
Ipratropium inhaled (Atrovent, Atrovent HFA)
Tiotropium, inhaled (Spiriva)

Glucocorticoids (Corticosteroids)

Inhaled
Beclomethasone dipropionate (Qvar)

Budesonide (Pulmicort Turbuhaler, Pulmicort Respules)
Ciclesonide (Alvescol)
Flunisolide (AeroBid)
Fluticasone propionate (Flovent HFA, Flovent Diskus)
Mometasone furoate (Asmanex Twisthaler)
Triamcinolone acetonide (Azmacort)

Oral
Prednisone
Prednisolone

Leukotriene Modifiers
Montelukast, oral (Singulair)
Zafirlukast, oral (Accolate)
Zileuton, oral (Zyflo, Zyflo CR)

Inhaled Nonsteroidal Antiallergy Agent
Cromolyn sodium, inhaled (Intal)

Monoclonal Antibody
Omalizumab (Xolair)

Adapted from Lehne, R. (2010). *Pharmacology for nursing care* (7th ed., p. 890). St. Louis: Saunders.

IV. GLUCOCORTICOIDS (CORTICOSTEROIDS) (see Box 50-1)

A. Glucocorticoids act as anti-inflammatory agents and reduce edema of the airways. They are used to treat asthma and other inflammatory respiratory conditions.

B. See Chapter 46 for information on glucocorticoids.

V. LEUKOTRIENE MODIFIERS (see Box 50-1)

A. Description
   1. Used in the prophylaxis and treatment of chronic bronchial asthma (not used for acute asthma episodes)
   2. Inhibit bronchoconstriction caused by specific antigens and reduce airway edema and smooth muscle constriction
   3. Contraindicated in clients with hypersensitivity and in breast-feeding mothers
   4. Should be used with caution in clients with impaired hepatic function
   5. Co-administration of inhaled glucocorticoids increases the risk of upper respiratory infection.

B. Side effects
   1. Headache
   2. Nausea and vomiting
   3. Dyspepsia
   4. Diarrhea

   5. Generalized pain, myalgia
   6. Fever
   7. Dizziness

C. Interventions
   1. Monitor vital signs.
   2. Check lung sounds for rhonchi and wheezing.
   3. Monitor liver function laboratory values.
   4. Monitor for cyanosis.
   5. The client is instructed to take medication 1 hour before or 2 hours after meals.
   6. The client is instructed to increase fluid intake.
   7. The client is instructed not to discontinue the medication and to take as prescribed, even during symptom-free periods.

VI. INHALED NONSTEROIDAL ANTIALLERGY AGENT (see Box 50-1)

A. Description
   1. Antiasthmatic, antiallergic, and mast cell stabilizers inhibit mast cell release after exposure to antigens.
   2. This medication is used to treat allergic rhinitis, bronchial asthma, and exercise-induced bronchospasm (see Box 50-1).
   3. It is contraindicated in clients with known hypersensitivity.
   4. Orally administered cromolyn sodium (Intal) is used with caution in clients with impaired hepatic or renal function.

B. Side effects
  1. Cough or bronchospasm after inhalation
  2. Nasal sting or sneezing after inhalation
  3. Unpleasant taste in the mouth
C. Interventions
  1. Monitor vital signs.
  2. Monitor respirations and check lung sounds for rhonchi or wheezing.
  3. Administer oral capsules at least 30 minutes before meals.
  4. The client is instructed not to discontinue the medication abruptly because a rebound asthmatic attack can occur.

⚠ The client taking inhaled medications is instructed to drink a few sips of water before and after inhalation to prevent a cough and an unpleasant taste in the mouth.

VII. MONOCLONAL ANTIBODY (see Box 50-1)

A. Description
  1. Omalizumab (Xolair) is a recombinant DNA-derived humanized immunoglobulin G (IgG) murine monoclonal antibody that selectively binds to IgE to limit the release of mediators in the allergic response.
  2. Used to treat allergy-related asthma; administered subcutaneously every 2 to 4 weeks
  3. Dose is titrated based on the serum IgE level and body weight.
  4. Contraindicated in those with hypersensitivity to the medication
B. Side effects
  1. Injection site reactions
  2. Viral infections
  3. Upper respiratory infections
  4. Sinusitis
  5. Headache
  6. Pharyngitis
  7. Anaphylaxis
  8. Malignancies
C. Interventions
  1. Monitor respiratory rate, rhythm, and depth and auscultate lung fields bilaterally.
  2. Check for allergies and/or allergic reaction symptoms such as rash or urticaria.
  3. The client is informed that respiratory improvement will not be immediate.
  4. The client is instructed not to stop taking or decrease the currently prescribed asthma medications unless instructed.
  5. Live virus vaccines are avoided for the duration of treatment.
  6. Medications for the treatment of severe hypersensitivity reactions are kept available during initial administration in case anaphylaxis occurs.

Box 50-2 Antihistamines

Cetirizine (Zyrtec)
Chlorpheniramine (Chlor-Trimeton, others)
Desloratadine (Clarinex)
Dimenhydrinate (Dramamine)
Diphenhydramine (Benadryl)
Fexofenadine (Allegra)
Levocetirizine (Xyzal)
Loratadine (Claritin, Alavert)
Olopatadine (Patanase)

VIII. ANTIHISTAMINES (Box 50-2)

A. Description
  1. Antihistamines are called histamine antagonists or H_1 blockers. These medications compete with histamine for receptor sites, thus preventing a histamine response.
  2. When the H_1 receptor is stimulated, the extravascular smooth muscles, including those lining the nasal cavity, are constricted.
  3. Antihistamines decrease nasopharyngeal, gastrointestinal, and bronchial secretions by blocking the H_1 receptor.
  4. Antihistamines are used for the common cold, rhinitis, nausea and vomiting, motion sickness, urticaria, and as a sleep aid.
  5. Can cause central nervous system (CNS) depression if taken with alcohol, opioids, hypnotics, or barbiturates
  6. Should be used with caution in clients with **chronic obstructive pulmonary disease** because of their drying effect
  7. Diphenhydramine (Benadryl) has an anticholinergic effect and should be avoided in clients with narrow-angle glaucoma.
B. Side effects
  1. Drowsiness and fatigue
  2. Dizziness
  3. Urinary retention
  4. Blurred vision
  5. Wheezing
  6. Constipation
  7. Dry mouth
  8. Gastrointestinal irritation
  9. Hypotension
  10. Hearing disturbances
  11. Photosensitivity
  12. Nervousness and irritability
  13. Confusion
  14. Nightmares
C. Interventions
  1. Monitor vital signs.
  2. Monitor for signs of urinary dysfunction.

3. This medication is administered with food or milk.

4. Subcutaneous injection is avoided; administered by intramuscular injection in a large muscle if the intramuscular route is prescribed.

5. The client is instructed to avoid hazardous activities, alcohol, and other CNS depressants.

6. The client taking the medication for motion sickness is instructed to take it 30 minutes before the event and then before meals and at bedtime during the event.

7. The client is instructed to suck on hard candy or ice chips for dry mouth.

IX. NASAL DECONGESTANTS (Box 50-3)

A. Description
1. Nasal decongestants include adrenergic, anticholinergic, and corticosteroid medications.
2. These medications shrink nasal mucosal membranes and reduce fluid secretion.
3. Are used for allergic rhinitis, hay fever, and acute coryza (profuse nasal discharge).
4. Contraindicated or used with extreme caution in clients with hypertension, cardiac disease, hyperthyroidism, or diabetes mellitus.

B. Side effects
1. Frequent use of decongestants, especially nasal sprays or drops, can result in tolerance and rebound nasal congestion (vasodilation) caused by irritation of the nasal mucosa.
2. Nervousness
3. Restlessness, insomnia
4. Hypertension
5. Hyperglycemia

⚠ Nasal decongestants can cause tolerance and rebound nasal congestion (vasodilation) as a result of irritation of the nasal mucosa. Therefore, the client needs to be informed that these medications should not be used for longer than 48 hours.

C. Interventions
1. The client is assessed for existing medical disorders.
2. Monitor for cardiac dysrhythmias.
3. Monitor blood glucose levels.
4. The client is instructed to avoid consuming caffeine in large amounts because it can increase restlessness and palpitations.
5. The client is instructed in the importance of limiting the use of nasal sprays and drops.

X. EXPECTORANTS AND MUCOLYTIC AGENTS (Box 50-4)

A. Description
1. Expectorants loosen bronchial secretions so that they can be eliminated with coughing. They are used for dry nonproductive cough and to stimulate bronchial secretions.
2. Mucolytic agents thin mucous secretions to help make the cough more productive.
3. Mucolytic agents with dextromethorphan should not be used by clients with **chronic obstructive pulmonary disease** because they suppress the cough.
4. Acetylcysteine (Mucomyst) can increase airway resistance and should not be used in clients with asthma.

B. Side effects
1. Gastrointestinal irritation
2. Skin rash
3. Oropharyngeal irritation

C. Interventions
1. The client is instructed to take the medication with a full glass of water to loosen mucus.
2. The client is instructed to maintain an adequate fluid intake.
3. The client is encouraged to cough and deep breathe.
4. Acetylcysteine (Mucomyst), administered by nebulization, should not be mixed with another medication.

Box 50-3 Nasal Decongestants

Nonglucocorticoids
Naphazoline (Privine)
Oxymetazoline (Afrin 12-Hour, others)
Phenylephrine hydrochloride (Neo-Synephrine, others)
Pseudoephedrine hydrochloride (Sudafed)
Tetrahydrozoline (Tyzine)
Xylometazoline (Natru-Vent, Otrivin)

Glucocorticoids
Beclomethasone (Beconase AQ)
Budesonide (Rhinocort Aqua)
Ciclesonide (Omnaris)
Flunisolide (Nasarel)
Fluticasone propionate (Flonase)
Fluticasone furoate (Veramyst)
Mometasone (Nasonex)
Triamcinolone (Nasacort AQ)

Box 50-4 Expectorants and Mucolytic Agents

Expectorants	Mucolytic
Guaifenesin (Humibid, Mucinex)	Acetylcysteine (Mucomyst)

5. If acetylcysteine is administered with a bronchodilator, the bronchodilator should be administered 5 minutes before the acetylcysteine.
6. Monitor for side effects of acetylcysteine such as nausea and vomiting, stomatitis, and runny nose.

XI. ANTITUSSIVES (Box 50-5)

A. Description: Act on the cough control center in the medulla to suppress the cough reflex; used for a cough that is nonproductive and irritating.

B. Side effects
1. Dizziness, drowsiness, sedation
2. Gastrointestinal irritation, nausea
3. Dry mouth
4. Constipation
5. Respiratory depression

C. Interventions
1. The client is instructed that if the cough lasts longer than 1 week and a fever or rash occurs to notify the HCP.
2. The client is encouraged to take adequate fluids with the medication.
3. The client is encouraged to sleep with the head of the bed elevated.
4. The client is encouraged to avoid hazardous activities.
5. Note that drug dependency can occur.
6. Administration to the client with a head injury or a postoperative cranial surgery client is avoided.
7. Administration to the client using opioids, sedative-hypnotics, barbiturates, or antidepressants is avoided because CNS depression can occur.
8. The client is instructed to avoid the use of alcohol.

XII. OPIOID ANTAGONISTS (Box 50-6)

A. Description
1. An opioid antagonist reverses respiratory depression in opioid overdose.
2. Avoid its use for nonopioid respiratory depression.

B. Side effects
1. CNS depression
2. Nausea, vomiting

Box 50-5 Antitussives

Opioids
Codeine phosphate, codeine sulfate
Hydrocodone

Nonopioids
Benzonatate (Tessalon)
Dextromethorphan
Diphenhydramine hydrochloride (Benadryl)

---

3. Tremors
4. Sweating
5. Increased blood pressure
6. Tachycardia

C. Interventions
1. Monitor vital signs, especially respirations.
2. For intravenous administration, the dose is titrated every 2 to 5 minutes as prescribed.
3. Have oxygen and resuscitative equipment available during administration.

XIII. TUBERCULOSIS MEDICATIONS (Box 50-7)

A. Description
1. **Tuberculosis** medications offer the most effective method for treating the disease and preventing transmission.
2. Treatment of identified lesions depends on whether the individual has active disease or has been exposed to the disease.
3. Treatment is difficult because the bacterium has a waxy substance on the capsule that makes penetration and destruction difficult.
4. The use of a multidrug regimen destroys organisms as quickly as possible and minimizes the emergence of drug-resistant organisms.

Box 50-6 Opioid Antagonists

Alvimopan (Entereg)
Methylnaltrexone (Relistor)
Nalmefene (Revex)
Naloxone (Narcan)
Naltrexone (ReVia, Depade)

Box 50-7 First- and Second-Line Medications for Tuberculosis

First-Line Agents
Isoniazid (INH, Nydrazid)
Rifampin (Rifadin)
Ethambutol (Myambutol)
Pyrazinamide
Rifabutin (Mycobutin)
Rifapentine (Priftin)

Second-Line Agents
Amikacin (Amikin)
Capreomycin sulfate (Capastat Sulfate)
Cycloserine (Seromycin)
Ethionamide (Trecator)
Kanamycin (Kantrex)
Levofloxacin (Levaquin)
Moxifloxacin (Avelox)
p-Aminosalicylic acid (Paser)
Streptomycin

5. Active **tuberculosis** is treated with a combination of medications to which the organism is susceptible.
6. Individuals with active **tuberculosis** are treated for 6 to 9 months. However, clients with human immunodeficiency virus (HIV) infection are treated for a longer period of time.
7. After the infected individual has received medication for 2 to 3 weeks, the risk of transmission is greatly reduced.
8. Most clients have negative sputum cultures after 3 months of compliance with medication therapy.
9. Individuals who have been exposed to active **tuberculosis** are treated with preventive isoniazid (INH) for 9 to 12 months.

B. First- or second-line medications
1. First-line medications provide the most effective antituberculosis activity.
2. Second-line medications are used in combination with first-line medications but are more toxic.
3. Current infecting organisms are proving resistant to standard first-line medications. The resistant organisms develop because individuals with the disease fail to complete the course of treatment, so surviving bacteria adapt to the medication and become resistant.
4. Multidrug therapies are instituted because of the resistant organisms.

C. Multidrug-resistant strain of tuberculosis (MDR-TB)
1. Resistance occurs when a client receiving two medications (first- and second-line medications) discontinues one of the medications.
2. The client briefly experiences some response from the single medication but then large numbers of resistant organisms begin to grow.
3. The client, infectious again, transmits the drug-resistant organism to other individuals.
4. As this event is repeated, an organism develops that is resistant to many of the first-line **tuberculosis** medications.

XIV. FIRST-LINE MEDICATIONS FOR TUBERCULOSIS (Box 50-7)

A. Isoniazid (INH)
1. Description
   a. Isoniazid is bactericidal.
   b. It inhibits the synthesis of mycolic acids and acts to kill actively growing organisms in the extracellular environment.
   c. It inhibits the growth of dormant organisms in the macrophages and caseating granulomas.
   d. It is active only during cell division and is used in combination with other antitubercular medications.

2. Contraindications and cautions
   a. Isoniazid is contraindicated in clients with hypersensitivity or with acute liver disease.
   b. Use with caution in clients with chronic liver disease, alcoholism, or renal impairment.
   c. Use with caution in clients taking nicotinic acid (niacin).
   d. Use with caution in clients taking hepatotoxic medications because the risk for hepatotoxicity increases.
   e. Alcohol increases the risk of hepatotoxicity.
   f. Isoniazid may increase the risk of toxicity of carbamazepine (Tegretol) and phenytoin (Dilantin).
   g. Isoniazid may decrease ketoconazole (Nizoral) concentrations.

3. Side effects
   a. Hypersensitivity reactions
   b. Peripheral neuritis
   c. Neurotoxicity
   d. Hepatotoxicity; increased liver function test levels
   e. Pyridoxine (vitamin B_6) deficiency
   f. Irritation at injection site with intramuscular administration
   g. Nausea and vomiting
   h. Dry mouth
   i. Dizziness
   j. Hyperglycemia
   k. Vision changes
   l. Hepatitis

4. Interventions
   a. Monitor for hypersensitivity.
   b. Monitor for hepatic dysfunction.
   c. Monitor for sensitivity to nicotinic acid.
   d. Monitor liver function test results.
   e. Monitor for signs of hepatitis, such as anorexia, nausea, vomiting, weakness, fatigue, dark urine, or jaundice. If these symptoms occur, withhold the medication and notify the registered nurse.
   f. Monitor for tingling, numbness, or burning of the extremities.
   g. Monitor mental status.
   h. Monitor for visual changes, and notify the registered nurse if they occur.
   i. Monitor for dizziness and initiate safety precautions.
   j. Monitor complete blood count (CBC) and blood glucose levels.
   k. Isoniazid is administered 1 hour before or 2 hours after a meal because food may delay absorption.
   l. Isoniazid is administered at least 1 hour before antacids, especially those antacids that contain aluminum.

m. Pyridoxine is administered as prescribed to reduce the risk of neurotoxicity.

⚠ Many tuberculosis medications can cause toxic effect such as hepatotoxicity, nephrotoxicity, neurotoxicity, optic neuritis, or ototoxicity. Teach the client about the signs of toxicity and inform the client that the HCP needs to be notified if any signs arise.

5. Client teaching
   a. The client is instructed not to skip doses and to take the medication for the full length of the prescribed therapy.
   b. The client is instructed not to take any other medication without consulting the HCP.
   c. The client is advised of the importance of follow-up HCP visits, vision testing, and laboratory tests.
   d. The client is instructed to avoid alcohol.
   e. The client is advised to take medication on an empty stomach with 8 oz of water 1 hour before or 2 hours after meals and to avoid taking antacids with the medication.
   f. The client is instructed to avoid tyramine-containing foods because they may cause a reaction such as red and itching skin, a pounding heartbeat, lightheadedness, a hot or clammy feeling, or a headache. If this does occur, the client should notify the HCP.
   g. The client is instructed in the signs of neurotoxicity, hepatitis, and hepatotoxicity.
   h. The client is instructed to notify the HCP if signs of neurotoxicity, hepatitis and hepatotoxicity, or visual changes occur.

B. Rifampin (Rifadin)
   1. Description
      a. Rifampin inhibits bacterial RNA synthesis.
      b. It binds to DNA-dependent RNA polymerase and blocks RNA transcription.
      c. It is used with at least one other antitubercular medication.
   2. Contraindications and cautions
      a. Rifampin is contraindicated in clients with hypersensitivity.
      b. It should be used with caution in clients with hepatic dysfunction or alcoholism.
      c. Use of alcohol or hepatotoxic medications may increase the risk of hepatotoxicity.
      d. Rifampin decreases the effects of several medications, including oral anticoagulants, oral hypoglycemics, chloramphenicol (Chloromycetin), digoxin (Lanoxin), disopyramide phosphate (Norpace), mexiletine (Mexitil), quinidine polygalacturonate, tocainide hydrochloride, fluconazole (Diflucan), methadone hydrochloride (Dolophine), phenytoin (Dilantin), and verapamil hydrochloride (Calan).

3. Side effects
   a. Hypersensitivity reaction, including fever, chills, shivering, headache, muscle and bone pain, and dyspnea
   b. Heartburn, nausea, vomiting, diarrhea
   c. Red-orange–colored body secretions
   d. Vision changes
   e. Hepatotoxicity and hepatitis
   f. Increased uric acid levels
   g. Blood dyscrasias
   h. Colitis
4. Interventions
   a. Monitor for hypersensitivity.
   b. Monitor CBC, uric acid, and liver function test results.
   c. Monitor for signs of hepatitis. If they occur, the medication is withheld and the HCP is notified.
   d. Monitor stools for signs of colitis.
   e. Monitor mental status.
   f. Monitor for visual changes.
5. Client teaching
   a. The client is instructed not to skip doses and to take medication for the full length of the prescribed therapy.
   b. The client is instructed not to take any other medication without consulting the HCP.
   c. The client is advised of the importance of follow-up HCP visits and laboratory tests.
   d. The client is instructed to avoid alcohol.
   e. The client is advised to take medication on an empty stomach with 8 oz of water 1 hour before or 2 hours after meals and to avoid taking antacids with the medication.
   f. The client is instructed that urine, feces, sweat, and tears will be red-orange and that soft contact lens can become permanently discolored.
   g. The client is instructed to notify the HCP if jaundice (yellow eyes or skin) develops or if weakness, fatigue, nausea, vomiting, sore throat, fever, or unusual bleeding occurs.

C. Ethambutol (Myambutol)
   1. Description
      a. Ethambutol is bacteriostatic.
      b. It interferes with cell metabolism and multiplication by inhibiting one or more metabolites in susceptible organisms.
      c. It inhibits bacterial RNA synthesis and is active only during cell division.
      d. Ethambutol is slow-acting and must be used with other bactericidal agents.
   2. Contraindications and cautions
      a. Ethambutol is contraindicated in clients with hypersensitivity or optic neuritis and children younger than 13 years.
      b. Used with caution in clients with renal dysfunction, gout, ocular defects, diabetic

retinopathy, cataracts, or ocular inflammatory conditions.

c. Used with caution in clients taking neurotoxic medications because the risk for neurotoxicity increases.

3. Side effects
   a. Hypersensitivity reactions
   b. Anorexia, nausea, vomiting
   c. Dizziness
   d. Malaise
   e. Mental confusion
   f. Joint pain
   g. Dermatitis
   h. Optic neuritis
   i. Peripheral neuritis
   j. Thrombocytopenia
   k. Increased uric acid levels
   l. Anaphylactoid reaction

4. Interventions
   a. Monitor the client for hypersensitivity.
   b. Monitor results of CBC, uric acid, and renal and liver function tests.
   c. Baseline visual acuity and color discrimination, especially to green, are obtained.
   d. Monitor for visual changes such as altered color perception and decreased visual acuity. If changes occur, the medication is withheld and the HCP is notified.
   e. Administered once every 24 hours and administered with food to decrease gastrointestinal upset.
   f. Monitor uric acid concentration and check for painful or swollen joints or signs of gout.
   g. Monitor intake and output and for adequate renal function.
   h. Monitor mental status.
   i. Monitor for dizziness and initiate safety precautions.
   j. Monitor for peripheral neuritis (numbness, tingling or burning of the extremities). If it occurs, the HCP is notified.

5. Client teaching
   a. The client is informed that he or she can prevent nausea related to the medication by taking the daily dose at bedtime or by taking the prescribed antinausea medications.
   b. The client is instructed not to skip doses and to take the medication for the full length of the prescribed therapy.
   c. The client is instructed not to take any other medication without consulting the HCP.
   d. The client is advised of the importance of follow-up HCP visits, vision testing, and laboratory tests.
   e. The client is instructed to notify the HCP immediately if any visual problems occur or

a rash, swelling and pain in the joints, or numbness, tingling, or burning in the hands or feet occurs.

D. Pyrazinamide
1. Description
   a. The exact mechanism of action of pyrazinamide is unknown.
   b. Pyrazinamide may be bacteriostatic or bactericidal, depending on its concentration at the infection site and susceptibility of infecting organism.
   c. It is used with at least one other antitubercular medication after failure or ineffectiveness of the primary medication(s).

2. Contraindications and cautions
   a. Pyrazinamide is contraindicated in clients with hypersensitivity.
   b. Used with caution in clients with diabetes mellitus, renal impairment, or gout, and in children.
   c. Pyrazinamide may decrease the effects of allopurinol (Zyloprim), colchicine, probenecid (Benemid), and sulfinpyrazone (Anturane).
   d. Cross-sensitivity is possible with isoniazid (INH), ethionamide (Trecator), or nicotinic acid.

3. Side effects
   a. Increases liver function tests and uric acid levels
   b. Arthralgia, myalgia
   c. Photosensitivity
   d. Hepatotoxicity
   e. Thrombocytopenia

4. Interventions
   a. Monitor for hypersensitivity.
   b. Monitor CBC, liver function test results, and uric acid levels.
   c. Observe for hepatotoxic effects. If they occur, the medication is withheld and the HCP is notified.
   d. Monitor for painful or swollen joints.
   e. Monitor blood glucose level because diabetes mellitus may be difficult to control while client is taking the medication.

5. Client teaching
   a. The client is instructed to take the medication with food to reduce gastrointestinal distress.
   b. The client is instructed to avoid sunlight or ultraviolet light until photosensitivity is determined.
   c. The client is instructed to notify the HCP if any side effects occur.
   d. The client is instructed not to skip doses and to take the medication for the full length of the prescribed therapy.
   e. The client is instructed not to take any other medication without consulting the HCP.

f. The client is advised of the importance of follow-up HCP visits and laboratory tests.

E. Rifabutin (Mycobutin)
1. Description
   a. Inhibits mycobacterial DNA-dependent RNA polymerase and suppresses protein synthesis.
   b. Used to prevent disseminated *Mycobacterium avium* complex (MAC) disease in clients with advanced HIV infection.
   c. Used to treat active MAC disease and **tuberculosis** in clients with HIV infection.
2. Cautions
   a. Can affect blood levels of some medications, including oral contraceptives and some medications used to treat HIV infection.
   b. A nonhormonal method of birth control should be used instead of an oral contraceptive.
3. Side effects
   a. Rash
   b. GI disturbances
   c. Neutropenia
   d. Red-orange–colored body secretions
   e. Uveitis
   f. Myositis
   g. Arthralgia
   h. Hepatitis
   i. Chest pain with dyspnea
   j. Flu-like syndrome
4. Interventions
   a. A medication history is obtained.
   b. Observe for hepatotoxic effects. If they occur, the medication is withheld and the HCP is notified.
   c. Monitor for painful or swollen joints.
   d. Monitor for ocular pain or blurred vision.
5. Client teaching
   a. The client is instructed that the medication can be taken without regard to food.
   b. The client is instructed to notify the HCP if any side effects occur.
   c. The client is instructed not to skip doses and to take the medication for the full length of the prescribed therapy.
   d. The client is instructed not to take any other medication without consulting the HCP.
   e. The client is advised of the importance of follow-up HCP visits and laboratory tests.

F. Rifapentine (Priftin)
1. Description: Used only for pulmonary **tuberculosis**
2. Cautions: Can affect blood levels of some medications, including oral contraceptives and warfarin (Coumadin), and some medications used to treat HIV infection
3. Side effects

a. Red-orange–colored body secretions
b. Hepatotoxicity
4. Interventions
   a. A medication history is obtained.
   b. Monitor baseline liver function studies and monitor throughout therapy.
   c. Observe for hepatotoxic effects; if they occur, the medication is withheld and the HCP is notified.
5. Client teaching
   a. The client is instructed that the medication can be taken without regard to food.
   b. The client is instructed to avoid sunlight or ultraviolet light until photosensitivity is determined.
   c. The client is instructed to notify the HCP if any side effects occur.
   d. The client is instructed not to skip doses and to take the medication for the full length of the prescribed therapy.
   e. The client is instructed not to take any other medication without consulting the HCP.
   f. The client is advised of the importance of follow-up HCP visits and laboratory tests.

⚠ Some tuberculosis medications can cause red-orange–colored body secretions. The client is informed that this is not a harmful effect, but that the secretions can stain and permanently discolor items.

XV. SECOND-LINE MEDICATIONS FOR TUBERCULOSIS (see Box 50-7)

A. Capreomycin sulfate (Capastat sulfate)
1. Description
   a. Mechanism of action for capreomycin is unknown.
   b. Used to treat MDR-TB when significant resistance to other medications is expected.
   c. Capreomycin must be given intramuscularly.
2. Contraindications and cautions
   a. The risk of nephrotoxicity, ototoxicity, and neuromuscular blockade is increased with the use of aminoglycosides or loop diuretics.
   b. Used with caution in clients with renal insufficiency, acoustic nerve impairment, hepatic disorder, myasthenia gravis, or parkinsonism.
   c. Not administered to clients receiving streptomycin.
3. Side effects
   a. Nephrotoxicity
   b. Ototoxicity
   c. Neuromuscular blockade
4. Interventions

a. Baseline audiometric testing is performed.
b. Renal, hepatic, and electrolyte levels are monitored before administration.
c. Monitor intake and output.
d. Reconstituted medication may be stored for 48 hours at room temperature.
e. Administered intramuscularly deep into a large muscle mass.
f. Injection sites are rotated.
g. Observe injection site for redness, excessive bleeding, and inflammation.

5. Client teaching
a. The client is instructed not to perform tasks that require mental alertness.
b. The client is instructed to report any hearing loss, balance disturbances, respiratory difficulty, weakness, or signs of hypersensitivity reactions.

B. Antibiotics
1. Description
a. Aminoglycoside antibiotics (kanamycin [Kantrex]; amikacin [Amikin]) or fluoroquinolones (levofloxacin [Levaquin]; moxifloxacin [Avelox]) are given with at least one other antitubercular medication.
b. These medications are bactericidal because of receptor-binding action interfering with protein synthesis in susceptible microorganisms.
c. Gastrointestinal disturbances are the most common side effect.
d. Fluoroquinolones are not recommended for use in children.

2. Contraindications and cautions
a. Contraindicated in clients with hypersensitivity, neuromuscular disorders, or eighth cranial nerve damage.
b. Used with caution in the older client, in neonates because of renal insufficiency and immaturity, and in young infants because it may cause CNS depression.
c. The risk of toxicity increases if taken with other aminoglycosides or nephrotoxicity- or ototoxicity-producing medications.

3. Side effects
a. Hypersensitivity
b. Pain and irritation at the injection site
c. Nephrotoxicity is indicated by increased blood urea nitrogen and serum creatinine levels.
d. Ototoxicity is indicated by tinnitus, dizziness, ringing or roaring in the ears, and reduced hearing.
e. Neurotoxicity is indicated by headache, dizziness, lethargy, tremors, and visual disturbances.
f. Superinfections

4. Interventions
a. Monitor for hypersensitivity.
b. Monitor for ototoxic, neurotoxic, and nephrotoxic reactions.
c. Monitor liver and renal function test results.
d. Baseline audiometric test is obtained and repeated every 1 to 2 months because the medication impairs the eighth cranial nerve.
e. Determine acuteness of hearing.
f. Monitor for visual changes.
g. Determine hydration status and maintain adequate hydration during therapy.
h. Monitor intake and output.
i. Monitor urinalysis results.
j. Monitor for superinfection.

5. Client teaching
a. The client is instructed not to skip doses and to take the medication for the full length of the prescribed therapy.
b. The client is instructed not to take any other medication without consulting the HCP.
c. The client is advised of the importance of follow-up HCP visits and laboratory tests.
d. The client is instructed to notify the HCP if hearing loss, changes in vision, or urinary problems occur.

C. Ethionamide (Trecator)
1. Description
a. Mechanism of action of ethionamide is unknown.
b. Ethionamide is used to treat MDR-TB when significant resistance to other medications is expected.

2. Contraindications and cautions
a. Ethionamide is contraindicated in clients with hypersensitivity.
b. Used with caution in clients with diabetes mellitus or renal dysfunction.

3. Side effects
a. Anorexia, nausea, vomiting
b. Metallic taste in the mouth
c. Orthostatic hypotension
d. Jaundice
e. Mental changes
f. Peripheral neuritis
g. Rash

4. Interventions
a. Monitor liver and renal function test results.
b. Monitor glucose levels in the client with diabetes mellitus.
c. Administered as prescribed to reduce the risk of neurotoxicity.

5. Client education
a. The client is instructed to take medication with food or meals to minimize gastrointestinal irritation.

b. The client is instructed to change positions slowly.

c. The client is instructed to report signs of a rash, which can progress to exfoliative dermatitis if the medication is not discontinued.

d. The client is instructed to avoid alcohol.

e. The client is instructed to report signs of jaundice and other side effects of the medication if they occur.

D. Aminosalicylic acid (Paser)

1. Description

a. Aminosalicylic acid inhibits folic acid metabolism in mycobacteria.

b. It is used to treat MDR-TB when significant resistance to other medications is expected.

2. Contraindications and cautions

a. Contraindicated with hypersensitivity to aminosalicylates, salicylates, or compounds containing the para-aminophenol group.

b. Aminobenzoates block the absorption of aminosalicylate sodium.

3. Side effects

a. Hypersensitivity

b. Bitter taste in the mouth

c. Gastrointestinal tract irritation

d. Exfoliative dermatitis

e. Blood dyscrasias

f. Crystalluria

g. Changes in thyroid function

4. Interventions

a. Monitor for hypersensitivity.

b. Offer clear water to rinse the mouth and chewing gum or hard candy to alleviate the bitter taste.

c. Encourage fluid intake to prevent crystalluria.

d. Monitor intake and output.

5. Client teaching

a. The client is instructed to discard the medication and obtain a new supply if a purplish-brown discoloration occurs.

b. The client is instructed to take the medication with food.

c. The client is informed that urine may turn red on contact with hypochlorite bleach if bleach was used to clean a toilet.

d. The client instructed not to take aspirin or over-the-counter medications without the HCP's approval.

e. The client is instructed to report signs of a blood dyscrasia, such as sore throat or mouth, malaise, fatigue, bruising, or bleeding.

E. Cycloserine (Seromycin)

1. Description

a. Cycloserine interferes with cell wall biosynthesis.

b. It is used to treat MDR-TB when significant resistance to other medications is expected.

2. Contraindications and cautions

a. Use of alcohol or ethionamide increases the risk of seizures.

b. Used with caution in clients with epilepsy, depression, severe anxiety, psychosis, or renal insufficiency, or the client who uses alcohol.

3. Side effects

a. Hypersensitivity

b. CNS reactions

c. Neurotoxicity

d. Seizures

e. Congestive heart failure

f. Headache

g. Vertigo

h. Altered level of consciousness

i. Irritability, nervousness, anxiety

j. Confusion

k. Mood changes, depression, thoughts of suicide

4. Interventions

a. Monitor level of consciousness.

b. Monitor for changes in mental status and thought processes.

c. Monitor renal and hepatic function tests.

d. Monitor serum drug level to avoid the risk of neurotoxicity. The peak concentration, measured 2 hours after dosing, should be 25 to 35 mcg/mL.

5. Client teaching

a. The client is instructed to take the medication after meals to prevent gastrointestinal upset.

b. The client is instructed to avoid alcohol.

c. The client is instructed to report signs of a rash or signs of CNS toxicity.

d. The client is instructed to avoid driving or performing tasks that require alertness until the reaction to the medication has been determined.

e. The client is advised of the need for monitoring serum drug levels weekly, as prescribed.

F. Streptomycin

1. Description

a. Streptomycin is an aminoglycoside antibiotic used with at least one other antitubercular medication.

b. It is bactericidal because of receptor-binding action that interferes with protein synthesis in susceptible organisms.

2. Contraindications and cautions

a. Streptomycin is contraindicated in clients with hypersensitivity, myasthenia gravis, parkinsonism, or eighth cranial nerve damage.

b. Use with caution in the older client, neonates because of renal insufficiency and immaturity, and young infants because the medication may cause CNS depression.

c. The risk of toxicity increases when streptomycin is taken with other aminoglycosides or nephrotoxicity- or ototoxicity-producing medications.

3. Side effects (Box 50-8)
   a. Hypersensitivity
   b. Visual changes
   c. Increased liver and renal function studies
   d. Peripheral neuritis, such as burning of the face or mouth

4. Interventions
   a. Monitor for hypersensitivity.
   b. Monitor liver and renal function test results.
   c. Monitor for ototoxic, neurotoxic, and nephrotoxic reactions.
   d. Baseline audiometric testing is performed and repeated every 1 to 2 months because the medication impairs the eighth cranial nerve.
   e. Check hearing acuity.
   f. Monitor for visual changes.
   g. Monitor hydration status and maintain adequate hydration during therapy.
   h. Monitor intake and output.
   i. Monitor urinalysis results.
   j. Monitor for signs of peripheral neuritis.

5. Client teaching
   a. The client is instructed not to skip doses and to take medication for the full length of the prescribed therapy.

b. The client is instructed not to take any other medication without consulting the HCP.

c. The client is advised of the importance of follow-up HCP visits and laboratory tests.

d. The client is instructed to notify the HCP if hearing loss, changes in vision, or urinary problems occur.

XVI. INFLUENZA MEDICATIONS

A. Vaccines (Box 50-9)
   1. Description
      a. Because the strain of influenza virus is different every year, annual vaccination is recommended (usually in October or November).
      b. Vaccine is available as inactivated influenza vaccine administered intramuscularly or as a live attenuated influenza vaccine, which is administered nasally.
      c. Future influenza vaccines will contain both seasonal and H1N1 vaccines in the same preparation.

   ⚠ Seasonal flu and the H1N1 (swine) flu vaccine are recommended for all individuals unless a contraindication to receiving them exists.

   2. Swine flu and the H1N1 vaccine
      a. Refer to Chapter 39 for additional information on the swine flu and its vaccine.
      b. The nasal spray vaccine is approved only for healthy people ages 2 to 49.
      c. The nasal spray vaccine is not approved for pregnant women.
      d. The flu shots, depending on the manufacturer, are approved for children as young as 6 months of age and are safe for pregnant women.
      e. The nasal spray contains a live flu virus that has been weakened to the point that it cannot cause the flu. Its advantage is that it may elicit a stronger immune response than the shot in children who have never before had the flu or a flu vaccine.

Box 50-8 Side Effects of Streptomycin

Nephrotoxicity
Changes in urine output
Decreased appetite
Increased thirst
Nausea, vomiting

Neurotoxicity
Muscle numbness
Seizures
Tingling
Twitching

Vestibular Ototoxicity
Clumsiness
Dizziness
Unsteadiness

Auditory Ototoxicity
A full feeling in the ears
Ringing in the ears
Loss of hearing

Box 50-9 Influenza Vaccines

Inactivated (Intramuscular Administration)
Afluria
Fluarix
FluLaval
Fluvirin
Fluzone

Live, Attenuated (Nasal Administration)
FluMist

f. The disadvantage of the nasal spray is that it may not be quite as protective as the flu shot for older people who have had the flu or flu vaccines before.

g. All individuals should receive an H1N1 vaccine. High-priority individuals include: pregnant women, household contacts and caregivers of children younger than 6 months of age; people age 6 months to 24 years are a priority; health care workers and emergency medical personnel; and many adults aged 25 to 64 with a medical condition, such as asthma, that increases risk of flu complications.

3. Contraindications and cautions
   a. Contraindications of the inactivated vaccine include hypersensitivity, chicken egg allergy, active infection, Guillain-Barré syndrome, active febrile illness, and children younger than 6 months.
   b. Contraindications of the live attenuated vaccine include age younger than 5 years or older than 50 years, pregnant women, children or adolescents on long-term aspirin therapy, and those with severe nasal congestion or long-term conditions such as asthma, diabetes mellitus, anemia or blood disorders, or heart, kidney, or lung disease.

4. Side effects
   a. Side effects of the inactivated vaccine include localized pain and swelling at the injection site, general body aches and pains, malaise, fever.
   b. Side effects of the attenuated vaccine include runny nose or nasal congestion, cough, headache, and sore throat.

5. Interventions
   a. The intramuscular route is recommended for the inactivated vaccine. Adults and older children should be vaccinated in the deltoid muscle.
   b. Monitor for side effects of the vaccine.
   c. Monitor for hypersensitivity reactions in clients receiving vaccination for the first time.

6. Client teaching
   a. The client is instructed about the importance of an annual vaccination.
   b. The client is instructed that the inactivated vaccine contains noninfectious killed viruses and cannot cause influenza.
   c. The client is instructed that any respiratory disease unrelated to influenza can occur after the vaccination.
   d. The client who has received the attenuated vaccine is instructed that the virus may be shed up to 2 days after vaccination.

e. The client is instructed that development of antibodies in adults takes approximately 2 weeks.

B. Antiviral medications (Box 50-10)
   1. Description
      a. Antiviral medication use during outbreaks of influenza depends on the current strain of influenza.
      b. Diagnosis of influenza should include rapid diagnostic tests because symptoms of infection from other pathogens may cause symptoms similar to those of influenza infection.
      c. Influenza antivirals may also be administered as prophylaxis against infection, but should not replace vaccination.
   2. Contraindication and cautions: Antiviral medications are contraindicated in hypersensitive clients.
   3. Side effects
      a. Common side effects include headache, dizziness, fatigue, and nausea and vomiting.
      b. Some side effects depend on the medication (Table 50-1).

Box 50-10 Antiviral Influenza Medications

Amantadine (Symmetrel)
Oseltamivir (Tamiflu)
Rimantadine (Flumadine)
Zanamivir (Relenza)

TABLE 50-1 Side Effects of Antiviral Influenza Medications

Antiviral Medications	Side Effects
Amantadine (Symmetrel)	Drowsiness, anxiety, psychosis, depression, hallucinations, tremors, confusion, insomnia, orthostatic hypotension, heart failure, blurred vision, constipation, dry mouth, urinary frequency and retention, leukopenia, photosensitivity, dermatitis
Oseltamivir (Tamiflu)	Insomnia, diarrhea, abdominal pain, cough
Rimantadine (Flumadine)	Depression, hallucinations, tremors, seizures, insomnia, poor concentration, asthenia, gait abnormalities, anxiety, confusion, pallor, palpitations, hypotension, edema, tinnitus, eye pain, constipation, dry mouth, anorexia, abdominal pain, diarrhea, dyspepsia, rash
Zanamivir (Relenza)	Ear, nose, throat infections, diarrhea, nasal symptoms, cough, sinusitis, bronchitis

4. Interventions
   a. Administered within 2 days of onset of symptoms and continue for the entire prescription.
   b. Monitor for side effects of specific medications.
5. Client teaching
   a. The client is taught that the medication may not prevent the transmission of influenza to others.
   b. The client is instructed to adjust activities if dizziness or fatigue occur.
   c. The client is instructed about management of side effects of various medications.
   d. The client is instructed to take medication exactly as prescribed and for the duration of prescription.

XVII. PNEUMOCOCCAL CONJUGATE VACCINE

A. Pneumococcal conjugate vaccine (PCV, Prevnar) is used for the prevention of invasive pneumococcal disease in infants and children.
B. Pneumococcal polysaccharide vaccine (Pneumovax 23) is used for adults and high-risk children older than 2 years.
C. Side effects may include erythema, swelling, pain, and tenderness at the injection site, fever, irritability, drowsiness, and reduced appetite.
D. See Chapter 39 for additional information about vaccines for pneumonia.

MORE QUESTIONS ON EVOLVE!

Practice Questions

511. A client is receiving acetylcysteine (Mucomyst), 20% solution diluted in 0.9% normal saline by nebulizer. The nurse should have which item available for possible use after giving this medication?
1. Ambu bag
2. Intubation tray
3. Nasogastric tube
4. Suction equipment

512. A client has a prescription to take guaifenesin (Humibid) every 4 hours, as needed. The nurse determines that the client understands the most effective use of this medication if the client states that he or she will:
1. Watch for irritability as a side effect
2. Take the tablet with a full glass of water
3. Take an extra dose if the cough is accompanied by fever
4. Crush the sustained-release tablet if immediate relief is needed

513. A postoperative client has received a dose of naloxone hydrochloride for respiratory depression shortly after transfer to the nursing unit from the postanesthesia care unit. After administration of the medication, the nurse checks the client for:
1. Pupillary changes
2. Scattered lung wheezes
3. Sudden increase in pain
4. Sudden episodes of diarrhea

514. A client has been taking isoniazid (INH) for 2 months. The client complains to a nurse about numbness, paresthesias, and tingling in the extremities. The nurse interprets that the client is experiencing:
1. Hypercalcemia
2. Peripheral neuritis
3. Small blood vessel spasm
4. Impaired peripheral circulation

515. A client is to begin a 6-month course of therapy with isoniazid (INH). A nurse plans to teach the client to:
1. Drink alcohol in small amounts only.
2. Report yellow eyes or skin immediately.
3. Increase intake of Swiss or aged cheeses.
4. Avoid vitamin supplements during therapy.

516. A client has been started on long-term therapy with rifampin (Rifadin). A nurse teaches the client that the medication:
1. Should always be taken with food or antacids
2. Should be double-dosed if one dose is forgotten
3. Causes orange discoloration of sweat, tears, urine, and feces
4. May be discontinued independently if symptoms are gone in 3 months

517. A nurse has given a client taking ethambutol (Myambutol) information about the medication. The nurse determines that the client understands the instructions if the client states that he or she will immediately report:
1. Impaired sense of hearing
2. Problems with visual acuity
3. Gastrointestinal (GI) side effects
4. Orange-red discoloration of body secretions

518. Cycloserine (Seromycin) is added to the medication regimen for a client with tuberculosis. Which of the following would the nurse include in the client-teaching plan regarding this medication?
1. To take the medication before meals
2. To return to the clinic weekly for serum drug–level testing

3. It is not necessary to call the health care provider (HCP) if a skin rash occurs.
4. It is not necessary to restrict alcohol intake with this medication.

519. A client with tuberculosis is being started on anti-tuberculosis therapy with isoniazid (INH). Before giving the client the first dose, a nurse ensures that which of the following baseline studies has been completed?
1. Electrolyte levels
2. Coagulation times
3. Liver enzyme levels
4. Serum creatinine level

520. Rifabutin (Mycobutin) is prescribed for a client with active *Mycobacterium avium* complex (MAC) disease and tuberculosis. The nurse monitors for which side effects of the medication? **Select all that apply**.
❒ 1. Signs of hepatitis
❒ 2. Flu-like syndrome
❒ 3. Low neutrophil count
❒ 4. Vitamin B$_6$ deficiency
❒ 5. Ocular pain or blurred vision
❒ 6. Tingling and numbness of the fingers

ANSWERS

511. 4
Rationale: Acetylcysteine can be given orally or by nasogastric tube to treat acetaminophen overdose, or it may be given by inhalation for use as a mucolytic. The nurse administering this medication as a mucolytic should have suction equipment available in case the client cannot manage to clear the increased volume of liquefied secretions.
Test-Taking Strategy: To answer this question, it is necessary to know that acetylcysteine may be given for either acetaminophen overdose or as a mucolytic agent. It is also necessary to know that the inhalation route is only used for mucolytic effects. With this in mind, options 1 and 2 are eliminated because the client does not need resuscitation. Option 3 is eliminated as well, because a nasogastric tube may be used in the client with acetaminophen overdose but is not necessary when used as a mucolytic. If you had difficulty with this question, review the purpose of this medication and the related nursing interventions.
Level of Cognitive Ability: Applying
Client Needs: Physiological Integrity
Integrated Process: Nursing Process/Implementation
Content Area: Pharmacology
References: Skidmore-Roth, pp. 42–43. 2009.
Workman, LaCharity, Kruchko, p. 338. 2011.

512. 2
Rationale: Guaifenesin is an expectorant. It should be taken with a full glass of water to decrease viscosity of secretions. Sustained-release preparations should not be broken open, crushed, or chewed. The medication may occasionally cause dizziness, headache, or drowsiness as side effects. The client should contact the health care provider if the cough lasts longer than 1 week or is accompanied by fever, rash, sore throat, or persistent headache.
Test-Taking Strategy: Use the process of elimination. Begin to answer this question by eliminating option 4 first. Sustained-release preparations are not crushed or broken. Option 3 is eliminated next, because fever indicates infection, and an "extra dose" of an expectorant is not helpful in treating infection. From the remaining options, recalling that increased fluids help liquefy secretions for more effective coughing will direct you to option 2. Review this medication if you had difficulty with this question.

Level of Cognitive Ability: Evaluating
Client Needs: Physiological Integrity
Integrated Process: Nursing Process/Evaluation
Content Area: Pharmacology
Reference: Skidmore-Roth, pp. 545–546. 2010.

513. 3
Rationale: Naloxone hydrochloride is an antidote to opioids and may also be given to the postoperative client to treat respiratory depression. When given to the postoperative client for respiratory depression, it may also reverse the effects of analgesics. Therefore, the nurse must check the client for a sudden increase in the level of pain experienced. Options 1, 2, and 4 are not associated with this medication.
Test-Taking Strategy: Use the process of elimination. Recalling that this medication is an antidote to opioid analgesics will assist in directing you to option 3. Remember that this medication will cause sudden pain in the postoperative client or return of pain in the client who received opioid analgesics. If you had difficulty with this question, review this medication.
Level of Cognitive Ability: Analyzing
Client Needs: Physiological Integrity
Integrated Process: Nursing Process/Data Collection
Content Area: Pharmacology
Reference: Hodgson, Kizior, pp. 802–803. 2011.

514. 2
Rationale: A common side effect of INH is peripheral neuritis. This is manifested by numbness, tingling, and paresthesias in the extremities. This side effect can be minimized by pyridoxine (vitamin B$_6$) intake. Options 1, 3, and 4 are incorrect.
Test-Taking Strategy: Use the process of elimination. Options 3 and 4 would not cause the symptoms presented in the question, but instead would cause pallor and coolness. From the remaining options, you should know either that peripheral neuritis is a side effect of the medication or that these signs and symptoms do not correlate with hypercalcemia. Review the side effects associated with INH if you had difficulty with this question.
Level of Cognitive Ability: Analyzing
Client Needs: Physiological Integrity
Integrated Process: Nursing Process/Data Collection
Content Area: Pharmacology
Reference: Hodgson, Kizior, pp. 629–631. 2011.

515. 2

Rationale: INH is hepatotoxic, and therefore the client is taught to report signs and symptoms of hepatitis immediately (which include yellow skin and sclera). For the same reason, alcohol should be avoided during therapy. The client should avoid intake of Swiss cheese, fish such as tuna, and foods containing tyramine because they may cause a reaction characterized by redness and itching of the skin, flushing, sweating, tachycardia, headache, or lightheadedness. The client can avoid developing peripheral neuritis by increasing the intake of pyridoxine (vitamin B$_6$) during the course of INH therapy.

Test-Taking Strategy: Use the process of elimination. Alcohol intake is avoided when the client is taking a prescribed medication, so option 1 should be eliminated first. Because the client receiving this medication typically is supplemented with vitamin B$_6$, option 4 is incorrect and is eliminated next. From the remaining options, recalling that the medication is hepatotoxic will direct you to option 2. If you had difficulty with this question, review this medication.

Level of Cognitive Ability: Applying
Client Needs: Physiological Integrity
Integrated Process: Teaching and Learning
Content Area: Pharmacology
Reference: Hodgson, Kizior, p. 631. 2011.

516. 3

Rationale: Rifampin should be taken exactly as directed. Doses should not be doubled or skipped. The client should not stop therapy until directed to do so by a health care provider. The medication should be administered on an empty stomach unless it causes gastrointestinal upset, and then it may be taken with food. Antacids, if prescribed, should be taken at least 1 hour before the medication. Rifampin causes orange-red discoloration of body secretions and will permanently stain soft contact lenses.

Test-Taking Strategy: Use the process of elimination. Use of general medication administration principles will assist in eliminating options 2 and 4. Eliminate option 1 next because of the closed-ended word "always." If you had difficulty with this question, review the side effects associated with this medication.

Level of Cognitive Ability: Applying
Client Needs: Physiological Integrity
Integrated Process: Teaching and Learning
Content Area: Pharmacology
Reference: Hodgson, Kizior, p. 1014. 2011.

517. 2

Rationale: Ethambutol causes optic neuritis, which decreases visual acuity and the ability to discriminate between the colors red and green. This poses a potential safety hazard when a client is driving a motor vehicle. The client is taught to report this symptom immediately. The client is also taught to take the medication with food if GI upset occurs. Impaired hearing results from antitubercular therapy with streptomycin. Orange-red discoloration of secretions occurs with rifampin (Rifadin).

Test-Taking Strategy: Use the process of elimination. Option 3 is the least likely symptom to report; rather, it should be managed by taking the medication with food. To select from the other options, it is necessary to know that this medication

causes optic neuritis, resulting in difficulty with red-green discrimination. If you had difficulty with this question, review antitubercular medications.

Level of Cognitive Ability: Evaluating
Client Needs: Physiological Integrity
Integrated Process: Nursing Process/Evaluation
Content Area: Pharmacology
Reference: Hodgson, Kizior, p. 443. 2011.

518. 2

Rationale: Cycloserine (Seromycin) is an antitubercular medication that requires weekly serum drug level determinations to monitor for the potential of neurotoxicity. Serum drug levels lower than 30 mcg/mL reduce the incidence of neurotoxicity. The medication must be taken after meals to prevent gastrointestinal irritation. The client must be instructed to notify the HCP if a skin rash or signs of central nervous system toxicity are noted. Alcohol must be avoided because it increases the risk of seizure activity.

Test-Taking Strategy: Use the process of elimination. Eliminate options 3 and 4 first, using guidelines related to general medication administration principles. From this point, knowing that the medication level needs to be monitored will assist in selecting the correct option. If you had difficulty with this question, review this medication.

Level of Cognitive Ability: Applying
Client Needs: Physiological Integrity
Integrated Process: Teaching and Learning
Content Area: Pharmacology
Reference: Lehne, pp. 819–820. 2010.

519. 3

Rationale: INH therapy can cause an elevation of hepatic enzyme levels and hepatitis. Therefore, liver enzyme levels are monitored when therapy is initiated and during the first 3 months of therapy. They may be monitored longer in the client who is greater than age 50 or abuses alcohol.

Test-Taking Strategy: Use the process of elimination. To answer this question correctly, it is necessary to know that this medication can be toxic to the liver. Review the adverse effects of the various antituberculosis medications if this is an area that is unfamiliar to you.

Level of Cognitive Ability: Analyzing
Client Needs: Physiological Integrity
Integrated Process: Nursing Process/Data Collection
Content Area: Pharmacology
Reference: Hodgson, Kizior, pp. 629–631. 2011.

520. 1, 2, 3, 5

Rationale: Rifabutin (Mycobutin) may be prescribed for a client with active MAC disease and tuberculosis. It inhibits mycobacterial DNA–dependent RNA polymerase and suppresses protein synthesis. Side effects include rash, gastrointestinal disturbances, neutropenia (low neutrophil count), red-orange body secretions, uveitis (blurred vision and eye pain), myositis, arthralgia, hepatitis, chest pain with dyspnea, and flu-like syndrome. Vitamin B$_6$ deficiency and numbness and tingling in the extremities are associated with the use of isoniazid (INH). Ethambutol (Myambutol) also causes peripheral neuritis.

Test-Taking Strategy: Focus on the name of the medication to assist in answering the question and use the process of elimination. Recalling that vitamin B_6 deficiency and numbness and tingling in the extremities are associated with the use of isoniazid (INH) will assist in answering. Review the side effects associated with rifabutin (Mycobutin) if you had difficulty with this question.

Level of Cognitive Ability: Analyzing
Client Needs: Physiological Integrity
Integrated Process: Nursing Process/Data Collection
Content Area: Pharmacology
Reference: Lehne, pp. 1050–1051. 2010.

The Adult Client with a Cardiovascular Disorder

PYRAMID TERMS

arterial anastomosis Ensures that when one of the blood-supplying arteries is damaged, flow is maintained from the other arteries; blood flow to the hands, feet, brain, and other organs is protected by arterial anastomosis

blood pressure (BP) Measures the force exerted by the blood against the walls of the blood vessels; if the BP falls too low, blood flow to the tissues, heart, brain, and other organs becomes inadequate; if the BP becomes too high, the risk of vessel rupture and damage increases

cardiac output The total volume of blood pumped through the heart in 1 minute; the normal cardiac output is 4 to 8 L/min; cardiac output = stroke volume × heart rate

contractility Refers to the inherent ability of the myocardium to alter contractile force and velocity; sympathetic stimulation increases myocardial contractility, thus increasing stroke volume; conditions that decrease myocardial contractility reduce stroke volume

diastole The phase of the cardiac cycle in which the heart relaxes between contractions; it represents the period when the two ventricles are dilated by the blood flowing into them

diastolic pressure The force of the blood exerted against the artery walls when the heart relaxes or fills

postural (orthostatic) hypotension A blood pressure decrease of more than 10 to 15 mm Hg of the systolic pressure or a decrease of more than 10 mm Hg of the diastolic pressure and a 10% to 20% increase in heart rate; occurs when the client's blood pressure is not adequately maintained when moving from a lying to a sitting or standing position

pulse pressure The difference between the systolic and diastolic pressures; normal pulse pressure is 30 to 40 mm Hg

systole The phase of contraction of the heart, especially of the ventricles, during which blood is forced into the aorta and pulmonary artery

systolic pressure The maximum pressure of blood exerted against the artery walls when the heart contracts

venous pressure The force exerted by the blood against the vein walls; normal venous pressures are highest in the extremities (5 to 14 cm H_2O in the arm), and lowest closest to the heart (6 to 8 cm H_2O in the inferior vena cava)

PYRAMID TO SUCCESS

Pyramid points focus on data collection related to cardiovascular risks, health screening and promotion, complications of the various cardiovascular disorders, emergency implementation measures, and client education. Focus on the findings in angina, myocardial infarction (MI), heart failure and pulmonary edema, hypertension, and arterial and vascular disorders. Focus also on the care of the client following diagnostic treatments and surgical procedures. Note appropriate and therapeutic client positions, particularly with arterial and venous disorders of the extremities. Focus on treatments and medications prescribed for the various cardiovascular disorders and client teaching related to prescribed treatment plans. Be familiar with the components related to cardiac rehabilitation.

CLIENT NEEDS

Safe and Effective Care Environment

- Consulting with members of the health care team
- Establishing priorities
- Initiating cardiovascular consultations and referrals

- Maintaining medical and surgical asepsis
- Maintaining standard and other precautions
- Obtaining informed consent related to treatments and procedures
- Upholding client rights

Health Promotion and Maintenance

- Discussing alterations in lifestyle
- Implementing cardiovascular data collection techniques
- Mobilizing appropriate community resources
- Promoting cardiac rehabilitation
- Providing health screening and health promotion programs
- Preventing cardiovascular disease
- Teaching related to diet, therapy, exercise, and medications

Psychosocial Integrity

- Assisting the client to accept lifestyle changes
- Considering religious, spiritual, and cultural influences on health

- Discussing grief and loss and end-of-life issues
- Discussing situational role changes
- Discussing unexpected body image changes
- Identifying coping mechanisms
- Identifying fear, anxiety, and denial
- Identifying support systems

Physiological Integrity

- Assisting with basic care measures
- Discussing activity limitations and promoting rest and sleep
- Monitoring for complications related to cardiovascular disorders
- Monitoring for therapeutic effects of medications
- Monitoring of cardiac enzymes, troponin levels, and other laboratory values related to the cardiovascular system
- Providing interventions required in emergencies
- Providing nonpharmacological and pharmacological comfort interventions
- Responding to medical emergencies

Cardiovascular Disorders

I. ANATOMY AND PHYSIOLOGY

A. Heart and heart wall layers
1. The heart is located in the left side of the mediastinum.
2. The heart consists of three layers.
   a. The epicardium is the outermost layer of the heart.
   b. The myocardium is the middle layer and actual contracting muscle of the heart.
   c. The endocardium is the innermost layer and lines the inner chambers and heart valves.

B. Pericardial sac
1. Encases and protects the heart from trauma and infection
2. Has two layers
   a. The parietal pericardium is the tough, fibrous outer membrane that attaches anteriorly to the lower half of the sternum, posteriorly to the thoracic vertebrae, and inferiorly to the diaphragm.
   b. The visceral pericardium is the thin, inner layer that closely adheres to the heart.
3. The pericardial space is between the parietal and visceral layers. It holds 5 to 20 mL of pericardial fluid, lubricates the pericardial surfaces, and cushions the heart.

C. There are four heart chambers.
1. The right atrium receives deoxygenated blood from the body via the superior and inferior vena cava.
2. The right ventricle receives blood from the right atrium and pumps it to the lungs via the pulmonary artery.
3. The left atrium receives oxygenated blood from the lungs via four pulmonary veins
4. The left ventricle is the largest and most muscular chamber. It receives oxygenated blood from the lungs via the left atrium and pumps blood into the systemic circulation via the aorta.

D. There are four valves in the heart.
1. There are two atrioventricular (AV) valves—the tricuspid and the mitral—that lie between the atria and ventricles.

a. The tricuspid valve is located on the right side of the heart.
b. The bicuspid (mitral) valve is located on the left side of the heart.
c. The AV valves close at the beginning of ventricular contraction and prevent blood from flowing back into the atria from the ventricles. These valves open when the ventricle relaxes.
2. There are two semilunar valves—the pulmonic and the aortic.
   a. The pulmonic semilunar valve lies between the right ventricle and the pulmonary artery.
   b. The aortic semilunar valve lies between the left ventricle and the aorta.
   c. The semilunar valves prevent blood from flowing back into the ventricles during relaxation. They open during ventricular contraction and close when the ventricles begin to relax.

E. Sinoatrial (SA) node
1. The main pacemaker that initiates each heart beat
2. Located at the junction of the superior vena cava and the right atrium.
3. The SA node generates electrical impulses at 60 to 100 times per minute and is controlled by the sympathetic and parasympathetic nervous systems.

F. Atrioventricular (AV) node
1. Located in the lower aspect of the atrial septum
2. Receives electrical impulses from the SA node
3. If the SA node fails, the AV node can initiate and sustain a heart rate of 40 to 60 beats/min.

G. The bundle of His
1. A continuation of the AV node and located at the interventricular septum
2. It branches into the right bundle branch, which extends down the right side of the interventricular septum, and the left bundle branch, which extends into the left ventricle.
3. The right and left bundle branches terminate into Purkinje fibers.

H. Purkinje fibers
1. Purkinje fibers are a diffuse network of conducting strands located beneath the ventricular endocardium.

2. These fibers spread the wave of depolarization through the ventricles.
3. Purkinje fibers can act as the pacemaker with a rate between 20 and 40 beats/min when higher pacemakers fail.

I. Coronary arteries: supply the capillaries of the myocardium with blood (Box 51-1)

⚠ The coronary arteries supply the capillaries of the myocardium with blood. If blockage occurs in these arteries, the client is at risk for myocardial infarction.

J. Heart sounds
1. The first heart sound (S_1) is heard as the AV valves close and is heard loudest at the apex of the heart.
2. The second heart sound (S_2) is heard when the semilunar valves close and is heard loudest at the base of the heart.
3. A third heart sound (S_3) may be heard if ventricular wall compliance is decreased and structures in the ventricular wall vibrate; this can occur in conditions such as congestive heart failure or valvular regurgitation. However, a third heart sound may be normal in individuals younger than 30 years.
4. A fourth heart sound (S_4) may be heard on atrial systole if resistance to ventricular filling is present; this is an abnormal finding, and the causes include cardiac hypertrophy, disease, or injury to the ventricular wall.

K. Heart rate
1. The faster the heart rate, the less time the heart has for filling, and the **cardiac output** decreases.
2. An increase in heart rate increases oxygen consumption.
3. The normal sinus heart rate is 60 to 100 beats/min.
4. Sinus tachycardia is a rate greater than 100 beats/min.
5. Sinus bradycardia is a rate less than 60 beats/min.

Box 51-1 Coronary Arteries

Right coronary artery (RCA): Supplies the right atrium and ventricle, the inferior portion of the left ventricle, the posterior septal wall, and the sinoatrial and atrioventricular nodes
Left coronary artery (LCA): Consists of two major branches—the left anterior descending (LAD) and the circumflex arteries
LAD artery: Supplies blood to the anterior wall of the left ventricle, the anterior ventricular septum, and the apex of the left ventricle
Circumflex artery: Supplies blood to the left atrium and the lateral and posterior surfaces of the left ventricle

---

L. Autonomic nervous system
1. Stimulation of sympathetic nerve fibers releases the neurotransmitter norepinephrine, producing an increased heart rate, increased conduction speed through the AV node, increased atrial and ventricular **contractility**, and peripheral vasoconstriction. Stimulation occurs when a decrease in pressure is detected.
2. Stimulation of the parasympathetic nerve fibers releases the neurotransmitter acetylcholine, which decreases the heart rate and lessens atrial and ventricular **contractility** and conductivity. Stimulation occurs when an increase in pressure is detected.

M. **Blood pressure (BP)** control
1. Baroreceptors, also called pressoreceptors, are located in the walls of the aortic arch and carotid sinuses.
2. Baroreceptors are specialized nerve endings that are affected by changes in the arterial **BP**.
3. Increases in arterial pressure stimulate baroreceptors, and the heart rate and arterial pressure decrease.
4. Decreases in arterial pressure reduce stimulation of the baroreceptors, and vasoconstriction and an increase in heart rate occur.
5. Stretch receptors, located in the vena cava and the right atrium, respond to pressure changes that affect circulatory blood volume.
6. When the **BP** decreases as a result of hypovolemia, a sympathetic response occurs, causing an increased heart rate and blood vessel constriction. When the **BP** increases as a result of hypervolemia, an opposite effect occurs.
7. Antidiuretic hormone (vasopressin) influences **BP** indirectly by regulating vascular volume.
8. Increases in blood volume result in decreased antidiuretic hormone release, increasing diuresis, and decreasing blood volume and thus decreasing **BP**.
9. Decreases in blood volume result in increased antidiuretic hormone release. This promotes an increase in blood volume and thus **BP**.
10. Renin, a potent vasoconstrictor, causes the **BP** to increase.
11. Renin converts angiotensinogen to angiotensin I. Angiotensin I is then converted to angiotensin II in the lungs.
12. Angiotensin II stimulates the release of aldosterone, which promotes water and sodium retention by the kidneys. This action increases blood volume and **BP**.

N. The vascular system
1. Arteries are vessels through which the blood passes away from the heart to various parts of the body. They convey highly oxygenated blood from the left side of heart to the tissues.

2. Arterioles control the blood flow into the capillaries.
3. Capillaries allow the exchange of fluid and nutrients between the blood and the interstitial spaces.
4. Venules receive blood from the capillary bed and move blood into the veins.
5. Veins transport deoxygenated blood from the tissues back to the right heart and then the lungs for oxygenation.
6. Valves help return blood to the heart against the force of gravity.
7. The lymphatics drain the tissues and return the tissue fluid to the blood.

II. DIAGNOSTIC TESTS AND PROCEDURES

A. Cardiac enzymes
  1. CK-MB (creatine kinase, myocardial muscle)
     a. An elevation in value indicates myocardial damage.
     b. An elevation occurs within 4 to 6 hours and peaks 18 to 24 hours following an acute ischemic attack.
     c. Normal value is 0% to 5% of total; total CK is 26 to 174 units/L.
  2. Lactic dehydrogenase (LDH)
     a. Elevations in LDH levels occur 24 hours following myocardial infarction and peak in 48 to 72 hours.
     b. Normally, LDH1 is lower than LDH2; when the serum concentration of LDH1 is higher than LDH2, the pattern is indicated as "flipped," signifying myocardial necrosis.
     c. The normal value of LDH in conventional units is 140 to 280 international units/L.
  3. Troponin
     a. Troponin is composed of three proteins— troponin C, cardiac troponin I, and cardiac troponin T.
     b. Troponin I especially has a high affinity for myocardial injury; it rises within 3 hours and persists for up to 7 days.
     c. Normal values are low, with troponin I being lower than 0.6 ng/mL and troponin T normally ranging from 0 to 0.2 ng/mL; thus, any rise can indicate myocardial cell damage.
  4. Myoglobin
     a. Myoglobin is an oxygen-binding protein found in cardiac and skeletal muscle.
     b. The level rises within 1 hour after cell death, peaks in 4 to 6 hours, and returns to normal within 24 to 36 hours (even faster in some clients).
B. Complete blood count
  1. The red blood cell count decreases in rheumatic heart disease and infective endocarditis and increases in conditions characterized by inadequate tissue oxygenation.

2. The white blood cell count increases in infectious and inflammatory diseases of the heart and after MI because large numbers of white blood cells are needed to dispose of the necrotic tissue resulting from the infarction.
  3. An elevated hematocrit can result from vascular volume depletion.
  4. Decreases in hematocrit and hemoglobin can indicate anemia.
C. Blood coagulation factors: An increase in coagulation factors can occur during and after MI, which places the client at greater risk of thrombophlebitis and extension of clots in the coronary arteries.
D. Serum lipids: used to assess the risk of developing coronary artery disease
  1. The lipid profile measures serum cholesterol, triglyceride, and lipoprotein levels.
  2. The lipid profile is used to assess the risk of developing coronary artery disease.
  3. The desirable range for serum cholesterol is lower than 200 mg/dL, with low-density lipoprotein cholesterol lower than 130 mg/dL and high-density lipoprotein cholesterol at 30 to 70 mg/dL.
  4. Lipoprotein-a or $Lp(a)$, a modified form of LDL, increases atherosclerotic plaques and increases clots; value should be less than 30 mg/dL.
E. Homocysteine: elevated levels may increase the risk of cardiovascular disease; level should be less than 14 mmol/dL.
F. Highly sensitive C-reactive protein (hsCRP): detects an inflammatory process such as that associated with the development of atherothrombosis; a level less than 1 mg/dL is considered low risk and a level over 3 mg/dL places the client at risk for heart disease.
G. Microalbuminuria: a small amount of protein in the urine has been a marker for endothelial dysfunction in cardiovascular disease.
H. Electrolytes
  1. Potassium
     a. Hypokalemia causes increased cardiac electrical instability, ventricular dysrhythmias, and increased risk of digoxin toxicity.
     b. In hypokalemia, the electrocardiogram would show flattening and inversion of the T wave, the appearance of a U wave, and ST depression.
     c. Hyperkalemia causes asystole and ventricular dysrhythmias.
     d. In hyperkalemia, the electrocardiogram may show tall peaked T waves, widened QRS complexes, prolonged PR intervals, or flat P waves.
  2. Sodium
     a. The serum sodium level decreases with the use of diuretics.
     b. The serum sodium level decreases in heart failure, indicating water excess.

I. Calcium
  1. Hypocalcemia can cause ventricular dysrhythmias, prolonged ST and QT interval, and cardiac arrest.
  2. Hypercalcemia can cause a shortened ST segment and widened T wave, AV block, tachycardia or bradycardia, digitalis hypersensitivity, and cardiac arrest.
J. Phosphorus level: Phosphorus levels should be interpreted with calcium levels because the kidneys retain or excrete one electrolyte in an inverse relationship to the other.
K. Magnesium
  1. A low magnesium level can cause ventricular tachycardia (VT) and fibrillation.
  2. Electrocardiographic changes that may be observed with hypomagnesemia include tall T waves and depressed ST segments.
  3. A high magnesium level can cause muscle weakness, hypotension, and bradycardia.
  4. Electrocardiographic changes that may be observed with hypermagnesemia include a prolonged PR interval and widened QRS complex.

⚠ Electrolyte and mineral imbalances can cause cardiac electrical instability that can result in life-threatening dysrhythmias.

L. Blood urea nitrogen: The blood urea nitrogen is elevated in heart disorders that adversely affect renal circulation, such as heart failure and cardiogenic shock.
M. Blood glucose: An acute cardiac episode can elevate the blood glucose.
N. B-type natriuretic peptide (BNP)
  1. BNP is released in response to atrial and ventricular stretch; serves as a marker for congestive heart failure.
  2. BNP levels should be less than 100 pg/mL. The higher the level, the more severe the congestive heart failure.
O. Chest x-ray film
  1. Description
    a. Radiography of the chest is done to determine the size, silhouette, and position of the heart.
    b. Specific pathological changes are difficult to determine via x-ray film, but anatomical changes can be seen.
  2. Interventions
    a. Prepare the client for x-ray film, explaining the purpose and procedure.
    b. Remove jewelry.
P. Electrocardiography
  1. Description: This common noninvasive diagnostic test records the electrical activity of the heart and is useful in detecting cardiac dysrhythmias, detecting location and extent of myocardial

infarction, cardiac hypertrophy, and for evaluation of the effectiveness of cardiac medications.
  2. Interventions
    a. Determine the client's ability to lie still. Advise the client to lie still, breathe normally, and refrain from talking during the test.
    b. Reassure the client that an electrical shock will not occur.
    c. Document any cardiac medications the client is taking.
Q. Holter monitoring
  1. Description
    a. In this noninvasive test, the client wears a Holter monitor and an electrocardiographic tracing is recorded continuously over a period of 24 hours or more while the client performs his activities of daily living.
    b. The Holter monitor identifies dysrhythmias if they occur and evaluates the effectiveness of antidysrhythmics or pacemaker therapy.
  2. Interventions
    a. Instruct the client to resume normal daily activities and to maintain a diary documenting activities and any symptoms that may develop for correlation to the electrocardiographic tracing.
    b. Instruct the client to avoid tub baths or showers because they will interfere with the electrocardiographic recorder device.
R. Echocardiography
  1. Description
    a. This noninvasive procedure is based on the principles of ultrasound and evaluates structural and functional changes in the heart.
    b. Heart chamber size is measured, ejection fraction is calculated, and flow gradient across the valves is determined.
    c. A transesophageal echocardiography may be done in which the echocardiogram is done through the esophagus; this is an invasive exam and requires pre- and post-procedure preparation and care is similar to endoscopy procedures.
  2. Interventions: Determine the client's ability to lie still, and advise the client to lie still, breathe normally, and refrain from talking during the test.
S. Exercise electrocardiography testing (stress test)
  1. Description
    a. This noninvasive test studies the heart during activity and detects and evaluates coronary artery disease.
    b. Treadmill testing is the most commonly used mode of stress testing.
    c. Stress testing may be used with myocardial radionuclide testing (perfusion imaging), at which point the procedure becomes invasive because a radionuclide must be injected.

d. If the client is unable to tolerate exercise, an intravenous (IV) infusion of dipyridamole (Persantine), dobutamine hydrochloride, or adenosine (Adenocard) is given to dilate the coronary arteries and simulate the effect of exercise.

e. An informed consent is required if a radionuclide is injected.

2. Preprocedure interventions
   a. Obtain an informed consent if required.
   b. Provide adequate rest the night before the procedure.
   c. Instruct the client to eat a light meal 1 to 2 hours before the procedure.
   d. Instruct the client to avoid smoking, alcohol, and caffeine before the procedure.
   e. Instruct the client to ask the health care provider (HCP) about taking prescribed medication on the day of the procedure. Theophylline products are usually held 12 hours before the test and calcium channel blockers and β-blockers are usually held for 24 hours.
   f. Instruct the client to wear nonconstrictive, comfortable clothing and supportive rubber-soled shoes for the exercise stress test.
   g. Instruct the client to notify the HCP if any chest pain, dizziness, or shortness of breath occurs during the procedure.

3. Postprocedure interventions: Instruct the client to avoid taking a hot bath or shower for at least 1 to 2 hours.

T. Digital subtraction angiography
1. Description
   a. This test combines x-ray techniques and a computerized subtraction technique with fluoroscopy for visualization of the cardiovascular system.
   b. A contrast medium (dye) is injected.
2. Preprocedure interventions
   a. Check for allergies to seafood, iodine, or radiopaque dyes. If allergic, the client may be premedicated with antihistamines and steroids to prevent a reaction.
   b. Obtain informed consent.
3. Postprocedure interventions
   a. Monitor vital signs.
   b. Monitor injection site for bleeding or discomfort.

U. Nuclear cardiology
1. Description
   a. Nuclear cardiology is the use of radionuclide techniques and scanning in cardiovascular assessment.
   b. The most common tests include technetium pyrophosphate scanning, thallium imaging, and multigated cardiac blood pool imaging;

can evaluate cardiac motion and calculate the ejection fraction.

2. Preprocedure interventions
   a. Obtain informed consent.
   b. Inform the client that a small amount of radioisotope will be injected and that the radiation exposure and risks are minimal.
3. Postprocedure interventions
   a. Monitor vital signs.
   b. Monitor injection site for bleeding or discomfort.
   c. Inform the client that fatigue is possible.

V. Magnetic resonance imaging (MRI)
1. Description
   a. This is a noninvasive diagnostic test that produces an image of the heart or great vessels through interaction of magnetic fields, radio waves, and atomic nuclei.
   b. It provides information on chamber size and thickness, valve and ventricular function, and blood flow through the great vessels and coronary arteries.
2. Preprocedure interventions
   a. Evaluate the client for the presence of a pacemaker or other implanted items that present a contraindication to the test.
   b. Ensure that the client has removed all metallic objects such as watches, jewelry, clothing with metal fasteners, and metal hair fasteners.
   c. Inform the client that he or she may experience claustrophobia while in the scanner.

W. Eletrophysiologic studies: An invasive procedure in which a programmed electrical stimulation of the heart is induced to cause dysrhythmias and conduction defects; assists in finding an accurate diagnosis and aids in determining treatment.

X. Electronic-Beam Computer Tomography Scan (EBCT): Determines whether calcifications are present in the arteries; coronary artery calcium (CAC) score is provided (a score higher than 400 requires intensive preventive treatment).

Y. Cardiac catheterization
1. Description
   a. An invasive test involving insertion of a catheter into the heart and surrounding vessels
   b. Obtains information about the structure and performance of the heart chambers and valves and the coronary circulation
2. Preprocedure interventions
   a. Obtain informed consent.
   b. Monitor for allergies to seafood, iodine, or radiopaque dyes. If allergic, the client may be premedicated with antihistamines and corticosteroids to prevent a reaction.
   c. Withhold solid food for 6 to 8 hours and liquids for 4 hours as prescribed to prevent vomiting and aspiration during the procedure.

d. Document the client's height and weight because these data will be needed to determine the amount of dye to be administered.

e. Document baseline vital signs and note the quality and presence of peripheral pulses for postprocedure comparison.

f. Inform the client that a local anesthetic will be administered before catheter insertion.

g. Inform the client that he or she may feel fatigued because of the need to lie still and quiet on a hard table for up to 2 hours.

h. Inform the client that he or she may feel a fluttery feeling as the catheter passes through the heart; a flushed, warm feeling when the dye is injected; a desire to cough; and palpitations caused by heart irritability.

i. Prepare the insertion site by shaving and cleaning with an antiseptic solution if prescribed.

j. Administer preprocedure medications such as sedatives if prescribed.

k. Insert an IV line if prescribed.

⚠ If a client taking metformin (Glucophage) is schedule to undergo a procedure requiring the administration of iodine dye, the metformin is withheld 48 hours prior because of the risk of lactic acidosis. The medication is not resumed until directed to do so by the HCP (usually 48 hours after the procedure or after renal function studies are done and the results are evaluated).

3. Postprocedure interventions
   a. Monitor vital signs and cardiac rhythm for dysrhythmias at least every 30 minutes for 2 hours initially.
   b. Monitor for chest pain. If dysrhythmias or chest pain occurs, notify the HCP.
   c. Monitor peripheral pulses and the color, warmth, and sensation of the extremity distal to the insertion site at least every 30 minutes for 2 hours initially.
   d. Notify the HCP if the client complains of numbness and tingling; the extremity becomes cool, pale, or cyanotic; or loss of the peripheral pulses occurs.
   e. Monitor the pressure dressing for bleeding or hematoma formation.
   f. Apply a sandbag or compression device to the insertion site to provide additional pressure if prescribed.
   g. Monitor for bleeding. If bleeding occurs, apply manual pressure immediately and notify the HCP.
   h. Monitor for hematoma. If a hematoma develops, notify the HCP.

i. Keep extremity extended for 4 to 6 hours, as prescribed, keeping the leg straight to prevent arterial occlusion.

j. Maintain strict bedrest for 6 to 12 hours, as prescribed; however, the client may turn from side to side. Do not elevate the head of the bed more than 15 degrees.

k. If the antecubital vessel was used, immobilize the arm with an armboard.

l. Encourage fluid intake, if not contraindicated, to promote renal excretion of the dye and replace fluid loss caused by the osmotic diuretic effect of the dye.

m. Monitor for nausea, vomiting, rash, or other signs of hypersensitivity to the dye.

n. Do not resume the administration of metformin (Glucophage) until directed by the HCP (usually 48 hours after catheterization).

III. THERAPEUTIC MANAGEMENT

A. Percutaneous transluminal coronary angioplasty (PTCA)
   1. Description (Figure 51-1)
      a. An invasive, nonsurgical technique in which one or more arteries is (are) dilated with a balloon catheter to open the vessel lumen and improve arterial blood flow.
      b. PTCA may be used alone for clients with an evolving MI or in combination with medications to achieve reperfusion.
      c. The client can experience reocclusion after the procedure; thus, the procedure may need to be repeated.
      d. Complications can include arterial dissection or rupture, immobilization of plaque fragments, spasm, and acute MI.
      e. A firm commitment is needed on the part of the client to stop smoking, adhere to dietary restrictions, lose weight, alter exercise patterns, and discontinue any behaviors that could lead to the progression of artery occlusion.
   2. Preprocedure interventions
      a. Maintain NPO status after midnight.
      b. Obtain informed consent and allergy assessment to iodine, and hold metformin (Glucophage), as with cardiac catheterization.
      c. Prepare the groin area with antiseptic soap and shave per institutional procedure and as prescribed.
      d. Monitor baseline vital signs and peripheral pulses.
      e. Instruct the client that chest pain may occur during balloon inflation and to report it if it does occur.

1. The balloon-tipped catheter is positioned in the artery.
2. The uninflated balloon is centered in the obstruction.
3. The balloon is inflated, which flattens plaque against the artery wall.
4. The balloon is removed, and the artery is left unoccluded.

▲ **FIGURE 51-1** Percutaneous transluminal coronary angioplasty. (From Ignatavicius, D., & Workman, M. [2010]. *Medical-surgical nursing: Patient-centered collaborative care* [6th ed.]. St. Louis: Saunders.)

3. Postprocedure interventions
   a. Monitor vital signs closely.
   b. Check distal pulses in both extremities.
   c. Maintain bedrest as prescribed, keeping the limb straight for 6 to 8 hours.
   d. Administer anticoagulants such as IV heparin and antiplatelet agents as prescribed to prevent thrombus formation.
   e. Intravenous nitroglycerin may be prescribed to prevent coronary artery vasospasm.
   f. Encourage fluids if not contraindicated to enhance renal excretion of dye.
   g. Instruct the client in the administration of nitrates, calcium channel blockers, antiplatelet agents, and anticoagulants as prescribed.
   h. Instruct the client to take acetylsalicylic acid (aspirin) daily permanently if prescribed.
   i. Assist the client with planning lifestyle modifications.

B. Laser-assisted angioplasty
   1. Description
      a. A laser probe is advanced through a cannula similar to that used for PTCA.
      b. Laser-assisted angioplasty is also used for clients with small occlusions in the distal superficial femoral, proximal popliteal, and common iliac arteries, as well as in the coronary arteries.
      c. Heat from the laser vaporizes the plaque to open the occluded artery.
   2. Preprocedure and postprocedure interventions
      a. Care is similar to that for PTCA.
      b. Monitor for complications of coronary dissection, acute occlusion, perforation, embolism, and myocardial infarction.

C. Coronary artery stents
   1. Description
      a. Coronary artery stents are used in conjunction with PTCA to provide a supportive scaffold to eliminate the risk of acute coronary vessel closure and improve long-term patency of the vessel.
      b. A balloon catheter bearing the stent is inserted into the coronary artery and positioned at the site of occlusion. Balloon inflation deploys the stent.
      c. When placed in the coronary artery, the stent reopens the blocked artery.
   2. Preprocedure and postprocedure interventions
      a. Care is similar to that for PTCA.
      b. Acute thrombosis is a major concern following the procedure, and the client is placed on antiplatelet therapy such as clopidogrel (Plavix) and acetylsalicylic acid (aspirin) for several months after the procedure.
      c. Monitor for complications of the procedure such as stent migration or occlusion, coronary artery dissection, and bleeding resulting from anticoagulation.

D. Atherectomy
   1. Description
      a. Atherectomy removes plaque from a coronary artery by the use of a cutting chamber on the inserted catheter or a rotating blade that pulverizes the plaque.
      b. Atherectomy is also used to improve blood flow to ischemic limbs in individuals with peripheral arterial disease.
   2. Preprocedure and postprocedure interventions
      a. Care is similar to that for PTCA.
      b. Monitor for complications of perforation, embolus, and reocclusion.

E. Transmyocardial revascularization
   1. Used for clients with widespread atherosclerosis involving vessels that are too small and numerous for replacement or balloon catheterization. The procedure is performed through a small chest incision.
   2. Transmyocardial revascularization uses a high-power laser that creates 20 to 24 channels through the muscle of the left ventricle and blood enters these small channels, providing the affected region of the heart with oxygenated blood.

3. The opening on the surface of the heart heals; however, the main channels remain and perfuse the myocardium.

F. Arterial revascularization
   1. Description
      a. Performed to increase arterial blood flow to the affected limb
      b. Inflow procedures involve bypassing the arterial occlusion above the superficial femoral arteries.
      c. Outflow procedures involve bypassing the arterial occlusions at or below the superficial femoral arteries.
      d. Graft material is sutured above and below the occlusion to facilitate blood flow around the occlusion.
   2. Preoperative interventions
      a. Monitor baseline vital signs and peripheral pulses.
      b. Insert an IV line and urinary catheter as prescribed.
      c. Maintain a central venous catheter and/or arterial line if inserted.
   3. Postoperative interventions
      a. Monitor vital signs.
      b. Monitor the **BP** and notify the HCP if changes occur.
      c. Monitor for hypotension, which may indicate hypovolemia.
      d. Monitor for hypertension, which may place stress on the graft and facilitate clot formation.
      e. Maintain bedrest for 24 hours as prescribed.
      f. Instruct the client to keep the affected extremity straight, limit movement, and avoid bending the knee and hip.
      g. Monitor for warmth, redness, and edema, which are often expected outcomes because of increased blood flow.
      h. Monitor for graft occlusion, which often occurs within the first 24 hours.
      i. Monitor peripheral pulses and for adverse changes in color and temperature of the extremity.
      j. Encourage coughing and deep breathing and the use of incentive spirometry.
      k. Maintain NPO status, with progression to clear liquids as prescribed.
      l. Use strict aseptic technique when in contact with the incision.
      m. Monitor the incision for drainage, warmth, or swelling.
      n. Monitor for excessive bleeding. (A small amount of bloody drainage is expected.)
      o. Monitor the area over the graft for hardness, tenderness, and warmth, which may indicate infection. If this occurs, notify the HCP immediately.
      p. Instruct the client about proper foot care and measures to prevent ulcer formation.
      q. Instruct the client to take medications as prescribed.
      r. Instruct the client on how to care for the incision.
      s. Assist the client in modifying lifestyle (such as diet) to prevent further plaque formation.

⚠ After arterial vascularization, monitor for a sharp increase in pain because pain is frequently the first indicator of postoperative graft occlusion. If signs of graft occlusion occur, notify the HCP immediately.

G. Coronary artery bypass graft
   1. Description
      a. The occluded coronary arteries are bypassed with the client's own venous or arterial blood vessels.
      b. The saphenous vein, internal mammary artery, or other arteries may be used to bypass lesions in the coronary arteries.
      c. Coronary artery bypass graft is performed when the client does not respond to medical management of coronary artery disease or when vessels are severely occluded.
   2. Preoperative interventions
      a. Familiarize the client and family with the cardiac surgical critical care unit.
      b. Inform the client to expect a sternal incision, possible arm or leg incision(s), one or two chest tubes, a Foley catheter, and several IV fluid catheters.
      c. Inform the client that an endotracheal tube will be in place and that he or she will be unable to speak.
      d. Advise the client that he or she will be on mechanical ventilation and to breathe with—and not fight—the ventilator.
      e. Instruct the client to inform the nurse of any postoperative pain because pain medication will be available.
      f. Instruct the client on how to splint the chest incision, cough and deep breathe, use the incentive spirometer, and perform arm and leg exercises.
      g. Encourage the client and family to discuss anxieties and fears related to surgery.
      h. Note that prescribed medications may be discontinued preoperatively (usually diuretics 2 to 3 days before surgery, digoxin 12 hours before surgery, and aspirin and anticoagulants 1 week before surgery).
      i. Administer medications as prescribed, which may include potassium chloride, antihypertensives, antidysrhythmics, and antibiotics.

3. Transfer from the cardiac surgical unit
   a. Monitor vital signs, level of consciousness, and peripheral perfusion.
   b. Monitor for dysrhythmias.
   c. Auscultate lungs and monitor respiratory status.
   d. Encourage the client to splint the incision, cough and deep breathe, and use the incentive spirometer to raise secretions and prevent atelectasis.
   e. Monitor temperature and white blood cell count, which indicate infection if elevated after 3 to 4 days.
   f. Provide adequate fluids and hydration as prescribed to liquefy secretions.
   g. Monitor suture line and chest tube insertion sites for redness, purulent discharge, and signs of infection.
   h. Monitor sternal suture line for instability, which may indicate an infection.
   i. Guide the client to gradually resume activity.
   j. Monitor the client for tachycardia, **postural (orthostatic) hypotension**, and fatigue before, during, and after activity.
   k. Discontinue activities if the **BP** drops more than 10 to 20 mm Hg or the pulse increases more than 10 beats/min.
   l. Monitor episodes of pain closely.
   m. See Box 51-2 for home care instructions.
H. Heart transplant
   1. A donor heart from an individual with a comparable body weight and ABO compatibility is transplanted into a recipient within 6 hours of procurement.
   2. The surgeon removes the diseased heart, leaving the posterior portion of the atria to serve as an anchor for the new heart.
   3. Because a remnant of the client's atria remains, two unrelated P waves are noted on the electrocardiogram.
   4. The transplanted heart is denervated and unresponsive to vagal stimulation. Because the heart is denervated, clients do not experience angina.

5. Symptoms of heart rejection include hypotension, dysrhythmias, weakness, fatigue, and dizziness.
6. Endomyocardial biopsies are performed at regular scheduled intervals and whenever rejection is suspected.
7. The client requires lifetime immunosuppressive therapy.
8. Strict aseptic technique and vigilant handwashing must be maintained when caring for the post-transplant client because of increased risk for infection from immunosuppression.
9. The heart rate approximates 100 beats/min and responds slowly to exercise or stress with regard to increases in heart rate, **contractility**, and **cardiac output**.

IV. CARDIAC DYSRHYTHMIAS

A. Normal sinus rhythm (Figure 51-2)
   1. Rhythm originates from the sinoatrial node
   2. Atrial and ventricular rhythms are regular at 60 to 100 beats/min.

Box 51-2 Home Care Instructions After Cardiac Surgery

Progressively return to activities at home.
Limit pushing or pulling activities for 6 weeks after discharge.
Maintain incisional care and record signs of redness, swelling, or drainage.
Sternotomy incision heals in about 6 to 8 weeks.
Avoid crossing legs. Wear elastic hose as prescribed until edema subsides, and elevate surgical limb when sitting in a chair.
Follow prescribed medications as instructed by the HCP.
Follow prescribed dietary measures such as avoiding saturated fat, cholesterol, and salt.
Sexual intercourse can be resumed on the advice of the HCP after exercise tolerance is assessed. If the client can walk one block or climb two flights of stairs without symptoms, he or she can resume sexual activity safely.

▲ **FIGURE 51-2** Normal sinus rhythm. (From Ignatavicius, D., Workman, M. [2010]. *Medical-surgical nursing: Patient-centered collaborative care* [6th ed.]. St. Louis: Saunders.)

B. Sinus bradycardia
1. Atrial and ventricular rates are regular and are less than 60 beats/min.
2. Note that a low heart rate may be normal for some individuals.
3. Treatment may be necessary if the client is symptomatic (signs of decreased cardiac output).
4. Treatment depends on the cause and may include holding a medication, oxygen, atropine sulfate, or a pacemaker; notify the registered nurse (RN).

C. Sinus tachycardia
1. Atrial and ventricular rhythms are regular.
2. Atrial and ventricular rates are 100 to 180 beats/min.
3. Treatment depends on the cause.

D. Atrial fibrillation
1. Multiple rapid impulses from many foci depolarize in the atria in a totally disorganized manner at a rate of 350 to 600 times per minute; the atria quiver, which can lead to the formation of thrombi.
2. No definitive P wave can be observed—only fibrillatory waves before each QRS.
3. Treatment includes oxygen, anticoagulants, cardiac medications, and possible cardioversion. Notify the RN.

E. Premature ventricular contractions (PVCs) (Box 51-3 and Figure 51-3)
1. Early ventricular complexes result from increased irritability of the ventricles.
2. Treatment depends on the cause and the RN nurse is notified if PVCs occur.

⚠ For the client experiencing PVCs, notify the HCP if the client complains of chest pain or if the PVCs increase in frequency, are multifocal, occur on the T wave (R on T), or occur in runs of ventricular tachycardia.

F. Ventricular tachycardia (VT) (Figure 51-4)
1. VT occurs because of a repetitive firing of an irritable ventricular ectopic focus at a rate of 140 to 250 beats/min or more and can lead to cardiac arrest. Notify the RN if VT occurs.
2. A stable client with sustained VT (with pulse and no signs or symptoms of decreased **cardiac output**) will be treated with oxygen and antidysrhythmics.
3. An unstable client with VT (with pulse and signs and symptoms of decreased **cardiac output**) will be treated with oxygen and antidysrhythmics and cough cardiopulmonary resuscitation (CPR) or possible synchronized cardioversion.
4. A pulseless client with VT will be treated with defibrillation and CPR.

G. Ventricular fibrillation (VF) (Figure 51-5)
1. Ventricular fibrillation is a chaotic rapid rhythm in which the ventricles quiver and there is no **cardiac output**.
2. Client lacks a pulse, **BP**, respirations, and heart sounds, and VF is fatal if not successfully terminated within 3 to 5 minutes
3. Treatment includes CPR and immediate defibrillation.

Box 51-3 Premature Ventricular Contractions (PVCs)

Bigeminy: PVC every other heartbeat
Trigeminy: PVC every third heartbeat
Quadrigeminy: PVC every fourth heartbeat
Couplet or pair: Two sequential PVCs
Unifocal: Uniform upward or downward deflection, arising from the same ectopic focus
Multifocal: Different shapes, with the impulse generation from different sites
R-on-T phenomenon: PVC falls on the T wave of the preceding beat and may precipitate ventricular fibrillation

▲ **FIGURE 51-3** Normal sinus rhythm with multifocal premature ventricular contractions (one negative and the other positive). (From Ignatavicius, D., & Workman, M. [2010]. *Medical-surgical nursing: Patient-centered collaborative care* [6th ed.]. St. Louis: Saunders.)

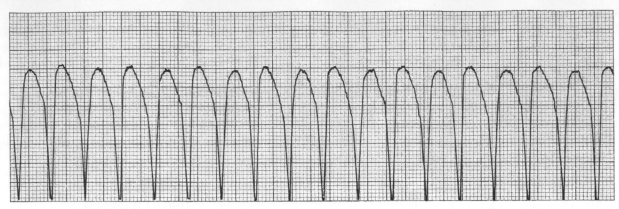

▲ **FIGURE 51-4** Ventricular tachycardia. (From Ignatavicius, D., & Workman, M. [2010]. *Medical-surgical nursing: Patient-centered collaborative care* [6th ed.]. St. Louis: Saunders.)

▲ **FIGURE 51-5** Ventricular fibrillation. (From Ignatavicius, D., & Workman, M. [2010]. *Medical-surgical nursing: Patient-centered collaborative care* [6th ed.]. St. Louis: Saunders.)

V. MANAGEMENT OF DYSRHYTHMIAS

A. Vagal maneuvers
1. Description: Vagal maneuvers induce vagal stimulation of the cardiac conduction system and are used to terminate supraventricular tachydysrhythmias.
2. Carotid sinus massage
   a. The HCP instructs the client to turn the head away from the side to be massaged.
   b. The HCP massages over one carotid artery for a few seconds to determine if a change in cardiac rhythm occurs.
   c. The client should be on a cardiac monitor and an electrocardiogram rhythm strip before, during, and after the procedure should be obtained and documented on the chart.
   d. Have a defibrillator and resuscitative equipment available.
   e. Monitor vital signs, cardiac rhythm, and level of consciousness after the procedure.
3. Valsalva's maneuver
   a. The HCP instructs the client to bear down or induces a gag reflex in the client to stimulate a vagal response.

   b. Monitor the heart rate, rhythm, and **BP**.
   c. Observe the cardiac monitor for a change in rhythm.
   d. Record an electrocardiographic rhythm strip before, during, and after the procedure.
   e. Provide an emesis basin if the gag reflex is stimulated, and initiate precautions to prevent aspiration.
   f. Have a defibrillator and resuscitative equipment available.

B. Cardioversion
1. Description
   a. Cardioversion is synchronized countershock to convert an undesirable rhythm to a stable rhythm.
   b. Cardioversion can be an elective procedure performed by the HCP for stable tachydysrhythmias resistant to medical therapies or an emergent procedure for hemodynamically unstable ventricular or supraventricular tachydysrhythmias.
   c. A lower amount of energy is used than with defibrillation.
   d. Defibrillator is synchronized to the client's R wave to avoid discharging the shock during the vulnerable period (T wave).

e. If the defibrillator were not synchronized, it could discharge on the T wave and cause VF.

2. Preprocedure interventions
   a. Obtain an informed consent if it is an elective procedure.
   b. Administer sedation as prescribed.
   c. If it is an elective procedure, hold digoxin (Lanoxin) 48 hours preprocedure as prescribed to prevent postcardioversion ventricular irritability.
   d. If it is an elective procedure for atrial fibrillation or atrial flutter, the client should receive anticoagulant therapy for 4 to 6 weeks preprocedure.

3. During the procedure
   a. Ensure that the skin is clean and dry in the area where the electrode paddles will be placed.
   b. Stop the oxygen during the procedure to avoid the hazard of fire.
   c. Be sure that no one is touching the bed or the client when delivering the countershock.

4. Postprocedure interventions
   a. Priority data collection includes the ability of the client to maintain airway and breathing.
   b. Resume oxygen administration as prescribed.
   c. Monitor the vital signs.
   d. Monitor the level of consciousness.
   e. Monitor the cardiac rhythm.
   f. Monitor for indications of successful response such as conversion to sinus rhythm, strong peripheral pulses, an adequate **BP**, and adequate urine output.
   g. Check the skin on the chest for evidence of burns from the edges of the paddles.

C. Defibrillation
1. Defibrillation is an asynchronous countershock used to terminate pulseless VT or VF.
2. Monophasic defibrillators deliver energy in one direction; includes an initial shock at 360 joules followed by immediate cardiopulmonary resuscitation beginning with chest compressions.
3. Biphasic defibrillators deliver energy in two directions; the first and any successive shocks are delivered at 120 to 200 joules.

⚠ Before defibrillating a client be sure that the oxygen is shut off to avoid the hazard of fire and be sure that no one is touching the bed or the client.

D. Use of paddle electrodes
1. Apply conductive pads.
2. One paddle is placed at the third intercostal space to the right of the sternum; the other is placed at the fifth intercostal space on the left midaxillary line.
3. Apply firm pressure of at least 25 lb to each of the paddles.

4. Be sure that no one is touching the bed or the client when delivering the countershock.

E. Automatic external defibrillator
1. An automatic external defibrillator is used by laypersons and emergency medical technicians for prehospital cardiac arrest.
2. Place the client on a firm dry surface.
3. Stop CPR.
4. Ensure that no one is touching the client to avoid motion artifact during rhythm analysis.
5. Place the electrode patches in the correct position on the client's chest.
6. Press the analyzer button to identify the rhythm, which may take 30 seconds. The machine will advise whether a shock is necessary.
7. Shocks are recommended for pulseless VT or VF only.
8. If shock is recommended, the shock initially is delivered at an energy of 200 J.
9. If unsuccessful, the shock is repeated at 200 to 300 J.
10. The third and subsequent shock is 360 J.
11. If unsuccessful, CPR is continued for 1 minute, and then another series of three shocks is delivered, each at 360 J.

F. Implantable cardioverter defibrillator (ICD)
1. Description
   a. An ICD monitors cardiac rhythm and detects and terminates episodes of VT and VF.
   b. The ICD senses VT or VF and delivers 25 to 30 J up to four times if necessary.
   c. An ICD is used in clients with episodes of spontaneous sustained VT or VF unrelated to an MI or in clients whose medication therapy has been unsuccessful in controlling life-threatening dysrhythmias.
   d. Transvenous electrode leads are placed in the right atrium and ventricle in contact with the endocardium. Leads are used for sensing, pacing, and delivery of cardioversion or defibrillation.
   e. The generator is most commonly implanted in the left pectoral region.
2. Client education
   a. Instruct the client in the basic functions of the ICD.
   b. Teach the client how to perform cough CPR.
   c. Know the rate cutoff of the ICD and the number of consecutive shocks that it will deliver.
   d. Wear loose-fitting clothing over the ICD generator site.
   e. Avoid contact sports to prevent trauma to the ICD generator and lead wires.
   f. Report any fever, redness, swelling, or drainage from the insertion site.
   g. Report symptoms of fainting, nausea, weakness, blackouts, and rapid pulse rates to the HCP.

h. During shock discharge, the client may feel faint or short of breath.

i. Instruct the client to sit or lie down if he or she feels a shock and to notify the HCP.

j. Advise the client to maintain a log of the date, time, and activity preceding the shock, the symptoms preceding the shock, and post-shock sensations.

k. Instruct the client and family in how to access the emergency medical system.

l. Encourage the family to learn CPR.

m. Instruct the client to avoid electromagnetic fields directly over the ICD because they can inactivate the device.

n. Instruct the client to move away from a magnetic field immediately if beeping tones are heard, and notify the HCP.

o. Keep an ICD identification card in the wallet and obtain and wear a Medic-Alert bracelet.

p. Inform all HCPs that an ICD has been inserted. Certain diagnostic tests, such as an MRI, and procedures using diathermy or electrocautery interfere with ICD function.

q. Advise the client of restrictions on activities such as driving and operating dangerous equipment.

VI. PACEMAKERS

A. Description: a temporary or permanent device that provides electrical stimulation and maintains the heart rate when the client's intrinsic pacemaker fails to provide a perfusing rhythm

B. Settings

1. A synchronous (demand) pacemaker senses the client's rhythm and paces only if the client's intrinsic rate falls below the set pacemaker rate to stimulate depolarization.

2. An asynchronous (fixed rate) pacemaker paces at a preset rate regardless of the client's intrinsic rhythm and is used when the client is asystolic or profoundly bradycardic.

3. Overdrive pacing suppresses the underlying rhythm in tachydysrhythmias so that the sinus node will regain control of the heart.

C. Spikes

1. When a pacing stimulus is delivered to the heart, a spike (straight vertical line) is seen on the monitor or electrocardiogram strip.

2. Spikes precede the chamber being paced. A spike preceding a P wave indicates that the atrium is being paced, and a spike preceding the QRS indicates the ventricle is being paced.

3. An atrial spike followed by a P wave indicates atrial depolarization, and a ventricular spike followed by a QRS represents ventricular depolarization. This is referred to as "capture."

4. If the electrode is in the atrium, the spike is before the P wave; if the electrode is in the ventricle, the spike is before the QRS complex.

D. Temporary pacemakers

1. Noninvasive transcutaneous pacing

a. Noninvasive transcutaneous pacing is used as a temporary emergency measure in the profoundly bradycardic or asystolic client until invasive pacing can be initiated.

b. Large electrode pads are placed on the client's chest and back and connected to an external pulse generator.

c. Wash the skin with soap and water before applying electrodes.

d. It is not necessary to shave the hair or apply alcohol or tinctures to the skin.

e. Place the posterior electrode between the spine and left scapula, behind the heart, avoiding placement over bone.

f. Place the anterior electrode between the V_2 and V_5 positions over the heart.

g. Do not place the anterior electrode over female breast tissue; rather, displace breast tissue and place under the breast.

h. Do not take the pulse or **BP** on the left side. The results will not be accurate because of the muscle twitching and electrical current.

i. Ensure that electrodes are in good contact with the skin.

j. If loss of "capture" occurs, check the skin contact of the electrodes and increase the current until "capture" is regained.

k. Evaluate the client for discomfort from cutaneous and muscle stimulation. Administer analgesics as needed.

2. Invasive transvenous pacing

a. Pacing lead wire is placed through the antecubital, femoral, jugular, or subclavian vein into the right atrium or right ventricle so that it is in direct contact with the endocardium.

b. Monitor cardiac rhythm continuously.

c. Monitor vital signs.

d. Monitor the pacemaker insertion site.

e. Restrict client movement to prevent lead wire displacement.

3. Invasive epicardial pacing: Applied by using a transthoracic approach. The lead wires are threaded loosely on the epicardial surface of the heart after cardiac surgery.

4. Reducing the risk of microshock

a. Use only inspected and approved equipment.

b. Insulate the exposed portion of wires with plastic or rubber material (fingers of rubber gloves) when wires are not attached to the pulse generator, and cover with nonconductive tape.

c. Ground all electrical equipment using a three-pronged plug.

    d. Wear gloves when handling exposed wires.

    e. Keep dressings dry.

E. Permanent pacemakers

1. The pulse generator is internal and surgically implanted in a subcutaneous pocket below the clavicle.

2. The leads are passed transvenously via the cephalic or subclavian vein to the endocardium on the right side of the heart. Postoperatively, limitation of arm movement on the operative side is required to prevent lead wire dislodgement.

3. Permanent pacemakers may be single chambered, in which the lead wire is placed in the chamber to be paced, or dual chambered, with lead wires placed in both the right atrium and ventricle.

4. A permanent pacemaker is programmed when inserted and can be reprogrammed if necessary by noninvasive transmission from an external programmer to the implanted generator.

5. Pacemakers are powered by a lithium battery that has an average life span of 10 years, are nuclear powered with a life span of 20 years or longer, or are designed to be recharged externally.

6. Pacemaker function can be checked in the HCP's office or clinic by a pacemaker interrogator or programmer or from home using telephone transmitter devices.

7. The client may be provided with a device that is placed over the pacemaker battery generator with an attachment to the telephone. The heart rate then can be transmitted to the clinic.

8. Provide client teaching as per Box 51-4.

VII. CORONARY ARTERY DISEASE

A. Description

1. Coronary artery disease is a narrowing or obstruction of one or more coronary arteries as a result of atherosclerosis, an accumulation of lipid-containing plaque in the arteries (Figure 51-6).

2. The disease causes decreased perfusion of myocardial tissue and inadequate myocardial oxygen supply, leading to hypertension, angina, dysrhythmias, MI, heart failure, and death.

3. Collateral circulation, more than one artery supplying a muscle with blood, is normally present in the coronary arteries, especially in older persons.

4. The development of collateral circulation takes time and develops when chronic ischemia occurs to meet the metabolic demands. Therefore an occlusion of a coronary artery in a younger individual is more likely to be lethal than in an older individual.

5. Symptoms occur when the coronary artery is occluded to the point that inadequate blood supply to the muscle occurs, causing ischemia.

6. Coronary artery narrowing is significant if the lumen diameter of the left main artery is reduced at least 50%, or any major branch is reduced at least 75%.

7. The goal of treatment is to alter the atherosclerotic progression.

B. Data collection

1. Possibly normal findings during asymptomatic periods

2. Chest pain

3. Palpitations

4. Dyspnea

Box 51-4 Pacemakers: Client Education

Instruct the client about the pacemaker, including the programmed rate.

Instruct the client on the signs of battery failure and when to notify the HCP.

Instruct the client to report any fever, redness, swelling, or drainage from the insertion site.

Report signs of dizziness, weakness or fatigue, swelling of the ankles or legs, chest pain, or shortness of breath.

Keep a pacemaker identification card in the wallet and obtain and wear a Medic-Alert bracelet.

Instruct the client on how to take the pulse, to take the pulse daily, and to maintain a diary of pulse rates.

Wear loose-fitting clothing over the pulse generator site.

Avoid contact sports.

Inform all HCPs that a pacemaker has been inserted.

Instruct the client to inform airport security that he or she has a pacemaker because the pacemaker may set off the security detector.

Instruct the client that most electrical appliances can be used without any interference with the functioning of the pacemaker; however, advise the client not to operate electrical appliances directly over the pacemaker site.

Avoid transmitter towers and antitheft devices in stores.

Instruct the client that if any unusual feelings occur when near any electrical devices to move 5 to 10 feet away and check the pulse.

Instruct the client about the methods of monitoring the function of the device.

Emphasize the importance of follow-up with the HCP.

Use cell phones on the side opposite to the pacemaker.

5. Syncope
6. Cough or hemoptysis
7. Excessive fatigue
C. Diagnostic studies
    1. Electrocardiography
        a. When blood flow is reduced and ischemia occurs, ST segment depression, T wave inversion, or both are noted. The ST segment returns to normal when the blood flow returns.
        b. With infarction, cell injury results in ST segment elevation, followed by T wave inversion and an abnormal Q wave.
    2. Cardiac catheterization
        a. Cardiac catheterization provides the most definitive source for diagnosis.
        b. Cardiac catheterization shows the presence of atherosclerotic lesions.
    3. Blood lipid levels
        a. Blood lipid levels may be elevated.

    b. Cholesterol-lowering medications may be prescribed to reduce the development of atherosclerotic plaques.
D. Interventions
    1. Instruct the client regarding the purpose of diagnostic medical and surgical procedures and the preprocedure and postprocedure expectations.
    2. Assist the client to identify risk factors that can be modified.
    3. Assist the client to set goals to promote lifestyle changes that will reduce the impact of risk factors.
    4. Assist the client to identify barriers to compliance with the therapeutic plan and to identify methods to overcome barriers.
    5. Instruct the client regarding a low-calorie, low-sodium, low-cholesterol, and low-fat diet, with an increase in dietary fiber.

▲ **FIGURE 51-6** Cross section of an atherosclerotic coronary artery. (From Ignatavicius, D., & Workman, M. [2010]. *Medical-surgical nursing: Patient-centered collaborative care* [6th ed.]. St. Louis: Saunders.)

6. Stress to the client that dietary changes are not temporary and must be maintained for life. Teach the client about prescribed medications.
7. Provide community resources to the client regarding exercise, smoking reduction, and stress reduction as appropriate.

E. Surgical procedures
1. PTCA to compress the plaque against the walls of the artery and dilate the vessel.
2. Laser angioplasty to vaporize the plaque
3. Atherectomy to remove the plaque from the artery
4. Vascular stent to prevent the artery from closing and to prevent restenosis
5. Coronary artery bypass graft to improve blood flow to the myocardial tissue that is at risk for ischemia or infarction because of the occluded artery

F. Medications
1. Nitrates to dilate the coronary arteries and decrease preload and afterload
2. Calcium channel blockers to dilate coronary arteries and reduce vasospasm
3. Cholesterol-lowering medications to reduce the development of atherosclerotic plaques
4. β-blockers to reduce the **BP** in individuals who are hypertensive

VIII. ANGINA

A. Description
1. Angina is chest pain resulting from myocardial ischemia caused by inadequate myocardial blood and oxygen supply.
2. Angina is caused by an imbalance between oxygen supply and demand.
3. Causes include obstruction of coronary blood flow because of atherosclerosis, coronary artery spasm, and conditions increasing myocardial oxygen consumption.

⚠ The goal of treatment for angina is to provide relief of the acute attack, correct the imbalance between myocardial oxygen supply and demand, and prevent the progression of the disease and further attacks to reduce the risk of MI.

B. Patterns of angina
1. Stable angina
   a. Also called exertional angina
   b. Occurs with activities that involve exertion or emotional stress and is relieved with rest or nitroglycerin
   c. Usually has a stable pattern of onset, duration, severity, and relieving factors
2. Unstable angina
   a. Also called preinfarction angina

b. Occurs with an unpredictable degree of exertion or emotion and increases in occurrence, duration, and severity over time
   c. Pain may not be relieved with nitroglycerin
3. Variant angina
   a. Also called Prinzmetal's or vasospastic angina
   b. Results from coronary artery spasm
   c. May occur at rest
   d. Attacks may be associated with ST segment elevation noted on the electrocardiogram.
4. Intractable angina is a chronic, incapacitating angina that is unresponsive to interventions.
5. Preinfarction angina: Is associated with acute coronary insufficiency and is characterized by chest pain that occurs days to weeks before an MI.

C. Data collection
1. Pain (Table 51-1)
2. Dyspnea
3. Pallor
4. Sweating
5. Palpitations and tachycardia
6. Dizziness and faintness
7. Hypertension
8. Digestive disturbances

D. Diagnostic studies
1. Electrocardiography: Readings are normal during rest, with ST depression and/or T wave inversion during an episode of pain.
2. Stress test: Chest pain or changes in the electrocardiogram or vital signs during testing may indicate ischemia.
3. Cardiac enzymes and troponins: Findings are normal in angina.
4. Cardiac catheterization: Catheterization provides a definitive diagnosis by providing information about the patency of the coronary arteries.

E. Interventions
1. Immediate management
   a. Monitor pain.
   b. Provide bedrest.

TABLE 51-1 Characteristics of Pain: Angina and Myocardial Infarction

Angina	Myocardial Infarction
Can develop slowly or quickly	Occurs without cause, primarily early in the morning
Usually described as mild or moderate pain	
Substernal, crushing, squeezing pain	Crushing substernal pain
	May radiate to the jaw, back, and left arm
May radiate to the shoulders, arms, jaw, neck, and back	Lasts 30 minutes or longer
Usually lasts less than 5 minutes; however, can last up to 15-20 minutes	Is unrelieved by rest or nitroglycerin, and relieved only by opioids
Relieved by nitroglycerin or rest	

c. Administer oxygen at 3 L/min by nasal cannula as prescribed.

d. Administer nitroglycerin as prescribed to dilate the coronary arteries, reduce the oxygen requirements of the myocardium, and relieve the chest pain.

e. Obtain a 12-lead electrocardiogram.

f. Provide continuous cardiac monitoring.

2. After the acute episode

a. Instruct the client regarding the purpose of diagnostic medical and surgical procedures and the preprocedure and postprocedure expectations.

b. Assist the client to identify angina-precipitating events.

c. Instruct the client to stop activity and rest if chest pain occurs and to take nitroglycerin as prescribed.

d. Instruct the client to seek medical attention if pain persists.

e. Instruct the client regarding prescribed medications.

f. Provide diet instructions to the client, stressing that dietary changes are not temporary and must be maintained for life.

g. Assist the client to identify risk factors that can be modified.

h. Assist the client to set goals that will promote changes in lifestyle to reduce the impact of risk factors.

i. Assist the client to identify barriers to compliance with therapeutic plan and to identify methods to overcome barriers.

j. Provide community resources to the client regarding exercise, smoking reduction, and stress reduction.

F. Surgical procedures: Refer to the "Coronary Artery Disease" section.

G. Medications

1. Refer to the "Coronary Artery Disease" section.

2. Antiplatelet therapy may be prescribed that inhibits platelet aggregation and reduces the risk of developing an acute MI.

IX. MYOCARDIAL INFARCTION

A. Description

1. Myocardial infarction occurs when myocardial tissue is abruptly and severely deprived of oxygen.

2. Ischemia can lead to necrosis of myocardial tissue if blood flow is not restored.

3. Infarction does not occur instantly but evolves over several hours.

4. Obvious physical changes do not occur in the heart until 6 hours after the infarction, when the infarcted area appears blue and swollen.

5. After 48 hours the infarct turns gray with yellow streaks as neutrophils invade the tissue.

6. By 8 to 10 days after infarction, granulation tissue forms.

7. Over 2 to 3 months, the necrotic area develops into a scar. Scar tissue permanently changes the size and shape of the entire left ventricle.

8. Not all clients experience the classic symptoms of an MI.

9. Women may experience atypical discomfort, shortness of breath, or fatigue.

10. An older client may experience shortness of breath, pulmonary edema, dizziness, altered mental status, or dysrhythmia.

B. Location of MI

1. Obstruction of the left anterior descending artery results in anterior or septal MI or both.

2. Obstruction of the circumflex artery results in posterior wall MI or lateral wall MI.

3. Obstruction of the right coronary artery results in inferior wall MI.

C. Risk factors

1. Atherosclerosis

2. Coronary artery disease

3. Elevated cholesterol levels

4. Smoking

5. Hypertension

6. Obesity

7. Physical inactivity

8. Impaired glucose tolerance

9. Stress

D. Diagnostic studies

1. Troponin level

a. Level rises within 3 hours

b. Level remains elevated for up to 7 days

2. Total creatine kinase level

a. Level rises within 4 hours after the onset of chest pain.

b. Level peaks within 24 hours after damage and death of cardiac tissue.

3. CK-MB isoenzyme

a. Peak elevation occurs 18 to 24 hours after the onset of chest pain.

b. Level returns to normal 48 to 72 hours later.

4. Myoglobin: Level rises within 1 hour after cell death, peaks in 4 to 6 hours, and returns to normal within 24 to 36 hours or less.

5. LDH level

a. Level rises 24 hours after MI.

b. Level peaks between 48 and 72 hours and falls to normal in 7 days.

c. Serum level of LDH_1 isoenzyme rises higher than serum level of LDH_2.

6. White blood cell count: An elevated white blood cell count of 10,000 to 20,000 cells/mm^3 appears on the second day after the MI and lasts up to a week.

7. Electrocardiogram
   a. Electrocardiogram shows either ST elevation MI (STEMI), T wave inversion, or non-ST elevation MI (NSTEMI); an abnormal Q wave may also be present.
   b. Hours to days after the MI, ST and T wave changes will return to normal but the Q wave usually remains permanently.
8. Diagnostic tests after the acute stage
   a. Exercise tolerance test or stress test may be prescribed to assess for electrocardiographic changes and ischemia and to evaluate for medical therapy or identify clients who may need invasive therapy.
   b. Thallium scans may be prescribed to assess for ischemia or necrotic muscle tissue.
   c. Multigated cardiac blood pool imaging scans may be used to evaluate left ventricular function.
   d. Cardiac catheterization is performed to determine the extent and location of obstructions of the coronary arteries.
E. Data collection
   1. Pain (see Table 51-1)
   2. Nausea and vomiting
   3. Diaphoresis
   4. Dyspnea
   5. Dysrhythmias
   6. Feelings of fear and anxiety
   7. Pallor, cyanosis, and coolness of extremities
F. Complications of MI (Box 51-5)
G. Interventions, acute stage

> ⚠ Pain relief increases oxygen supply to the myocardium. Morphine sulfate is administered as a priority in managing pain in the client having an MI.

   1. Obtain a description of the chest discomfort.
   2. Institute pain relief measures (morphine, nitroglycerin as prescribed).

Box 51-5 Complications of Myocardial Infarction

Dysrhythmias
Heart failure
Pulmonary edema
Cardiogenic shock
Thrombophlebitis
Pericarditis
Mitral valve insufficiency
Postinfarction angina
Ventricular rupture
Dressler's syndrome (a combination of pericarditis, pericardial effusion, and pleural effusion, which can occur several weeks to several months after a myocardial infarction)

---

3. Administer oxygen by nasal cannula as prescribed.
4. Monitor vital signs and cardiovascular status and maintain cardiac monitoring.
5. Ensure bedrest and place the client in a semi-Fowler's position to enhance comfort and tissue oxygenation.
6. Assist to establish an IV access route.
7. Obtain a 12-lead ECG.
8. Assist to administer antidysrhythmics as prescribed.
9. Assist to administer thrombolytic therapy, which may be prescribed within the first 6 hours of the coronary event.
10. Monitor for signs of bleeding if the client is receiving thrombolytic therapy.
11. Monitor laboratory values as prescribed.
12. Administer β-blockers as prescribed to slow the heart rate and increase myocardial perfusion while reducing the force of myocardial contraction.
13. Monitor for complications related to the MI.
14. Monitor for cardiac dysrhythmias because tachycardia and PVCs frequently occur in the first few hours after MI.
15. Monitor distal peripheral pulses and skin temperature because poor **cardiac output** may be identified by cool diaphoretic skin and diminished or absent pulses.
16. Monitor intake and output.
17. Monitor respiratory rate and breath sounds for signs of heart failure, as indicated by the presence of crackles or wheezes or dependent edema.
18. Monitor the **BP** closely after the administration of medications. If the **BP** is less than 100 systolic or 25 mm Hg lower than the previous reading, lower the head of the bed and notify the HCP.
19. Provide reassurance to the client and family.
H. Interventions after the acute episode
   1. Maintain bedrest for the first 24 to 36 hours as prescribed.
   2. Allow the client to stand to void or use a bedside commode if prescribed.
   3. Provide range-of-motion exercises to prevent thrombus formation and maintain muscle strength.
   4. Progress to dangling legs at the side of the bed or out of bed to the chair for 30 minutes three times a day as prescribed.
   5. Progress to ambulation in the client's room and to the bathroom and then in the hallway three times a day.
   6. Monitor for complications.
   7. Encourage the client to verbalize feelings regarding the MI.

I. Cardiac rehabilitation: Process of actively assisting the client with cardiac disease to achieve and maintain a vital and productive life within the limitations of the heart disease

 X. HEART FAILURE

A. Description
1. Heart failure is the inability of the heart to maintain adequate **cardiac output** to meet the metabolic needs of the body owing to impaired pumping ability.
2. Diminished **cardiac output** results in inadequate peripheral tissue perfusion.
3. Congestion of the lungs and periphery may occur. The client can develop acute pulmonary edema.

B. Classification
1. Acute heart failure occurs suddenly.
2. Chronic heart failure develops over time; however, a client with chronic heart failure can develop an acute episode.

C. Types of heart failure
1. Right ventricular failure/left ventricular failure
   a. Because the two ventricles of the heart represent two separate pumping systems, it is possible for one to fail alone for a short period.
   b. Most heart failure begins with left ventricular failure and progresses to failure of both ventricles.
   c. Acute pulmonary edema—a medical emergency—results from left ventricular failure.
   d. If pulmonary edema is not treated, death will occur from suffocation because the client literally drowns in his or her own fluids.
2. Forward failure/backward failure
   a. In forward failure, an inadequate output of the affected ventricle causes decreased perfusion to vital organs.
   b. In backward failure, blood backs up behind the affected ventricle, causing increased pressure in the atrium behind the affected ventricle.
3. Low output/high output
   a. In low-output failure, not enough **cardiac output** is available to meet the demands of the body.
   b. High-output failure occurs when a condition causes the heart to work harder to meet the demands of the body.
4. Systolic failure/diastolic failure
   a. Systolic failure leads to problems with contraction and the ejection of blood.
   b. Diastolic failure leads to problems with the heart relaxing and filling with blood.

D. Compensatory mechanisms
1. Compensatory mechanisms act to restore **cardiac output** to near-normal levels.

2. Initially these mechanisms increase **cardiac output**; however, they eventually have a damaging effect on pump action.
3. Compensatory mechanisms contribute to an increase in myocardial oxygen consumption; when this occurs, myocardial reserve is exhausted and clinical manifestations of heart failure develop.
4. Compensatory mechanisms include increased heart rate, improved **stroke volume**, arterial vasoconstriction, sodium and water retention, and myocardial hypertrophy.

⚠ Signs of left ventricular failure are evident in the pulmonary system. Signs of right ventricular failure are evident in the systemic circulation.

E. Data collection
1. Right ventricular failure: Signs of right ventricular failure are evident in the systemic circulation (Table 51-2).
2. Left ventricular failure: Signs of left ventricular failure are evident in the pulmonary system (see Table 51-2).
3. Acute pulmonary edema
   a. Severe dyspnea and orthopnea
   b. Pallor
   c. Tachycardia
   d. Expectoration of large amounts of blood-tinged, frothy sputum
   e. Wheezing and crackles on auscultation
   f. Bubbling respirations
   g. Acute anxiety, apprehension, and restlessness
   h. Profuse sweating
   i. Cold, clammy skin
   j. Cyanosis
   k. Nasal flaring
   l. Use of accessory breathing muscles

TABLE 51-2 Clinical Manifestations of Right-Sided and Left-Sided Heart Failure

Right-Sided Heart Failure	Left-Sided Heart Failure
Dependent edema (legs and sacrum)	Signs of pulmonary congestion
	Dyspnea
Jugular venous distention	Tachypnea
Abdominal distention	Crackles in the lungs
Hepatomegaly	Dry, hacking cough
Splenomegaly	Paroxysmal nocturnal dyspnea
Anorexia and nausea	Increased BP (from fluid volume excess) or decreased BP (from pump failure)
Weight gain	
Nocturnal diuresis	
Swelling of the fingers and hands	
Increased BP (from fluid volume excess) or decreased BP (from pump failure)	

m. Tachypnea
  n. Hypocapnia, evidenced by muscle cramps, weakness, dizziness, and paresthesias
F. Immediate management (see Priority Nursing Actions)

■■■ PRIORITY NURSING ACTIONS! ■■■

Actions to Take if a Client Develops Pulmonary Edema

1. Place the client in a high Fowler's position.
2. Administer oxygen.
3. Check the client quickly, including checking lung sounds.
4. Ensure an intravenous access device is in place.
5. Prepare for the administration of a diuretic and morphine sulfate.
6. Insert a Foley catheter as prescribed.
7. Prepare for intubation and ventilator support, if required.
8. Document the event, actions taken, and the client's response.

Pulmonary edema is a life-threatening event that can result from severe heart failure. In pulmonary edema, the left ventricle fails to eject sufficient blood, and pressure increases in the lungs because of the accumulated blood. The client is immediately placed in a high Fowler's position, with the legs in a dependent position, to reduce pulmonary congestion and relieve edema. Oxygen is always prescribed, usually in high concentrations by mask or cannula to improve gas exchange and pulmonary function; the goal is to keep the oxygen saturation above 90%. The client is then checked quickly, including checking the lung sounds. Next it is important to ensure that an IV access device is in place for the administration of a diuretic and morphine sulfate. Furosemide, a rapid-acting diuretic, will eliminate accumulated fluid. Morphine sulfate reduces venous return (preload), decreases anxiety, and also reduces the work of breathing. A Foley catheter is inserted to measure output accurately. The nurse then prepares for intubation and ventilator support, if required. The nurse stays with the client and provides reassurance. Vital signs are monitored and a cardiac monitor is used to monitor the heart rate and for dysrhythmias. The lung sounds are monitored for crackles, decreased breath sounds, and for a response to treatment. A weight measurement will also determine a response to treatment. Other interventions may include the administration of digoxin to increase ventricular contractility and improve cardiac output, bronchodilators for severe bronchospasm or bronchoconstriction, medications to facilitate myocardial contractility and enhance stroke volume, and vasodilators to reduce afterload, increase the capacity of the systemic venous bed, and decrease venous return to the heart. The nurse finally documents the event, actions taken, and the client's response.

Reference: Ignatavicius, D., & Workman, M. (2010). *Medical-surgical nursing: Patient-centered collaborative care* (6th ed., p. 775). St. Louis: Saunders.

G. After the acute episode
  1. Encourage the client to verbalize feelings about the lifestyle changes required as a result of the heart failure.
  2. Assist the client to identify precipitating risk factors of heart failure and methods of eliminating these risk factors.
  3. Instruct the client in the prescribed medication regimen, which may include digoxin (Lanoxin), a diuretic, angiotensin-converting enzyme (ACE) inhibitors, low-dose β-blockers, and vasodilators.
  4. Advise the client to notify the HCP if side effects occur from the medications.
  5. Advise the client to avoid over-the-counter medications.
  6. Instruct the client to contact the HCP if he or she is unable to take medications because of illness.
  7. Instruct the client to avoid large amounts of caffeine, found in coffee, tea, cocoa, chocolate, and some carbonated beverages.
  8. Instruct the client about the prescribed low-sodium, low-fat, and low-cholesterol diet.
  9. Provide the client with a list of potassium-rich foods because diuretics can cause hypokalemia (except for potassium-sparing diuretics).
  10. Instruct the client regarding fluid restriction, if prescribed, advising the client to spread the fluid out during the day and to suck on hard candy to reduce thirst.
  11. Instruct the client to balance periods of activity and rest.
  12. Advise the client to avoid isometric activities, which increase pressure in the heart.
  13. Instruct the client to monitor daily weight.
  14. Instruct the client to report signs of fluid retention such as edema or weight gain.

XI. CARDIOGENIC SHOCK (Box 51-6)

XII. INFLAMMATORY DISEASES OF THE HEART

A. Pericarditis
  1. Description
      a. Pericarditis is an acute or chronic inflammation of the pericardium.

Box 51-6 Cardiogenic Shock

Failure of the heart to pump adequately, thereby reducing cardiac output and compromising tissue perfusion

Necrosis of more than 40% of the left ventricle, usually as a result of occlusion of major coronary vessels

Goal of treatment: to maintain tissue oxygenation and perfusion and improve the pumping ability of the heart

    b. Chronic pericarditis, a chronic inflammatory thickening of the pericardium, constricts the heart, causing compression.

    c. The pericardial sac becomes inflamed.

    d. Pericarditis can result in loss of pericardial elasticity or an accumulation of fluid within the sac.

    e. Heart failure or cardiac tamponade may result.

  2. Data collection

    a. Precordial pain in the anterior chest that radiates to the left side of the neck, shoulder, or back.

    b. Pain is grating and is aggravated by breathing (particularly inspiration), coughing, and swallowing.

    c. Pain is worse when in the supine position and may be relieved by leaning forward.

    d. Pericardial friction rub (scratchy, high-pitched sound) heard on auscultation and produced by the rubbing of the inflamed pericardial layers

    e. Fever and chills

    f. Fatigue and malaise

    g. Elevated white blood cell count

    h. Electrocardiogram changes with acute pericarditis; ST segment elevation with the onset of inflammation; atrial fibrillation is common

    i. Signs of right ventricular failure in clients with chronic constrictive pericarditis

  3. Interventions

    a. Monitor the nature of the pain.

    b. Position the client in the high Fowler's position, or upright and leaning forward.

    c. Administer analgesics, nonsteroidal anti-inflammatory drugs, or corticosteroids for pain as prescribed.

    d. Auscultate for a pericardial friction rub.

    e. Check results of blood culture to identify causative organism.

    f. Administer antibiotics for bacterial infection as prescribed.

    g. Administer diuretics and digoxin (Lanoxin) as prescribed to the client with chronic constrictive pericarditis. Surgical incision of the pericardium (pericardiectomy) may be necessary.

    h. Monitor for signs of cardiac tamponade, which include pulsus paradoxus, jugular vein distention with clear lung sounds, muffled heart sounds, narrowed **pulse pressure**, tachycardia, and decreased **cardiac output**.

    i. Notify the HCP if signs of cardiac tamponade occur.

B. Myocarditis

  1. Description: an acute or chronic inflammation of the myocardium as a result of pericarditis, systemic infection, or allergic response

  2. Data collection

    a. Fever

    b. Pericardial friction rub

    c. A gallop rhythm

    d. A murmur that sounds like fluid passing an obstruction

    e. Pulsus alternans

    f. Signs of heart failure

    g. Fatigue

    h. Dyspnea

    i. Tachycardia

    j. Chest pain

  3. Interventions

    a. Assist the client to a position of comfort such as sitting up and leaning forward.

    b. Administer analgesics, salicylates, and nonsteroidal anti-inflammatory drugs as prescribed to reduce fever and pain.

    c. Administer oxygen as prescribed.

    d. Provide adequate rest periods.

    e. Limit activities to avoid overexertion and to decrease the workload of the heart.

    f. Administer digoxin (Lanoxin) as prescribed, and monitor for signs of digoxin toxicity.

    g. Administer antidysrhythmics as prescribed.

    h. Administer antibiotics as prescribed to treat the causative organism.

    i. Monitor for complications, which can include thrombus, heart failure, or cardiomyopathy.

C. Endocarditis

  1. Description

    a. Endocarditis is an inflammation of the inner lining of the heart and valves.

    b. Occurs primarily in clients who are IV drug abusers, have had valve replacements, or have mitral valve prolapse or other structural defects.

    c. Ports of entry for the infecting organism include the oral cavity (especially if the client had a dental procedure in the previous 3 to 6 months), cutaneous invasion, infections, or invasive procedures or surgery.

  2. Data collection

    a. Fever

    b. Anorexia

    c. Weight loss

    d. Fatigue

    e. Cardiac murmurs

    f. Heart failure

    g. Embolic complications from vegetation fragments traveling through the circulation

    h. Petechiae

    i. Splinter hemorrhages in the nail beds

    j. Osler's nodes (reddish tender lesions) on the pads of the fingers, hands, and toes

    k. Janeway lesions (nontender hemorrhagic lesions) on the fingers, toes, nose, or ear lobes

l. Splenomegaly

m. Clubbing of the fingers

3. Interventions

a. Provide adequate rest balanced with activity to prevent thrombus formation.

b. Maintain antiembolism stockings.

c. Monitor cardiovascular status.

d. Monitor for signs of heart failure.

e. Monitor for signs of emboli.

f. Monitor for splenic emboli, as evidenced by sudden abdominal pain radiating to the left shoulder, and the presence of rebound abdominal tenderness on palpation.

g. Monitor for renal emboli, as evidenced by flank pain radiating to the groin, hematuria, and pyuria.

h. Monitor for confusion, aphasia, or dysphasia, which may indicate central nervous system emboli.

i. Monitor for pulmonary emboli as evidenced by pleuritic chest pain, dyspnea, and cough.

j. Monitor skin, mucous membranes, and conjunctiva for petechiae.

k. Monitor nail beds for splinter hemorrhages.

l. Monitor for Osler's nodes on the pads of the fingers, hands, and toes.

m. Monitor for Janeway lesions on the fingers, toes, nose, or ear lobes.

n. Monitor for clubbing of the fingers.

o. Evaluate blood culture results.

p. Administer antibiotics intravenously as prescribed.

q. Plan and arrange for discharge, providing resources required for the continued administration of antibiotics intravenously.

4. Client education (Box 51-7)

XIII. CARDIAC TAMPONADE (Box 51-8)

⚠ Acute cardiac tamponade can occur when small volumes (20 to 50 mL) of fluid accumulate rapidly in the pericardium.

XIV. VALVULAR HEART DISEASE

A. Description

1. Valvular heart disease occurs when the heart valves cannot fully open (stenosis) or close completely (insufficiency or regurgitation).

2. Valvular heart disease prevents efficient blood flow through the heart.

B. Types

1. Mitral stenosis: Valvular tissue thickens and narrows the valve opening, preventing blood flow from the left atrium to left ventricle.

Box 51-7 Home Care Instructions for the Client with Infective Endocarditis

Teach the client to maintain aseptic technique during set-up and administration of IV antibiotics.

Instruct the client to administer IV antibiotics at scheduled times to maintain the blood level.

Instruct the client to monitor IV catheter sites for signs of infection and report immediately to the HCP.

Instruct the client to record his or her temperature daily for up to 6 weeks and report fever.

Encourage oral hygiene at least twice a day with a soft toothbrush and rinse well with water after brushing.

Client should avoid use of oral irrigation devices and flossing to avoid bacteremia.

Teach the client to thoroughly cleanse any skin lacerations thoroughly and apply an antibiotic ointment as prescribed.

Client should inform all HCPs of a history of endocarditis and request prophylactic antibiotics prior to every invasive procedure, including dental procedures.

Teach the client to observe for signs and symptoms of embolic phenomena and heart failure.

Box 51-8 Cardiac Tamponade

A pericardial effusion occurs when the space between the parietal and visceral layers of the pericardium fills with fluid.

Pericardial effusion places the client at risk for cardiac tamponade, an accumulation of fluid in the pericardial cavity.

Tamponade restricts ventricular filling, and cardiac output drops. Distant, muffled heart sounds are heard.

Acute tamponade occurs when a small volume (20 to 50 mL) of fluid accumulates quickly in the pericardium.

---

2. Mitral insufficiency/regurgitation: The valve is incompetent, preventing complete valve closure during **systole**.

3. Mitral valve prolapse: Valve leaflets protrude into the left atrium during **systole**.

4. Aortic stenosis: Valvular tissue thickens and narrows the valve opening, preventing blood flow from the left ventricle into the aorta.

5. Aortic insufficiency: Valve is incompetent, preventing complete valve closure during **diastole**.

C. Repair procedures

1. Balloon valvuloplasty

a. Balloon valvuloplasty is an invasive, nonsurgical procedure.

b. A balloon catheter is passed from the femoral vein through the atrial septum to the mitral valve or through the femoral artery to the aortic valve.

c. The balloon is inflated to enlarge the orifice.

d. Institute precautions for arterial puncture if appropriate.

e. Monitor for bleeding from the catheter insertion site.

f. Monitor for signs of systemic emboli.

g. Monitor for signs of a regurgitant valve by monitoring cardiac rhythm, heart sounds, and **cardiac output**.

2. Mitral annuloplasty: tightening and suturing the malfunctioning valve annulus to eliminate or greatly reduce regurgitation

3. Commissurotomy/valvotomy
   a. The procedure is accomplished with cardiopulmonary bypass during open heart surgery.
   b. The valve is visualized, thrombi are removed from the atria, fused leaflets are incised, and calcium is débrided from the leaflets, thus widening the orifice.

D. Valve replacement procedures
   1. Mechanical prosthetic valves: These prosthetic valves are durable.

⚠ Thromboembolism is a problem after valve replacement with a mechanical prosthetic valve, and lifetime anticoagulant therapy is required.

   2. Bioprosthetic valves
      a. Biological grafts are xenografts (valves from other species): porcine valves (pig), bovine valves (cow), or homografts (human cadavers).
      b. The risk of clot formation is small; therefore long-term anticoagulation is not indicated.
   3. Preoperative interventions: Consult with the HCP regarding discontinuing anticoagulants 72 hours before surgery.
   4. Postoperative interventions
      a. Monitor closely for signs of bleeding.
      b. Monitor **cardiac output** and for signs of heart failure.
      c. Administer digoxin (Lanoxin) as prescribed to maintain **cardiac output** and prevent atrial fibrillation.
      d. Provide client teaching (Box 51-9).

XV. CARDIOMYOPATHY

A. Cardiomyopathy is a subacute or chronic disorder of the heart muscle.

B. Treatment is palliative, not curative, and the client needs to deal with numerous lifestyle changes and a shortened life span.

C. Types, signs and symptoms, and treatment: Refer to Table 51-3.

Box 51-9 Client Instructions After Valve Replacement

Adequate rest is important, and fatigue is common.

Anticoagulant therapy is necessary if a mechanical prosthetic valve was inserted.

Instruct the client concerning hazards related to anticoagulant therapy and to notify the HCP if bleeding or excessive bruising occurs.

Instruct the client concerning the importance of good oral hygiene to reduce the risk of infective endocarditis.

Brush teeth twice daily with a soft toothbrush, followed by oral rinses.

Avoid irrigation devices, electric toothbrushes, and flossing because these activities can cause the gums to bleed, allowing bacteria to enter the mucous membranes and bloodstream.

Monitor incision and report any drainage or redness.

Avoid any dental procedures for 6 months.

Heavy lifting (greater than 10 lb) is to be avoided, and be cautious when in an automobile to prevent injury to the sternal incision.

If a prosthetic valve was inserted, a soft audible clicking sound may be heard.

Instruct the client concerning the importance of prophylactic antibiotics before any invasive procedure and the importance of informing all HCPs of the valvular disease history.

Obtain and wear a Medic-Alert bracelet.

XVI. VASCULAR DISORDERS

A. Venous thrombosis
   1. Description
      a. Thrombus can be associated with an inflammatory process.
      b. When a thrombus develops, inflammation occurs, thickening the vein wall and leading to embolization.
   2. Types
      a. Thrombophlebitis: A thrombus associated with inflammation
      b. Phlebothrombosis: A thrombus without inflammation
      c. Phlebitis: Vein inflammation associated with invasive procedures such as IV lines
      d. Deep vein thrombophlebitis: More serious than a superficial thrombophlebitis because of the risk for pulmonary embolism
   3. Risk factors for thrombus formation
      a. Venous stasis from varicose veins, heart failure, and immobility
      b. Hypercoagulability disorders
      c. Injury to the venous wall from IV injections; administration of vessel irritants (chemotherapy, hypertonic solutions)
      d. After surgery, particularly orthopedic and abdominal surgery

TABLE 51-3 Pathophysiology, Signs and Symptoms, and Treatment of Cardiomyopathies

| Dilated Cardiomyopathy | Hypertrophic Cardiomyopathy | | Restrictive Cardiomyopathy |
	Nonobstructed	Obstructed	
PATHOPHYSIOLOGY			
Fibrosis of myocardium and endocardium Dilated chambers Mural wall thrombi prevalent	Hypertrophy of the walls Hypertrophied septum Relatively small chamber size	Same as for nonobstructed except for obstruction of left ventricular outflow tract associated with the hypertrophied septum and mitral valve incompetence	Mimics constrictive pericarditis Fibrosed walls cannot expand or contract Chambers narrowed; emboli common
SIGNS AND SYMPTOMS			
Fatigue and weakness Heart failure (left side) Dysrhythmias or heart block Systemic or pulmonary emboli S_3 and S_4 gallops Moderate to severe cardiomegaly	Dyspnea Angina Fatigue, syncope, palpitations Mild cardiomegaly S_4 gallop Ventricular dysrhythmias Sudden death common Heart failure	Same as for nonobstructed except with mitral regurgitation murmur Atrial fibrillation	Dyspnea and fatigue Heart failure (right sided) Mild to moderate cardiomegaly S_3 and S_4 gallops Heart block Emboli
TREATMENT			
Symptomatic treatment of heart failure Vasodilators Control of dysrhythmias Surgery: heart transplant	For both: Symptomatic treatment β-Blockers Conversion of atrial fibrillation Surgery: ventriculomyotomy or muscle resection with mitral valve replacement Digoxin, nitrates, and other vasodilators contraindicated with the obstructed form		Supportive treatment of symptoms Treatment of hypertension Conversion from dysrhythmias Exercise restrictions Emergency treatment of acute pulmonary edema

From Ignatavicius, D., & Workman, M. (2010). *Medical-surgical nursing: Patient-centered collaborative care* (6th ed.). St. Louis: Saunders.

e. Pregnancy

f. Ulcerative colitis

g. Use of oral contraceptives

h. Certain malignancies

i. Fractures or other injuries of the pelvis or lower extremities

B. Phlebitis

1. Data collection

a. Red, warm area radiating up the vein of an extremity

b. Pain and soreness

c. Swelling

2. Interventions

a. Apply warm moist soaks as prescribed to dilate the vein and promote circulation (check temperature of soak before applying).

b. Monitor for signs of complications such as tissue necrosis, infection, or pulmonary embolus.

C. Deep vein thrombophlebitis

1. Data collection

a. Calf or groin tenderness or pain with or without swelling

b. Positive Homans' sign may be noted; however, false-positive results are common.

c. Warm skin that is tender to touch

2. Interventions

a. Provide bedrest as prescribed.

b. Elevate the affected extremity above the level of the heart as prescribed.

c. Avoid using the knee gatch or a pillow under the knees.

d. Do not massage the extremity.

e. Provide thigh-high or knee-high antiembolism stockings as prescribed to reduce venous stasis and to assist in the venous return of blood to the heart.

f. Administer intermittent or continuous warm, moist compresses as prescribed.

g. Palpate the site gently, monitoring for warmth and edema.

h. Measure and record the circumferences of the thighs and calves.

i. Monitor for shortness of breath and chest pain, which can indicate pulmonary emboli.

j. Administer thrombolytic therapy (tissue plasminogen activator) if prescribed, which must be initiated within 5 days after the onset of symptoms.

k. Administer heparin therapy as prescribed to prevent enlargement of the existing clot and prevent the formation of new clots.

l. Monitor activated partial thromboplastin time during heparin therapy.

m. Administer warfarin (Coumadin) as prescribed after heparin therapy when the symptoms of deep vein thrombophlebitis have resolved.

n. Monitor prothrombin time and international normalized ratio during warfarin (Coumadin) therapy.

o. Monitor for the hazards and side effects associated with anticoagulant therapy.

p. Administer analgesics as prescribed to reduce pain.

q. Administer diuretics as prescribed to reduce lower extremity edema.

r. Provide client teaching (Box 51-10).

D. Venous insufficiency

1. Description

a. Venous insufficiency results from prolonged venous hypertension, which stretches the veins and damages the valves.

b. The resultant edema and venous stasis cause venous stasis ulcers, swelling, and cellulitis.

c. Treatment focuses on decreasing edema and promoting venous return from the affected extremity.

d. Treatment for venous stasis ulcers focuses on healing the ulcer and preventing stasis and ulcer recurrence.

2. Data collection

a. Stasis dermatitis or brown discoloration along the ankles and extending up to the calf

b. Edema

c. Ulcer formation: Edges are uneven, ulcer bed is pink, and granulation is present.

3. Interventions

 For venous insufficiency, leg elevation is usually prescribed to assist with the return of the blood to the heart.

Box 51-10 Instructions for the Client with Deep Vein Thrombophlebitis

Instruct the client concerning the hazards of anticoagulation therapy.

Recognize the signs and symptoms of bleeding.

Avoid prolonged sitting or standing, constrictive clothing, or crossing legs when seated.

Elevate the legs for 10 to 20 minutes every few hours each day.

Plan a progressive walking program.

Inspect the legs for edema, and measure the circumference of the legs.

Wear antiembolism stockings as prescribed.

Avoid smoking.

Avoid any medications unless prescribed by the HCP.

Instruct the client concerning the importance of follow-up HCP visits and laboratory studies.

Obtain and wear a Medic-Alert bracelet.

---

a. Instruct the client to wear elastic or compression stockings during the day and evening as prescribed. (Instruct the client to put on elastic stockings upon awakening before getting out of bed.)

b. Advise the client to put on a clean pair of elastic stockings each day and that it will probably be necessary to wear the stockings for the rest of his or her life.

c. Instruct the client to avoid prolonged sitting or standing, constrictive clothing, or crossing legs when seated.

d. Instruct the client to elevate the legs for 10 to 20 minutes every few hours each day.

e. Instruct the client to elevate legs above the level of the heart when in bed.

f. Instruct the client in the use of an intermittent sequential pneumatic compression system, if prescribed. Instruct the client to apply the compression system twice daily for 1 hour in the morning and evening.

g. Advise the client with an open ulcer that the compression system is applied over a dressing.

4. Wound care

a. Provide care to the wound as prescribed by the HCP.

b. Monitor the client's ability to care for the wound, and initiate home care resources as necessary.

c. If an Unna boot (a dressing constructed of gauze moistened with zinc oxide) is prescribed, the HCP will change it weekly.

d. The wound is cleansed with normal saline before application of the Unna boot. Povidone-iodine (Betadine) and hydrogen peroxide are not used because they destroy granulation tissue.

e. The Unna boot is covered with an elastic wrap that hardens to promote venous return and prevent stasis.

f. Monitor for signs of arterial occlusion from an Unna boot that may be too tight.

g. Keep tape off the client's skin.

h. Occlusive dressings such as polyethylene film or hydrocolloid dressings may be used to cover the ulcer.

5. Medications

a. Apply topical agents to the wound as prescribed to débride the ulcer, eliminate necrotic tissue, and promote healing.

b. When applying topical agents, apply an oil-based agent such as petroleum jelly (Vaseline) on surrounding skin, because débriding agents can injure healthy tissue.

c. Administer antibiotics as prescribed if infection or cellulitis occurs.

E. Varicose veins

1. Description

a. Distended, protruding veins that appear darkened and tortuous are evident.

b. Vein walls weaken and dilate, and valves become incompetent.

2. Data collection

a. Pain in the legs with dull aching after standing

b. A feeling of fullness in the legs

c. Ankle edema

3. Trendelenburg's test

a. Place the client in a supine position with the legs elevated.

b. When the client sits up, if varicosities are present, veins fill from the proximal end. Veins normally fill from the distal end.

4. Interventions

a. Assist with Trendelenburg's test.

b. Emphasize the importance of antiembolism stockings as prescribed.

c. Instruct the client to elevate the legs as much as possible.

d. Instruct the client to avoid constrictive clothing and pressure on the legs.

e. Prepare the client for sclerotherapy or vein stripping as prescribed.

5. Sclerotherapy

a. A solution is injected into the vein, followed by the application of a pressure dressing.

b. An incision and drainage of the trapped blood in the sclerosed vein are performed 14 to 21 days after the injection, followed by the application of a pressure dressing for 12 to 18 hours.

6. Vein stripping

a. Varicose veins are removed if they are larger than 4 mm in diameter or are in clusters.

b. Preoperatively assist the HCP with vein marking.

c. Evaluate pulses as a baseline for comparison postoperatively.

d. Maintain elastic (Ace) bandages on the client's legs postoperatively.

e. Monitor the groin and leg for bleeding through the elastic bandages.

f. Monitor the extremity for edema, warmth, color, and pulses.

g. Check for paresthesias, which could include saphenous nerve damage.

h. Elevate the legs above the level of the heart postoperatively.

i. Encourage range-of-motion exercises of the legs.

j. Instruct the client to avoid leg dangling or chair sitting.

k. Instruct the client to elevate the legs when sitting.

l. Emphasize the importance of wearing elastic stockings after bandage removal.

7. Laser therapy: A laser fiber is used to heat and close the main vessel contributing to the varicosity.

XVII. ARTERIAL DISORDERS

A. Peripheral arterial disease

1. Description

a. A chronic disorder in which partial or total arterial occlusion deprives the lower extremities of oxygen and nutrients

b. Tissue damage occurs below the level of the arterial occlusion.

c. Atherosclerosis is the most common cause of peripheral arterial disease.

2. Data collection

a. Intermittent claudication (pain in the muscles resulting from an inadequate blood supply).

b. Rest pain, characterized by numbness, burning, or aching in the distal portion of the lower extremities, which awakens the client at night and is relieved by placing the extremity in a dependent position

c. Lower back or buttock discomfort

d. Loss of hair and dry scaly skin on the lower extremities

e. Thickened toenails

f. Cold and gray-blue skin in the lower extremities

g. Elevational pallor and dependent rubor in the lower extremities

h. Decreased or absent peripheral pulses

i. Signs of arterial ulcer formation occurring on or between the toes or on the upper aspect of the foot that are characterized as painful

j. **BP** measurements at the thigh, calf, and ankle are lower than the brachial pressure (Normally **BP** readings in the thigh and calf are higher than those in the upper extremities.)

3. Interventions

⚠ Because swelling in the extremities prevents arterial blood flow, the client with peripheral arterial disease is instructed to elevate the feet at rest but to refrain from elevating them above the level of the heart because extreme elevation slows arterial blood flow to the feet. In severe cases of peripheral arterial disease, clients with edema may sleep with the affected limb hanging from the bed or they may sit upright (without leg elevation) in a chair for comfort.

a. Monitor pain.
b. Monitor the extremities for color, motion and sensation, and pulses.
c. Obtain **BP** measurements.
d. Monitor for signs of ulcer formation or signs of gangrene.
e. Assist in developing an individualized exercise program, which is initiated gradually and slowly increased.
f. Encourage prescribed exercise, which will improve arterial flow through the development of collateral circulation.
g. Instruct the client to walk to the point of claudication, stop and rest, and then walk a little farther.
h. Because swelling in the extremities prevents arterial blood flow, instruct the client to elevate the feet at rest but to refrain from elevating them above the level of the heart because extreme elevation slows arterial blood flow to the feet.
i. In severe cases of peripheral arterial disease, clients with edema may sleep with the affected limb hanging from the bed or sit upright in a chair for comfort.
j. Instruct the client with peripheral arterial disease to avoid crossing the legs, which interferes with blood flow.
k. Instruct the client to avoid exposure to cold (causes vasoconstriction) to the extremities and to wear socks or insulated shoes for warmth at all times.
l. Instruct the client never to apply direct heat to the limb, such as with a heating pad or hot water, because the decreased sensitivity in the limb will cause burning.
m. Instruct the client to inspect the skin on the extremities daily and report any signs of skin breakdown.
n. Instruct the client to avoid tobacco and caffeine because of their vasoconstrictive effects.
o. Instruct the client in the use of hemorheologic and antiplatelet medications as prescribed.
p. Inform the client of the importance of taking all medications prescribed by the HCP.

4. Procedures to improve arterial blood flow
a. Percutaneous transluminal angioplasty with or without intravascular stent
b. Laser-assisted angioplasty
c. Atherectomy
d. Bypass surgery: Inflow procedures bypass the occlusion above the superficial femoral arteries and include aortoiliac, aortofemoral, and axillofemoral bypasses. Outflow procedures bypass the occlusion at or below the superficial femoral arteries and include femoropopliteal and femorotibial bypasses.

B. Raynaud's disease
1. Description
a. Raynaud's disease is vasospasm of the arterioles and arteries of the upper and lower extremities.
b. Vasospasm causes constriction of the cutaneous vessels.
c. Attacks are intermittent and occur with exposure to cold or stress.
d. Primarily affects fingers, toes, ears, and cheeks
2. Data collection
a. Blanching of the extremity, followed by cyanosis during vasoconstriction
b. Reddened tissue when the vasospasm is relieved
c. Numbness, tingling, swelling, and a cold temperature at the affected body part
3. Interventions
a. Monitor pulses.
b. Administer vasodilators as prescribed.
c. Instruct the client regarding medication therapy.
d. Assist the client to identify and avoid precipitating factors such as cold and stress.
e. Instruct the client to avoid smoking.
f. Instruct the client to wear warm clothing, socks, and gloves in cold weather.
g. Advise the client to avoid injuries to fingers and hands.

C. Buerger's disease (thromboangiitis obliterans)
1. Description
a. Buerger's disease is an occlusive disease of the median and small arteries and veins.
b. The distal upper and lower limbs are affected most commonly.
2. Data collection
a. Intermittent claudication
b. Ischemic pain occurring in the digits while at rest
c. Aching pain that is more severe at night
d. Cool, numb, or tingling sensation
e. Diminished pulses in the distal extremities
f. Extremities that are cool and red in the dependent position
g. Development of ulcerations in the extremities

3. Interventions
   a. Instruct the client to stop smoking.
   b. Monitor pulses.
   c. Instruct the client to avoid injury to the upper and lower extremities.
   d. Administer vasodilators as prescribed.
   e. Instruct the client regarding medication therapy.

XVIII. AORTIC ANEURYSMS

A. Description
1. An aortic aneurysm is an abnormal dilation of the arterial wall caused by localized weakness and stretching in the medial layer or wall of an artery.
2. The aneurysm can be located anywhere along the abdominal aorta.
3. The goal of treatment is to limit the progression of the disease by modifying risk factors, controlling the **BP** to prevent strain on the aneurysm, recognizing symptoms early, and preventing rupture.

B. Types of aortic aneurysm
1. Fusiform: Diffuse dilation that involves the entire circumference of the arterial segment
2. Saccular: Distinct localized outpouching of the artery wall
3. Dissecting: Created when blood separates the layers of the artery wall, forming a cavity between them
4. False (pseudoaneurysm)
   a. Pseudoaneurysm occurs when the clot and connective tissue are outside the arterial wall.
   b. Pseudoaneurysm occurs as a result of vessel injury or trauma to all three layers of the arterial wall.

C. Data collection
1. Thoracic aneurysm
   a. Pain extending to neck, shoulders, lower back, or abdomen
   b. Syncope
   c. Dyspnea
   d. Increased pulse
   e. Cyanosis
   f. Weakness
   g. Hoarseness/difficulty swallowing because of pressure from the aneurysm
2. Abdominal aneurysm
   a. Prominent, pulsating mass in the abdomen, at or above the umbilicus
   b. Systolic bruit over the aorta
   c. Tenderness on deep palpation
   d. Abdominal or lower back pain
3. Rupturing aneurysm
   a. Severe abdominal or back pain
   b. Lumbar pain radiating to the flank and groin
   c. Hypotension
   d. Increased pulse rate
   e. Signs of shock
   f. Hematoma at flank area

4. Diagnostic tests
   a. Diagnostic tests are done to confirm the presence, size, and location of the aneurysm.
   b. Tests include abdominal ultrasound, computed tomography scan, and arteriography.
5. Interventions
   a. Monitor vital signs.
   b. Check risk factors for the arterial disease process.
   c. Obtain information regarding back or abdominal pain.
   d. Question the client regarding the sensation of pulsation in the abdomen.
   e. Inspect the skin for the presence of vascular disease or breakdown.
   f. Check peripheral circulation, including pulses, temperature, and color.
   g. Observe for signs of rupture.
   h. Note any tenderness over the abdomen.
   i. Monitor for abdominal distention.
6. Nonsurgical interventions
   a. Modify the risk factors.
   b. Instruct the client regarding the procedure for monitoring **BP**.
   c. Instruct the client on the importance of regular HCP visits to follow the size of the aneurysm.
   d. Instruct the client to notify the HCP immediately if any of the following occur: severe back or abdominal pain or fullness, soreness over the umbilicus, sudden development of discoloration in the extremities, or a persistent elevation of **BP**.

⚠ Instruct the client with an aortic aneurysm to report immediately the occurrence of chest or back pain, shortness of breath, difficulty swallowing, or hoarseness.

D. Pharmacological interventions
1. Administer antihypertensives to maintain the **BP** within normal limits and prevent strain on the aneurysm.
2. Instruct the client on the purpose of the medications.
3. Instruct the client about the side effects and schedule of the medications.

E. Abdominal aortic aneurysm resection
1. Description: Surgical resection or excision of the aneurysm. The excised section is replaced with a graft that is sewn end to end.
2. Preoperative interventions
   a. Monitor all peripheral pulses as a baseline for postoperative comparison.
   b. Instruct the client on coughing and deep-breathing exercises.
   c. Administer bowel preparation as prescribed.

3. Postoperative interventions
   a. Monitor the vital signs.
   b. Monitor peripheral pulses distal to the graft site.
   c. Monitor for signs of graft occlusion, including changes in pulses, cool to cold extremities below the graft, white or blue extremities or flanks, severe pain, or abdominal distention.
   d. Limit elevation of the head of the bed to 45 degrees to prevent flexion of the graft.
   e. Monitor for hypovolemia and renal failure resulting from significant blood loss during surgery.
   f. Monitor urine output hourly, and notify the HCP if it is less than 30 to 50 mL/hour.
   g. Monitor serum creatinine and blood urea nitrogen daily.
   h. Monitor respiratory status and auscultate breath sounds to identify respiratory complications.
   i. Encourage turning, coughing, and deep breathing, as well as splinting of the incision.
   j. Ambulate as prescribed.
   k. Maintain nasogastric tube to low suction until bowel sounds return.
   l. Monitor bowel sounds and report their return to the HCP.
   m. Monitor for pain and administer medication as prescribed.
   n. Monitor incision site for bleeding or signs of infection.
   o. Prepare the client for discharge by providing instructions regarding pain management, wound care, and activity restrictions.
   p. Instruct the client not to lift objects heavier than 15 to 20 lb for 6 to 12 weeks.
   q. Advise the client to avoid activities requiring pushing, pulling, or straining.
   r. Instruct the client not to drive a vehicle until approved by the HCP.

F. Thoracic aneurysm repair
   1. Description
      a. A thoracotomy or median sternotomy approach is used to enter the thoracic cavity.
      b. The aneurysm is exposed and excised, and a graft or prosthesis is sewn onto the aorta.
      c. Total cardiopulmonary bypass is necessary for excision of aneurysms in the ascending aorta.
      d. Partial cardiopulmonary bypass is used for clients with an aneurysm in the descending aorta.
   2. Postoperative interventions
      a. Monitor the vital signs, and neurological and renal status.
      b. Monitor for signs of hemorrhage, such as a drop in **BP** and increased pulse rate and respirations, and report to the HCP immediately.
      c. Monitor chest tubes for an increase in chest drainage, which may indicate bleeding or separation at the graft site.
      d. Monitor sensation and motion of all extremities and notify the HCP if deficits occur, which can be caused by a lack of blood supply to the spinal cord during surgery.
      e. Monitor respiratory status and auscultate breath sounds to identify respiratory complications.
      f. Encourage turning, coughing, and deep breathing while splinting the incision.
      g. Monitor cardiac status for dysrhythmias.
      h. Monitor for pain and administer medication as prescribed.
      i. Monitor the incision site for bleeding or signs of infection.
      j. Prepare the client for discharge by providing instructions regarding pain management, wound care, and activity restrictions.
      k. Instruct the client not to lift objects heavier than 15 to 20 lb for 6 to 12 weeks.
      l. Advise the client to avoid activities requiring pushing, pulling, or straining.
      m. Instruct the client not to drive a vehicle until approved by the HCP.

XIX. EMBOLECTOMY

A. Description
   1. Embolectomy is removal of an embolus from an artery using a catheter.
   2. A patch graft may be required to close the artery.

B. Preoperative interventions
   1. Obtain a baseline vascular assessment.
   2. Administer anticoagulants as prescribed.
   3. Administer thrombolytics as prescribed.
   4. Place a bed cradle on the bed.
   5. Avoid bumping or jarring the bed.
   6. Maintain the extremity in slightly dependent position.

C. Postoperative interventions
   1. Monitor cardiac, respiratory, and neurological status.
   2. Monitor the affected extremity for color, temperature, and pulse.
   3. Monitor sensory and motor function of the affected extremity.
   4. Monitor for signs and symptoms of new thrombi or emboli.
   5. Administer oxygen as prescribed.
   6. Monitor pulse oximetry.
   7. Monitor for complications caused by reperfusion of the artery, such as spasms and swelling of the skeletal muscles.
   8. Monitor for signs of swollen skeletal muscles such as edema, pain on passive movement, poor capillary refill, numbness, and muscle tenseness.

9. Maintain bedrest initially, with the client in a semi-Fowler's position.
10. Place a bed cradle on the bed.
11. Check incision site for bleeding or hematoma.
12. Administer anticoagulants as prescribed.
13. Instruct the client to recognize the signs and symptoms of infection and edema.
14. Instruct the client to avoid prolonged sitting or crossing the legs when sitting.
15. Instruct the client to elevate the legs when sitting.
16. Instruct the client to wear antiembolism stockings as prescribed and how to remove and reapply the stockings.
17. Instruct the client to ambulate daily.
18. Instruct the client about anticoagulant therapy and the hazards associated with anticoagulants.

XX. VENA CAVAL FILTER AND LIGATION OF INFERIOR VENA CAVA

A. Vena cava filter: insertion of an intracaval filter (umbrella) that partially occludes the inferior vena cava and traps emboli to prevent pulmonary emboli
B. Ligation: suturing or placing clips on the inferior vena cava to prevent pulmonary emboli; performed via abdominal laparotomy
C. Preoperative interventions: If the client has been taking an anticoagulant, consult with the HCP regarding discontinuation of the medication to prevent hemorrhage
D. Postoperative interventions
   1. Maintain a semi-Fowler's position.
   2. Avoid hip flexion.
   3. Refer to postoperative interventions for embolectomy.

XXI. HYPERTENSION

A. Description
   1. For an adult (ages 18 and older), a normal **BP** is a systolic **BP** below 120 mm Hg and a diastolic below 80 mm Hg.
   2. The classification of prehypertension describes an individual with a systolic **BP** between 120 and 139 mm Hg or a **diastolic pressure** between 80 and 89 mm Hg.
   3. Stage 1 hypertension can be classified as a systolic **BP** between 140 and 159 mm Hg or a **diastolic pressure** between 90 and 99 mm Hg.
   4. Stage 2 hypertension can be classified as a systolic **BP** equal to or greater than 160 mm Hg or a **diastolic pressure** equal to or greater than 100 mm Hg.
   5. Hypertension is a major risk factor for coronary, cerebral, renal, and peripheral vascular disease.
   6. The disease is initially asymptomatic.

7. The goals of treatment include reducing the **BP** and preventing or lessening the extent of organ damage (Table 51-4).
8. Nonpharmacological approaches, such as lifestyle changes, may be prescribed initially; if the **BP** cannot be decreased after a reasonable period (1 to 3 months), the client may require pharmacological treatment.

B. Primary or essential hypertension
   1. No known cause
   2. Risk factors
      a. Aging
      b. Family history
      c. Black race, with higher prevalence in males
      d. Obesity
      e. Smoking
      f. Stress
      g. Excessive alcohol
      h. Hyperlipidemia
      i. Increased intake of salt or caffeine

C. Secondary hypertension
   1. Treatment depends on the cause and the organs involved.
   2. Secondary hypertension occurs as a result of other disorders or conditions.
   3. Precipitating disorders or conditions
      a. Cardiovascular disorders
      b. Renal disorders
      c. Endocrine system disorders
      d. Pregnancy
      e. Medications (such as estrogens, glucocorticoids, and mineralocorticoids)

D. Data collection
   1. May be asymptomatic
   2. Headache
   3. Visual disturbances
   4. Dizziness
   5. Chest pain
   6. Tinnitus
   7. Flushed face
   8. Epistaxis

E. Interventions
   1. Goals
      a. One treatment goal is to reduce the **BP**.
      b. Another treatment goal is to prevent or lessen the extent of organ damage.

TABLE 51-4 Hypertension

Organ Involvement	Complications
Eyes	Visual changes
Brain	Stroke
Cardiovascular system	Heart failure
Kidneys	Hypertensive crisis
	Renal failure

2. Question the client regarding the signs and symptoms indicative of hypertension.
3. Obtain the **BP** two or more times on both arms with the client supine and standing.
4. Compare the **BP** with prior documentation.
5. Determine family history of hypertension.
6. Identify current medication therapy.
7. Obtain weight.
8. Evaluate dietary patterns and sodium intake.
9. Monitor for visual changes or retinal damage.
10. Monitor for cardiovascular changes such as distended neck veins, increased heart rate, and dysrhythmias.
11. Evaluate chest x-ray film for heart enlargement.
12. Monitor neurological system.
13. Evaluate renal function.
14. Evaluate results of diagnostic and laboratory studies.

F. Nonpharmacological interventions
1. Weight reduction, if necessary, or maintenance of ideal weight
2. Dietary sodium restriction to 2 g daily as prescribed
3. Moderate intake of alcohol and caffeine-containing products
4. Initiation of a regular exercise program
5. Avoidance of smoking
6. Relaxation techniques and biofeedback therapy
7. Elimination of unnecessary medications that may contribute to the hypertension

G. Pharmacological Interventions
1. Medication therapy is individualized for each client and the selection of the medication is based on such factors as client's age, culture, presence of coexisting conditions, severity of hypertension, and client's preferences.
2. See Chapter 52 for medications to treat hypertension.

H. See Box 51-11 for client education.

XXII. HYPERTENSIVE CRISIS

A. Description
1. A hypertensive crisis is any clinical condition requiring immediate reduction in **BP**.
2. A hypertensive crisis is an acute and life-threatening condition.
3. The accelerated hypertension requires emergency treatment because target organ damage (brain, heart, kidneys, retina of the eye) can occur quickly.
4. Death can be caused by stroke, renal failure, or cardiac disease.

B. Data collection
1. An extremely high **BP** and usually the **diastolic pressure** is greater than 120 mm Hg
2. Headache
3. Drowsiness and confusion
4. Blurred vision
5. Changes in neurological status
6. Tachycardia and tachypnea
7. Dyspnea
8. Cyanosis
9. Seizures

C. Interventions
1. Maintain a patent airway.
2. IV antihypertensive medications may be prescribed.

Box 51-11 Client Education for Hypertension

Describe the importance of compliance with the treatment plan.

Describe the disease process, explaining that symptoms usually do not develop until organs have suffered damage.

Initiate and assist the client in planning a regular exercise program, avoiding heavy weight lifting and isometric exercises.

Emphasize the importance of beginning the exercise program gradually.

Encourage the client to express feelings about daily stress.

Assist the client to identify ways to reduce stress.

Teach relaxation techniques.

Instruct the client on how to incorporate relaxation techniques into the daily living pattern.

Instruct the client and family in the technique for monitoring blood pressure.

Instruct the client to maintain a diary of blood pressure readings.

Emphasize the importance of lifelong medication and the need for follow-up treatment.

Instruct the client and family about the dietary restrictions, which may include sodium, fat, calories, and cholesterol.

Instruct the client on how to shop for and prepare low-sodium meals.

Provide a list of products that contain sodium.

Instruct the client to read labels of products to determine sodium content, focusing on substances listed as sodium, NaCl, or MSG (monosodium glutamate).

Instruct the client to bake, roast, or boil foods. Avoid salt in preparation of foods; and avoid using salt at the table.

Instruct the client that fresh foods are best to consume and to avoid canned foods.

Instruct the client about the actions, side effects, and scheduling of medications.

Advise the client that if uncomfortable side effects occur to contact the HCP and not to stop the medication.

Instruct the client to avoid over-the-counter medications.

Stress the importance of follow-up care.

3. Monitor vital signs, checking the **BP** every 5 minutes.
4. Monitor for hypotension during the administration of antihypertensives. Place the client in a supine position if hypotension occurs.
5. Have emergency medications and resuscitation equipment readily available.
6. Maintain bedrest, with the head of the bed elevated at 45 degrees.
7. Monitor IV therapy, monitoring for fluid overload.
8. Monitor I&O.
9. Insert a Foley catheter as prescribed.
10. Monitor urinary output, and if oliguria or anuria occurs, notify the HCP.

MORE QUESTIONS ON EVOLVE!

Practice Questions

521. A postcardiac surgery client with a blood urea nitrogen (BUN) level of 45 mg/dL and a serum creatinine level of 2.2 mg/dL has a total 2-hour urine output of 25 mL. The nurse understands that the client is at risk for:
1. Hypovolemia
2. Acute renal failure
3. Glomerulonephritis
4. Urinary tract infection

522. A nurse is preparing to ambulate a postoperative client after cardiac surgery. The nurse plans to do which of the following to enable the client to best tolerate the ambulation?
1. Provide the client with a walker.
2. Remove the telemetry equipment.
3. Encourage the client to cough and deep breathe.
4. Premedicate the client with an analgesic before ambulating.

523. A client is wearing a continuous cardiac monitor, which begins to alarm at the nurse's station. The nurse sees no electrocardiographic complexes on the screen. The nurse would first:
1. Call a code blue.
2. Call the health care provider.
3. Check the client status and lead placement.
4. Press the recorder button on the ECG console.

524. A client with a diagnosis of rapid rate atrial fibrillation asks the nurse why the health care provider is going to perform carotid massage. The nurse responds that this procedure may stimulate the:
1. Vagus nerve to slow the heart rate
2. Vagus nerve to increase the heart rate

3. Diaphragmatic nerve to slow the heart rate
4. Diaphragmatic nerve to increase the heart rate

525. A nurse is caring for a client on a cardiac monitor who is alone in a room at the end of the hall. The client has a short burst of ventricular tachycardia (VT) followed by ventricular fibrillation (VF). The client suddenly loses consciousness. Which intervention should the nurse do first?
1. Go to the nurse's station quickly and call a code.
2. Run to get a defibrillator from an adjacent nursing unit.
3. Call for help and initiate cardiopulmonary resuscitation (CPR).
4. Start oxygen by cannula at 10 L/minute and lower the head of the bed.

526. A nurse is monitoring a client following cardioversion. Which of the following observations would be of highest priority to the nurse?
1. Blood pressure
2. Status of airway
3. Oxygen flow rate
4. Level of consciousness

527. A nurse is planning to use an external cardiac defibrillator on a client. Which one of the following actions should the nurse perform to check the cardiac rhythm?
1. Holding the defibrillator paddles firmly against the chest
2. Applying the adhesive patch electrodes to the skin and moving away from the client
3. Connecting standard electrocardiographic electrodes to a transtelephonic monitoring device
4. Applying standard electrocardiographic monitoring leads to the client and observing the rhythm

528. The nurse is caring for the client immediately after insertion of a permanent demand pacemaker via the right subclavian vein. The nurse prevents dislodgement of the pacing catheter by implementing which intervention?
1. Limiting movement and abduction of the left arm
2. Limiting movement and abduction of the right arm
3. Assisting the client to get out of bed and ambulate with a walker
4. Having the physical therapist do active range of motion to the right arm

529. A client diagnosed with thrombophlebitis 1 day ago suddenly complains of chest pain and shortness of breath, and the client is visibly anxious.

The nurse understands that a life-threatening complication of this condition is:
1. Pneumonia
2. Pulmonary edema
3. Pulmonary embolism
4. Myocardial infarction

530. A 24-year-old man seeks medical attention for complaints of claudication in the arch of the foot. The nurse also notes superficial thrombophlebitis of the lower leg. The nurse would next check the client for:
1. Smoking history
2. Recent exposure to allergens
3. History of recent insect bites
4. Familial tendency toward peripheral vascular disease

531. A nurse has given instructions to the client with Raynaud's disease about self-management of the disease process. The nurse determines that the client needs further instructions if the client states that:
1. Smoking cessation is very important.
2. Moving to a warmer climate should help.
3. Sources of caffeine should be eliminated from the diet.
4. Taking nifedipine (Procardia) as prescribed will decrease vessel spasm.

532. A client with myocardial infarction suddenly becomes tachycardic, shows signs of air hunger, and begins coughing frothy, pink-tinged sputum. A nurse listens to breath sounds, expecting to hear bilateral:
1. Rhonchi
2. Crackles
3. Wheezes
4. Diminished breath sounds

533. A nurse is collecting data on a client with a diagnosis of right-sided heart failure. The nurse would expect to note which specific characteristic of this condition?
1. Dyspnea
2. Hacking cough
3. Dependent edema
4. Crackles on lung auscultation

534. A nurse is checking the neurovascular status of a client who returned to the surgical nursing unit 4 hours ago after undergoing aortoiliac bypass graft. The affected leg is warm, and the nurse notes redness and edema. The pedal pulse is palpable and unchanged from admission. The nurse interprets that the neurovascular status is:
1. Moderately impaired, and the surgeon should be called
2. Normal, caused by increased blood flow through the leg
3. Slightly deteriorating, and should be monitored for another hour
4. Adequate from an arterial approach, but venous complications are arising

535. A nurse in a medical unit is caring for a client with heart failure. The client suddenly develops extreme dyspnea, tachycardia, and lung crackles, and the nurse suspects pulmonary edema. The nurse immediately notifies the registered nurse and expects which interventions to be prescribed? **Select all that apply.**
❏ 1. Administering oxygen
❏ 2. Inserting a Foley catheter
❏ 3. Administering furosemide (Lasix)
❏ 4. Administering morphine sulfate intravenously
❏ 5. Transporting the client to the coronary care unit
❏ 6. Placing the client in a low Fowler's side-lying position

ANSWERS

521. 2
Rationale: The client who undergoes cardiac surgery is at risk for acute renal failure from poor perfusion, hemolysis, low cardiac output, or vasopressor medication therapy. Renal failure is signaled by a decreased urine output and increased BUN and creatinine levels. The client may need medications to increase renal perfusion and could need peritoneal dialysis or hemodialysis.
Test-Taking Strategy: Use the process of elimination. The question provides no evidence of any infection, so eliminate options 3 and 4 first. Noting the laboratory values in question will assist with eliminating option 1. Review laboratory values and postcardiac surgery complications if you had difficulty with this question.
Level of Cognitive Ability: Understanding
Client Needs: Physiological Integrity

Integrated Process: Nursing Process/Data Collection
Content Area: Adult Health/Cardiovascular
References: Black, Hawks, p. 675–676, 1426. 2009. Ignatavicius, Workman, p. 290. 2010.

522. 4
Rationale: The nurse should encourage regular use of pain medication for the first 48 to 72 hours after cardiac surgery, because analgesia will promote rest, decrease myocardial oxygen consumption caused by pain, and allow better participation in activities such as coughing, deep breathing, and ambulation.
Test-Taking Strategy: Use the process of elimination. The question asks for the best action of the nurse to help a client tolerate ambulation. Coughing and deep breathing will not actively help endurance, so eliminate option 3. Eliminate option 2 because removal of telemetry equipment is contraindicated

unless prescribed. From the remaining options, noting that the client is postoperative will direct you to option 4. Review postoperative nursing care if you had difficulty with this question.
Level of Cognitive Ability: Applying
Client Needs: Physiological Integrity
Integrated Process: Nursing Process/Planning
Content Area: Adult Health/Cardiovascular
References: Black, Hawks, p. 1428. 2009.
Linton, p. 690. 2012.

523. 3
Rationale: Sudden loss of electrocardiographic complexes indicates ventricular asystole or possibly electrode displacement. Checking of the client and equipment is the first action by the nurse.
Test-Taking Strategy: Use the steps of the nursing process and remember that data collection is the first step. Options 1 and 2 are incorrect because they indicate calling for assistance before collecting data. Option 4 may sound reasonable, but the electrocardiographic monitor automatically starts recording when an alarm sounds. Option 3 is the best option because you should always check the client directly before taking any action. Review care of a client on a cardiac monitor if you had difficulty with this question.
Level of Cognitive Ability: Applying
Client Needs: Physiological Integrity
Integrated Process: Nursing Process/Implementation
Content Area: Adult Health/Cardiovascular
Reference: Christensen, Kockrow, pp. 309–310. 2011. *Adult health nursing.*

524. 1
Rationale: Carotid sinus massage is one maneuver used for vagal stimulation to decrease a rapid heart rate and possibly terminate a tachydysrhythmia. The other maneuvers are the Valsalva maneuver of inducing the gag reflex and asking the client to strain or bear down. Medication therapy is often needed as an adjunct to keep the rate down or maintain the normal rhythm.
Test-Taking Strategy: Use the process of elimination. Eliminate options 2 and 4 first because these options indicate increasing an already rapid rate. From the remaining options, use knowledge of anatomy and physiology. A rapid-rate dysrhythmia would need to be slowed, which is the function of the vagus nerve. The diaphragmatic nerve affects respiration. If you are unfamiliar with the functions of these nerves, review this content.
Level of Cognitive Ability: Understanding
Client Needs: Physiological Integrity
Integrated Process: Nursing Process/Implementation
Content Area: Adult Health/Cardiovascular
Reference: Ignatavicius, Workman, p. 754. 2010.

525. 3
Rationale: When VF occurs, the nurse remains with the client and initiates CPR until a defibrillator is available and attached to the client. Options 1, 2, and 4 are incorrect.
Test-Taking Strategy: Use the process of elimination. Eliminate options 1 and 2 first because you would never leave the client alone. From the remaining options, lowering the head of bed is appropriate (for resuscitation), but the oxygen by cannula at 10 L/minute is incorrect. Option 3 is the correct choice.

Review care of the client with VF if you had difficulty with this question.
Level of Cognitive Ability: Applying
Client Needs: Physiological Integrity
Integrated Process: Nursing Process/Implementation
Content Area: Adult Health/Cardiovascular
References: Christensen, Kockrow, p. 317. 2011. *Adult health nursing.*
deWit, p. 472. 2009.

526. 2
Rationale: Nursing responsibilities after cardioversion include maintenance of a patent airway, oxygen administration, assessment of vital signs and level of consciousness, and dysrhythmia detection. Airway is the priority.
Test-Taking Strategy: Use the ABCs—airway, breathing, and circulation—to answer the question. This will direct you to option 2. Remember, airway comes first. Review care of the client after cardioversion if you had difficulty with this question.
Level of Cognitive Ability: Analyzing
Client Needs: Physiological Integrity
Integrated Process: Nursing Process/Data Collection
Content Area: Adult Health/Cardiovascular
Reference: deWit, p. 478. 2009.
Linton, pp. 688–689. 2012.

527. 2
Rationale: The nurse or rescuer puts two large adhesive patch electrodes on the client's chest in the usual defibrillator position. The nurse stops cardiopulmonary resuscitation and orders anyone near the client to move away and not touch the client. The defibrillator then analyzes the rhythm, which may take up to 30 seconds. The machine then indicates if it is necessary to defibrillate. Although automatic external defibrillation can be done transtelephonically, it is done through the use of patch electrodes (not standard electrocardiographic electrodes) that interact via telephone lines to a base station that controls any actual defibrillation. It is not necessary to hold defibrillator paddles against the client's chest with this device.
Test-Taking Strategy: If you are not familiar with this piece of equipment, look first at the word "automatic" in the name. This implies that someone is not as involved in the process as with a conventional defibrillator and thus may help you eliminate option 1. Because standard electrocardiographic monitoring leads are not used (options 3 and 4), you can eliminate these comparable or alike, and incorrect, options. Although automatic external defibrillation can be done transtelephonically, it is done through the use of patch electrodes. Review the use of this device if you had difficulty with this question.
Level of Cognitive Ability: Applying
Client Needs: Physiological Integrity
Integrated Process: Nursing Process/Implementation
Content Area: Adult Health/Cardiovascular
References: Christensen, Kockrow, p. 740. 2011. *Foundations of nursing.*
deWit, pp. 1085, 1087–1088. 2009.

528. 2
Rationale: In the first several hours after insertion of either a permanent or temporary pacemaker, the most common complication is pacing electrode dislodgment. The nurse helps prevent this complication by limiting the client's activities.

Test-Taking Strategy: Use the process of elimination. The question tells you that the pacemaker was inserted on the right side. Therefore, to prevent pacing electrode dislodgment, motion must be limited on that side. Options 3 and 4 involve movement of the right arm. Limiting the movement of the left arm (option 1) is of no benefit to the client. Thus, option 2 is correct. Review care of the client following pacemaker insertion if you had difficulty with this question.
Level of Cognitive Ability: Applying
Client Needs: Physiological Integrity
Integrated Process: Nursing Process/Implementation
Content Area: Adult Health/Cardiovascular
Reference: Linton, p. 687. 2012.

529. 3
Rationale: Pulmonary embolism is a life-threatening complication of deep vein thrombosis and thrombophlebitis. Chest pain is the most common symptom, which is sudden in onset and may be aggravated by breathing. Other signs and symptoms include dyspnea, cough, diaphoresis, and apprehension.
Test-Taking Strategy: Use the process of elimination. This question tests your ability to analyze signs and symptoms of pulmonary embolism in a client at risk. Options 2 and 4 should be eliminated because myocardial infarction and pulmonary edema are cardiac-related problems and are therefore comparable or alike. Eliminate option 1 because pneumonia is an infectious process. Review the complications of thrombophlebitis if you had difficulty with this question.
Level of Cognitive Ability: Understanding
Client Needs: Physiological Integrity
Integrated Process: Nursing Process/Data Collection
Content Area: Adult Health/Cardiovascular
Reference: Christensen, Kockrow, pp. 362–364. 2011. *Adult health nursing.*

530. 1
Rationale: The mixture of arterial and venous manifestations (claudication and phlebitis, respectively) in the young male client suggests thromboangiitis obliterans (Buerger's disease). This is a relatively uncommon disorder, characterized by inflammation and thrombosis of smaller arteries and veins. This disorder is typically found in young men who smoke. The cause is unknown but is suspected to have an autoimmune component.
Test-Taking Strategy: Use the process of elimination. You can first eliminate options 2 and 3 because they would most likely cause local skin reactions. The question asks which item you should check "next." It is often better to assess a modifiable factor before a nonmodifiable one. This will direct you to option 1. Review the causes of Buerger's disease if you had difficulty with this question.
Level of Cognitive Ability: Analyzing
Client Needs: Health Promotion and Maintenance
Integrated Process: Nursing Process/Data Collection
Content Area: Adult Health/Cardiovascular
Reference: Christensen, Kockrow, pp. 360–361. 2011. *Adult health nursing.*
Linton, p. 742. 2012.

531. 2
Rationale: Raynaud's disease responds favorably to the elimination of nicotine and caffeine. Medications such as calcium channel blockers may inhibit vessel spasm and prevent symptoms.

Avoiding exposure to cold through a variety of means is very important. However, moving to a warmer climate may not necessarily be beneficial, because the symptoms could still occur with the use of air conditioning and during periods of cooler weather.
Test-Taking Strategy: Note the strategic words "needs further instructions." These words indicate a negative event query and the need to select the incorrect client statement. All of the options seem reasonable. However, when you analyze each of them, note that relocation is the least favorable of all the options, from the viewpoints of practicality and encountering new environmental concerns. Review treatment measures for this disorder if you had difficulty with this question.
Level of Cognitive Ability: Evaluating
Client Needs: Health Promotion and Maintenance
Integrated Process: Teaching and Learning
Content Area: Adult Health/Cardiovascular
Reference: Christensen, Kockrow, pp. 361–362. 2011. *Adult health nursing.*

532. 2
Rationale: Pulmonary edema is characterized by extreme breathlessness, dyspnea, air hunger, and production of frothy, pink-tinged sputum. Auscultation of the lungs reveals crackles. Wheezes, rhonchi, and diminished breath sounds are not associated with pulmonary edema.
Test-Taking Strategy: Use the process of elimination. Recall that fluid produces sounds that are called crackles. This will assist in eliminating the incorrect options. If you had difficulty with this question, review the manifestations found in pulmonary edema.
Level of Cognitive Ability: Analyzing
Client Needs: Physiological Integrity
Integrated Process: Nursing Process/Data Collection
Content Area: Adult Health/Cardiovascular
Reference: Christensen, Kockrow, pp. 340, 415–416. 2011. *Adult health nursing.*

533. 3
Rationale: Right-sided heart failure is characterized by signs of systemic congestion that occur as a result of right ventricular failure, fluid retention, and pressure buildup in the venous system. Edema develops in the lower legs and ascends to the thighs and abdominal wall. Other characteristics include jugular (neck vein) congestion, enlarged liver and spleen, anorexia and nausea, distended abdomen, swollen hands and fingers, polyuria at night, and weight gain. Left-sided heart failure produces pulmonary signs. These include dyspnea, crackles on lung auscultation, and a hacking cough.
Test-Taking Strategy: Focus on the subject: right-sided heart failure. Eliminate options 1, 2, and 4 because they are comparable or alike and are pulmonary signs. Review the signs of right- and left-sided heart failure if you had difficulty with this question.
Level of Cognitive Ability: Analyzing
Client Needs: Physiological Integrity
Integrated Process: Nursing Process/Data Collection
Content Area: Adult Health/Cardiovascular
Reference: Christensen, Kockrow, pp. 333–334. 2011. *Adult health nursing.*

534. 2
Rationale: An expected outcome of surgery is warmth, redness, and edema in the surgical extremity cause by increased blood flow. Options 1, 3, and 4 are incorrect.

Test-Taking Strategy: Use the process of elimination. Option 1 can be eliminated because the pedal pulse is unchanged. Venous complications from immobilization caused by surgery would not be apparent within 4 hours, so eliminate option 4 next. To choose between options 2 and 3, think about the effects of sudden reperfusion in an ischemic limb. There would be redness from new blood flow and edema from the sudden change in pressure in the blood vessels. Thus, option 2 is correct. Review the expected findings after aortoiliac bypass graft if you had difficulty with this question.

Level of Cognitive Ability: Analyzing
Client Needs: Physiological Integrity
Integrated Process: Nursing Process/Data Collection
Content Area: Adult Health/Cardiovascular
References: deWit, pp. 444–445. 2009.
Lewis, Dirksen, Heitkemper, Bucher, Camera, pp. 878–879. 2011.

❖ **535. 1, 2, 3, 4**
Rationale: Pulmonary edema is a life-threatening event that can result from severe heart failure. In pulmonary edema the left ventricle fails to eject sufficient blood, and pressure increases in the lungs because of the accumulated blood. Oxygen is always prescribed, and the client is placed in a high Fowler's position to ease the work of breathing. Furosemide, a rapid-acting diuretic, will eliminate accumulated fluid. A Foley catheter is inserted to accurately measure output. Intravenously administered morphine sulfate reduces venous return (preload), decreases anxiety, and reduces the work of breathing. Transporting the client to the coronary care unit is not a priority intervention. In fact, this may not be necessary at all if the client's response to treatment is successful.

Test-Taking Strategy: Note the strategic words "priority interventions" and focus on the client's diagnosis. Recalling the pathophysiology associated with pulmonary edema and using the ABCs—airway, breathing, and circulation—will assist in determining the priority interventions. Review priority interventions for the client with pulmonary edema if you had difficulty with this question.

Level of Cognitive Ability: Analyzing
Client Needs: Physiological Integrity
Integrated Process: Nursing Process/Implementation
Content Area: Delegating/Prioritizing
Reference: Christensen, Kockrow, p. 340. 2011. *Adult health nursing.*
Linton, p. 701. 2012.

52

Cardiovascular Medications

I. ANTICOAGULANTS (Box 52-1)

A. Description (Box 52-2)

1. Anticoagulants prevent the extension and formation of clots by inhibiting factors in the clotting cascade and decreasing blood coagulability.
2. Anticoagulants are administered when there is evidence of or likelihood of clot formation—myocardial infarction, unstable angina, atrial fibrillation, deep vein thrombosis, pulmonary embolism, and the presence of mechanical heart valves.
3. Anticoagulants are contraindicated with active bleeding (except for disseminated intravascular coagulation), bleeding disorders or blood dyscrasias, ulcers, liver and kidney disease, and hemorrhagic brain injuries.

B. Side effects

1. Hemorrhage
2. Hematuria
3. Epistaxis
4. Ecchymosis
5. Bleeding gums
6. Thrombocytopenia
7. Hypotension

C. Heparin sodium

1. Description
   a. Heparin prevents thrombin from converting fibrinogen to fibrin.
   b. Heparin prevents thromboembolism.
   c. The therapeutic dose does not dissolve clots but prevents new thrombus formation.
2. Blood levels
   a. The normal activated partial thromboplastin time (aPTT) is 20 to 36 seconds in most laboratories but may be as high as 40 seconds.
   b. To maintain a therapeutic level of anticoagulation when the client is receiving a continuous infusion of heparin, the aPTT should be 1.5 to 2.5 times the normal value.
   c. Activated partial thromboplastin time therapy should be measured every 4 to 6 hours during initial continuous infusion therapy and then daily.

   d. If the aPTT is too long (longer than 80 seconds), the dosage should be lowered.
   e. If aPTT is too short (less than 60 seconds), the dosage should be increased.
3. Interventions
   a. Monitor aPTT.
   b. Monitor platelet count.
   c. Observe for bleeding gums, bruises, nosebleeds, hematuria, hematemesis, occult blood in the stool, and petechiae.
   d. When heparin is administered subcutaneously, it is injected into the abdomen with a ⅝-inch needle (25 to 28 gauge) at a 90-degree angle; do not aspirate or rub the injection site.
   e. Continuous infusions must be run on an infusion pump to ensure precise rate of delivery.
   f. The client is instructed regarding measures to prevent bleeding.
   g. The antidote to heparin is protamine sulfate.

D. Enoxaparin (Lovenox)—low-molecular-weight heparin

1. Description: Enoxaparin has the same mechanism of action and use as heparin but is not interchangeable. It has a longer half-life than heparin.
2. Interventions
   a. Administered by subcutaneous injection only to the recumbent client in the anterolateral or posterolateral abdominal wall. Do not expel the air bubble from the prefilled syringe or aspirate during injection.
   b. Monitor the same laboratory values as for heparin and observe for bleeding.
   c. The antidote to enoxaparin is protamine sulfate.

E. Warfarin sodium (Coumadin)

1. Description
   a. Warfarin suppresses coagulation by acting as an antagonist of vitamin K by inhibiting four dependent clotting factors (X, IX, VII, and II).
   b. Warfarin prolongs clotting time and is monitored by the prothrombin time (PT).
   c. It is used for long-term anticoagulation and is used mainly to prevent thromboembolic

conditions such as thrombophlebitis, pulmonary embolism, and embolism formation caused by atrial fibrillation, thrombosis, myocardial infarction, or heart valve damage.

2. Blood levels
   a. The normal PT is 9.6 to 11.8 seconds.
   b. Warfarin sodium prolongs the PT. The therapeutic range is 1.5 to 2 times the control value.

3. International normalized ratio (INR)
   a. The normal INR is 1.3 to 2.0.
   b. The INR is determined by multiplying the observed PT ratio (the ratio of the client's PT to a control PT) by a correction factor specific to a particular thromboplastin preparation used in the testing.
   c. The treatment goal is to raise the INR to an appropriate value.
   d. An INR of 2 to 3 is appropriate for most clients, although for some clients the target INR is 3 to 4.5.
   e. If the INR is below the recommended range, warfarin sodium should be increased.
   f. If the INR is above the recommended range, warfarin sodium should be reduced.

4. Interventions
   a. Monitor PT and INR.
   b. Observe for bleeding gums, bruises, nosebleeds, hematuria, hematemesis, occult blood in the stool, and petechiae.
   c. The client is instructed regarding measures to prevent bleeding.
   d. The antidote for warfarin is phytonadione (vitamin K).

II. THROMBOLYTIC MEDICATIONS (Box 52-3)

A. Description
   1. Thrombolytic medications activate plasminogen. Plasminogen generates plasmin (the enzyme that dissolves clots).
   2. Thrombolytic medications are used early in the course of myocardial infarction (within 4 to 6 hours of the onset of the infarct) to restore blood flow, limit myocardial damage, preserve left ventricular function, and prevent death.
   3. Thrombolytics are also used in arterial thrombosis, deep vein thrombosis, occluded shunts or catheters, and pulmonary emboli.

B. Contraindications
   1. Active internal bleeding
   2. History of hemorrhagic brain attack (stroke)
   3. Intracranial problems, including trauma
   4. Intracranial or intraspinal surgery within the previous 2 months
   5. History of thoracic, pelvic, or abdominal surgery in the previous 10 days
   6. History of hepatic or renal disease
   7. Uncontrolled hypertension
   8. Recently required, prolonged cardiopulmonary resuscitation
   9. Known allergy to the specific product or any of its preservatives

C. Side effects
   1. Bleeding
   2. Dysrhythmias
   3. Fever
   4. Allergic reactions

D. Interventions
   1. Determine aPTT, PT, fibrinogen level, hematocrit, and platelet count.
   2. Monitor the vital signs.
   3. Check the pulses.
   4. Monitor for bleeding.

Box 52-1 Anticoagulants

Oral
Warfarin sodium (Coumadin)

Parenteral
Argatroban (Acova)
Bivalirudin (Angiomax)
Dalteparin (Fragmin)
Desirudin (Iprivask)
Enoxaparin (Lovenox)
Fondaparinux (Arixtra)
Heparin sodium
Tinzaparin (Innohep)
Lepirudin (Refludan)

Box 52-2 Substances to Avoid with Anticoagulants

Allopurinol (Zyloprim)
Cimetidine (Tagamet)
Corticosteroids
Green leafy vegetables and foods high in vitamin K
Nonsteroidal anti-inflammatory drugs
Oral hypoglycemic agents
Phenytoin (Dilantin)
Salicylates
Sulfonamides
Gingko and ginseng (herbs)

Box 52-3 Thrombolytic Medications

Alteplase (Activase, tPA)
Reteplase (Retavase)
Streptokinase (Streptase)
Tenecteplase (TNKase)

5. Monitor all excretions for occult blood.
6. Monitor for neurological changes such as slurred speech, lethargy, confusion, and hemiparesis.
7. Monitor for hypotension and tachycardia.
8. Injections are avoided if possible.
9. Direct pressure is applied over a puncture site for 20 to 30 minutes.
10. The client is handled as little as possible when moving.
11. The client is instructed to use an electric razor for shaving and brush teeth gently.
12. The medication is withheld if bleeding develops, and the health care provider (HCP) is notified.
13. Antidote
    a. Aminocaproic acid (Amicar) is the antidote for streptokinase.
    b. Used only in acute, life-threatening conditions

⚠ Bleeding is the primary concern for a client taking an anticoagulant, thrombolytic, or antiplatelet medication.

III. ANTIPLATELET MEDICATIONS (Box 52-4)

A. Description
1. Antiplatelet medications inhibit the aggregation of platelets in the clotting process, thereby prolonging the bleeding time.
2. Antiplatelet medications may be used with anticoagulants.
3. Used in the prophylaxis of long-term complications after myocardial infarction, coronary revascularization, stents, and brain attacks (stroke).
4. These medications are contraindicated in those with bleeding disorders and known sensitivity.

B. Side effects
1. Gastrointestinal bleeding
2. Bruising
3. Hematuria
4. Tarry stools

C. Interventions
1. Sensitivity is determined before administration.
2. Monitor the vital signs.
3. The client is instructed to take medication with food if gastrointestinal upset occurs.

Box 52-4 Antiplatelet Medications

Abciximab (ReoPro)
Aspirin (acetylsalicylic acid, ASA)
Cilostazol (Pletal)
Clopidogrel (Plavix)
Dipyridamole (Persantine)
Dipyridamole; aspirin (Aggrenox)
Eptifibatide (Integrilin)
Ticlopidine (Ticlid)
Tirofiban (Aggrastat)

---

4. Monitor the bleeding time.
5. Monitor for side effects related to bleeding.
6. The client is instructed in the use of the medication.
7. The client is instructed to monitor for side effects related to bleeding and the measures to prevent bleeding.

IV. CARDIAC GLYCOSIDES (Box 52-5)

A. Description
1. Cardiac glycosides inhibit the sodium-potassium pump, thus increasing intracellular calcium, which causes the heart muscle fibers to contract more efficiently.
2. Cardiac glycosides produce a positive inotropic action, which increases the force of myocardial contractions.
3. Cardiac glycosides produce a negative chronotropic action, which slows the heart rate.
4. Cardiac glycosides produce a negative dromotropic action that slows conduction velocity through the atrioventricular (AV) node.
5. The increase in myocardial **contractility** increases cardiac, peripheral, and kidney function by increasing **cardiac output**, decreasing preload, improving blood flow to the periphery and kidneys, decreasing edema, and increasing fluid excretion. As a result, fluid retention in the lungs and extremities is decreased.
6. Cardiac glycosides are used for heart failure and cardiogenic shock, atrial tachycardia, atrial fibrillation, and atrial flutter (Figure 52-1).
7. These medications are contraindicated in those with ventricular dysrhythmias and second- or third-degree heart block and should be used with caution in clients with renal disease, hypothyroidism, and hypokalemia.

B. Side effects and toxic effects
1. Anorexia, nausea, vomiting, diarrhea
2. Headache
3. Visual disturbances: Diplopia, blurred vision, yellow-green halos, photophobia
4. Drowsiness
5. Bradycardia
6. Fatigue, weakness

⚠ Early signs of digoxin toxicity present as gastrointestinal manifestations (anorexia, nausea, vomiting, diarrhea). Then heart rate abnormalities and visual disturbances appear.

Box 52-5 Cardiac Glycoside

Digoxin (Lanoxicaps, Lanoxin)

C. Interventions

1. Monitor for toxicity as evidenced by anorexia, nausea, vomiting, visual disturbances, confusion, bradycardia, heart block, premature ventricular contractions, and tachydysrhythmias.
2. Monitor serum digoxin level, electrolyte levels, and renal function test results.
3. The therapeutic digoxin range is 0.5 to 2 ng/mL. Levels greater than 2 ng/mL are toxic.
4. An increased risk of toxicity exists in clients with hypercalcemia, hypokalemia, hypomagnesemia, or hypothyroidism.
5. Monitor the potassium level. If hypokalemia occurs (potassium lower than 3.5 mEq/L), notify the HCP.
6. The client is instructed to avoid over-the-counter medications.
7. Monitor the client taking a potassium-wasting diuretic or corticosteroids closely for hypokalemia because the hypokalemia can cause digoxin toxicity.
8. Note that older clients are more sensitive to digoxin toxicity.
9. Advise the client to eat foods high in potassium, such as fresh and dried fruits, fruit juices, vegetables, and potatoes.
10. Monitor the apical pulse for 1 full minute.
11. If the apical pulse rate is lower than 60 beats/min, the medication should be withheld and the HCP notified.
12. The client is taught how to measure the pulse.
13. The client is taught to notify the HCP if the pulse rate is lower than 60 or higher than 100 beats/min.
14. The client is taught the signs and symptoms of toxicity.
15. Antidote: Digoxin immune Fab (Digibind) is used in extreme toxicity.

V. ANTIHYPERTENSIVE MEDICATIONS (Box 52-6)

A. Thiazide diuretics (Box 52-7)
1. Description
   a. Thiazide diuretics increase sodium and water excretion by inhibiting sodium reabsorption in the distal tubule of the kidney.
   b. Used for hypertension and peripheral edema
   c. Not effective for immediate diuresis
   d. Used in clients with normal renal function (contraindicated in clients with renal failure)
   e. Thiazide diuretics should be used with caution in the client taking lithium because lithium toxicity can occur in the client taking digoxin, corticosteroids, or hypoglycemic medications.
2. Side effects
   a. Hypercalcemia, hyperglycemia, hyperuricemia
   b. Hypokalemia, hyponatremia
   c. Hypovolemia
   d. Hypotension
   e. Headaches
   f. Nausea, vomiting
   g. Constipation
   h. Rashes
   i. Photosensitivity
   j. Blood dyscrasias

Box 52-6 Classifications of Diuretics

Loop diuretics
Osmotic diuretics
Potassium-sparing diuretics
Thiazide diuretics

Box 52-7 Thiazide and Thiazide-like Diuretics

Bendroflumethiazide
Benzthiazide
Chlorothiazide
Chlorthalidone (Hygroton, Thalitone)
Hydrochlorothiazide (HydroDIURIL)
Hydroflumethiazide (Saluron)
Indapamide (Lozol)
Methyclothiazide (Enduron)
Metolazone (Zaroxolyn)
Polythiazide
Quinethazone
Trichlormethiazide

▲ **FIGURE 52-1** The vicious cycle of maladaptive compensatory responses to a failing heart. (From Lehne, R. [2010]. *Pharmacology for nursing care* [7th ed.]. St. Louis: Saunders.)

3. Interventions
   a. Monitor vital signs.
   b. Monitor the weight.
   c. Monitor the urine output.
   d. Monitor electrolyte, glucose, calcium, blood urea nitrogen (BUN), creatinine, and uric acid levels.
   e. Check peripheral extremities for edema.
   f. Instruct the client to take the medication in the morning to avoid nocturia and sleep interruption.
   g. Instruct the client in how to record the **blood pressure (BP)**.
   h. The client is instructed to eat foods high in potassium.
   i. The client is instructed in how to take potassium supplements if prescribed.
   j. The client is instructed to take medication with food to avoid gastrointestinal upset.
   k. The client is instructed to change positions slowly to prevent **orthostatic hypotension**.
   l. The client is instructed to use sunscreen when in direct sunlight because of increased photosensitivity.
   m. The client with diabetes mellitus is instructed to have the blood glucose level checked periodically.

B. Loop diuretics (Box 52-8)
   1. Description
      a. Loop diuretics inhibit sodium and chloride reabsorption from the loop of Henle and the distal tubule.
      b. Loop diuretics have little effect on the blood glucose level; however, they cause depletion of water and electrolytes, increased uric acid levels, and the excretion of calcium.
      c. Loop diuretics are more potent than thiazide diuretics, causing rapid diuresis, and thus decreasing vascular fluid volume, **cardiac output**, and **BP**.
      d. Loop diuretics are used for hypertension, pulmonary edema, edema associated with heart failure, hypercalcemia, and renal disease.
      e. Use loop diuretics with caution in the client taking digoxin or lithium and the client on aminoglycosides, anticoagulants, corticosteroids, or amphotericin B.
   2. Side effects
      a. Hypokalemia, hyponatremia, hypocalcemia, hypomagnesemia
      b. Hypochloremia

Box 52-8 Loop Diuretics

Bumetanide
Ethacrynic acid (Edecrin)
Furosemide (Lasix)
Torsemide (Demadex)

---

   c. Thrombocytopenia
   d. Hyperuricemia
   e. **Orthostatic hypotension**
   f. Skin disturbances
   g. Ototoxicity and deafness
   h. Thiamine deficiency
   i. Dehydration
3. Interventions
   a. Monitor vital signs.
   b. Monitor the weight.
   c. Monitor the urine output.
   d. Monitor electrolyte, calcium, magnesium, BUN, creatinine, and uric acid levels.
   e. Check the peripheral extremities for edema.
   f. Monitor for signs of digoxin or lithium toxicity if the client is on these medications.
   g. The client is instructed to take the medication in the morning to avoid nocturia and sleep interruption.
   h. The client is instructed in how to record the **BP**.
   i. The client is instructed to eat foods high in potassium.
   j. The client is instructed in how to take potassium supplements if prescribed.
   k. The client is instructed to take medication with food to avoid gastrointestinal upset.
   l. The client is instructed to change positions slowly to prevent **orthostatic hypotension**.
   m. IV furosemide (Lasix) is administered slowly because hearing loss can occur if injected rapidly.

C. Osmotic diuretics
   1. See Chapter 58 for information regarding osmotic diuretics.
   2. Box 52-9 lists osmotic diuretics.

D. Potassium-sparing diuretics (Box 52-10)
   1. Description
      a. Potassium-sparing diuretics act on the distal tubule to promote sodium and water excretion and potassium retention.

Box 52-9 Osmotic Diuretics

Mannitol (Osmitrol)
Urea (Ureaphil)

Box 52-10 Potassium-Sparing Diuretics

Amiloride (Midamor)
Amiloride hydrochloride; hydrochlorothiazide (Moduretic)
Spironolactone (Aldactone)
Spironolactone; hydrochlorothiazide (Aldactazide)
Triamterene (Dyrenium)

Aldosterone-Receptor Blocker
Eplerenone (Inspra)

b. Used for edema and hypertension, to increase urine output, and to treat fluid retention and overload associated with heart failure, ascites resulting from cirrhosis or nephrotic syndrome, and diuretic-induced hypokalemia.

c. Potassium-sparing diuretics are contraindicated in severe kidney or hepatic disease and severe hyperkalemia.

d. Potassium-sparing diuretics should be used with caution in the client with diabetes mellitus, taking antihypertensives or lithium, taking angiotensin-converting enzyme inhibitors because hyperkalemia can result, or taking potassium supplements.

⚠ The primary concern with administering potassium-sparing diuretics is hyperkalemia.

2. Side effects
   a. Hyperkalemia
   b. Nausea, vomiting, diarrhea
   c. Rash
   d. Dizziness, weakness
   e. Headache
   f. Dry mouth
   g. Photosensitivity
   h. Anemia
   i. Thrombocytopenia
3. Interventions
   a. Monitor the vital signs.
   b. Monitor the urine output.
   c. Monitor for signs and symptoms of hyperkalemia such as nausea, diarrhea, abdominal cramps, tachycardia followed by bradycardia, tall peaked T wave on the electrocardiogram, and oliguria.
   d. Monitor for a potassium level greater than 5.1 mEq/L, which indicates hyperkalemia.
   e. The client is instructed to avoid foods high in potassium.
   f. The client is instructed to avoid exposure to direct sunlight.
   g. The client is instructed to monitor for signs of hyperkalemia.
   h. The client is instructed to avoid salt substitutes because they contain potassium.
   i. The client is instructed to take with or after meals to decrease gastrointestinal irritation.

VI. PERIPHERALLY ACTING α-ADRENERGIC BLOCKERS (Box 52-11)

A. Description
1. These medications decrease sympathetic vasoconstriction by reducing the effects of norepinephrine at peripheral nerve endings, resulting in vasodilation and decreased **BP**.

2. These medications are used to maintain renal blood flow.
3. These medications are used to treat hypertension.

B. Side effects
1. **Orthostatic hypotension**
2. Reflex tachycardia
3. Sodium and water retention
4. Gastrointestinal disturbances
5. Nausea
6. Drowsiness
7. Nasal congestion
8. Edema
9. Weight gain

C. Interventions
1. Monitor vital signs.
2. Monitor for fluid retention and edema.
3. The client is instructed to change positions slowly to prevent **orthostatic hypotension**.
4. The client is instructed in how to monitor the **BP**.
5. The client is instructed to monitor for edema.
6. The client is instructed to decrease salt intake.
7. The client is instructed to avoid over-the-counter medications.

VII. CENTRALLY ACTING SYMPATHOLYTICS (ADRENERGIC BLOCKERS) (Box 52-12)

A. Description
1. Centrally acting sympatholytics stimulate alpha receptors in the central nervous system to inhibit vasoconstriction, thus reducing peripheral resistance.
2. Used to treat hypertension
3. Contraindicated in impaired liver function

B. Side effects
1. Sodium and water retention
2. Drowsiness, dizziness
3. Dry mouth
4. Bradycardia

Box 52-11 Peripherally Acting α-Adrenergic Blockers

Doxazosin (Cardura)
Prazosin (Minipress)
Terazosin (Hytrin)

Box 52-12 Centrally Acting Sympatholytics

Clonidine (Catapres)
Methyldopa (Aldomet)
Guanabenz (Wytensin)
Guanfacine (Tenex)

5. Edema
6. Impotence
7. Hypotension
8. Depression

C. Interventions
1. Monitor vital signs.
2. The client is instructed not to discontinue medication because abrupt withdrawal can cause severe rebound hypertension.
3. Monitor liver function tests.

VIII. ANGIOTENSIN-CONVERTING ENZYME (ACE) INHIBITORS AND ANGIOTENSIN II RECEPTOR BLOCKERS (ARBs) (Box 52-13)

A. Description
1. ACE inhibitors prevent peripheral vasoconstriction by blocking conversion of angiotensin I to angiotensin II (AII).
2. ARBs prevent peripheral vasoconstriction and secretion of aldosterone and block the binding of AII to type 1 AII receptors.
3. These medications are used to treat hypertension and heart failure. ACE inhibitors are administered for their cardioprotective effect after myocardial infarction.
4. Use with potassium supplements and potassium-sparing diuretics is avoided.

B. Side effects
1. Nausea, vomiting, diarrhea
2. Persistent dry cough (ACE inhibitors only)
3. Hypotension
4. Hyperkalemia

Box 52-13 Angiotensin-Converting Enzyme Inhibitors and Angiotensin Receptor Blockers

Angiotensin-Converting Enzyme Inhibitors
Benazepril (Lotensin)
Captopril (Capoten)
Enalapril (Vasotec)
Fosinopril (Monopril)
Lisinopril (Prinivil, Zestril)
Moexipril (Univasc)
Perindopril (Aceon)
Quinapril (Accupril)
Ramipril (Altace)
Trandolapril (Mavik)

Angiotensin II Receptor Blockers
Candesartan (Atacand)
Eprosartan (Teveten)
Irbesartan (Avapro)
Losartan (Cozaar)
Olmesartan (Benicar)
Telmisartan (Micardis)
Valsartan (Diovan)

---

5. Tachycardia
6. Headache
7. Dizziness, fatigue
8. Insomnia
9. Hypoglycemic reaction in the client with diabetes mellitus
10. Bruising, petechiae, bleeding
11. Diminished taste (ACE inhibitors)

⚠ A persistent dry cough is a common complaint for those taking an ACE inhibitor. The client is instructed to contact the HCP if this side effect occurs and persists.

C. Interventions
1. Monitor vital signs.
2. Monitor white blood cells, and protein, albumin, BUN, creatinine, and potassium levels.
3. Monitor for hypoglycemic reactions in the client with diabetes mellitus.
4. The client is instructed to take captopril (Capoten) 20 to 60 minutes before a meal.
5. Monitor for bruising, petechiae, or bleeding with captopril.
6. The client is instructed not to discontinue medications because rebound hypertension can occur.
7. The client is instructed not to take over-the-counter medications.
8. The client is instructed in how to take the **BP**.
9. The client is instructed that if dizziness or any other side effects occur and persist to notify the HCP.
10. The client is informed that the taste of food may be diminished during the first month of therapy.
11. The client is instructed to report the side effect of angioedema immediately to the HCP.

IX. ANTIANGINAL MEDICATIONS (Box 52-14)

A. Nitrates (see Priority Nursing Actions)
1. Description
a. Nitrates produce vasodilation.

Box 52-14 Antianginal Medications (Organic Nitrates)

Amyl nitrate inhalant
Isosorbide dinitrate (Isordil, Isordil Titradose, Dilitrate-SR)
Isosorbide mononitrate (Imdur, Monoket, ISMO, Isotrate ER)
Nitroglycerin, sublingual (Nitrostat, NitroQuick, Nitrotab)
Nitroglycerin, translingual (Nitrolingual Pumpspray)
Nitroglycerin, transmucosal (Nitrogard)
Nitroglycerin, transdermal patches (Minitran, Nitro-Dur, Nitrodisc, Nitrek, Transderm-Nitro)
Nitroglycerin ointment (Nitro Bid)
Intravenous nitroglycerin (Nitro-Bid IV, Tridil)

b. Nitrates decrease preload and afterload and reduce myocardial oxygen consumption.

c. Contraindicated in the client with significant hypotension, increased intracranial pressure, severe anemia, and in clients taking medication for sexual dysfunction (because of the risk for severe hypotension)

d. Should be used with caution with severe renal or hepatic disease

e. Abrupt withdrawal of long-acting preparations is avoided to prevent the rebound effect of severe pain from myocardial ischemia.

◼◼◼ PRIORITY NURSING ACTIONS! ◼◼◼

Actions to Take if a Hospitalized Client with Cardiac Disease Complains of Chest Pain

1. The client is quickly assessed, specifically characteristics of pain, heart rate and rhythm, and blood pressure (BP).
2. A nitroglycerin tablet is administered.
3. The client should not be left alone.
4. The client is reassessed in 5 minutes.
5. Another nitroglycerin tablet is administered if pain is not relieved and the BP is stable.
6. The client is reassessed in 5 minutes.
7. A third nitroglycerin tablet is administered if pain is not relieved and the BP is stable.
8. The client is reassessed in 5 minutes. The HCP is contacted if the third nitroglycerin tablet does not relieve the pain.
9. The event, actions taken, and the client's response to treatment are documented.

The usual guidelines for administering nitroglycerin tablets for chest pain include administering one tablet every 5 minutes PRN for chest pain, for a total dose of three tablets. If the client does not obtain relief after taking a third dose of nitroglycerin, the HCP is notified. Before administering the first dose of nitroglycerin, the nurse quickly assesses the client, specifically the characteristics of the pain, the heart rate and rhythm, and blood pressure (BP). The nurse always stays with the client during the event to provide reassurance and relieve anxiety. Additionally the nurse must be present if a life-threatening situation develops. The nurse assesses the client before administering each subsequent dose of nitroglycerin and pays particular attention to the BP because nitroglycerin causes hypotension. The nurse must lower the head of the bed and contact the HCP before administering another nitroglycerin if hypotension occurs. Agency protocols for this type of event should also be followed. The nurse documents the event, actions taken, and the client's response to treatment.

References: Ignatavicius, D., & Workman, M. (2010). *Medical-surgical nursing: Patient-centered collaborative care* (6th ed., p. 856). St. Louis: Saunders; and Kee, J., Hayes, E., & McCuistion, L. (2009). *Pharmacology: A nursing process approach* (6th ed., p. 926). St. Louis: Saunders.

2. Side effects
   a. Headache
   b. **Orthostatic hypotension**
   c. Dizziness, weakness
   d. Faintness
   e. Nausea, vomiting
   f. Flushing or pallor
   g. Confusion
   h. Rash
   i. Dry mouth
   j. Reflex tachycardia
3. Sublingual medications
   a. Monitor the vital signs.
   b. Offer sips of water before giving because dryness may inhibit medication absorption.
   c. The client is instructed to place under the tongue and leave until fully dissolved.
   d. The client is instructed not to swallow the medication.
   e. In the hospitalized client, the nurse should administer one tablet for chest pain and repeat every 5 minutes, for a total of three doses and follow agency protocols for a client experiencing chest pain.
   f. For the client who is at home, the client is instructed to seek medical help immediately (call emergency medical services) if pain is not relieved in 5 minutes after taking one dose of the nitroglycerin.
   g. The client is informed that a stinging or burning sensation may indicate that the tablet is fresh.
   h. The client is instructed to store medication in a dark, tightly closed bottle.
   i. The client is instructed to take acetaminophen (Tylenol) for a headache.
4. Translingual medications (spray)
   a. The client is instructed to direct the spray against the oral mucosa.
   b. The client is instructed to avoid inhaling the spray.
5. Sustained-released medications: The client is instructed to swallow and not chew or crush the medication.
6. Transmucosal-buccal medications
   a. The client is instructed to place the medication between the upper lip and gum or in the buccal area between the cheek and gum.
   b. The client is informed that the medication will adhere to the oral mucosa and slowly dissolve.
7. Transdermal patch
   a. The client is instructed to apply the patch to a hairless area, using a new patch and different site each day.
   b. As prescribed, the client is instructed to remove the patch after 12 to 14 hours, allowing 10 to 12 "patch-free" hours each day to prevent tolerance.

8. Topical ointments
   a. The client is instructed to remove the ointment on the skin from the previous dose.
   b. The client is instructed to squeeze a ribbon of ointment of the prescribed length onto the applicator paper.
   c. The client is instructed to spread the ointment over a 6 × 6-inch area, using the chest, back, abdomen, upper arm, or anterior thigh (avoiding hairy areas), and cover with a plastic wrap.
   d. The client is instructed to rotate sites and avoid touching the ointment when applying.
9. Patches and ointments
   a. Wear gloves when applying.
   b. Do not apply on the chest in the area of defibrillator-cardioverter paddle placement because skin burns can result if the paddles need to be used.

⚠ Instruct the client using nitroglycerin tablets to check the expiration date on the medication bottle because expiration may occur within 6 months of obtaining the medication. The tablets will not relieve the chest pain if they have expired.

X. β-ADRENERGIC BLOCKERS (Box 52-15)

A. Description
1. β-Adrenergic blockers inhibit response to β-adrenergic stimulation, thus decreasing **cardiac output**.
2. β-Adrenergic blockers block the release of catecholamines, epinephrine, and norepinephrine, thus decreasing the heart rate and **BP**.

Box 52-15 β-Adrenergic Blockers

Nonselective (Block β_1 and β_2)
Carteolol (Cartrol Filmtab)
Carvedilol (Coreg Tiltab)
Labetalol (Trandate)
Nadolol (Corgard)
Nebivolol (Bystolic)
Penbutolol (Levatol)
Pindolol (Visken)
Propranolol (Inderal)
Sotalol (Betapace)
Timolol (Blocadren)

Cardioselective (Block β_1)
Acebutolol (Sectral)
Atenolol (Tenormin)
Betaxolol (Kerlone)
Bisoprolol (Zebeta)
Metoprolol (Lopressor, Toprol XL)

---

3. β-Adrenergic blockers decrease the workload of the heart and decrease oxygen demands.
4. Used for angina, dysrhythmias, hypertension, migraine headaches, prevention of myocardial infarction, and glaucoma.
5. β-Adrenergic blockers are contraindicated in the client with asthma, bradycardia, heart failure (with exceptions), severe renal or hepatic disease, hyperthyroidism, or brain attack (stroke). Carvedilol, metoprolol, and bisoprolol have been approved for use in heart failure once the client has been stabilized with ACE inhibitor and diuretic therapy.
6. β-Adrenergic blockers should be used with caution in the client with diabetes mellitus because the medication may mask the symptoms of hypoglycemia.
7. β-Adrenergic blockers should be used with caution in the client taking antihypertensive medications.

B. Side effects
1. Bradycardia
2. Bronchospasm
3. Hypotension
4. Weakness, fatigue
5. Nausea, vomiting
6. Dizziness
7. Hyperglycemia
8. Agranulocytosis
9. Behavioral or psychotic response
10. Depression
11. Nightmares

C. Interventions
1. Monitor the vital signs.
2. Hold the medication if the pulse or **BP** is not within the prescribed parameters.
3. Monitor for signs of heart failure or worsening heart failure.
4. Check for respiratory distress and for signs of wheezing and dyspnea.
5. The client is instructed to report dizziness, lightheadedness, or nasal congestion.
6. The client is instructed not to stop the medication because rebound hypertension, rebound tachycardia, or an anginal attack can occur.
7. The client taking insulin is advised that the β-adrenergic blocker can mask early signs of hypoglycemia, such as tachycardia and nervousness.
8. The client taking insulin is instructed to monitor the blood glucose level.
9. The client is instructed in how to take pulse and **BP**.
10. The client is instructed to change positions slowly to prevent **orthostatic hypotension**.
11. The client is instructed to avoid over-the-counter cold medications and nasal decongestants.

XI. CALCIUM CHANNEL BLOCKERS (Box 52-16)

A. Description
1. Calcium channel blockers decrease cardiac **contractility** (negative inotropic effect by relaxing smooth muscle) and the workload of the heart, thus decreasing the need for oxygen.
2. Calcium channel blockers promote vasodilation of the coronary and peripheral vessels.
3. Used for angina, dysrhythmias, or hypertension
4. Should be used with caution in the client with CHF, bradycardia, or atrioventricular block

B. Side effects
1. Bradycardia
2. Hypotension
3. Reflex tachycardia as a result of hypotension
4. Headache
5. Dizziness, light-headedness
6. Fatigue
7. Peripheral edema
8. Constipation
9. Flushing of the skin
10. Changes in liver and kidney function

C. Interventions
1. Monitor vital signs.
2. Monitor for signs of heart failure.
3. Monitor liver enzyme levels.
4. Monitor kidney function tests.
5. The client is instructed not to discontinue the medication.
6. The client is instructed in how to take a pulse.
7. The client is instructed to notify the HCP if dizziness or fainting occurs.
8. The client is instructed not to crush or chew sustained-release tablets.

XII. PERIPHERAL VASODILATORS (Box 52-17)

A. Description
1. Peripheral vasodilators decrease peripheral resistance by exerting a direct action on the arteries or the arteries and the veins.

2. Peripheral vasodilators increase blood flow to the extremities and are used in peripheral vascular disorders of venous and arterial vessels.
3. Peripheral vasodilators are most effective for disorders resulting from vasospasm (Raynaud's disease).
4. These medications may decrease some symptoms of cerebral vascular insufficiency.

B. Side effects
1. Light-headedness, dizziness
2. **Orthostatic hypotension**
3. Tachycardia
4. Palpitations
5. Flushing
6. Gastrointestinal distress

C. Interventions
1. Monitor the vital signs, especially the **BP** and heart rate.
2. Monitor for **orthostatic hypotension** and tachycardia.
3. Monitor for signs of inadequate blood flow to the extremities, such as pallor, feeling cold, and pain.
4. The client is instructed that it may take up to 3 months for a desired therapeutic response.
5. The client is advised not to smoke because smoking increases vasospasm.
6. The client is instructed to avoid aspirin or aspirin-like compounds unless approved by the HCP.
7. The client is instructed to take the medication with meals if gastrointestinal disturbances occur.
8. The client is instructed to avoid alcohol because it may cause a hypotensive reaction.
9. The client is encouraged to change positions slowly to avoid **orthostatic hypotension**.

Vasodilators cause orthostatic hypotension. The client is instructed about safety measures when taking these medications, such as the need to rise from a lying to a sitting or standing position slowly.

Box 52-16 Calcium Channel Blockers

Amlodipine (Norvasc)
Clevidipine (Cleviprex)
Diltiazem (Cardizem, Dilacor XR)
Felodipine (Plendil)
Isradipine (DynaCirc)
Nicardipine (Cardene)
Nifedipine (Adalat, Nifedical, Nifediac, Procardia)
Nimodipine
Nisoldipine (Sular)
Verapamil (Calan, Isoptin SR, Covera-HS, Verelan)

Box 52-17 Peripheral Vasodilators

α-Adrenergic Blockers
Prazosin (Minipress)
Terazosin (Hytrin)

Calcium Channel Blockers
Diltiazem (Cardizem, Dilacor XR, others)
Nifedipine (Adalat, Nifedical, Nifediac, Procardia)
Nimodipine (Nimotop)
Verapamil (Calan, Isoptin SR, Covera-HS, Verelan)

Hemorheological
Pentoxifylline (Trental; increases microcirculation and tissue perfusion)

XIII. ANTILIPEMIC MEDICATIONS

A. Description
  1. Antilipemic medications reduce serum levels of cholesterol, triglycerides, or low-density lipoprotein.
  2. When cholesterol, triglyceride, and low-density lipoprotein levels are elevated, the client is at increased risk for coronary artery disease.
  3. In many cases, diet alone will not lower blood lipid levels; therefore antilipemic medications will be prescribed.

B. Bile sequestrants (Box 52-18)
  1. Description
     a. Bind with acids in the intestines, which prevents reabsorption of cholesterol
     b. Should not be used as the only therapy in clients with elevated triglyceride levels because they may raise triglyceride levels.
  2. Side effects
     a. Constipation
     b. Gastrointestinal disturbances: Heartburn, nausea, belching, bloating
  3. Interventions
     a. Cholestyramine (Questran) comes in a gritty powder that must be mixed thoroughly in juice or water before administration.
     b. Monitor the client for early signs of peptic ulcer such as nausea and abdominal discomfort followed by abdominal pain and distention.
     c. The client is instructed that the medication must be taken with and followed by sufficient fluids.

C. HMG-CoA reductase inhibitors (Box 52-19)
  1. Description
     a. Lovastatin (Mevacor) is highly protein-bound and should not be administered with anticoagulants.
     b. Lovastatin should not be administered with gemfibrozil (Lopid).
     c. Lovastatin is administered with caution to the client taking immunosuppressive medications.
  2. Side effects
     a. Nausea
     b. Diarrhea or constipation
     c. Abdominal pain or cramps
     d. Flatulence
     e. Dizziness
     f. Headache
     g. Blurred vision
     h. Rash
     i. Pruritus
     j. Elevated liver enzyme levels
     k. Muscle cramps and fatigue
  3. Interventions
     a. Monitor serum liver enzyme levels.
     b. The client is instructed to receive an annual eye examination because the medications can cause cataract formation.
     c. If lovastatin is not effective in lowering the lipid level after 3 months, it should be discontinued.

⚠ The client who is taking an antilipemic medication is instructed to report any unexplained muscular pain to the HCP immediately.

D. Other antilipemic medications (Box 52-20)
  1. Description
     a. Gemfibrozil should not be taken with anticoagulants because they compete for protein sites. If the client is taking an anticoagulant, the anticoagulant dose should be reduced during antilipemic therapy and the INR should be monitored closely.
     b. Do not administer gemfibrozil with HMG-CoA reductase inhibitors because it increases the risk for myositis, myalgias, and rhabdomyolysis.
     c. Fish oil supplements have been associated with a decreased risk for cardiovascular heart disease. Plant stanol and sterol esters and Cholestin have been associated with reducing cholesterol levels.

Box 52-19 HMG-CoA Reductase Inhibitors

Atorvastatin (Lipitor)
Fluvastatin (Lescol)
Lovastatin (Mevacor)
Pravastatin (Pravachol)
Rosuvastatin (Crestor)
Simvastatin (Zocor)

Box 52-20 Other Antilipemic Medications

Ezetimibe (Zetia)
Ezetimibe; simvastatin (Vytorin)
Fenofibrate
Gemfibrozil (Lopid)
Nicotinic acid (Niacin)
Probucol

Box 52-18 Bile Acid Sequestrants

Cholestyramine (Questran)
Colesevelam (WelChol)
Colestipol (Colestid)

2. Interventions
   a. Monitor vital signs.
   b. Monitor the liver enzyme levels.
   c. Monitor the serum cholesterol and triglyceride levels.
   d. The client is instructed to restrict intake of fats, cholesterol, carbohydrates, and alcohol.
   e. The client is instructed to follow an exercise program.
   f. The client is instructed that it will take several weeks before the lipid level declines.
   g. The client is instructed to have an annual eye examination and report any changes in vision.
   h. The client with diabetes mellitus who is taking gemfibrozil is instructed to monitor blood glucose levels regularly.
   i. The client is instructed to increase fluid intake.
   j. Note that nicotinic acid has numerous side effects, including gastrointestinal disturbances, flushing of the skin, elevated liver enzyme levels, hyperglycemia, and hyperuricemia.
   k. The client is instructed that aspirin or nonsteroidal anti-inflammatory drugs taken 30 minutes before may assist in reducing the side effect of cutaneous flushing from nicotinic acid.
   l. The client is instructed to take nicotinic acid with meals to reduce gastrointestinal discomfort.

MORE QUESTIONS ON EVOLVE!

Practice Questions

536. A nurse reinforces discharge instructions to a postoperative client who is taking warfarin sodium (Coumadin). Which statement, if made by the client, reflects the need for further teaching?
   1. "I will take my pills every day at the same time."
   2. "I will be certain to avoid alcohol consumption."
   3. "I have already called my family to pick up a Medic-Alert bracelet."
   4. "I will take Ecotrin (enteric-coated aspirin) for my headaches because it is coated."

537. A client who is receiving digoxin (Lanoxin) daily has a serum potassium level of 3.0 mEq/L and is complaining of anorexia. A health care provider prescribes a digoxin level to rule out digoxin toxicity. A nurse checks the results, knowing that which of the following is the therapeutic serum level (range) for digoxin?
   1. 3 to 5 ng/mL
   2. 0.5 to 2 ng/mL
   3. 1.2 to 2.8 ng/mL
   4. 3.5 to 5.5 ng/mL

538. Heparin sodium is prescribed for the client. The nurse expects that the health care provider will prescribe which of the following to monitor for a therapeutic effect of the medication?
   1. Hematocrit level
   2. Hemoglobin level
   3. Prothrombin time (PT)
   4. Activated partial thromboplastin time (aPTT)

539. A nurse is monitoring a client who is taking propranolol (Inderal LA). Which data collection finding would indicate a potential serious complication associated with propranolol?
   1. The development of complaints of insomnia
   2. The development of audible expiratory wheezes
   3. A baseline blood pressure of 150/80 mm Hg followed by a blood pressure of 138/72 mm Hg after two doses of the medication
   4. A baseline resting heart rate of 88 beats/min followed by a resting heart rate of 72 beats/min after two doses of the medication

540. Isosorbide mononitrate (Imdur) is prescribed for a client with angina pectoris. The client tells the nurse that the medication is causing a chronic headache. The nurse appropriately suggests that the client:
   1. Cut the dose in half.
   2. Discontinue the medication.
   3. Take the medication with food.
   4. Contact the health care provider (HCP).

541. A client is diagnosed with an acute myocardial infarction and is receiving tissue plasminogen activator, alteplase (Activase, tPA). Which action is a priority nursing intervention?
   1. Monitor for renal failure.
   2. Monitor psychosocial status.
   3. Monitor for signs of bleeding.
   4. Have heparin sodium available.

542. A nurse is planning to administer hydrochlorothiazide (HydroDIURIL) to a client. The nurse understands that which of the following are concerns related to the administration of this medication?
   1. Hypouricemia, hyperkalemia
   2. Increased risk of osteoporosis
   3. Hypokalemia, hyperglycemia, sulfa allergy
   4. Hyperkalemia, hypoglycemia, penicillin allergy

543. A home health care nurse is visiting a client with elevated triglyceride levels and a serum cholesterol level of 398 mg/dL. The client is taking cholestyramine (Questran). Which of the following

statements, if made by the client, indicates the need for further education?
1. "Constipation and bloating might be a problem."
2. "I'll continue to watch my diet and reduce my fats."
3. "Walking a mile each day will help the whole process."
4. "I'll continue my nicotinic acid from the health food store."

544. A client is on nicotinic acid (niacin) for hyperlipidemia and the nurse provides instructions to the client about the medication. Which statement by the client would indicate an understanding of the instructions?
1. "It is not necessary to avoid the use of alcohol."
2. "The medication should be taken with meals to decrease flushing."
3. "Clay-colored stools are a common side effect and should not be of concern."
4. "Ibuprofen (Motrin) taken 30 minutes before the nicotinic acid should decrease the flushing."

545. A client with coronary artery disease complains of substernal chest pain. After checking the client's heart rate and blood pressure, a nurse administers nitroglycerin, 0.4 mg, sublingually. After 5 minutes, the client states, "My chest still hurts." Select the appropriate actions that the nurse should take. **Select all that apply.**
❑ 1. Call a code blue.
❑ 2. Contact the registered nurse.
❑ 3. Contact the client's family.
❑ 4. Assess the client's pain level.
❑ 5. Check the client's blood pressure.
❑ 6. Administer a second nitroglycerin, 0.4 mg, sublingually.

ANSWERS

536. 4
Rationale: Ecotrin is an aspirin-containing product and should be avoided. Alcohol consumption should be avoided by a client taking warfarin sodium. Taking prescribed medication at the same time each day increases client compliance. The Medic-Alert bracelet provides health care personnel emergency information.
Test-Taking Strategy: Use the process of elimination and note the strategic words "need for further teaching." These words indicate a negative event query and ask you to select an option that is an incorrect statement. Recalling that warfarin (Coumadin) is an anticoagulant and that Ecotrin is an aspirin-containing product will direct you to the correct option. Review client teaching points related to warfarin if you had difficulty with this question.
Level of Cognitive Ability: Evaluating
Client Needs: Physiological Integrity
Integrated Process: Teaching and Learning
Content Area: Pharmacology
Reference: Lehne, p. 606. 2010.

537. 2
Rationale: Therapeutic levels for digoxin range from 0.5 to 2 ng/mL. Therefore, options 1, 3, and 4 are incorrect.
Test-Taking Strategy: Knowledge of the therapeutic serum digoxin level will direct you to the correct option. If you had difficulty with this question, learn the therapeutic level for digoxin.
Level of Cognitive Ability: Understanding
Client Needs: Physiological Integrity
Integrated Process: Nursing Process/Data Collection
Content Area: Pharmacology
Reference: Lehne, p. 525. 2010.

538. 4
Rationale: The PT will assess for the therapeutic effect of warfarin sodium (Coumadin) and the aPTT will assess the therapeutic effect of heparin sodium. Heparin sodium doses are determined based on these laboratory results. The hemoglobin and hematocrit values assess red blood cell concentrations.
Test-Taking Strategy: Use the process of elimination. Eliminate options 1 and 2 because these laboratory values are unrelated to heparin sodium therapy. From the remaining options, knowledge of the appropriate test for monitoring therapeutic values of both heparin sodium and warfarin sodium is required to answer this question. Review this content if you had difficulty with this question.
Level of Cognitive Ability: Understanding
Client Needs: Physiological Integrity
Integrated Process: Nursing Process/Data Collection
Content Area: Pharmacology
Reference: Lehne, p. 616. 2010.

539. 2
Rationale: Audible expiratory wheezes may indicate a serious adverse reaction, bronchospasm. β-Blockers may induce this reaction, particularly in clients with chronic obstructive pulmonary disease or asthma. Normal decreases in blood pressure and heart rate are expected. Insomnia is a frequent mild side effect and should be monitored.
Test-Taking Strategy: Use the process of elimination, eliminating options 3 and 4 because these are expected effects from the medication. Note the strategic words "potential serious complication." These strategic words will direct you to option 2. Review the adverse effects of this medication if you had difficulty with this question.
Level of Cognitive Ability: Analyzing
Client Needs: Physiological Integrity
Integrated Process: Nursing Process/Data Collection
Content Area: Pharmacology
References: Hodgson, Kizior, p. 975. 2011.
Kee, Hayes, McCuistion, p. 666. 2009.

540. 3
Rationale: Isosorbide mononitrate is an antianginal medication. Headache is a frequent side effect of isosorbide mononitrate and usually disappears during continued therapy. If a headache occurs during therapy, the client should be instructed to take the medication with food or meals. It is not necessary to contact the HCP unless the headaches persist with therapy. It is not appropriate to instruct the client to discontinue therapy or adjust the dosages.
Test-Taking Strategy: Use the process of elimination. Eliminate options 1 and 2 first because it is not within the scope of nursing practice to instruct a client to discontinue or adjust dosages. From the remaining options, recalling that the headache can be relieved with the administration of food with the medication will assist in directing you to option 3. Review this medication if you had difficulty with this question.
Level of Cognitive Ability: Applying
Client Needs: Physiological Integrity
Integrated Process: Teaching and Learning
Content Area: Pharmacology
Reference: Hodgson, Kizior, p. 633. 2011.

541. 3
Rationale: Tissue plasminogen activator is a thrombolytic. Hemorrhage is a complication of any type of thrombolytic medication. The client is monitored for bleeding. Monitoring for renal failure and monitoring the client's psychosocial status are important but are not the most critical interventions. Heparin is given after thrombolytic therapy, but the question is not asking about follow-up medications.
Test-Taking Strategy: Use the process of elimination and note the strategic word "priority." Remember that bleeding is a priority. Review care of the client on tissue plasminogen activator if you had difficulty with this question.
Level of Cognitive Ability: Applying
Client Needs: Physiological Integrity
Integrated Process: Nursing Process/Implementation
Content Area: Pharmacology
Reference: Lehne, p. 618. 2010.

542. 3
Rationale: Thiazide diuretics such as hydrochlorothiazide are sulfa-based medications, and a client with a sulfa allergy is at risk for an allergic reaction. Also, clients are at risk for hypokalemia, hyperglycemia, hypercalcemia, hyperlipidemia, and hyperuricemia.
Test-Taking Strategy: Use the process of elimination. Recalling that thiazide diuretics carry a sulfa ring will direct you to the correct option. Review the nursing considerations related to administering this medication if you had difficulty with this question.
Level of Cognitive Ability: Analyzing
Client Needs: Physiological Integrity
Integrated Process: Nursing Process/Data Collection
Content Area: Pharmacology
References: Hodgson, Kizior, pp. 566–567. 2011. Lehne, pp. 453–454. 2010.

543. 4
Rationale: Nicotinic acid, even an over-the-counter form, should be avoided because it may lead to liver abnormalities.

All lipid-lowering medications also can cause liver abnormalities, so a combination of nicotinic acid and cholestyramine resin is to be avoided. Constipation and bloating are the two most common side effects. Walking and the reduction of fats in the diet are therapeutic measures to reduce cholesterol and triglyceride levels.
Test-Taking Strategy: Use the process of elimination and note the strategic words "need for further education." These words indicate a negative event query and ask you to select an option that is an incorrect statement. Remembering that over-the-counter medications should be avoided when a client is taking a prescription medication will direct you to the correct option. Review client teaching points related to this medication if you had difficulty with this question.
Level of Cognitive Ability: Evaluating
Client Needs: Physiological Integrity
Integrated Process: Teaching and Learning
Content Area: Pharmacology
Reference: Lehne, pp. 577–578. 2010.

544. 4
Rationale: Flushing is a side effect of this medication. Aspirin or a nonsteroidal anti-inflammatory drug can be taken 30 minutes before taking the medication to decrease flushing. Alcohol consumption needs to be avoided because it will enhance this side effect. The medication should be taken with meals; this will decrease gastrointestinal upset. Taking the medication with meals has no effect on the flushing. Clay-colored stools are a sign of hepatic dysfunction and should be immediately reported to the health care provider (HCP).
Test-Taking Strategy: Use the process of elimination. Option 1 can be eliminated because alcohol must be abstained from. Option 2 can be eliminated because taking the medication with meals helps decrease the gastrointestinal symptoms. The clay-colored stools in option 3 are a sign of hepatic dysfunction and should be immediately reported to the HCP. Review the client teaching points related to this medication if you had difficulty with this question.
Level of Cognitive Ability: Evaluating
Client Needs: Physiological Integrity
Integrated Process: Nursing Process/Evaluation
Content Area: Pharmacology
Reference: Lehne, p. 578. 2010.

545. 2, 4, 5, 6
Rationale: The usual guideline for administering nitroglycerin tablets for a hospitalized client with chest pain is to administer one tablet every 5 minutes PRN for chest pain, for a total dose of three tablets. The registered nurse should be notified of the client's condition, who will then notify the health care provider as appropriate. Because the client is still complaining of chest pain, the nurse would administer a second nitroglycerin tablet. The nurse would assess the client's pain level and check the client's blood pressure before administering each nitroglycerin dose. There are no data in the question that indicate the need to call a code blue. In addition, it is not necessary to contact the client's family unless the client has requested this.
Test-Taking Strategy: Focus on the data in the question. Use the steps of the nursing process to determine that assessing the client's pain level and checking the client's blood pressure are appropriate actions. Next, recalling the usual guidelines for

administering nitroglycerin tablets will assist in determining that an appropriate action is to administer a second nitroglycerin, 0.4 mg, sublingually. Review care of the client with chest pain and the guidelines for the administration of nitroglycerin if you had difficulty with this question.

Level of Cognitive Ability: Analyzing
Client Needs: Physiological Integrity
Integrated Process: Nursing Process/Implementation
Content Area: Pharmacology
Reference: Hodgson, Kizior, pp. 834–837. 2011.

The Adult Client with a Renal Disorder

PYRAMID TERMS

acute renal failure (ARF) The sudden loss of kidney function caused by renal cell damage from ischemia or toxic substances; occurs abruptly and can be reversible; leads to hypoperfusion, cell death, and a deterioration in renal function; prognosis depends on the cause and the condition of the client; near-normal or normal kidney function may resume gradually

anuria Urine output of less than 100 mL/day

arterial steal syndrome Can develop after the insertion of an arteriovenous (AV) fistula when too much blood is diverted to the vein and arterial perfusion to the hand is compromised

azotemia The retention of nitrogenous waste products in the blood.

chronic renal failure (CRF) The progressive loss and ongoing deterioration in kidney function that occurs slowly over a period of time; irreversible and results in uremia or end-stage renal disease; requires dialysis or kidney transplantation to maintain life

disequilibrium syndrome A rapid change in the composition of the extracellular fluid (ECF) occurs during hemodialysis; solutes are removed from the blood faster than from the cerebrospinal fluid (CSF) and brain; fluid is pulled into the brain, causing cerebral edema

hemodialysis The process of cleansing the client's blood; the diffusion of dissolved particles from one fluid compartment into another across a semipermeable membrane; the client's blood flows through one fluid compartment and the dialysate is in another fluid compartment

internal arteriovenous fistula (AV fistula) Created surgically in which an artery in the arm is anastomosed to a vein, thus creating an opening, or fistula, between a large artery and a large vein; the flow of arterial blood into the venous system causes the vein to become engorged (maturity); maturity is necessary so that the engorged vein can be punctured with a large-bore needle for the dialysis procedure

nephrolithiasis The formation of kidney stones, which are formed in the renal parenchyma

oliguria Urine output of less than 400 mL/day

peritoneal dialysis The peritoneum is the dialyzing membrane (semipermeable membrane) and substitutes for kidney function during kidney failure; works on the principles of diffusion and osmosis; the dialysis occurs via the transfer of fluid and solute from the bloodstream through the peritoneum

renal failure The loss of kidney function. The types of renal failure include acute and chronic renal failure; the signs and symptoms are caused by the retention of wastes, the retention of fluids, and the inability of the kidneys to regulate electrolytes

uremia Accumulation of nitrogenous waste products in the blood caused by kidneys' inability to filter out these waste products

urolithiasis Refers to the formation of urinary stones or calculi; urinary calculi are formed in the ureter

PYRAMID TO SUCCESS

Pyramid points focus on the preprocedure and postprocedure care of the client undergoing diagnostic tests and procedures related to the renal system. Be familiar with renal failure, dialysis procedures such as hemodialysis and continuous ambulatory peritoneal dialysis (CAPD), dialysis access devices, and postoperative care after urinary or renal surgery. Be familiar with urinary diversions, care of the client after prostatectomy, and treatment measures for the client with urinary or renal calculi. In addition, pyramid points address measures that promote urinary elimination, prevent infection, and maintain skin integrity.

CLIENT NEEDS

Safe and Effective Care Environment

- Consulting with members of the health care team
- Establishing priorities
- Identifying the guidelines related to renal organ donation
- Maintaining confidentiality related to the renal disorder
- Maintaining asepsis related to wound care and dialysis access devices
- Obtaining informed consent related to diagnostic and surgical procedures
- Preventing injury related to complications associated with the disorder
- Maintaining standard and other precautions related to care of the client
- Upholding client rights

Health Promotion and Maintenance

- Discussing expected body image changes
- Performing data collection techniques specific to the renal system
- Providing client instructions regarding care of a urinary diversion, dialysis access device, and dialysis procedures
- Providing client instructions regarding postoperative management
- Providing client instructions regarding prescribed treatments related to urinary or renal disorder
- Providing client instructions regarding the prevention of the recurrence of a urinary and renal disorder

Psychosocial Integrity

- Assisting the client to use appropriate coping mechanisms
- Discussing body-image disturbances
- Discussing the loss of function of a body part that occurs in clients with a renal disorder
- Identifying appropriate community resources
- Identifying grief and loss and end-of-life issues
- Identifying religious and spiritual influences on health
- Identifying support systems

Physiological Integrity

- Ensuring elimination measures
- Informing the client about diagnostic tests and laboratory results
- Monitoring for fluid and electrolyte and acid-base disorders
- Monitoring for data indicating rejection of renal transplant
- Preventing complications arising as a result of dialysis
- Providing adequate rest and sleep
- Providing preoperative and postoperative care related to renal transplantation
- Providing care related to dialysis access devices
- Providing care related to hemodialysis and peritoneal dialysis
- Providing care to the client after prostatectomy
- Providing comfort interventions
- Providing pharmacological therapy
- Providing treatment measures for the client with urinary or renal calculi or the client with a urinary diversion
- Teaching the client about the prescribed nutrition and fluid measures

53

Renal System

I. ANATOMY AND PHYSIOLOGY

A. Kidney anatomy
1. Each person has two kidneys; one is attached to the left abdominal wall and one to the right abdominal wall at the level of the last thoracic and first three lumbar vertebrae.
2. The kidneys are enclosed in the renal capsule.
3. The renal cortex is the outer layer of the renal capsule, which contains blood-filtering mechanisms.
4. The renal medulla is the inner region, which contains the renal pyramids.
5. Together the renal cortex, pyramids, and medulla constitute the parenchyma or functional unit of the kidneys.
6. Nephron
   a. The functional unit of the kidney; located within the parenchyma
   b. Composed of glomerulus and tubules
   c. Selectively secretes and reabsorbs ions and filtrates including fluid, wastes, electrolytes, acids, and bases

 The nephrons are the functional unit of the kidney.

7. Glomerulus
   a. Each nephron contains tuft of capillaries that filters large plasma protein and blood cells
   b. Blood flows into the glomerular capillaries from the afferent arteriole and flows out of the glomerular capillaries into the efferent arteriole
8. Bowman's capsule
   a. Thin double-walled capsule that surrounds the glomerulus
   b. Fluid and particles from the blood, such as electrolytes, glucose, amino acids, and metabolic waste (glomerular filtrate), are filtered through the glomerular membrane into a fluid-filled space in Bowman's capsule (Bowman's space) and then enter the proximal convoluted tubule (PCT).
9. Tubules
   a. The tubules include the PCT, Henle's loop, and the distal convoluted tubule (DCT).

b. The PCT receives filtrate from the glomerular capsule and reabsorbs water and electrolytes through active and passive transport.
c. The descending loop of Henle passively reabsorbs water from the filtrate.
d. The ascending loop of Henle passively reabsorbs sodium and chloride from the filtrate and helps to maintain osmolality.
e. The DCT actively and passively removes sodium and water.
f. The filtered fluid is converted to urine in the tubules, and then the urine moves to the pelvis of the kidney.
g. The urine flows from the pelvis of the kidneys through the ureters and empties into the bladder.

B. Functions of kidneys
1. Maintain acid-base balance.
2. Excrete end products of body metabolism.
3. Control fluid and electrolyte balance.
4. Excrete bacterial toxins, water-soluble drugs, and drug metabolites.
5. Secrete renin and erythropoietin, which play a role in the function of the parathyroid hormones and vitamin D.
6. Synthesizes vitamin D for calcium absorption and regulation of the parathyroid hormones.

C. Urine production
1. As fluid flows through the tubules, water, electrolytes, and solutes are reabsorbed and other solutes such as creatinine, hydrogen ions, and potassium are secreted.
2. Water and solutes that are not reabsorbed become urine.
3. The process of selective reabsorption determines the amount of water and solutes to be secreted.

D. Homeostasis of water
1. The antidiuretic hormone (ADH) is primarily responsible for the reabsorption of water by the kidneys.
2. ADH is produced by the hypothalamus and secreted from the posterior lobe of the pituitary gland.

3. Secretion of ADH is stimulated by dehydration or high sodium intake and a decrease in blood volume.
4. ADH makes the DCTs and collecting duct permeable to water.
5. Water is drawn out of the tubules by osmosis and returns to the blood. Concentrated urine remains in the tubule to be excreted.
6. When ADH is lacking, the client develops diabetes insipidus (DI).
7. Clients with DI produce large amounts of dilute urine. Treatment is necessary because the client cannot drink sufficient water to survive.

E. Homeostasis of sodium
1. When the amount of sodium increases, extra water is retained to preserve osmotic pressure.
2. An increase in sodium and water produces an increase in the blood volume and blood pressure (BP).
3. When BP increases, glomerular filtration increases, and extra water and sodium are lost; blood volume is reduced, returning the BP to normal.
4. Reabsorption of sodium in the DCTs is controlled by the renin-angiotensin system.
5. Renin, an enzyme, is released from the nephron when the BP or fluid concentration in the DCT is low.
6. Renin catalyzes the splitting of angiotensin I from angiotensinogen. Angiotensin I converts to angiotensin II as blood flows through the lung.
7. Angiotensin II, a potent vasoconstrictor, stimulates the secretion of aldosterone.
8. Aldosterone stimulates the distal convoluted tubules to reabsorb sodium and secrete potassium.
9. The additional sodium increases water reabsorption and increases blood volume and BP, returning the BP to normal. The stimulus for the secretion of renin is then removed.

F. Homeostasis of potassium
1. Increases in serum potassium stimulate the secretion of aldosterone.
2. Aldosterone stimulates the distal convoluted tubules to secrete potassium. This action returns the serum potassium concentration to normal.

G. Homeostasis of acidity (pH)
1. Blood pH is controlled by maintaining the concentration of buffer systems.
2. Carbonic acid and sodium bicarbonate form the most important buffers for neutralizing acids in the plasma.
3. The concentration of carbonic acid is controlled by the respiratory system.
4. The concentration of sodium bicarbonate is controlled by the kidneys.
5. Normal arterial pH is 7.35 to 7.45, maintained by keeping the ratio of concentrations of sodium bicarbonate to carbon dioxide constant at 20:1.

6. Strong acids are neutralized by sodium bicarbonate to produce carbonic acid and the sodium salts of the strong acid. This process quickly restores the ratio and thus blood pH.
7. The carbonic acid dissociates into carbon dioxide and water. Because the concentration of carbon dioxide is maintained at a constant level by the respiratory system, the excess carbonic acid is rapidly excreted.
8. Sodium combined with the strong acid is actively reabsorbed in the DCTs in exchange for hydrogen or potassium ions. The strong acid is neutralized by ammonia and excreted as ammonia or potassium salts.

H. Adrenal glands (refer to Chapter 45 for information about the adrenal glands)
1. One adrenal gland is on top of each kidney.
2. Influence blood pressure and sodium and water retention.

I. Bladder
1. The bladder detrusor muscle, composed of smooth muscle, distends during bladder filling and contracts during bladder emptying.
2. The ureterovesical sphincter prevents reflux of urine from the bladder to the ureter.
3. The total bladder capacity is 1 L. Normal adult urine output is 1500 mL/day.

J. Prostate gland
1. The prostate gland surrounds the male urethra.
2. The prostate gland contains a duct that opens into the prostatic portion of the urethra and secretes the alkaline portion of seminal fluid, which protects passing sperm.

K. Risk factors associated with renal disorders (Box 53-1)

II. DIAGNOSTIC TESTS

A. Refer to Chapter 11 for information regarding normal values for renal function studies.
B. Determination of serum creatinine level

Box 53-1 Risk Factors Associated with Renal Disorders

Chemical or environmental toxin exposure
Contact sports
Diabetes mellitus
Family history of renal disease
Frequent urinary tract infections
Heart failure
High-sodium diet
Hypertension
Medications
Trauma

1. Description: A test that measures the amount of creatinine in the serum; creatinine is an end-product from protein and muscle metabolism
2. Analysis
   a. Creatinine level reflects glomerular filtration rate.
   b. Renal disease is the only pathological condition that increases the serum creatinine level.
   c. Serum creatinine increases only when at least 50% of renal function is lost.

C. Determination of blood urea nitrogen (BUN) level
1. Description: A serum test that measures the amount of nitrogenous urea, a by-product of protein metabolism in the liver
2. Analysis
   a. BUN levels indicate the extent of renal clearance of urea nitrogenous waste products.
   b. An elevation does not always mean renal disease is present.
   c. Some factors that can elevate the BUN include dehydration, poor renal perfusion, intake of a high-protein diet, infection, stress, corticosteroid use, or gastrointestinal (GI) bleeding, and factors that cause muscle breakdown.
   d. When the BUN and serum creatinine increase at the same rate and the ratio of the BUN/creatinine remains constant, the elevated serum creatinine and BUN levels suggest renal dysfunction.

D. Glomerular filtration rate (GFR): A blood test that checks how well the kidneys are working by estimating how much blood passes through the glomeruli every minute

E. Urinalysis
1. Description: A urine test for evaluation of the renal system and determination of renal disease
2. Interventions
   a. Wash perineal area and use a clean container for collection.
   b. Obtain 10 to 15 mL of the first morning voiding.
   c. Refrigerated samples may alter the specific gravity.
   d. If the client is menstruating, note this on the laboratory requisition form.

F. Specific gravity determination
1. Description: A urine test that measures the ability of the kidneys to concentrate urine
2. Interventions
   a. Specific gravity can be measured by a multiple-test dipstick method (most common method), refractometer (an instrument used in the laboratory setting), or urinometer (least accurate method).
   b. Factors that interfere with an accurate reading include radiopaque contrast agents, glucose, and proteins.

c. Cold specimens may produce a false high reading.
d. Normal value is 1.016 to 1.022 (may vary depending on the laboratory).
e. An increase in specific gravity (more concentrated urine) occurs with insufficient fluid intake, decreased renal perfusion, or increased ADH.
f. A decrease in specific gravity (less concentrated urine) occurs with increased fluid intake or diabetes insipidus; it may also indicate renal disease or the kidneys' inability to concentrate urine.

G. Urine culture and sensitivity testing
1. Description: A urine test that identifies the presence of microorganisms and determines the specific antibiotics to treat the existing microorganism appropriately
2. Interventions
   a. Clean the perineal area and urinary meatus with a bacteriostatic solution.
   b. Collect the midstream sample in a sterile container.
   c. Send the collected specimen to the laboratory immediately.
   d. Identify any sources of potential contaminants during the collection of the specimen, such as the hands, skin, clothing, hair, or vaginal or rectal secretions.
   e. Urine from the client who drank a very large amount of fluids may be too dilute to provide a positive culture.

H. Creatinine clearance test
1. Description
   a. The creatinine clearance test evaluates how well the kidneys remove creatinine from the blood.
   b. The test includes obtaining a blood sample and timed urine specimens.
   c. Blood is drawn at the start of the test and when the urine specimen collection is complete.
   d. The urine specimen for the creatinine clearance is usually collected for 24 hours, but shorter periods (8 or 12 hours) could be prescribed.

⚠️ The creatinine clearance test provides the best estimate of the glomerular filtration rate (GFR); the normal GFR is 125 mL/min.

2. Interventions
   a. Encourage fluids before and during the test.
   b. Instruct the client to avoid tea, coffee, and as prescribed, to withhold medications during testing.
   c. Check with the health care provider (HCP) regarding the administration of any prescribed medications during testing.
   d. Instruct the client about the urine collection.

e. At the start time, ask the client to void (or empty the tubing and drainage bag if the client has an indwelling urinary catheter) and discard that sample.

f. Collect all urine for the prescribed time.

g. Keep the urine specimen on ice or refrigerated and check with the laboratory regarding adding a preservative to the specimen during collection.

h. At the end of the prescribed time, ask the client to empty the bladder (or empty the tubing and drainage bag if the client has an indwelling urinary catheter catheter) and add that urine to the collection container.

i. Send the labeled urine specimen to the laboratory in a biohazard bag along with the requisition.

j. Document specimen collection, time started and completed, and other pertinent data.

I. Uric acid test

1. Description: A 24-hour urine collection to diagnose gout and kidney disease

2. Interventions

a. Encourage fluid intake and a regular diet during testing.

b. Follow the same procedure for urine collection as with the creatinine clearance test.

J. Vanillylmandelic acid (VMA) test

1. Description

a. The test is a 24-hour urine collection to diagnose pheochromocytoma, a tumor of the adrenal gland.

b. The test identifies an assay of urinary catecholamines in the urine.

2. Interventions

a. Check with the laboratory regarding medication restrictions.

b. Instruct the client to avoid foods such as caffeine, cocoa, vanilla, cheese, gelatin, licorice, and fruits for at least 2 days before and during urine collection and to check with the HCP regarding the administration of any prescribed medications before or during testing.

c. Instruct the client to avoid stress and encourage adequate food and fluid intake during the test.

d. Follow the same procedure for urine collection as with the creatinine clearance test.

K. KUB (kidneys, ureters, and bladder) radiography

1. Description: An x-ray film of the urinary system and adjacent structures used to detect urinary calculi.

2. Interventions: No specific preparation is necessary.

L. Bladder ultrasonography (bladder scan)

1. Bladder ultrasonography is a noninvasive method for measuring the volume of urine in the bladder.

2. Bladder ultrasonography may be performed for evaluating urinary frequency, inability to urinate, or residual urine (the amount of urine remaining in the bladder after voiding).

M. Computed tomography and magnetic resonance imaging

1. Description: These imaging methods provide cross-sectional views of the kidney and urinary tract.

2. Interventions (see Chapter 57)

N. Intravenous pyelography

1. Description: An x-ray procedure in which an intravenous injection of a radiopaque dye is used to visualize and identify abnormalities in the renal system.

2. Preprocedure interventions

a. Obtain an informed consent.

b. Check the client for allergies to iodine, seafood, and radiopaque dyes.

c. Withhold food and fluids after midnight on the night before the test.

d. Administer laxatives if prescribed.

e. Inform the client about possible throat irritation, flushing of the face, warmth, or a salty taste during the test.

3. Postprocedure interventions

a. Monitor the vital signs.

b. Instruct the client to drink at least 1 L of fluid unless contraindicated.

c. Monitor the venipuncture site for bleeding.

d. Monitor urinary output.

e. Monitor for signs of a possible allergic reaction to the dye used during the test and instruct the client to notify the HCP if any signs of an allergic reaction occur.

O. Renal angiography

1. Description: an injection of a radiopaque dye through a catheter inserted into the femoral artery to examine the renal blood vessels and renal arterial supply

2. Preprocedure interventions

a. Obtain an informed consent.

b. Check the client for allergies to iodine, seafood, and radiopaque dyes.

c. Inform the client about a possible feeling of burning or heat along the vessel when the dye is injected.

d. Withhold food and fluids after midnight on the night before the test.

e. Instruct the client to void immediately before the procedure.

f. Administer enemas if prescribed.

g. Shave injection sites as prescribed.

h. Check and mark the peripheral pulses.

3. Postprocedure interventions

a. Check the vital signs and peripheral pulses frequently as prescribed.

b. Maintain bedrest and apply a sandbag or other device that will provide pressure to prevent bleeding, if prescribed, at the insertion site for 4 to 8 hours.

c. Instruct the client to maintain a supine position with the leg straight (the head of the bed should not be elevated greater than 20 degrees for 8 hours or as prescribed).

d. Check the color, temperature, sensation, and movement (CMS) of the toes of the involved extremity with each vital sign check.

e. Inspect the catheter insertion site for bleeding or swelling with each vital sign check.

⚠ The dye used in a renal angiography may be nephrotoxic; therefore encourage increased fluids unless contraindicated, and monitor urinary output.

P. Renal scanning
1. Description: An intravenous (IV) injection of a radioisotope for visual imaging of renal blood flow, glomerular filtration, tubular function, and excretion
2. Preprocedure interventions
   a. Obtain an informed consent.
   b. Check for allergies.
   c. Inform the client that the test requires no dietary or activity restrictions.
   d. Assist with administering the radioisotope as necessary.
   e. Instruct the client to remain motionless during the test.
   f. Instruct the client that imaging may be repeated at various intervals before the test is complete.
3. Postprocedure interventions
   a. Encourage fluid intake unless contraindicated.
   b. Monitor the client for signs of delayed allergic reaction such as itching and hives.
   c. The radioactivity is eliminated in 24 hours. Wear gloves for excretion precautions.
   d. Follow standard precautions when caring for incontinent clients and double-bag client linens per agency policy.

Q. Cystoscopy and biopsy of the bladder
1. Description: The bladder mucosa is examined for inflammation, calculi, or tumors by means of a cystoscope. A biopsy may be obtained.
2. Preprocedure interventions
   a. Obtain an informed consent.
   b. If a biopsy is planned, withhold food and fluids after midnight the night before the test.
   c. If a cystoscopy alone is planned, no special preparation is necessary, and the procedure may be performed in the HCP's office.

3. Postprocedure interventions after biopsy
   a. Monitor the vital signs
   b. Increase fluid intake as prescribed.
   c. Monitor intake and output.
   d. Encourage deep-breathing exercises to relieve bladder spasms.
   e. Administer analgesics as prescribed.
   f. Administer sitz or tub baths for back and abdominal pain.
   g. Note that leg cramps are common because of the lithotomy position maintained during the procedure.
   h. Monitor the urine for color and consistency.
   i. Inform the client that burning on urination, pink-tinged or tea-colored urine, and urinary frequency are common after cystoscopy and resolve in a few days.
   j. Monitor for bright red urine or clots, and notify the HCP if this occurs.

R. Renal biopsy
1. Description: Insertion of a needle into the kidney to obtain a sample of tissue for examination; usually done percutaneously
2. Preprocedure interventions
   a. Check the vital signs.
   b. Check baseline coagulation studies. Notify the HCP if abnormal results are noted.
   c. Obtain an informed consent.
   d. Withhold food and fluids after midnight the night before the test.
3. Interventions during the procedure: Position the client prone with a pillow under the abdomen and shoulders.
4. Postprocedure interventions
   a. Monitor the vital signs, especially for hypotension and tachycardia, which could indicate bleeding.
   b. Provide pressure to the biopsy site for 30 minutes.
   c. Monitor the hemoglobin and hematocrit levels for decreases, which could indicate bleeding.
   d. Place the client in the supine position and on bedrest for 8 hours as prescribed.
   e. Check the biopsy site and under the client for bleeding.
   f. Encourage fluid intake of 1500 to 2000 mL as prescribed.
   g. Observe the urine for gross and microscopic bleeding.
   h. Instruct the client to avoid heavy lifting and strenuous activity for 2 weeks.
   i. Instruct the client to notify the health care provider if either a temperature greater than 100 degrees or hematuria occurs after the first 24 hours postprocedure.

III. ACUTE RENAL FAILURE

A. Description
1. **Acute renal failure (ARF)** is the rapid loss of kidney function from renal cell damage.
2. This occurs abruptly and can be reversible.
3. **Acute renal failure** leads to hypoperfusion, cell death, and decompensation of renal function.
4. The prognosis depends on the cause and the condition of the client.
5. Near-normal or normal kidney function may resume gradually.

B. Causes
1. Prerenal: Outside the kidney; caused by intravascular volume depletion, dehydration, decreased cardiac output, decreased peripheral vascular resistance, decreased renovascular blood flow, and prerenal infection or obstruction.
2. Intrarenal: Within the parenchyma of the kidney; caused by tubular necrosis, prolonged prerenal ischemia, intrarenal infection or obstruction, and nephrotoxicity.
3. Postrenal: Between the kidney and urethral meatus such as bladder neck obstruction, bladder cancer, calculi, and postrenal infection.

C. Phases of **acute renal failure** and interventions (Box 53-2)
1. Onset: Begins with precipitating event

Box 53-2 Acute Renal Failure Phases and Laboratory Findings

Onset
Begins with precipitating event

Oliguric Phase
Elevated blood urea nitrogen and serum creatinine
Decreased urine specific gravity (prerenal causes) or normal (intrarenal causes)
Decreased glomerular filtration rate
Hyperkalemia
Normal or decreased serum sodium
Hypervolemia
Hypocalcemia
Hyperphosphatemia

Diuretic Phase
Gradual decline in blood urea nitrogen and serum creatinine, but still elevated
Low creatinine clearance
Hypokalemia
Hyponatremia
Hypovolemia

Recovery Phase (Convalescent)
Increased glomerular filtration rate
Stabilization or continual decline in blood urea nitrogen and serum creatinine levels toward normal
Complete recovery may take 1 to 2 years

---

2. Oliguric phase
a. For some clients, **oliguria** does not occur and the urine output is normal; otherwise the duration of **oliguria** is 8 to 15 days; the longer the duration, the less chance of recovery.
b. Sudden decrease in urine output. Urine output is less than 400 mL/day.
c. Signs of excess fluid volume: Hypertension, edema, pleural and pericardial effusions, dysrhythmias, congestive heart failure (CHF), and pulmonary edema.
d. Signs of uremia: anorexia, nausea, vomiting, and pruritus
e. Signs of metabolic acidosis: Kussmaul's respirations
f. Signs of neurological changes: tingling of extremities, drowsiness progressing to disorientation, and then coma
g. Signs of pericarditis: friction rub, chest pain with inspiration, and low-grade fever
h. Laboratory analysis (see Box 53-2)
i. Restrict fluid intake. If hypertension is present, daily fluid allowances may be 400 mL to 1000 mL plus the measured urinary output.
j. Administer medications as prescribed such as diuretics (furosemide [Lasix]) to increase renal blood flow and diuresis.

3. Diuretic phase
a. Urine output rises slowly, followed by diuresis (4 to 5 L/day).
b. Excessive urine output indicates that damaged nephrons are recovering their ability to excrete wastes but not to concentrate urine.
c. Dehydration, hypovolemia, hypotension, and tachycardia can occur.
d. Level of consciousness improves
e. Laboratory analysis (see Box 53-2)
f. Administer IV fluids as prescribed, which may contain electrolytes to replace losses.

4. Recovery phase (convalescent)
a. Recovery is a slow process. Complete recovery may take 1 to 2 years.
b. Urine volume returns to normal.
c. Memory improves.
d. Strength increases.
e. The older adult is less likely than a younger adult to regain full kidney function.
f. Laboratory analysis (see Box 53-2)
g. **Acute renal failure** can progress to **chronic renal failure**.

 The signs and symptoms of acute renal failure are primarily caused by the retention of nitrogenous wastes, the retention of fluids, and the inability of the kidneys to regulate electrolytes.

D. Data collection: Obtain objective and subjective data noted in the phases of **ARF** (see Box 53-2).

E. Other interventions

1. Monitor the vital signs, especially for signs of hypertension, tachycardia, tachypnea, and an irregular heart rate.

2. Monitor urine and intake and output (hourly in **ARF**) and urine color and characteristics.

3. Monitor daily weight (same scale, same time of the day), noting that an increase of ½ to 1 lb daily indicates fluid retention.

4. Monitor for changes in the BUN, serum creatinine, and serum electrolyte values.

5. Monitor for acidosis (may be treated with sodium bicarbonate).

6. Monitor urinalysis for protein level, hematuria, casts, and specific gravity.

7. Monitor for altered level of consciousness caused by uremia.

8. Monitor for signs of infection because the client may not experience an elevated temperature or an increased white blood cell count.

9. Monitor the lungs for wheezes and rhonchi and monitor for edema, which can indicate fluid overload.

10. Administer prescribed diet, which is usually a moderate-protein (to decrease the work load on the kidneys) and a high-carbohydrate diet.

11. Restrict potassium and sodium intake as prescribed based on the electrolyte level.

12. Administer medications as prescribed. Be alert to the mechanism for metabolism and excretion of all prescribed medications.

13. Be alert to nephrotoxic medications, which may be prescribed.

14. Be alert to the HCP's adjustment of medication dosages for **renal failure**.

15. Prepare the client for dialysis if prescribed. Continuous renal replacement therapy (CRRT) may be used in **ARF** to treat fluid volume overload or rapidly developing **azotemia** and metabolic acidosis.

16. Provide emotional support by allowing opportunities for the client to express concerns and fears and encouraging family interactions.

17. Promote consistency in caregivers.

18. Also refer to the section in this chapter on special problems in **renal failure** and interventions.

IV. CHRONIC RENAL FAILURE (CRF)

A. Description

1. **Chronic renal failure (also known as chronic kidney disease)** is a slow, progressive, irreversible loss in kidney function with a GFR less than or equal to 60 mL/min for 3 months or longer.

2. Occurs in stages and results in uremia or end-stage renal disease (Table 53-1)

3. Hypervolemia can occur because of the kidneys' inability to excrete sodium and water, or hypovolemia can occur because of the kidneys' inability to conserve sodium and water.

⚠ Chronic renal failure affects all major body systems and requires dialysis or kidney transplantation to maintain life.

B. Primary causes

1. May follow **acute renal failure**

2. Diabetes mellitus and other metabolic disorders

3. Hypertension

4. Chronic urinary obstruction

5. Recurrent infections

6. Renal artery occlusion

7. Autoimmune disorders

C. Data collection

1. Monitor body systems for the manifestations of **chronic renal failure** (Box 53-3).

2. Monitor psychological changes, which could include emotional lability, withdrawal, depression, anxiety, suicidal behavior, denial, dependence/independence conflict, and changes in body image.

D. Interventions

1. Same as the interventions for **ARF**

2. Administer prescribed diet, which is usually a moderate protein (to decrease the workload on the kidneys) and a high-carbohydrate, low-potassium, and low-phosphorus diet.

3. Provide oral care to prevent stomatitis and reduce discomfort from mouth sores.

4. Provide skin care to prevent pruritus.

5. Teach the client about fluid and dietary restrictions and the importance of daily weights.

TABLE 53-1 Progression of Chronic Kidney Disease

Signs of CKD	Estimated GRF
At risk; normal kidney function (early kidney disease may or may not be present)	Greater than 90 mL/min
Mild CKD	60-89 mL/min
Moderate CKD	30-59 mL/min
Severe CKD	15-29 mL/min
ESKD	Less than 15 mL/min

CDK, Chronic kidney disease; *ESKD*, end-stage kidney disease; *GFR*, glomerular filtration rate.
From Ignatavicius, D., & Workman, M. (2010). *Medical-surgical nursing: Patient-centered collaborative care* (6th ed., p. 1609). St. Louis: Saunders.

Box 53-3   Essential Features of Chronic Renal Failure

Neurological Manifestations
- Lethargy and daytime drowsiness
- Inability to concentrate or decreased attention span
- Seizures
- Coma
- Slurred speed
- Asterixis
- Tremors, twitching, or jerky movements
- Myoclonus
- Ataxia (alteration in gait)
- Paresthesias

Cardiovascular Manifestations
- Cardiomyopathy
- Hypertension
- Peripheral edema
- Heart failure
- Uremic pericarditis
- Pericardial effusion
- Pericardial friction rub
- Cardiac tamponade

Respiratory Manifestations
- Uremic halitosis
- Tachypnea
- Deep sighing, yawning
- Kussmaul respirations
- Uremic pneumonitis
- Shortness of breath
- Pulmonary edema
- Pleural effusion
- Depressed cough reflex
- Crackles

Hematological Manifestations
- Anemia
- Abnormal bleeding and bruising

Gastrointestinal Manifestations
- Anorexia
- Nausea
- Vomiting

- Metallic taste in mouth
- Changes in taste acuity and sensation
- Uremic colitis (diarrhea)
- Constipation
- Uremic gastritis (possible gastrointestinal bleeding)
- Uremic fetor
- Stomatitis
- Diarrhea

Urinary Manifestations
- Polyuria, nocturia (early)
- Oliguria, anuria (later)
- Proteinuria
- Hematuria
- Diluted, strawlike appearance

Integumentary Manifestations
- Decreased skin turgor
- Yellow-gray pallor
- Dry skin
- Pruritus
- Ecchymosis
- Purpura
- Soft tissue calcifications
- Uremic frost (late, premorbid)

Musculoskeletal Manifestations
- Muscle weakness and cramping
- Bone pain
- Pathological fractures
- Renal osteodystrophy

Reproductive Manifestations
- Decreased fertility
- Infrequent or absent menses
- Decreased libido
- Impotence

From Ignatavicius, D., & Workman, M. (2010). *Medical-surgical nursing: Patient-centered collaborative care* (5th ed). St. Louis: Saunders.

6. Provide support to promote acceptance of the chronic illness and prepare the client for long-term dialysis and transplantation. Note that the client may choose to decline **dialysis** or transplantation.

E. Special problems in **renal failure** and interventions
   1. Activity intolerance and insomnia
      a. Fatigue results from anemia and the buildup of wastes from the diseased kidneys.
      b. Provide adequate rest periods.
      c. Teach the client to plan activities to avoid fatigue.
      d. Administer mild central nervous system (CNS) depressants as prescribed to promote rest.

   2. Anemia
      a. Anemia results from the decreased secretion of erythropoietin and decreased production of red blood cells as a result of the kidney disease.
      b. Monitor for decreased hemoglobin and hematocrit levels.
      c. Administer epoetin alfa (Epogen, Procrit) or darbepoetin alfa (Aranesp), or hematopoietics, as prescribed to stimulate the production of red blood cells.
      d. Administer folic acid (vitamin B_9) as prescribed.
      e. Administer iron orally as prescribed, but not at the same time as phosphate binders.

f. Administer stool softeners as prescribed because of the constipating effects of iron.

g. Be alert that oral iron is not well absorbed by the gastrointestinal tract in **chronic renal failure** and causes nausea and vomiting. Parenteral iron (iron sucrose [Venofer] or sodium ferric gluconate complex [Ferrlecit]) may be used if iron deficiencies persist despite folic acid or oral iron administration.

h. Administer blood transfusions if prescribed. Blood transfusions are prescribed only when necessary (acute blood loss, symptomatic anemia) because they decrease the stimulus to produce red blood cells. Note that certain religious beliefs such as Jehovah's Witnesses may refuse blood and blood products.

i. Blood transfusions also cause the development of antibodies against human tissues, which can make matching for organ transplantation difficult.

3. Gastrointestinal bleeding
   a. Urea is broken down by the intestinal bacteria to ammonia. Ammonia irritates the gastrointestinal mucosa, causing ulceration and bleeding.
   b. Monitor for decreasing hemoglobin and hematocrit levels.
   c. Monitor stools for occult blood.
   d. Instruct the client to use a soft toothbrush.
   e. Avoid the administration of acetylsalicylic acid (aspirin) because it is excreted by the kidneys. If administered, aspirin toxicity can occur and prolong the bleeding time.

4. Hyperkalemia
   a. Monitor the vital signs for hypertension or hypotension and the apical heart rate. An irregular heart rate could indicate dysrhythmias.
   b. Monitor the serum potassium level. A serum potassium level above 6 mEq/L can cause tall peaked T waves, flat P waves, a widened QRS complex, and a prolonged PR interval; decreased cardiac output; heart blocks; fibrillation; or asystole (Figure 53-1).
   c. Provide a low-potassium diet, avoiding foods high in potassium. (Refer to Chapter 9 for a listing of foods that are high in potassium.)
   d. Administer electrolyte-binding and -excreting medications such as oral or rectal sodium polystyrene sulfonate (Kayexalate) as prescribed to lower the serum potassium level.
   e. Administer prescribed medications: 50% dextrose and insulin may be prescribed to shift potassium into the cell. Calcium gluconate IV may be prescribed to reduce myocardial irritability from hyperkalemia, and sodium bicarbonate IV may be prescribed to correct acidosis.

Serum Potassium Levels

A. Normal (3.5-5.1 mEq/L)
B. About 7.0 mEq/L
C. 8.0-9.0 mEq/L
D. >10.0 mEq/L

▲ **FIGURE 53-1** Cardiac rhythm changes with hyperkalemia. (From Huszar, R. J. [2007]. *Basic dysrhythmias: Interpretation & management* [3rd ed]. St. Louis: Mosby.)

f. Administer prescribed loop diuretics to excrete potassium.

g. Avoid potassium-sparing medications such as spironolactone (Aldactone) and triamterene (Dyrenium), because these medications will increase the potassium level.

h. Prepare the client for **peritoneal** or **hemodialysis** as prescribed.

⚠ Place the client with renal failure on continuous cardiac monitoring. The client can develop hyperkalemia and is at risk for dysrhythmias.

5. Hypermagnesemia
   a. Results from decreased renal excretion of magnesium.
   b. Monitor cardiac manifestations of bradycardia, peripheral vasodilation, and hypotension.
   c. Monitor CNS manifestations of decreased nerve impulse transmission such as drowsiness or lethargy.
   d. Monitor neuromuscular manifestations such as reduced or absent deep tendon reflexes or weak or absent voluntary skeletal muscle contractions.

e. Administer loop diuretics as prescribed such as furosemide (Lasix).

f. Administer calcium as prescribed for resulting cardiac problems.

g. Avoid medications that contain magnesium such as antacids, laxatives, or enemas.

h. During severe elevations, avoid foods that increase magnesium levels. (Refer to Chapter 9 for a listing of foods that are high in magnesium.)

6. Hyperphosphatemia

a. As the phosphorus level rises, the calcium level drops; this leads to the stimulation of parathyroid hormone, causing bone demineralization.

b. Treatment is aimed at lowering the serum phosphorus levels.

c. Administer phosphate binders such as calcium carbonate (TUMS), calcium acetate (PhosLo), or sevelamer (Renagel) as prescribed with meals to lower serum phosphate levels.

d. Aluminum hydroxide preparations are avoided for use as phosphate binders because they are associated with dementia and osteomalacia.

e. Administer stools softeners and laxatives as prescribed because phosphate binders are constipating.

f. Teach the client about the need to limit the intake of foods high in phosphorus. (See Chapter 9 for a listing of foods that are high in phosphorus.)

7. Hypertension

a. Caused by failure of the kidneys to maintain BP homeostasis

b. Monitor the vital signs for elevated blood pressure.

c. Maintain fluid and sodium restrictions as prescribed.

d. Administer diuretics and antihypertensives as prescribed.

e. Administer propranolol (Inderal)—a β-adrenergic antagonist—as prescribed. Propranolol decreases renin release (renin causes vasoconstriction and subsequent hypertension).

8. Hypervolemia

a. Monitor the vital signs for an elevated blood pressure.

b. Monitor intake and output and daily weight for indications of fluid retention.

c. Monitor for periorbital, sacral, and peripheral edema.

d. Monitor the serum electrolytes.

e. Monitor for hypertension, and notify the HCP for sustained elevations.

f. Monitor for signs of CHF and pulmonary edema such as restlessness, heightened anxiety, tachycardia, dyspnea, basilar lung crackles, and blood-tinged sputum. Notify the HCP immediately if signs occur.

g. Maintain fluid restriction.

h. Avoid the administration of large amounts of IV fluids.

i. Administer diuretics such as furosemide (Lasix) as prescribed.

j. Teach the client to maintain a low-sodium diet.

k. Teach the client to avoid antacids or cold remedies containing sodium bicarbonate.

9. Hypocalcemia

a. Results from the high phosphorus level and the inability of the diseased kidney to activate vitamin D.

b. The absence of vitamin D causes poor calcium absorption from the intestinal tract.

c. Monitor the serum calcium level.

d. Administer calcium supplements as prescribed.

e. Administer activated vitamin D as prescribed.

f. See Chapter 9 for a listing of foods that are high in calcium.

10. Hypovolemia

a. Monitor the vital signs for hypotension and tachycardia.

b. Monitor for decreasing intake and output and a reduction in the daily weight.

c. Monitor for dehydration.

d. Monitor the electrolytes.

e. Provide replacement therapy based on the serum electrolyte results.

f. Provide sodium supplements as prescribed, based on the serum electrolyte value.

11. Infection

a. The client is at risk for infection because of a suppressed immune system, dialysis access site, and possible malnutrition.

b. Monitor for signs of infection.

c. Avoid urinary catheters when possible; if used, provide catheter care.

d. Provide strict asepsis during urinary catheter insertion and other invasive procedures.

e. Instruct the client to avoid fatigue, which decreases body resistance.

f. Instruct the client to avoid persons with infections.

g. Administer antibiotics as prescribed, monitoring for nephrotoxic effects.

12. Metabolic acidosis

a. The kidneys are unable to excrete hydrogen ions or manufacture bicarbonate, resulting in acidosis.

b. Administer alkalizers such as sodium bicarbonate as prescribed.

c. Note that clients with **chronic renal failure** adjust to low bicarbonate levels and do not become acutely ill.

13. Muscle cramps
   a. Occur from electrolyte imbalances and the effects of uremia on peripheral nerves.
   b. Monitor the serum electrolytes.
   c. Administer electrolyte replacements and medications to control muscle cramps as prescribed.
   d. Administer heat and massage as prescribed.

14. Neurological changes
   a. The buildup of active particles and fluids causes changes in the brain cells and leads to confusion and impairment in decision-making ability.
   b. Peripheral neuropathy results from the effects of uremia on peripheral nerves.
   c. Monitor the level of consciousness and for confusion.
   d. Monitor for restless leg syndrome, which is also common during dialysis treatments.
   e. Teach the client to examine areas of decreased sensation for signs of injury.

15. Ocular irritation
   a. Calcium deposits in the conjunctiva cause burning and watering of the eyes.
   b. Administer medications to control the calcium and phosphate levels as prescribed.
   c. Administer lubricating eye drops.
   d. Protect the client from injury.
   e. Provide a safe and hazard-free environment.
   f. Use side rails as needed.

16. Potential for injury
   a. The client is at risk for fractures because of alterations in the absorption of calcium and the excretion of phosphate and altered vitamin D metabolism.
   b. Provide for a safe environment.
   c. Avoid injury; tissue breakdown causes increased serum potassium levels.

17. Pruritus
   a. To rid the body of excess wastes, urate crystals are excreted through the skin, causing pruritus.
   b. The deposit of urate crystals (uremic frost) occurs in advanced stages of **renal failure**.
   c. Monitor for skin breakdown, rash, and uremic frost.
   d. Provide meticulous skin care and oral hygiene.
   e. Avoid the use of soaps.
   f. Administer antihistamines and antipruritics as prescribed to relieve itching.
   g. Teach the client to keep the nails trimmed to prevent local infection from scratching.

18. Psychosocial problems
   a. Listen to the client's concerns to determine how he or she is handling the situation.
   b. Allow the client time to mourn the loss of kidney function.
   c. With the client's permission, include the family members in discussions of the client's concerns.
   d. Reinforce education about treatment options and support their decision.
   e. Offer information about support groups.
   f. Provide end-of-life care for the client with end-stage renal disease.

V. UREMIC SYNDROME

A. Description
   1. The accumulation of nitrogenous waste products in the blood caused by the kidneys' inability to filter out these waste products.
   2. Uremic syndrome may occur as a result of **acute** or **chronic renal failure**.

B. Data collection
   1. **Oliguria**
   2. The presence of protein, red blood cells, and casts in the urine
   3. A urine specific gravity of 1.010
   4. Elevated levels of urea, uric acid, potassium, and magnesium in the urine
   5. Hypotension or hypertension
   6. Alterations in the level of consciousness
   7. Electrolyte imbalances
   8. Stomatitis
   9. Nausea or vomiting from **azotemia**
   10. Diarrhea or constipation

C. Interventions
   1. Monitor the vital signs for hypertension, tachycardia, and an irregular heart rate.
   2. Monitor serum electrolyte levels.
   3. Monitor intake and output and for **oliguria**.
   4. Provide a limited, but high-quality, protein diet as prescribed.
   5. Provide a limited sodium, nitrogen, potassium, and phosphate diet as prescribed.
   6. Assist the client to cope with body-image disturbances caused by uremic syndrome.

VI. HEMODIALYSIS

A. Description
   1. **Hemodialysis** is the process of cleansing the client's blood
   2. It involves the diffusion of dissolved particles from one fluid compartment into another across a semipermeable membrane. The client's blood flows through one fluid compartment of a dialysis filter, and the dialysate is in another fluid compartment.

B. Functions of **hemodialysis**

1. Cleanses the blood of accumulated waste products
2. Removes the by-products of protein metabolism such as urea, creatinine, and uric acid from the blood
3. Removes excess body fluids
4. Maintains or restores the buffer system of the body
5. Maintains or restores electrolyte levels in the body

C. Principles of **hemodialysis**

1. The semipermeable membrane is made of thin, porous cellophane.
2. The pore size of the membrane allows small particles to pass through, such as urea, creatinine, uric acid, and water molecules.
3. Proteins, bacteria, and some blood cells are too large to pass through the membrane.
4. The client's blood flows into the dialyzer. The movement of substances occurs from the blood to the dialysate by the principles of osmosis and diffusion.
5. Diffusion is the movement of particles from an area of greater concentration to one of lower concentration.
6. Osmosis is the movement of fluids across a semipermeable membrane from an area of lower concentration of particles to an area of higher concentration of particles.
7. Ultrafiltration is the movement of fluid across a semipermeable membrane as a result of an artificially created pressure gradient.

D. Dialysate bath

1. Composed of water and major electrolytes
2. Dialysate need not be sterile because bacteria and viruses are too large to pass through the pores of the semipermeable membrane; however, the dialysate must meet specific standards, and water is treated to ensure a safe water supply.

E. Interventions

1. Monitor vital signs before, during, and after dialysis; the client's temperature may elevate because of slight warming of the blood from the dialysis machine. (Notify the HCP about excessive temperature elevations because this could indicate sepsis; obtain samples for blood culture as prescribed for excessive temperature elevations.)
2. Monitor laboratory values before, during, and after dialysis.
3. Monitor the client for fluid overload before dialysis and fluid volume deficit after dialysis.
4. Weigh the client before and after dialysis to determine fluid loss.
5. Monitor the patency of the blood access device before, during, and after dialysis.

6. Monitor for bleeding. Heparin is added to the dialysis bath to prevent clots from forming within the dialyzer or the blood tubing.
7. Monitor for hypovolemia and shock during dialysis, which can occur from blood loss or excess fluid and electrolyte removal.
8. Provide adequate nutrition. The client may eat before or during dialysis.
9. Identify the client's reactions to the treatment and support coping mechanisms. Encourage independence and involvement in care.

⚠ Withhold antihypertensives and other medications that can affect the blood pressure or result in hypotension until after the hemodialysis treatment. Also withhold medications that could be removed by dialysis, such as water-soluble vitamins, certain antibiotics, and digoxin (Lanoxin).

VII. ACCESS FOR HEMODIALYSIS

A. Subclavian and femoral catheter (Figure 53-2)

1. Description
   a. A subclavian (subclavian vein) or femoral (femoral vein) catheter may be inserted for short-term or temporary use in **ARF**.
   b. The catheter is used until a fistula or graft matures or develops or may be required when the client's fistula or graft access has failed because of infection or clotting.
2. Interventions
   a. Monitor the insertion site for hematoma, bleeding, catheter dislodgement, and infection.
   b. These catheters should only be used for dialysis treatments.
   c. Maintain an occlusive dressing over the catheter insertion site.
3. Subclavian vein catheter
   a. The catheter is usually filled with heparin and capped to maintain patency between dialysis treatments.
   b. The catheter should not be uncapped except for dialysis treatments.
   c. The catheter may be left in place for up to 6 weeks if complications do not occur.
4. Femoral vein catheter
   a. Monitor the extremity for circulation, temperature, and pulses.
   b. Prevent pulling or disconnecting of the catheter when giving care.
   c. Because the groin is not a clean site, meticulous perineal care is required.
   d. Use an IV infusion pump or controller with microdrip tubing if a heparin infusion through the catheter to maintain patency is prescribed.

▲ **FIGURE 53-2** Common means for gaining vascular access for hemodialysis include **A,** arteriovenous fistula, and **B,** arteriovenous graft. (From Monahan, F., Sands, J., Neighbors, M., et al. [2007]. *Phipps' medical-surgical nursing: Health and illness perspectives* [8th ed.]. St. Louis: Mosby.)

⚠ The client with a femoral vein catheter should not sit up more than 45 degrees or lean forward, because the catheter may kink and occlude.

B. External arteriovenous shunt (see Figure 53-2)
  1. Description
     a. Two Silastic cannulas are surgically inserted into an artery and a vein in either the forearm or the leg to form an external blood path.
     b. The cannulas are connected to form a U shape. Blood flows from the client's artery through the shunt into the vein.
     c. A tube leading to the membrane compartment of the dialyzer is connected to the arterial cannula.
     d. Blood fills the membrane compartment, passes through the dialyzer, and is returned back to the client by way of a tube connected to the venous cannula.
     e. When dialysis is complete, the cannulas are clamped and reattached, reforming the U shape.
  2. Advantages
     a. The external arteriovenous shunt can be used immediately after its creation.
     b. No venipuncture is necessary for dialysis.
  3. Disadvantages
     a. Disconnection or dislodgment of the external shunt
     b. Risk of hemorrhage, infection, or clotting
     c. Potential for skin erosion around the catheter site
  4. Interventions
     a. Avoid getting the shunt wet.
     b. Wrap a dressing completely around the shunt and keep it dry and intact.
     c. Keep cannula clamps at the client's bedside or attached to the arteriovenous dressing for use in the event of accidental disconnection.

     d. Teach the client that the shunt extremity should not be used for monitoring BP, drawing blood, placing IV lines, or administering injections.
     e. Fold back the dressing to expose the shunt tubing and check for signs of hemorrhage, infection, or clotting.
     f. Monitor skin integrity around the insertion site.
     g. Auscultate for a bruit and palpate for a thrill, although a bruit may not be heard with the shunt.
     h. Notify the HCP immediately if signs of clotting, hemorrhage, or infection occur.
  5. Signs of clotting
     a. Fibrin-white flecks noted in the tubing
     b. Separation of serum and cells
     c. Thrill absent on palpation
     d. The absence of a previously heard bruit
     e. Coolness of the tubing or extremity
     f. Client complaints of a tingling sensation

C. Internal arteriovenous fistula (see Figure 53-2)
  1. Description
     a. The access of choice for the client with **CRF** requiring dialysis
     b. The fistula is created surgically by anastomosis of a large artery and a large vein in the arm.
     c. The flow of arterial blood into the venous system causes the vein to become engorged (matured or developed).
     d. Maturity takes about 1 to 2 weeks depending on the client's ability to do hand-flexing exercises such as "ball squeezing," which will help the fistula mature.
     e. The fistula is required to be mature before it can be used because the engorged vein is punctured with a large-bore needle for the dialysis procedure.

f. Subclavian or femoral catheters, **peritoneal dialysis**, or an external arteriovenous shunt can be used for dialysis while the fistula is maturing or developing.

2. Advantages
   a. Because the fistula is internal, the risk of clotting and bleeding is low.
   b. The fistula can be used indefinitely.
   c. Fistulas have a decreased incidence of infection.
   d. Once healing has occurred, no external dressing is required.
   e. The fistula allows freedom of movement.

3. Disadvantages
   a. The fistula cannot be used immediately after insertion so planning ahead for alternate access for dialysis is important.
   b. Needle insertions through the skin and tissues to the fistula are required for dialysis.
   c. Infiltration of the needles during dialysis can occur and cause hematomas.
   d. An aneurysm can form in the fistula.
   e. Congestive heart failure (CHF) can occur from the increased blood flow in the venous system.

⚠ Arterial steal syndrome can develop in a client with an internal arteriovenous fistula. In this complication, too much blood is diverted to the vein, and arterial perfusion to the hand is compromised.

D. Internal arteriovenous graft (see Figure 53-2)
   1. Description
      a. The internal graft is used primarily for chronic dialysis clients who do not have adequate blood vessels for the creation of a fistula.
      b. An artificial graft made of Gore-Tex or a bovine (cow) carotid artery is used to create an artificial vein for blood flow.
      c. The procedure involves the anastomosis of an artery to a vein using an artificial graft.
      d. The graft can be used 2 weeks after insertion.
      e. Complications of the graft include clotting, aneurysms, and infection.
   2. Advantages
      a. Because the graft is internal, the risk of clotting and bleeding is low.
      b. The graft can be used indefinitely.
      c. The graft has a decreased incidence of infection.
      d. Once healing has occurred, no external dressing is required.
      e. The graft allows freedom of movement.
   3. Disadvantages
      a. The graft cannot be used immediately after insertion.
      b. Needle insertions through the skin and tissues to the graft are required for dialysis.

c. Infiltration of the needles during dialysis can occur and cause hematomas.
d. An aneurysm can form in the graft; additionally grafts clot more frequently than **arteriovenous fistulas**.
e. **Arterial steal syndrome** can develop (too much blood is diverted to the vein, and arterial perfusion to the hand is compromised).
f. Congestive heart failure can occur from the increased blood flow in the venous system.

E. Interventions for an **arteriovenous fistula** and arteriovenous graft
   1. Teach the client that the shunt extremity should not be used for monitoring blood pressure, drawing blood, placing IV lines, or administering injections.
   2. Teach the client with an **arteriovenous fistula** hand-flexing exercises such as "ball squeezing" to promote graft maturity.
   3. Note the temperature and capillary refill of the extremity.
   4. Palpate pulses below the fistula or graft, and monitor for hand swelling as an indication of ischemia.
   5. Note the temperature and capillary refill of the extremity.
   6. Monitor for clotting.
      a. Complaints of tingling or discomfort in the extremity
      b. Inability to palpate a thrill or auscultate a bruit over the fistula or graft
   7. Monitor for **arterial steal syndrome**.
   8. Monitor for infection.
   9. Monitor lung and heart sounds for signs of CHF.
   10. Notify the HCP immediately if signs of clotting, infection, or **arterial steal syndrome** occur.

⚠ To ensure patency, palpate for a thrill or auscultate for a bruit over the fistula or graft. Notify the HCP if a thrill or bruit is absent.

VIII. COMPLICATIONS OF HEMODIALYSIS (Box 53-4)

A. Air embolus
   1. Description
      a. Introduction of air into the circulatory system
      b. Results in cardiopulmonary complications
   2. Data collection
      a. Dyspnea and tachypnea
      b. Chest pain
      c. Hypotension
      d. Reduced oxygen saturation
      e. Cyanosis
      f. Anxiety
      g. Changes in sensorium
   3. Interventions (see Priority Nursing Actions)

Box 53-4 Complications of Hemodialysis

Air embolus
Disequilibrium syndrome
Electrolyte alterations
Encephalopathy
Hemorrhage
Hepatitis
Hypotension
Sepsis
Shock

■■■ PRIORITY NURSING ACTIONS! ■■■

Actions to Take if a Client Receiving Hemodialysis Develops an Air Embolism
1. Stop the hemodialysis.
2. Turn the client on the left side, with the head down (Trendelenburg's).
3. Notify the HCP.
4. Administer oxygen.
5. Check the vital signs and pulse oximetry.
6. Document the event, actions taken, and the client's response.

Air embolism occurs when air enters the catheter system and is a complication of hemodialysis. The signs of air embolism include dyspnea, tachypnea, chest pain, hypotension, reduced oxygen saturation, cyanosis, anxiety, and changes in sensorium. Air embolism is a critical situation and if it is suspected, hemodialysis is stopped immediately and the client should be placed in a left side-lying position with the head lower than the feet. This position is used to try to prevent the air from traveling as a bolus to the lungs by trapping it in the right side of the heart. The HCP is notified immediately and oxygen is administered. Vital signs are checked, including the pulse oximetry and other prescribed interventions are done. The event, actions taken, and the client's response are documented.

References: Ignatavicius, D., & Workman, M. (2010). *Medical-surgical nursing: Patient-centered collaborative care* (6th ed., p. 231). St. Louis: Saunders; and Perry, A., & Potter, P. (2010). *Clinical nursing skills & techniques* (7th ed., p. 850). St. Louis: Mosby.

B. Disequilibrium syndrome
  1. Description
     a. A rapid change in the composition of the extracellular fluid occurs during **hemodialysis**.
     b. Solutes are removed from the blood faster than from the cerebrospinal fluid and brain; fluid is pulled into the brain, causing cerebral edema.
     c. Occurs more frequently in a new client during the initial onset of hemodialysis.
  2. Data collection
     a. Nausea and vomiting
     b. Headache

c. Hypertension
d. Restlessness and agitation
e. Muscle cramps
f. Confusion
g. Seizures
  3. Interventions
     a. Slow or stop the dialysis.
     b. Notify the HCP if signs of **disequilibrium syndrome** occur.
     c. Reduce environmental stimuli.
     d. Prepare to administer IV hypertonic saline solution, albumin, or mannitol (Osmitrol) if prescribed.
     e. Prepare to dialyze the client for a shorter period at reduced flow rates to prevent the occurrence.

C. Dialysis encephalopathy
  1. Description: aluminum toxicity from dialysate water sources containing aluminum or from ingestion of aluminum-containing antacids (phosphate binders).
  2. Data collection
     a. Progressive neurological impairment
     b. Mental cloudiness
     c. Speech disturbances
     d. Dementia
     e. Muscle incoordination
     f. Bone pain
     g. Seizures
  3. Interventions
     a. Monitor for the signs of dialysis encephalopathy.
     b. Notify the HCP if signs of **dialysis** encephalopathy occur.
     c. Administer aluminum-chelating agents as prescribed so that aluminum is released and dialyzed from the body.

IX. PERITONEAL DIALYSIS

A. Description
  1. The peritoneum acts as the dialyzing membrane (semipermeable membrane) to achieve dialysis during kidney failure.
  2. **Peritoneal dialysis (PD)** works on the principles of osmosis, diffusion and ultrafiltration; PD occurs via the transfer of fluid and solute from the bloodstream through the peritoneum into the dialysate solution.
  3. The peritoneal membrane is large and porous, allowing solutes and fluid to move via osmosis from an area of higher concentration in the body to an area of lower concentration in the dialyzing fluid.
  4. The peritoneal cavity is rich in capillaries; therefore, it provides a ready access to the blood supply.

B. Contraindications to **peritoneal dialysis**
   1. Peritonitis
   2. Recent abdominal surgery
   3. Abdominal adhesions
   4. Other gastrointestinal problems such as diverticulosis

C. Access for **peritoneal dialysis** (Figure 53-3)
   1. A siliconized rubber catheter such as a Tenckhoff catheter is surgically inserted into the client's peritoneal cavity to allow infusion of dialysis fluid.
   2. The preferred insertion site is 3 to 5 cm below the umbilicus. This area is relatively avascular and has less fascial resistance.
   3. The catheter is tunneled under the skin, through the fat and muscle tissue to the peritoneum. It is stabilized with Dacron cuffs in the muscle and under the skin.
   4. Over a period of 1 to 2 weeks after insertion, fibroblasts and blood vessels grow around the cuffs, fixing the catheter in place and providing an extra barrier against dialysate leakage and bacterial invasion.
   5. If the client is scheduled for transplant surgery, the **peritoneal dialysis** catheter may either be removed or left in place if the need for **dialysis** is suspected post-transplantation.

D. Dialysate solution
   1. Solution is sterile
   2. All dialysis solutions are prescribed by the HCP; the solution contains electrolytes and minerals and has a specific osmolarity, specific glucose concentration, and other medication additives as prescribed.
   3. The higher the glucose concentration, the greater the hypertonicity and the amount of fluid removed during a **peritoneal dialysis** exchange.
   4. Increasing the glucose concentration increases the concentration of active particles that cause osmosis, the rate of ultrafiltration, and the amount of fluid removed.
   5. If hyperkalemia is not a problem, potassium may be added to each bag of dialysate solution.
   6. Heparin is added to the dialysate solution to prevent clotting of the catheter.
   7. Prophylactic antibiotics may be added to the dialysate solution to prevent peritonitis.
   8. Insulin may be added to the dialysate solution for the client with diabetes mellitus.

E. **Peritoneal dialysis** infusion
   1. Description
      a. One infusion (fill), dwell, and drain is considered one exchange.
      b. Fill: The infusion of 1 to 2 L of dialysate as prescribed is infused by gravity into the peritoneal space, which usually takes 10 to 20 minutes.
      c. Dwell time: The amount of time that the dialysate solution remains in the peritoneal cavity is prescribed by the HCP and can last 20 to 30 minutes to 8 or more hours depending on the type of dialysis used.
      d. Drain (outflow): Fluid drains out of body by gravity into the drainage bag.
   2. Interventions before treatment
      a. Monitor the vital signs.
      b. Obtain weight.

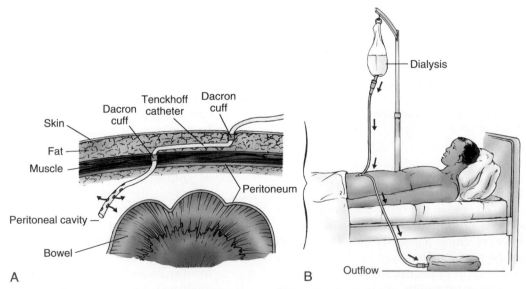

▲ **FIGURE 53-3** Manual peritoneal dialysis via an implanted abdominal catheter (Tenckhoff catheter). **A,** Implanted abdominal catheter. **B,** Dialysate inflow and outflow through implanted abdominal catheter. (From Ignatavicius, D., & Workman, M. [2010]. *Medical-surgical nursing: Patient-centered collaborative care* [6th ed.]. St. Louis: Saunders.)

c. Have the client void, if possible.

d. Monitor electrolyte and glucose levels.

3. Interventions during treatment

a. Monitor the vital signs.

b. Monitor for respiratory distress, pain, or discomfort.

c. Monitor for signs of pulmonary edema.

d. Monitor for hypotension and hypertension.

e. Monitor for malaise, nausea, and vomiting.

f. Monitor the catheter site dressing for wetness or bleeding.

g. Monitor dwell time as prescribed by the HCP.

h. Do not allow dwell time to extend beyond the HCP's order because this increases the risk for hyperglycemia.

i. Initiate outflow; turn the client from side to side if the outflow is slow to start.

j. Monitor outflow, which should be a continuous stream after the clamp is opened.

k. Monitor outflow for color and clarity.

l. Monitor intake and output accurately. If outflow is less than inflow, the difference is equal to the amount absorbed or retained by the client during dialysis and should be counted as intake.

m. An outflow greater than inflow should be reported to the HCP, as should the appearance of frank blood or cloudiness in outflow.

F. Types of **peritoneal dialysis**

1. Continuous ambulatory **peritoneal dialysis** (CAPD)

a. Closely resembles renal function because it is a continuous process.

b. Does not require a machine for the procedure.

c. Promotes client independence.

d. The client performs self-dialysis 24 hours a day, 7 days a week.

e. Four dialysis cycles are usually administered in a 24-hour period, including an overnight 8-hour dwell time.

f. Dialysate, 1.5 to 2 L is instilled into the abdomen 4 times daily and allowed to dwell as prescribed.

g. Between exchanges, the catheter is clamped; an empty bag is reconnected for outflow and a new bag of dialysate attached at each exchange time.

h. After dwell, the bag is placed lower than the insertion site so that fluid drains by gravity flow.

i. When full, the bag is changed, new dialysate is instilled into the abdomen, and the process continues.

2. Automated **peritoneal dialysis**

a. Automated dialysis requires a peritoneal cycling machine.

b. Automated dialysis can be done as intermittent **peritoneal dialysis**, continuous cycling **peritoneal dialysis**, or nightly **peritoneal dialysis**.

c. The exchanges are automated instead of manual.

X. COMPLICATIONS OF PERITONEAL DIALYSIS (Box 53-5)

⚠ Infection is a concern with peritoneal dialysis. Sites of infection are either the catheter insertion site or in the peritoneum causing peritonitis.

A. Peritonitis

1. Monitor for symptoms of peritonitis: fever, cloudy outflow, rebound abdominal tenderness, abdominal pain, general malaise, nausea, and vomiting.

2. Cloudy or opaque outflow is an early sign of peritonitis.

3. If peritonitis is suspected, obtain a culture of the outflow to determine the infective organism.

4. Administer antibiotics as prescribed.

5. Avoid infections by maintaining meticulous sterile technique when connecting and disconnecting **PD** solution bags and when caring for the catheter insertion site.

6. Prevent the catheter insertion site dressing from becoming wet during care of the client or the dialysis procedure; change the dressing if wet or soiled.

7. Follow institutional procedure for connecting and disconnecting **PD** solution bags, which may include scrubbing the connection sites with an antiseptic solution.

B. Abdominal pain

1. Peritoneal irritation during inflow commonly causes pain during the first few exchanges. The pain usually disappears after 1 to 2 weeks of dialysis treatments.

2. Warm the dialysate before administration using a special dialysate warmer pad because the cold temperature of the dialysate can cause discomfort.

Box 53-5 Complications of Peritoneal Dialysis

Abdominal pain
Bladder or bowel perforation
Insufficient outflow
Leakage around the catheter site
Peritonitis

C. Abnormal outflow characteristics indicative of complications
  1. Bloody outflow after the first few exchanges indicates vascular complications (the outflow should be clear and colorless after the initial exchanges).
  2. Brown outflow indicates bowel perforation.
  3. Urine-colored outflow indicates bladder perforation.
  4. Cloudy outflow indicates peritonitis.

D. Insufficient outflow
  1. The main cause of insufficient outflow is a full colon. Encourage a high-fiber diet (because constipation can cause inflow and outflow problems) and administer stool softeners as prescribed.
  2. Insufficient outflow may also be caused by catheter migration out of the peritoneal area. If this occurs, an x-ray will be prescribed to evaluate catheter position.
  3. Maintain the drainage bag below the client's abdomen.
  4. Check for kinks in the tubing.
  5. Check for fibrin clots in the tubing and milk the tubing to dislodge the clot as prescribed.
  6. Change the client's outflow position by turning the client to a side-lying position or ambulating the client.

E. Leakage around the catheter site
  1. Clear fluid that leaks from the catheter exit site will be noted.
  2. It takes 1 to 2 weeks after insertion of the catheter before fibroblasts and blood vessels grow into the catheter cuffs, fixing it in place and providing an extra barrier against dialysate leakage and bacterial invasion.
  3. Smaller amounts of dialysate need to be used and it may take up to 2 weeks for the client to tolerate a full 2-L exchange without leaking around the catheter site.

XI. CONTINUOUS RENAL REPLACEMENT THERAPY (CRRT)

A. Description
  1. Continuous renal replacement therapy (CRRT) provides continuous ultrafiltration of extracellular fluid and clearance of urinary toxins over a period of 8 to 24 hours; used primarily for clients in **ARF** or critically ill clients with **CRF** who cannot tolerate hemodialysis.
  2. Water, electrolytes, and other solutes are removed as the client's blood passes through a hemofilter.
  3. Because rapid shifts in fluids and electrolytes typically do not occur, hemofiltration is usually well tolerated by critically ill clients.
  4. There are five variations of CRRT, some requiring a **hemodialysis** machine whereas others rely on the client's blood pressure to power the system.

XII. KIDNEY TRANSPLANTATION

A. Description
  1. A human kidney from a compatible donor is implanted into a recipient.
  2. Kidney transplantation is performed for irreversible kidney failure; specific criteria are established for eligibility for a transplant.
  3. The recipient must take immunosuppressive medications for life.

B. Living related donors
  1. The most desirable source of kidneys for transplant is living related donors who closely match the client.
  2. Donors are screened for ABO blood group, tissue-specific antigen, human leukocyte antigen suitability, mixed lymphocyte culture index (histocompatibility), and the presence of any communicable diseases and undergo a complete medication evaluation as well as a nephrology consultation.
  3. The donor must be in excellent health with two properly functioning kidneys.
  4. The emotional well-being of the donor is determined.
  5. Complete understanding on the part of the donor of the donation process and outcome is necessary.

C. Cadaver donors
  1. Cadaver donors must meet the criteria of brain death.
  2. Cadaver donors usually need to be less than 70 years of age.
  3. Cadaver donors must have normal renal function, although "marginal" donor organs have been used with the consent of the recipient.
  4. No malignant disease outside of the central nervous system can be present.
  5. No generalized infection or communicable disease can be present.
  6. No renal trauma can be present.
  7. The potential donor must be negative for communicable diseases at the time of donation.
  8. Once cerebral death has been established for a potential donor, restoration of intravascular volume, weaning from vasopressors, and establishing diuresis are crucial; management of the donor is determined by organ bank personnel.
  9. Continuous ventilation, a normal blood pressure, and heart rate are maintained until the kidneys are surgically removed.

D. Preoperative interventions
  1. Verify the histocompatibility tests of the identical twin or family member.
  2. Administer immunosuppressive medications to the recipient as prescribed for 2 days before the transplantation, if possible.
  3. Maintain protective isolation for the recipient.

4. Verify that **hemodialysis** of the recipient was completed 24 hours before the transplant.
5. Ensure that the recipient is free of any infections.
6. Monitor renal function studies.
7. Encourage discussion of feelings of the donor and the recipient.
8. Provide psychological support to the live donor or cadaver donor family and the recipient.

E. Postoperative interventions for the recipient
1. Urine output usually begins immediately if the donor was a living donor. It is usually delayed for a few days or more with a cadaver kidney.
2. **Hemodialysis** is performed until adequate kidney function is established.
3. Monitor the vital signs, central venous pressure (CVP), and pulse oximetry for signs of complications.
4. Monitor urine output hourly. Immediately report a urine output less than 100 mL/hr.
5. Monitor IV fluids closely; for the first 12 to 24 hours, IV fluid volume includes replacement per milliliter of hourly urine output.
6. Administer prescribed diuretics and osmotic agents.
7. Monitor daily weight to evaluate fluid status.
8. Monitor daily laboratory results to evaluate renal function including hematocrit, BUN, serum creatinine levels, and urine for blood and specific gravity.
9. Position the client in the semi-Fowler's position to promote gas exchange, turning from the back to the nonoperative side.
10. Monitor indwelling urinary catheter patency. The indwelling urinary catheter remains in the bladder for 3 to 5 days to allow for anastomosis healing.
11. Note that urine is pink and bloody initially, but gradually returns to normal within several days to weeks.
12. Notify the HCP if gross hematuria and clots are noted in the urine.
13. Monitor the three-way bladder irrigation, if present, for clots; irrigate only if a HCP's prescription is present.
14. Remove the indwelling urinary catheter as soon as possible to prevent infection.
15. Maintain aseptic technique and monitor for bowel sounds and for the passage of flatus; initiate a specific diet and oral fluids as prescribed when flatus and bowel sounds return (usually, fluids, sodium, and potassium are restricted if the client is oliguric).
16. Maintain strict aseptic technique with wound care.
17. Maintain good oral hygiene, monitoring for stomatitis and bacterial and fungal infections.
18. Encourage coughing and deep-breathing exercises.
19. Administer medications as prescribed, which may include antifungal medications, antibiotics, immunosuppressive agents, and corticosteroids.
20. The client is usually ambulated after 24 hours.
21. Monitor for signs of organ rejection.
22. Promote live donor and recipient relationship.
23. Monitor both the donor and recipient for depression.
24. Provide the recipient with instructions following the kidney transplant (Box 53-6).
25. Assist the recipient to cope with the body-image disturbances that occur from long-term use of immunosuppressants.
26. Advise the recipient of available support groups.

F. Graft rejection: Except for identical twin donor and recipient, the major postoperative complication is graft rejection.
1. Data collection (Box 53-7)
2. Hyperacute rejection
   a. Hyperacute rejection occurs immediately after surgery to 48 hours postoperatively.
   b. Interventions: removal of rejected kidney
3. Acute rejection
   a. Most common type; occurs most frequently within 6 weeks postoperatively but can occur any time post-transplant.

Box 53-6 Client Instructions after Kidney Transplant

Avoid prolonged periods of sitting.
Monitor intake and output.
Recognize the signs and symptoms of infection and rejection.
Use medications as prescribed, and maintain immunosuppressive therapy for life.
Avoid contact sports.
Avoid exposure to persons with infections.
Know the signs and symptoms that require the need to contact the HCP.
Ensure follow-up care.

Box 53-7 Clinical Signs of Renal Transplant (Graft) Rejection

Fever greater than 100° F (37.7° C)
Pain or tenderness over the grafted kidney
A 2- to 3-lb weight gain in 24 hours
Edema
Hypertension
Malaise
Elevated BUN and serum creatinine
Decreased creatinine clearance
Elevated white blood cell count
Rejection indicated by ultrasound or biopsy

b. Interventions: It is potentially reversible with an increase in immunosuppression, or administering high doses of corticosteroids or monoclonal antibodies if corticosteroids are ineffective.
4. Chronic rejection
   a. Occurs slowly months to years after transplant and mimics **CRF**.
   b. Interventions: immunosuppressive medications and retransplantation if necessary.

⚠ Except for identical twin donors and recipients, the major postoperative complication after renal transplant is graft rejection.

XIII. CYSTITIS/URINARY TRACT INFECTIONS (UTI)

A. Description
1. An inflammation of the bladder from an infection, obstruction of the urethra, or other irritants (Box 53-8)
2. The most common causative organisms are *Escherichia coli, Enterobacter, Pseudomonas,* and *Serratia* species.
3. Cystitis is more common in women because women have a shorter urethra than men and the location of the urethra in the woman is close to the rectum.
4. Sexually active and pregnant women are most vulnerable to cystitis.

B. Data collection
1. Frequency and urgency
2. Burning on urination
3. Voiding in small amounts
4. Inability to void

Box 53-8 Causes of Cystitis

Allergens or irritants, such as soaps, sprays, bubble bath, and perfumed sanitary napkins
Bladder distention
Calculus
Hormonal changes, influencing alterations in vaginal flora
Indwelling urethral catheters
Invasive urinary tract procedures
Loss of bactericidal properties of prostatic secretions in the male
Microorganisms
Poor-fitting vaginal diaphragms
Sexual intercourse
Synthetic underwear and pantyhose
Urinary stasis
Use of spermicides
Wet bathing suits

---

5. Incomplete emptying of the bladder
6. Lower abdominal discomfort or back discomfort
7. Cloudy, dark, foul-smelling urine
8. Hematuria
9. Bladder spasms
10. Malaise, chills, and fever
11. Nausea and vomiting
12. WBC count greater than 100,000 cells/mm^3 on urinalysis.
13. An elevated specific gravity and pH may be noted on urinalysis.

⚠ Altered mentation is a sign of a urinary tract infection in older adults; frequency and urgency may not be specific symptoms of UTI because of urinary elimination changes that occur with aging.

C. Interventions
1. Before administering prescribed antibiotics, obtain a urine specimen for culture and sensitivity, if prescribed, to identify bacterial growth.
2. Encourage the client to increase fluids up to 3000 mL/day, especially if the client is taking a sulfonamide. Sulfonamides can form crystals in concentrated urine.
3. Administer prescribed medications, which may include analgesics, antiseptics, antispasmodics, antibiotics, and antimicrobials.
4. Maintain an acid urine pH (5.5). Instruct the client about foods to consume to maintain acidic urine.
5. Provide heat to the abdomen or sitz baths for complaints of discomfort.
6. Note that if the client is prescribed an aminoglycoside, a sulfonamide, or nitrofurantoin (Macrodantin), the actions of these medications are diminished by acidic urine.
7. Use sterile technique when inserting a urinary catheter.
8. Maintain closed urinary drainage systems for the client with an indwelling catheter and avoid elevating the urinary drainage bag above the level of the bladder.
9. Provide meticulous perineal care for the client with an indwelling catheter.
10. Discourage caffeine products such as coffee, tea, and cola.
11. Client education
    a. Avoid alcohol.
    b. Take medications as prescribed.
    c. Take antibiotics on schedule and complete the entire course of medications as prescribed, which may be 10 to 14 days.
    d. Repeat the urine culture after treatment.
    e. Prevent recurrence of cystitis (Box 53-9).

XIV. UROSEPSIS

A. Description
1. Urosepsis is a gram-negative bacteremia originating in the urinary tract.
2. The most common responsible organism is *Escherichia coli*.
3. The most common cause is infection from an indwelling urinary catheter or an untreated UTI in a client who is immunocompromised.
4. The major problem is the ability of this bacterium to develop resistant strains.
5. Urosepsis can lead to septic shock if not treated aggressively.

B. Data collection: Fever is the most common and earliest manifestation.

C. Interventions
1. Obtain a urine specimen for urine culture and sensitivity before administering antibiotics.
2. Administer IV antibiotics as prescribed, usually until the client has been afebrile for 3 to 5 days.
3. Administer oral antibiotics as prescribed after the 3- to 5-day afebrile period.

XV. URETHRITIS

A. Description
1. An inflammation of the urethra commonly associated with sexually transmitted infections and may occur with cystitis.
2. In men, urethritis most often is caused by gonorrhea or chlamydial infection.
3. In women, urethritis is most often caused by feminine hygiene sprays, perfumed toilet paper or sanitary napkins, spermicidal jelly, UTIs, or changes in the vaginal mucosal lining.

B. Data collection
1. Pain or burning on urination
2. Frequency and urgency
3. Nocturia
4. Difficulty voiding

Box 53-9 Teaching for Prevention of Cystitis

Use good perineal care, wiping front to back.
Avoid bubble baths, tub baths, and vaginal deodorants or sprays.
Void every 2 to 3 hours.
Wear cotton pants and avoid wearing tight clothes or panty-hose with slacks.
Avoid sitting in a wet bathing suit for prolonged periods.
If pregnant, void every 2 hours.
If menopausal, use estrogen vaginal creams to restore pH.
Use water-soluble lubricants for intercourse, especially after menopause.
Void and drink a glass of water after intercourse.

---

5. Males may have clear to mucopurulent discharge from the penis.
6. Females may have lower abdominal discomfort.

C. Interventions
1. Encourage fluid intake.
2. Prepare the client for testing to determine if a sexually transmitted infection (STI) is present.
3. Administer antibiotics as prescribed.
4. Instruct the client in the administration of sitz or tub baths.
5. If stricture occurs, prepare the client for dilation of the urethra and instillation of an antiseptic solution.
6. Instruct the female client to avoid the use of perfumed toilet paper or sanitary napkins and feminine hygiene sprays.
7. Instruct the client to avoid intercourse until the symptoms subside or treatment of the STI is complete.
8. Instruct the client on STIs if this is the cause.
   a. Prevent STIs by the use of latex condoms or abstinence.
   b. All sexual partners during the 30 days before diagnosis with chlamydial infection should be notified, examined, and treated if indicated.
   c. Chlamydial infection often coexists with gonorrhea; diagnostic testing is done for both STIs.
   d. Treatment for STIs includes antibiotics, as prescribed, to treat the causative organism.
   e. The most serious complication of chlamydial infection is sterility.
   f. Follow-up culture may be requested in 4 to 7 days to evaluate the effectiveness of medications.

XVI. URETERITIS

A. Ureteritis
1. Description: an inflammation of the ureter commonly associated with bacterial or viral infections and pyelonephritis
2. Data collection
   a. Dysuria
   b. Frequent urination
   c. Clear to mucopurulent penile discharge in males
3. Interventions
   a. Treatment includes identifying and treating the underlying cause and providing symptomatic relief.
   b. Administer metronidazole (Flagyl) or clotrimazole (Mycelex) as prescribed for treating *Trichomonas* infection.
   c. Administer nystatin (Mycostatin) or fluconazole (Diflucan) as prescribed for treating monilial infections.
   d. Doxycycline (Vibramycin) or azithromycin (Zithromax) may be prescribed for treating chlamydial infections.

XVII. PYELONEPHRITIS

A. Description
1. An inflammation of the renal pelvis and the parenchyma commonly caused by bacterial invasion
2. Acute pyelonephritis often occurs after bacterial contamination of the urethra or an invasive procedure of the urinary tract.
3. Chronic pyelonephritis most commonly occurs after chronic urinary flow obstruction with reflux.
4. *Escherichia coli* is the most common bacterial causative organism.

B. Acute pyelonephritis
1. Acute pyelonephritis occurs as a new infection or recurs as a relapse of a previous infection.
2. It can progress to bacteremia or chronic pyelonephritis.
3. Data collection
   a. Fever and chills
   b. Nausea
   c. Flank pain on the affected side
   d. Costovertebral angle tenderness
   e. Headache
   f. Dysuria
   g. Frequency and urgency
   h. Cloudy, bloody, or foul-smelling urine
   i. Increased white blood cells in the urine

C. Chronic pyelonephritis
1. A slow, progressive disease usually associated with recurrent acute attacks
2. Causes contraction of the kidney and dysfunctioning of the nephrons, which are replaced by scar tissue
3. Causes the ureter to become fibrotic and narrowed by strictures
4. Can lead to **renal failure**
5. Data collection
   a. Frequently diagnosed incidentally when a client is being evaluated for hypertension
   b. Poor urine-concentrating ability
   c. Pyuria
   d. **Azotemia**
   e. Proteinuria

D. Interventions
1. Monitor the vital signs, especially for elevated temperature.
2. Encourage fluid intake up to 3000 mL/day to reduce fever and prevent dehydration.
3. Monitor intake and output (ensure that output is a minimum of 1500 mL/24 hr).
4. Monitor weight.
5. Encourage adequate rest.
6. Instruct the client in a high-calorie, low-protein diet.
7. Provide warm, moist compresses to the flank area to help relieve pain.
8. Encourage the client to take warm baths for pain relief.
9. Administer analgesics, antipyretics, antibiotics, urinary antiseptics, and antiemetics as prescribed.
10. Monitor for signs of **renal failure**.
11. Encourage follow-up urine culture.

XVIII. GLOMERULONEPHRITIS (refer to Chapter 35 for information on this disorder)

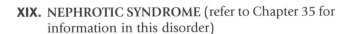

XIX. NEPHROTIC SYNDROME (refer to Chapter 35 for information in this disorder)

XX. POLYCYSTIC KIDNEY DISEASE

A. Description
1. A cystic formation and hypertrophy of the kidneys, which leads to cystic rupture, infection, formation of scar tissue, and damaged nephrons
2. There is no specific treatment to arrest the progress of the destructive cysts.
3. The ultimate result of this disease is **renal failure**.

B. Types
1. Infantile polycystic disease: an inherited autosomal recessive trait that results in the death of the infant within a few months after birth
2. Adult polycystic disease: an autosomal dominant trait that manifests between 30 and 40 years of age and results in end-stage renal disease

C. Data collection
1. Often asymptomatic before the ages of 30 to 40 years
2. Flank, lumbar, or abdominal pain that worsens with activity and is relieved when lying down
3. Fever and chills
4. Recurrent urinary tract infections
5. Hematuria, proteinuria, and pyuria
6. Calculi
7. Hypertension
8. Palpable abdominal masses and enlarged kidneys

D. Interventions
1. Monitor for gross hematuria, which indicates cyst rupture.
2. Increase sodium and water intake because sodium loss rather than retention occurs.
3. Provide bedrest if ruptured cysts and bleeding occur.
4. Prepare the client for percutaneous cyst puncture for relief of obstruction or draining an abscess.
5. Administer antihypertensives as prescribed.
6. Prevent and/or treat urinary tract infections.

7. Prepare the client for dialysis or renal transplantation.
8. Encourage the client to seek genetic counseling.
9. Provide psychological support to the client and family.
10. Provide psychosocial support and genetic counseling for family who may want to donate a kidney.

XXI. HYDRONEPHROSIS (Figure 53-4)

A. Description
1. The distention of the renal pelvis and calices caused by an obstruction of normal urine flow
2. The urine becomes trapped proximal to the obstruction.
3. The causes include calculus, tumors, scar tissue, ureter obstructions, and hypertrophy of the prostate.

B. Data collection
1. Hypertension
2. Headache
3. Colicky or dull flank pain that radiates to the groin

C. Interventions
1. Monitor the vital signs frequently.
2. Monitor for fluid and electrolyte imbalances, including dehydration after the obstruction is relieved.

▲ **FIGURE 53-4** Hydronephrosis and hydroureter. (From Ignatavicius, D., & Workman, M. [2010]. *Medical-surgical nursing: Patient-centered collaborative care* [6th ed.]. St. Louis: Saunders.)

3. Monitor for diuresis, which can lead to fluid depletion.
4. Monitor weight daily.
5. Monitor urine for specific gravity, albumin, and glucose levels.
6. Administer fluid replacement as prescribed.
7. Prepare the client for insertion of a nephrostomy tube or a surgical procedure to relieve the obstruction if prescribed.

XXII. RENAL CALCULI

A. Description
1. Calculi are stones that can form anywhere in the urinary tract; however, the most frequent site is the kidneys.
2. Problems resulting from calculi are pain, obstruction, tissue trauma, secondary hemorrhage, and infection.
3. Stone location can be determined through a kidneys, ureters, and bladder film; intravenous pyelogram; computed tomography scan; and renal ultrasonography.
4. A stone analysis will be performed after passage to determine the type of stone and assist in determining treatment.
5. **Urolithiasis** refers to the formation of urinary calculi; these form in the ureters.
6. **Nephrolithiasis** refers to the formation of kidney calculi; these form in the renal parenchyma.
7. When a calculus occludes the ureter and blocks the flow of urine, the ureter dilates, producing hydroureter (see Figure 53-4).
8. If the obstruction is not removed, urinary stasis results in infection, impairment of renal function on the side of the blockage, hydronephrosis (see Figure 53-4), and irreversible kidney damage.

B. Causes
1. Family history of stone formation
2. Diet high in calcium, vitamin D, milk, protein, oxalate, purines, or alkali
3. Obstruction and urinary stasis
4. Dehydration
5. Use of diuretics, which can cause volume depletion
6. UTIs and prolonged urinary catheterization
7. Immobilization
8. Hypercalcemia and hyperparathyroidism
9. Elevated uric acid level, such as in gout

C. Data collection
1. Renal colic, which originates in the lumbar region and radiates around the side and down toward the testicle in men and to the bladder in women
2. Ureteral colic, which radiates toward the genitalia and thigh

3. Sudden onset of sharp, severe pain
4. Dull, aching pain in the kidney
5. Nausea and vomiting, pallor, and diaphoresis during acute pain
6. Urinary frequency with alternating retention
7. Signs of a urinary tract infection
8. Low-grade fever
9. High numbers of red blood cells, white blood cells, and bacteria in the urinalysis
10. Hematuria

D. Interventions
1. Monitor the vital signs, especially the temperature, for signs of infection.
2. Monitor intake and output.
3. Monitor for fever, chills, and infection.
4. Monitor for nausea, vomiting, and diarrhea.
5. Encourage fluid intake up to 3000 mL/day, unless contraindicated, to facilitate the passage of the stone and prevent infection.
6. Administer fluids intravenously as prescribed if unable to take fluids orally or in adequate amounts to increase the flow of urine and facilitate the passage of the stone.
7. Provide warm baths and heat to the flank area (massage therapy should be avoided).
8. Administer analgesics at regularly scheduled intervals as prescribed to relieve pain.
9. Monitor the client's response to pain medication.
10. Assist the client in performing relaxation techniques to assist in relieving pain.
11. Encourage client ambulation if stable to promote the passage of the stone.
12. Turn and reposition the immobilized client to promote the passage of the stone.
13. Instruct the client in the diet specific to the stone composition if prescribed.
14. Prepare the client for surgical procedures if prescribed.

⚠ For the client with renal calculi, strain all urine for the presence of stones and send the stones to the laboratory for analysis.

E. Stone composition
1. A special diet, such as an alkaline ash or acid ash, may be prescribed, depending on the HCP's preference
2. Calcium phosphate stones
   a. Caused by supersaturation of urine with calcium and phosphate
   b. Diet includes acid-ash foods because calcium stones are alkaline.
   c. Dietary prescription may include decreasing intake of foods high in calcium and phosphate to reduce urinary calcium content and avoiding excess vitamin D intake to prevent stones from forming.
   d. Medications prescribed for calcium stones may include phosphates, thiazide diuretics, and allopurinol (Zyloprim).
3. Calcium oxalate stones
   a. Caused by supersaturation of urine with calcium and oxalate
   b. Diet includes acid-ash foods because calcium stones are alkaline.
   c. Dietary prescription may include decreasing the intake of foods high in calcium and avoiding oxalate food sources to reduce urinary oxalate content and stone formation.
   d. Oxalate-rich food sources include tea, almonds, cashews, chocolate, cocoa, beans, spinach, and rhubarb.
   e. Allopurinol (Zyloprim), pyridoxine (vitamin B_6), or magnesium oxide may be prescribed for clients with oxalate stones.
4. Struvite stones
   a. Also called triple phosphate stones; composed of magnesium and ammonium phosphate
   b. Caused by urea-splitting bacteria and tend to form in alkaline urine
   c. Diet includes acid-ash foods and includes limiting high-phosphate foods such as dairy products, red and organ meats, and whole grains to reduce urinary phosphate content
   d. Treatment includes controlling infection with antibiotics (long-term antibiotic use may be prescribed).
5. Uric acid stones
   a. Caused by excess dietary purine or gout
   b. Tend to form in acidic urine
   c. Dietary prescription to reduce urinary purine content may include alkaline-ash foods and decreased intake of high purine foods such as organ meats, gravies, red wines, and sardines.
   d. Allopurinol (Zyloprim) may be prescribed to lower uric acid levels
6. Cystine stones
   a. Caused by cystine crystal formation and tend to form in acidic urine
   b. Diet includes alkaline-ash foods, and dietary prescription may also include a low intake of methionine, an essential amino acid that forms cystine. The client would be instructed to avoid meat, milk, cheese, and eggs.
   c. Dietary measures also focus on encouraging fluid intake up to 3 L/day, unless contraindicated, to help dilute the urine and prevent cystine crystals from forming.
   d. Long-term antibiotic use may be prescribed for clients with cystine stones.

XXIII. TREATMENT OPTIONS FOR RENAL CALCULI (Figure 53-5)

A. Cystoscopy
1. Cystoscopy may be done for stones located in the bladder or lower ureter.
2. No incision is made.
3. One or two ureteral catheters are inserted past the stone. The stone may be manipulated and dislodged by the procedure and the catheters may guide the stones mechanically downward as they are removed.
4. The catheters are left in place for 24 hours to drain the urine trapped proximal to the stone and dilate the ureter.
5. A continuous chemical irrigation may be prescribed to dissolve the stone.

B. Extracorporeal shock wave lithotripsy (ESWL)
1. A noninvasive mechanical procedure for breaking up stones located in the kidney or upper ureter so that they can pass spontaneously or be removed by other methods
2. No incision is made and no drains are placed. A stent may be placed to promote passing stone fragments.
3. Fluoroscopy is used to visualize the stone, and ultrasonic waves are delivered to the areas of the stone to disintegrate it.
4. The stones are passed in the urine within a few days.
5. Preprocedure: Maintain the client on an NPO status for 8 hours before the procedure.
6. Postprocedure
   a. Monitor the vital signs, especially for hypotension and tachycardia, which could indicate bleeding.
   b. Monitor intake and output.
   c. Monitor for bleeding.
   d. Monitor for pain and signs of urinary obstruction.
   e. Instruct the client that the ureteral stent placed to promote passage of the stone is usually removed in 1 to 2 weeks.
   f. Instruct the client to increase fluid intake to flush out the stone fragments.
   g. Inform the client that ambulation is important.

C. Percutaneous lithotripsy
1. Performed for stones in the bladder, ureter, or kidney
2. An invasive procedure in which a guide is inserted under fluoroscopy near the area of the stone; an ultrasonic wave is aimed at the stone to break it into fragments.
3. Percutaneous lithotripsy may be performed via cystoscopy or nephroscopy.
4. No incision is required for cystoscopy; a small flank incision is needed for nephroscopy.
5. The client may possibly have a bladder indwelling catheter.
6. A nephrostomy tube may be placed to administer chemical irrigations to break up the stone. The nephrostomy tube may remain in place for 1 to 5 days.
7. Encourage the client to drink 3000 to 4000 mL of fluid/day after the procedure.
8. Monitor for and instruct the client to monitor for complications of infection, hemorrhage, and extravasation of fluid into the retroperitoneal cavity.

D. Ureterolithotomy
1. An open surgical procedure is performed if lithotripsy is not effective for removal of a stone in the ureter.

PROXIMAL URETER
• ESWL
• Retrograde ureteroscopy
• Antegrade nephrostoureterolithotomy
• Stenting alone
• Percutaneous ureterolithotomy or nephrolithotomy

DISTAL URETER
• ESWL/ureteroscopy
• Antegrade nephrostoureterolithotomy
• Stenting alone
• Open ureterolithotomy

MIDURETER
• Retrograde ureteroscopy
• ESWL
• Antegrade nephrostoureterolithotomy
• Open ureterolithotomy

▲ **FIGURE 53-5** Treatment options for ureteral stones. ESWL, Extracorporeal shockwave lithotripsy. (From Ignatavicius, D., & Workman, M. [2010]. *Medical-surgical nursing: Patient-centered collaborative care* [6th ed.]. St. Louis: Saunders. Adapted from Singal, R. K., & Denstedt, J. D. [1997]. Contemporary management of ureteral stones. *Urologic Clinics of North America, 24*[1], 59–70.)

2. An incision is made through the lower abdomen or flank and then into the ureter to remove the stone.
3. The client may have a Penrose drain, a ureteral stent catheter, and an indwelling bladder catheter.

E. Pyelolithotomy and nephrolithotomy
1. Pyelolithotomy is an incision into the renal pelvis to remove a stone. A large flank incision is required and the client may have a Penrose drain and an indwelling bladder catheter.
2. Nephrolithotomy is an incision into the kidney made to remove a stone. A large flank incision is required and the client may have a nephrostomy tube and an indwelling bladder catheter.

F. Partial or total nephrectomy
1. Performed for extensive kidney damage, renal infection, severe obstruction from stones or tumors, and the prevention of stone recurrence
2. Postoperative interventions
   a. The plan of care depends on the incision location and the type of drainage tubes present.
   b. Monitor the incision, particularly if a Penrose drain is in place, because it will drain large amounts of urine.
   c. Protect the skin from urinary drainage, changing dressings frequently if necessary.
   d. Place an ostomy pouch over the Penrose drain to protect the skin if urinary drainage is excessive.
   e. Monitor the nephrostomy tube, which may be attached to a drainage bag, for a continuous flow of urine.
   f. Do not irrigate the nephrotomy tube or bladder catheter unless specifically prescribed.
   g. Monitor the indwelling bladder (indwelling urinary catheter) catheter for drainage.
   h. Encourage fluid intake to ensure a urine output of 2500 to 3000 mL or more/day.
   i. Measure intake and output accurately.
   j. If a stone was removed, determine its composition from laboratory analysis.

XXIV. KIDNEY TUMORS

A. Description
1. Kidney tumors may be benign or malignant, bilateral or unilateral.
2. Common sites of metastasis include bone, lungs, liver, spleen, or other kidney.
3. The exact cause of renal carcinoma is unknown.

B. Data collection for those with advanced disease
1. Dull flank pain
2. Palpable renal mass
3. Painless gross hematuria

C. Radical nephrectomy
1. Description
   a. The surgical removal of the entire kidney, adjacent adrenal gland, and renal artery and vein
   b. Radiation therapy and possibly chemotherapy may follow radical nephrectomy.
   c. Before surgery, radiation may be used to embolize (occlude) the arteries supplying the kidney to reduce bleeding during nephrectomy.
2. Postoperative interventions
   a. Monitor the vital signs for indicators of bleeding (hypotension and tachycardia).
   b. Monitor for abdominal distention, decreases in urinary output, and alterations in level of consciousness as additional signs indicative of bleeding. Check the client's bed linens for bleeding.
   c. Monitor for signs of adrenal insufficiency, which include a large urinary output followed by hypotension and subsequent **oliguria**.
   d. Administer fluids and packed red blood cells intravenously as prescribed.
   e. Monitor intake and output and daily weight.
   f. Monitor for a urinary output of 30 to 50 mL/hour to ensure adequate renal function.
   g. Monitor urine specific gravity.
   h. Maintain a semi-Fowler's position.
   i. Monitor for signs of respiratory complications related to surgery; encourage coughing and deep-breathing exercises.
   j. Monitor for passing of flatus and bowel sounds (lack of flatus and bowel sounds can indicate paralytic ileus).
   k. Apply antiembolism stockings as prescribed.
   l. If a nephrostomy tube is in place, do not irrigate (unless specifically prescribed) or manipulate the tube.
   m. Administer pain medications as prescribed.

XXV. EPIDIDYMITIS

A. Description
1. An acute or chronic inflammation of the epididymis that occurs as a result of a UTI, STI, or prostatitis, or from long-term use of an indwelling urinary catheter.
2. The infective organism travels upward through the urethra and ejaculatory duct and along the vas deferens to the epididymis.

B. Data collection
1. Scrotal pain
2. Groin pain
3. Swelling in the scrotum and groin
4. Pus and bacteria in the urine
5. Fever and chills
6. Abscess development

C. Interventions
 1. Encourage fluid intake.
 2. Encourage bedrest with the scrotum elevated to prevent traction on the spermatic cord, facilitate drainage, and relieve pain.
 3. Instruct the client in the intermittent application of cold compresses to the scrotum.
 4. Instruct the client in the use of tub or sitz baths.
 5. Instruct the client in the administration of antibiotics for self and sexual partner if the cause is chlamydial or gonorrheal infection.
 6. Instruct the client to avoid lifting and straining and sexual contact until the infection subsides.
 7. Instruct the client to limit the force of the stream because organisms can be forced into the vas deferens and epididymis from strain or pressure during voiding.
 8. Teach the client that condom use can help prevent urethritis and epididymitis.
 9. Teach the client measures to prevent UTI or STI recurrence.

XXVI. PROSTATITIS

A. Description
 1. Inflammation of the prostate gland commonly caused by an infectious agent; may be acute or chronic.
 2. The bacterial type occurs as a result of the organism reaching the prostate via the urethra, bladder, bloodstream, or lymphatic channels.
 3. The abacterial type usually occurs after a viral illness or a decrease in sexual activity.
B. Data collection
 1. Bacterial prostatitis
    a. Client becomes acutely ill
    b. Fever and chills
    c. Frequency and urgency of urination; dysuria
    d. Perineal and low back pain
    e. Urethral discharge
    f. Prostate is tender, indurated, and warm to touch
    g. Urethral discharge on palpation of prostate
    h. White blood cells found in prostatic secretions
    i. Urine culture is usually positive for gram negative bacteria, especially after prostate massage.
 2. Abacterial prostatitis
    a. Backache
    b. Dysuria
    c. Perineal pain
    d. Frequency
    e. Hematuria
    f. Irregularly enlarged, firm, and tender prostate
C. Interventions
 1. Encourage adequate fluid intake.
 2. Instruct the client in the use of tub or sitz baths to promote comfort.

 3. Administer antibiotics, analgesics, antispasmodics, and stool softeners as prescribed.
 4. Inform the client of activities to drain the prostate, such as intercourse, masturbation, and prostatic massage.
 5. Instruct the client to avoid spicy foods, coffee, alcohol, prolonged automobile rides, and sexual intercourse during an acute inflammation.

XXVII. BENIGN PROSTATIC HYPERTROPHY OR HYPERPLASIA (BPH)

A. Description
 1. A slow enlargement of the prostate gland, with hypertrophy and hyperplasia of normal tissue
 2. Enlargement compresses the urethra, resulting in partial or complete obstruction.
 3. Usually occurs in men older than 50 years
 4. Possible causes include stimulation from excessive dihydroxytestosterone, estrogen, or local growth hormone.
B. Data collection
 1. Diminished size and force of urinary stream (early sign of BPH)
 2. Urinary urgency and frequency
 3. Nocturia
 4. Inability to start (hesitancy) or continue a urinary stream
 5. Feelings of incomplete bladder emptying
 6. Postvoid dribbling from overflow incontinence (later sign)
 7. Urinary retention and bladder distention
 8. Hematuria
 9. Urinary stasis
 10. Dysuria and bladder pain
 11. UTIs
C. Interventions
 1. Encourage fluid intake of up to 2000 to 3000 mL/day unless contraindicated.
 2. Prepare for urinary catheterization to drain the bladder and prevent distention.
 3. Avoid administering medications that cause urinary retention, such as anticholinergics, antihistamines, decongestants, and antidepressants.
 4. Administer medications as prescribed to shrink the prostate gland and improve urine flow.
 5. Administer medications as prescribed to relax prostatic smooth muscle and improve urine flow.
 6. Instruct the client to decrease intake of caffeine and artificial sweeteners and limit spicy or acidic foods.
 7. Instruct the client to follow a timed voiding schedule.
 8. Prepare the client for surgery or invasive procedures as prescribed (Box 53-10).
D. Surgical interventions and postoperative care (see Chapter 43)

Box 53-10 Surgical and Invasive Procedures for Prostatic Hyperplasia

Transurethral resection of the prostate (TURP): Removal of benign prostatic tissue surrounding the urethra with use of a resectoscope introduced through the urethra; there is little risk of impotence and is most commonly used for benign prostatic hypertrophy (BPH)

Transurethral incision of the prostate (TUIP): Removal of prostatic tissue through an incision made in the bladder neck

Transurethral microwave thermotherapy: Application of heat to destroy the hypertrophied tissue

Transurethral needle ablation of the prostate (TUNA): Placement of interstitial radiofrequency needles through the urethra and into the lateral lobes of the prostate, causing heat-induced coagulation necrosis of the prostate for treating BPH

Laser prostatectomy: Ablation of the enlarged prostate using laser instead of radiofrequency waves

Transurethral electrovaporization of the prostate: Placement of a special metal instrument that emits a high-frequency electrical current that cuts and vaporizes excess tissue and seals the remaining tissue to prevent bleeding; especially useful for men on anticoagulants and those at risk for complications

Perineal prostatectomy: Removal of prostatic tissue (may be performed for prostatic cancer) low in the pelvic region through an incision between the scrotum and rectum; impotence and incontinence usually result

Retropubic prostatectomy: Removal of hypertrophied prostatic tissue high in the pelvic region through a low abdominal incision; the bladder is not incised

Suprapubic prostatectomy: Removal of prostatic tissue mass through a low midline incision; an incision into the bladder and urethral mucosa to the anterior aspect of the prostate is made

Urethral stents: Application of stents or coils in the urethra where it is narrowed by the prostate

---

XXVIII. BLADDER CANCER (see Chapter 43)

XXIX. BLADDER TRAUMA

A. Description
1. Occurs after a blunt or penetrating injury to the lower abdomen
2. Penetrating wounds occur as a result of a stabbing, gunshot wound, or other objects piercing the abdominal wall.
3. A fractured pelvis that results in bone fragments puncturing the bladder is a common cause of bladder trauma.
4. Blunt trauma causes compression of the abdominal wall and the bladder.

B. Data collection
1. **Anuria**
2. Hematuria
3. Pain below the level of the umbilicus; can radiate to the shoulders
4. Nausea and vomiting

C. Interventions
1. Monitor the vital signs.
2. Monitor for hematuria, bleeding, and signs of shock.
3. Promote bedrest.
4. Monitor the pain level.
5. If blood is seen at the meatus, avoid urinary catheterization until a retrograde urethrogram can be performed.
6. Prepare the client for insertion of a suprapubic catheter to aid in urinary drainage if prescribed.
7. Prepare the client for surgical repair of the laceration if prescribed.

MORE QUESTIONS ON EVOLVE!

Practice Questions

546. A nurse is caring for the client with epididymitis. The nurse understands that which treatment modality could increase swelling in the affected area?
1. Bedrest
2. Sitz bath
3. Heating pad
4. Scrotal elevation

547. A client has epididymitis as a complication of urinary tract infection (UTI). The nurse is giving the client instructions to prevent a recurrence. The nurse determines that the client needs further instruction if the client states the intention to:
1. Drink increased amounts of fluids.
2. Limit the force of the stream during voiding.
3. Continue to take antibiotics until all symptoms are gone.
4. Use condoms to eliminate risk from chlamydia and gonorrhea.

548. A nurse is collecting data from a client who has had benign prostatic hyperplasia (BPH) in the past. To determine if the client is currently experiencing exacerbation of BPH, the nurse asks the client about the presence of which early symptom?
1. Nocturia
2. Urinary retention
3. Urge incontinence
4. Decreased force in the stream of urine

549. A client newly diagnosed with chronic renal failure has recently begun hemodialysis. Knowing that the client is at risk for disequilibrium syndrome, the nurse monitors the client during dialysis for:
1. Hypertension, tachycardia, and fever
2. Hypotension, bradycardia, and hypothermia
3. Restlessness, irritability, and generalized weakness
4. Headache, deteriorating level of consciousness, and twitching

550. A client with chronic renal failure has been on dialysis for 3 years. The client is receiving the usual combination of medications for the disease, including aluminum hydroxide as a phosphate-binding agent. The client now has mental cloudiness, dementia, and complaints of bone pain. The nurse interprets that these data are compatible with:
1. Advancing uremia
2. Phosphate overdose
3. Folic acid deficiency
4. Aluminum intoxication

551. A hemodialysis client with a left arm fistula is at risk for arterial steal syndrome. The nurse monitors this client for which manifestation of this disorder?
1. Warmth, redness, and pain in the left hand
2. Aching pain, pallor, and edema of the left arm
3. Edema and purpura of the left arm
4. Pallor, diminished pulse, and pain in the left hand

552. A nurse is reviewing the medical record of a client with a diagnosis of pyelonephritis. Which disorder, if noted on the client's record, would the nurse identify as a risk factor for this disorder?
1. Hypoglycemia
2. Diabetes mellitus
3. Coronary artery disease
4. Orthostatic hypotension

553. A nurse is reviewing the client's record and notes that the health care provider has documented that the client has a renal disorder. On review of the laboratory results, the nurse would most likely expect to note which of the following?
1. Decreased hemoglobin level
2. Decreased red blood cell (RBC) count
3. Decreased white blood cell (WBC) count
4. Elevated blood urea nitrogen (BUN) level

554. A client is scheduled for intravenous pyelography (IVP). Before the test, the priority nursing action would be to:
1. Restrict fluids.

2. Administer a sedative.
3. Determine a history of allergies.
4. Administer an oral preparation of radiopaque dye.

555. After a renal biopsy, the client complains of pain at the biopsy site, which radiates to the front of the abdomen. Based on this complaint, the nurse further monitors the client for:
1. Bleeding
2. Infection
3. Renal colic
4. Normal, expected pain

556. A nurse is monitoring an older client suspected of having a urinary tract infection (UTI) for signs of the infection. The nurse would be alert to the presence of:
1. Fever
2. Urgency
3. Confusion
4. Frequency

557. A nurse is collecting data on a newly admitted client with a diagnosis of bladder cancer. While collecting data on this client the nurse would most likely expect to note:
1. Urgency
2. Frequency
3. Hematuria
4. Burning on urination

558. A client with benign prostatic hypertrophy (BPH) undergoes a transurethral resection of the prostate (TURP) and is receiving continuous bladder irrigations postoperatively. The nurse monitors the client for signs of transurethral resection (TUR) syndrome, including:
1. Tachycardia and diarrhea
2. Bradycardia and confusion
3. Increased urinary output and anemia
4. Decreased urinary output and bladder spasms

559. A client with prostatitis resulting from kidney infection has received instructions on management of the condition at home and prevention of recurrence. The nurse determines that the client understood the instructions if the client has verbalized that he will:
1. Stop antibiotic therapy when pain subsides.
2. Exercise as much as possible to stimulate circulation.
3. Use warm sitz baths and analgesics to increase comfort.
4. Keep fluid intake to a minimum to decrease the need to void.

❖ **560.** The nurse monitoring a client receiving peritoneal dialysis notes that the client's outflow is less than the inflow. The nurse should take which actions? **Select all that apply.**

❏ 1. Contact the health care provider (HCP).
❏ 2. Check the level of the drainage bag.
❏ 3. Reposition the client to his or her side.
❏ 4. Place the client in good body alignment.
❏ 5. Check the peritoneal dialysis system for kinks.
❏ 6. Increase the flow rate of the peritoneal dialysis solution.

ANSWERS

546. 3

Rationale: Common interventions used in the treatment of epididymitis include bedrest, elevation of the scrotum, ice packs, sitz baths, analgesics, and antibiotics. A heating pad would not be used because direct application of heat could increase blood flow to the area and increase the swelling.

Test-Taking Strategy: Note the strategic words "could increase swelling." Eliminate options 1 and 4 because they are obviously the most helpful in the care of the client. Note that both remaining options address the application of heat to the client. A sitz bath provides heat that is moist and soothing. Knowing that direct heat may increase inflammation in tissue that is already at risk will guide you to option 3 as the item that could increase swelling. Review care of the client with epididymitis if you had difficulty with this question.

Level of Cognitive Ability: Understanding
Client Needs: Physiological Integrity
Integrated Process: Nursing Process/Implementation
Content Area: Adult Health/Renal
Reference: Christensen, Kockrow, p. 584. 2011. *Adult health nursing.*

547. 3

Rationale: The client who experiences epididymitis from UTI should increase intake of fluids to flush the urinary system. Because organisms can be forced into the vas deferens and epididymis from strain or pressure during voiding, the client should limit the force of the stream. Condom use can help prevent urethritis and epididymitis from sexually transmitted infections. Antibiotics are always taken until the full course of therapy is completed.

Test-Taking Strategy: Note the strategic words "needs further instruction." These words indicate a negative event query and the need to select the incorrect client statement. Because option 1 is consistent with good practices in the prevention of UTI, this option can be eliminated first. From the remaining options, it is necessary to know that the force of stream should be limited to prevent backflow into the epididymis, and that condoms are helpful in preventing this disorder from occurring as a complication of a sexually transmitted infection. Remember that antibiotics are not stopped when symptoms subside but must be taken until the full course of therapy is completed. Review care of the client with epididymitis if you had difficulty with this question.

Level of Cognitive Ability: Evaluating
Client Needs: Physiological Integrity
Integrated Process: Teaching and Learning
Content Area: Adult Health/Renal
Reference: Ignatavicius, Workman, p. 1734. 2010.
Lewis, Dirksen, Heitkemper, Bucher, Camera, p. 1395. 2011.

548. 4

Rationale: Decreased force in the stream of urine is an early sign of BPH. The stream later becomes weak and dribbling. The client may then develop hematuria, frequency, urgency, urge incontinence, and nocturia. If untreated, complete obstruction and urinary retention can occur.

Test-Taking Strategy: Note the strategic words "early symptom." Option 2 identifies the most severe symptom and therefore is eliminated first. From the remaining options, focusing on the strategic words and recalling the pathophysiology related to BPH will direct you to option 4. Review the signs of benign prostatic hypertrophy if you had difficulty with this question.

Level of Cognitive Ability: Understanding
Client Needs: Physiological Integrity
Integrated Process: Nursing Process/Data Collection
Content Area: Adult Health/Renal
Reference: Linton, p. 1137. 2012.

549. 4

Rationale: Disequilibrium syndrome is characterized by headache, mental confusion, decreasing level of consciousness, nausea and vomiting, twitching, and possible seizure activity. It is caused by rapid removal of solutes from the body during hemodialysis. At the same time, the blood-brain barrier interferes with the efficient removal of wastes from brain tissue. As a result, water goes into cerebral cells because of the osmotic gradient, causing brain swelling and onset of symptoms. It most often occurs in clients who are new to dialysis and is prevented by dialyzing for shorter times or at reduced blood flow rates.

Test-Taking Strategy: Use the process of elimination. Noting the relation between the words "disequilibrium syndrome" and the signs in option 4 will direct you to this option. Review this syndrome if you had difficulty with this question.

Level of Cognitive Ability: Analyzing
Client Needs: Physiological Integrity
Integrated Process: Nursing Process/Data Collection
Content Area: Adult Health/Renal
Reference: Ignatavicius, Workman, p. 1626. 2010.

550. 4

Rationale: Aluminum intoxication may occur when there is accumulation of aluminum, an ingredient in many phosphate-binding antacids. It results in mental cloudiness, dementia, and bone pain from infiltration of the bone with aluminum. This condition was formerly known as dialysis dementia. It may be treated with aluminum-chelating agents, which make aluminum available to be dialyzed from the body. It can be prevented by avoiding or limiting the use of phosphate-binding agents that contain aluminum.

Test-Taking Strategy: Use the process of elimination. Note the relation between the medication name in the question and

option 4. Review the signs of aluminum intoxication if you had difficulty with this question.
Level of Cognitive Ability: Analyzing
Client Needs: Physiological Integrity
Integrated Process: Nursing Process/Data Collection
Content Area: Adult Health/Renal
Reference: Ignatavicius, Workman, p. 1619. 2010.

551. 4
Rationale: Arterial steal syndrome results from vascular insufficiency after creation of a fistula. The client exhibits pallor and diminished pulse distal to the fistula and complains of pain distal to the fistula, which is caused by tissue ischemia. Warmth, redness, and pain would more likely characterize a problem with infection. Options 2 and 3 are not characteristics of steal syndrome.
Test-Taking Strategy: Use the process of elimination. Recalling that arterial steal syndrome results from vascular insufficiency will direct you to the correct option. Review these signs if you had difficulty with this question.
Level of Cognitive Ability: Analyzing
Client Needs: Physiological Integrity
Integrated Process: Nursing Process/Data Collection
Content Area: Adult Health/Renal
Reference: Ignatavicius, Workman, p. 1623. 2010.

552. 2
Rationale: Risk factors associated with pyelonephritis include diabetes mellitus, hypertension, chronic renal calculi, chronic cystitis, structural abnormalities of the urinary tract, presence of urinary stones, and indwelling or frequent urinary catheterization.
Test-Taking Strategy: Use the process of elimination. Eliminate options 1 and 4 first as least likely being associated as risk factors. From the remaining options, remember that diabetes mellitus can cause renal complications. This will direct you to the correct option. Review these risk factors if you had difficulty with this question.
Level of Cognitive Ability: Analyzing
Client Needs: Health Promotion and Maintenance
Integrated Process: Nursing Process/Data Collection
Content Area: Adult Health/Renal
Reference: Christensen, Kockrow, p. 455. 2011. *Adult health nursing.*

553. 4
Rationale: BUN testing is a frequently used laboratory test to determine renal function. The BUN level starts to rise when the glomerular filtration rate falls below 40% to 60%. A decreased hemoglobin and RBC count may be noted if bleeding from the urinary tract occurs or if erythropoietic function by the kidney is impaired. An increased WBC is most likely to be noted in renal disease.
Test-Taking Strategy: Use the process of elimination. Focus on the client's diagnosis and note the strategic words "most likely expect to note." Eliminate option 3 first because it is unassociated with the renal system. Although options 1 and 2 may be noted in some renal disorders, option 4 is the most likely laboratory finding. Remember that the BUN level is a frequently used laboratory test to determine renal function.

Review the laboratory tests to determine renal function if you had difficulty with this question.
Level of Cognitive Ability: Understanding
Client Needs: Physiological Integrity
Integrated Process: Nursing Process/Data Collection
Content Area: Adult Health/Renal
Reference: deWit, p. 855. 2009.

554. 3
Rationale: An iodine-based dye may be used during the IVP and can cause allergic reactions such as itching, hives, rash, tight feeling in the throat, shortness of breath, and bronchospasm. Checking for allergies is the priority. Options 1, 2, and 4 are unnecessary.
Test-Taking Strategy: Note the strategic word "priority," and use the nursing process as a guide. Options 1, 2, and 4 address implementation. Option 3 is the only option that addresses data collection. Review this test if you had difficulty with this question.
Level of Cognitive Ability: Applying
Client Needs: Physiological Integrity
Integrated Process: Nursing Process/Implementation
Content Area: Adult Health/Renal
Reference: Pagana, Pagana, p. 568. 2009.

555. 1
Rationale: If pain originates at the biopsy site and begins to radiate to the flank area and around the front of the abdomen, bleeding should be suspected. Hypotension, a decreasing hematocrit, and gross or microscopic hematuria would also indicate bleeding. Signs of infection would not appear immediately after a biopsy. Pain of this nature is not normal. There are no data to support the presence of renal colic.
Test-Taking Strategy: Use the process of elimination. Focusing on the data in the question will assist in eliminating options 3 and 4. Recalling that signs of infection may not appear immediately after biopsy will assist in directing you to option 1 from the remaining options. Review the complications following renal biopsy if you had difficulty with this question.
Level of Cognitive Ability: Analyzing
Client Needs: Physiological Integrity
Integrated Process: Nursing Process/Data Collection
Content Area: Adult Health/Renal
Reference: Pagana, Pagana, pp. 802–803. 2009.

556. 3
Rationale: In an older client, the only symptom of a UTI may be something as vague as increasing mental confusion or frequent unexplained falls. Frequency and urgency may commonly occur in an older client, and fever can be associated with a variety of conditions.
Test-Taking Strategy: Use the process of elimination. Note the client's age in the question. Eliminate options 2 and 4 because they may commonly occur in an older client. Eliminate option 1 next, because fever can be associated with a variety of conditions. Review the clinical manifestations of UTI that occur in the older client if you had difficulty with this question.
Level of Cognitive Ability: Understanding
Client Needs: Physiological Integrity
Integrated Process: Nursing Process/Data Collection

Content Area: Adult Health/Renal
Reference: Black, Hawks, p. 732. 2009.

557. 3

Rationale: Gross, painless hematuria is most frequently the first manifestation of bladder cancer. As the disease progresses, the client may experience burning, frequency, and urgency.
Test-Taking Strategy: Use the process of elimination and focus on the subject—a manifestation of bladder cancer. Eliminate options 1, 2, and 4 because they are common signs of a urinary tract infection. Review the specific manifestations associated with bladder cancer if you had difficulty with this question.
Level of Cognitive Ability: Understanding
Client Needs: Physiological Integrity
Integrated Process: Nursing Process/Data Collection
Content Area: Adult Health/Renal
Reference: Linton, p. 909. 2012.

558. 2

Rationale: TUR syndrome is caused by increased absorption of nonelectrolyte irrigating fluid used during surgery. The client may show signs of cerebral edema and increased intracranial pressure such as increased blood pressure, bradycardia, confusion, disorientation, muscle twitching, visual disturbances, and nausea and vomiting.
Test-Taking Strategy: Knowledge regarding TUR syndrome is required to answer this question. Recalling that increased intracranial pressure is the concern will direct you to option 2. Review this disorder if you had difficulty with this question.
Level of Cognitive Ability: Analyzing
Client Needs: Physiological Integrity
Integrated Process: Nursing Process/Data Collection
Content Area: Adult Health/Renal
Reference: Black, Hawks, p. 879. 2009.

559. 3

Rationale: Treatment of prostatitis includes medication with antibiotics, analgesics, and stool softeners. The client is also taught to rest, increase fluid intake, and use sitz baths for

comfort. Antimicrobial therapy is always continued until the prescription is completely finished.
Test-Taking Strategy: Use the process of elimination. Eliminate option 1 first, because stopping medication therapy before the end of the course is contraindicated. Option 4 is also eliminated, because fluid intake should be increased. From the remaining options, it is necessary to understand that sitz baths provide comfort and that rest is helpful in the healing process. Knowledge of either of these concepts will direct you to option 3. Review the measures to prevent prostatitis if you had difficulty with this question.
Level of Cognitive Ability: Evaluating
Client Needs: Physiological Integrity
Integrated Process: Nursing Process/Evaluation
Content Area: Adult Health/Renal
Reference: Christensen, Kockrow, pp. 454–455. 2011. *Adult health nursing.*

560. 2, 3, 4, 5

Rationale: If outflow drainage is inadequate, the nurse attempts to stimulate outflow by changing the client's position. Turning the client to the other side or making sure that the client is in good body alignment may assist with outflow drainage. The drainage bag needs to be lower than the client's abdomen to enhance gravity drainage. The connecting tubing and the peritoneal dialysis system is also checked for kinks or twisting, and the clamps on the system are checked to ensure that they are open. There is no reason to contact the HCP. Increasing the flow rate is an inappropriate action and is unassociated with the amount of outflow solution.
Test-Taking Strategy: Use the principles related to gravity flow and preventing obstruction to flow to answer this question. This will assist in determining the correct interventions. Review the nursing interventions related to insufficient flow of dialysate if you had difficulty with this question.
Level of Cognitive Ability: Applying
Client Needs: Physiological Integrity
Integrated Process: Nursing Process/Implementation
Content Area: Adult Health/Renal
Reference: Ignatavicius, Workman, p. 1630. 2010.

Renal Medications

I. URINARY TRACT ANTISEPTICS

A. Description
1. Urinary tract antiseptics inhibit the growth of bacteria in the urine (Box 54-1).
2. Act as disinfectants within the urinary tract
3. Used to treat acute cystitis or urinary tract infections (UTIs)
4. Urinary tract antiseptics do not achieve effective antibacterial concentrations in blood or tissues and therefore cannot be used for infections outside the urinary tract.

B. Side effects and nursing considerations
1. Cinoxacin (Cinobac)
   a. The side effects are similar to those of nalidixic acid.
   b. The dosage should be reduced in clients with renal impairment. Failure to do so could result in accumulation of the medication to toxic levels.
2. Methenamine (Mandelamine, Hiprex, Urex)
   a. Used to treat chronic UTIs, but not recommended for acute infections
   b. Administer after meals and at bedtime to minimize gastric distress.
   c. Chronic high-dose therapy can cause bladder irritation.
   d. Methenamine can cause crystalluria and should not be used in clients with renal impairment.
   e. Decomposition of the medication generates ammonia; therefore it should not be used for clients with liver dysfunction.
   f. Methenamine requires acidic urine with a pH of 5.5 or lower.
   g. Increasing fluid intake reduces antibacterial effects by diluting the medication and raising urine pH.
   h. Methenamine should not be combined with sulfonamides because of the risk of crystalluria and urinary tract injury.
   i. Clients taking this medication should avoid alkalinizing agents, including over-the-counter (OTC) antacids containing sodium bicarbonate or sodium carbonate.

3. Nalidixic acid (NegGram)
   a. Gastrointestinal side effects include anorexia, nausea, vomiting, and diarrhea.
   b. Skin side effects include rash and photosensitivity.
   c. Central nervous system (CNS) side effects include visual disturbances and insomnia.
   d. Nalidixic acid may produce intracranial hypertension in pediatric clients and should not be administered to children younger than 3 months.
   e. When nalidixic acid is used for more than 2 weeks, complete blood cell counts and liver function tests should be performed.
   f. Nalidixic acid can intensify the effects of orally administered anticoagulants.
   g. Nalidixic acid is contraindicated in clients with a history of seizure disorders.
4. Nitrofurantoin (Furadantin, Macrodantin, Macrobid)
   a. Gastrointestinal side effects include anorexia, nausea, vomiting, and diarrhea; administration with milk or meals minimizes gastrointestinal distress.
   b. Pulmonary reactions include dyspnea, chest pain, chills, fever, cough, and alveolar infiltrates. These resolve in 2 to 4 days after cessation of treatment.
   c. Hematological side effects include agranulocytosis, leukopenia, thrombocytopenia, and megaloblastic anemia.
   d. Peripheral neuropathy side effects include muscle weakness, tingling sensations, and numbness.
   e. Neurological side effects include headache, vertigo, drowsiness, and nystagmus.
   f. Allergic reactions include anaphylaxis, hives, rash, and tingling sensations around the mouth.
   g. Nitrofurantoin may produce a harmless brown color to the urine.
   h. Nitrofurantoin is contraindicated in clients with renal impairment.

Box 54-1 Urinary Tract Antiseptics

Cinoxacin (Cinobac)
Methenamine (Mandelamine, Hiprex, Urex)
Nalidixic acid (NegGram)
Nitrofurantoin (Furadantin, Macrodantin, Macrobid)

    i. Instruct the client about the expected side effects and the signs warranting notification of the health care provider (HCP).

II. FLUOROQUINOLONES (Box 54-2)

A. Description: Suppress bacterial growth by inhibiting an enzyme necessary for DNA synthesis; active against a broad spectrum of microbes

B. Side effects and nursing considerations

1. Significant side effects include dizziness, drowsiness, gastric distress, diarrhea, vaginitis (trovafloxacin), nausea, and vomiting.
2. Adverse effects include psychoses, hallucinations, confusion, tremors, hypersensitivity, and interstitial nephritis.
3. Fluoroquinolones should be used with caution in clients with hepatic, renal, or central nervous system disorders.
4. Monitor client for side effects and adverse effects.
5. Enoxacin and Norfloxacin (Noroxin) are to be taken on an empty stomach.
6. Ciprofloxacin (Cipro), lomefloxacin (Maxaquin), and ofloxacin (Floxin) may be taken with or without food.
7. Intravenously administered ciprofloxacin and ofloxacin are infused slowly over 60 minutes to minimize discomfort and vein irritation.
8. The client is advised to report dizziness, lightheadedness, visual disturbances, increased light sensitivity, and feelings of depression, because these signs could indicate central nervous system toxicity.

Box 54-2 Fluoroquinolones

Ciprofloxacin (Cipro)
Enoxacin
Gemifloxacin (Factive)
Levofloxacin (Levaquin)
Lomefloxacin (Maxaquin)
Moxifloxacin (Avelox)
Norfloxacin (Noroxin)
Ofloxacin (Floxin)
Sparfloxacin
Trovafloxacin (Trovan)

9. The client is informed of signs of hepatic and renal toxicity and the importance of reporting these signs to the HCP.

 Fluoroquinolones are administered with a full glass of water, and the client is taught that it is necessary to maintain a urine output of at least 1200 to 1500 mL daily to minimize the development of crystalluria.

III. SULFONAMIDES (Box 54-3)

A. Description: Suppress bacterial growth by inhibiting the synthesis of folic acid; active against a broad spectrum of microbes; used primarily to treat acute urinary tract infections

B. Side effects and nursing considerations

1. Hypersensitivity reactions include rash, fever, and photosensitivity.
2. Stevens-Johnson syndrome, the most severe hypersensitivity response, produces symptoms that include widespread lesions of the skin and mucous membranes, fever, malaise, and toxemia.
3. Sulfonamides can cause hemolytic anemia, agranulocytosis, leukopenia, and thrombocytopenia. The client is instructed to notify the HCP if sore throat or fever occurs.
4. Sulfonamides are administered with caution in clients with renal impairment.
5. Sulfonamides are contraindicated if hypersensitivity exists to sulfonamides, sulfonylureas, or thiazide or loop diuretics.
6. Sulfonamides are contraindicated in infants younger than 2 months and in pregnant women or mothers who are breast-feeding.
7. Sulfonamides can potentiate the effects of warfarin sodium (Coumadin), phenytoin (Dilantin), and orally administered hypoglycemics such as tolbutamide (Orinase). When combined with sulfonamides, these medications may require a reduction in dosage.
8. The client is instructed to take the medication on an empty stomach with a full glass of water.
9. The client is instructed to complete the entire course of antibiotics prescribed.

Box 54-3 Sulfonamides

Sulfadiazine
Sulfamethizole
Sulfamethoxazole
Sulfisoxazole
Trimethoprim (Proloprim, Trimpex)
Trimethoprim-sulfamethoxazole (TMP-SMZ) (Bactrim, Cotrim)

10. The client is instructed to avoid prolonged exposure to sunlight, wear protective clothing, and apply a sunscreen to exposed skin.
11. The client should maintain a daily urine output of 1200 mL by consuming 8 to 10 glasses of water each day to minimize the risk of renal damage from the medication.
12. The client is informed that some combination medications of sulfonamides can cause the urine to turn dark brown or red.
13. The sulfonamide combination of trimethoprim-sulfamethoxazole (TMP-SMZ; Bactrim, Cotrim) is more effective than either medication alone because it inhibits the sequential steps in bacterial folic acid synthesis.
14. TMP-SMZ is used cautiously with clients experiencing impaired kidney function, folate deficiency, severe allergy, or bronchial asthma.
15. An intravenous dose of TMP-SMZ is administered over 60 to 90 minutes and is not mixed with other medications.

⚠ Sulfonamides should be withheld if a rash is noted. The client is informed to contact the HCP if a rash appears.

IV. URINARY TRACT ANALGESIC (Box 54-4)

A. Description
1. Phenazopyridine is a urinary tract analgesic used to treat pain from urinary tract irritation or infection.
2. A urinary tract analgesic is administered with an antibiotic because the analgesic only treats pain, not the infection.

B. Side effects
1. Nausea
2. Headache
3. Vertigo

C. Nursing considerations
1. The client is instructed that the urine will turn red or orange and stain clothing.
2. A urinary tract analgesic is contraindicated in clients with renal or hepatic disease.
3. The medication interferes with accurate urine testing for glucose and ketones.

V. ANTICHOLINERGICS-ANTISPASMODICS (Box 54-5)

A. Description: Used for overactive bladder (urge incontinence)

Box 54-4 Urinary Tract Analgesic

Phenazopyridine (Pyridium, Azo-Standard, Pyridiate, Urogesic)

Box 54-5 Anticholinergics-Antispasmodics

Darifenacin (Enablex)
Oxybutynin chloride (Ditropan, Ditropan XL)
Solifenacin (Vesicare)
Tolterodine (Detrol, Detrol LA)
Trospium (Sanctura, Sanctura XR)

B. Side effects
1. Anorexia, nausea, vomiting, and dry mouth
2. Blurred vision
3. Confusion in older clients
4. Constipation
5. Decreased sweating
6. Dizziness
7. Drowsiness
8. Dry eyes
9. Gastric distress
10. Headache
11. Tachycardia
12. Urinary retention

C. Nursing considerations
1. Extended-release capsules should not be split, chewed, or crushed.
2. Detrol LA should be used cautiously in clients with narrow-angle glaucoma.
3. Oxybutynin is not administered to clients with known hypersensitivity, gastrointestinal or genitourinary obstruction, glaucoma, severe colitis, or myasthenia gravis.
4. The client is instructed to avoid hazardous activities because of the side effects of dizziness and drowsiness.
5. Monitor intake and output.
6. Provide gum or hard candy for dry mouth.
7. Monitor for signs of toxicity (central nervous system stimulation) such as hypotension, hypertension, confusion, tachycardia, flushed or red face, signs of respiratory depression, nervousness, restlessness, hallucinations, and irritability.

VI. CHOLINERGIC (Box 54-6)

A. Description: Bethanechol chloride (Urecholine) is a cholinergic used to increase bladder tone and function and to treat nonobstructive urinary retention and neurogenic bladder.

B. Side effects
1. Headache
2. Hypotension
3. Flushing and sweating

Box 54-6 Cholinergic

Bethanechol chloride (Urecholine)

4. Increased salivation
5. Abdominal cramps
6. Nausea and vomiting
7. Diarrhea
8. Urinary urgency
9. Bronchoconstriction
10. Transient complete heart block

C. Nursing considerations
1. Administered on an empty stomach, 1 hour before or 2 hours after meals to lessen nausea and vomiting
2. Never administered by the intramuscular or intravenous (IV) routes
3. Monitor intake and output.
4. Monitor for increased bladder tone and function.
5. Monitor for cholinergic overdose (excessive salivation, sweating, involuntary urination and defecation, bradycardia, and severe hypotension).
6. Have atropine sulfate (antidote) readily available for IV or subcutaneous administration.

⚠ A cholinergic such as bethanechol chloride (Urecholine) is not given to a client who has a urinary stricture or obstruction.

VII. MEDICATIONS FOR PREVENTING ORGAN REJECTION (Box 54-7)

A. Medications include immunosuppressants, corticosteroids, cytotoxic medications, and antibodies

B. Some medications may be used in combination with one another to produce different actions on the immune system. Combination therapy also allows for administration of the medications in lower doses, reducing the possibility of side effects.

Box 54-7 Preventing Organ Rejection

Immunosuppressants
Cyclosporine (Sandimmune, Gengraf, Neoral)
Tacrolimus (Prograf)
Sirolimus (Rapamune)

Glucocorticoid
Prednisone

Cytotoxic Medications
Azathioprine (Imuran)
Mycophenolate mofetil (CellCept)

Antibodies
Basiliximab (Simulect)
Daclizumab (Zenapax)
Antithymocyte globulin, equine (Atgam)
Muromonab-CD3 (Orthoclone OKT3)

C. Cyclosporine (Sandimmune, Gengraf, Neoral)
1. Cyclosporine inhibits calcineurin and acts on T lymphocytes to suppress the production of interleukin-2, interferon-γ, and other cytokines.
2. Cyclosporine may be used to prevent rejection of allogeneic kidney, liver, and heart transplants.
3. Prednisone may be administered concurrently.
4. Oral administration of cyclosporine is preferred. Intravenous administration is reserved for clients who cannot take the medication orally.
5. Blood levels of the medication should be measured regularly because of its nephrotoxic effects.
6. The most common adverse effects are nephrotoxicity, infection, hypertension, tremor, and hirsutism.
7. The client is assured that hirsutism is reversible and instructed in the use of a depilatory.
8. Other adverse effects include neurotoxicity, gastrointestinal effects, hyperkalemia, and hyperglycemia.
9. The risk of infection and lymphomas is increased with the use of cyclosporine.
10. Cyclosporine is contraindicated in the presence of hypersensitivity, pregnancy and breastfeeding, recent inoculation with live virus vaccines, and recent contact with an active infection such as chickenpox or herpes zoster.
11. Cyclosporine is embryotoxic, and women of childbearing age should use a mechanical form of contraception and avoid oral contraceptives.
12. The client should be informed about the possibility of renal damage and liver damage and the need for periodic liver function tests and determination of coagulation factors and blood urea nitrogen, serum creatinine, serum potassium, and blood glucose levels.
13. The client should be instructed to monitor for early signs of infection and report these signs immediately.
14. Available in a pill form. If the client is unable to swallow the pill, the client is instructed to dispense the oral liquid medication into a glass container by using a specially calibrated pipette, mix well, and drink immediately; rinse the glass container with diluent and drink it to ensure ingestion of the complete dose; dry the outside of the pipette and return to its cover for storage.
15. To promote palatability, the client is instructed to mix the liquid medication with milk, chocolate milk, or orange juice just before administration.
16. Consuming grapefruit juice is prohibited because it raises cyclosporine levels and increases the risk of toxicity.
17. Ketoconazole (Nizoral), erythromycin, and amphotericin B deoxycholate can elevate cyclosporine levels.

18. Phenytoin (Dilantin), phenobarbital, rifampin (Rifadin), and trimethoprim-sulfamethoxazole can decrease cyclosporine levels.
19. Renal damage can be intensified by the concurrent use of other nephrotoxic medications.

D. Sirolimus (Rapamune)
1. Sirolimus is used for the prevention of renal transplant rejection by inhibiting the response of helper T lymphocytes and B lymphocytes to cytokinesis.
2. It may be used with cyclosporine or tacrolimus (Prograf) and corticosteroids.
3. Increases the risk of infection, increases the risk of renal injury, increases the risk of lymphocele (a complication of renal transplant surgery), and raises cholesterol and triglyceride levels
4. Side effects include rash, acne, anemia, thrombocytopenia, joint pain, diarrhea, and hypokalemia.

E. Tacrolimus (Prograf)
1. Tacrolimus inhibits calcineurin and thereby prevents T cells from producing interleukin-2, interferon-γ, and other cytokines.
2. Tacrolimus is more effective than cyclosporine, but is more toxic.
3. Adverse effects are similar to those of cyclosporine and include nephrotoxicity, infection, hypertension, tremor, hirsutism, neurotoxicity, gastrointestinal effects, hyperkalemia, and hyperglycemia.
4. Tacrolimus should be used cautiously in immunosuppressed clients and those with renal, hepatic, or pancreatic impairment.
5. Tacrolimus is contraindicated for clients hypersensitive to cyclosporine.
6. Blood glucose levels are monitored, and prescribed insulin or oral hypoglycemics are administered.

F. Prednisone
1. Prednisone is a glucocorticoid that inhibits accumulation of inflammatory cells at inflammation sites.
2. Hyperglycemia and hypokalemia can occur with prednisone use. Monitor glucose and serum potassium levels.
3. See Chapter 46 for additional information about prednisone.

G. Azathioprine (Imuran)
1. Azathioprine suppresses cell-mediated and humoral immune responses by inhibiting the proliferation of B and T lymphocytes.
2. Not used routinely since the advent of newer medications that suppress transplant rejection.
3. Can cause neutropenia and thrombocytopenia from bone marrow suppression
4. Contraindicated in pregnancy; associated with an increased incidence of neoplasms

5. Monitor hematocrit, white blood cell count, platelet count, liver enzyme levels, and coagulation factors.

H. Mycophenolate mofetil (CellCept)
1. Mycophenolate mofetil causes selective inhibition of B- and T-lymphocyte proliferation.
2. May be used with cyclosporine or tacrolimus and glucocorticoids for prophylaxis against organ rejection
3. Major adverse effects include diarrhea, severe neutropenia, vomiting, and sepsis.
4. Mycophenolate mofetil is associated with an increased risk of infection and malignancies.
5. Absorption is decreased by the use of magnesium and aluminum antacids and cholestyramine (Questran, Prevalite).
6. It is contraindicated in pregnancy and during breast-feeding.
7. The client is instructed to take the medication on an empty stomach and not to open or crush capsules.
8. The client is instructed to contact the HCP for unusual bleeding or bruising, sore throat, mouth sores, abdominal pain, or fever.

I. Daclizumab (Zenapax) and basiliximab (Simulect)
1. Daclizumab and basiliximab bind to interleukin-2 receptors on lymphocytes, resulting in diminished cell-mediated immune reactions.
2. Used primarily as an induction agent at the time of transplantation; may be used with other immunosuppressants to prevent acute rejection of transplanted kidneys
3. Administered by the intravenous route
4. Daclizumab (Zenapax)
   a. The initial dose is administered within 24 hours before transplantation.
   b. Side effects include chest pain, gastrointestinal distress, edema, shortness of breath, pain in the joints, and slow wound healing.
5. Basiliximab (Simulect)
   a. The initial dose is administered within 2 hours before transplantation.
   b. Side effects are similar to those for daclizumab; in addition, headache, insomnia, dizziness, and tremors can occur.

J. Antithymocyte globulin, equine (Atgam)
1. Antithymocyte globulin, equine, causes a decrease in the number and activity of thymus-derived lymphocytes and is used to suppress organ rejection following renal, liver, bone marrow, and heart transplantation.
2. It is used primarily to treat acute rejection episodes.
3. Before the first infusion, the client should undergo intradermal skin testing to determine hypersensitivity.

4. Because this product is made using equine and human blood components, it may carry a risk of transmitting infectious agents, such as viruses.
5. Monitor the platelet count and report it if below 100,000 cells/mm^3.
6. Arrange for outpatient referral for repeated infusions after discharge.

K. Muromonab-CD3 (Orthoclone OKT3)
1. Blocks all T-cell functions; used to prevent acute allograft rejection of kidney transplants
2. Adverse reactions include fever, chills, dyspnea, chest pain, and nausea and vomiting.
3. Administered via the IV route. The client is pretreated with IV glucocorticoid.

VIII. HEMATOPOIETIC GROWTH FACTORS
(Box 54-8)

A. Erythropoietic growth factors
1. Stimulate the production of red blood cells
2. Used to treat anemia of **chronic renal failure**, chemotherapy-induced anemia, anemia caused by zidovudine (AZT), and anemia in clients requiring surgery
3. Initial effects can be seen within 1 to 2 weeks, and the hematocrit reaches normal levels (30% to 33%) in 2 to 3 months.
4. Side effect: The major side effect is hypertension.
5. Other effects can include heart failure, thrombotic effects such as stroke or myocardial infarction, and cardiac arrest.

B. Leukopoietic growth factors
1. Stimulate the production of white blood cells (leukocytes)
2. Used for clients undergoing myelosuppressive chemotherapy or bone marrow transplantation and those with severe chronic neutropenia.
3. Can cause bone pain, leukocytosis, and elevation of plasma uric acid, lactate dehydrogenase, and alkaline phosphatase levels. Long-term therapy has caused splenomegaly.

C. Thrombopoietic growth factor
1. Stimulates the production of platelets

Box 54-8 Hematopoietic Growth Factors

Erythropoietic Growth Factors
Epoetin alfa (Epogen, Procrit)
Darbepoetin alfa (Aranesp)
MPEG-epoetin beta (Mircera)

Leukopoietic Growth Factors
Filgrastim (Neupogen)
Pegfilgrastim (Neulasta)
Sargramostim (Leukine)

Thrombopoietic Growth Factor
Oprelvekin (Neumega)

---

2. Used for clients undergoing myelosuppressive chemotherapy to minimize thrombocytopenia and decrease the need for platelet transfusions
3. Adverse effects include fluid retention, cardiac dysrhythmias, conjunctival infection, visual blurring, and papilledema.

MORE QUESTIONS ON EVOLVE!

Practice Questions

561. The client who has a cold is seen in the emergency department with an inability to void. Because the client has a history of benign prostatic hyperplasia, the nurse determines that the client should be questioned about the use of which of the following medications?
   1. Diuretics
   2. Antibiotics
   3. Antitussives
   4. Decongestants

562. Nalidixic acid (NegGram) is prescribed for a client with a urinary tract infection. On review of the client's record, the nurse notes that the client is taking warfarin sodium (Coumadin) daily. Which prescription should the nurse anticipate for this client?
   1. Discontinuation of warfarin sodium (Coumadin)
   2. A decrease in the warfarin sodium (Coumadin) dosage
   3. An increase in the warfarin sodium (Coumadin) dosage
   4. A decrease in the usual dose of nalidixic acid (NegGram)

563. A nurse is reinforcing discharge instructions to a client receiving sulfisoxazole. Which of the following should be included in the list of instructions?
   1. Restrict fluid intake.
   2. Maintain a high fluid intake.
   3. If the urine turns dark brown, call the health care provider (HCP) immediately.
   4. Decrease the dosage when symptoms are improving to prevent an allergic response.

564. Trimethoprim-sulfamethoxazole (TMP-SMZ) is prescribed for a client. A nurse should instruct the client to report which symptom if it developed during the course of this medication therapy?
   1. Nausea
   2. Diarrhea
   3. Headache
   4. Sore throat

565. Phenazopyridine hydrochloride (Pyridium) is prescribed for a client for symptomatic relief of pain resulting from a lower urinary tract infection. The nurse reinforces to the client:
1. To take the medication at bedtime
2. To take the medication before meals
3. To discontinue the medication if a headache occurs
4. That a reddish orange discoloration of the urine may occur

566. Bethanechol chloride (Urecholine) is prescribed for a client with urinary retention. Which disorder would be a contraindication to the administration of this medication?
1. Gastric atony
2. Urinary strictures
3. Neurogenic atony
4. Gastroesophageal reflux

567. A nurse who is administering bethanechol chloride (Urecholine) is monitoring for acute toxicity associated with the medication. The nurse checks the client for which sign of toxicity?
1. Dry skin
2. Dry mouth
3. Bradycardia
4. Signs of dehydration

568. Oxybutynin chloride (Ditropan XL) is prescribed for a client with neurogenic bladder. Which sign would indicate a possible toxic effect related to this medication?
1. Pallor
2. Drowsiness
3. Bradycardia
4. Restlessness

569. After kidney transplantation, cyclosporine (Sandimmune) is prescribed for a client. Which laboratory result would indicate an adverse effect from the use of this medication?
1. Decreased creatinine level
2. Decreased hemoglobin level
3. Elevated blood urea nitrogen level
4. Decreased white blood cell count

570. Cinoxacin (Cinobac), a urinary antiseptic, is prescribed for the client. The nurse reviews the client's medical record and should contact the health care provider regarding which documented finding to verify the prescription?

CHART/EXHIBIT
CLIENT'S MEDICAL RECORD
Laboratory Test Result: Blood glucose, 102 mg/dL
Diagnostic Test Result: Chest x-ray: normal
Client's History: Renal insufficiency
Medication History: Folic acid (vitamin B$_6$) 0.5 mg, orally daily

1. Renal insufficiency
2. Chest x-ray: normal
3. Blood glucose, 102 mg/dL
4. Folic acid (vitamin B$_6$) 0.5 mg, orally daily

ANSWERS

561. 4
Rationale: In the client with benign prostatic hyperplasia, episodes of urinary retention can be triggered by certain medications, such as decongestants, anticholinergics, and antidepressants. The client should be questioned about the use of these medications if he or she has urinary retention. Retention also can be precipitated by other factors, such as alcoholic beverages, infection, bedrest, and becoming chilled.
Test-Taking Strategy: Use the process of elimination. The question is asking about medications that could exacerbate or contribute to urinary retention in the client with benign prostatic hyperplasia. Diuretics should help voiding; therefore readily eliminate option 1. Antibiotics should have no effect at all; thus eliminate option 2. From the remaining options, recalling that medications that contain anticholinergics may cause urinary retention will direct you to option 4. Review the factors that can precipitate urinary retention in the client with benign prostatic hyperplasia if you had difficulty with this question.
Level of Cognitive Ability: Analyzing
Client Needs: Physiological Integrity
Integrated Process: Nursing Process/Data Collection
Content Area: Adult Health/Renal
Reference: Black, Hawks, p. 878. 2009.

562. 2
Rationale: Nalidixic acid can intensify the effects of oral anticoagulants by displacing these agents from binding sites on plasma protein. When an oral anticoagulant is combined with nalidixic acid, a decrease in the anticoagulant dosage may be needed.
Test-Taking Strategy: Knowledge about the medication interactions associated with the use of nalidixic acid is needed to answer this question. Remember that nalidixic acid can intensify the effects of oral anticoagulants. Review these interactions if you had difficulty with this question.
Level of Cognitive Ability: Analyzing
Client Needs: Physiological Integrity
Integrated Process: Nursing Process/Planning
Content Area: Pharmacology
References: Kee, Hayes, McCuistion, p. 490. 2009. Lehne, p. 1036. 2010.

563. 2

Rationale: Each dose of sulfisoxazole should be administered with a full glass of water, and the client should maintain a high fluid intake. The medication is more soluble in alkaline urine. The client should not be instructed to taper or discontinue the dose. Some forms of sulfisoxazole cause urine to turn dark brown or red. This does not indicate the need to notify the HCP.

Test-Taking Strategy: Use the process of elimination. Recalling that this medication is used to treat urinary tract infections will direct you to the correct option. Review client instructions regarding this medication if you had difficulty with this question.

Level of Cognitive Ability: Applying
Client Needs: Physiological Integrity
Integrated Process: Teaching and Learning
Content Area: Pharmacology
Reference: Lehne, p. 1030. 2010.

564. 4

Rationale: Clients taking trimethoprim-sulfamethoxazole (TMP-SMZ) should be informed about early signs of blood disorders that can occur from this medication. These include sore throat, fever, and pallor, and the client should be instructed to notify the physician if these symptoms occur. The other options do not require health care provider notification.

Test-Taking Strategy: Use the process of elimination. Knowledge that this medication can cause blood dyscrasias will direct you to option 4. If you are unfamiliar with this medication, review this content.

Level of Cognitive Ability: Applying
Client Needs: Physiological Integrity
Integrated Process: Teaching and Learning
Content Area: Pharmacology
Reference: Lehne, p. 1031. 2010.

565. 4

Rationale: The nurse should instruct the client that a reddish-orange discoloration of urine may occur. The nurse also should instruct the client that this discoloration can stain fabric. The medication should be taken after meals to reduce the possibility of gastrointestinal upset. A headache is an occasional side effect of the medication and does not warrant discontinuation of the medication.

Test-Taking Strategy: Use the process of elimination. Eliminate options 1 and 2 first because they are comparable or alike in that they address time schedules for the administration of the medication. From the remaining options, eliminate option 3 because the nurse would not advise the client to discontinue this medication. Review client instructions regarding this medication if you had difficulty with this question.

Level of Cognitive Ability: Applying
Client Needs: Physiological Integrity
Integrated Process: Teaching and Learning
Content Area: Pharmacology
Reference: Hodgson, Kizior, p. 921. 2012.

566. 2

Rationale: Bethanechol chloride (Urecholine) can be harmful to clients with urinary tract obstruction or weakness of the bladder wall. The medication has the ability to contract the bladder and thereby increase pressure within the urinary tract. Elevation of pressure within the urinary tract could rupture the bladder in clients with these conditions.

Test-Taking Strategy: Use the process of elimination. Noting that the medication is used for urinary retention may assist in directing you to the correct option. Review the contraindications associated with this medication if you had difficulty with this question.

Level of Cognitive Ability: Analyzing
Client Needs: Physiological Integrity
Integrated Process: Nursing Process/Data Collection
Content Area: Pharmacology
Reference: Hodgson, Kizior, pp. 123–124. 2012.

567. 3

Rationale: Toxicity (overdose) produces manifestations of excessive muscarinic stimulation such as salivation, sweating, involuntary urination and defecation, bradycardia, and severe hypotension. Treatment includes supportive measures and the administration of atropine sulfate subcutaneously or intravenously.

Test-Taking Strategy: Use the process of elimination. Noting the similarity in options 1, 2, and 4 will assist in eliminating these options. Review the signs of toxicity if you had difficulty with this question.

Level of Cognitive Ability: Analyzing
Client Needs: Physiological Integrity
Integrated Process: Nursing Process/Data Collection
Content Area: Pharmacology
References: Hodgson , Kizior, pp. 123–124. 2012.
Lehne, pp. 122, 130. 2010.

568. 4

Rationale: Toxicity (overdosage) of this medication produces central nervous system excitation, such as nervousness, restlessness, hallucinations, and irritability. Other signs of toxicity include hypotension or hypertension, confusion, tachycardia, flushed or red face, and signs of respiratory depression. Drowsiness is a frequent side effect of the medication but does not indicate overdosage.

Test-Taking Strategy: Knowledge regarding the manifestations related to toxicity is required to answer this question. Remember that restlessness is a sign of toxicity. Review the signs that indicate toxicity if you had difficulty with this question.

Level of Cognitive Ability: Analyzing
Client Needs: Physiological Integrity
Integrated Process: Nursing Process/Data Collection
Content Area: Pharmacology
Reference: Hodgson, Kizior, p. 878–880. 2012.

569. 3

Rationale: Nephrotoxicity can occur from the use of cyclosporine (Sandimmune). Nephrotoxicity is evaluated by monitoring for elevated blood urea nitrogen and serum creatinine levels. Cyclosporine does not depress the bone marrow.

Test-Taking Strategy: Use the process of elimination. Eliminate options 2 and 4 first because they are unrelated to renal function. Next, eliminate option 1 because the creatinine level would be elevated, not decreased. Option 3 is the only option that indicates an increased level of a renal function test. Review

the adverse effects related to this medication if you had difficulty with this question.
Level of Cognitive Ability: Analyzing
Client Needs: Physiological Integrity
Integrated Process: Nursing Process/Data Collection
Content Area: Pharmacology
Reference: Hodgson, Kizior, p. 291. 2012.

❖ **570. 1**
Rationale: Cinoxacin should be administered with caution in clients with renal impairment. The dosage should be reduced, and failure to do so could result in accumulation of cinoxacin to toxic levels. Therefore the nurse would verify the prescription if the client had a documented history of renal insufficiency. The laboratory and diagnostic test results are normal findings. Folic acid (vitamin B_6) may be prescribed for a client with renal insufficiency to prevent anemia.
Test-Taking Strategy: Focus on the subject—the need to contact the physician. Eliminate options 2 and 3 because the laboratory and diagnostic test results are normal findings. From the remaining options, note the disorder in the client's history. This directs you to option 1. Review the contraindications associated with this medication if you had difficulty with this question.
Level of Cognitive Ability: Analyzing
Client Needs: Physiological Integrity
Integrated Process: Nursing Process/Data Collection
Content Area: Pharmacology
References: Kee, Hayes, McCuistion, pp. 488–489. 2009. Lehne, p. 1036. 2010.

The Adult Client with an Eye or Ear Disorder

PYRAMID TERMS

accommodation Process by which a clear visual image is maintained as the gaze is shifted from a distant to a near point

astigmatism A condition that results from an uneven curvature of the cornea or lens in which light rays do not focus on a single point on the retina

cataract An opacity of the lens that distorts the image projected onto the retina and that can progress to blindness

conductive hearing loss A mechanical dysfunction or blockage of sound waves to the inner ear fibers because of external ear or middle ear disorders; the blockage can be caused by impacted cerumen, foreign bodies, pus, or serum in the middle ear; disorders can often be corrected with no damage to hearing or minimal permanent hearing loss

cycloplegia The paralysis of the ciliary muscles by medications that block muscarinic receptors; cycloplegia causes blurred vision because the shape of the lens can no longer be adjusted to near vision

fenestration Removal of the stapes with a small hole drilled in the footplate and connection of a prosthesis between the incus and footplate; sounds cause the prosthesis to vibrate in the same manner as did the stapes

glaucoma Increased intraocular pressure as a result of inadequate drainage of aqueous humor from the canal of Schlemm or overproduction of aqueous humor; the condition damages the optic nerve and can result in blindness

hyperopia Farsightedness; objects converge to a point behind the retina; vision beyond 20 feet is normal, but near vision is poor; correction is done by a convex lens

legally blind The best visual acuity with corrective lenses in the better eye of 20/200 or less, or visual acuity of less than 20 degrees of the visual field in the better eye

macular degeneration A blurred central vision caused by progressive degeneration of the center of the retina; condition may be atrophic or age related, or dry or exudative (wet)

Ménière's syndrome A syndrome also called endolymphatic hydrops that refers to dilation of the endolymphatic system by overproduction or decreased reabsorption of endolymphatic fluid; the syndrome is characterized by tinnitus, unilateral sensorineural hearing loss, and vertigo

miosis A constricted and fixed pupil achieved primarily by stimulation of the muscarinic receptors of the sphincter muscles; occurs with the use of pilocarpine drops when treating glaucoma, the use of opioids, or if there is brain damage of the pons

miotics Medications that cause contraction of the pupil

mydriasis A dilated pupil achieved by blockage of the muscarinic receptors of the sphincter muscles or stimulation of the alpha receptors of the dilator muscles; enlarged pupils occur with stimulation of the sympathetic nervous system, use of dilating drops, acute glaucoma, or past or recent trauma

mydriatics Medications that dilate the pupil

myopia Nearsightedness; rays coming from an object are focused in front of the retina; near vision is normal, but distant vision is defective; a biconcave lens is used for correction

otosclerosis Disease of the labyrinthine capsule of the middle ear that results in a bony overgrowth of tissue surrounding the ossicles; causes the development of irregular areas of new bone formation and causes fixation of the bones; stapes fixation leads to a conductive hearing loss

presbycusis Gradual nerve degeneration associated with aging; a common cause of sensorineural hearing loss

retinal detachment Separation of the layers of the retina because of the accumulation of fluid between them or because both retinal layers elevate away from the choroid as a result of a tumor; partial separation becomes complete if untreated; when detachment becomes complete, blindness occurs

sensorineural hearing loss A pathological process of the inner ear or the sensory fibers that lead to the cerebral cortex; such hearing loss is often permanent, and measures must be taken to reduce further damage or attempt to amplify sound as a means of improving hearing to some degree

PYRAMID TO SUCCESS

Pyramid points focus on nursing interventions for clients with impairment in sight or hearing and on the nursing care related to disorders such as cataracts, glaucoma, and retinal detachment. Pyramid points also focus on emergency interventions for eye and ear disorders and injuries. Review nursing care related to organ donation for the donor and recipient. Pyramid points also focus on client instructions related to medication administration, sensory perceptual alterations and safety issues, and available support systems.

CLIENT NEEDS

Safe and Effective Care Environment

- Caring for the recipient of a tissue (corneal) donation
- Consulting with members of the health care team
- Establishing priorities
- Maintaining asepsis with procedures and treatments
- Maintaining standard and other precautions
- Obtaining informed consent for invasive procedures
- Preventing accidents that can occur as a result of sensory impairments
- Upholding client rights

Health Promotion and Maintenance

- Discussing changes that occur with the aging process
- Discussing expected body image changes and self-care deficits

- Implementing measures for the prevention and early detection of health problems and diseases related to the eye and ear
- Performing data collection techniques for eye and ear disorders
- Providing home care instructions after procedures related to the eye and ear
- Providing instructions regarding the administration of eye and ear medications
- Providing instructions regarding activity limitations or postoperative activities
- Teaching the importance of compliance to the prescribed therapy

Psychosocial Integrity

- Assessing the client's ability to cope with feelings of isolation, fear, or anxiety regarding a possible change in vision and/or hearing status, and loss of independence
- Discussing role changes
- Identifying family support systems
- Informing the client about available community resources
- Monitoring for sensory perceptual alterations
- Using appropriate communication techniques for impaired vision and hearing

Physiological Integrity

- Monitoring for complications related to procedures
- Monitoring for expected responses to therapy
- Providing care to assistive devices such as glasses, contact lenses, and hearing aids
- Taking action in medical emergencies

55

The Eye and the Ear

I. ANATOMY AND PHYSIOLOGY OF THE EYE

A. The eye
1. Is 1 inch in diameter and is located in the anterior portion of the orbit
2. The orbit is the bony structure of the skull that surrounds the eye and offers protection to the eye.

B. Layers of the eye
1. External layer
   a. The fibrous coat that supports the eye
   b. Contains the sclera, which is an opaque white tissue
   c. Contains the cornea, which is a dense transparent layer
2. Middle layer
   a. Called the uveal tract
   b. Consists of the choroid, the ciliary body, and the iris
   c. The choroid is the dark brown membrane located between the sclera and the retina that has dark pigmentation to prevent light from reflecting internally.
   d. The choroid lines most of the sclera and is attached to the retina but can detach easily from the sclera.
   e. The choroid contains many blood vessels and supplies nutrients to the retina.
   f. The ciliary body connects the choroid with the iris and secretes aqueous humor that helps give the eye its shape. The muscles of the ciliary body control the thickness of the lens.
   g. The iris is the colored portion of the eye, is located in front of the lens, and has a central circular opening called the pupil. The pupil controls the amount of light admitted into the retina (darkness produces dilation and light produces constriction).
3. Internal layer
   a. Consists of the retina, a thin, delicate structure in which the fibers of the optic nerve are distributed
   b. The retina is bordered externally by the choroid and sclera and internally by the vitreous.
   c. The retina is the visual receptive layer of the eye in which light waves are changed into nerve impulses and contains blood vessels and photoreceptors called rods and cones.

C. Vitreous body
1. Contains a gelatinous substance that occupies the vitreous chamber, which is the space between the lens and the retina
2. The vitreous body transmits light and gives shape to the posterior eye.

D. Vitreous
1. Gel-like substance that maintains the shape of the eye
2. Provides additional physical support to the retina

E. Rods and cones
1. Rods are responsible for peripheral vision and function at reduced levels of illumination.
2. Cones function at bright levels of illumination and are responsible for color vision and central vision.

F. Optic disk
1. The optic disk is a creamy pink to white depressed area in the retina.
2. The optic nerve enters and exits the eyeball at this area.
3. This area is called the blind spot because it contains only nerve fibers, lacks photoreceptor cells, and is insensitive to light.

G. Macula lutea
1. A small, oval, yellowish-pink area located lateral and temporal to the optic disc
2. The central depressed part of the macula is the fovea centralis, the area of sharpest and keenest vision, where most acute vision occurs.

H. Aqueous humor
1. The aqueous humor is a clear watery fluid that fills the anterior and posterior chambers of the eye.
2. The aqueous humor is produced by the ciliary processes, and the fluid drains into the canal of Schlemm.
3. The anterior chamber lies between the cornea and the iris.
4. The posterior chamber lies between the iris and the lens.

I. Canal of Schlemm: A passageway that extends completely around the eye that permits fluid to drain out of the eye into the systemic circulation so that a constant intraocular pressure is maintained

J. Lens
1. A transparent convex structure behind the iris and in front of the vitreous body
2. The lens bends rays of light so that the light falls on the retina.
3. The curve of the lens changes to focus on near or distant objects.

K. Conjunctiva: The thin transparent mucous membrane of the eye that lines the posterior surface of each eyelid and is located over the sclera

L. Lacrimal gland
1. The lacrimal gland produces tears.
2. Tears are drained through the punctum into the lacrimal duct and sac.

M. Eye muscles
1. Muscles do not work independently but work with the muscle that produces the opposite movement
2. Rectus muscles exert their pull when the eye turns temporally.
3. Oblique muscles exert their pull when the eye turns nasally.

N. Nerves
1. Cranial nerve II: Optic nerve (nerve of sight)
2. Cranial nerve III: Oculomotor
3. Cranial nerve IV: Trochlear
4. Cranial nerve VI: Abducens

O. Blood vessels
1. The ophthalmic artery is the major artery supplying the structures in the eye.
2. The ophthalmic veins drain the blood from the eye.

II. ASSESSMENT OF VISION (refer to Chapter 29 for information on assessment)

III. DIAGNOSTIC TESTS FOR THE EYE

A. Fluorescein angiography
1. Description
   a. A detailed imaging and recording of ocular circulation by a series of photographs after the administration of a dye
   b. This test is useful for assessing problems with retinal circulation, such as those that occur in diabetic retinopathy, retinal bleeding, and **macular degeneration,** or to rule out intraocular tumors.
2. Preprocedure interventions
   a. Check the client for allergies and previous reactions to dyes.
   b. Obtain informed consent.
   c. A **mydriatic** medication, which causes pupil dilation, is instilled into the eye 1 hour before the test.
   d. The dye is injected into a vein of the client's arm.
   e. Inform the client that the dye may cause the skin to appear yellow for several hours after the test and is eliminated gradually through the urine.
   f. The client may experience nausea, vomiting, sneezing, paresthesia of the tongue, or pain at the injection site.
   g. If hives appear, orally or intramuscularly administered antihistamines such as diphenhydramine (Benadryl) are given as prescribed.
3. Postprocedure interventions
   a. Encourage rest.
   b. Encourage fluid intake to assist in eliminating the dye from the client's system.
   c. Remind the client that the yellow skin appearance will disappear.
   d. Inform the client that the urine will appear bright green until the dye is excreted.
   e. Advise the client to avoid direct sunlight for a few hours after the test and to wear sunglasses if staying inside is not possible.
   f. Inform the client that the photophobia will continue until pupil size returns to normal.

B. Computed tomography (CT)
1. Description
   a. The test is performed to examine the eyes, the bony structures around the eye, and the extraocular muscles.
   b. A beam of x-rays scans the skull and orbits of the eye.
   c. A cross-sectional image is formed by the use of a computer.
   d. Contrast material may be used unless eye trauma is suspected.
2. Interventions
   a. No special client preparation or follow-up care is required.
   b. Instruct the client that he or she will be positioned in a confined space and will need to keep his or her head still during the procedure.

C. Slit lamp
1. Description
   a. A slit lamp allows examination of the anterior ocular structures under microscopic magnification.
   b. The client leans on a chin rest to stabilize the head while a narrowed beam of light is aimed so that it illuminates only a narrow segment of the eye.
2. Interventions
   a. Explain the procedure the client.

b. Advise the client about the brightness of the light and the need to look forward at a point over the examiner's ear.

D. Corneal staining
1. Description
   a. A topical dye is instilled into the conjunctival sac to outline irregularities of the corneal surface that are not easily visible.
   b. The eye is viewed through a blue filter, and a bright green color indicates areas of a nonintact corneal epithelium.
2. Interventions
   a. If the client wears contact lenses, the lenses must be removed.
   b. The client is instructed to blink after the dye has been applied to distribute the dye evenly across the cornea.

E. Tonometry
1. Description: The test is used primarily to assess for an increase of intraocular pressure and potential **glaucoma**.
2. Noncontact tonometry measurement
   a. No direct contact with the client's cornea is needed and no topical eye anesthetic is needed.
   b. A puff of air is directed at the cornea to indent the cornea, which can be unpleasant and may startle the client.
   c. It is a less accurate method of measurement as compared with contact tonometry.
3. Contact tonometry measurement
   a. Requires a topical anesthetic
   b. A flattened cone is brought in contact with the cornea, and the amount of pressure needed to flatten the cornea is measured.
   c. The client must be instructed to avoid rubbing the eye after the examination if the eye has been anesthetized because of the potential for scratching the cornea.

⚠ Normal intraocular pressure is 10 to 21 mm Hg. Intraocular pressure varies throughout the day and is normally higher in the morning. Always document the time of intraocular measurement.

F. Ultrasound: Procedure is similar to an ultrasound procedure done in other parts of the body and is done to detect lesions or tumors in the eye.
G. Magnetic resonance imaging (MRI): Similar to an MRI done in other parts of the body; refer to Chapter 57 for additional information on MRI.

IV. DISORDERS OF THE EYE

A. Risk factors related to eye disorders (Box 55-1)
D. Refractive errors
1. Description

Box 55-1 Risk Factors of Eye Disorders

Aging process	Hereditary
Congenital	Medications
Diabetes mellitus	Trauma

a. Refraction is the bending of light rays. Any problem associated with either eye length or refraction can lead to refractive errors.
b. **Myopia** (nearsightedness): Refractive ability of the eye is too strong for the eye length; images are bent and fall in front of, not on, the retina.
c. **Hyperopia** (farsightedness): Refractive ability of the eye is too weak; images are focused behind the retina.
d. Presbyopia: Loss of lens elasticity caused by aging; less able to focus the eye for close work and images fall behind the retina.
e. **Astigmatism**: Occurs because of the irregular curvature of the cornea; image does not focus on the retina.

2. Data collection
   a. Refractive errors are diagnosed through a process called refraction.
   b. The client views an eye chart while various lenses of different strengths are systematically placed in front of the eye and is asked whether each lens sharpens or worsens the vision.
3. Nonsurgical interventions: Eyeglasses or contact lenses
4. Surgical interventions
   a. Radial keratotomy: Incisions are made through the peripheral cornea to flatten the cornea, which allows the image to be focused closer to the retina; used to treat **myopia**.
   b. Photorefractive keratotomy: A laser beam is used to remove small portions of the corneal surface to reshape the cornea to focus an image properly on the retina; used to treat **myopia** and **astigmatism**.
   c. Laser in-situ keratomileusis (LASIK): The superficial layers of the cornea are lifted as a flap, a laser reshapes the deeper corneal layers, and then the corneal flap is replaced; used to treat **hyperopia**, **myopia**, and **astigmatism**.
   d. Intrastromal corneal rings (Intacs): The shape of the cornea is changed by placing a flexible ring in the outer edges of the cornea; used to treat **myopia**.

C. Legally blind
1. Description: The best visual acuity with corrective lenses in the better eye of 20/200 or less or the visual field is no greater than 20 degrees in its widest diameter in the better eye
2. Interventions

a. When speaking to the client who has limited sight or is blind, the nurse uses a normal tone of voice.

b. Alert the client when approaching.

c. Orient the client to the environment.

d. Use a focal point and provide further orientation to the environment from that focal point.

e. Allow the client to touch objects in the room.

f. Use the clock placement of foods on the meal tray to orient the client.

g. Promote independence as much as possible.

h. Provide radios, televisions, and clocks that give the time orally, or provide a Braille watch.

i. When ambulating, allow the client to grasp the nurse's arm at the elbow. The nurse keeps his or her arm close to the body so that the client can detect the direction of movement.

j. Instruct the client to remain one step behind the nurse when ambulating.

k. Instruct the client in the use of the cane used for the blind client, which is differentiated from other canes by its straight shape and white color with red tip.

l. Instruct the client that the cane is held in the dominant hand several inches off the floor.

m. Instruct the client that the cane sweeps the ground where the client's foot will be placed next to determine the presence of obstacles.

D. Cataracts (Figure 55-1)

1. Description

a. A **cataract** is opacity of the lens that distorts the image projected onto the retina and that can progress to blindness.

b. Causes include the aging process (senile **cataracts**), heredity (congenital **cataracts**), and injury (traumatic **cataracts**). Cataracts can also result from another eye disease (secondary cataracts).

c. Causes of secondary **cataracts** include diabetes mellitus, maternal rubella, severe **myopia**, ultraviolet light exposure, and medications such as corticosteroids.

d. Intervention is indicated when visual acuity has been reduced to a level that the client finds to be unacceptable or adversely affects lifestyle.

2. Data collection

a. Blurred vision and decreased color perception are early signs.

b. Diplopia, reduced visual acuity, absence of the red reflex, and the presence of a white pupil are late signs.

c. Pain or eye redness is associated with age-related **cataract** formation.

d. Loss of vision is gradual.

3. Interventions

▲ **FIGURE 55-1** The cloudy appearance of a lens affected by cataract. (From Black, J., & Hawks, J. [2009]. *Medical-surgical nursing: Clinical management for positive outcomes* [8th ed.]. St. Louis: Saunders. Courtesy of Ophthalmic Photography at the University of Michigan W.K. Kellogg Eye Center, Ann Arbor, MI.)

a. Surgical removal of the lens, one eye at a time, is performed.

b. With extracapsular extraction, the lens is lifted out without removing the lens capsule. The procedure may be performed by phacoemulsification, in which the lens is broken up by ultrasonic vibrations and is extracted.

c. With intracapsular extraction, the lens and capsule are removed completely.

d. A partial iridectomy may be performed with the lens extraction to prevent acute secondary **glaucoma**.

e. A lens implantation may be performed at the time of the surgical procedure.

4. Preoperative interventions

a. Instruct the client regarding the postoperative measures to prevent or decrease intraocular pressure, such as bending over, coughing, straining, and rubbing the eye.

b. Stress to the client that care after surgery requires instillation of different types of eye drops several times a day for 2 to 4 weeks.

c. Administer eye medications preoperatively, including **mydriatics** and cycloplegics as prescribed.

5. Postoperative interventions

a. Elevate the head of the bed 30 to 45 degrees.

b. Turn the client to the back or nonoperative side.

c. Provide an eye patch as prescribed. Orient the client to the environment.

d. Position the client's personal belongings to the nonoperative side.

e. Use side rails for safety.

f. Assist with ambulation.

6. Client education (Box 55-2)

Box 55-2 Client Education After Cataract Surgery

Avoid eye straining.

Avoid rubbing or placing pressure on the eyes.

Avoid rapid movements, straining, sneezing, coughing, bending, vomiting, or lifting objects of more than 5 lb.

Take measures to prevent constipation.

Follow instructions for dressing changes and prescribed eye drops and medications.

Wipe excess drainage or tearing with a sterile wet cotton ball from the inner to the outward canthus.

Use an eye shield at bedtime.

If a lens implant is not performed, accommodation is affected and glasses must be worn at all times.

Cataract glasses act as magnifying glasses and replace central vision only.

Because cataract glasses magnify, objects appear closer; therefore the client needs to accommodate, judge distance, and climb stairs carefully.

Contact lenses provide sharp visual acuity, but dexterity is needed to insert them.

Contact the health care provider (HCP) for any decrease in vision, severe eye pain, or increase in eye discharge.

E. Glaucoma

1. Description
   a. A group of ocular diseases resulting in increased intraocular pressure
   b. Intraocular pressure is the fluid (aqueous humor) pressure within the eye. (Normal intraocular pressure is 10 to 21 mm Hg.)
   c. Increased intraocular pressure results from inadequate drainage of aqueous humor from the canal of Schlemm or overproduction of aqueous humor.
   d. The condition damages the optic nerve and can result in blindness.
   e. The gradual loss of visual fields may go unnoticed because central vision is unaffected.
2. Types
   a. Primary open-angle **glaucoma** (POAG) results from obstruction to outflow of aqueous humor, is the most common type, is painless, and vision changes are slow; results in "tunnel" vision.
   b. Primary angle-closure **glaucoma** (PACG) results from blocking the outflow of aqueous humor into the trabecular meshwork; causes include lens or pupil dilation from medications or sympathetic stimulation. Symptoms include blurred vision, halos around lights, and ocular erythemia.
3. Data collection
   a. Early signs include diminished **accommodation** and increased intraocular pressure.
   b. Primary open-angle **glaucoma** (POAG): painless, and vision changes are slow; results in "tunnel" vision.

   c. Primary angle-closure **glaucoma** (PACG): blurred vision, halos around lights, and ocular erythema.
4. Interventions for acute **glaucoma**

⚠️ Acute angle-closure glaucoma is a medical emergency that causes sudden eye pain and possible nausea and vomiting.

   a. Treat acute **glaucoma** as a medical emergency.
   b. Administer medications as prescribed to lower intraocular pressure.
   c. Prepare the client for peripheral iridectomy, which allows aqueous humor to flow from the posterior to the anterior chamber.
5. Interventions for chronic **glaucoma**
   a. Instruct the client on the importance of medications (**miotics**) to constrict the pupils, carbonic anhydrase inhibitors to decrease the production of aqueous humor, and β-blockers to decrease the production of aqueous humor and intraocular pressure.
   b. Instruct the client on the need for lifelong medication use.
   c. Instruct the client to wear a Medic-Alert bracelet.
   d. Instruct the client to avoid anticholinergic medications.
   e. Instruct the client to report eye pain, halos around the eyes, and changes in vision to the HCP.
   f. Instruct the client that when maximal medical therapy has failed to halt the progression of visual field loss and optic nerve damage, surgery will be recommended.
   g. Instruct the client to contact the health care provider before taking medications, including over-the-counter medications.
   h. Prepare the client for trabeculoplasty as prescribed to facilitate aqueous humor drainage.
   i. Prepare the client for trabeculectomy as prescribed, which allows drainage of aqueous humor into the conjunctival spaces by the creation of an opening.

F. Retinal detachment

1. Description
   a. Detachment or separation of the retina from the epithelium
   b. **Retinal detachment** occurs when the layers of the retina separate because of the accumulation of fluid between them, or when both retinal layers elevate away from the choroid as a result of a tumor.
   c. Partial detachment becomes complete if untreated.
   d. When detachment becomes complete, blindness occurs.

2. Data collection
   a. Flashes of light
   b. Floaters or black spots (signs of bleeding)
   c. Increase in blurred vision
   d. Sense of a curtain being drawn over the eye
   e. Loss of a portion of the visual field; painless loss of central or peripheral vision
3. Immediate interventions
   a. Provide bedrest.
   b. Cover both eyes with patches as prescribed to prevent further detachment.
   c. Speak to the client before approaching.
   d. Position the client's head as prescribed.
   e. Protect the client from injury.
   f. Avoid jerky head movements.
   g. Minimize eye stress.
   h. Prepare the client for a surgical procedure as prescribed.
4. Surgical procedures
   a. Draining fluid from the subretinal space so that the retina can return to the normal position
   b. Sealing retinal breaks by cryosurgery, a cold probe applied to the sclera, to stimulate an inflammatory response leading to adhesions
   c. Diathermy, the use of an electrode needle and heat through the sclera, to stimulate an inflammatory response
   d. Laser therapy, to stimulate an inflammatory response and to seal small retinal tears before the detachment occurs
   e. Scleral buckling, to hold the choroid and retina together with a splint until scar tissue forms and closes the tear (Figure 55-2)
   f. Insertion of gas or silicone oil to promote reattachment. These agents float against the retina to hold it in place until healing occurs.
5. Postoperative interventions
   a. Maintain eye patches as prescribed.
   b. Monitor for hemorrhage.
   c. Prevent nausea and vomiting and monitor for restlessness, which can cause hemorrhage.
   d. Monitor for sudden, sharp eye pain (notify the HCP).
   e. Encourage deep breathing but avoid coughing.
   f. Provide bedrest for 1 to 2 days as prescribed.
   g. Position the client as prescribed. (Positioning depends on the location of the detachment.)
   h. Administer eye medications as prescribed.
   i. Assist the client with activities of daily living.
   j. Avoid sudden head movements or anything that increases intraocular pressure.
   k. Instruct the client to limit reading for 3 to 5 weeks.
   l. Instruct the client to avoid squinting, straining and constipation, lifting heavy objects, and bending from the waist.

▲ **FIGURE 55-2** The scleral buckling procedure for repair of retinal detachment. (From Ignatavicius, D., & Workman, M. [2010]. *Medical surgical nursing: Patient-centered collaborative care* [6th ed.]. St. Louis: Saunders.)

   m. Instruct the client to wear dark glasses during the day and an eye patch at night.
   n. Encourage follow-up care because of the danger of recurrence or occurrence in the other eye.
G. Macular degeneration
   1. A deterioration of the macula, the area of central vision
   2. Can be atrophic (age related or dry) or exudative (wet)
   3. Age-related: caused by gradual blocking of retinal capillaries leading to an ischemic and necrotic macula; rods and cones photoreceptors die.
   4. Exudative: serous detachment of pigment epithelium in the macula occurs and fluid and blood collect under the macula, resulting in scar formation and visual distortion.
   5. Interventions are aimed at maximizing the remaining vision.
   6. Data collection
      a. A decline in central vision
      b. Blurred vision and distortion
   7. Interventions
      a. Initiate strategies to assist in maximizing remaining vision and maintaining independence.
      b. Provide referrals to community organizations.

c. Laser therapy or photodynamic therapy may be prescribed to seal the leaking blood vessels in or near the macula.

H. Ocular melanoma
1. Most common malignant eye tumor in adults
2. Tumor usually found in the uveal tract and can spread easily because of rich blood supply
3. Data collection
   a. Tumor can be discovered during routine examination.
   b. If macular area is invaded, blurring of vision occurs.
   c. Increased intraocular pressure is present if the canal of Schlemm is invaded.
   d. Change of iris color is noted if the tumor invades the iris.
   e. Ultrasonography may be performed to detect the tumor size and location.
4. Interventions
   a. Enucleation: The entire eyeball is removed surgically and a ball implant is inserted to provide a base for socket prosthesis.
   b. Radiation via a radioactive plaque that is sutured to the sclera. The radioactive plaque remains in place until the prescribed radiation dose is delivered.

I. Enucleation and exenteration
1. Description
   a. Enucleation is the removal of the entire eyeball.
   b. Exenteration is the removal of the eyeball and surrounding tissues and bone.
   c. The procedures are performed for the removal of ocular tumors.
   d. After the eye is removed, a ball implant is inserted to provide a firm base for socket prosthesis and facilitate the best cosmetic result.
   e. A prosthesis is fitted about 1 month after surgery.
2. Preoperative interventions
   a. Provide emotional support to the client.
   b. Encourage the client to verbalize feelings related to loss.
3. Postoperative interventions
   a. Monitor the vital signs.
   b. Monitor a pressure patch or dressing as prescribed.
   c. Report changes in vital signs or the presence of bright red drainage on the pressure patch or dressing.

J. Hyphema
1. Description
   a. The presence of blood in the anterior chamber that occurs as a result of an injury
   b. The condition usually resolves in 5 to 7 days.
2. Interventions
   a. Encourage rest with the client in the semi-Fowler's position.

b. Avoid sudden eye movements for 3 to 5 days to decrease the likelihood of bleeding.
c. Administer cycloplegic eye drops as prescribed to relax the eye muscles and place the eye at rest.
d. Instruct the client in the use of eye shields or eye patches as prescribed.
e. Instruct the client to restrict reading and limit watching television.

K. Contusions
1. Description
   a. Bleeding into the soft tissue as a result of an injury
   b. A contusion causes a black eye, and the discoloration disappears in about 10 days.
   c. Pain, photophobia, edema, and diplopia may occur.
2. Interventions
   a. Place ice on the eye immediately.
   b. Instruct the client to receive a thorough eye examination.

L. Foreign bodies
1. Description: An object such as dust or dirt that enters the eye and causes irritation
2. Interventions
   a. Have the client look upward, expose the lower lid, wet a cotton-tipped applicator with sterile normal saline, and gently twist the swab over the particle, and remove it.
   b. If the particle cannot be seen, have the client look downward, place a cotton applicator horizontally on the outer surface of the upper eye lid, grasp the lashes, and pull the upper lid outward and over the cotton applicator. If the particle is seen, gently twist a swab over it to remove.

M. Penetrating objects
1. Description: An injury that occurs to the eye in which an object penetrates the eye
2. Interventions
   a. Never remove the object because it may be holding ocular structures in place. The object must be removed by the HCP.
   b. Cover the object with a cup.
   c. Do not allow the client to bend over or lie flat.
   d. Do not place pressure on the eye.
   e. The client must be seen by a HCP immediately.
   f. X-rays and computed tomography (CT) scans of the orbit are usually performed.
   g. Magnetic resonance imaging (MRI) is contraindicated because of the possibility of metal-containing projectile movement during the procedure.

N. Chemical burns (see Priority Nursing Actions)
1. Description: An eye injury in which a caustic substance enters the eye
2. Interventions

▰▰▰ PRIORITY NURSING ACTIONS! ▰▰▰

Actions to Take if a Client Sustains a Chemical Eye Injury

1. Irrigate the eye.
2. Check the pH of the eye.
3. Assess visual acuity.
4. Document the event, actions taken, and the client's response.

Emergency care after a chemical burn to the eye includes irrigating the eye immediately with sterile normal saline or ocular irrigating solution. If the injury occurred outside the hospital, the eye is irrigated immediately with tap water and then the client is brought to the emergency department. In the emergency department, the irrigation should be maintained for at least 10 minutes (and at least 1 liter should be used to irrigate). After irrigation, the pH of the eye is checked and, if a pH of 6 to 7 has not returned, the irrigation should be continued. Some HCP's prefer the use of lactated Ringer's solution for irrigation because its pH is 6 to 7.5, which is closer to the pH of tears (7.1) than that of normal saline, which may range from 4.5 to 7. After this emergency treatment, visual acuity is assessed. It is also important for the nurse to find out what chemical splashed into the eye.

Finally, the event is documented, as well as the actions taken and the client's response.

References: Black, J., & Hawks, J. (2009). *Medical-surgical nursing: Clinical management for positive outcomes* (8th ed., pp. 1252, 2206). St. Louis: Saunders; and Proehl, J. (2009). *Emergency nursing procedures* (4th ed., p. 756). St. Louis: Saunders.

⚠ If a chemical splash to the eye occurs, treatment should begin immediately. Immediately flush the eyes at the scene of the injury with water for at least 15 to 20 minutes.

   a. At the scene of the injury, obtain a sample of the chemical involved.
   b. At the emergency department, the eye is irrigated with normal saline solution or an ophthalmic irrigation solution for at least 10 minutes.
   c. The solution is directed across the cornea and toward the lateral canthus.
   d. Prepare for visual acuity assessment.
   e. Apply an antibiotic ointment as prescribed.
   f. Cover the eye with a patch as prescribed.

O. Eye (tissue) donation
   1. Donor eyes
      a. Donor eyes are obtained from cadavers.
      b. Donor eyes must be enucleated soon after death because of rapid endothelial cell death.
      c. Donor eyes must be stored in a preserving solution.
      d. Storage, handling, and coordination of donor tissue with surgeons are provided by a network of state eye bank associations.

   2. Care to the deceased client as a potential eye donor
      a. Discuss the option of eye donation with the HCP and family.
      b. Raise the head of the bed 30 degrees.
      c. Instill antibiotic eye drops as prescribed.
      d. Close the eyes and apply sterile gauze and a small ice pack to the closed eyes.
   3. Preoperative care to the recipient of the cornea
      a. Recipient may be told of the tissue (cornea) availability only several hours to 1 day before the surgery.
      b. Assist in alleviating client anxiety.
      c. Assess the recipient's eye for signs of infection.
      d. Report the presence of any redness, watery or purulent drainage, or edema around the recipient's eye to the HCP.
      e. Instill antibiotic drops into the recipient's eye as prescribed to reduce the number of microorganisms.
      f. Administer fluids and medications intravenously as prescribed.
   4. Postoperative care to the recipient
      a. The eye is covered with a pressure patch and protective shield that is left in place for 1 day.
      b. Do not remove or change the dressing without a HCP's prescription.
      c. Monitor the vital signs.
      d. Monitor the level of consciousness.
      e. Monitor the eye dressing.
      f. Position the client with the head elevated and on the nonoperative side to reduce intraocular pressure.
      g. Orient the client frequently.
      h. Monitor for complications of bleeding, wound leakage, infection, and tissue rejection.
      i. Instruct the client on how to apply a patch and eye shield.
      j. Instruct the client to wear the eye shield at night for 1 month and whenever around small children or pets.
      k. Advise the client not to rub the eye.
   5. Graft rejection
      a. Rejection can occur at any time.
      b. Inform the client of the signs of rejection.
      c. Signs include *r*edness, *s*welling, *d*ecreased vision, and *p*ain (RSVP).
      d. The eye is treated with topical corticosteroids.

V. ANATOMY AND PHYSIOLOGY OF THE EAR

A. Functions
   1. Hearing
   2. Maintenance of balance
B. External ear (pinna)
   1. The external ear is embedded in the temporal bone bilaterally at the level of the eyes.

2. The external ear extends from the auricle through the external canal to the tympanic membrane or eardrum.
3. The external ear includes the mastoid process, which is the bony ridge located over the temporal bone.

C. Middle ear
1. The middle ear consists of the medial side of the tympanic membrane.
2. The middle ear contains three bony ossicles.
   a. Malleus
   b. Incus
   c. Stapes
3. Functions of the middle ear
   a. Conduct sound vibrations from the outer ear to the central hearing apparatus in the inner ear
   b. Protect the inner ear by reducing the amplitude of loud sounds
   c. The eustachian tube allows equalization of air pressure on each side of the tympanic membrane so that the membrane does not rupture.

D. Inner ear
1. The inner ear contains the semicircular canals, the cochlea, and the distal end of the eighth cranial nerve.
2. The semicircular canals contain fluid and hair cells connected to sensory nerve fibers of the vestibular portion of the eighth cranial nerve.
3. The inner ear maintains sense of balance or equilibrium.
4. The cochlea is the spiral-shaped organ of hearing.
5. The organ of Corti (within the cochlea) is the receptor and organ of hearing.
6. Eighth cranial nerve
   a. The cochlear branch of the nerve transmits neuroimpulses from the cochlea to the brain, where they are interpreted as sound.
   b. The vestibular branch maintains balance and equilibrium.

E. Hearing and equilibrium
1. The external ear conducts sound waves to the middle ear.
2. The middle ear, also called the tympanic cavity, conducts sound waves to the inner ear.
3. The middle ear is filled with air, which is kept at atmospheric pressure by the opening of the auditory canal.
4. The inner ear contains sensory receptors for sound and for equilibrium.
5. The receptors in the inner ear transmit sound waves and changes in body position to the nerve impulses.

VI. ASSESSMENT OF THE EAR (refer to Chapter 29 for information on ear assessment)

VII. DIAGNOSTIC TESTS FOR THE EAR

A. Tomography
1. Description
   a. Tomography may be performed with or without contrast medium.
   b. Tomography assesses the mastoid, middle ear, and inner ear structures.
   c. Multiple radiographs of the head are obtained.
   d. Tomography is especially helpful in the diagnosis of acoustic tumors.
2. Interventions
   a. All jewelry is removed.
   b. Lead eye shields are used to cover the cornea to diminish the radiation dose to the eyes.
   c. The client must remain still in a supine position.
   d. No follow-up care is required.

B. Audiometry
1. Description
   a. Audiometry measures hearing acuity.
   b. Audiometry uses two types: pure tone audiometry and speech audiometry.
   c. Pure tone audiometry is used to identify problems with hearing, speech, music, and other sounds in the environment.
   d. In speech audiometry, the client's ability to hear spoken words is measured.
   e. After testing, audiogram patterns are depicted on a graph to determine the type and level of the hearing loss.
2. Interventions
   a. Inform the client regarding the procedure.
   b. Instruct the client to identify the sounds as they are heard.

C. Electronystagmography (ENG)
1. Description
   a. ENG is a vestibular test that evaluates spontaneous and induced eye movements known as nystagmus.
   b. ENG is used to distinguish between normal nystagmus and medication-induced nystagmus or nystagmus caused by a lesion in the central or peripheral vestibular pathway.
   c. ENG records changing electrical fields with the movement of the eye, as monitored by electrodes placed on the skin around the eye.
2. Interventions
   a. The client is instructed to remain NPO for 3 hours before testing and to avoid caffeine-containing beverages for 24 to 48 hours before the test.
   b. Unnecessary medications are omitted for 24 hours before testing.
   c. Instruct the client that this is a long and tiring procedure.
   d. The client should bring prescription eyeglasses to the examination.

e. The client sits and is instructed to gaze at lights, focus on a moving pattern, focus on a moving point, and then close the eyes.

f. While sitting in a chair, the client may be rotated to provide information about vestibular function.

g. In addition, the client's ears are irrigated with cool and warm water, which may cause nausea and vomiting.

h. After the procedure, the client begins taking clear fluids slowly and cautiously because nausea and vomiting may occur.

i. Assistance with ambulation may also be necessary after the procedure.

D. Magnetic resonance imaging (MRI): Refer to Chapter 57 for information on MRI.

VIII. DISORDERS OF THE EAR

A. Risk factors related to ear disorders (Box 55-3)

B. Conductive hearing loss

1. Description

a. **Conductive hearing loss** occurs when sound waves are blocked to the inner ear fibers because of external ear or middle ear disorders.

b. Disorders can often be corrected with no damage to hearing or with minimal permanent hearing loss.

2. Causes

a. Any inflammatory process or obstruction of the external or middle ear

b. Tumors

c. **Otosclerosis**

d. A buildup of scar tissue on the ossicles from previous middle ear surgery

C. Sensorineural hearing loss

1. Description

a. **Sensorineural hearing loss** is a pathological process of the inner ear or of the sensory fibers that lead to the cerebral cortex.

b. **Sensorineural hearing loss** is often permanent, and measures must be taken to reduce further damage.

2. Causes

a. Damage to the inner ear structures

b. Damage to the eighth cranial nerve

c. Prolonged exposure to loud noise

d. Medications

e. Trauma

f. Inherited disorders

g. Metabolic and circulatory disorders

h. Infections

i. Surgery

j. **Ménière's syndrome**

k. Diabetes mellitus

l. Myxedema

D. Mixed hearing loss

1. Mixed hearing loss also is known as **conductive-sensorineural hearing loss**.

2. Client has **sensorineural** and **conductive hearing loss**.

E. Central hearing loss: Involves the inability to interpret sound, including speech, due to a problem in the brain.

F. Signs of hearing loss and facilitating communication (Boxes 55-4 and 55-5)

Box 55-4 Signs of Hearing Loss

Frequently asking others to repeat statements
Straining to hear
Turning head or leaning forward to favor one ear
Shouting in conversation
Ringing in the ears
Failing to respond when not looking in the direction of the sound
Answering questions incorrectly
Raising the volume of the television or radio
Avoiding large groups
Better understanding of speech when in small groups
Withdrawing from social interactions

Box 55-5 Facilitation of Communication

Using written words if the client is able to see, read, and write
Providing plenty of light in the room
Getting the attention of the client before beginning to speak
Facing the client when speaking
Talking in a room without distracting noises
Moving close to the client and speaking slowly and clearly
Keeping hands and other objects away from the mouth when talking to the client
Talking in normal volume and lower pitch, since shouting is not helpful and higher frequencies are less easily heard
Rephrasing sentences and repeating information
Validating with the client the understanding of statements made by asking the client to repeat what was said
Using lip-reading
Encouraging the client to wear glasses when talking to someone to improve vision for lip reading
Using sign language, which combines speech with hand movements that signify letters, words, or phrases
Using telephone amplifiers
Using flashing lights that are activated by ringing of the telephone or doorbell
Using specially trained dogs that help the client to be aware of sound and to alert the client to potential dangers

---

Box 55-3 Risk Factors of Ear Disorders

Aging process	Ototoxicity
Infection	Trauma
Medications	Tumors

G. Cochlear implantation (Figure 55-3)

1. Cochlear implants are used for **sensorineural hearing loss**.
2. A small computer converts sound waves into electrical impulses.
3. Electrodes are placed by the internal ear with a computer device attached to the external ear.
4. Electronic impulses directly stimulate nerve fibers.

H. Hearing aids

1. Hearing aids are used for the client with **conductive hearing loss**.
2. Hearing aids have limited value for the client with **sensorineural hearing loss**, because they only make sounds louder, not clearer.
3. A difficulty that exists in the use of hearing aids is the amplification of background noise and voices.
4. Client education (Box 55-6)

I. Presbycusis

1. Description
   a. **Presbycusis** is a **sensorineural hearing loss** associated with aging.

Box 55-6 Client Education Regarding a Hearing Aid

Encourage the client to begin using the hearing aid slowly to adjust to the device.

Adjust the volume to the minimal hearing level to prevent feedback squeaking.

Teach the client to concentrate on the sounds that are to be heard and filter out background noise.

Instruct the client to clean the ear mold with mild soap and water.

Avoid excessive wetting of the hearing aid, and try to keep the hearing aid dry.

Clean the ear cannula of the hearing aid with a toothpick or pipe cleaner.

Turn off the hearing aid before removing from the ear to prevent squealing feedback. Remove the battery when not in use.

Keep extra batteries on hand.

Keep the hearing aid in a safe place.

Prevent hair sprays, oils, or other hair and face products from coming in contact with the receiver of the hearing aid.

---

1 Sound enters the system through a tiny microphone behind the ear.

2 The sound is sent from the microphone to the speech processor through the thin cord that connects them.

3 The speech processor selects and codes the elements of sound that are most useful for understanding speech.

4 These electronic codes are sent back up through the thin cable to the transmitter.

5 The transmitting coil, a plastic-covered ring about 1 inch in diameter, sends the codes across the skin to the receiver/stimulator.

6 The receiver/stimulator contains an integrated circuit that converts the codes into special electrical signals and sends them along the electrode array. The electrode array is a set of 22 tiny electrode bands arranged in a row around a piece of tapered flexible tubing. Each electrode has a wire connecting it to the receiver/stimulator. The coded electrical signals are sent to specific electrodes. Each electrode is programmed separately to deliver signals that can vary in loudness and pitch. These electrodes then stimulate different hearing nerve fibers, which send the messages on to the brain.

7 The brain receives the signals and interprets them as sound.

▲ FIGURE 55-3 Cochlear implant to restore hearing. (From Black, J., & Hawks, J. [2009]. *Medical-surgical nursing: Clinical management for positive outcomes* [8th ed.]. St. Louis: Saunders.)

b. **Presbycusis** leads to degeneration or atrophy of the ganglion cells in the cochlea and a loss of elasticity of the basilar membranes.

c. **Presbycusis** leads to compromise of the vascular supply to the inner ear with changes in several areas of the ear structure.

2. Data collection

a. Hearing loss is gradual and bilateral.

b. The client states that he or she has no problem with hearing but cannot understand what the words are.

c. The client thinks that the speaker is mumbling.

J. External otitis

1. Description

a. External otitis is an infective inflammatory or allergic response involving the structure of the external auditory canal or the auricles.

b. An irritating or infective agent comes in contact with the epithelial layer of the external ear.

c. Contact leads to an allergic response or signs and symptoms of an infection.

d. The skin becomes red, swollen, and tender to touch on movement.

e. The extensive swelling of the canal can lead to **conductive hearing loss** because of obstruction.

f. External otitis is more common in children, is termed "swimmer's ear," and occurs more often in hot, humid environments.

g. Prevention includes the elimination of irritating or infecting agents.

2. Data collection

a. Pain

b. Itching

c. Plugged feeling in the ear

d. Redness and edema

e. Exudate

f. Hearing loss

3. Interventions

a. Apply heat locally for 20 minutes three times a day.

b. Encourage rest to assist in reducing pain.

c. Administer antibiotics or corticosteroids as prescribed.

d. Administer analgesics such as aspirin or acetaminophen (Tylenol) for the pain as prescribed.

e. Instruct the client that the ears should be kept clean and dry.

f. Instruct the client to use earplugs for swimming.

g. Instruct the client that cotton-tipped applicators should not be used to dry ears because their use can lead to trauma to the canal.

h. Instruct the client that irritating agents such as hair products or headphones should be discontinued.

Box 55-7 Client Education After Myringotomy

Avoid strenuous activities.

Avoid rapid head movements, bouncing, or bending.

Avoid straining on bowel movement.

Avoid drinking through a straw.

Avoid traveling by air.

Avoid forceful coughing.

Avoid contact with persons with colds.

Avoid washing hair, showering, or getting the head wet for 1 week as prescribed.

Instruct the client that if he or she needs to blow the nose, to blow one side at a time with the mouth open.

Instruct the client to keep ears dry by keeping a ball of cotton coated with petroleum jelly in the ear and to change the cotton ball daily.

Instruct the client to report excessive ear drainage to the HCP.

K. Otitis media: See Chapter 32

1. Myringotomy: See Chapter 32

2. Client education (Box 55-7)

L. Chronic otitis media

1. Description

a. Chronic otitis media is a chronic infective, inflammatory, or allergic response involving the structure of the middle ear.

b. Frequent removal of debris from the canal may be required.

c. Myringoplasty can reconstruct the tympanic membrane and ossicles and improve **conductive hearing loss**.

d. Mastoidectomy may be performed if the infection has spread to involve the mastoid bone.

 Monitor the client with otitis media closely for response to treatment. Otic and systemic antibiotics may be used to treat the infection, but often the organism is resistant.

2. Preoperative interventions

a. Administer antibiotic drops as prescribed.

b. Clean the ear of debris as prescribed. Irrigate the ear with a solution as prescribed to restore the normal pH of the ear.

c. Instruct the client to avoid persons with upper respiratory infections.

d. Instruct the client to obtain adequate rest, eat a balanced diet, and drink adequate fluids.

e. Instruct the client in deep breathing and coughing. Forceful coughing, which increases pressure in the middle ear, is to be avoided postoperatively.

3. Postoperative interventions

a. Inform the client that initial hearing after surgery is diminished because of the packing in the ear canal and that hearing improvement will occur after the packing is removed.

b. Keep the dressing clean and dry.

c. Keep the client flat with the operative ear up for at least 12 hours as prescribed.

d. Administer antibiotics as prescribed.

M. Mastoiditis

1. Description

a. Mastoiditis may be acute or chronic and results from untreated or inadequately treated chronic or acute otitis media.

b. The pain is not relieved by myringotomy.

2. Data collection

a. Swelling behind the ear and pain with minimal movement of the head

b. Cellulitis on the skin or external scalp over the mastoid process

c. A reddened, dull, thick, immobile tympanic membrane with or without perforation

d. Tender and enlarged postauricular lymph nodes

e. Low-grade fever

f. Malaise

g. Anorexia

3. Interventions

a. Prepare the client for surgical removal of infected material.

b. Monitor for complications.

c. Simple or modified radical mastoidectomy with tympanoplasty is the most common treatment.

d. Once infected tissue is removed, the tympanoplasty is performed to reconstruct the ossicles and the tympanic membranes in an attempt to restore normal hearing.

4. Complications

a. Damage to the abducens and facial cranial nerves

b. Damage exhibited by inability to look laterally (cranial nerve VI, abducens) and a drooping of the mouth on the affected side (cranial nerve VII, facial)

c. Meningitis

d. Brain abscess

e. Chronic purulent otitis media

f. Wound infections

g. Vertigo, if the infection spreads into the labyrinth

5. Postoperative interventions

a. Monitor for dizziness.

b. Monitor for signs of meningitis as evidenced by a stiff neck and vomiting.

c. Prepare for a wound dressing change 24 hours postoperatively.

d. Monitor the surgical incision for edema, drainage, and redness.

e. Position the client flat with the operative side up.

f. Restrict the client to bed with bedside commode privileges for 24 hours as prescribed.

g. Assist the client with getting out of bed to prevent falling or injuries from dizziness.

h. With reconstruction of the ossicles via a graft, take precautions to prevent dislodging of the graft.

N. **Otosclerosis**

1. Description

a. **Otosclerosis** is a disease of the labyrinthine capsule of the middle ear that results in a bony overgrowth of the tissue surrounding the ossicles.

b. **Otosclerosis** causes the development of irregular areas of new bone formation and causes the fixation of the bones.

c. Stapes fixation leads to a **conductive hearing loss**.

d. If the disease involves the inner ear, **sensorineural hearing loss** is present.

e. Bilateral involvement is not uncommon, although hearing loss may be worse in one ear.

f. It is thought to be a hereditary autosomal dominant disorder; is most commonly seen in young women.

g. Nonsurgical intervention promotes the improvement of hearing through amplification.

h. Surgical intervention involves removal of the bony growth that is causing the hearing loss.

i. A partial stapedectomy or complete stapedectomy with prosthesis (**fenestration**) may be performed surgically.

2. Data collection

a. Slowly progressing **conductive hearing loss**

b. Bilateral hearing loss

c. A ringing or roaring type of constant tinnitus

d. Loud sounds heard in the ear when chewing

e. Pinkish discoloration (Schwartze's sign) of the tympanic membrane, which indicates vascular changes within the ear

f. Negative Rinne test

g. Weber test that shows lateralization of sound to the ear with the most **conductive hearing loss**

O. **Fenestration**

1. Description

a. **Fenestration** is removal of the stapes, with a small hole drilled in the footplate; a prosthesis is connected between the incus and footplate.

b. Sounds cause the prosthesis to vibrate in the same manner as did the stapes.

c. Complications include complete hearing loss, prolonged vertigo, infection, or facial nerve damage.

2. Preoperative interventions

a. Instruct the client on measures to prevent middle ear or external ear infections.

b. Instruct the client to avoid excessive nose blowing.

c. Instruct the client not to clean the ear canal with cotton-tipped applicators and to avoid trauma or injury to the ear canal.

3. Postoperative interventions

a. Inform the client that hearing is initially worse after the surgical procedure because of swelling and that no noticeable improvement in hearing may occur for as long as 6 weeks.

b. Inform the client that the Gelfoam ear packing interferes with hearing but is used to decrease bleeding.

c. Assist with ambulating during the first 1 to 2 days after surgery.

d. Provide side rails when the client is in bed.

e. Administer antibiotics, antivertiginous, and pain medications as prescribed.

f. Monitor for facial nerve damage, weakness, changes in tactile sensation, changes in taste sensation, vertigo, nausea, and vomiting.

g. Instruct the client to move the head slowly when changing positions to prevent vertigo.

h. Instruct the client to avoid persons with upper respiratory tract infections.

i. Instruct the client to avoid showering and getting the head and wound wet.

j. Instruct the client to avoid using small objects (cotton-tipped applicators) to clean the external ear canal.

k. Instruct the client to avoid rapid, extreme changes in pressure caused by quick head movements, sneezing, nose blowing, straining, and changes in altitude.

l. Instruct the client to avoid changes in middle ear pressure because they could dislodge the graft or prosthesis.

P. Labyrinthitis

1. Description: Infection of the labyrinth that occurs as a complication of acute or chronic otitis media

2. May result from growth of a cholesteatoma—benign overgrowth of squamous cell epithelium

3. Data collection

a. Hearing loss that may be permanent on the affected side

b. Tinnitus

c. Spontaneous nystagmus to the affected side

d. Vertigo

e. Nausea and vomiting

4. Interventions

a. Monitor for signs of meningitis, the most common complication, as evidenced by headache, stiff neck, and lethargy.

b. Administer systemic antibiotics as prescribed.

c. Advise the client to rest in bed in a darkened room.

d. Administer antiemetics and antivertiginous medications as prescribed.

e. Instruct the client that the vertigo subsides as the inflammation resolves.

f. Instruct the client that balance problems that persist may require gait training through physical therapy.

Q. Ménière's syndrome

1. Description

a. **Ménière's syndrome** is also called endolymphatic hydrops and refers to dilation of the endolymphatic system by overproduction or decreased reabsorption of endolymphatic fluid.

b. The syndrome is characterized by tinnitus, unilateral **sensorineural hearing loss**, and vertigo.

c. Symptoms occur in attacks and last for several days, and the client becomes totally incapacitated during the attacks.

d. Initial hearing loss is reversible but as the frequency of attacks continues, hearing loss becomes permanent.

⚠ A priority nursing intervention in the care of a client with Ménière's syndrome is instituting safety measures.

2. Causes

a. Any factor that increases endolymphatic secretion in the labyrinth

b. Viral and bacterial infections

c. Allergic reactions

d. Biochemical disturbances

e. Vascular disturbance producing changes in the microcirculation in the labyrinth

f. Long-term stress may be a possible contributing factor

3. Data collection

a. Feelings of fullness in the ear

b. Tinnitus, as a continuous low-pitched roar or humming sound, that is present much of the time but worsens just before and during severe attacks

c. Hearing loss that is worse during an attack

d. Vertigo, as periods of whirling, that might cause the client to fall to the ground

e. Vertigo that is so intense that even while lying down, the client holds the bed or ground in an attempt to prevent the whirling

f. Nausea and vomiting

g. Nystagmus

h. Severe headaches

4. Nonsurgical interventions

a. Prevent injury during vertigo attacks.

b. Provide bedrest in a quiet environment.

c. Provide assistance with walking.

d. Instruct the client to move the head slowly to prevent worsening of the vertigo.

e. Initiate sodium and fluid restrictions as prescribed.

f. Instruct the client to stop smoking.

g. Instruct the client to avoid watching television because the flickering of lights may exacerbate symptoms.

h. Administer nicotinic acid (niacin) as prescribed for its vasodilatory effect.

i. Administer antihistamines as prescribed, which will reduce the production of histamine and the inflammation.

j. Administer antiemetics as prescribed.

k. Administer tranquilizers and sedatives as prescribed to calm the client and allow him or her to rest and to control vertigo, nausea, and vomiting.

l. Mild diuretics may be prescribed to decrease endolymph volume.

m. Inform the client about vestibular rehabilitation as prescribed.

5. Surgical interventions

a. Surgery is performed when medical therapy is ineffective and the functional level of the client has decreased significantly.

b. Endolymphatic drainage and insertion of a shunt may be performed early in the course of the disease to assist with the drainage of excess fluids.

c. A resection of the vestibular nerve or total removal of the labyrinth or a labyrinthectomy may be performed.

6. Postoperative interventions

a. Monitor packing and dressing on the ear.

b. Speak to the client on the side of the unaffected ear.

c. Perform neurological assessments.

d. Maintain side rails.

e. Assist with ambulating.

f. Encourage the client to use a bedside commode rather than ambulating to the bathroom.

g. Administer antivertiginous and antiemetic medications as prescribed.

R. Acoustic neuroma

1. Description

a. Acoustic neuroma is a benign tumor of the vestibular or acoustic nerve.

b. The tumor may cause damage to hearing and to facial movements and sensations.

c. Treatment includes surgical removal of the tumor via craniotomy.

d. Care is taken to preserve the function of the facial nerve.

e. The tumor rarely recurs after surgical removal.

f. Postoperative nursing care is similar to postoperative craniotomy care.

2. Data collection

a. Symptoms usually begin with tinnitus and progress to gradual **sensorineural hearing loss**.

b. As the tumor enlarges, damage to adjacent cranial nerves occurs.

S. Trauma

1. Description

a. The tympanic membrane has a limited stretching ability and gives way under high pressure.

b. Foreign objects placed in the external canal may exert pressure on the tympanic membrane and cause perforation.

c. If the object continues through the canal, the bony structure of the stapes, incus, and malleus may be damaged.

d. A blunt injury to the basal skull and ear can damage the middle ear structures through fractures extending to the middle ear.

e. Excessive nose blowing and rapid changes of pressure that occur with nonpressurized air flights can increase pressure in the middle ear.

f. Depending on the damage to the ossicles, hearing loss may or may not return.

2. Interventions

a. Tympanic membrane perforations usually heal within 24 hours.

b. Surgical reconstruction of the ossicles and tympanic membrane through tympanoplasty or myringoplasty may be performed to improve hearing.

T. Cerumen and foreign bodies

1. Description

a. Cerumen or wax is the most common cause of impacted canals.

b. Foreign bodies can include vegetables, beads, pencil erasers, insects, or other objects.

2. Data collection

a. Sensation of fullness in the ear with or without hearing loss

b. Pain, itching, or bleeding

3. Cerumen

a. Removal of wax by irrigation may be a slow process.

b. Irrigation is contraindicated in clients with a history of tympanic membrane perforation or otitis media.

c. To soften cerumen, add three drops of glycerin or mineral oil to the ear at bedtime, and three drops of hydrogen peroxide twice a day as prescribed.

d. After several days, irrigate the ear.

e. The maximal amount of solution that should be used for irrigation is 50 to 70 mL.

Inform the client that ear candles should never be used to remove cerumen. Their use can cause burns and a vacuum effect, causing a perforation in the tympanic membrane.

4. Foreign bodies
   a. With a foreign object of vegetable matter, irrigation is used with care because this material expands with hydration.
   b. Insects are killed before removal, unless they can be coaxed out by flashlight or a humming noise.
   c. Mineral oil or diluted alcohol is instilled to suffocate the insect, which then is removed using ear forceps.
   d. Use a small ear forceps to remove the object and avoid pushing the object farther into the canal and damaging the tympanic membrane.

MORE QUESTIONS ON EVOLVE!

Practice Questions

571. A client is diagnosed with glaucoma. Which data gathered by the nurse indicate a risk factor associated with glaucoma?
    1. Cardiovascular disease
    2. A history of migraine headaches
    3. Frequent urinary tract infections
    4. Frequent upper respiratory infections

572. A nurse is assisting in developing a teaching plan for the client with glaucoma. Which instruction should the nurse suggest to include in the plan of care?
    1. Decrease the amount of salt in the diet.
    2. Decrease fluid intake to control the intraocular pressure.
    3. Avoid reading the newspaper and watching television.
    4. Eye medications will need to be administered for the rest of your life.

573. A nurse is assigned to care for a client with a detached retina. Which finding would the nurse expect to be documented in the client's record?
    1. Blurred vision
    2. Pain in the effected eye
    3. A yellow discoloration of the sclera
    4. A sense of a curtain falling across the field of vision

574. A nurse is assigned to care for a client with a diagnosis of detached retina. Which finding would indicate that bleeding has occurred as a result of retinal detachment?

    1. Total loss of vision
    2. A reddened conjunctiva
    3. A sudden sharp pain in the eye
    4. Complaints of a burst of black spots or floaters

575. A client arrives in the emergency department after an automobile crash. The client's forehead hit the steering wheel and a hyphema has been diagnosed. The nurse would prepare to position the client:
    1. Flat on bedrest
    2. On bedrest in a semi-Fowler's position
    3. In lateral position on the unaffected side
    4. In the lateral position on the affected side

576. A client sustains a contusion of the eyeball after a traumatic injury with a blunt object. The nurse takes which action immediately?
    1. Notifies the health care provider (HCP)
    2. Applies ice to the affected eye
    3. Irrigates the eye with cool water
    4. Accompanies the client to the emergency department

577. A client sustains a chemical eye injury from a splash of battery acid. The nurse prepares the client for which immediate measure?
    1. Checking visual acuity
    2. Covering the eye with a pressure patch
    3. Swabbing the eye with antibiotic ointment
    4. Irrigating the eye with sterile normal saline

578. A nurse is caring for a client after enucleation and notes the presence of bright red drainage on the dressing. The nurse takes which appropriate action?
    1. Documents the finding
    2. Continues to monitor vital signs
    3. Reports the finding to the registered nurse (RN)
    4. Marks the drainage on the dressing and monitors for any increase in bleeding

579. A nurse is preparing to administer ear drops to an adult client. The nurse administers the ear drops by:
    1. Pulling the pinna up and back
    2. Pulling the earlobe down and back
    3. Tilting the client's head forward and down
    4. Instructing the client to stand and lean to one side

580. A nurse is caring for a client who is hearing-impaired and takes which approach to facilitate communication?
    1. Speaks loudly
    2. Speaks frequently

3. Speaks in a normal tone
4. Speaks directly into the impaired ear

581. A client arrives at the emergency department with a foreign body in the left ear that has been determined to be an insect. Which intervention would the nurse anticipate to be prescribed initially?
1. Irrigation of the ear
2. Instillation of antibiotic ear drops
3. Instillation of corticosteroid ointment
4. Instillation of mineral oil or diluted alcohol

582. A nurse notes that the health care provider has documented a diagnosis of presbycusis on the client's chart. The nurse understands that this condition is accurately described as:
1. Tinnitus that occurs with aging
2. Nystagmus that occurs with aging
3. A conductive hearing loss that occurs with aging
4. A sensorineural hearing loss that occurs with aging

583. A client with Ménière's disease is experiencing severe vertigo. The nurse instructs the client to do which of the following to assist in controlling the vertigo?
1. Increase sodium in the diet.
2. Lie still and watch television.

3. Avoid sudden head movements.
4. Increase fluid intake to 3000 mL/day.

584. A nurse is assigned to care for a client hospitalized with Ménière's disease. The nurse expects that which of the following would most likely be prescribed for the client?
1. Low-fat diet
2. Low-sodium diet
3. Low-cholesterol diet
4. Low-carbohydrate diet

585. The nurse is preparing a teaching plan for a client ❖ who is undergoing cataract extraction with intraocular implant. Which home care measures will the nurse include in the plan? **Select all that apply.**
❑ 1. To avoid activities that require bending over
❑ 2. To contact the surgeon if eye scratchiness occurs
❑ 3. To place an eye shield on the surgical eye at bedtime
❑ 4. That episodes of sudden severe pain in the eye are expected
❑ 5. To contact the surgeon if a decrease in visual acuity occurs
❑ 6. To take acetaminophen (Tylenol) for minor eye discomfort

ANSWERS

571. 1
Rationale: Hypertension, cardiovascular disease, diabetes mellitus, and obesity are associated with the development of glaucoma. Smoking, ingestion of caffeine or large amounts of alcohol, illicit drugs, corticosteroids, altered hormone levels, posture, and eye movements may cause varying transient increases in intraocular pressure.
Test-Taking Strategy: Use knowledge regarding the risk factors associated with glaucoma to answer this question. Remember, cardiovascular disease is associated with the development of glaucoma. If you had difficulty with this question, review the risk factors associated with this disorder.
Level of Cognitive Ability: Analyzing
Client Needs: Health Promotion and Maintenance
Integrated Process: Nursing Process/Data Collection
Content Area: Adult Health/Eye
References: Black, Hawks, p. 1700. 2009.
Ignatavicius, Workman, p. 1095. 2010.

572. 4
Rationale: The administration of eye drops is a critical component of the treatment plan for the client with glaucoma. The client needs to be instructed that medications will need to be taken for the rest of his or her life. Limiting fluids and reducing salt will not decrease intraocular pressure. Option 3 is not necessary.

Test-Taking Strategy: Use the process of elimination. Knowing that medications are an integral component of the treatment plan will assist in directing you to the correct option. Review the treatment associated with the care of the client with glaucoma if you had difficulty with this question.
Level of Cognitive Ability: Applying
Client Needs: Health Promotion and Maintenance
Integrated Process: Teaching and Learning
Content Area: Adult Health/Eye
References: Christensen, Kockrow, p. 627. 2011. *Adult health nursing.*
deWit, p. 649. 2009.

573. 4
Rationale: A characteristic clinical manifestation of retinal detachment described by clients is the feeling that a shadow or curtain is falling across the field of vision. There is no pain associated with detachment of the retina. A retinal detachment is an ophthalmic emergency and even more so if visual acuity is still normal. Options 1 and 3 are not specifically associated with a detached retina.
Test-Taking Strategy: Use the process of elimination. Remember that a characteristic clinical manifestation is the feeling that a shadow or curtain is falling across the field of vision. Retinal detachment can occur suddenly and is an ophthalmic emergency. Review the clinical manifestations associated with this condition if you had difficulty with this question.
Level of Cognitive Ability: Understanding

Client Needs: Physiological Integrity
Integrated Process: Nursing Process/Data Collection
Content Area: Adult Health/Eye
Reference: Christensen, Kockrow, p. 622. 2011. *Adult health nursing.*

574. 4

Rationale: Complaints of a sudden burst of black spots or floaters indicate that bleeding has occurred as a result of the detachment. Options 1, 2, and 3 are not specifically associated with bleeding as a result of detached retina.
Test-Taking Strategy: Use the process of elimination. Hemorrhage is a serious complication associated with retinal detachment. Remember, complaints of a sudden burst of black spots or floaters indicate that bleeding has occurred as a result of the detachment. Review the clinical manifestations associated with the complications of a detached retina if you had difficulty with this question.
Level of Cognitive Ability: Analyzing
Client Needs: Physiological Integrity
Integrated Process: Nursing Process/Data Collection
Content Area: Adult Health/Eye
Reference: deWit, p. 650. 2009.

575. 2

Rationale: A hyphema is the presence of blood in the anterior chamber. It is produced when a force is sufficient to break the integrity of the blood vessels in the eye. It can be caused by direct injury, such as penetrating injury from a BB pellet, or indirectly, such as from striking the forehead on a steering wheel during an accident. The client is treated by bedrest in a semi-Fowler's position to assist gravity in keeping the hyphema away from the optical center of the cornea.
Test-Taking Strategy: Use the process of elimination. Eliminate options 1, 3, and 4 because they are comparable or alike. Placing the client flat will produce an increase in pressure at the injured site. Review care of the client with hyphema if you had difficulty with this question.
Level of Cognitive Ability: Applying
Client Needs: Physiological Integrity
Integrated Process: Nursing Process/Implementation
Content Area: Adult Health/Eye
Reference: Ignatavicius, Workman, p. 1103. 2010.

576. 2

Rationale: Treatment for a contusion begins at the time of injury. Ice is applied immediately. The client should receive a thorough eye examination to rule out the presence of other eye injuries. Eye irrigation is not indicated in a contusion. Options 1 and 4 will delay immediate treatment. After the application of ice, the HCP would be notified.
Test-Taking Strategy: Use the process of elimination, noting the strategic word "immediately." Noting that the client sustained a contusion to the eye will direct you to option 2. Review immediate treatment of an eye contusion if you had difficulty with this question.
Level of Cognitive Ability: Applying
Client Needs: Physiological Integrity
Integrated Process: Nursing Process/Implementation
Content Area: Adult Health/Eye

Reference: Christensen, Kockrow, p. 160. 2011. *Adult health nursing.*

577. 4

Rationale: Emergency care after a chemical burn to the eye includes irrigating the eye immediately with sterile normal saline or ocular irrigating solution. The irrigation should be maintained for at least 10 minutes. After this emergency treatment, visual acuity is assessed. Options 2 and 3 are not immediate measures.
Test-Taking Strategy: Use the process of elimination. Read the question carefully, noting the type of injury to the eye. The question asks about emergency care; therefore in this type of injury, it is necessary to irrigate the eye first. Review this content if you had difficulty with this question.
Level of Cognitive Ability: Applying
Client Needs: Physiological Integrity
Integrated Process: Nursing Process/Implementation
Content Area: Adult Health/Eye
References: deWit, p. 641. 2009.
Kunz Howard, Steinmann, p. 609. 2010.

578. 3

Rationale: If the nurse notes the presence of bright red drainage on the dressing, it must be reported to the registered nurse, because this can indicate hemorrhage. Options 1, 2, and 4 will delay necessary treatment.
Test-Taking Strategy: Note the strategic words "bright red." Bright red drainage indicates active bleeding. The registered nurse needs to be notified if this type of drainage occurs. Review postoperative complications associated with an enucleation if you had difficulty with this question.
Level of Cognitive Ability: Applying
Client Needs: Physiological Integrity
Integrated Process: Nursing Process/Implementation
Content Area: Adult Health/Eye
Reference: Linton, p. 1238. 2012.

579. 1

Rationale: The nurse tilts the client's head slightly away and pulls the pinna up and back. Asking the client to stand and lean to one side is inappropriate and unsafe.
Test-Taking Strategy: Use the process of elimination, noting that the question addresses an adult client. Use basic knowledge regarding the administration of ear medications in selecting the correct option. In the adult, the pinna is pulled up and back. Review this procedure if you had difficulty with this question.
Level of Cognitive Ability: Applying
Client Needs: Physiological Integrity
Integrated Process: Nursing Process/Implementation
Content Area: Adult Health/Ear
References: Christensen, Kockrow, pp. 708, 710. 2011. *Foundations of nursing.*
Linton, p. 1246. 2012.

580. 3

Rationale: It is important to speak in a normal tone to the client with impaired hearing and avoid shouting. The nurse should talk directly to the client while facing the client and speak clearly. If the client does not seem to understand what is said, the nurse should express it differently. Moving closer to the client and toward the better ear may facilitate communication, but it is important to avoid talking directly into the impaired ear.

Test-Taking Strategy: Knowledge regarding effective communication techniques for the hearing impaired is required to answer this question. Thinking about the effect of each action identified in the options will direct you to the correct option. If you had difficulty with this question, review these techniques.

Level of Cognitive Ability: Applying
Client Needs: Psychosocial Integrity
Integrated Process: Communication and Documentation
Content Area: Adult Health/Ear
Reference: Christensen, Kockrow, p. 633. 2011. *Adult health nursing.*

581. 4

Rationale: Insects are killed before removal unless they can be coaxed out by a flashlight or a humming noise. Mineral oil or diluted alcohol is instilled into the ear to suffocate the insect, which is then removed by using ear forceps. When the foreign object is vegetable matter, irrigation is not used because this material expands with hydration and the impaction becomes worse. Options 1, 2, and 3 may be prescribed after the initial treatment if necessary and if inflammation or infection is a concern.

Test-Taking Strategy: Use the process of elimination and knowledge regarding care of the client with a foreign body in the ear to answer this question. Remember, insects are killed before removal with mineral oil or diluted alcohol. If you had difficulty with this question, review the treatment for this occurrence.

Level of Cognitive Ability: Understanding
Client Needs: Physiological Integrity
Integrated Process: Nursing Process/Planning
Content Area: Adult Health/Ear
References: Christensen, Kockrow, pp. 639–640. 2011. *Adult health nursing.*
Linton, p. 1252. 2012.

582. 4

Rationale: Presbycusis is a type of hearing loss that occurs with aging. It is a gradual sensorineural loss caused by nerve degeneration in the inner ear or auditory nerve. Options 1, 2, and 3 are not accurate descriptions.

Test-Taking Strategy: Knowledge regarding the description of presbycusis is required to answer this question. Remember presbycusis is a sensorineural hearing loss that occurs with aging. If you are unfamiliar with this condition, review this age-related disorder.

Level of Cognitive Ability: Understanding
Client Needs: Physiological Integrity
Integrated Process: Nursing Process/Data Collection
Content Area: Adult Health/Ear
Reference: Linton, pp. 1258–1259. 2012.

583. 3

Rationale: The nurse instructs the client to make slow head movements to prevent worsening of the vertigo. Dietary changes such as salt and fluid restrictions that reduce the amount of endolymphatic fluid are sometimes prescribed. Watching television can increase the vertigo.

Test-Taking Strategy: Identify the subject of the question. The subject is severe vertigo. Note the relation between severe vertigo and the correct option, avoiding sudden head movements. If you had difficulty with this question, review measures that will reduce vertigo in the client with Ménière's disease.

Level of Cognitive Ability: Applying
Client Needs: Physiological Integrity
Integrated Process: Teaching and Learning
Content Area: Adult Health/Ear
Reference: Linton, pp. 1256–1258. 2012.

584. 2

Rationale: Dietary changes such as salt and fluid restrictions that reduce the amount of endolymphatic fluid are sometimes prescribed. Options 1, 3, and 4 are not specific dietary prescriptions for this condition.

Test-Taking Strategy: Use the process of elimination. Recalling the pathophysiology related to Ménière's disease will direct you to the correct option. Review the pathophysiology related to this condition and the treatment if you had difficulty with this question.

Level of Cognitive Ability: Understanding
Client Needs: Physiological Integrity
Integrated Process: Nursing Process/Planning
Content Area: Adult Health/Ear
Reference: Linton, pp. 1256–1257. 2012.

585. 1, 3, 5, 6

Rationale: After eye surgery, some scratchiness and mild eye discomfort may occur in the operative eye and is usually relieved by mild analgesics. If the eye pain becomes severe, the client should notify the surgeon because this may indicate hemorrhage, infection, or increased intraocular pressure. The nurse would also instruct the client to notify the surgeon of purulent drainage, increased redness, or any decrease in visual acuity. The client is instructed to place an eye shield over the operative eye at bedtime to protect the eye from injury during sleep and to avoid activities that increase intraocular pressure such as bending over.

Test-Taking Strategy: Note that the client has had eye surgery. Recalling that the eye needs to be protected and that a concern is increased intraocular pressure will assist in determining the home care measures to be included in the plan. Review these measures if you had difficulty with this question.

Level of Cognitive Ability: Applying
Client Needs: Physiological Integrity
Integrated Process: Teaching and Learning
Content Area: Adult health/Eye
References: Christensen, Kockrow, p. 619. 2011. *Adult health nursing.*
deWit, pp. 643–644. 2009.

Ophthalmic and Otic Medications

I. OPHTHALMIC MEDICATION ADMINISTRATION

A. Guidelines for the use of eye medications

1. Eye medications are usually in the form of drops or ointments.
2. To prevent overflow of medication into the nasal and pharyngeal passages, thus reducing systemic absorption, the client is instructed to apply pressure over the inner canthus next to the nose for 30 to 60 seconds after administration of the medication. The client is instructed to close the eye gently to help distribute the medication.
3. If both an eye drop and an eye ointment are scheduled to be administered at the same time, the eye drop is administered first.
4. Hands should be washed and gloves donned before administering eye medications to avoid contaminating the eye or medication dropper or applicator.
5. A separate bottle or tube of medication is used for each client to avoid accidental cross-contamination.
6. The prescribed dose of eye medication is placed in the lower conjunctival sac, never directly onto the cornea.
7. Touching any part of the eye with the dropper or applicator is avoided.
8. Glucocorticoid preparations are administered before other medications.
9. Monitor the pulse of the client receiving an ophthalmic β-blocker. The client is instructed to do the same. If the pulse is less than 50 to 60 beats/min (adult), the next dose of eye medication is withheld and the health care provider (HCP) is notified.
10. The client is instructed in how to instill medication correctly and instillation is supervised until he or she can do it safely.
11. The client is instructed to read the medication labels carefully to ensure administration of the correct medication and correct strength.
12. The client is reminded to keep these medications out of the reach of children.
13. The client is instructed to avoid driving or operating hazardous equipment if vision is blurred.
14. The client is informed that he or she may be unable to drive home after eye examinations when a medication to dilate the pupil (**mydriatic**) or to paralyze the ciliary muscle (**cycloplegic**) is used.
15. If photophobia occurs, the client is instructed to wear sunglasses and avoid bright lights.
16. The client is instructed to administer a missed dose of the eye medication as soon as it is remembered, unless the next dose is scheduled to be administered in 1 to 2 hours.
17. The client with **glaucoma** is informed that the disorder cannot be cured, only controlled.
18. Reinforce the importance of using medications to treat **glaucoma** as prescribed and not to discontinue these medications without consulting the HCP.
19. The client is informed that medications used to treat **glaucoma** may cause pain and blurred vision, especially when therapy is begun.
20. The client is instructed to report the development of any eye irritation.
21. The client using eye gel is instructed to store the gel at room temperature or in the refrigerator, but not to freeze it.
22. The client is instructed to discard unused eye gel kept at room temperature as recommended by the HCP and/or the pharmacist.
23. The client is informed that soft contact lenses may absorb certain eye medications and that preservatives in eye medications may discolor the contact lenses.
24. The client wearing contact lenses is advised to question the HCP carefully about special precautions to observe with eye medications.
25. In infants, the parents are informed that atropine sulfate eye drops may contribute to abdominal distention.
26. The parents are instructed to keep a record of the infant's bowel movements if atropine sulfate eye drops are being administered.
27. Bowel sounds of the infant or child receiving atropine sulfate eye drops are auscultated.

Because the timing of medication administration is critical, eye medications are administered at precise intervals. Instillation is separated by 3 to 5 minutes if two medications must be administered at the same time in the same eye(s).

B. Instillation of eye medications
  1. Drops
     a. Wash hands.
     b. Put on gloves.
     c. Check the name, strength, and expiration date of the medication.
     d. Instruct the client to tilt the head backward, open the eyes, and look up.
     e. Pull the lower lid down against the cheekbone.
     f. Hold the bottle like a pencil, with the tip downward.
     g. Holding the bottle, gently rest the wrist of the hand on the client's cheek.
     h. Squeeze the bottle gently to allow the drop to fall into the conjunctival sac.
     i. Instruct the client to close the eyes gently and not to squeeze the eyes shut.
     j. Wait 3 to 5 minutes before instilling another drop; if more than one drop is prescribed, to promote maximal absorption of the medication.
     k. Do not allow the medication bottle, dropper, or applicator to come into contact with the eyelid or conjunctival sac.
     l. To prevent systemic absorption of the medication, apply gentle pressure with a clean tissue to the client's nasolacrimal duct for 30 to 60 seconds.
  2. Ointments
     a. Instruct the client to lie down or tilt head backward and look up.
     b. Hold the ointment tube near, but not touching, the eye or eyelashes.
     c. Squeeze a thin ribbon of ointment along the lining of the lower conjunctival sac from the inner to the outer canthus.
     d. Instruct the client to close the eyes gently, rolling the eyeball in all directions (which increases contact area of medication to eye).
     e. Instruct the client that vision may be blurred by the ointment.
     f. If possible, apply ointment just before bedtime.

II. MYDRIATIC-CYCLOPLEGIC AND ANTICHOLINERGIC MEDICATIONS (Box 56-1)

A. Description (Figure 56-1)
  1. **Mydriatics** and cycloplegics dilate the pupils and relax the ciliary muscles (**cycloplegia**).

Box 56-1 Mydriatic and Cycloplegic Medications

Atropine (Isopto Atropine)
Cyclopentolate (AK-Pentolate, Cyclogyl, Pentolair)
Homatropine (Isopto Homatropine)
Scopolamine (Isopto Hyoscine)
Tropicamide (Mydriacyl, Tropicacyl, Opticyl)

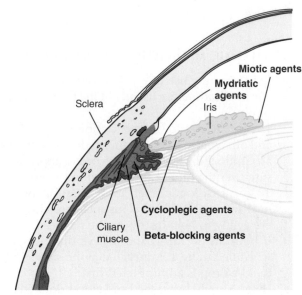

▲ **FIGURE 56-1** Sites of action of mydriatic, β-blocking, cycloplegic, and miotic agents. (From Black, J., & Hawks, J. [2009]. *Medical-surgical nursing: Clinical management for positive outcomes* [8th ed.]. St. Louis: Saunders.)

  2. Anticholinergics block responses of the sphincter muscle in the ciliary body, producing **mydriasis** and **cycloplegia**.
  3. These medications are used preoperatively or for eye examinations to produce **mydriasis**.
  4. **Mydriatics** are contraindicated in cardiac dysrhythmias and cerebral atherosclerosis and should be used with caution in the older client and in those with prostatic hypertrophy, diabetes mellitus, or parkinsonism.

B. Side effects
  1. Tachycardia
  2. Photophobia
  3. Conjunctivitis
  4. Dermatitis
  5. Elevated blood pressure

C. Atropine toxicity
  1. Dry mouth
  2. Blurred vision
  3. Photophobia
  4. Tachycardia
  5. Fever
  6. Urinary retention
  7. Constipation

8. Headache, brow pain
9. Confusion
10. Hallucinations, delirium
11. Coma
12. Worsening of **glaucoma**

D. Systemic reactions of anticholinergics
1. Dry mouth and skin
2. Fever
3. Thirst
4. Confusion
5. Hyperactivity

E. Interventions
1. Monitor for allergic response.
2. Determine risk for injury.
3. Check for constipation and urinary retention.
4. The client is instructed that a burning sensation may occur on instillation.
5. The client is instructed not to drive or perform hazardous activities for 24 hours after instillation of the medication unless otherwise directed by the HCP.
6. The client is instructed to wear sunglasses until the effects of the medication wear off.
7. The client is instructed to notify the HCP if blurring of vision, loss of sight, difficulty breathing, sweating, or flushing occurs.
8. The client is instructed to report eye pain to the HCP.

⚠ Mydriatics are contraindicated in clients with glaucoma because of the risk of increased intraocular pressure.

III. ANTI-INFECTIVE EYE MEDICATIONS
(Box 56-2)

A. Description: Anti-infective medications kill or inhibit the growth of bacteria, fungi, and viruses.

B. Side effects
1. Superinfection
2. Global irritation

C. Interventions
1. Determine risk for injury.
2. The client is instructed how to apply the eye medication. The client is reminded to clean exudates from the eyes before administering drops.
3. The importance of completing the prescribed medication regimen is reinforced.
4. The client is instructed to wash the hands thoroughly and frequently.
5. The client is advised that if improvement does not occur to notify the HCP.

IV. ANTI-INFLAMMATORY EYE MEDICATIONS
(Box 56-3)

A. Description

Box 56-2 Anti-infective Eye Medications

Antibacterial
Chloramphenicol (Chloromycetin powder)
Erythromycin (Ilotycin)

Aminoglycosides
Gentamicin sulfate (Garamycin, Genoptic)
Tobramycin (Tobrex)

Antifungal
Natamycin (Natacyn)

Antiviral
Idoxuridine
Trifluridine (Viroptic)
Vidarabine (Vira-A)

Sulfonamide
Sulfacetamide (Bleph-10, Sodium Sulamyd)

Box 56-3 Anti-inflammatory Eye Medications

Antiallergic Agents
Cromolyn sodium (Crolom, Opticrom)
Lodoxamide (Alomide)
Nedocromil sodium (Alocril)
Pemirolast potassium (Alamast)

Corticosteroids
Dexamethasone (Maxidex, others)
Fluorometholone; sulfacetamide (FML-S eye drop suspension)
Loteprednol etabonate (Alrex, Lotemax)
Prednisolone; gentamicin (Pred-G, Pred Forte, others)

Nonsteroidal Anti-Inflammatory Agents
Cyclosporine (Restasis)
Diclofenac (Voltaren)
Flurbiprofen sodium (Ocufen)
Ketorolac tromethamine (Acular)

Mast-Cell Stabilizers/H1 Blockers
Azelastine hydrochloride (Optivar)
Epinastine (Elestat)
Ketotifen fumarate (Zaditor, Alaway)
Olopatadine hydrochloride (Patanol)

H_1 Receptor Blocker
Emedastine difumarate (Emadine)

---

1. Anti-inflammatory medications control inflammation, thereby reducing vision loss and scarring.
2. Anti-inflammatory medications are used for uveitis, allergic conditions, and inflammation of the conjunctiva, cornea, and lids.

B. Side effects
1. **Cataracts**
2. Increased intraocular pressure
3. Impaired healing
4. Masking signs and symptoms of infection

C. Interventions
1. Interventions are the same as for anti-infective medications.
2. Note that dexamethasone (Maxidex) should not be used for eye abrasions and wounds.

V. TOPICAL EYE ANESTHETICS

A. Description
1. Topical anesthetics produce corneal anesthesia.
2. Topical anesthetics are used for anesthesia for eye examinations and surgery or to remove foreign bodies from the eye.
3. Do not use discolored solution and store the bottle tightly closed.
4. Medication: proparacaine hydrochloride (Ophthetic)

B. Side effects
1. Temporary stinging or burning of the eye
2. Temporary loss of corneal reflex

C. Interventions
1. Determine risk for injury.
2. Note that the medications should not be given to the client for home use and are not to be self-administered by the client.
3. The client is instructed not to rub or touch the eye while it is anesthetized.
4. Note that the blink reflex is lost temporarily and that the corneal epithelium must be protected.
5. An eye patch is provided to protect the eye from injury until the corneal reflex returns.

VI. EYE LUBRICANTS (Box 56-4)

A. Description
1. Replace tears or add moisture to the eyes.
2. Moisten contact lenses or an artificial eye and protect the eyes during surgery or diagnostic procedures.
3. Used for keratitis, during anesthesia, or for a disorder that results in unconsciousness or decreased blinking.

B. Side effects
1. Burning on instillation
2. Discomfort or pain on instillation

C. Interventions
1. The client is informed that burning may occur on instillation.
2. Be alert to allergic responses to the preservatives in the lubricants.

Box 56-4 Eye Lubricants

Hydroxypropyl methylcellulose (Lacril, Isopto Plain)
Petroleum-based ointment (Artificial Tears)
Polyvinyl alcohol (Liquifilm Tears)

VII. MEDICATIONS TO TREAT GLAUCOMA
(Box 56-5; also see Figure 56-1)

A. Description
1. These medications reduce intraocular pressure by constricting the pupil and contracting the ciliary muscle, thereby increasing the blood flow to the retina and decreasing retinal damage and loss of vision.
2. These medications open the anterior chamber angle and increase the outflow of aqueous humor.
3. Cholinergic medications reduce intraocular pressure by mimicking the action of acetylcholine.
4. Acetylcholine inhibitors reduce intraocular pressure by inhibiting the action of cholinesterase.
5. Some may be used to achieve **miosis** during eye surgery.
6. Contraindicated in clients with **retinal detachment**, adhesions between the iris and lens, or inflammatory diseases.
7. Used with caution in clients with asthma, hypertension, corneal abrasion, hyperthyroidism, coronary vascular disease, urinary tract obstruction, gastrointestinal obstruction, ulcer disease, parkinsonism, and bradycardia.

Box 56-5 Medications to Treat Glaucoma

Miotics
Echothiophate
Pilocarpine hydrochloride (Isopto Carpine)

β-Adrenergic Blocking Eye Medications
Betaxolol hydrochloride (Betoptic)
Carteolol hydrochloride (Ocupress)
Levobetaxolol (Betaxon)
Levobunolol hydrochloride (Betagan Liquifilm)
Metipranolol (OptiPranolol)
Timolol maleate (Timoptic)

α-Adrenergic Agonists
Apraclonidine (Iopidine)
Brimonidine (Alphagan)

Prostaglandin Analogs
Latanoprost (Xalatan)
Travoprost (Travatan)
Bimatoprost (Lumigan)

Cholinergic Agonists
Pilocarpine hydrochloride (Isopto Carpine, others)
Echothiophate iodide (Phospholine Iodide)

Carbonic Anhydrase Inhibitors
Dorzolamide (Trusopt)
Brinzolamide (Azopt)

Nonselective Adrenergic Agonists
Dipivefrin (Propine)

B. Side effects
1. **Myopia**
2. Headache
3. Eye pain
4. Decreased vision in poor light
5. Local irritation
6. Systemic effects
   a. Flushing
   b. Diaphoresis
   c. Gastrointestinal upset and diarrhea
   d. Frequent urination
   e. Increased salivation
   f. Muscle weakness
   g. Respiratory difficulty
7. Toxicity
   a. Vertigo and syncope
   b. Bradycardia
   c. Hypotension
   d. Cardiac dysrhythmias
   e. Tremors
   f. Seizures

C. Interventions
1. Monitor the vital signs.
2. Determine risk for injury.
3. Monitor the client for the degree of diminished vision.
4. Monitor for side effects and toxic effects.
5. Monitor for postural hypotension, and instruct the client to change positions slowly.
6. Check breath sounds for wheezes and rhonchi because cholinergic medications can cause bronchospasms and increased bronchial secretions.
7. Maintain oral hygiene because of the increase in salivation.
8. Have atropine sulfate available as an antidote for pilocarpine.
9. The client or family is instructed regarding the correct administration of eye medications.
10. The client is instructed not to stop the medication suddenly.
11. The client is instructed to avoid activities such as driving while vision is impaired.

⚠ The client with glaucoma is instructed to read labels on over-the-counter medications and avoid atropine-like medications because atropine increases intraocular pressure.

VIII. β-ADRENERGIC BLOCKER EYE MEDICATIONS (see Box 56-5)

A. Description (see Figure 56-1)
1. These medications reduce intraocular pressure by decreasing sympathetic impulses and decreasing aqueous humor production without affecting **accommodation** or pupil size.
2. These medications are used to treat **glaucoma**.

3. These medications are contraindicated in the client with asthma or chronic obstructive pulmonary disease because systemic absorption can cause increased airway resistance.
4. These medications are used with caution in the client receiving oral β-blockers.

B. Side effects
1. Ocular irritation
2. Visual disturbances
3. Bradycardia
4. Hypotension
5. Bronchospasm

C. Interventions
1. Monitor the vital signs, especially blood pressure and pulse, before administering medication.
2. If the pulse is 60 beats/min or less or if the systolic blood pressure is less than 90 mm Hg, the medication is withheld and the HCP is contacted.
3. Monitor for shortness of breath.
4. Determine risk for injury.
5. Monitor intake and output (I&O).
6. The client is instructed to notify the health care provider if shortness of breath occurs.
7. The client is instructed not to discontinue the medication abruptly.
8. The client is instructed to change positions slowly because of the potential for orthostatic hypotension.
9. The client is instructed to avoid hazardous activities.
10. The client is instructed to avoid over-the-counter medications without the HCP's approval.
11. Clients with diabetes mellitus using β-adrenergic blockers are instructed to monitor blood glucose levels frequently.

IX. CARBONIC ANHYDRASE INHIBITORS (see Box 56-5)

A. Description
1. Carbonic anhydrase inhibitors interfere with the production of carbonic acid, which leads to decreased aqueous humor formation and decreased intraocular pressure.
2. These medications are used for long-term treatment of **glaucoma**.
3. These medications are contraindicated in the client allergic to sulfonamides.
4. Used with caution for clients with severe renal or liver disease.

B. Side effects
1. Appetite loss
2. Gastrointestinal upset
3. Paresthesias in the fingers, toes, and face
4. Polyuria

5. Hypokalemia
6. Renal calculi
7. Photosensitivity
8. Lethargy and drowsiness
9. Depression

C. Interventions
1. Monitor the vital signs.
2. Check visual acuity.
3. Determine risk for injury.
4. Monitor intake and output.
5. Monitor weight.
6. Maintain oral hygiene.
7. Monitor for side effects such as lethargy, anorexia, drowsiness, polyuria, nausea, and vomiting.
8. Monitor electrolyte levels for hypokalemia.
9. Fluid intake is increased unless contraindicated.
10. The client is advised to avoid prolonged exposure to sunlight.
11. The use of artificial tears for dry eyes is encouraged.
12. The client is instructed not to discontinue the medication abruptly.
13. The client is instructed to avoid hazardous activities while vision is impaired.
14. The client is taught not to wear contact lenses during or within 15 minutes of instilling these medications.

X. OCUSERT SYSTEM

A. Description
1. A thin eye wafer (disk) is impregnated with a time-release dose of pilocarpine (Ocusert Pilo-20).
2. The Ocusert system was devised to overcome the frequent application of pilocarpine.
3. It is placed in the upper or lower cul-de-sac of the eye.
4. The pilocarpine is released over 1 week.
5. The disk is replaced every 7 days.
6. Drawbacks of its use include sudden leakage of pilocarpine, migration of the system over the cornea, and unnoticed loss of the system.

B. Interventions
1. Determine the client's ability to insert the medication disk.
2. Store the medication in the refrigerator.
3. The client is instructed to discard damaged or contaminated disks.
4. The client is informed that temporary stinging is expected, but to notify the HCP if blurred vision or brow pain occurs.
5. The client is instructed to check for the presence of the disk in the conjunctival sac daily at bedtime and on arising.
6. Because vision may change in the first few hours after the eye system is inserted, the client is instructed to replace the disk at bedtime.

XI. OSMOTIC MEDICATIONS (Box 56-6)

A. Description
1. Lower intraocular pressure.
2. Used in emergency treatment of **glaucoma.**
3. Used preoperatively and postoperatively to decrease vitreous humor volume.

B. Side effects
1. Headache
2. Nausea, vomiting, diarrhea, dehydration
3. Disorientation
4. Electrolyte imbalances

C. Interventions
1. Monitor the vital signs.
2. Check visual acuity.
3. Determine risk for injury.
4. Monitor intake and output.
5. Monitor weight.
6. Monitor electrolyte imbalances.
7. Increase fluid intake unless contraindicated.
8. Monitor for changes in level of orientation.

XII. MEDICATIONS TO TREAT MACULAR DEGENERATION (Box 56-7)

A. Description
1. Age-related macular degeneration (ARMD) can be either dry ARMD (atrophic ARMD) or wet ARMD (neovascular).
2. Dry is more common; macular photoreceptors undergo gradual breakdown, leading to gradual blurring of central vision.
3. Wet progresses faster and macular degeneration is caused by growth of new subretinal blood vessels that leads to fluid leakage that lifts the macula and causes permanent injury.
4. Characterized by the presence of drusen (yellow deposits under the retina).

B. Side effects
1. Endophthalmitis (eye inflammation caused by bacterial, viral, or fungal infection)

Box 56-6 Osmotic Medications for the Eye

Glycerin (Osmoglyn)
Mannitol (Osmitrol)

Box 56-7 Medications to Treat Macular Degeneration

Pegaptanib (Macugen)
Ranibizumab (Lucentis)
Bevacizumab (Avastin)

2. Blurred vision
3. Cataracts
4. Corneal edema
5. Eye discomfort and discharge
6. Conjunctival hemorrhage
7. Increased intraocular pressure
8. Reduced visual acuity

C. Interventions
1. The client is taught about administration of the medications.
2. The client is taught about the side effects and the need to notify the HCP.

XIII. OTIC MEDICATION ADMINISTRATION
(Box 56-8)

A. Instillation of ear drops
1. In an adult, pull the pinna up and back to straighten the external canal to instill ear drops.
2. Tilt the client's head in the opposite direction of the affected ear and apply the drops into the ear.
3. With the head tilted, gently move the head back and forth five times.
4. Pull the pinna down and back for infants and children younger than 3 years, up and back for older children.

B. Irrigation of the ear
1. Irrigation of the ear needs to be prescribed by the HCP.
2. Ensure direct visualization of the tympanic membrane.
3. Warm irrigating solution to 98° F because solution temperature not close to the client's body temperature will cause ear injury, nausea, and vertigo.
4. Irrigation must be done gently to avoid damage to the eardrum.

5. When irrigating, do not direct irrigation solution directly toward the eardrum.

⚠ If a perforation of the eardrum is suspected, do not perform ear irrigation.

XIV. ANTI-INFECTIVE EAR MEDICATIONS
(Box 56-9)

A. Description
1. Anti-infective medications kill or inhibit the growth of bacteria and are used for otitis media or otitis externa.
2. Anti-infective medications are contraindicated if a prior hypersensitivity exists.

B. Side effects: Overgrowth of nonsusceptible organisms

C. Interventions
1. Monitor the vital signs.
2. Check for allergies.
3. Monitor for pain.
4. Monitor for nephrotoxicity.
5. The client is instructed to report dizziness, fatigue, fever, or sore throat, which may indicate a superimposed infection.
6. The client is instructed to complete the entire course of the medication.
7. The client is instructed to keep ear canals dry.

XV. ANTIHISTAMINES AND DECONGESTANTS
(Box 56-10)

A. Description
1. These medications produce vasoconstriction.
2. These medications stimulate the receptors of the respiratory mucosa.

Box 56-8 Medications That Affect Hearing

Antibiotics
Amikacin (Amikin)
Chloramphenicol
Erythromycin (ERYC, Ery-Tab, PCE Dispertab, Ilotycin)
Gentamicin (Garamycin)
Streptomycin sulfate
Tobramycin sulfate (Nebcin)
Vancomycin (Vancocin)

Diuretics
Ethacrynic acid (Edecrin)
Furosemide (Lasix)

Others
Cisplatin (Platinol)
Nitrogen mustard
Quinine
Quinidine

Box 56-9 Anti-infective Ear Medications

Acetic acid; aluminum acetate (Otic Domeboro)
Amoxicillin (Amoxil)
Ampicillin (Principen)
Cefaclor (Ceclor)
Chloramphenicol
Clarithromycin (Biaxin)
Clindamycin hydrochloride (Cleocin)
Erythromycin (Ilotycin)
Gentamicin sulfate otic solution (Garamycin)
Penicillin V potassium (Veetids)
Trimethoprim; sulfamethoxazole (Bactrim, Cotrim)

Box 56-10 Antihistamines and Decongestants

Cetirizine (Zyrtec)
Chlorpheniramine (Chlor-Trimeton)
Naphazoline hydrochloride (Allerest, others)

3. These medications reduce respiratory tissue hyperemia and edema to open obstructed eustachian tubes.
4. These medications are used for acute otitis media.

B. Side effects
1. Drowsiness
2. Blurred vision
3. Dry mucous membranes

C. Interventions
1. The client is informed that drowsiness, blurred vision, and a dry mouth may occur.
2. The client is instructed to increase fluid intake unless contraindicated and suck on hard candy to alleviate the dry mouth.
3. The client is instructed to avoid hazardous activities if drowsiness occurs.

XVI. LOCAL ANESTHETICS

A. Description
1. Local anesthetics block nerve conduction at or near the application site to control pain.
2. Local anesthetics are used for pain associated with ear infections.

B. Medication: Benzocaine-antipyrine-phenylephrine (Tympagesic)

C. Side effects
1. Allergic reaction
2. Irritation

D. Interventions
1. Monitor for effectiveness if used for pain relief.
2. Check for irritation or allergic reaction.

XVII. CERUMINOLYTIC MEDICATIONS
(Box 56-11)

A. Description
1. Ceruminolytic medications emulsify and loosen cerumen deposits.
2. Ceruminolytic medications are used to loosen and remove impacted wax from the ear canal.

B. Side effects
1. Irritation
2. Redness or swelling of the ear canal

C. Interventions
1. The client is instructed not to use drops more often than prescribed.
2. A cotton plug is moistened with medication before insertion.

Box 56-11 Ceruminolytic Medications

Boric acid (Ear-Dry)
Carbamide peroxide (Debrox)
Trolamine polypeptide oleate-condensate (Cerumenex)

---

3. Keep the container tightly closed and away from moisture.
4. Touching the ear with the dropper is avoided.
5. Thirty minutes after instillation, the ear is gently irrigated as prescribed with warm water, using a soft rubber bulb ear syringe.
6. Irrigation may be done with hydrogen peroxide solution as prescribed to flush cerumen deposits out of the ear canal.
7. For a chronic cerumen impaction, one or two drops of mineral oil will soften the wax.
8. The client is instructed to notify the health care provider if redness, pain, or swelling persists.

MORE QUESTIONS ON EVOLVE!

Practice Questions

586. Betaxolol hydrochloride (Betoptic SR) eye drops have been prescribed for the client with glaucoma. Which nursing action is most appropriate related to monitoring for the side effects of this medication?
1. Monitoring temperature
2. Monitoring blood pressure
3. Checking peripheral pulses
4. Checking the blood glucose level

587. The nurse prepares the client for ear irrigation as prescribed by the health care provider. In performing the procedure, the nurse:
1. Warms the irrigating solution to 98° F
2. Positions the client with the affected side up after the irrigation
3. Directs a slow steady stream of irrigation solution toward the eardrum
4. Assists the client to turn his or her head so that the ear to be irrigated is facing upward

588. In preparation for cataract surgery, the nurse is to administer cyclopentolate (Cyclogyl) eye drops. The nurse administers the eye drops, knowing that the purpose of this medication is to:
1. Produce miosis of the operative eye.
2. Dilate the pupil of the operative eye.
3. Provide lubrication to the operative eye.
4. Constrict the pupil of the operative eye.

589. The nurse is providing instructions to a client who will be self-administering eye drops. To minimize the systemic effects that eye drops can produce, the client is instructed to:
1. Eat before instilling the drops.
2. Swallow several times after instilling the drops.
3. Blink vigorously to encourage tearing after instilling the drops.
4. Occlude the nasolacrimal duct with a finger over the inner canthus for 30 to 60 seconds after instilling the drops.

590. The client is receiving an eye drop and an eye ointment to the right eye. The nurse should:
1. Administer the eye drop first, followed by the eye ointment.
2. Administer the eye ointment first, followed by the eye drop.
3. Administer the eye drop, wait 10 minutes, and administer the eye ointment.
4. Administer the eye ointment, wait 10 minutes, and administer the eye drop.

591. The nurse is caring for a client with glaucoma. Which of the following medications, if prescribed for the client, would the nurse question?
1. Betaxolol (Betoptic)
2. Pilocarpine (Ocusert Pilo-20)
3. Atropine sulfate (Isopto Atropine)
4. Pilocarpine hydrochloride (Isopto Carpine)

592. A miotic medication has been prescribed for the client with glaucoma. The client asks the nurse about the purpose of the medication. The nurse tells the client that:
1. "The medication will help dilate the eye to prevent an increase in eye pressure."
2. "The medication will relax the muscles of the eyes and prevent blurred vision."
3. "The medication causes the pupil to constrict and will lower the pressure in the eye."
4. "The medication will help block the responses that are sent to the muscles in the eye."

593. A client was just admitted to the hospital to rule out a gastrointestinal (GI) bleed. The client has brought several bottles of medications prescribed by different specialists. During the admission assessment, the client states, "Lately, I have been hearing some roaring sounds in my ears, especially when I am alone." Which medication would the nurse determine could be the cause of the client's complaint?
1. Doxycycline (Vibramycin)
2. Acetylsalicylic acid (aspirin)
3. Atropine sulfate (Isopto Atropine)
4. Diltiazem hydrochloride (Cardizem)

594. Pilocarpine hydrochloride (Isopto Carpine) is prescribed for the client with glaucoma. Which medication does the nurse plan to have available in the event of systemic toxicity?
1. Atropine sulfate
2. Timolol maleate (Timoptic)
3. Metipranolol (OptiPranolol)
4. Carteolol hydrochloride (Ocupress)

595. The nurse is preparing to administer eye ❖ drops. Select the interventions that the nurse takes to administer the drops. **Select all that apply**.
❏ 1. Wash hands.
❏ 2. Put on gloves.
❏ 3. Place the drop in the conjunctival sac.
❏ 4. Pull the lower lid down against the cheek bone.
❏ 5. Instruct the client to squeeze the eyes shut after instilling the eye drop.
❏ 6. Instruct the client to tilt the head forward, open the eyes, and look down.

ANSWERS

586. 2
Rationale: Hypotension, dizziness, nausea, diaphoresis, headache, fatigue, constipation, and diarrhea are systemic effects of the medication. Nursing interventions include monitoring the blood pressure for hypotension and assessing the pulse for strength, weakness, irregular rate, and bradycardia. Options 1, 3, and 4 are not specifically associated with this medication.
Test-Taking Strategy: Use the ABCs—airway, breathing, and circulation—to direct you to option 2. Although option 3, peripheral pulses, also is related to circulation monitoring, the blood pressure is the umbrella choice. Review the side effects of this medication if you had difficulty with this question.
Level of Cognitive Ability: Applying
Client Needs: Physiological Integrity
Integrated Process: Nursing Process/Data Collection
Content Area: Adult Health/Eye
References: Hodgson, Kizior, pp. 124–125. 2011. Lehne, pp. 172–173. 2010.

587. 1
Rationale: Irrigation solutions that are not close to the client's body temperature can be uncomfortable and may cause injury, nausea, and vertigo. The client is positioned so that the ear to be irrigated is facing downward, because this allows gravity to assist in the removal of the ear wax and solution. After the irrigation, the client is to lie on the affected side to finish draining the irrigating solution. A slow steady stream of solution should be directed toward the upper wall of the ear canal and not toward the eardrum. Too much force could cause the tympanic membrane to rupture.
Test-Taking Strategy: Use the process of elimination. Read each option carefully and remember that the nurse's concern is to prevent damage to the tympanic membrane. Additionally, remember that the client should be positioned with the affected side downward to allow drainage of the irrigation solution. Review the procedure for performing ear irrigation if you had difficulty with this question.
Level of Cognitive Ability: Applying
Client Needs: Physiological Integrity
Integrated Process: Nursing Process/Implementation

Content Area: Adult Health/Ear
References: deWit, p. 656. 2009.
Linton, p. 1246. 2012.

588. 2
Rationale: Cyclopentolate is a rapidly acting mydriatic and cycloplegic medication. Cyclopentolate is effective in 25 to 75 minutes, and accommodation returns in 6 to 24 hours. Cyclopentolate is used for preoperative mydriasis.
Test-Taking Strategy: Use the process of elimination. Options 1 and 4 are comparable or alike and are eliminated first. Miosis refers to a constricted pupil. Note that the question identifies a client being prepared for eye surgery. The pupil would need to be dilated for the surgical procedure. Review the action and purpose of this medication if you had difficulty with this question.
Level of Cognitive Ability: Understanding
Client Needs: Physiological Integrity
Integrated Process: Nursing Process/Implementation
Content Area: Adult Health/Eye
Reference: Lehne, pp. 1222–1223. 2010.

589. 4
Rationale: Applying pressure on the nasolacrimal duct prevents systemic absorption of the medication. Options 1, 2, and 3 will not prevent systemic absorption.
Test-Taking Strategy: Use the process of elimination. Eating and swallowing are comparative options and are not related to the systemic absorption of an eye medication. Blinking vigorously to produce tearing may result in the loss of the administered medication. Review the procedure for administering eye drops to prevent systemic absorption if you had difficulty with this question.
Level of Cognitive Ability: Applying
Client Needs: Physiological Integrity
Integrated Process: Teaching and Learning
Content Area: Adult Health—Eye
Reference: Workman, LaCharity, Kruchko, p. 470. 2011.

590. 1
Rationale: When an eye drop and an eye ointment are scheduled to be administered at the same time, the eye drop is administered first. Options 2, 3, and 4 are incorrect.
Test-Taking Strategy: Use the process of elimination. Recalling the guidelines for administering eye medications will direct you to the correct option. Review these guidelines if you had difficulty with this question.
Level of Cognitive Ability: Applying
Client Needs: Physiological Integrity
Integrated Process: Nursing Process/Implementation
Content Area: Adult Health/Eye
Reference: Perry, Potter, p. 549. 2010.

591. 3
Rationale: Options 1, 2, and 4 are miotic agents used to treat glaucoma. Option 3 is a mydriatic and cycloplegic medication, and its use is contraindicated in clients with glaucoma. Mydriatic medications dilate the pupil and can cause an increase in intraocular pressure in the eye.
Test-Taking Strategy: Use the process of elimination. Knowledge regarding the classifications of the medications identified in the options will assist in answering the question. Remember that mydriatics dilate, and that these medications are contraindicated in glaucoma. Review the contraindications related to medications for the client with glaucoma if you had difficulty with this question.
Level of Cognitive Ability: Analyzing
Client Needs: Safe and Effective Care Environment
Integrated Process: Nursing Process/Implementation
Content Area: Adult Health/Eye
References: Kee, Hayes, McCuistion, p. 750. 2009.
Lehne, pp. 124, 1222-1223. 2010.

592. 3
Rationale: Miotics cause pupillary constriction and are used to treat glaucoma. They lower the intraocular pressure, thereby increasing blood flow to the retina and decreasing retinal damage and loss of vision. Miotics cause a contraction of the ciliary muscle and a widening of the trabecular meshwork. Options 1, 2, and 4 are incorrect.
Test-Taking Strategy: Use the process of elimination. Note that the client has glaucoma. Recall that prevention of increased intraocular pressure is the goal in the client with glaucoma. Options 1, 2, and 4 describe actions related to mydriatic medications, which primarily dilate the pupils and relax the ciliary muscles. Review the action of a miotic medication if you had difficulty with this question.
Level of Cognitive Ability: Understanding
Client Needs: Physiological Integrity
Integrated Process: Nursing Process/Implementation
Content Area: Adult Health/Eye
References: Edmunds, p. 396. 2010.
Kee, Hayes, McCuistion, pp. 743–744. 2009.

593. 2
Rationale: Aspirin is contraindicated for gastrointestinal bleed and is potentially ototoxic. The client should be advised to notify the prescribing health care provider so the medication can be discontinued and/or a substitute that is less toxic to the ear can be taken instead. Options 1, 2, and 4 do not have side effects that are potentially associated with hearing difficulties.
Test-Taking Strategy: Focus on the client's complaint. Review the classifications and/or therapeutic effects as well as the side effects of each medication in the options. Of the medications identified, only aspirin can cause ototoxicity. Additionally, it is contraindicated for GI bleed as well. Review medications that can cause ototoxicity if you had difficulty with this question.
Level of Cognitive Ability: Analyzing
Client Needs: Physiological Integrity
Integrated Process: Nursing Process/Data Collection
Content Area: Adult Health/Ear
Reference: Hodgson, Kizior, pp. 86–88. 2012.

594. 1
Rationale: Systemic absorption of pilocarpine hydrochloride can produce toxicity and includes manifestations of vertigo, bradycardia, tremors, hypotension, and seizures. Atropine sulfate must be available in the event of systemic toxicity. Pindolol, timolol maleate, and carteolol hydrochloride are β-blockers.

Test-Taking Strategy: Note that options 2, 3, and 4 are comparable or alike and are β-blockers. Also remember that atropine sulfate is the antidote for systemic reactions that occur with pilocarpine hydrochloride. Review antidotes if you had difficulty with this question.
Level of Cognitive Ability: Applying
Client Needs: Physiological Integrity
Integrated Process: Nursing Process/Implementation
Content Area: Adult Health/Eye
Reference: Kee, Hayes, McCuistion, p. 746. 2009.

❖ **595. 1, 2, 3, 4**
Rationale: To administer eye medications, the nurse would wash hands and put on gloves. The client is instructed to tilt the head backward, open the eyes, and look up. The nurse pulls the lower lid down against the cheekbone and holds the bottle like a pencil with the tip downward. Holding the bottle, the nurse gently rests the wrist of the hand on the client's cheek and squeezes the bottle gently to allow the drop to fall into the conjunctival sac. The client is instructed to close the eyes gently and not to squeeze the eyes shut to prevent the loss of medication.

Test-Taking Strategy: Use guidelines related to standard precautions and visualize this procedure. This will assist in determining the correct interventions. If you are unfamiliar with the procedure for administering eye medications, review these guidelines.
Level of Cognitive Ability: Applying
Client Needs: Physiological Integrity
Integrated Process: Nursing Process/Implementation
Content Area: Adult Health/Eye
References: Edmunds, p. 129. 2010.
Kee, Hayes, McCuistion, p. 34. 2009.
Perry, Potter, pp. 545–549. 2010.

The Adult Client with a Neurological Disorder

PYRAMID TERMS

agnosia The inability to recognize familiar objects or persons

apraxia The inability to carry out a purposeful activity

autonomic dysreflexia Also known as hyperreflexia; characterized by paroxysmal hypertension, bradycardia, excessive sweating, facial flushing, nasal congestion, pilomotor responses, and headache; occurs with spinal lesions above T6 after the period of spinal shock is complete; causes include visceral distention from a distended bladder or impacted rectum; the syndrome is a neurological emergency and must be treated immediately to prevent a hypertensive stroke

Babinski's reflex Dorsiflexion of the ankle and great toe with fanning of the other toes elicited by firmly stroking the lateral aspect of the sole of the foot; indicates a disruption of the pyramidal tract

Brudzinski's sign Flexion of the head that causes flexion of both thighs at the hips and knee flexion and indicates meningeal irritation

decerebrate posturing Stiff extension of one or both arms and possibly the legs that indicates a brainstem lesion

decorticate posturing Flexure of one or both arms on the chest and possibly stiff extension of the legs that indicates a nonfunctioning cortex

flaccid posturing No motor response display in any extremity

Glasgow Coma Scale A method of assessing a client's neurological condition; a scoring system based on a scale of 1 to 15 points; a score of less than 8 indicates that coma is present; eye-opening is the most important indicator

halo traction Insertion of pins or screws into the client's skull and application of a circular fixation device and halo jacket or cast; used to immobilize the cervical spine

hemianopsia Blindness in half of the visual field

homonymous hemianopsia Blindness in the same visual field of both eyes

increased intracranial pressure (ICP) An increase in intracranial pressure caused by trauma, hemorrhage, growths or tumors, hydrocephalus, edema, or inflammation; can impede circulation to the brain and absorption of cerebrospinal fluid and can affect the functioning of nerve cells and lead to brainstem compression and death

Kernig's sign Loss of the ability to straighten the leg completely when it is fully flexed at the knee and hip: indicates meningeal irritation

neurogenic shock Occurs from an injury at T5 or above and usually is experienced soon after the injury (within 30 minutes) lasting up to 6 weeks. Massive vasodilation occurs leading to pooling of the blood in blood vessels, tissue hypoperfusion, and impaired cellular metabolism

nuchal rigidity Stiff neck; flexion of the neck onto the chest causes intense pain

skull tongs Tongs inserted into the outer aspect of the client's skull, just above the ears, with application of traction; a method for applying skeletal traction in the treatment of injuries of the cervical spine. Some types include Gardner-Wells, Barton, and Crutchfield tongs

spinal shock A sudden depression of reflex activity in the spinal cord below the level of injury (areflexia) that occurs within the first hour of injury and lasts days to months; the muscles become completely paralyzed and flaccid, and reflexes are absent

unconscious client A state of depressed cerebral functioning with unresponsiveness to sensory and motor function; causes include head trauma, cerebral toxins, shock, hemorrhage, tumor, and infections

unilateral neglect Also known as neglect syndrome; an inability to recognize a physical impairment that occurs most commonly in clients who have had a right cerebral stroke

PYRAMID TO SUCCESS

Pyramid points related to neurological disorders focus on safety issues; care of the unconscious client; monitoring for increased intracranial pressure; monitoring level of consciousness; positioning clients; nursing interventions during a seizure, head injury, brain attack (stroke), spinal cord injury, Parkinson's disease, and meningitis; and care of the client with myasthenia gravis. Altered body image and psychosocial issues that occur as a result of the neurological disorder are also a focus of the Pyramid to Success.

CLIENT NEEDS

Safe and Effective Care Environment

- Acting as a client advocate
- Consulting with members of the health care team
- Ensuring advance directives are in the client's medical record
- Establishing priorities
- Initiating referrals to appropriate services
- Maintaining asepsis with procedures and treatments
- Maintaining confidentiality
- Maintaining standard and other precautions
- Obtaining informed consent for invasive procedures
- Preventing accidents that can occur as a result of neurological deficits
- Upholding client rights

Health Promotion and Maintenance

- Discussing expected and unexpected body image changes resulting from neurological deficits

- Performing neurological data collection techniques
- Preventing and detecting health problems associated with neurological deficits
- Providing home care instructions regarding care related to the neurological disorder
- Teaching about the importance of prescribed therapy

Psychosocial Integrity

- Acknowledging end-of-life issues and grief and loss issues
- Assessing the ability to cope with feelings of isolation and loss of independence
- Considering the cultural, religious, and spiritual influences of the client when planning care
- Identifying sensory and perceptual alterations
- Identifying support systems and encouraging the use of community resources
- Mobilizing coping mechanisms

Physiological Integrity

- Administering pharmacological therapy
- Monitoring for alterations in body systems
- Monitoring for complications related to procedures
- Monitoring for fluid and electrolyte imbalances
- Providing assistive devices for mobility
- Providing emergency care
- Providing measures to promote comfort
- Promoting normal elimination patterns
- Promoting self-care measures

57

Neurological System

I. ANATOMY AND PHYSIOLOGY OF THE BRAIN AND SPINAL CORD

A. Cerebrum
1. The cerebrum consists of the right and left hemispheres.
2. Each hemisphere receives sensory information from the opposite side of the body and controls the skeletal muscles of the opposite side.
3. The cerebrum governs sensory and motor activity and thought and learning.

B. Cerebral cortex (Box 57-1)
1. The cerebral cortex is the outer gray layer and it is divided into five lobes.
2. It is responsible for the conscious activities of the cerebrum.

C. Basal ganglia: cell bodies in white matter that assist the cerebral cortex in producing smooth voluntary movements

D. Diencephalon
1. Thalamus
   a. Relays sensory impulses to the cortex
   b. Provides a pain gate
   c. Is part of the reticular activating system
2. Hypothalamus
   a. Regulates autonomic responses of the sympathetic and parasympathetic nervous systems
   b. Regulates the stress response, sleep, appetite, body temperature, fluid balance, and emotions
   c. Is responsible for the production of hormones secreted by the pituitary gland and the hypothalamus

E. Brainstem
1. Midbrain
   a. Responsible for motor coordination
   b. Contains the visual reflex and auditory relay centers
2. Pons: Contains the respiratory centers and regulates breathing
3. Medulla oblongata
   a. Contains all afferent and efferent tracts and contains cardiac, respiratory, vomiting, and vasomotor centers
   b. Controls heart rate, respiration, blood vessel diameter, sneezing, swallowing, vomiting, and coughing

F. Cerebellum: Coordinates smooth muscle movement, posture, equilibrium, and muscle tone

G. Spinal cord
1. Provides neuron and synapse networks to produce involuntary responses to sensory stimulation
2. Controls body movement and regulates visceral function
3. Carries sensory information to and motor information from the brain
4. Extends from the first cervical to the second lumbar vertebra
5. Is protected by the meninges, cerebrospinal fluid (CSF), and adipose tissue
6. Horns
   a. Inner column of gray matter contains two anterior and two posterior horns
   b. Posterior horns connect with afferent (sensory) nerve fibers
   c. Anterior horns contain efferent (motor) nerve fibers
7. Nerve tracts
   a. White matter contains the nerve tract
   b. Ascending tracts (sensory pathway)
   c. Descending tract (motor pathway)

H. Meninges
1. Dura mater is the tough and fibrous membrane.
2. Arachnoid membrane is the delicate membrane and contains subarachnoid fluid.
3. Pia mater is the vascular membrane.
4. Subarachnoid space is formed by the arachnoid membrane and the pia mater.

I. Cerebrospinal fluid (CSF)
1. Clear, colorless, and odorless fluid secreted in the ventricles and circulates in the subarachnoid space and through the ventricles to the subarachnoid layer of the meninges, where it is reabsorbed
2. Acts as a protective cushion and aids in the exchange of nutrients and wastes

Box 57-1 Cerebral Cortex

Frontal Lobe
Broca's area for speech
Motor cortex for voluntary motor function, voluntary eye movement, memory storage, morals, emotions, reasoning and judgment, concentration, and abstraction

Parietal Lobe
Interpretation of taste, pain, touch, temperature, and pressure
Spatial perception

Temporal Lobe
Auditory center
Wernicke's area for sensory and speech

Occipital Lobe
Visual area

Limbic Lobe
Emotional and visceral patterns for survival
Learning and memory

  3. Normal pressure is 50 to 175 mm H_2O in the lateral recumbent position, and 200 to 350 mm H_2O in the sitting position.
  4. Normal volume is 125 to 150 mL
J. Ventricles
  1. Four ventricles
  2. The ventricles communicate between the subarachnoid spaces and produce and circulate CSF
K. Blood supply
  1. Right and left internal carotids
  2. Right and left vertebral arteries
  3. These arteries supply the brain via an anastomosis at the base of the brain called the circle of Willis.
L. Neurotransmitters
  1. Acetylcholine
  2. Norepinephrine
  3. Dopamine
  4. Serotonin
  5. Amino acids
  6. Polypeptides
M. Neurons
  1. The neuron consists of cell body, axons, and dendrites.
  2. The cell body contains the nucleus.
  3. Neurons carrying impulses to the central nervous system (CNS) are called sensory neurons.
  4. Neurons carrying impulses away from the CNS are called motor neurons.
  5. Synapse is the chemical transmission of impulses from one neuron to another.
N. Axons and dendrites
  1. The axon conducts impulses from the cell body.
  2. The dendrites receive stimuli from the body and transmit them to the axon.

  3. The neurons are protected and insulated by Schwann cells.
  4. The Schwann cell sheath is called the neurilemma.
  5. Neurons do not reproduce after the neonatal period.
  6. If an axon or dendrite is damaged, it will die and be replaced slowly only if the neurilemma is intact and the cell body has not died.
O. Spinal nerves
  1. Human beings have 31 pairs of spinal nerves.
  2. Mixed nerve fibers are formed by the joining of the anterior motor and posterior sensory roots.
  3. Posterior roots contain afferent (sensory) nerve fibers.
  4. Anterior roots contain efferent (motor) nerve fibers.
P. Autonomic nervous system
  1. Sympathetic (adrenergic) fibers dilate pupils, increase heart rate and rhythm, contract blood vessels, and relax smooth muscles of the bronchi.
  2. Parasympathetic (cholinergic) fibers produce the opposite effect.

II. DIAGNOSTIC TESTS

A. Skull and spinal radiography
  1. Description
    a. Radiographs of the skull reveal the size and shape of the skull bones, suture separation in infants, fractures or bony defects, erosion, or calcification.
    b. Spinal radiographs identify fractures, dislocation, compression, curvature, erosion, narrowed spinal cord, and degenerative processes.
  2. Preprocedure interventions
    a. Provide nursing support for the confused, combative, or ventilator-dependent client.
    b. Maintain immobilization of the neck if a spinal fracture is suspected.
    c. Remove metal items from body parts.
    d. If the client has thick and heavy hair, this should be documented because it may affect interpretation of the x-ray film.
  3. Postprocedure intervention: Maintain immobilization until results are known.

 Always check with the client about the possibility of pregnancy before any radiographic procedures are done.

B. Computed tomography (CT) scan of the brain
  1. Description
    a. CT is a type of brain scanning that may or may not require injection of a dye.
    b. It is used to detect intracranial bleeding, space-occupying lesions, cerebral edema, infarctions, hydrocephalus, cerebral atrophy, and shifts of brain structures.

2. Preprocedure interventions
   a. Obtain an informed consent if a dye is used.
   b. Assess for allergies to iodine, contrast dyes, or shellfish if a dye is used.
   c. Instruct the client on the need to lie still and flat during the test.
   d. Instruct the client to hold his or her breath when requested.
   e. Initiate an IV line if prescribed.
   f. Remove objects from the head, such as wigs, barrettes, earrings, and hairpins.
   g. Inform the client that there may be a hot, flushed sensation and a metallic taste in the mouth when the dye is injected.
   h. Note that some clients may be given the dye even if they report an allergy and are treated with an antihistamine and corticosteroids before the injection to reduce the severity of a reaction.

   ⚠ Assess the need to withhold metformin (Glucophage) if iodinated contrast dye is used for a diagnostic procedure because of the risk for metformin-induced lactic acidosis.

3. Postprocedure interventions
   a. Provide replacement fluids because diuresis from the dye is expected.
   b. Monitor for an allergic reaction to the dye.
   c. Assess dye injection site for bleeding or hematoma, and monitor the extremity for color, warmth, and the presence of distal pulses.

C. Magnetic resonance imaging (MRI)
   1. Description
      a. MRI is a noninvasive procedure that identifies types of tissues, tumors, and vascular abnormalities.
      b. It is similar to the CT scan but provides more detailed pictures.
   2. Preprocedure interventions
      a. Remove all metal objects from the client.
      b. Determine whether the client has a pacemaker, implanted defibrillator, or other metal implants such as a hip prosthesis or vascular clips because these clients cannot have this test performed.
      c. Remove IV fluid pumps during the test.
      d. Provide precautions for the client who is attached to pulse oximeter because it can cause a burn during testing if coiled around the body or a body part.
      e. Assess for claustrophobia (unless an open MRI machine is used).
      f. Inform the client of possible mechanical noises as the scanning occurs.
      g. Administer medication as prescribed for the client with claustrophobia.

   h. Determine if a contrast agent is to be used, and follow the prescription related to the administration of food, fluids, and medications.
   i. Instruct the client that he or she will need to remain still during the procedure.

   ⚠ An MRI is contraindicated in a pregnant woman because the increase in amniotic fluid temperature that occurs during the procedure may be harmful to the fetus.

3. Postprocedure interventions
   a. Client may resume normal activities.
   b. Expect diuresis if a contrast agent was used.

D. Lumbar puncture
   1. Description
      a. Insert a spinal needle through the L3-L4 interspace into the lumbar subarachnoid space to check for CNS infection, SDH, obtain CSF, measure CSF fluid or decrease pressure, or instill air, dye, or administer medications.
      b. The test is contraindicated in clients with **increased intracranial pressure (ICP)** because the procedure will cause a rapid decrease in pressure within the CSF around the spinal cord, leading to brain herniation.
      c. May also be used in the treatment for idiopathic intracranial hypertension.
   2. Preprocedure interventions
      a. Obtain an informed consent.
      b. Have the client empty the bladder.
   3. Interventions during the procedure
      a. Position the client in a lateral recumbent position and have the client draw the knees up to the abdomen and the chin onto the chest. (the prone position may be required for radiologically guided punctures)
      b. Assist with the collection of specimens. (Label the specimens in sequence.)
      c. Maintain strict asepsis.
   4. Postprocedure interventions
      a. Monitor vital signs, headache, and neurological signs that may indicate leakage of CSF; monitor injection site for leakage of CSF.
      b. Position the client flat as prescribed.
      c. Encourage fluids to replace CSF obtained from the specimen collection or from leakage.
      d. Monitor intake and output (I&O).

E. Cerebral angiography
   1. Description: Injection of a contrast material through the femoral artery into the carotid arteries to visualize the cerebral arteries and assess for lesions
   2. Preprocedure interventions
      a. Obtain an informed consent.
      b. Assess the client for allergies to iodine and shellfish.

c. Encourage hydration for 2 days before the test.

d. Maintain the client on NPO status 4 to 6 hours before the test as prescribed.

e. Obtain a baseline neurological assessment.

f. Mark the peripheral pulses.

g. Remove metal items from the hair.

h. Administer premedication as prescribed.

3. Postprocedure interventions

a. Monitor neurological status and vital signs frequently until stable.

b. Monitor for swelling in the neck and for difficulty swallowing, and notify the health care provider (HCP) if these symptoms occur.

c. Maintain bedrest for 12 hours as prescribed.

d. Elevate the head of the bed 15 to 30 degrees only if prescribed.

e. Keep the bed flat if the femoral artery is used, as prescribed.

f. Assess peripheral pulses.

g. Apply sandbags or another device to immobilize the limb and a pressure dressing to the injection site to decrease bleeding, as prescribed.

h. Place ice on the puncture site as prescribed.

i. Encourage fluid intake.

F. Electroencephalography

1. Description: A graphic recording of the electrical activity of the superficial layers of the cerebral cortex

2. Preprocedure interventions

a. Wash the client's hair.

b. Inform the client that electrodes are attached to the head and that electricity does not enter the head.

c. Withhold stimulants, such as coffee, tea, and caffeine beverages; antidepressants; tranquilizers; and possibly anticonvulsants for 24 to 48 hours before the test as prescribed.

d. Allow the client to have breakfast if prescribed.

e. Premedicate for sedation as prescribed.

3. Postprocedure interventions

a. Wash the client's hair.

b. Maintain side rails and safety precautions, if the client was sedated.

G. Caloric testing (oculovestibular reflex)

1. Description: Caloric testing provides information about the function of the vestibular portion of the eighth cranial nerve and aids in the diagnosis of cerebellum and brainstem lesions.

2. Procedure

a. Patency of the external auditory canal is confirmed.

b. The client is positioned supine with the head of the bed elevated 30 degrees.

c. Water that is warmer or cooler than body temperature is infused into the ear.

d. A normal response is the onset of vertigo and nystagmus (involuntary eye movements) within 20 to 30 seconds.

e. Absent or dysconjugate eye movements indicate brainstem damage.

III. NEUROLOGICAL DATA COLLECTION (refer to Chapter 29 for information on neurological data collection techniques)

A. Risk factors

1. Trauma
2. Hemorrhage
3. Tumors
4. Infection
5. Toxicity
6. Metabolic disorders
7. Hypoxic conditions
8. Hypertension
9. Cerebral artery disease
10. Cigarette smoking
11. Aging process
12. Chemicals, either ingestion or environmental exposure

⚠ Level of consciousness is the most sensitive indicator of neurological status.

B. Vital signs: Monitor for blood pressure or pulse changes, which may indicate increased **ICP** (rise in blood pressure with widening pulse pressure, slowing of the pulse, elevated temperature, abnormal respirations).

C. Respirations (Box 57-2)

Box 57-2 Data Collection: Respirations

Cheyne-Stokes
Rhythmic with periods of apnea
Can indicate a metabolic dysfunction or dysfunction in the cerebral hemisphere or basal ganglia

Neurogenic Hyperventilation
Regular rapid and deep sustained respirations
Indicates a dysfunction in the low midbrain and middle pons

Apneustic
Irregular respirations with pauses at the end of inspiration and expiration
Indicates a dysfunction in the middle or caudal pons

Ataxic
Totally irregular in rhythm and depth
Indicates a dysfunction in the medulla

Cluster
Clusters of breaths with irregularly spaced pauses
Indicates a dysfunction in the medulla and pons

D. Temperature
1. An elevated temperature increases the metabolic rate of the brain.
2. An elevation in temperature may indicate a dysfunction of the hypothalamus or brainstem.
3. A slow rise in temperature may indicate infection.

E. Pupils (see Figure 57-1)
1. Unilateral pupil dilation indicates compression of the third cranial nerve
2. Midposition fixed pupil indicates midbrain injury
3. Pinpoint fixed pupil indicates pontine damage
4. See Figure 57-2 for checking extraocular eye movements.

F. Motor function
1. Check muscle tone, including strength and equality
2. Check for voluntary and involuntary movements and purposeful and nonpurposeful movements

G. Posturing (see Figure 31-1)
1. Posturing indicates a deterioration of the condition.
2. Flexor (**decorticate posturing**)
   a. The client flexes one or both arms on the chest and may extend the legs stiffly.

b. Flexor posturing indicates a nonfunctioning cortex.
3. Extensor (**decerebrate posturing**)
   a. The client stiffly extends one or both arms and possibly the legs.
   b. Extensor posturing indicates a brainstem lesion.
4. **Flaccid posturing**: The client displays no motor response in any extremity.

H. Reflexes (Box 57-3)
I. Meningeal irritation (Box 57-4)

Box 57-3 Data Collection: Reflexes

Babinski's Reflex
Dorsiflexion of the ankle and great toe with fanning of the other toes when firmly stroking the lateral aspect of the sole of the foot
Indicates a disruption of the pyramidal tract

Corneal Reflex
Loss of the blink reflex
Indicates a dysfunction of cranial nerve V

Gag Reflex
Loss of the gag reflex
Indicates a dysfunction of cranial nerves IX and X

Box 57-4 Data Collection: Meningeal Irritation

General Findings
Irritability
Nuchal rigidity
Severe, unrelenting headaches
Generalized muscle aches and pains
Nausea and vomiting
Fever and chills
Tachycardia
Photophobia
Nystagmus
Abnormal pupil reaction and eye movement

Brudzinski's Sign
Flexion of the head causes flexion of both thighs at the hips and knee flexion

Kernig's Sign
Flexion of the thigh and knee to right angles and when the limbs are extended, it causes stiffness and spasm of the hamstring and pain

Motor Response
Hemiparesis, hemiplegia, and decreased muscle tone
Cranial nerve dysfunction, especially cranial nerves III, IV, VI, VII, and VIII

Memory Changes
Short attention span
Personality and behavioral changes
Bewilderment

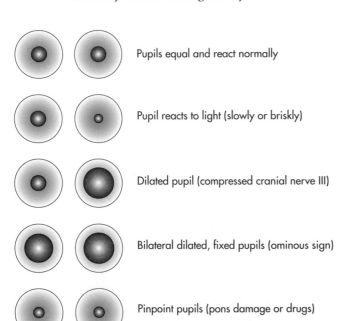

Pupils equal and react normally

Pupil reacts to light (slowly or briskly)

Dilated pupil (compressed cranial nerve III)

Bilateral dilated, fixed pupils (ominous sign)

Pinpoint pupils (pons damage or drugs)

▲ **FIGURE 57-1** Pupillary check for size and response. (From Lewis, S., Heitkemper, M., & Dirksen, S. [2011]. *Medical-surgical nursing: Assessment and management of clinical problems* [8th ed.]. St. Louis: Mosby.)

▲ **FIGURE 57-2** Checking extraocular eye movements. (From Ignatavicius, D., & Workman, M. [2010]. *Medical-surgical nursing: Patient-centered collaborative care* [6th ed.]. St. Louis: Saunders.)

J. Autonomic system
1. Sympathetic functions/adrenergic responses
   a. Increased pulse and blood pressure
   b. Dilated pupils
   c. Decreased peristalsis
   d. Increased perspiration
2. Parasympathetic function/cholinergic responses
   a. Decreased pulse and blood pressure
   b. Constricted pupils
   c. Increased salivation
   d. Increased peristalsis
   e. Dilated blood vessels
   f. Bladder contraction

K. Sensory function: Assess touch, pressure, pain, bladder control, and bowel control

L. Glasgow Coma Scale (Box 57-5)
1. The scale is a method of assessing a client's neurological condition.
2. The scoring system is based on a scale of 1 to 15 points.
3. A score of less than 8 indicates coma is present.
4. Eye opening is the most important indicator.

IV. THE UNCONSCIOUS CLIENT

A. Description
1. The **unconscious client** is in a state of depressed cerebral functioning with unresponsiveness to sensory and motor function.

Box 57-5 Glasgow Coma Scale

Score
The highest possible score is 15 points

Motor Response Points
Obeys a simple response = 6
Localizes painful stimuli = 5
Normal flexion (withdrawal) = 4
Abnormal flexion (decorticate posturing) = 3
Extensor response (decerebrate posturing) – 2
No motor response to pain = 1

Verbal Response Points
Oriented – 5
Confused conversation = 4
Inappropriate words = 3
Responds with incomprehensible sounds = 2
No verbal response = 1

Eye-Opening Points
Spontaneous = 4
In response to sound – 3
In response to pain = 2
No response even to painful stimuli = 1

Adapted from Ignatavicius, D., & Workman, M. (2010). *Medical-surgical nursing: Patient-centered collaborative care* (6th ed.). St. Louis: Saunders.

---

2. Some of the causes include head trauma, cerebral toxins, shock, hemorrhage, tumor, and infection.

B. Data collection
1. Unarousable
2. Primitive or no response to painful stimuli
3. Altered respirations
4. Decreased cranial nerve and reflex activity

C. Interventions (Box 57-6)

V. INCREASED INTRACRANIAL PRESSURE (ICP)

A. Description
1. An increase in **ICP** may be caused by trauma, hemorrhage, growths or tumors, hydrocephalus, edema, or inflammation.
2. Increased **ICP** can impede circulation to the brain, hinder the absorption of CSF, affect the functioning of nerve cells, and lead to brainstem compression and death.

B. Data collection
1. Altered LOC, which is the most sensitive and earliest indication of increasing **ICP**
2. Headache
3. Abnormal respirations (see Box 57-2)
4. Rise in blood pressure with widening pulse pressure
5. Slowing of pulse
6. Elevated temperature
7. Vomiting
8. Pupil changes
9. Late signs of increased **ICP**, including increased systolic blood pressure, widened pulse pressure, and slowed heart rate
10. Other late signs include changes in motor function from weakness to hemiplegia, a positive **Babinski's reflex**, **decorticate** or **decerebrate posturing**, and seizures.

C. Interventions
1. Monitor respiratory status and prevent hypoxia.
2. Avoid the administration of morphine sulfate to prevent the occurrence of hypoxia.
3. Maintain mechanical ventilation as prescribed; maintaining the $Paco_2$ at 30 to 35 mm Hg will result in vasoconstriction of the cerebral blood vessels, decreased blood flow, and therefore decreased **ICP**.
4. Maintain body temperature.
5. Prevent shivering, which can increase **ICP**.
6. Decrease environmental stimuli.
7. Monitor electrolyte levels and acid-base balance.
8. Monitor intake and output.
9. Limit fluid intake to 1200 mL/day.
10. Instruct the client to avoid straining activities, such as coughing and sneezing.
11. Instruct the client to avoid Valsalva's maneuver.

⚠ For the client with increased intracranial pressure, elevate the head of the bed 30 to 40 degrees, avoid the Trendelenburg's position, and prevent flexion of the neck and hips.

D. Medications (Box 57-7)

E. Surgical intervention: See Chapter 31 for additional information on ventriculoperitoneal shunt.

Box 57-6 Care of the Unconscious Client

Monitor patency of the airway and keep airway and emergency equipment at the bedside.

Monitor blood pressure, pulse, and heart sounds.

Monitor respiratory and circulatory status.

Maintain a patent airway and ventilation because a high CO_2 level increases intracranial pressure.

Check lung sounds for the accumulation of secretions.

Suction fluids from the airway as needed.

Monitor neurological status, including level of consciousness, pupillary reactions, and motor and sensory function, using the Glasgow Coma Scale.

Place the client in a semi-Fowler's position.

Change position of the client every 2 hours, avoiding injury when turning.

Avoid Trendelenburg's position.

Use side rails at all times.

Monitor for edema.

Monitor for dehydration.

Monitor intake and output and daily weight.

Maintain NPO status until consciousness returns.

Maintain nutrition as prescribed, and monitor fluid and electrolyte balance.

Check the gag and swallow reflex before resuming a diet, and begin the diet with ice chips and fluids when the client becomes alert.

Provide intravenous or enteral feedings as prescribed.

Check bowel sounds.

Monitor elimination patterns.

Monitor for constipation, impaction, and paralytic ileus.

Maintain urinary output to prevent stasis, infection, and calculus formation.

Monitor the status of skin integrity.

Initiate measures to prevent skin breakdown.

Provide frequent mouth care.

Remove dentures and contact lenses.

Check the eyes for the presence of a corneal reflex and irritation, and instill artificial tears or cover the eyes with eye patches.

Monitor drainage from the ears or nose for the presence of cerebrospinal fluid.

Assume that the unconscious client can hear.

Avoid restraints.

Do not leave the client unattended if unstable.

Initiate seizure precautions if necessary.

Provide range-of-motion exercises to prevent contractures.

Use a footboard or high-top sneakers to prevent foot drop.

Use splints to prevent wrist deformities.

Initiate physical therapy as appropriate.

Box 57-7 Medications for Intracranial Pressure

Anticonvulsants

Anticonvulsants may be given prophylactically to prevent seizures.

Seizures increase metabolic requirements and cerebral blood flow and volume, thus increasing intracranial pressure.

Antipyretics and Muscle Relaxants

Temperature reduction decreases metabolism, cerebral blood flow, and thus intracranial pressure.

Antipyretics prevent temperature elevations.

Muscle relaxants prevent shivering.

Blood Pressure Medication

Blood pressure medication may be required to maintain cerebral perfusion at a normal level.

Notify the HCP if the blood pressure range is less than 100 or greater than 150 mm Hg systolic.

Corticosteroids

Corticosteroids stabilize the cell membrane and reduce the leakiness in the blood-brain barrier.

Corticosteroids decrease cerebral edema.

A histamine blocker may be administered to counteract the excess gastric secretion that occurs with the corticosteroid.

Clients must be withdrawn slowly from corticosteroid therapy to reduce the risk of adrenal crisis.

Intravenous Fluids

Fluids are administered intravenously via an infusion pump to control the amount administered.

Hypertonic intravenous solutions are usually avoided because of the risk of promoting additional cerebral edema.

Mannitol (Osmitrol)

Mannitol is a hyperosmotic agent that increases intravascular pressure by drawing fluid from the interstitial spaces and from the brain cells.

Monitor renal function.

Diuresis is expected.

VI. HYPERTHERMIA

A. Description
1. A temperature greater than 105° F, which increases the cerebral metabolism and increases the risk of hypoxia
2. The causes include infection, heat stroke, exposure to high environmental temperatures, and dysfunction of the thermoregulatory center.

B. Data collection
1. Temperature greater than 105° F
2. Shivering
3. Nausea and vomiting

C. Interventions
1. Maintain a patent airway.
2. Initiate seizure precautions.
3. Monitor the I&O and assess the skin and mucous membranes for signs of dehydration.
4. Monitor lung sounds.
5. Monitor for dysrhythmias.
6. Assess peripheral pulses for systemic blood flow.
7. Induce normothermia with fluids, cool baths, fans, or a hypothermia blanket.

D. Inducement of normothermia
1. Prevent shivering, which will increase **ICP** and oxygen consumption.
2. Administer medications as prescribed to prevent shivering.
3. Monitor neurological status.
4. Monitor for infection and respiratory complications because hypothermia may mask the signs of infection.
5. Monitor for cardiac dysrhythmias.
6. Monitor the I&O.
7. Prevent trauma to the skin and tissues.
8. Apply lotion to the skin frequently.
9. Inspect for frostbite if a hypothermia blanket is used.

VII. HEAD INJURY

A. Description
1. Head injury is trauma to the scalp, skull, or brain resulting in injury.
2. Immediate complications include cerebral bleeding, hematomas, uncontrolled **ICP**, infections, and seizures.
3. Changes in personality or behavior, cranial nerve deficits, and any other residual deficits depend on the area of the brain damage and the extent of the damage.

B. Types of head injuries (Box 57-8)
1. Open
   a. Scalp lacerations
   b. Fractures in the skull
   c. Interruption of the dura mater
2. Closed
   a. Concussions
   b. Contusions
   c. Fractures

C. Hematoma
1. Description: Hematoma can occur as a result of a subarachnoid hemorrhage, subdural hemorrhage, or intracerebral hemorrhage.
2. Data collection
   a. Findings depend on the injury
   b. Clinical manifestations usually result from increased **ICP**
   c. Changing neurological signs in the client
   d. Changes in LOC
   e. Airway and breathing pattern changes
   f. Vital signs changes reflecting increasing **ICP**
   g. Headache, nausea, and vomiting
   h. Visual disturbances, pupillary changes, and papilledema
   i. **Nuchal rigidity** (not tested until spinal cord injury is ruled out)

Box 57-8 Types of Head Injuries

Concussion
Concussion is a jarring of the brain within the skull with temporary loss of consciousness.

Contusion
Contusion is a bruising of brain tissue.
Contusion may occur with subdural or extradural collections of blood.

Skull Fractures
Linear
Depressed
Compound
Comminuted

Epidural Hematoma
As the most serious type of hematoma, epidural hematoma forms rapidly and results from arterial bleeding.

Epidural hematoma forms between the dura and the skull from a tear in the meningeal artery.
Often associated with temporary loss of consciousness, followed by a lucid period, that rapidly progresses to coma.
Epidural hematoma is a surgical emergency.

Subdural Hematoma
Subdural hematoma forms slowly and results from a venous bleed.
Subdural hematoma occurs under the dura as a result of tears in the veins crossing the subdural space.

Intracerebral Hemorrhage
Multiple hemorrhages occur around a contused area.

Subarachnoid Hemorrhage
Bleeding occurs directly into the brain, the ventricles, or the subarachnoid space.

j. CSF drainage from the ears or nose

k. Weakness and paralysis

l. Posturing

m. Decreased sensation or absence of feeling

n. Reflex activity changes

o. Seizure activity

⚠ CSF can be distinguished from other fluids by the presence of concentric rings (clear or bloody fluid surrounded by a yellow stain) when the fluid is placed on a white sterile background, such as a gauze pad. Clear CSF also tests positive for glucose when tested using a strip test (blood will normally test positive for glucose; therefore if the fluid is bloody, testing for glucose is not a reliable indicator of the presence of CSF).

3. Interventions

a. Monitor respiratory status and maintain a patent airway because increased CO_2 levels increase cerebral edema.

b. Monitor neurological status and vital signs, including temperature.

c. Monitor for increased **ICP**.

d. Maintain head elevation to reduce venous pressure.

e. Protect cervical spine, maintain neutral head position and prevent neck flexion.

f. Initiate normothermia measures for increased temperature and prevent shivering.

g. Assess cranial nerve function, reflexes, and motor and sensory function.

h. Initiate seizure precautions.

i. Monitor for pain and restlessness.

j. Morphine sulfate may be prescribed to decrease agitation and control restlessness caused by pain for the head-injured client on a ventilator. Administer with caution because it is a respiratory depressant and may increase **ICP**.

k. Monitor for drainage from the nose or ears because this fluid may be CSF.

l. Do not attempt to clean the nose, suction, or allow the client to blow the nose if drainage occurs.

m. Do not clean the ear if drainage is noted, but apply a loose, dry sterile dressing.

n. Check drainage for the presence of CSF.

o. Notify the HCP if drainage from the ears or nose is noted and the drainage tests positive for CSF.

p. Instruct the client to avoid coughing because this increases **ICP**.

q. Monitor for signs of infection.

r. Turn and position every 2 hours and prevent complications of immobility.

D. Craniotomy

1. Description

a. A surgical procedure that involves an incision through the cranium to remove accumulated blood or a tumor

b. Complications of the procedure include increased **ICP** from cerebral edema, hemorrhage, or obstruction of normal flow of CSF.

c. Additional complications include hematomas, hypovolemic shock, hydrocephalus, respiratory and neurogenic complications, pulmonary edema, and wound infections.

d. Complications related to fluid and electrolyte imbalances include diabetes insipidus and inappropriate secretion of antidiuretic hormone.

2. Preoperative interventions

a. Explain the procedure to the client and family.

b. Ensure that an informed consent has been obtained.

c. Prepare to shave the client's head as prescribed (usually done in the operating room) and cover the head with appropriate covering.

d. Stabilize the client before surgery.

3. Postoperative interventions (Box 57-9)

4. Postoperative positioning (Box 57-10)

VIII. SPINAL CORD INJURY

A. Description

1. Trauma to the spinal cord causes partial or complete disruption of the nerve tracts and neurons.

2. The injury can involve contusion, laceration, or compression of the cord.

3. Spinal cord edema develops, and necrosis of the spinal cord can develop as a result of compromised capillary circulation and venous return.

4. Loss of motor function, sensation, reflex activity, and bowel and bladder control may result.

5. The most common causes include motor vehicle accidents, falls, sporting and industrial accidents, and gunshot or stab wounds.

6. Complications related to the injury include respiratory failure, **autonomic dysreflexia**, **spinal shock**, further cord damage, and death.

B. Most frequently involved vertebrae

1. Cervical: C5, C6, and C7

2. Thoracic: T12

3. Lumbar: L1

C. Transection of the cord

1. Complete disruption of the cord. The spinal cord is severed completely, with total loss of sensation, movement, and reflex activity below the level of injury.

2. Partial transection of the cord

a. The spinal cord is damaged or severed partially.

Box 57-9 Nursing Care After Craniotomy

Monitor vital signs and neurological status every 30 minutes to 1 hour.

Monitor for increased intracranial pressure.

Monitor for decreased level of consciousness, motor weakness or paralysis, aphasia, visual changes, and personality changes.

Maintain mechanical ventilation and slight hyperventilation for the first 24 to 48 hours as prescribed to prevent increased intracranial pressure.

Check the HCP's prescriptions regarding client positioning.

Avoid extreme hip or neck flexion, and maintain the head in a midline neutral position.

Provide a quiet environment.

Monitor the head dressing frequently for signs of drainage.

Mark any area of drainage at least once each nursing shift for baseline comparison.

Monitor the Hemovac or Jackson-Pratt drain, which may be in place for 24 hours.

Maintain suction on the Hemovac or Jackson-Pratt drain.

Measure drainage from the Hemovac or Jackson-Pratt drain every 8 hours, and record the amount and color.

Notify the HCP if drainage is greater than the normal of 30 to 50 mL per shift.

Notify the HCP immediately of excessive amounts of drainage or a saturated head dressing.

Provide basic hygiene.

Record strict measurement of hourly intake and output.

Maintain fluid restriction at 1500 mL/day as prescribed.

Monitor labs and electrolyte values.

Monitor for dysrhythmias, which may occur as a result of fluid and electrolyte imbalance.

Apply ice packs or cool compresses as prescribed. Expect periorbital edema and ecchymosis of one or both eyes, which is not an unusual occurrence.

Turn and position every 2 hours and provide range-of-motion exercises every 8 hours.

Prevent development of DVT and place antiembolism stockings on the client as prescribed.

Administer anticonvulsants, antacids, corticosteroids, and antibiotics as prescribed.

Administer analgesics such as codeine sulfate and acetaminophen (Tylenol) as prescribed for pain.

Box 57-10 Client Positioning After Craniotomy

Positions prescribed after craniotomy vary with the type of surgery and the specific postoperative HCP's prescriptions.

Always check the HCP's prescriptions regarding client positioning.

Incorrect positioning may cause serious and possibly fatal complications.

Removal of a Bone Flap for Decompression

To facilitate brain expansion, the client should be turned from the back to the nonoperative side, but not to the side of the operation.

Posterior Fossa Surgery

To protect the operative site from pressure and to minimize tension on the suture line, position the client on the side, with a pillow under the head for support and not on the back.

Infratentorial Surgery

Infratentorial surgery involves surgery below the tentorium of the brain.

The HCP may prescribe a flat position without head elevation or may prescribe the head of the bed to be elevated at 30 to 45 degrees.

Do not elevate the head of the bed in the acute phase of care after surgery without a HCP's prescription.

Supratentorial Surgery

Supratentorial surgery involves surgery above the tentorium of the brain.

The HCP may prescribe the head of the bed to be elevated at 30 degrees to promote venous outflow through the jugular veins.

Do not lower the head of the bed in the acute phase of care after surgery without a HCP's prescription.

    b. The symptoms depend on the extent and location of the damage.

    c. If the cord has not suffered irreparable damage, early treatment is needed to prevent partial damage from developing into total and permanent damage.

D. Types of injuries (Figure 57-3)

    1. Central cord syndrome

       a. Central cord syndrome occurs from a lesion in the central portion of the spinal cord.

       b. Loss of motor function is more pronounced in the upper extremities, and varying degrees and patterns of sensation remain intact.

    2. Anterior cord syndrome

       a. Anterior cord syndrome is caused by damage to the anterior portion of the gray and white matter of the spinal cord.

       b. Motor function, pain, and temperature sensation are lost below the level of injury; however, the sensations of position, vibration, and touch remain intact.

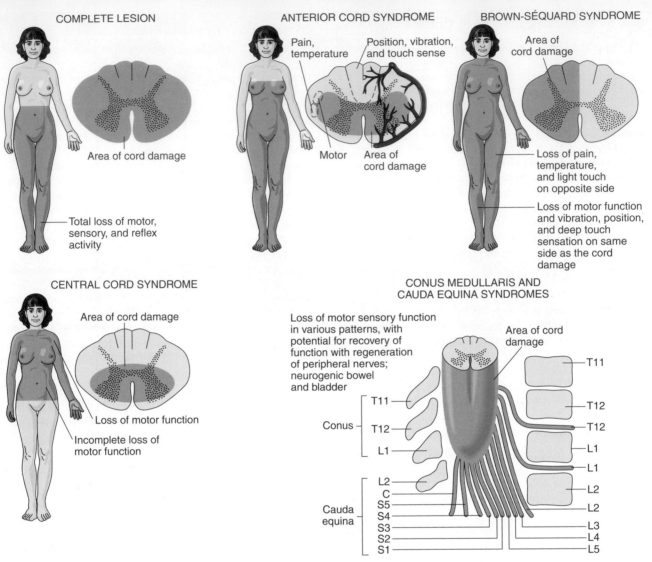

▲ **FIGURE 57-3** Common spinal cord syndromes. (From Ignatavicius, D., & Workman, M. [2010]. *Medical-surgical nursing: Patient-centered collaborative care* [6th ed.]. St. Louis: Saunders.)

3. Posterior cord syndrome
   a. Posterior cord syndrome is caused by damage to the posterior portion of the gray and white matter of the spinal cord.
   b. Motor function remains intact, but the client experiences a loss of vibratory sense, crude touch, and position sensation.
4. Brown-Séquard's syndrome
   a. Brown-Séquard's syndrome results from penetrating injuries that cause hemisection of the spinal cord or injuries that affect half of the cord.
   b. Motor function, vibration, proprioception, and deep touch sensations are lost on the same side of the body (ipsilateral) as the lesion or cord damage.
   c. On the opposite side of the body (contralateral) from the lesion or cord damage, the

sensations of pain, temperature, and light touch are affected.
5. Conus medullaris syndrome
   a. Conus medullaris syndrome follows damage to the lumbar nerve roots and conus medullaris in the spinal cord.
   b. Client experiences bowel and bladder areflexia and flaccid lower extremities.
   c. If damage is limited to the upper sacral segments of the spinal cord, bulbospongiosus penile (erection) and micturition reflexes will remain.
6. Cauda equina syndrome
   a. Cauda equina syndrome occurs from injury to the lumbosacral nerve roots below the conus medullaris.
   b. The client experiences areflexia of the bowel, bladder, and lower reflexes.

E. Data collection: Spinal cord injuries (Box 57-11)
1. Dependent on the level of the cord injury
2. The level of spinal cord injury: the lowest spinal cord segment with intact motor and sensory function
3. Respiratory status changes
4. Motor and sensory changes below the level of injury
5. Total sensory loss and motor paralysis below the level of injury
6. Loss of reflexes below the level of injury
7. Loss of bladder and bowel control
8. Urinary retention and bladder distention
9. Presence of sweat, which does not occur on paralyzed areas

F. Cervical injuries
1. Injury at C2 to C3 is usually fatal.
2. C4 is the major innervation to the diaphragm by the phrenic nerve.
3. Involvement above C4 causes respiratory difficulty and paralysis of all four extremities.
4. Client may have movement in the shoulder if the injury is at C5 or below.
5. Client at risk for developing **autonomic dysreflexia**.

G. Thoracic level injuries
1. Loss of movement of the chest, trunk, bowel, bladder, and legs may occur, depending on the level of injury.
2. Leg paralysis (paraplegia) may occur.
3. **Autonomic dysreflexia** with lesions or injuries above T6 and in cervical lesions may occur.
4. Visceral distention from a noxious stimulus such as a distended bladder or impacted rectum may cause reactions such as sweating, bradycardia, hypertension, nasal stuffiness, and goose flesh.

H. Lumbar and sacral level injuries
1. Loss of movement and sensation of the lower extremities may occur.
2. S2 and S3 center on micturition; therefore, below this level, the bladder will contract but not empty (neurogenic bladder).
3. Injury above S2 in males allows them to have an erection, but they are unable to ejaculate because of sympathetic nerve damage.
4. Injury between S2 and S4 damages the sympathetic and parasympathetic response, preventing erection or ejaculation.

⚠ Always suspect spinal cord injury when trauma occurs until this injury is ruled out. Immobilize the client on a spinal backboard with the head in a neutral position to prevent an incomplete injury from becoming complete.

I. Emergency interventions
1. Emergency management is critical because improper movement can cause further damage and loss of neurological function.

Box 57-11 Effects of Spinal Cord Injury

Tetraplegia (Quadriplegia)
Injury occurring between C1 and C8
Paralysis involving all four extremities

Paraplegia
Injury occurring between T1 and L4
Paralysis involving only the lower extremities

---

2. Assess the respiratory pattern and maintain a patent airway.
3. Prevent head flexion, rotation, or extension.
4. During immobilization, maintain traction and alignment on the head by placing hands on either side of the head by the ears.
5. Maintain an extended position.
6. Logroll the client.
7. No part of the body should be twisted or turned, and the client is not allowed to assume a sitting position.
8. In the emergency department, a client who has sustained a severe cervical fracture should be placed immediately in skeletal traction via **skull tongs** or **halo traction** to immobilize the cervical spine and reduce the fracture and dislocation.

J. Interventions during hospitalization
1. Respiratory system
   a. Monitor respiratory status because paralysis of the intercostal and abdominal muscles occurs with C4 injuries.
   b. Monitor arterial blood gases and maintain mechanical ventilation if prescribed to prevent respiratory arrest, especially with cervical injuries.
   c. Encourage deep breathing and the use of an incentive spirometer.
   d. Monitor for signs of infection, particularly pneumonia.
2. Cardiovascular system
   a. Monitor for cardiac dysrhythmias.
   b. Monitor for signs of hemorrhage or bleeding around the fracture site.
   c. Monitor for signs of shock, such as hypotension, tachycardia, and a weak and thready pulse.
   d. Monitor the lower extremities for deep vein thrombosis.
   e. Measure circumferences of the calf and thigh to identify increases in size.
   f. Apply thigh high antiembolism stockings or sequential compression devices (SCDs) as prescribed.
   g. Remove antiembolism stockings and SCDs daily to assess the skin.
   h. Monitor for orthostatic hypotension when repositioning the client.

3. Neuromuscular system
   a. Monitor neurological status.
   b. Monitor motor and sensory status to determine the level of injury.
   c. Monitor motor ability by testing the client's ability to squeeze hands, spread the fingers, move the toes, and turn the feet.
   d. Check for absent sensation, hyposensation, or hypersensation by pinching the skin or pricking it with a pin, starting at the toes and working upward.
   e. Monitor for signs of **autonomic dysreflexia** and **spinal shock**.
   f. Immobilize the client to promote healing and prevent further injury.
   g. Monitor pain.
   h. Initiate measures to reduce pain.
   i. Administer analgesics as prescribed.
   j. Monitor for complications of immobility.
   k. Prepare the client for decompression laminectomy, spinal fusion, or insertion of instrumentation or rods if prescribed.
   l. Collaborate with the physical therapist and occupational therapist to determine appropriate exercise techniques, assess the need for hand and wrist splints, and develop an appropriate plan to prevent footdrop.
4. Gastrointestinal system
   a. Check abdomen for distention and hemorrhage.
   b. Monitor bowel sounds and assess for paralytic ileus.
   c. Prevent bowel retention.
   d. Initiate a bowel control program as appropriate.
   e. Maintain adequate nutrition and a high-fiber diet.
5. Renal system
   a. Prevent urinary retention.
   b. Initiate a bladder control program as appropriate.
   c. Maintain fluid and electrolyte balance.
   d. Maintain adequate fluid intake of 2000 mL/day.
   e. Monitor for urinary tract infection and calculi.
6. Integumentary system
   a. Check skin integrity.
   b. Turn the client every 2 hours.
7. Psychosocial integrity
   a. Monitor psychosocial status.
   b. Encourage the client to express feelings of anger and depression.
   c. Discuss the sexual concerns of the client.
   d. Promote self-care, setting realistic goals based on the client's potential functional level
   e. Encourage contact with appropriate community resources.

K. Spinal shock and **neurogenic shock**
1. Description
   a. **Spinal shock** is a transient condition that occurs after a spinal cord injury; voluntary and reflex neurological activity below the level of injury is absent.
   b. **Neurogenic shock** occurs from an injury at T5 or above and usually is experienced soon after the injury (within 30 minutes) lasting up to 6 weeks. Massive vasodilation occurs leading to pooling of the blood in blood vessels, tissue hypoperfusion, and impaired cellular metabolism.
2. Data collection (Box 57-12)
3. Interventions
   a. Monitor for signs of **spinal shock** after a spinal cord injury.
   b. Monitor for hypotension and bradycardia.
   c. Monitor for reflex activity.
   d. Check bowel sounds.
   e. Monitor for bowel and urinary retention.
   f. Provide supportive measures as prescribed, based on the presence of symptoms.
   g. Monitor for the return of reflexes.
L. Autonomic dysreflexia
1. Description
   a. **Autonomic dysreflexia** is also known as autonomic hyperreflexia.
   b. **Autonomic dysreflexia** generally occurs after the period of **spinal shock** is resolved and occurs with lesions or injuries above T6 and in cervical lesions.

Box 57-12 Neurogenic Shock, Spinal Shock, and Autonomic Dysreflexia

Neurogenic Shock
Hypotension
Bradycardia

Spinal Shock
Flaccid paralysis
Loss of reflex activity below the level of injury
Bradycardia
Paralytic ileus
Hypotension

Autonomic Dysreflexia
Sudden onset of severe, throbbing headache
Severe hypertension and bradycardia
Flushing above the level of the lesion
Pale extremities below the level of injury
Nasal stuffiness
Nausea
Dilated pupils or blurred vision
Sweating
Piloerection (goose bumps)
Restlessness and a feeling of apprehension

Actions to Take for a Spinal Cord Injury Client Who Develops Autonomic Dysreflexia

1. Raise the head of the bed.
2. Loosen tight clothing on the client.
3. Check for bladder distention or other noxious stimulus.
4. Administer an antihypertensive medication.
5. Document the occurrence, treatment, and response.

Autonomic dysreflexia is characterized by severe hypertension, bradycardia, severe headache, nasal stuffiness, and flushing. The cause is a noxious stimulus, most often a distended bladder or constipation. Autonomic dysreflexia is a neurological emergency and must be treated promptly to prevent a hypertensive stroke. Immediate nursing actions are to sit the client up in bed in a high Fowler's position and remove the noxious stimulus. The nurse would loosen any tight clothing and then check for bladder distention. If the client has a Foley catheter, the nurse would check for kinks in the tubing. The nurse also would check for a fecal impaction and disimpact the client, if necessary. The HCP is contacted. The nurse checks the environment to ensure that it is not too cool or too drafty and also monitors vital signs, particularly the blood pressure, every 15 minutes. Antihypertensive medication may be prescribed by the HCP to minimize cerebral hypertension. Finally the nurse documents the occurrence, treatment, and client response.

Reference: Ignatavicius, D., & Workman, M. (2010). *Medical-surgical nursing: Patient-centered collaborative care* (6th ed., p. 998). St. Louis: Saunders.

c. It is commonly caused by visceral distention from a distended bladder or impacted rectum.
d. It is a neurological emergency and must be treated immediately to prevent a hypertensive stroke.
2. Data collection (see Box 57-12)
3. Interventions (see Priority Nursing Actions)
M. Cervical spine traction for cervical injuries
1. Description
a. Skeletal traction is used to stabilize fractures or dislocations of the cervical or upper thoracic spine.
b. Two types of equipment used for cervical traction are **skull** (cervical) **tongs** and **halo traction** (halo fixation device).
2. **Skull tongs**
a. **Skull tongs** are inserted into the outer aspect of the client's skull, and traction is applied.
b. Weights are attached to the tongs, and the client is used as countertraction.
c. Monitor the neurological status of the client.
d. Determine the amount of weight prescribed to be added to the traction.
e. Ensure that weights hang securely and freely at all times.

f. Ensure that the ropes for the traction remain within the pulley.
g. Maintain body alignment and maintain care of the client on a special bed (such as a Roto-Rest bed, Stryker, or Foster frame) as prescribed.
h. Turn the client every 2 hours.
i. Check insertion site of the tongs for infection.
j. Provide sterile pin site care as prescribed.
3. **Halo traction**
a. **Halo traction** is a static traction device that consists of a headpiece with four pins—two anterior and two posterior—inserted into the client's skull.
b. The metal halo ring may be attached to a vest (jacket) or cast when the spine is stable, allowing increased client mobility.
c. Monitor the client's neurological status for changes in movement or decreased strength.
d. Never move or turn the client by holding or pulling on the **halo traction** device.
e. Check tightness of the jacket by ensuring that one finger can be placed under the jacket.
f. Check skin integrity to ensure that the jacket or cast is not causing pressure.
g. Provide sterile pin site care as prescribed.
4. Client education for **halo traction** device (Box 57-13)
5. Initiate interventions in support of the client's self-image.
6. Teach the client and family pin care, care of the vest, and signs and symptoms of infection to report to his or her HCP.
N. Interventions for thoracic and lumbar/sacral injuries
1. Bedrest
2. Immobilize with a body cast if prescribed.
3. Monitor for respiratory impairment and paralytic ileus, as possible complications of the body cast.
4. Use a brace or corset when the client is out of bed.
O. Surgical interventions for thoracic and lumbar/sacral injuries
1. Decompressive laminectomy
a. Removal of one or more laminae
b. Allows for cord expansion from edema and is performed if conventional methods fail to prevent neurological deterioration
2. Spinal fusion
a. Spinal fusion is used for thoracic spinal injuries.
b. Bone is grafted between the vertebrae for support and to strengthen the back.
3. Postoperative interventions
a. Monitor for respiratory impairment.
b. Monitor vital signs, motor function, sensation, and circulatory status in the lower extremities.

c. Encourage breathing exercises.

d. Assess for signs of fluid and electrolyte imbalance.

e. Observe for complications of immobility.

f. Keep the client in a flat position as prescribed.

g. Provide cast care if the client is in a full body cast.

h. Turn and reposition frequently by logrolling side to back to side, using turning sheets and pillows between the legs to maintain alignment.

i. Administer pain medication as prescribed.

j. Maintain an NPO status until the client is passing flatus.

k. Monitor bowel sounds.

l. Provide the use of a fracture bedpan.

m. Monitor the I&O.

n. Maintain nutritional status.

P. Medications

1. Dexamethasone (Decadron)
   a. Used for its anti-inflammatory and edema-reducing effects
   b. May interfere with healing

2. Dextran: A plasma expander used to increase capillary blood flow within the spinal cord and to prevent or treat hypotension

3. Dantrolene (Dantrium)/Baclofen (Lioresal): These medications are used for clients with upper motor neuron injuries to control muscle spasticity.

IX. CEREBRAL ANEURYSM

A. Description

1. A dilation of the walls of a weakened cerebral artery
2. Aneurysm can lead to rupture

B. Data collection

1. Headache and pain
2. Irritability
3. Diplopia

4. Blurred vision

5. Tinnitus

6. Hemiparesis

7. **Nuchal rigidity**

8. Seizures

C. Interventions

1. Maintain a patent airway (suction only with a HCP's prescription).
2. Administer oxygen as prescribed.
3. Monitor vital signs and for hypertension or dysrhythmias.
4. Avoid taking temperatures via the rectum.
5. Initiate aneurysm precautions (Box 57-14).

Box 57-14 Aneurysm Precautions

Maintain bedrest in a semi-Fowler's or side-lying position.

Maintain a darkened room (subdued lighting and no direct, bright, artificial lights) without stimulation (a private room is optimal).

Provide a quiet environment (avoid activities or startling noises); telephone in the room is not usually allowed.

Reading, watching television, and listening to music are permitted, provided they do not overstimulate the client.

Limit visitors.

Maintain fluid restrictions.

Provide diet as prescribed; avoid stimulants in the diet.

Prevent any activities that initiate the Valsalva maneuver (straining at stooling, coughing); provide stool softeners to prevent straining.

Administer care gently (e.g., the bath, back rub, range of motion).

Limit invasive procedures.

Maintain normothermia.

Prevent hypertension.

Provide sedation.

Provide pain control.

Administer prophylactic anticonvulsant medications.

Provide deep vein thrombosis (DVT) prophylaxis as prescribed.

Box 57-13 Client Education for a Halo Fixation Device

Notify the HCP if the halo vest (jacket) or ring bolts loosen.

Use fleece or foam inserts to relieve pressure points.

Keep the vest lining dry.

Clean the pin site daily.

Notify the HCP if redness, swelling, drainage, open areas, pain, tenderness, or a clicking sound occurs from the pin site.

A sponge bath or tub bath is allowed. Showers are prohibited.

Check the skin under the vest daily for breakdown, using a flashlight.

Do not use any products other than shampoo on the hair.

When shampooing the hair, cover the vest with plastic.

When getting out of bed, roll onto the side and push on the mattress with the arms.

Never use the metal frame for turning or lifting.

Use a rolled towel or pillowcase between the back of the neck and the bed or next to the cheek when lying on the side, and raise the head of the bed to increase sleep comfort.

Adapt clothing to fit over the halo device.

Eat foods high in protein and calcium to promote bone healing.

Have the correct-size wrench available at all times for an emergency.

If cardiopulmonary resuscitation is required, the anterior portion of the vest will be loosened and the posterior portion will remain in place to provide stability.

X.   SEIZURES

A. Description

1. Seizures are an abnormal, sudden, excessive discharge of electrical activity within the brain.
2. Epilepsy is a disorder characterized by chronic seizure activity and indicates brain or CNS irritation.
3. Causes include genetic factors, trauma, tumors, circulatory or metabolic disorders, toxicity, and infections.
4. Status epilepticus involves a rapid succession of epileptic spasms without intervals of consciousness. It is a potential complication that can occur with any type of seizure, and brain damage may result.

B. Types of seizures (Box 57-15)

1. Generalized seizures
2. Partial seizures

C. Data collection

1. Seizure history
2. Type of seizure
3. Occurrences before, during, and after the seizure
4. Prodromal signs, such as mood changes, irritability, and insomnia
5. Aura: a sensation that warns the client of the impending seizure
6. Loss of motor activity or bowel and bladder function or loss of consciousness during the seizure
7. Occurrences during the postictal state, such as headache, loss of consciousness, sleepiness, and impaired speech or thinking

D. Interventions

 If the client is having a seizure, maintain a patent airway. Do not force the jaws open or place anything in the client's mouth.

1. Note the time and duration of the seizure.
2. Assess behavior at the onset of the seizure. Note if the client experienced an aura, a change in facial expression occurred, or a sound or cry occurred from the client.
3. If the client is standing, place him or her on the floor and protect the head and body.
4. Support the ABCs—airway, breathing, and circulation.
5. Administer oxygen.
6. Prepare to suction secretions from the airway.
7. Turn the client to the side, to allow secretions to drain, while maintaining the airway.
8. Prevent injury during the seizure.
9. Remain with the client.
10. Do not restrain the client.
11. Loosen restrictive clothing.
12. Note the type, character, and progression of the movements during the seizure.
13. Monitor for incontinence.
14. Administer IV medications as prescribed to stop the seizure.
15. Document the characteristics of the seizure.
16. Provide privacy, if possible.
17. Monitor behavior after the seizure, such as the state of consciousness, motor ability, and speech ability.

Box 57-15 Types of Seizures

Generalized Seizures

Tonic-Clonic
Tonic-clonic seizures may begin with an aura.
The tonic phase involves the stiffening or rigidity of the muscles of the arms and legs and usually lasts 10 to 20 seconds, followed by loss of consciousness.
The clonic phase consists of hyperventilation and jerking of the extremities and usually lasts about 30 seconds.
Full recovery from the seizure may take several hours.

Absence
Brief seizure lasts seconds, and the individual may or may not lose consciousness.
No loss or change in muscle tone occurs.
Seizures may occur several times during a day.
The victim appears to be daydreaming.
This type of seizure is more common in children.

Myoclonic
Myoclonic seizures present as a brief generalized jerking or stiffening of extremities.

The victim may fall to the ground from the seizure.

Atonic or Akinetic (Drop Attacks)
An atonic seizure is a sudden momentary loss of muscle tone.
The victim may fall to the ground as a result of the seizure.

Partial Seizures

Simple Partial
The simple partial seizure produces sensory symptoms accompanied by motor symptoms that are localized or confined to a specific area.
The client remains conscious and may report an aura.

Complex Partial
The complex partial seizure is a psychomotor seizure.
The area of the brain most involved is the temporal lobe.
The seizure is characterized by periods of altered behavior of which the client is not aware.
The client loses consciousness for a few seconds.

18. Instruct the client about the importance of life-long medication and the need for follow-up medication blood levels.
19. Instruct the client to avoid alcohol, excessive stress, fatigue, and strobe lights.
20. Encourage the client to contact available community resources, such as the Epilepsy Foundation of America.
21. Encourage the client to wear a Medic-Alert bracelet.

XI. STROKE (BRAIN ATTACK)

A. Description
1. A stroke or brain attack, formerly known as a cerebrovascular accident (CVA), is a sudden focal neurological deficit caused by cerebrovascular disease.
2. A stroke is a syndrome in which the cerebral circulation is interrupted, causing neurological deficits.
3. Cerebral anoxia lasting longer than 10 minutes causes cerebral infarction with irreversible change.
4. Cerebral edema and congestion cause further dysfunction.
5. Diagnosis is determined by CT scan, electroencephalogram, cerebral arteriography, and MRI.
6. The permanent disability cannot be determined until the cerebral edema subsides.
7. The order in which function may return is facial, swallowing, lower limb, speech, and arms.
8. Carotid endarterectomy is a surgical intervention used in stroke management and is targeted at stroke prevention, especially in clients with symptomatic carotid stenosis.

⚠ A transient ischemic attack (TIA) may be a warning sign of an impending stroke.

B. Causes
1. Thrombosis
2. Embolism
3. Hemorrhage from rupture of a vessel
4. Transient ischemic attack

C. Risk factors
1. Atherosclerosis
2. Hypertension
3. Anticoagulation therapy
4. Diabetes mellitus
5. Stress
6. Obesity
7. Oral contraceptives

⚠ A critical factor in the early intervention and treatment of stroke is the accurate identification of stroke manifestations and establishing the onset of the manifestations. Stroke screening scales may be used to quickly identify stroke manifestations.

D. Data collection (Boxes 57-16 and 57-17 and Figure 57-4)
1. Findings depend on the area of the brain affected.
2. Lesions in the cerebral hemisphere result in manifestations on the contralateral side, which is the side of the body opposite the stroke.
3. Airway patency is always a priority.
4. Pulse (may be slow and bounding)
5. Respirations (Cheyne-Stokes)
6. Blood pressure (hypertension)
7. Headache, nausea, and vomiting
8. Facial drooping
9. **Nuchal rigidity**
10. Visual changes
11. Ataxia
12. Dysarthria
13. Dysphagia
14. Speech changes
15. Decreased sensation to pressure, heat, and cold
16. Bowel and bladder dysfunctions
17. Paralysis

Box 57-16 Neurological Data Collection: Stroke

Changes in level of consciousness
Signs of increasing intracranial pressure
Assessment of cranial nerves V, VII, IX, X, and XII
Cranial nerve V: difficulty with chewing
Cranial nerve VII: facial paralysis or paresis
Cranial nerves IX and X: dysphagia
Cranial nerve IX: absent gag reflex
Cranial nerve XII: impaired tongue movement

Box 57-17 Data Collection Findings: Stroke

Agnosia
Inability to recognize and use an object correctly

Apraxia
Inability to carry out a purposeful activity

Hemianopsia
Blindness in half of the visual field

Homonymous Hemianopsia
Blindness in the same visual field of both eyes

Neglect Syndrome (Unilateral Neglect)
Client unaware of the existence of his or her paralyzed side

Proprioception Alterations
Altered position sense that places the client at increased risk of injury

With visual problems, the client must turn the head to scan the complete range of vision.

E. Aphasia
1. Expressive
   a. Damage occurs in Broca's area of the frontal brain.
   b. The client understands what is said but is unable to communicate verbally.
2. Receptive
   a. The injury involves Wernicke's area in the temporoparietal area.
   b. The client is unable to understand the spoken and often the written word.
3. Global or mixed: Language dysfunction occurs in expression and reception.
4. Interventions for aphasia
   a. Provide repetitive directions.
   b. Break tasks down to one step at a time.
   c. Repeat names of objects frequently used.
   d. Allow time for the client to communicate.
   e. Use a picture board, communication board, or computerized technologies.

F. Interventions during the acute phase of stroke
1. Maintain a patent airway and administer oxygen as prescribed.
2. Monitor the vital signs.
3. Maintain a blood pressure of 150/100 mm Hg or as prescribed to maintain cerebral perfusion.

Right-brain damage (stroke on right side of the brain)	**Left-brain damage** (stroke on left side of the brain)
• Paralyzed left side: hemiplegia	• Paralyzed right side: hemiplegia
• Left-sided neglect	• Impaired speech/language aphasias
• Spatial-perceptual deficits	• Impaired right/left discrimination
• Tends to deny or minimize problems	• Slow performance, cautious
• Rapid performance, short attention span	• Aware of deficits: depression, anxiety
• Impulsive, safety problems	• Impaired comprehension related to language, math
• Impaired judgment	
• Impaired time concepts	

▲ **FIGURE 57-4** Manifestations of right brain and left brain stroke. (From Lewis, S., Heitkemper, M., & Dirksen, S. [2011]. *Medical-surgical nursing: Assessment and management of clinical problems* [8th ed.]. St. Louis: Mosby.)

4. Suction secretions as prescribed, but never suction nasally and for longer than 10 seconds to prevent increasing **ICP**.
5. Monitor for increasing **ICP** because the client is at most risk during the first 72 hours after the stroke.
6. Position the client on the side, with the head of the bed elevated 15 to 30 degrees as prescribed.
7. Monitor LOC, pupillary response, motor and sensory response, cranial nerve function, and reflexes.
8. Maintain a quiet environment, and provide minimal handling of the client to prevent further bleeding.
9. Insert a Foley catheter as prescribed.
10. Monitor prescribed IV fluids closely.
11. Maintain fluid and electrolyte balance.
12. Prepare to administer anticoagulants, antiplatelets, diuretics, antihypertensives, and anticonvulsants as prescribed.
13. Establish a form of communication.

G. Interventions in the postacute phase of a stroke
1. Continue with interventions from the acute phase.
2. Position the client 2 hours on the unaffected side, 20 minutes on the affected side.
3. Position the client in the prone position if prescribed, for 30 minutes three times daily.
4. Provide skin, mouth, and eye care.
5. Perform passive range-of-motion exercises to prevent contractures.
6. Place sequential compression devices (SCDs) or antiembolism stockings on the client.
7. Measure the thighs and calves for an increase in size.
8. Monitor the gag reflex and ability to swallow.
9. Provide sips of fluids and slowly advance the diet to foods that are easy to chew and swallow.
10. Provide soft and semisoft foods and flavored, cool or warm, thickened fluids rather than thin liquids because the stroke client is better able to tolerate these types of foods. Speech therapists may do swallow studies to recommend consistency of food and fluids.
11. When the client is eating, position him or her sitting in a chair or sitting up in bed, with the head and neck positioned slightly forward and flexed.
12. Place food in the back of the mouth on the unaffected side to prevent trapping of food in the affected cheek.

H. Interventions in the chronic phase of stroke
1. Neglect syndrome
   a. The client is unaware of the existence of the paralyzed side (**unilateral neglect**), which places him or her at risk for injury.
   b. Teach the client to touch and use both sides of the body.

2. **Hemianopsia**
   a. The client has blindness in half of the visual field.
   b. **Homonymous hemianopsia** is blindness in the same visual field of both eyes.
   c. Encourage the client to turn the head to scan the complete range of vision; otherwise, he or she does not see half of the visual field.
3. Approach the client from the unaffected side.
4. Place the client's personal objects within the visual field.
5. Provide eye care for visual deficits.
6. Place a patch over the affected eye if the client has diplopia.
7. Increase mobility as tolerated.
8. Encourage fluid intake and a high-fiber diet.
9. Monitor for pain.
10. Administer stool softeners as prescribed.
11. Encourage the client to express his or her feelings.
12. Encourage independence in activities of daily living.
13. Assess the need for assistive devices such as a cane, walker, splints, or braces.
14. Assess for safety in bed and chair and prevent falls.
15. Teach transfer technique from bed to chair and chair to bed.
16. Provide gait training.
17. Initiate physical and occupational therapy.
18. Refer the client to a speech and language pathologist as prescribed.
19. Encourage the client and family to contact available community resources.

XII. MULTIPLE SCLEROSIS

A. Description
1. Multiple sclerosis is a chronic, progressive, noncontagious, degenerative disease of the CNS characterized by demyelinization of the neurons.
2. It usually occurs between the ages of 20 and 40 and consists of periods of remissions and exacerbations.
3. The causes are unknown, but the disease is thought to be a result of an autoimmune response or viral infection.
4. Precipitating factors include pregnancy, fatigue, stress, infection, and trauma.
5. Electroencephalogram findings are abnormal.
6. A lumbar puncture indicates increased gamma-globulin, but the serum globulin level is normal.

B. Data collection
1. Fatigue and weakness
2. Ataxia and vertigo
3. Tremors and spasticity of the lower extremities
4. Paresthesias
5. Blurred vision, diplopia, and transient blindness
6. Nystagmus

7. Dysphasia
8. Decreased perception to pain, touch, and temperature
9. Bladder and bowel disturbances, including urgency, frequency, retention, and incontinence
10. Abnormal reflexes, including hyperreflexia, absent reflexes, and a positive **Babinski's reflex**
11. Emotional changes such as apathy, euphoria, irritability, and depression
12. Memory changes and confusion

C. Interventions
1. Provide bedrest during exacerbation.
2. Protect the client from injury by providing safety measures.
3. Place an eye patch on the eye for diplopia.
4. Monitor for potential complications such as urinary tract infections, calculi, pressure ulcers, respiratory tract infections, and contractures.
5. Promote regular elimination by bladder and bowel training.
6. Encourage independence.
7. Assist the client to establish a regular exercise and rest program.
8. Instruct the client to balance moderate activity with rest periods.
9. Assess the need for and provide assistive devices.
10. Initiate physical and speech therapy.
11. Instruct the client to avoid fatigue, stress, infection, overheating, and chilling.
12. Instruct the client to increase fluid intake and eat a balanced diet, including low-fat, high-fiber foods and foods high in potassium.
13. Instruct the client on safety measures related to sensory loss, such as regulating the temperature of bath water and avoiding heating pads.
14. Instruct the client on safety measures related to motor loss, such as avoiding the use of scatter rugs and using assistive devices.
15. Instruct the client in the self-administration of prescribed medications.
16. Provide information about the National Multiple Sclerosis Society.

XIII. MYASTHENIA GRAVIS

A. Description
1. Myasthenia gravis is a neuromuscular disease that is characterized by considerable weakness and abnormal fatigue of the voluntary muscles.
2. A defect in the transmission of nerve impulses at the myoneural junction occurs.
3. Causes include insufficient secretion of acetylcholine, excessive secretion of cholinesterase, and unresponsiveness of the muscle fibers to acetylcholine.

B. Data collection
1. Weakness and fatigue

2. Difficulty chewing and swallowing
3. Dysphagia
4. Ptosis
5. Diplopia
6. Weak, hoarse voice
7. Difficulty breathing
8. Diminished breath sounds
9. Respiratory paralysis and failure

C. Interventions
1. Monitor respiratory status and ability to cough and deep breathe adequately.
2. Monitor for respiratory failure.
3. Maintain suctioning and emergency equipment at the bedside.
4. Monitor the vital signs.
5. Monitor speech and swallowing abilities to prevent aspiration.
6. Encourage the client to sit up when eating.
7. Assess muscle status.
8. Instruct the client to conserve strength.
9. Plan short activities that coincide with times of maximal muscle strength.
10. Monitor for myasthenic and cholinergic crises.
11. Administer anticholinesterase medications as prescribed.
12. Instruct the client to avoid stress, infection, fatigue, and over-the-counter medications.
13. Instruct the client to wear a Medic-Alert bracelet.
14. Inform the client about services from the Myasthenia Gravis Foundation.

D. Anticholinesterase medications: Increase levels of acetylcholine at the myoneural junction (see Chapter 58)

E. Myasthenic crisis
1. Description
   a. Myasthenic crisis is an acute exacerbation of the disease.
   b. The crisis is caused by a rapid, unrecognized progression of the disease; an inadequate amount of medication; infection; fatigue; or stress.
2. Data collection
   a. Increased pulse, respirations, and blood pressure
   b. Respiratory distress and cyanosis
   c. Bowel and bladder incontinence
   d. Decreased urine output
   e. Absent cough and swallow reflex
3. Interventions
   a. Assess for signs of myasthenic crisis.
   b. Increase anticholinesterase medication, as prescribed.

F. Cholinergic crisis
1. Description
   a. Cholinergic crisis results in depolarization of the motor end plates.
   b. The crisis is caused by overmedication with anticholinesterase.

2. Data collection
   a. Abdominal cramps
   b. Nausea, vomiting, and diarrhea
   c. Blurred vision
   d. Pallor
   e. Facial muscle twitching
   f. Hypotension
   g. Pupillary miosis
3. Interventions
   a. Hold anticholinesterase medication.
   b. Prepare to administer the antidote, atropine sulfate, if prescribed.

G. Edrophonium (Enlon) test

⚠ Have atropine sulfate available when performing the edrophonium test.

1. Description: The edrophonium test is performed to diagnose myasthenia gravis and differentiate between myasthenic crisis and cholinergic crisis.
2. To diagnose myasthenia gravis
   a. An edrophonium (Enlon) injection is administered to the client.
   b. Positive for myasthenia gravis: The client shows improvement in muscle strength after the administration of edrophonium.
   c. Negative for myasthenia gravis: The client shows no improvement in muscle strength, and strength may even deteriorate after injection of edrophonium.
3. To differentiate crisis
   a. Myasthenic crisis: Edrophonium is administered; if strength improves, the client needs more medication.
   b. Cholinergic crisis: Edrophonium is administered; if the client's weakness is more severe, then the client is overmedicated. Administer atropine sulfate, which is the antidote, as prescribed.

XIV. PARKINSON'S DISEASE

A. Description
1. Parkinson's disease is a degenerative disease caused by the depletion of dopamine, which interferes with the inhibition of excitatory impulses, resulting in a dysfunction of the extrapyramidal system.
2. It is a slow, progressive disease that results in a crippling disability.
3. The debilitation can result in falls, self-care deficits, failure of body systems, and depression.
4. Mental deterioration occurs late in the progression of disease.

B. Data collection
1. Bradykinesia, abnormal slowness of movement, and sluggishness of physical and mental responses

2. Akinesia
3. Monotonous speech
4. Handwriting that becomes progressively smaller
5. Tremors in hands and fingers at rest (pill rolling)
6. Tremors increasing when fatigued and decreasing with purposeful activity or sleep
7. Rigidity with jerky movements
8. Restlessness and pacing
9. Blank facial expression; masklike facies
10. Drooling
11. Difficulty swallowing and speaking
12. Loss of coordination and balance
13. Shuffling steps, stooped position, and propulsive gait

C. Interventions
1. Monitor neurological status.
2. Check ability to swallow and chew.
3. Provide a high-calorie, high-protein, high-fiber soft diet with small, frequent feedings.
4. Increase fluid intake to 2000 mL/day.
5. Monitor for constipation.
6. Promote independence along with safety measures.
7. Avoid rushing the client with activities.
8. Assist with ambulation and provide assistive devices.
9. Instruct the client to rock back and forth to initiate movement.
10. Instruct the client to wear low-heeled shoes.
11. Encourage the client to lift his or her feet when walking and to avoid prolonged sitting.
12. Provide a firm mattress, and position the client prone, without a pillow, to facilitate proper posture.
13. Instruct in proper posture by teaching the client to hold the hands behind the back to keep the spine and neck erect.
14. Promote physical therapy and rehabilitation.
15. Administer antiparkinsonian medications to increase the level of dopamine in the CNS.
16. Instruct the client to avoid foods high in vitamin B_6 because they block the effects of antiparkinsonian medications.
17. Instruct the client to avoid monoamine oxidase inhibitors because they precipitate hypertensive crisis.
18. See Chapter 58 regarding medication to treat Parkinson's disease.

XV. TRIGEMINAL NEURALGIA

A. Description
1. Trigeminal neuralgia is a sensory disorder of the trigeminal or cranial nerve V.
2. It results in severe, recurrent, sharp, facial pain along the trigeminal nerve.

B. Data collection
1. The client has severe pain on the lips, gums, or nose, or across the cheeks.
2. Situations that stimulate symptoms include cold, washing the face, chewing, or food or fluids of extreme temperatures.

C. Interventions
1. Instruct the client to avoid hot or cold foods and fluids.
2. Provide small feedings of liquid and soft foods.
3. Instruct the client to chew food on the unaffected side.
4. Administer medications as prescribed (see Chapter 58).

D. Surgical interventions
1. Microvascular decompression: Surgical relocation of the artery that compresses the trigeminal nerve as it enters the pons may relieve pain without compromising facial sensation.
2. Radiofrequency wave forms: Creates lesions that provide relief from pain without compromising touch or motor function
3. Rhizotomy: Resection of the root of the nerve to relieve pain
4. Glycerol injection: Destroys the myelinated fibers of the trigeminal nerve (may take up to 3 weeks for pain relief to occur)

XVI. BELL'S PALSY (FACIAL PARALYSIS)

A. Description
1. Bell's palsy is caused by a lower motor neuron lesion of cranial nerve VII that may result from infection, trauma, hemorrhage, meningitis, or a tumor.
2. It results in paralysis of one side of the face.
3. Recovery usually occurs in a few weeks without residual effects.

B. Data collection
1. Flaccid facial muscles
2. Inability to raise the eyebrows, frown, smile, close the eyelids, or puff out the cheeks
3. Upward movement of the eye when attempting to close the eyelid
4. Loss of taste

C. Interventions
1. Encourage the client to do facial exercises to prevent the loss of muscle tone. (A face sling may be prescribed to prevent stretching of weak muscles.)
2. Protect the eyes from dryness and prevent injury.
3. Promote frequent oral care.
4. Instruct the client to chew on the unaffected side.

XVII. GUILLAIN-BARRÉ SYNDROME

A. Description
1. Guillain-Barré syndrome is an acute infectious neuronitis of the cranial and peripheral nerves.

2. The immune system overreacts to the infection and destroys the myelin sheath.
3. The syndrome is usually preceded by a mild upper respiratory infection or gastroenteritis.
4. Recovery is a slow process and can take years.

⚠ The major concern in Guillain-Barré syndrome is difficulty breathing. Monitor respiratory status closely.

B. Data collection
1. Paresthesias
2. Pain and/or hypersensitivity such as with the weight of bed sheets or other items touching the body
3. Weakness of lower extremities
4. Gradual progressive weakness of the upper extremities and facial muscles
5. Possible progression to respiratory failure
6. Cardiac dysrhythmias
7. CSF that reveals an elevated protein level
8. Abnormal electroencephalogram

C. Interventions
1. Direct care toward the treatment of symptoms.
2. Monitor respiratory status.
3. Provide respiratory treatments.
4. Prepare to initiate respiratory support.
5. Monitor cardiac status.
6. Assess for complications of immobility.
7. Provide the client and family with support.

XVIII. AMYOTROPHIC LATERAL SCLEROSIS

A. Description
1. Amyotrophic lateral sclerosis is also known as Lou Gehrig's disease.
2. It is a progressive degenerative disease involving the motor system.
3. The sensory and autonomic systems are not involved, and mental status changes do not result from the disease.
4. The cause of the disease may be related to an excess of glutamate, a chemical responsible for relaying messages between the motor neurons.
5. As the disease progresses, muscle weakness and atrophy develop until a flaccid quadriplegia develops.
6. Eventually the respiratory muscles become affected, leading to respiratory compromise, pneumonia, and death.
7. No cure is known, and the treatment is symptomatic.

B. Data collection
1. Fatigue (including while talking)
2. Respiratory distress
3. Muscle weakness and atrophy
4. Tongue atrophy
5. Dysphagia
6. Weakness of the hands and arms

7. Fasciculations of the face
8. Nasal quality of speech
9. Dysarthria

C. Interventions
1. Care is directed toward the treatment of symptoms.
2. Monitor the respiratory status.
3. Provide respiratory treatments.
4. Prepare to initiate respiratory support.
5. Assess for complications of immobility.
6. Provide the client and family with support.

XIX. ENCEPHALITIS

A. Description
1. Encephalitis is an inflammation of the brain parenchyma and often the meninges.
2. It affects the cerebrum, brainstem, and cerebellum.
3. It is most often caused by a viral agent, although bacteria, fungi, or parasites may also be involved.
4. Viral encephalitis is almost always preceded by a viral infection.

B. Transmission
1. Arboviruses can be transmitted to human beings through the bite of an infected mosquito or tick.
2. Echovirus, coxsackievirus, poliovirus, herpes zoster, and viruses that cause mumps and chickenpox are common enteroviruses associated with encephalitis.
3. Herpes simplex type 1 virus can cause viral encephalitis.
4. The organism that causes amebic meningoencephalitis can enter the nasal mucosa of persons swimming in warm freshwater ponds and lakes.

C. Data collection
1. Presence of cold sores, lesions, or ulcerations of the oral cavity
2. History of insect bites and swimming in freshwater
3. Exposure to infectious diseases
4. Travel to areas where the disease is prevalent
5. Fever
6. Nausea and vomiting
7. **Nuchal rigidity**
8. Changes in LOC and mental status
9. Signs of increased **ICP**
10. Motor dysfunction and focal neurological deficits

D. Interventions
1. Monitor vital and neurological signs.
2. Assess LOC using the **Glasgow Coma Scale**.
3. Assess for mental status changes and personality and behavior changes.
4. Assess for signs of increased **ICP**.
5. Assess for the presence of **nuchal rigidity** and a positive **Kernig's sign** or **Brudzinski's sign**, indicating meningeal irritation.

6. Assist the client to turn, cough, and deep breathe frequently.
7. Elevate the head of the bed 30 to 45 degrees.
8. Assess for muscle and neurological deficits.
9. Administer acyclovir (Zovirax) as prescribed (medication of choice for herpes encephalitis).
10. Initiate rehabilitation as needed for motor dysfunction or neurological deficits.

XX. WEST NILE VIRUS

A. Description
1. West Nile virus is a potentially serious illness that affects the CNS.
2. The virus is contracted primarily by the bite of an infected mosquito. (Mosquitoes become carriers when they feed on infected birds.)
3. Symptoms typically develop between 3 and 14 days after being bitten by the infected mosquito.
4. Neurological effects can be permanent.

B. Data collection
1. Many individuals will not experience any symptoms.
2. Mild symptoms include fever, headache and body aches, nausea, vomiting, swollen glands, or a rash on the chest, stomach, or back.
3. Severe symptoms include a high fever, headache, neck stiffness, stupor, disorientation, tremors, muscle weakness, vision loss, numbness, paralysis, seizures, or coma.

C. Interventions are supportive. There is no specific treatment for the virus.

D. Prevention
1. Use insect repellents containing DEET (*N*, *N*-diethyl-meta-toluamide) when outdoors and wear long sleeves and pants and light-colored clothing.
2. Stay indoors at dusk and dawn when mosquitoes are most active.
3. Ensure that mosquito breeding sites are eliminated, such as standing water and water in bird baths, and keep wading pools empty and on their sides when not in use.

XXI. MENINGITIS

A. Description
1. Meningitis is inflammation of the arachnoid and pia mater of the brain and spinal cord
2. It is caused by bacterial and viral organisms, although fungal and protozoal meningitis also occurs.
3. Predisposing factors include skull fractures, brain or spinal surgery, sinus or upper respiratory infections, the use of nasal sprays, and individuals with a compromised immune system.

4. CSF is analyzed to determine the diagnosis and the type of meningitis. In meningitis, CSF is cloudy, with increased protein, increased white blood cells, and decreased glucose counts

B. Transmission: Occurs in areas of high-population density and crowded living areas such as college dormitories, and prisons.

⚠️ Transmission of meningitis is by direct contact, including droplet spread.

C. Data collection (see Box 57-4)
1. Mild lethargy; photophobia
2. Deterioration in the level of consciousness
3. Signs of meningeal irritation such as **nuchal rigidity** and positive **Kernig's sign** and **Brudzinski's sign**
4. Red, macular rash with meningococcal meningitis
5. Abdominal and chest pain with viral meningitis

D. Interventions
1. Monitor vital signs and neurological signs.
2. Assess for signs of increasing **ICP**.
3. Initiate seizure precautions.
4. Monitor for seizure activity.
5. Monitor for signs of meningeal irritation.
6. Perform cranial nerve assessment.
7. Check peripheral vascular status. (Septic emboli may block circulation.)
8. Maintain isolation precautions as necessary with bacterial meningitis.
9. Maintain urine and stool precautions with viral meningitis.
10. Maintain respiratory isolation for the client with pneumococcal meningitis.
11. Elevate the head of the bed 30 degrees, and avoid neck flexion and extreme hip flexion.
12. Prevent stimulation and restrict visitors.
13. Administer analgesics as prescribed.
14. Administer antibiotics as prescribed.

MORE QUESTIONS ON EVOLVE!

Practice Questions

596. A client is having a lumbar puncture (LP) performed. The nurse would place the client in which position for the procedure?
1. Supine, in semi-Fowler's
2. Prone, in slight Trendelenburg's
3. Prone, with a pillow under the abdomen
4. Side-lying, with legs pulled up and head bent down onto the chest

597. A client has just undergone computed tomography (CT) scanning with a contrast medium. The nurse determines that the client understands

postprocedure care if the client verbalizes that he or she will:
1. Drink extra fluids for the day.
2. Hold medications for at least 4 hours.
3. Eat lightly for the remainder of the day.
4. Rest quietly for the remainder of the day.

598. A nurse is caring for a client with increased intracranial pressure (ICP). The nurse should monitor for which of the following trends in vital signs that would occur if ICP is rising?
1. Increasing temperature, decreasing pulse, decreasing respirations, increasing blood pressure (BP)
2. Decreasing temperature, decreasing pulse, increasing respirations, decreasing BP
3. Decreasing temperature, increasing pulse, decreasing respirations, increasing BP
4. Increasing temperature, increasing pulse, increasing respirations, decreasing BP

599. A nurse is positioning the client with increased intracranial pressure (ICP). Which position should the nurse avoid?
1. Head midline
2. Head turned to the side
3. Neck in neutral position
4. Head of bed elevated 30 to 45 degrees

600. A client recovering from a head injury is arousable and participating in care. The nurse determines that the client understands measures to prevent elevations in intracranial pressure (ICP) if the nurse observes the client doing which of the following activities?
1. Blowing the nose
2. Isometric exercises
3. Coughing vigorously
4. Exhaling during repositioning

601. A client has clear fluid leaking from the nose after a basilar skull fracture. The nurse determines that this is cerebrospinal fluid (CSF) if the fluid:
1. Is grossly bloody in appearance and has a pH of 6
2. Clumps together on the dressing and has a pH of 7
3. Is clear in appearance and tests negative for glucose
4. Separates into concentric rings and tests positive for glucose

602. A client is admitted to the hospital for observation with a probable minor head injury after an automobile crash. The nurse would plan on leaving the cervical collar in place until:
1. The family comes to visit.

2. The nurse needs to do physical care.
3. The result of spinal x-rays is known.
4. The health care provider makes rounds.

603. A client was seen and treated in the emergency department for treatment of a concussion. The nurse determines that the family needs further discharge instructions if they say to bring the client back to the emergency department if which of the following occurs?
1. Vomiting
2. Minor headache
3. Difficulty speaking
4. Difficulty awakening

604. A nurse is caring for a client who has undergone craniotomy with a supratentorial incision. The nurse should plan to place the client in which position postoperatively?
1. Head of bed flat, head and neck midline
2. Head of bed flat, head turned to the nonoperative side
3. Head of bed elevated 30 to 45 degrees, head and neck midline
4. Head of bed elevated 30 to 45 degrees, head turned to the operative side

605. A client with a cervical spine injury has Crutchfield tongs applied in the emergency department. The nurse should avoid which of the following when planning care for this client?
1. Using a Stryker frame bed
2. Removing the weights to reposition the client
3. Assessing the integrity of the weights and pulleys
4. Comparing the amount of prescribed traction with the amount in use

606. A nurse has provided discharge instructions to a client with an application of a halo device. The nurse determines that the client needs further clarification of the instructions if the client states that he or she will:
1. Use a straw for drinking.
2. Drive only during the daytime.
3. Use caution, because the device alters balance.
4. Wash the skin daily under the lamb's wool liner of the vest.

607. A nurse is caring for the client who has suffered spinal cord injury. The nurse further monitors the client for signs of autonomic dysreflexia and suspects this complication if which of the following is noted?
1. Sudden tachycardia
2. Pallor of the face and neck
3. Severe, throbbing headache
4. Severe and sudden hypotension

608. A client with spinal cord injury is prone to experiencing autonomic dysreflexia. The nurse should avoid which measure to minimize the risk of recurrence?
   1. Strict adherence to a bowel retraining program
   2. Keeping the linen wrinkle-free under the client
   3. Avoiding unnecessary pressure on the lower limbs
   4. Limiting bladder catheterization to once every 12 hours

609. A client with spinal cord injury suddenly experiences an episode of autonomic dysreflexia. After checking vital signs, the nurse immediately:
   1. Raises the head of the bed and removes the noxious stimulus
   2. Lowers the head of the bed and removes the noxious stimulus
   3. Lowers the head of the bed and administers an antihypertensive agent
   4. Removes the noxious stimulus and administers an antihypertensive agent

610. The client with a spinal cord injury suddenly experiences an episode of autonomic dysreflexia. After checking the client's vital signs, number the nurse's actions in order of priority, with the first selected action being of highest priority and the last selected action of lowest priority. (Number 1 is the first priority action and number 6 is the last priority action.) ❖
   ___ Contact the health care provider (HCP).
   ___ Raise the head of the bed.
   ___ Check for bladder distention.
   ___ Loosen tight clothing on the client.
   ___ Administer an antihypertensive medication.
   ___ Document the occurrence, treatment, and response.

ANSWERS

596. 4
Rationale: The client undergoing LP is positioned lying on the side, with the legs pulled up to the abdomen and the head bent down onto the chest. This position helps open the spaces between the vertebrae.
Test-Taking Strategy: Use the process of elimination. Recalling that an LP is the introduction of a needle into the subarachnoid space, it is reasonable that the position of the client must facilitate this. The correct answer is the only position that flexes the vertebrae for easier needle insertion. Review positioning procedures for an LP if you had difficulty with this question.
Level of Cognitive Ability: Applying
Client Needs: Physiological Integrity
Integrated Process: Nursing Process/Implementation
Content Area: Adult Health/Neurological
References: deWit, p. 519. 2009.
Pagana, Pagana, pp. 614–616. 2009.

597. 1
Rationale: After CT scanning, the client may resume all usual activities. The client should be encouraged to take in extra fluids to replace those lost with diuresis from the contrast dye. Options 2, 3, and 4 are unnecessary.
Test-Taking Strategy: Use the process of elimination. Recalling that there is no special aftercare following this procedure and noting the words "contrast medium" in the question will direct you to the correct option. Review the procedure related to CT scanning if you had difficulty with this question.
Level of Cognitive Ability: Evaluating
Client Needs: Physiological Integrity
Integrated Process: Nursing Process/Evaluation
Content Area: Adult Health/Neurological
Reference: Christensen, Kockrow, p. 116. 2011. *Adult health nursing.*

598. 1
Rationale: A change in vital signs may be a late sign of increased ICP. Trends include increasing temperature and blood pressure and decreasing pulse and respirations. Respiratory irregularities may also arise.
Test-Taking Strategy: Use the process of elimination. This question looks complex but can be answered logically. If you remember that temperature rises, you are able to eliminate options 2 and 3. If you know that the client becomes bradycardic, or know that the BP rises, you are able to select the correct option. Review the signs of increased ICP if you had difficulty with this question.
Level of Cognitive Ability: Analyzing
Client Needs: Physiological Integrity
Integrated Process: Nursing Process/Data Collection
Content Area: Adult Health/Neurological
Reference: Linton, p. 448. 2012.

599. 2
Rationale: The head of the client with increased ICP should be positioned so that the head is in a neutral, midline position. The nurse should avoid flexing or extending the neck or turning the head side to side. The head of the bed should be raised to 30 to 45 degrees. Use of proper positions promotes venous drainage from the cranium to keep ICP down.
Test-Taking Strategy: Note the strategic word "avoid." This word indicates a negative event query and the need to select the incorrect position. This would be one that interferes with arterial circulation to the brain or with venous drainage from the brain. The only position that meets one of those criteria is option 2. Review client positioning with ICP if you had difficulty with this question.
Level of Cognitive Ability: Applying
Client Needs: Physiological Integrity
Integrated Process: Nursing Process/Implementation
Content Area: Adult Health/Neurological
Reference: Christensen, Kockrow, pp. 671–672. 2011. *Adult health nursing.*

600. 4

Rationale: Activities that increase intrathoracic and intra-abdominal pressures cause indirect elevation of the ICP. Some of these activities include isometric exercises, Valsalva maneuver, coughing, sneezing, and blowing the nose. Exhaling during activities such as repositioning or pulling up in bed opens the glottis, which prevents intrathoracic pressure from rising.

Test-Taking Strategy: Use the process of elimination. Evaluate each option in terms of the tension it puts on the body to help you eliminate each of the incorrect options. Review the measures that will reduce or prevent increased intracranial pressure if you had difficulty with this question.

Level of Cognitive Ability: Evaluating
Client Needs: Physiological Integrity
Integrated Process: Nursing Process/Evaluation
Content Area: Adult Health/Neurological
Reference: deWit, pp. 548–549. 2009.

601. 4

Rationale: Leakage of CSF from the ears or nose may accompany basilar skull fracture. It can be distinguished from other body fluids because the drainage will separate into bloody and yellow concentric rings on dressing material, which is known as the halo sign. It also tests positive for glucose. Options 1, 2, and 3 are not characteristics of CSF.

Test-Taking Strategy: Use the process of elimination. Recalling that CSF contains glucose, whereas other secretions such as mucus do not, will direct you to option 4. Also, remember that CSF separates into rings. Review testing for CSF fluid if you had difficulty with this question.

Level of Cognitive Ability: Analyzing
Client Needs: Physiological Integrity
Integrated Process: Nursing Process/Data Collection
Content Area: Adult Health/Neurological
References: deWit, pp. 542, 544. 2009.
Ignatavicius, Workman, p. 1055. 2010.

602. 3

Rationale: There is a significant association between cervical spine injury and head injury. For this reason, the nurse leaves any form of spinal immobilization in place until lateral cervical spine x-rays rule out fracture or other damage.

Test-Taking Strategy: Focus on the data in the question and note the client's injury. Remember that the reason for spinal immobilization is to protect the spine from movement, which could cause further damage if the cervical spine were injured. If x-ray results are negative, there is no reason to leave the collar in place. Review emergency care of the client with a suspected cervical injury if this question was difficult.

Level of Cognitive Ability: Applying
Client Needs: Physiological Integrity
Integrated Process: Nursing Process/Implementation
Content Area: Adult Health/Neurological
Reference: Christensen, Kockrow, p. 712. 2011. *Adult health nursing.*

603. 2

Rationale: A concussion after head injury is a temporary loss of consciousness (from a few seconds to a few minutes) without evidence of structural damage. After concussion, the family is taught to monitor the client and call the health care provider or return the client to the emergency department if certain signs and symptoms are noted. These include confusion, difficulty awakening or speaking, one-sided weakness, vomiting, or severe headache. Minor headache is expected.

Test-Taking Strategy: Note the strategic words "needs further discharge instructions." These words indicate a negative event query and the need to select the incorrect family statement. Noting the word "minor" in option 2 will direct you to this option. Review care of the client with a concussion if you had difficulty with this question.

Level of Cognitive Ability: Evaluating
Client Needs: Physiological Integrity
Integrated Process: Teaching and Learning
Content Area: Adult Health/Neurological
Reference: deWit, p. 546. 2009.

604. 3

Rationale: Following supratentorial surgery, the head of the bed is kept at a 30- to 45-degree angle. The head and neck should not be angled either anteriorly or laterally, but rather should be kept in a neutral (midline) position. This will promote venous return through the jugular veins, which will help prevent a rise in intracranial pressure.

Test-Taking Strategy: This question tests knowledge of differences in positioning the craniotomy client with an infratentorial versus supratentorial incision. If you remember that with "supra-" one should "keep the head up," and with "infra-" one should "keep the head down," options 1 and 2 can be eliminated. Knowing how to position the head for optimal venous drainage helps you select option 3 over option 4. Review client positioning after craniotomy if you had difficulty with this question.

Level of Cognitive Ability: Applying
Client Needs: Physiological Integrity
Integrated Process: Nursing Process/Planning
Content Area: Adult Health/Neurological
References: deWit, p. 544. 2009.
Ignatavicius, Workman, p. 1063. 2010.

605. 2

Rationale: Crutchfield tongs are applied after drilling holes in the client's skull under local anesthesia. Weights are attached to the tongs, which exert pulling pressure on the longitudinal axis of the cervical spine. Serial x-rays of the cervical spine are taken, with weights being added gradually until radiography reveals that the vertebral column is realigned. Weights then may be gradually reduced to a point that maintains alignment. The client with Crutchfield tongs is placed on a Stryker frame or Roto-Rest bed. The nurse ensures that weights hang freely and the amount of weight matches the current prescription. The nurse also inspects the integrity and position of the ropes and pulleys. The nurse does not remove the weights to administer care.

Test-Taking Strategy: Note the strategic word "avoid." This word indicates a negative event query and the need to select the item that would be contraindicated. Recalling the basics of traction and recalling that weights are not removed will direct you to the correct option. Review nursing care related to the client with cervical tongs if you had difficulty with this question.

Level of Cognitive Ability: Applying
Client Needs: Physiological Integrity
Integrated Process: Nursing Process/Planning
Content Area: Adult Health/Neurological
References: deWit, p. 553. 2009.
Linton, pp. 527–528. 2012.

606. 2

Rationale: The halo device alters balance and can cause fatigue because of its weight. The client should cleanse the skin daily under the vest or the device to protect the skin from ulceration and should use powder or lotions sparingly or not at all. The wool liner should be changed if odor becomes a problem. The client should have food cut into small pieces to facilitate chewing and use a straw for drinking. Pin care is done as instructed. The client should not drive because the device impairs the range of vision.
Test-Taking Strategy: Note the strategic words "needs further clarification." These words indicate a negative event query and the need to select the incorrect client statement. Recall that a halo device is used to allow mobility for the client who needs continuous cervical traction; it maintains the head and spine in a neutral position. With this in mind, it will be easy to select option 2 as the correct answer as stated. The inability to turn the head without turning the torso would contraindicate driving. Review client-teaching points related to a halo device if you had difficulty with this question.
Level of Cognitive Ability: Evaluating
Client Needs: Safe and Effective Care Environment
Integrated Process: Teaching and Learning
Content Area: Adult Health/Neurological
Reference: Ignatavicius, Workman, p. 1000. 2010.

607. 3

Rationale: The client with spinal cord injury above the level of T7 is at risk for autonomic dysreflexia. It is characterized by severe, throbbing headache, flushing of the face and neck, bradycardia, and sudden severe hypertension. Other signs include nasal stuffiness, blurred vision, nausea, and sweating. It is a life-threatening syndrome triggered by a noxious stimulus below the level of the injury.
Test-Taking Strategy: Use the process of elimination. To answer this question correctly, it is necessary to know what causes autonomic dysreflexia. Remember, it results from the sudden exaggerated response of the sympathetic nervous system to a noxious stimulus. A massive sympathetic nervous system response causes severe hypertension. This would account for the throbbing headache (the correct answer) and cause flushing of the face and neck. Baroreceptors sense the sudden hypertension, causing a reflex bradycardia. Also, remember that the pulse and blood pressure changes with autonomic dysreflexia are actually the opposite of what would occur with hypovolemic shock. Review the signs of autonomic dysreflexia if you had difficulty with this question.
Level of Cognitive Ability: Analyzing
Client Needs: Physiological Integrity
Integrated Process: Nursing Process/Data Collection
Content Area: Adult Health/Neurological
Reference: Christensen, Kockrow, pp. 710, 712. 2011. *Adult health nursing.*

608. 4

Rationale: The most frequent cause of autonomic dysreflexia is a distended bladder. Straight catheterization should be performed every 4 to 6 hours, and Foley catheters should be checked frequently for kinks in the tubing. Constipation and fecal impaction are other causes, so maintaining bowel regularity is important. Other causes include stimulation of the skin from tactile, thermal, or painful stimuli. The nurse administers care to minimize risk in these areas.
Test-Taking Strategy: Note the strategic word "avoid." Remember that autonomic dysreflexia is caused by noxious stimuli to the bowel, bladder, or skin. With this in mind, you can eliminate each of the incorrect options. Review the measures to minimize the risk of autonomic dysreflexia if you had difficulty with this question.
Level of Cognitive Ability: Applying
Client Needs: Physiological Integrity
Integrated Process: Nursing Process/Implementation
Content Area: Adult Health/Neurological
References: deWit, p. 554. 2009.
Linton, p. 533. 2012.

609. 1

Rationale: Key nursing actions are to sit the client up in bed, remove the noxious stimulus, and bring the blood pressure under control with antihypertensive medication per protocol. The nurse can also clearly label the client's chart identifying the risk for autonomic dysreflexia. Client and family should be taught to recognize, and later manage, the signs and symptoms of this syndrome.
Test-Taking Strategy: Note the strategic word "immediately" in the question. This is a clue that the first item in each option must be the first action. If you know to raise the head of the client's bed first (to try to minimize cerebral hypertension), then this eliminates each of the incorrect options. Review immediate nursing interventions for the client experiencing autonomic dysreflexia if you had difficulty with this question.
Level of Cognitive Ability: Applying
Client Needs: Physiological Integrity
Integrated Process: Nursing Process/Implementation
Content Area: Adult Health/Neurological
References: deWit, p. 554. 2009.
Linton, p. 533. 2012.

610. 4, 1, 3, 2, 5, 6

Rationale: Autonomic dysreflexia is characterized by severe hypertension, bradycardia, severe headache, nasal stuffiness, and flushing. The cause is a noxious stimulus, most often a distended bladder or constipation. Autonomic dysreflexia is a neurological emergency and must be treated promptly to prevent a hypertensive stroke. Immediate nursing actions are to sit the client up in bed in a high-Fowler's position and remove the noxious stimulus. The nurse would loosen any tight clothing and then check for bladder distention. If the client has a Foley catheter, the nurse would check for kinks in the tubing. The nurse would also check for a fecal impaction and disimpact the client if necessary. The HCP is contacted especially if these actions do not relieve the signs and symptoms. Antihypertensive medication may be prescribed by the HCP to minimize cerebral hypertension. Finally, the nurse documents the occurrence, treatment, and client response.

Test-Taking Strategy: Recalling that this syndrome causes severe hypertension will assist you in determining that elevating the head of the bed is the first action. Next, recalling that the syndrome is caused by a noxious stimulus will assist you in determining that loosening tight clothing and checking for bladder distention would be the next actions. Because loosening any tight clothing would take less time than checking for bladder distention, this action would be taken next. Antihypertensives require a HCP's prescription; therefore, calling the HCP would be the next action. Review immediate nursing interventions for the client experiencing autonomic dysreflexia if you had difficulty with this question.

Level of Cognitive Ability: Applying
Client Needs: Physiological Integrity
Integrated Process: Nursing Process/Implementation
Content Area: Critical Care
References: deWit, p. 554. 2009.
Ignatavicius, Workman, p. 998. 2010.

Neurological Medications

 I. ANTIMYASTHENIC MEDICATIONS

A. Description

1. Antimyasthenic, also called anticholinesterase, medications relieve muscle weakness associated with myasthenia gravis by blocking acetylcholine breakdown at the neuromuscular junction.
2. Antimyasthenic medications are used to treat or diagnose myasthenia gravis or distinguish cholinergic crisis from myasthenic crisis.
3. Neostigmine bromide (Prostigmin), pyridostigmine (Mestinon), and ambenonium chloride (Mytelase) are used to control myasthenic symptoms.
4. Edrophonium chloride (Enlon) is used to diagnose myasthenia gravis and distinguish cholinergic crisis from myasthenic crisis.

B. Medications (Box 58-1)

C. Side effects: Cholinergic crisis (Box 58-2)

D. Interventions

1. Monitor neuromuscular status, including reflexes, muscle strength, and gait.
2. Monitor the client for signs and symptoms of medication overdose (cholinergic crisis) and underdose (myasthenic crisis).
3. The client is instructed to take medications on time to maintain therapeutic blood level, thus preventing weakness, because weakness can impair the client's ability to breathe and swallow.
4. The client is instructed to take the medication with a small amount of food to prevent gastrointestinal symptoms.
5. The client is instructed to eat 45 to 60 minutes after taking medications to decrease the risk for aspiration.
6. The client is instructed to wear a Medic-Alert bracelet.
7. Note that antimyasthenic therapy is lifelong therapy.
8. Evaluate for medication effectiveness, which is based on the improvement of neuromuscular symptoms or strength without cholinergic signs and symptoms.

9. When administering edrophonium chloride, have emergency resuscitation equipment on hand and atropine sulfate available for cholinergic crisis.

E. Edrophonium (Enlon) test

1. Edrophonium (Enlon) is injected intravenously.
2. The edrophonium (Enlon) can cause bronchospasm, laryngospasm, hypotension, bradycardia, and cardiac arrest.
3. Atropine sulfate is the antidote for overdose.
4. Diagnosis of myasthenia gravis: Most myasthenic clients show a significant improvement in muscle tone within 30 to 60 seconds after injection, and the muscle improvement lasts 4 to 5 minutes.
5. The test is used to diagnose cholinergic crisis (overdose with anticholinesterase) or myasthenic crisis (undermedication).
   a. In cholinergic crisis, muscle tone does not improve after the administration of edrophonium, and muscle twitching may be noted around the eyes and face.
   b. An edrophonium injection makes the client in cholinergic crisis temporarily worse (negative test).
   c. An edrophonium injection temporarily improves the condition when the client is in myasthenic crisis (positive test).

II. ANTIPARKINSONIAN MEDICATIONS

A. Description

1. Antiparkinsonian medications restore the balance of the neurotransmitters acetylcholine and dopamine in the central nervous system (CNS), decreasing the signs and symptoms of Parkinson's disease to maximize the client's functional abilities.
2. These medications include the dopaminergics, which stimulate the dopamine receptors, and the anticholinergics, which block the cholinergic receptors.
3. Antiparkinsonian medications are used for drug-induced parkinsonism, in which neuroleptic agents block dopamine receptors in the CNS, leading to functional loss of dopamine activity.

Box 58-1 Antimyasthenic Medications

Ambenonium chloride (Mytelase)
Edrophonium chloride (Enlon)
Neostigmine bromide (Prostigmin)
Pyridostigmin (Mestinon)

Box 58-2 Signs of Cholinergic Crisis

Abdominal cramps
Nausea, vomiting, and diarrhea
Pupillary miosis
Hypotension and dizziness
Increased bronchial secretions
Increased tearing and salivation
Increased perspiration
Increased bronchial secretions
Bronchospasm, wheezing, and bradycardia

Box 58-3 Medications to Treat Parkinson's Disease

Medications Affecting the Amount of Dopamine
Amantadine (Symmetrel)
Bromocriptine (Parlodel)
Carbidopa; levodopa (Sinemet)
Levodopa (Larodopa)
Pramipexole (Mirapex)
Ropinirole (Requip)
Selegiline hydrochloride (Carbex, Eldepryl)

Anticholinergics
Benztropine mesylate (Cogentin)
Biperiden hydrochloride (Akineton)
Procyclidine hydrochloride (Kemadrin)
Trihexyphenidyl hydrochloride

Catechol O-Methyltransferase (COMT) Inhibitors
Entacapone (Comtan)
Tolcapone (Tasmar)

4. Antiparkinsonian medications are used for Parkinson's disease, in which dopamine-containing neurons in the basal ganglia are destroyed or deficient, which causes loss of fine motor control.

B. Dopaminergic medications

1. Description

   a. Dopaminergic medications stimulate the dopamine receptors and increase the amount of dopamine available in the CNS or enhance neurotransmission of dopamine.

   b. Dopaminergic medications are contraindicated in clients with cardiac, renal, or psychiatric disorders.

⚠ Levodopa taken with a monoamine oxidase inhibitor antidepressant can cause a hypertensive crisis.

2. Medications (Box 58-3 and Figure 58-1)

3. Side effects

   a. Dyskinesia

   b. Involuntary body movements

   c. Chest pain

   d. Nausea and vomiting

   e. Urinary retention

   f. Constipation

   g. Sleep disturbances, insomnia, or periods of sedation

   h. Orthostatic hypotension and dizziness

   i. Confusion

   j. Mood changes, especially depression

   k. Hallucinations

   l. Dry mouth

4. Interventions

   a. Monitor the vital signs.

   b. Determine the risk for injury.

▲ **FIGURE 58-1** Steps leading to alteration of central nervous system function by levodopa. To produce its beneficial effects in Parkinson's disease (PD), levodopa must be (1) transported across the blood-brain barrier; (2) taken up by dopaminergic nerve terminals in the striatum; (3) converted into dopamine (DA); (4) released into the synaptic space; and (5) bound to DA receptors on striatal GABAergic neurons, causing them to fire at a slower rate. Note that DA itself is unable to cross the blood-brain barrier, and hence cannot be used to treat PD. (From Lehne, R. [2010]. *Pharmacology for nursing care* [7th ed.]. St. Louis: Saunders.)

   c. The client is instructed to take the medication with food if nausea or vomiting occurs.

   d. Check for signs and symptoms of parkinsonism, such as rigidity, tremors, akinesia, and bradykinesia, a stooped forward posture, shuffling gait, and masked facies.

e. Monitor for signs of dyskinesia.

f. The client is instructed to report side effects and symptoms of dyskinesia.

g. Monitor the client for improvement in signs and symptoms of parkinsonism without the development of severe side effects from the medications.

h. The client is instructed to change positions slowly to minimize orthostatic hypotension.

i. The client is instructed not to discontinue the medication abruptly.

j. The client is instructed to avoid alcohol.

k. The client is informed that urine or perspiration may be discolored and that this is harmless, but may stain the clothing.

l. The client with diabetes mellitus is advised that glucose testing should not be done by urine testing because the results will not be reliable.

m. The client taking carbidopa-levodopa (Sinemet) is instructed to divide the total daily prescribed protein intake among all meals of the day. High-protein diets interfere with medication availability to the CNS.

n. When administering levodopa, the client is instructed to avoid excessive vitamin B_6 intake to prevent medication reactions.

C. Anticholinergic medications

1. Description

a. Anticholinergic medications block the cholinergic receptors in the CNS, thereby suppressing acetylcholine activity.

b. Anticholinergic medications reduce tremors and drooling, but have a minimal effect on bradykinesia, rigidity, and balance abnormalities.

c. Anticholinergic medications are contraindicated in clients with glaucoma.

d. The client with chronic obstructive lung disease can develop dry, thick mucus secretions.

2. Medications (see Box 58-3)

3. Side effects

a. Blurred vision

b. Dryness of the nose, mouth, throat, and respiratory secretions

c. Increased pulse rate, palpitations, and dysrhythmias

d. Constipation

e. Urinary retention

f. Restlessness, confusion, depression, and hallucinations

g. Photophobia

4. Interventions

a. Monitor the vital signs.

b. Determine the risk for injury.

c. Monitor the client for improvement in signs and symptoms.

d. Check the client's bowel and urinary function and monitor for urinary retention, constipation, and paralytic ileus.

e. Monitor for involuntary movements.

f. The client is encouraged to avoid alcohol, smoking, caffeine, and aspirin to decrease gastric acidity.

g. The client is instructed to consult with the health care provider (HCP) before taking any nonprescription medications.

h. The client is instructed to minimize dry mouth by increasing fluid intake and using ice chips, hard candy, or gum.

i. The client is instructed to prevent constipation by increasing fluids and fiber in the diet.

j. The client is instructed to use sunglasses in direct sunlight because of possible photophobia.

k. The client is instructed to have routine eye examinations to assess for intraocular pressure.

⚠ If an anticholinergic medication is discontinued abruptly, the signs and symptoms of parkinsonism, such as rigidity, tremors, akinesia, and bradykinesia, a stooped forward posture, shuffling gait, and masked facies may be intensified.

III. ANTICONVULSANT MEDICATIONS

A. Description

1. Anticonvulsant medications are used to depress abnormal neuronal discharges and prevent the spread of seizures to adjacent neurons.

2. Anticonvulsant medications should be used with caution in clients taking anticoagulants, aspirin, sulfonamides, cimetidine (Tagamet), and antipsychotic drugs.

3. Absorption is decreased with the use of antacids, calcium preparations, and antineoplastic medications.

B. Interventions for clients on anticonvulsants

1. Initiate seizure precautions.

2. Monitor urinary output.

3. Monitor liver and renal function tests and medication blood serum levels (Table 58-1).

4. Monitor for signs of medication toxicity, which would include CNS depression, ataxia, nausea, vomiting, drowsiness, dizziness, restlessness, and visual disturbances.

5. If a seizure occurs, monitor seizure activity, including location and duration.

6. Protect the client from hazards in the environment during a seizure.

C. Client education (Box 58-4)

D. Hydantoins (Box 58-5)
 1. Hydantoins are used to treat partial and generalized tonic-clonic seizures.
 2. Phenytoin (Dilantin) also is used to treat dysrhythmias.

TABLE 58-1 Anticonvulsant Medications

Medication	Therapeutic Serum Range
Amobarbital (Amytal)	1-5 mcg/mL
Carbamazepine (Tegretol)	3-14 mcg/mL
Clonazepam (Klonopin)	20-80 ng/mL
Ethosuximide (Zarontin)	40-100 mcg/mL
Ethotoin (Peganone)	10-50 mcg/mL
Lorazepam (Ativan)	50-240 ng/mL
Mephobarbital (Mebaral)	15-40 mcg/mL
Phenobarbital (Luminal)	15-40 mcg/mL
Phenytoin (Dilantin)	10-20 mcg/mL

Box 58-4 Client Education: Anticonvulsants

- Take the prescribed medication in the prescribed dose and frequency.
- Take anticonvulsants with food to decrease gastrointestinal irritation, but avoid milk and antacids, which impair absorption.
- If taking liquid medication, shake well before ingesting.
- Do not discontinue the medications.
- Avoid alcohol.
- Avoid over-the-counter medications.
- Wear a Medic-Alert bracelet.
- Use caution when driving or performing activities that require alertness.
- Maintain good oral hygiene and use a soft toothbrush.
- Maintain preventive dental checkups.
- Maintain follow-up health care visits with periodic blood studies related to determining toxicity.
- Monitor serum glucose levels (diabetes mellitus).
- Urine may be a harmless pink-red or red-brown in color.
- Report symptoms of sore throat, bruising, and nosebleeds, which may indicate a blood dyscrasia.
- Inform the HCP if adverse reactions occur, such as gingivitis, nystagmus, slurred speech, rash, or dizziness.

Box 58-5 Hydantoins

Ethotoin (Peganone)
Fosphenytoin (Cerebyx)
Phenytoin (Dilantin)

3. Side effects
 a. Gingival hyperplasia (reddened gums that bleed easily)
 b. Slurred speech
 c. Confusion
 d. Sedation and drowsiness
 e. Nausea and vomiting
 f. Blurred vision and nystagmus
 g. Headaches
 h. Blood dyscrasias: Decreased platelet count and decreased white blood cell count
 i. Elevated blood glucose level
 j. Alopecia or hirsutism
 k. Skin rash or pruritus
4. Interventions
 a. Oral tube feedings may interfere with the absorption of orally administered phenytoin and diminish the effectiveness of the medication; therefore feedings should be scheduled as far as possible from the time of phenytoin administration.
 b. Monitor therapeutic serum levels to assess for toxicity.
 c. Monitor for signs of toxicity.
 d. When phenytoin is administered intravenously, it is diluted in normal saline because dextrose causes the medication to precipitate.
 e. When phenytoin is administered intravenously to treat status epilepticus, it is infused no faster than 25 to 50 mg/min; otherwise, hypotension and cardiac dysrhythmias can occur.
 f. Monitor for ataxia (staggering gait).
 g. The client is instructed to consult with the health care provider before taking other medications to ensure compatibility with anticonvulsants.

 Phenytoin decreases the effectiveness of some birth control pills and can have teratogenic effects if taken during pregnancy.

E. Barbiturates (Box 58-6)
 1. Barbiturates are used for tonic-clonic seizures and acute episodes of seizures caused by status epilepticus.
 2. Barbiturates also may be used as adjuncts to anesthesia.
 3. Side effects
  a. Sedation, ataxia, and dizziness during initial treatment

Box 58-6 Barbiturates

Amobarbital (Amytal)
Mephobarbital (Mebaral)
Phenobarbital (Luminal)

b. Mood changes
c. Hypotension
d. Respiratory depression
e. Tolerance to the medication

F. Benzodiazepines (Box 58-7)
1. Benzodiazepines are used to treat absence seizures.
2. Diazepam (Valium) and lorazepam (Ativan) are used to treat status epilepticus, anxiety, and skeletal muscle spasms.
3. Clorazepate (Tranxene) is used as adjunctive therapy for partial seizures.
4. Side effects
   a. Sedation, drowsiness, dizziness, blurred vision
   b. Bradycardia can occur when administered rapidly by the intravenous route.
   c. Medication tolerance and drug dependency
   d. Blood dyscrasias: Decreased platelet count and decreased white blood cell count
   e. Hepatotoxicity

⚠ Flumazenil (Romazicon) reverses the effects of benzodiazepines. It should not be administered to clients with increased intracranial pressure or status epilepticus who were treated with benzodiazepines because these problems may recur with reversal.

G. Succinimides (Box 58-8)
1. Succinimides are used to treat absence seizures.
2. Side effects
   a. Anorexia, nausea, vomiting
   b. Blood dyscrasias
H. Oxazolidinediones (Box 58-9)
1. Oxazolidinediones are used for absence seizures.

Box 58-7 Benzodiazepines

Clonazepam (Klonopin)
Clorazepate (Tranxene)
Diazepam (Valium)
Lorazepam (Ativan)
Zolpidem (Ambien)

Box 58-8 Succinimides

Ethosuximide (Zarontin)
Methsuximide (Celontin)

Box 58-9 Oxazolidinedione

Trimethadione (Troxidone)

2. Side effects
   a. Sedation, drowsiness, fatigue
   b. Headache
   c. Photophobia
   d. Blood dyscrasias

I. Valproates (Box 58-10)
1. Valproates are used to treat tonic-clonic, partial, myoclonic, and psychomotor seizures.
2. Side effects
   a. Transient nausea, vomiting, and indigestion
   b. Sedation, drowsiness, and dizziness
   c. Pancreatitis
   d. Blood dyscrasias: Decreased platelet count and decreased white blood cell count
   e. Hepatotoxicity

J. Iminostilbenes
1. Iminostilbenes are used to treat seizure disorders that have not responded to other anticonvulsants (Box 58-11).
2. Iminostilbenes are used to treat trigeminal neuralgia.
3. Side effects
   a. Drowsiness
   b. Dizziness
   c. Nausea and vomiting
   d. Constipation or diarrhea
   e. Rash
   f. Visual abnormalities
   g. Dry mouth
   h. Headache

IV. CENTRAL NERVOUS SYSTEM STIMULANTS

A. Description
1. Amphetamines and caffeine stimulate the cerebral cortex of the brain (Box 58-12).
2. Amphetamines have a high potential for abuse.

Box 58-10 Valproates

Valproic acid (Depakene, Depacon)
Divalproex sodium (Depakote ER)

Box 58-11 Other Anticonvulsants

Carbamazepine (Tegretol)
Gabapentin (Neurontin)
Lamotrigine (Lamictal)
Levetiracetam (Keppra)
Oxcarbazepine (Trileptal)
Pregabalin (Lyrica)
Tiagabine (Gabitril Filmtab)
Topiramate (Topamax)
Zonisamide (Zonogran)
Vigabatrin (Sabril)

3. Analeptics and caffeine act on the brainstem and medulla to stimulate respiration.
4. Anorexiants act on the cerebral cortex and hypothalamus to suppress appetite (Box 58-13).
5. Central nervous system stimulants are used to treat narcolepsy and attention-deficit/hyperactivity disorders.
6. Central nervous system stimulants are used as adjunctive therapy for exogenous obesity.
7. Other central nervous system stimulants (Box 58-14)

B. Side effects
   1. Irritability
   2. Restlessness
   3. Tremors
   4. Insomnia
   5. Heart palpitations
   6. Tachycardia and dysrhythmias
   7. Hypertension
   8. Dry mouth
   9. Anorexia and weight loss
   10. Abdominal cramping
   11. Diarrhea or constipation
   12. Hepatic failure
   13. Psychoses
   14. Impotence
   15. Dependence and tolerance

C. Interventions
   1. Monitor the vital signs.
   2. Monitor the mental status.
   3. The degree of inattention, impulsivity, hyperactivity, and periods of sleepiness is documented.

Box 58-12 Amphetamines

Amphetamine sulfate
Amphetamine; dextroamphetamine (Adderall)
Atomoxetine (Strattera)
Methylphenidate hydrochloride (Ritalin, Concerta)

Box 58-13 Anorexiants

Benzphetamine hydrochloride (Didrex)
Orlistat (Xenical)
Phendimetrazine (Bontril, Melfiat-105)
Phentermine hydrochloride (Adipex-P, Ionamin)
Sibutramine (Meridia)

Box 58-14 Other Central Nervous System Stimulants

Doxapram (Dopram)
Theobromine
Theophylline

---

4. Check the height, weight, and growth of the child.
5. Monitor the complete blood count and white blood cell and platelet counts before and during therapy.
6. Monitor for side effects.
7. Monitor the sleep patterns.
8. Monitor for withdrawal symptoms such as nausea, vomiting, weakness, and headache.
9. The client is instructed to take the medication before meals.
10. The client is instructed to avoid foods and beverages containing caffeine to prevent additional stimulation.
11. The client is instructed not to chew or crush long-acting forms of the medications.
12. The client is instructed to read labels on over-the-counter products because many contain caffeine.
13. The client is instructed to avoid alcohol.
14. The client is instructed not to discontinue the medication abruptly.
15. The client is instructed to take the last daily dose of the CNS stimulant at least 6 hours before bedtime to prevent insomnia.
16. Monitor for drug dependence and abuse with amphetamines.
17. If a child is taking a CNS stimulant, instruct the parents to notify the school nurse.
18. Monitor for calming effects of CNS stimulants within 3 to 4 weeks on children with attention-deficit/hyperactivity disorder.
19. Monitor growth in the child on long-term therapy with methylphenidate hydrochloride (Ritalin) or other medication to treat attention-deficit/hyperactivity disorder.

V. NONOPIOID ANALGESICS

A. Nonsteroidal anti-inflammatory drugs (NSAIDs) (Box 58-15)
   1. Description
      a. NSAIDs are aspirin and aspirin-like medications that inhibit the synthesis of prostaglandins.
      b. The medications act as an analgesic to relieve pain, as an antipyretic to reduce body temperature, and as an anticoagulant to inhibit platelet aggregation.
      c. NSAIDs are used to relieve inflammation and pain and treat rheumatoid arthritis, bursitis, tendinitis, osteoarthritis, and acute gout.
      d. NSAIDs are contraindicated in clients with hypersensitivity or liver or renal disease.
      e. Clients taking anticoagulants should not take aspirin or NSAIDs.
      f. Aspirin and an NSAID should not be taken together because aspirin decreases the blood

level and the effectiveness of the NSAID and can increase the risk of bleeding.

g. NSAIDs can increase the effects of warfarin (Coumadin), sulfonamides, cephalosporins, and phenytoin (Dilantin).

h. Hypoglycemia can result if ibuprofen (Motrin) is taken with insulin or an oral hypoglycemic medication.

i. A high risk of toxicity exists if ibuprofen is taken concurrently with calcium blockers.

⚠️ Adolescents and children with flu symptoms, viral illnesses, and varicella should not take aspirin because of the risk of Reye's syndrome.

2. Side effects (Box 58-16)
3. Interventions
   a. Check client for allergies.
   b. Obtain a medication history on the client.
   c. Check for history of gastric upset or bleeding or liver or renal disease.
   d. Monitor the client for gastrointestinal upset during medication administration.
   e. Monitor for edema.
   f. Monitor serum salicylate (aspirin) level when the client is taking high doses.

g. Monitor for signs of bleeding such as tarry stools, bleeding gums, petechiae, ecchymosis, and purpura.

h. The client is instructed to take the medication with water, milk, or food.

i. An enteric-coated or buffered form of aspirin can be taken to decrease gastric distress.

j. The client is instructed that enteric-coated tablets cannot be crushed or broken.

k. Clients taking aspirin should sit upright for 20 to 30 minutes after taking the dose.

l. The client is advised to inform other health care professionals if he or she is taking high doses of aspirin.

m. Note that aspirin should be discontinued 3 to 7 days before surgery to reduce the risk of bleeding.

n. The client is instructed to avoid alcoholic beverages.

B. Acetaminophen (Tylenol)
   1. Description
      a. Acetaminophen inhibits prostaglandin synthesis.
      b. Acetaminophen is used to decrease pain and fever.

Box 58-15 Nonopioid Analgesics

Acetaminophen
Acetaminophen (Tylenol)

Aspirin
Aspirin (acetylsalicylic acid) (ASA, Aspergum, Bayer Aspirin, Ecotrin)
Aspirin (acetylsalicylic acid), buffered (Alka-Seltzer, Bufferin, others)

Nonsteroidal Anti-Inflammatory Drugs
Fenoprofen (Nalfon)
Ibuprofen (Motrin, Advil)
Naproxen (Advil, Anaprox, Naprosyn, Aleve, Naprelan)
Oxaprozin (Daypro)

Cyclooxygenase-2 (COX-2) Inhibitor
Celecoxib (Celebrex)

Other Nonsteroidal Anti-Inflammatory Drugs
Diclofenac (Voltaren)
Diflunisal (Dolobid)
Etodolac (Lodine)
Indomethacin (Indocin)
Ketorolac
Meclofenamate
Mefenamic acid (Ponstel)
Meloxicam (Mobic)
Piroxicam (Feldene)
Sulindac (Clinoril)

Box 58-16 Side Effects of Aspirin and Nonsteroidal Anti-Inflammatory Drugs

Aspirin
Allergic reactions (anaphylaxis, laryngeal edema)
Bleeding (anemia, hemolysis, increased bleeding time)
Dizziness
Drowsiness
Flushing
Gastrointestinal symptoms (distress, heartburn, nausea, vomiting)
Headaches
Decreased renal function
Tinnitus
Visual changes

Nonsteroidal Anti-Inflammatory Drugs
Dysrhythmias
Blood dyscrasias
Cardiovascular thrombotic events
Dizziness
Gastric irritation
Hepatotoxicity
Hypotension
Pruritus
Decreased renal function
Sodium and water retention
Tinnitus

2. Side effects
   a. Anorexia, nausea, vomiting
   b. Rash
   c. Hypoglycemia
   d. Oliguria
   e. Hepatotoxicity
3. Interventions
   a. Monitor the vital signs.
   b. Check the client for a history of liver and renal dysfunction, alcoholism, and malnutrition.
   c. Monitor for hepatic damage, which includes nausea, vomiting, diarrhea, and abdominal pain.
   d. Monitor the liver enzyme test results.
   e. The client is instructed that self-medication should not be used longer than 10 days for an adult and 5 days for a child.
   f. Note that the antidote for acetaminophen is acetylcysteine (Mucomyst).
   g. Evaluate for the effectiveness of the medication.

⚠ Acetaminophen is contraindicated in clients with hepatic or renal disease, alcoholism, and/or hypersensitivity.

VI. OPIOID ANALGESICS

A. Description
1. Opioid analgesics suppress pain impulses but can suppress respiration and coughing by acting on the respiratory and cough center in the medulla of the brainstem.
2. Opioid analgesics can produce euphoria and sedation and cause physical dependence.
3. Opioid analgesics are used for relief of mild, moderate, or severe pain.
B. Medications (Box 58-17)
1. Codeine sulfate
   a. Codeine sulfate also is an effective cough suppressant at low doses.
   b. Codeine sulfate can cause constipation.
2. Hydromorphone hydrochloride (Dilaudid)
   a. Hydromorphone can decrease respiration.
   b. Hydromorphone can cause constipation.
3. Meperidine hydrochloride (Demerol)
   a. Meperidine can cause hypotension, dizziness, and urinary retention.
   b. Meperidine may be used for acute pain and as a preoperative medication.
   c. Meperidine can increase intracranial pressure in clients with head injuries.
   d. Meperidine is contraindicated in clients with head injuries and **increased intracranial pressure**, respiratory disorders, hypotension, shock, and severe hepatic and renal disease and in clients taking monoamine oxidase inhibitors.

e. Meperidine should not be taken with alcohol or a sedative-hypnotic because it may increase the CNS depression.
   f. Meperidine should be used cautiously in children and adults with a seizure disorder or a history of seizures because it decreases the seizure threshold.
4. Morphine sulfate
   a. Morphine can cause respiratory depression, orthostatic hypotension, and constipation.
   b. Morphine may cause nausea and vomiting because of increased vestibular sensitivity.
   c. Morphine is used for acute pain caused by myocardial infarction or cancer, for dyspnea caused by pulmonary edema, surgery, and as a preoperative medication.
   d. Morphine is contraindicated in clients with severe respiratory disorders, head injuries, **increased intracranial pressure**, severe renal, hepatic, or pulmonary disease, or seizure activity.
   e. Morphine is used with caution in clients with shock or blood loss.

⚠ Respiratory depression is the priority concern with morphine sulfate.

5. Oxycodone with aspirin (Percodan)
   a. Percodan should not be taken by a client allergic to aspirin.
   b. Percodan can cause gastric irritation and should be taken with food or plenty of liquids.

Box 58-17 Opioid Analgesics

Acetaminophen/hydrocodone (Lortab)
Buprenorphine hydrochloride (Buprenex)
Butorphanol tartrate (Stadol)
Codeine sulfate, codeine phosphate
Fentanyl (Duragesic, Sublimaze)
Hydrocodone (Hycodan)
Hydromorphone hydrochloride (Dilaudid)
Levorphanol tartrate (Levo-Dromoran)
Meperidine hydrochloride (Demerol)
Methadone hydrochloride (Dolophine, Methadose)
Morphine sulfate (Duramorph, MS Contin, Kadian, Oramorph SR)
Nalbuphine hydrochloride (Nubain)
Oxycodone (Roxicodone, OxyContin)
Oxycodone hydrochloride; acetaminophen (Percocet)
Oxycodone; aspirin (Percodan)
Oxymorphone hydrochloride (Numorphan)
Propoxyphene napsylate (Darvon-N)
Remifentanil (Ultiva)
Sufentanil (Sufenta)
Tramadol (Ultram)

6. Propoxyphene hydrochloride (Darvon) and propoxyphene napsylate (Darvon-N)
   a. Darvon compounds contain aspirin and should not be taken by a client allergic to aspirin.
   b. Darvocet-N contains acetaminophen.
7. Nalbuphine hydrochloride (Nubain) is preferable for treating the pain of a myocardial infarction because it reduces the oxygen needs of the heart without reducing blood pressure.
8. Methadone hydrochloride (Dolophine)
   a. Doses of oral concentrate are diluted with at least 90 mL of water.
   b. Dispersible tablets are diluted in at least 120 mL of water, orange juice, or acidic fruit beverage.
   c. Methadone is used as a replacement medication for opiate dependence and to facilitate withdrawal.
9. Hydrocodone (Hycodan) frequently is used for cough suppression.

C. Interventions for opioid analgesics
   1. Monitor the vital signs.
   2. Check the client thoroughly before administering pain medication.
   3. Initiate nursing measures such as massage, distraction, deep breathing and relaxation exercises, the application of heat or cold as prescribed, and providing care and comfort before administration of the opioid analgesic.
   4. Medications are administered 30 to 60 minutes before painful activities.
   5. Monitor respiratory rate and, if the rate is less than 12 breaths/min in an adult, the medication is withheld unless ventilatory support is being provided.
   6. Monitor pulse and, if bradycardia develops, the dose is held and the HCP is notified.
   7. Monitor the blood pressure for hypotension.
   8. Auscultate breath sounds because opioid analgesics suppress the cough reflex.
   9. Activities such as turning, deep breathing, and incentive spirometry to prevent atelectasis and pneumonia are encouraged.
   10. Monitor the level of consciousness.
   11. Initiate safety precautions such as side rails, a night light, and supervised ambulation.
   12. Monitor the intake and output (I&O).
   13. Monitor for urinary retention.
   14. The client is instructed to take oral doses with milk or a snack to reduce gastric irritation.
   15. The client is instructed to avoid alcohol.
   16. The client is instructed to avoid activities that require alertness.
   17. Monitor bowel function for constipation, abdominal distention, and decreased peristalsis.

18. The effectiveness of medication is evaluated.
19. Have the opioid antagonist, oxygen, and resuscitation equipment available.

D. Morphine sulfate
   1. Side effects
      a. Respiratory depression
      b. Orthostatic hypotension
      c. Urinary retention
      d. Nausea and vomiting
      e. Constipation
      f. Sedation, confusion, and hallucinations
      g. Cough suppression
      h. Reduction in pupillary size
      i. Miosis
   2. Interventions
      a. Have naloxone (Narcan) available for overdose.
      b. Monitor the vital signs and level of consciousness.
      c. Compare the rate and depth of respirations to the baseline.
      d. The medication is withheld if the respiratory rate is less than 12 breaths/min. Respirations of less than 10 breaths/min can indicate respiratory distress.
      e. Monitor urinary output, which should be at least 30 mL/hr.
      f. Monitor bowel sounds for decreased peristalsis because constipation can occur.
      g. Monitor for pupil changes because pinpoint pupils can indicate morphine overdose.
      h. The client is instructed to avoid alcohol or CNS depressants because they can cause respiratory depression.
      i. The client is instructed to report dizziness or difficulty breathing.
      j. If taking sustained-release morphine, the client may need short-acting opioid doses for breakthrough pain.
      k. To administer morphine intravenously, it is diluted in at least 5 mL of sterile water for injection and administered at a rate of 15 mg or less over 4 to 5 minutes.
      l. How and when to administer morphine and how to care for infusion equipment is explained to the client and his or her family.

E. Meperidine hydrochloride (Demerol)
   1. Side effects
      a. Respiratory depression
      b. Hypotension and dizziness
      c. Tachycardia
      d. Drowsiness and confusion
      e. Constipation
      f. Urinary retention
      g. Nausea and vomiting
      h. Seizures
      i. Tremors

2. Interventions
   a. Monitor the vital signs.
   b. Monitor for respiratory depression and hypotension.
   c. Have naloxone available for overdose.
   d. Monitor for urinary retention.
   e. Monitor bowel sounds and for constipation.
   f. To administer meperidine intravenously, the medication is diluted in at least 5 mL of sterile water or normal saline for injection and the dose is administered over 4 to 5 minutes.

VII. OPIOID ANTAGONISTS

A. Opioid antagonists (Box 58-18) are used to treat respiratory depression from opioid overdose.

B. Interventions
   1. Monitor blood pressure, pulse, and respiratory rate every 5 minutes initially, tapering to every 15 minutes, and then every 30 minutes until the client is stable.
   2. Place the client on a cardiac monitor and monitor cardiac rhythm.
   3. Auscultate breath sounds.
   4. Have resuscitation equipment available.
   5. Do not leave the client unattended.
   6. Monitor the client closely for several hours because when the effects of the antagonist wear off, the client may again display signs of opioid overdose.

VIII. OSMOTIC DIURETICS

A. Description
   1. Osmotic diuretics (Box 58-19) increase osmotic pressure of the glomerular filtrate, inhibiting reabsorption of water and electrolytes.
   2. Osmotic diuretics are used for oliguria and to prevent renal failure, decrease intracranial pressure, and decrease intraocular pressure in clients with narrow-angle glaucoma.
   3. Mannitol is used with chemotherapy to induce diuresis.

Box 58-18 Opioid Antagonists

Naloxone hydrochloride (Narcan)
Naltrexone (ReVia)

Box 58-19 Osmotic Diuretics

Mannitol (Osmitrol)
Urea (Ureaphil)

B. Side effects
   1. Fluid and electrolyte imbalances
   2. Pulmonary edema from the rapid shifts of fluid
   3. Nausea and vomiting
   4. Headache
   5. Tachycardia from the rapid fluid loss
   6. Hyponatremia and dehydration

C. Interventions
   1. Monitor the vital signs.
   2. Monitor the weight.
   3. Monitor the urine output.
   4. Monitor the electrolyte levels.
   5. Monitor the lungs and heart sounds for signs of pulmonary edema.
   6. Monitor for signs of dehydration.
   7. Monitor the neurological status.
   8. Monitor for increased intraocular pressure.
   9. Check for signs of decreasing intracranial pressure if appropriate.
   10. Change the client's position slowly to prevent orthostatic hypotension.
   11. Monitor for crystallization in the vial of mannitol before administering the medication. If crystallization is noted, do not administer the medication from that vial.

MORE QUESTIONS ON EVOLVE!

Practice Questions

611. A client with myasthenia gravis is suspected of having cholinergic crisis. Which of the following indicate that this crisis exists?
   1. Ataxia
   2. Mouth sores
   3. Hypotension
   4. Hypertension

612. A client with myasthenia gravis is receiving pyridostigmine (Mestinon). The nurse monitors for signs and symptoms of cholinergic crisis caused by overdose of the medication. The nurse checks the medication supply to ensure that which medication is available for administration if a cholinergic crisis occurs?
   1. Vitamin K
   2. Atropine sulfate
   3. Protamine sulfate
   4. Acetylcysteine (Mucomyst)

613. A client with myasthenia gravis becomes increasingly weak. The health care provider prepares to identify whether the client is reacting to an overdose of the medication (cholinergic crisis) or increasing severity of the disease (myasthenic crisis). An injection of edrophonium (Enlon) is

administered. Which of the following indicates that the client is in cholinergic crisis?
1. No change in the condition
2. Complaints of muscle spasms
3. An improvement of the weakness
4. A temporary worsening of the condition

614. Carbidopa-levodopa (Sinemet) is prescribed for a client with Parkinson's disease, and the nurse monitors the client for adverse reactions to the medication. Which of the following indicates that the client is experiencing an adverse reaction?
1. Pruritus
2. Tachycardia
3. Hypertension
4. Impaired voluntary movements

615. Phenytoin (Dilantin), 100 mg orally three times daily, has been prescribed for a client for seizure control. The nurse reinforces instructions regarding the medication to the client. Which statement by the client indicates an understanding of the instructions?
1. "I will use a soft toothbrush to brush my teeth."
2. "It's all right to break the capsules to make it easier for me to swallow them."
3. "If I forget to take my medication, I can wait until the next dose and eliminate that dose."
4. "If my throat becomes sore, it's a normal effect of the medication and it's nothing to be concerned about."

616. A client is taking phenytoin (Dilantin) for seizure control and a sample for a serum drug level is drawn. Which of the following indicates a therapeutic serum drug range?
1. 5 to 10 mcg/mL
2. 10 to 20 mcg/mL
3. 20 to 30 mcg/mL
4. 30 to 40 mcg/mL

617. Ibuprofen (Advil) is prescribed for a client. The nurse tells the client to take the medication:
1. With 8 oz of milk
2. In the morning after arising
3. 60 minutes before breakfast
4. At bedtime on an empty stomach

618. A nurse is caring for a client who is taking phenytoin (Dilantin) for control of seizures. During data collection, the nurse notes that the client is taking birth control pills. Which of the following information should the nurse provide to the client?
1. Pregnancy should be avoided while taking phenytoin (Dilantin).
2. The client may stop taking the phenytoin (Dilantin) if it is causing severe gastrointestinal effects.
3. The potential for decreased effectiveness of the birth control pills exists while taking phenytoin (Dilantin).
4. The increased risk of thrombophlebitis exists while taking phenytoin (Dilantin) and birth control pills together.

619. A client with trigeminal neuralgia is being treated with carbamazepine (Tegretol). Which laboratory result would indicate that the client is experiencing an adverse reaction to the medication?
1. Sodium level, 140 mEq/L
2. Uric acid level, 5.0 mg/dL
3. White blood cell count, 3000 cells/mm^3
4. Blood urea nitrogen (BUN) level, 15 mg/dL

620. A client is receiving meperidine hydrochloride (Demerol) for pain. Which of the following are side effects of this medication. **Select all that apply**.
☐ 1. Diarrhea
☐ 2. Tremors
☐ 3. Drowsiness
☐ 4. Hypotension
☐ 5. Urinary frequency
☐ 6. Increased respiratory rate

ANSWERS

611. 4
Rationale: Cholinergic crisis occurs as a result of an overdose of medication. Indications of cholinergic crisis include gastrointestinal disturbances, nausea, vomiting, diarrhea, abdominal cramps, increased salivation and tearing, miosis, hypertension, sweating, and increased bronchial secretions.
Test-Taking Strategy: Use the process of elimination. Note that options 3 and 4 identify opposite effects. This indicates that one of them may be the correct option. Remember,

hypertension occurs with cholinergic crisis. Review both cholinergic and myasthenic crisis if you had difficulty with this question.
Level of Cognitive Ability: Analyzing
Client Needs: Physiological Integrity
Integrated Process: Nursing Process/Data Collection
Content Area: Pharmacology
References: Kee, Hayes, McCuistion, p. 345. 2009.
Lehne, pp. 136, 138. 2010.

612. 2

Rationale: The antidote for cholinergic crisis is atropine sulfate. Vitamin K is the antidote for warfarin (Coumadin). Protamine sulfate is the antidote for heparin, and acetylcysteine (Mucomyst) is the antidote for acetaminophen (Tylenol).
Test-Taking Strategy: Knowledge regarding antidotes for various medications is needed to answer this question. Remember that atropine sulfate is the antidote for cholinergic crisis. Review antidotes if you had difficulty with this question.
Level of Cognitive Ability: Applying
Client Needs: Physiological Integrity
Integrated Process: Nursing Process/Implementation
Content Area: Pharmacology
Reference: Lehne, p. 136. 2010.

613. 4

Rationale: An edrophonium (Enlon) injection makes the client in cholinergic crisis temporarily worse. This is known as a negative test. An improvement of weakness would occur if the client were experiencing myasthenia gravis. Options 1 and 2 would not occur in either crisis.
Test-Taking Strategy: Focus on the data in the question. Noting the words "overdose of the medication (cholinergic crisis)" will direct you to option 4. It makes sense that administering additional medication will worsen the condition. Review this diagnostic test and the differences between cholinergic and myasthenic crisis if you had difficulty with this question.
Level of Cognitive Ability: Analyzing
Client Needs: Physiological Integrity
Integrated Process: Nursing Process/Data Collection
Content Area: Pharmacology
References: Kee, Hayes, McCuistion, p. 347. 2009. Lehne, pp. 136–138. 2010.

614. 4

Rationale: Dyskinesia and impaired voluntary movement may occur with high levodopa dosages. Nausea, anorexia, dizziness, orthostatic hypotension, bradycardia, and akinesia (the temporary muscle weakness that lasts 1 minute to 1 hour, also known as the "on-off phenomenon") are frequent side effects of the medication.
Test-Taking Strategy: Use the process of elimination. Options 2 and 3 are cardiac-related options, so these options can be eliminated first. Note that the question asks for an adverse reaction; therefore select option 4 over option 1 as the correct answer. Review the adverse effects of carbidopa and levodopa if you had difficulty with this question.
Level of Cognitive Ability: Analyzing
Client Needs: Physiological Integrity
Integrated Process: Nursing Process/Data Collection
Content Area: Pharmacology
Reference: Lehne, pp. 195–196. 2010.

615. 1

Rationale: Phenytoin (Dilantin) is an anticonvulsant. Gingival hyperplasia, bleeding, swelling, and tenderness of the gums can occur with the use of this medication. The client needs to be taught good oral hygiene, gum massage, and the need for regular dentist visits. The client should not skip medication doses, because this could precipitate a seizure. Capsules should not be chewed or broken and they must be swallowed. The client needs to be instructed to report a sore throat, fever, glandular swelling, or any skin reaction, because this indicates hematological toxicity.
Test-Taking Strategy: Use the process of elimination. Note the strategic words "an understanding of the instructions." Eliminate option 3 because the client needs to be encouraged to take medications on time. Also, eliminate option 4 because the client needs to report these symptoms to the health care provider. From the remaining options, recalling that capsules should not be broken will direct you to option 1. Review the side effects related to phenytoin (Dilantin) if you had difficulty with this question.
Level of Cognitive Ability: Evaluating
Client Needs: Physiological Integrity
Integrated Process: Nursing Process/Evaluation
Content Area: Pharmacology
Reference: Hodgson, Kizior, p. 924. 2011.

616. 2

Rationale: The therapeutic serum drug level range for phenytoin (Dilantin) is 10 to 20 mcg/mL. Therefore, options 1, 3, and 4 are incorrect.
Test-Taking Strategy: Knowledge regarding the therapeutic serum range of this medication is required to answer the question. A helpful hint may be to remember that the theophylline therapeutic range and the acetaminophen (Tylenol) therapeutic range are the same as the phenytoin (Dilantin) therapeutic range. Remembering this may assist you when answering questions related to any of these three medications. Review this therapeutic level if you had difficulty with this question.
Level of Cognitive Ability: Understanding
Client Needs: Physiological Integrity
Integrated Process: Nursing Process/Data Collection
Content Area: Pharmacology
Reference: Hodgson, Kizior, p. 924. 2011.

617. 1

Rationale: Ibuprofen is a nonsteroidal anti-inflammatory drug (NSAID). NSAIDs should be given with milk or food to prevent gastrointestinal irritation. Options 2, 3, and 4 are incorrect.
Test-Taking Strategy: Use the process of elimination. Note that options 2, 3, and 4 are comparable or alike. Each of these options indicates administering the medication without food. Remember, NSAIDs can cause gastric irritation. Review this medication if you had difficulty with this question.
Level of Cognitive Ability: Applying
Client Needs: Physiological Integrity
Integrated Process: Teaching and Learning
Content Area: Pharmacology
Reference: Hodgson, Kizior, p. 586. 2011.

618. 3

Rationale: Phenytoin (Dilantin) enhances the rate of estrogen metabolism, which can decrease the effectiveness of some birth control pills. Options 1, 2, are 4 are not accurate.
Test-Taking Strategy: Use the process of elimination. Option 4 would cause anxiety in the client. A client should not be instructed to stop anticonvulsant medication. Pregnancy does not need to be "avoided." Review medication interactions related to phenytoin (Dilantin) if you had difficulty with this question.

Level of Cognitive Ability: Applying
Client Needs: Health Promotion and Maintenance
Integrated Process: Nursing Process/Implementation
Content Area: Pharmacology
Reference: Lehne, p. 225. 2010.

619. 3
Rationale: Adverse effects of carbamazepine (Tegretol) appear as blood dyscrasias, including aplastic anemia, agranulocytosis, thrombocytopenia, leukopenia, cardiovascular disturbances, thrombophlebitis, dysrhythmias, and dermatological effects. Options 1, 2, and 4 identify normal laboratory values.
Test-Taking Strategy: Use the process of elimination. If you are familiar with normal laboratory values, you will note that the only option that indicates an abnormal value is option 3. Review the signs of adverse reactions related to this medication if you had difficulty with this question.
Level of Cognitive Ability: Understanding
Client Needs: Physiological Integrity

Integrated Process: Nursing Process/Data Collection
Content Area: Pharmacology
Reference: Lehne, pp. 226, 237. 2010.

620. 2, 3, 4
Rationale: Meperidine hydrochloride is an opioid analgesic. Side effects include respiratory depression, drowsiness, hypotension, constipation, urinary retention, nausea, vomiting, and tremors.
Test-Taking Strategy: Focus on the name of the medication. Recalling that this medication is an opioid analgesic and recalling the effects of an opioid analgesic will assist in identifying the side effects. Review the side effects of this medication if you had difficulty with this question.
Level of Cognitive Ability: Analyzing
Client Needs: Physiological Integrity
Integrated Process: Nursing Process/Data Collection
Content Area: Pharmacology
Reference: Hodgson, Kizior, p. 727. 2011.

UNIT 17

The Adult Client with a Musculoskeletal Disorder

PYRAMID TERMS

cast Stiff dressing or casting, made of plaster of Paris or synthetic material, to stabilize a part or parts of the body until healing occurs.

compartment syndrome Condition in which pressure increases in a confined anatomical space that leads to decreased blood flow, ischemia, and dysfunction of these tissues; initial ischemia with pain, pallor, paresthesia, muscle weakness, and loss of pulses may progress to necrosis and permanent muscle cellular dysfunction.

external fixation Stabilization of a fracture by the use of an external frame, with multiple pins applied through the bone.

fat embolism Sudden dislodgement of a fat globule that is freed into the circulation where it can lodge in a blood vessel and obstruct blood flow to tissue that is distal to the obstruction.

internal fixation Stabilization of a fracture that involves the application of screws, plates, pins, or nails to hold the fragments in alignment.

reduction Correction or realignment of a bone fracture or joint dislocation.

traction Exertion of a pulling force to a fractured bone or dislocated joint to establish and maintain correct alignment for healing and to decrease muscle spasms and pain.

PYRAMID TO SUCCESS

The Pyramid to Success focuses on the emergency care for a client who sustains a fracture or other musculoskeletal injury, monitoring for complications related to fractures, and interventions if complications occur. Nursing care related to casts and traction is emphasized. Skill related to instructing the client on the use of an assistive device such as a cane, walker, or crutches is a pyramid point. Pyramid points also include postoperative care following hip surgery or amputation, as well as care of the client with rheumatoid arthritis or osteoporosis.

Focus on the points related to the psychosocial effects as a result of the musculoskeletal disorder, such as unexpected body-image changes, and the appropriate and available support services needed for the client.

CLIENT NEEDS

Safe and Effective Care Environment

- Establishing priorities
- Handling hazardous and infectious materials safely
- Maintaining asepsis related to wounds
- Maintaining confidentiality regarding the disorder and plan of care
- Maintaining standard and other precautions
- Preventing accidents and injuries
- Providing a dietary consultation
- Providing informed consent for diagnostic treatments and surgical procedures
- Providing physical therapy and occupational therapy referrals
- Upholding client rights

Health Promotion and Maintenance

- Discussing expected body-image changes
- Performing physical assessment related to the musculoskeletal system
- Promoting health related to diet and activity
- Preventing diseases that occur as a result of the aging process
- Providing home care instructions regarding care related to the musculoskeletal disorder
- Reinforcing the importance of prescribed therapy

Psychosocial Integrity

- Assessing available support systems and use of community resources
- Assessing the client's ability to cope with feelings of isolation and loss of independence
- Considering cultural, religious, and spiritual influences
- Discussing grief and loss related to mobility limitations and restrictions
- Discussing situational role changes as a result of the musculoskeletal disorder
- Identifying unexpected body-image changes as a result of injury or disease
- Identifying sensory and perceptual alterations
- Mobilizing coping mechanisms

Physiological Integrity

- Identifying complications of a fracture
- Identifying complications related to procedures or injuries
- Providing care related to casts and traction
- Promoting normal elimination patterns
- Promoting self-care measures
- Providing emergency care for a fracture or other injury
- Providing measures to promote comfort
- Teaching about the use of assistive devices for mobility such as canes, walkers, and crutches
- Teaching pharmacological therapy

Musculoskeletal System

I. ANATOMY AND PHYSIOLOGY

A. Skeleton
  1. Axial portion
     a. Cranium
     b. Vertebrae
     c. Ribs
  2. Appendicular portion
     a. Limbs
     b. Shoulders
     c. Hips
B. Types of bones
  1. Types include long, short, flat, and irregular
  2. Spongy bone
     a. Is located in the ends of long bones and the center of flat and irregular bones
     b. Can withstand forces applied in many directions
  3. Dense (compact) bone
     a. Covers spongy bone
     b. Forms a cylinder around a central marrow cavity
     c. Can withstand force predominantly in one direction
  4. Characteristics of the bones
     a. Support and protect structures of the body
     b. Provide attachments for muscles, tendons, and ligaments
     c. Contain tissue in the central cavities, which aids in the formation of blood cells
     d. Assist in regulating calcium and phosphate concentrations
  5. Bone growth
     a. The length of bone growth results from the ossification of the epiphyseal cartilage at the ends of bones, and bone growth stops between the ages of 18 and 25 years.
     b. The width of bone growth results from the activity of osteoblasts and occurs throughout life but does slow down with aging.
C. Types of joints (Table 59-1)
  1. Characteristics of the joints
     a. Allow the movement between bones
     b. Are formed where two bones join
     c. Surfaces are covered with cartilage.
     d. Are enclosed in a capsule
     e. Contain a cavity filled with synovial fluid
     f. Ligaments hold the bone and joint in the correct position.
     g. Articulation is the meeting point of two or more bones.
  2. Synovial fluid
     a. Is found in the joint capsule
     b. Is formed by the synovial membrane, which lines the joint capsule
     c. Lubricates the cartilage
     d. Provides a cushion against shocks
D. Muscles
  1. Characteristics of muscles
     a. Are made up of bundles of muscle fibers
     b. Provide the force to move bones
     c. Assist in maintaining posture
     d. Assist with heat production
  2. The process of contraction and relaxation
     a. Muscle contraction and relaxation require large amounts of adenosine triphosphate.
     b. Contraction also requires calcium, which functions as a catalyst.
     c. Acetylcholine released by the motor end plate of the motor neuron initiates an action potential.
     d. Acetylcholine is then destroyed by acetylcholinesterase.
     e. Calcium is required to contract muscle fibers and acts as a catalyst for the enzyme needed for the sliding-together action of actin and myosin.
     f. Following contraction, adenosine triphosphate transports calcium out to allow actin and myosin to separate and to allow the muscle to relax.
  3. Skeletal muscles
     a. Skeletal muscles are attached to two bones and cross at least one joint.
     b. The point of origin is the point of attachment on the bone closest to the trunk.
     c. The point of insertion is the point of attachment on the bone farthest from the trunk.

TABLE 59-1 Types of Joints

Type	Description
Amphiarthrosis	Cartilaginous joints Slightly movable joints
Condyloid	Freely movable joints Allow frictionless, painless movement
Diarthrosis	Synovial joints Ball-and-socket joints
Synarthrosis	Fibrous or fixed joints No movement associated with these joints

Box 59-1 Risk Factors Associated with Musculoskeletal Disorders

Autoimmune disorders
Calcium deficiency
Falls
Hyperuricemia
Infection
Medications
Metabolic disorders
Neoplastic disorders
Obesity
Postmenopausal states
Trauma and injury

    d. Skeletal muscles act in groups.
    e. Prime movers contract to produce movement.
    f. Antagonists relax skeletal muscles.
    g. Synergists contract to stabilize body movement.
    h. Nerves activate and control the muscles.
E. Bone healing
    1. Description: Bone union or healing is the process that occurs after the integrity of a bone is interrupted.
    2. Three stages
      a. The fracture causes soft tissue edema and bleeding because of the vascularity of the bone, and this blood solidifies into a hematoma over 48 to 72 hours.
      b. After injury, the blood supply is interrupted, leading to ischemia and necrosis of the bone around the injury site.
      c. Dead cells promote migration of osteoblasts and fibroblasts to the area, and healing starts with the formation of fibrocartilage.
      d. Bone union begins as a callus forms with vascular and cellular proliferation surrounding the fracture site; this loose fibrous tissue or "callus" changes into bone over the next 3 to 6 months.
      e. Remodeling occurs as the excess bone tissue of the callus resorbs as time passes and weight-bearing activities are gradually increased; the time required for complete healing varies and is related to variables such as age, bone type, trauma severity, infection, and blood supply.

II. RISK FACTORS ASSOCIATED WITH MUSCULOSKELETAL DISORDERS (Box 59-1)

III. DIAGNOSTIC TESTS

A. Radiographs (x-rays)
    1. Description: Radiography is a commonly used procedure to diagnose disorders of the musculoskeletal system.

    2. Interventions
      a. Handle injured areas carefully and support extremities above and below the joint.
      b. Administer analgesics as prescribed before the procedure, particularly if the client is in pain.
      c. Remove any radiopaque objects, such as jewelry.
      d. Shield client's testes, ovaries, or pregnant abdomen (may be contraindicated in pregnancy).
      e. Instruct the client to lie still during a radiograph.
      f. Inform the client that exposure to radiation is minimal and not dangerous.
      g. Wear a lead apron if staying in the room with the client.
B. Arthrocentesis
    1. Description: Arthrocentesis is used to diagnose joint inflammation and infection.
      a. Arthrocentesis involves aspirating synovial fluid, blood, or pus via a needle inserted into a joint cavity.
      b. Medication, such as corticosteroids, may be instilled into the joint if necessary to alleviate inflammation.
    2. Interventions
      a. Obtain an informed consent.
      b. Apply an elastic compression bandage postprocedure as prescribed.
      c. Use ice to decrease pain and swelling.
      d. Pain may worsen after aspirating fluid from the joint.
      e. Pain can continue up to 2 days after administration of corticosteroids into a joint.
      f. Instruct the client to rest the joint for 8 to 24 hours postprocedure as prescribed.
      g. Instruct the client to notify the health care provider if a fever, increased redness, or swelling of the joint occurs.
C. Arthrography
    1. Description: Arthrography is used in unexplained joint pain or inflammation.
      a. Arthrography is a radiographic examination of the soft tissues of the joint structures and is used to diagnose trauma to the joint capsule or ligaments.
      b. A local anesthetic is used for the procedure.

c. A contrast medium or air is injected into the joint cavity, and the joint is moved through range of motion as a series of x-ray films are taken.

2. Interventions

a. Instruct the client to fast from food and fluids for 8 hours before the procedure as prescribed.

b. Assess the client for allergies to iodine or shellfish before the procedure.

c. Obtain an informed consent.

d. Inform the client of the need to remain as still as possible, except when asked to reposition.

e. Minimize the use of the joint for 12 hours after the procedure as prescribed.

f. Instruct the client that the joint may be edematous and tender for 1 to 2 days after the procedure and may be treated with ice packs and analgesics as prescribed.

g. Instruct the client to notify the health care provider (HCP) if edema and tenderness last longer than 2 days.

h. If knee arthrography was performed, an elastic compression wrap over the knee may be prescribed for 3 to 4 days and ice applied to decrease pain and swelling.

i. If air was used for injection, crepitus may be felt in the joint for up to 2 days.

D. Arthroscopy

1. Description: Arthroscopy is used to diagnose acute and chronic disorders of the joint.

a. Arthroscopy provides an endoscopic examination of various joints.

b. Articular cartilage abnormalities can be assessed, loose bodies can be removed, and the cartilage can be trimmed.

c. A biopsy may be performed during the procedure.

2. Interventions

a. Instruct the client to fast for 8 to 12 hours before the procedure.

b. Obtain an informed consent.

c. Administer pain medication as prescribed postprocedure.

d. Assess the neurovascular status of the affected extremity.

e. An elastic compression bandage should be worn for 2 to 4 days as prescribed postprocedure.

f. Instruct the client that walking without weight bearing is usually permitted after sensation returns but to limit activity for 1 to 4 days as prescribed postprocedure.

g. Instruct the client to elevate the extremity as often as possible for 2 days following the procedure and to place ice on the site to minimize swelling.

h. Reinforce instructions regarding the use of crutches, which may be used for 5 to 7 days postprocedure for walking.

i. Advise the client to notify the HCP if fever or increased knee pain occurs or if edema continues for more than 3 days postprocedure.

E. Bone mineral density measurements

1. Dual energy x-ray absorptiometry

a. Measures bone mass of the spine, other bones, and the total body

b. Radiation exposure is minimal.

c. Used to diagnose metabolic bone disease and to monitor changes in bone density with treatment

d. Inform the client that the procedure is painless.

e. All metallic objects are removed before the test.

2. Quantitative ultrasound

a. Quantitative ultrasound evaluates strength, density, and elasticity of various bones using ultrasound rather than radiation.

b. Inform the client that the procedure is painless.

F. Bone scan

1. Description: A bone scan is used to identify, evaluate, and stage bone cancer before and after treatment.

a. Radioisotope is injected intravenously and will collect in areas that indicate abnormal bone metabolism and some fractures, if they exist.

b. The isotope is excreted in the urine and feces within 48 hours and is not harmful to others.

2. Interventions

a. Hold fluids for 4 hours before the procedure.

b. Obtain an informed consent.

c. Remove all jewelry and metal objects.

d. Following the injection of the radioisotope, the client must drink 32 oz of water (if not contraindicated) to promote renal filtering of the excess isotope.

e. From 1 to 3 hours after the injection, have the client void to clear excess isotope from the bladder before the scanning procedure is completed.

f. Inform the client of the need to lie supine during the procedure and that the procedure is not painful.

g. Monitor the injection site for redness and swelling.

h. Encourage oral fluid intake after the procedure.

⚠ No special precautions are required after a bone scan, because a minimal amount of radioactivity exists in the radioisotope used for the procedure.

G. Bone or muscle biopsy
   1. Description: A biopsy may be performed during surgery or through aspiration or punch or needle biopsy.
   2. Interventions
      a. Obtain an informed consent.
      b. Monitor for bleeding, swelling, hematoma, or severe pain.
      c. Elevate the site for 24 hours following the procedure to reduce edema.
      d. Apply ice packs as prescribed following the procedure to prevent the development of a hematoma and to decrease site discomfort.
      e. Monitor for signs of infection following the procedure.
      f. Inform the client that mild to moderate discomfort is normal following the procedure.
H. Electromyography (EMG)
   1. Description: An EMG is used to evaluate muscle weakness.
      a. Electromyography measures electrical potential associated with skeletal muscle contractions.
      b. Needles are inserted into the muscle, and recordings of muscular electrical activity are traced on recording paper through an oscilloscope.
   2. Interventions
      a. Obtain an informed consent.
      b. Instruct the client that the needle insertion is uncomfortable.
      c. Instruct the client not to take any stimulants or sedatives for 24 hours before the procedure.
      d. Inform the client that slight bruising may occur at the needle insertion sites.
      e. Mild analgesics can be used for the pain.

IV. INJURIES

A. Strains
   1. Strains are an excessive stretching of a muscle or tendon.
   2. Management involves cold and heat applications, exercise with activity limitations, anti-inflammatory medications, and muscle relaxants.
   3. Surgical repair may be required for a severe strain (ruptured muscle or tendon).
B. Sprains
   1. Sprains are an excessive stretching of a ligament, usually caused by a twisting motion, such as in a fall or step on an uneven surface.
   2. Sprains are characterized by pain and swelling.
   3. Management involves RICE (rest, ice, a compression bandage, and elevation) to reduce swelling and provide joint support.
   4. Casting may be required for moderate sprains to allow the tear to heal.
   5. Surgery may be necessary for severe ligament damage.

C. Rotator cuff injuries
   1. Musculotendinous or rotator cuff of the shoulder sustains a tear, usually as a result of trauma.
   2. Injury is characterized by shoulder pain and the inability to maintain abduction of the arm at the shoulder (drop arm test).
   3. Management involves nonsteroidal anti-inflammatory drugs (NSAIDs), physical therapy, sling support, and ice/heat applications.
   4. Surgery may be required if medical management is unsuccessful or for those who have a complete tear.

V. FRACTURES

A. Description: A fracture is a break in the continuity of the bone caused by trauma, twisting as a result of muscle spasm or indirect loss of leverage, or bone decalcification and disease that result in osteopenia.
B. Types of fractures (Box 59-2)
C. Data collection: fracture of an extremity
   1. Pain or tenderness over the involved area
   2. Decrease or loss of muscular strength or function
   3. Obvious deformity of affected area
   4. Crepitation, erythema, edema, or bruising
   5. Muscle spasm and neurovascular impairment
D. Initial care of a fracture of an extremity
   1. Immobilize affected extremity with **cast** or splint
   2. If a compound (open) fracture exists, splint extremity and cover wound with a sterile dressing

---

Box 59-2 Types of Fractures

Closed or simple: Skin over the fractured area remains intact.
Comminuted: The bone is splintered or crushed, with three or more fragments.
Complete: The bone is separated completely by a break into two parts.
Compression: A fractured bone is compressed by other bone.
Depressed: Bone fragments are driven inward.
Greenstick: One side of the bone is broken and the other is bent; these fractures occur most commonly in children.
Impacted: A part of the fractured bone is driven into another bone.
Incomplete: The bone is partially broken.
Oblique: The break extends in an oblique direction.
Open or compound: The bone is exposed to air through a break in the skin, and soft tissue injury and infection are common.
Pathological: The fracture results from weakening of the bone structure by pathological processes such as neoplasia or osteomalacia; also called spontaneous fracture.
Spiral: The break partially encircles bone.
Transverse: The bone is fractured straight across.

3. Assess neurovascular status of the extremity
4. Interventions for a fracture include **reduction**, fixation, **traction**, and casting

⚠ If a compound (open) fracture exists, splint the extremity and cover the wound with a sterile dressing.

E. **Reduction** restores the bone to proper alignment.
   1. Closed **reduction** is a nonsurgical intervention that is performed by manual manipulation.
      a. Closed **reduction** may be performed under local or general anesthesia.
      b. A **cast** may be applied following **reduction**.
   2. Open **reduction** involves a surgical intervention.
      a. Fracture may be treated with **internal fixation** devices.
      b. The client may be placed in **traction** or a **cast** following the procedure.
F. Fixation
   1. **Internal fixation** follows an open **reduction** (Figure 59-1)
      a. **Internal fixation** involves the application of screws, plates, pins, or intramedullary rods to hold the fragments in alignment.
      b. **Internal fixation** may involve the removal of damaged bone and replacement with a prosthesis.
      c. **Internal fixation** provides immediate bone strength.
   2. **External fixation** is the use of an external frame to stabilize a fracture by attaching skeletal pins through bone fragments to a rigid external support.

▲ **FIGURE 59-1** A compression hip screw used for open reduction with internal fixation. (From Ignatavicius, D., & Workman, M. [2010]. *Medical-surgical nursing: Patient-centered collaborative care* [6th ed.]. St. Louis: Saunders.)

a. **External fixation** provides more freedom of movement than with **traction**.
b. Monitor pin stability and provide pin care to decrease infection risks.
c. Risk of infection exists with both fixation methods.
d. **External fixation** is commonly used when massive tissue trauma is present.
G. **Traction** (Figure 59-2)
   1. Description
      a. **Traction** is the exertion of a pulling force applied in two directions to reduce and immobilize a fracture.
      b. **Traction** provides proper bone alignment and reduces muscle spasms.
   2. Interventions
      a. Maintain proper body alignment.
      b. Ensure that the weights hang freely and do not touch the floor.
      c. Do not remove or lift the weights without a HCP's prescription.
      d. Ensure that pulleys are not obstructed and that ropes in the pulleys move freely.
      e. Place knots in the ropes to prevent slipping.
      f. Check the ropes for fraying.
H. Skeletal **traction** (Figure 59-3)
   1. Description: **Traction** is applied mechanically to the bone with pins, wires, or tongs.
   2. Interventions
      a. Monitor color, motion, and sensation of the affected extremity.
      b. Monitor the insertion sites for redness, swelling, drainage, or increased pain.
      c. Provide insertion site care as prescribed.
   3. Cervical tongs and a halo fixation device (refer to Chapter 57 regarding care of the client with these types of devices)
I. Skin **traction**
   1. Description: Skin **traction** is applied by using elastic bandages or adhesive; types include Buck's, cervical, pelvic, and Russell's.
   2. Cervical skin **traction** relieves muscle spasms and compression in the upper extremities and neck (see Figure 59-2).
      a. Cervical skin **traction** uses a head halter and a chin pad to attach the **traction**.
      b. Use powder to protect the ears from friction rub.
      c. Position the client with the head of the bed elevated 30 to 40 degrees, and attach the weights to a pulley system over the head of the bed.
   3. Buck's (extension) skin **traction** is used to alleviate muscle spasms and immobilize a lower limb by maintaining a straight pull on the limb with the use of weights (see Figure 59-2).

▲ **FIGURE 59-2** Types of traction. **A,** Buck's traction. **B,** Russell's traction. **C,** Head halter traction. **D,** Pelvic sling traction. **E,** Balanced suspension traction. (From Lewis, S., Heitkemper, M., & Dirksen, S. [2007]. *Medical-surgical nursing: Assessment and management of clinical problems* [7th ed.]. St. Louis: Mosby.)

Tibial pin for skeletal traction

▲ **FIGURE 59-3** Balanced suspension with a Thomas splint and Pearson attachment. The apparatus can be used alone or, as in this case, with skeletal traction. (From Monahan, F., Sands, J., Neighbors, M., et al. [2007]. *Phipps' medical-surgical nursing: Concepts and clinical practice* [8th ed.]. St. Louis: Mosby.)

a. A boot appliance is applied to attach to the **traction**.

b. Weight is attached to a pulley; allow the weights to hang freely over the edge of bed.

c. Not more than 8 to 10 lb of weight should be applied.

d. Elevate the foot of the bed to provide the **traction**.

4. Russell's skin **traction** (refer to Chapter 37 regarding information related to these types of **traction**)

5. Pelvic skin (sling) **traction** is used to relieve low back, hip, or leg pain or to reduce muscle spasm (see Figure 59-2).

a. Apply the **traction** snugly over the pelvis and iliac crest and attach to the weights.

b. Use measures as prescribed to prevent the client from slipping down in bed.

J. Balanced suspension **traction** (see Figure 59-2 and 59-3)

1. Description

a. Balanced suspension **traction** is used with skin or skeletal **traction**.

b. It is used to approximate fractures of the femur, tibia, or fibula.

c. Balanced suspension **traction** is produced by a counterforce other than the client.

2. Interventions

a. Position the client in a low Fowler's position on either the side or the back.

b. Maintain a 20-degree angle from the thigh to the bed.

c. Protect the skin from breakdown.

d. Provide pin care if pins are used with the skeletal **traction**.

e. Clean the pin sites with sterile normal saline and hydrogen peroxide or povidone-iodine (Betadine) as prescribed or per agency policy.

K. Dunlop's **traction**

1. Description: horizontal **traction** is used to align fractures of the humerus; vertical **traction** maintains the forearm in proper alignment.

2. Interventions: nursing care is similar to that for Buck's skin **traction**.

L. Casts

1. Description: plaster or fiberglass **casts** are used to immobilize bones and joints into correct alignment after a fracture or injury.

2. Interventions

a. Keep the **cast** and extremity elevated.

b. Allow a wet **cast** 24 to 72 hours to dry (synthetic **casts** dry in 20 minutes).

c. Handle a wet **cast** with the palms of the hands until dry.

d. Turn the extremity every 1 to 2 hours, unless contraindicated to allow air circulation and promote drying of the **cast**.

e. Cool setting on a hair dryer can be used to dry a plaster **cast**. (Heat cannot be used on a plaster **cast**, because the **cast** heats up and burns the skin.)

f. Prepare for bivalving or cutting the **cast** if circulatory impairment occurs.

g. Petal the **cast**; maintain smooth edges around the **cast** to prevent crumbling of the **cast** material.

h. Monitor for signs of infection such as temperature, hot spots on the **cast**, foul odor or changes in pain.

i. If an open draining area exists on the affected extremity, the HCP will make a cutout portion of the **cast** or a window.

j. Instruct the client not to stick objects inside the **cast**.

k. Teach the client to keep the **cast** clean and dry.

l. Instruct the client on isometric exercises to prevent muscle atrophy.

 Monitor a casted extremity for circulatory impairment such as pain, swelling, discoloration, tingling, numbness, coolness, or diminished pulse. Notify the HCP immediately if circulatory compromise occurs.

VI.   COMPLICATIONS OF FRACTURES (Box 59-3)

A. Fat embolism

1. Description: a **fat embolism** originates in the bone marrow and occurs after a fracture when a fat globule is released into the blood stream.

a. Clients with long bone fractures are at the greatest risk for the development of **fat embolism**.

b. **Fat embolism** can occur within the first 48 to 72 hours following the injury or when surgical manipulation occurs following surgery.

2. Data collection: Findings often suggest pulmonary embolism.

a. Restlessness, hypoxemia, or mental status changes

b. Tachycardia and hypotension

c. Dyspnea and tachypnea

d. Petechial rash over the upper chest and neck

Box 59-3 Complications of Fractures

Fat embolism
Compartment syndrome
Infection and osteomyelitis
Avascular necrosis
Pulmonary embolism

3. Interventions (see Priority Nursing Actions).

PRIORITY NURSING ACTIONS!

Actions to Take if the Client Develops a Fat Embolism

1. Notify the HCP.
2. Administer oxygen.
3. Administer intravenous fluids.
4. Monitor vital signs and respiratory status.
5. Prepare for intubation and mechanical ventilation if necessary.
6. Document the event, actions taken, and the client's response.

A fat embolism originates in the bone marrow and occurs after a fracture when a fat globule is released into the bloodstream. Fat embolism can occur within the first 48 to 72 hours after the injury, and clients with long bone fractures are at the greatest risk for the development of a fat embolism. Findings are similar to those noted with pulmonary embolism and include restlessness, hypoxemia, mental status changes, dyspnea, tachypnea, tachycardia, and hypotension. Additionally, a petechial rash may present over the upper chest and neck. The HCP is notified immediately while initiating emergency care. The client is maintained on bedrest and is repositioned only as necessary and gently. Oxygen is administered and IV hydration is administered to prevent hypovolemic shock. Vital signs and respiratory status are monitored closely and the client is prepared for intubation and mechanical ventilation if necessary. Corticosteroids may also be prescribed for the client. The nurse then documents the event, actions taken, and the client's response.

Reference: Ignatavicius, D., & Workman, M. (2010). *Medical-surgical nursing: Patient-centered collaborative care* (6th ed., p. 1182). St. Louis: Saunders.

B. Compartment syndrome
   1. Description
      a. Tough fascia surrounds muscle groups, forming compartments from which arteries, veins, and nerves enter and exit opposite ends.
      b. **Compartment syndrome** occurs when pressure increases within one or more compartments, leading to decreased blood flow, tissue ischemia, and neurovascular impairment.
      c. It may also occur when a dressing or **cast** is too tight.
      d. Within 4 to 6 hours after the onset of **compartment syndrome**, neurovascular damage is irreversible if not treated.
   2. Data collection
      a. Unrelieved or increased pain in the limb
      b. Tissue that is distal to the involved area becomes pale, dusky, or edematous.

c. Pain with passive movement and joint dysfunction
      d. Loss of sensation (paresthesia)
      e. Pulselessness (a late sign)
   3. Interventions
      a. Notify the HCP immediately and prepare to assist the HCP.
      b. If severe, assist the HCP with fasciotomy to relieve pressure and restore tissue perfusion.
      c. Loosen tight dressings or bivalve restrictive **cast** as prescribed.
C. Infection and osteomyelitis
   1. Description: Infection and osteomyelitis (inflammatory response in bone tissue) can be caused by the introduction of organisms into bones initially leading to localized bone infection.
   2. Data collection
      a. Tachycardia and fever (usually above 101 ° F)
      b. Erythema and pain in the area surrounding the infection
      c. Leukocytosis and elevated erythrocyte sedimentation rate (ESR)
   3. Interventions
      a. HCP notification
      b. Initiation of aggressive, long-term IV antibiotic therapy
      c. Hyperbaric oxygen therapy to promote client healing
      d. Surgery for resistant osteomyelitis with sequestrectomy and/or bone grafts
D. Avascular necrosis
   1. Description: occurs when a fracture interrupts the blood supply to a section of bone, leading to bone death
   2. Data collection
      a. Pain
      b. Decreased sensation
   3. Interventions
      a. Notify the HCP if pain or numbness occurs.
      b. Prepare the client for removal of necrotic tissue because it serves as a focus for infection.
E. Pulmonary embolism (see Priority Nursing Actions in Chapter 49)

VII. CRUTCH WALKING

A. Description
   1. An accurate measurement of the client for crutches is important, because an incorrect measurement could damage the brachial plexus.
   2. The distance between the axillae and the arm pieces on the crutches should be two to three finger widths in the axilla space
   3. The elbows should be slightly flexed, 20 to 30 degrees, when the client is walking.

TABLE 59-2 Crutch Gaits

Type of Gait	Use	Procedure
Two-point gait	Used with partial weight-bearing limitations and with bilateral lower extremity prostheses	The crutch on one side and the opposite foot are advanced at the same time.
Three-point gait	Used for partial weight bearing or no weight bearing on the affected leg; requires that the client have strength and balance	Both crutches and the foot of the affected extremity are advanced together, followed by the foot of the unaffected extremity.
Four-point gait	Used if weight bearing is allowed and one foot can be placed in front of the other	The right crutch is advanced, then the left foot, then the left crutch, then the right foot.
Swing-to gait	Used when there is adequate muscle power and balance in the arms and legs	Both crutches are advanced together, then both legs are lifted and placed down on a spot behind the crutches; the feet and crutches form a tripod.
Swing-through gait	Used when there is adequate muscle power and balance in the arms and legs	Both crutches are advanced together, then both legs are lifted through and beyond the crutches and placed down again at a point in front of the crutches.

Adapted from Linton, A., & Maebius, N. (2003). *Introduction to medical-surgical nursing* (3rd ed.). Philadelphia: Saunders.

4. When ambulating with the client, stand on the affected side.
5. Instruct the client never to rest the axilla on the axillary bars.
6. Instruct the client to look up and outward when ambulating and to place the crutches 6 to 10 inches diagonally in front of the foot.
7. Instruct the client to stop ambulation if numbness or tingling in the hands or arms occurs.

B. Crutch gaits (Table 59-2)

C. Assisting the client with crutches to sit and stand.
1. Place the unaffected leg against the front of the chair.
2. Move the crutches to the affected side, and grasp the arm of the chair with the hand on the unaffected side.
3. Flex the knee of the unaffected leg to lower oneself into the chair while placing the affected leg straight out in front.
4. Reverse the steps to move from a sitting to a standing position.

D. Going up and down stairs
1. Up the stairs
   a. The client moves the unaffected leg up first.
   b. The client moves the affected leg and the crutches up.
2. Down the stairs
   a. The client moves the crutches and the affected leg down.
   b. The client moves the unaffected leg down.

VIII. CANES AND WALKERS

A. Description: Canes and walkers are made of a lightweight material with a rubber tip at the bottom.

B. Interventions
1. Stand at the affected side of the client when ambulating.
2. The handle should be at the level of the client's greater trochanter.
3. The client's elbow should be flexed at a 15- to 30-degree angle.
4. Instruct the client to hold the cane 4 to 6 inches to the side of the foot.
5. Instruct the client to hold the cane in the hand on the unaffected side so that the cane and weaker leg can work together with each step.
6. Instruct the client to move the cane at the same time as the affected leg.
7. Instruct the client to inspect the rubber tips regularly for worn places.

C. Hemicanes or quadripod canes
1. Hemicanes or quadripod canes are used for clients who have the use of only one upper extremity.
2. Hemicanes provide more security than a quadripod cane; however, both types provide more security than a single-tipped cane.
3. Position the cane at the client's unaffected side, with the straight, nonangled side adjacent to the body.
4. Position the cane 6 inches from client's side, with the handgrips level with the greater trochanter.

D. Walker
1. Stand adjacent to the client on the affected side.
2. Instruct the client to put all four points of the walker flat on the floor before putting weight on the handpieces.
3. Instruct the client to move the walker forward and to walk into it.

⚠ Safety is the priority concern when the client uses an assistive device such as a cane, walker, or crutches. Be sure that the client demonstrates correct use of the device.

IX. FRACTURED HIP

A. Types

1. Intracapsular (femoral head is broken within the joint capsule)

   a. Femoral head and neck receives decreased blood supply and heals slowly.

   b. Skin **traction** is applied preoperatively to reduce fracture, immobilize bone, and help with muscle spasms.

   c. Treatment includes a total hip replacement or open **reduction internal fixation** (ORIF) with femoral head replacement.

   d. To prevent hip displacement postoperatively, avoid extreme hip flexion.

2. Extracapsular (fracture is outside the joint capsule)

   a. Fracture can occur at the greater trochanter or can be an intertrochanteric fracture.

   b. Trochanteric fracture is outside the joint.

   c. Preoperative treatment includes balanced suspension **traction** or skin **traction** to relieve muscle spasms and reduce pain.

   d. Avoid extreme hip flexion to prevent joint displacement.

   e. Surgical treatment includes ORIF with nail plate, screws, pins, or wires.

B. Postoperative interventions

1. Maintain leg and hip in proper alignment and prevent internal or external rotation; crossing over the midline with the operative leg needs to be avoided to prevent dislocation.

2. Turn the client to the unaffected side; turn to the affected side only if prescribed by the HCP.

3. Elevate the head of the bed 30 to 45 degrees for meals only.

4. Weight bearing is usually avoided on the affected leg as prescribed; instruct the client on the use of a walker to avoid weight bearing.

5. Keep the operative leg extended, supported, and elevated when getting client out of bed.

6. Avoid hip flexion greater than 90 degrees (or above the hip) and avoid low chairs when out of bed: when sitting the client needs to keep the knees below the hips and avoid leaning forward.

7. Monitor for wound infection or hemorrhage.

8. Perform neurovascular assessment of affected extremity: check color, pulses, capillary refill, movement, and sensation.

9. Maintain the compression of the Hemovac or Jackson-Pratt drain to facilitate wound drainage if present.

10. Monitor and record drainage amount, which decreases consistently about 80 mL every 8 hours until 48 hours postoperatively.

11. Postoperative blood salvage may be done to collect, filter, and reinfuse salvaged blood into the client.

12. Use antiembolism stockings or sequential compression stockings and encourage the client to flex and extend the feet to reduce the risk of deep vein thrombosis (DVT).

13. Instruct the client to avoid crossing the legs and activities that require bending over.

14. Physical therapy will be instituted postoperatively with progressive ambulation as prescribed by the HCP.

⚠ Always check the HCP's postoperative prescriptions regarding positioning and activity restrictions following hip surgery. Restrictions may vary depending on the type of surgery, surgical approach (anterior or posterior), and HCP preference.

X. TOTAL KNEE REPLACEMENT

A. Description: Total knee replacement is the implantation of a device to substitute for the femoral condyles and the tibial joint surfaces.

B. Postoperative interventions

1. Monitor surgical incision for drainage and infection.

2. Maintain the Hemovac or Jackson-Pratt drain if in place.

3. Begin continuous passive motion 24 to 48 hours postoperatively as prescribed to exercise the knee and provide moderate flexion and extension.

4. Administer analgesics before continuous passive motion to decrease pain.

5. The leg should not be dangled to prevent dislocation.

6. Prepare the client for out-of-bed activities as prescribed.

7. Avoid weight bearing and instruct the client in crutch walking.

8. Postoperative blood salvage to collect, filter, and reinfuse salvaged blood into the client may be prescribed.

XI. JOINT DISLOCATION AND SUBLUXATION

A. Dislocation: Injury of the ligaments surrounding a joint that leads to displacement or separation of the articular surfaces of the joint

B. Subluxation: Incomplete displacement of joint surfaces when forces disrupt the soft tissue that surrounds the joints

C. Data collection

1. Asymmetry of the contour of affected body parts

2. Pain, tenderness, dysfunction, and swelling

3. Complications include neurovascular compromise, avascular necrosis, and open joint injuries.

4. X-rays are completed to determine joint shifting.

D. Interventions

1. Focus of treatment includes pain relief, joint support, and joint protection.

2. Immediate treatment is done to reduce the dislocation and realign the dislocated joint.

3. Open or closed **reduction** is done with a postprocedural joint immobilization.

4. IV conscious sedation, local, or general anesthesia is used during joint manipulation.

5. Initial activity restriction is followed by gentle range of motion and a gradual return of activities to normal levels while supporting the affected joint.

6. A weakened joint is prone to recurrent dislocation and may require extended activity restriction.

XII. HERNIATION: INTERVERTEBRAL DISK

A. Description: The nucleus of the disk protrudes into the annulus, causing nerve compression.

B. Cervical disk herniation occurs at C5-C6 and C6-C7 interspaces.

1. Cervical disk herniation causes pain radiation to shoulders, arms, hands, scapula, and pectoral muscles.

2. Motor and sensory deficits can include paresthesia, numbness, and weakness of the upper extremities.

3. Interventions

  a. Use conservative management unless the client develops signs of neurological deterioration.

  b. Advocate bedrest to decrease pressure, inflammation, and pain

  c. Immobilize the cervical area with a cervical collar, **traction**, or brace.

  d. Apply heat to reduce muscle spasms; apply ice to reduce inflammation and swelling.

  e. Maintain the head and spine in alignment.

  f. Instruct the client in the use of analgesics, sedatives, anti-inflammatory agents, and corticosteroids as prescribed.

  g. Prepare the client for a corticosteroid injection into the epidural space if prescribed.

  h. Assist and instruct client in the use of a cervical collar or cervical **traction** as prescribed.

4. A cervical collar is used for cervical disk herniation.

  a. A cervical collar limits neck movement and holds the head in a neutral or slightly flexed position.

  b. The cervical collar may be worn intermittently or 24 hours a day.

  c. Inspect skin under the collar for irritation.

  d. When approved for use and after pain decreases, exercises are prescribed to strengthen the muscles.

5. Client education related to cervical disk conditions

  a. Avoid flexing, extending, and rotating the neck.

  b. Avoid the prone position, and maintain the neck, spine, and hips in neutral position while sleeping.

  c. Minimize long periods of sitting.

  d. Instruct the client regarding medications such as analgesics, sedatives, anti-inflammatory agents, and corticosteroids.

C. Lumbar disk herniation most often occurs at L4-L5 or L5-S1 interspaces.

1. Herniation produces muscle weakness, sensory deficits, and diminished tendon reflexes.

2. The client experiences pain and muscle spasms in the lower back, with radiation of the pain into one hip and down the leg (sciatica).

3. Pain is relieved by bedrest and aggravated by movement, lifting, straining, and coughing.

4. Interventions

  a. Conservative management is indicated unless neurological deterioration or bowel and bladder dysfunction occurs.

  b. Apply moist heat to decrease muscle spasms and apply ice to decrease inflammation.

  c. Instruct the client to sleep on the side, with the knees and hips flexed, and place a pillow between the legs.

  d. Apply pelvic **traction** as prescribed to relieve muscle spasms and decrease pain.

  e. Begin progressive ambulation as inflammation, edema, and pain subside.

5. Client education related to lumbar disk conditions

  a. Instruct the client in the use of prescribed medications such as analgesics, muscle relaxants, anti-inflammatory agents, or corticosteroids.

  b. Instruct the client about application techniques for corsets or braces to maintain immobilization and proper spine alignment.

  c. Instruct the client on correct posture while sitting, standing, walking, and working.

  d. Instruct the client on the correct technique to use when lifting objects such as bending knees, maintaining a straight back, and avoiding lifting objects above the elbow.

  e. Instruct in weight control program as prescribed.

  f. Instruct the client in an exercise program to strengthen back and abdominal muscles as prescribed.

D. Disk surgery is used when spinal cord compression is suspected or client symptoms do not respond to conservative or minimally invasive treatment (Box 59-4).

1. Preoperative interventions

  a. Provide routine preoperative instructions related to postoperative care.

  b. Instruct the client about logrolling and range-of-motion exercises.

Box 59-4 Types of Disk Surgery

Diskectomy: Removal of herniated disk tissue and related matter
Diskectomy with fusion: Fusion of vertebrae with bone graft
Laminectomy: Excision of part of the vertebrae (lamina) to remove the disk
Laminotomy: Division of the lamina of a vertebra

2. Postoperative interventions: Cervical disk
   a. Monitor for respiratory difficulty from inflammation or hematoma.
   b. Encourage coughing, deep breathing, and early ambulation as prescribed.
   c. Monitor for hoarseness and inability to cough effectively, because this may indicate laryngeal nerve damage.
   d. Use throat sprays or lozenges for sore throat, avoiding anesthetic lozenges that may numb the throat and increase choking risks.
   e. Monitor the surgical wound for infection, swelling, redness, drainage, or pain
   f. Provide a soft diet if the client complains of dysphagia.
   g. Monitor for sudden return of radicular pain, which may indicate cervical spine instability.

3. Postoperative interventions: lumbar disk
   a. Monitor for wound hemorrhage and presence of any cerebrospinal fluid (CSF).
   b. Monitor lower extremities for sensation, movement, color, temperature, and paresthesia.
   c. Monitor for urinary retention, paralytic ileus, and constipation, which can result from decreased movement, opioid administration, or spinal cord compression.
   d. Prevent constipation by encouraging a high-fiber diet, increased fluid intake, and stool softeners, as prescribed.
   e. Administer opioids and sedatives as prescribed to relieve pain and anxiety.
   f. Assist and instruct the client to apply a prescribed back brace or corset with cotton underwear to prevent skin irritation.

4. Postoperative lumbar disk positioning concerns
   a. In the immediate postoperative period, the client may be expected to lie supine or have other activity restrictions depending on specific surgical intervention.
   b. Instruct the client to avoid spinal flexion or twisting and that the spine should be kept aligned.
   c. Instruct the client to minimize sitting, which may place a strain on the surgical site.
   d. When the client is lying supine, place a pillow under the neck and slightly flex the knees.
   e. Avoid extreme hip flexion when lying on side.

▲ **FIGURE 59-4** Common levels of lower-extremity amputation. (From Ignatavicius, D., & Workman, M. [2010]. *Medical-surgical nursing: Patient-centered collaborative care* [6th ed.]. St. Louis: Saunders.)

⚠ Following disk surgery, instruct the client in correct logrolling techniques for turning and repositioning and for getting out of bed.

XIII. AMPUTATION OF A LOWER EXTREMITY (Figure 59-4)

A. Description: Amputation is the surgical removal of a limb or part of the limb.
B. Postoperative interventions
   1. Monitor vital signs.
   2. Monitor for infection and hemorrhage.
   3. Mark bleeding and drainage on the dressing if it occurs.
   4. Have a surgical tourniquet readily available and notify the HCP immediately if bleeding occurs.
   5. Observe for and prevent contractures, which can result from prolonged residual limb elevation.
   6. Monitor for signs of infection, necrosis, and neuroma.
   7. Evaluate for phantom limb sensation and pain; explain sensation and pain to the client, and medicate the client as prescribed.
   8. First 24 hours: Elevate the foot of the bed to reduce edema, then keep the bed flat to prevent hip flexion contractures, if prescribed by the HCP.
   9. After 24 to 48 hours postoperatively, position the client prone to stretch the muscles and prevent hip flexion contractures, if prescribed.
   10. To prevent hip flexion contractures, do not elevate the residual limb on a pillow.

11. Maintain surgical application of dressing, elastic compression wrap, or elastic stump (residual limb) shrinker, as prescribed, to reduce swelling, minimize pain, and mold the residual limb in preparation for prosthesis.

12. Wash the residual limb with mild soap and water and dry completely.

13. Massage the skin toward the suture line to mobilize scar and prevent its adherence to underlying bone.

14. Prepare for the prosthesis and instruct the client in progressive resistive techniques by gently pushing the residual limb against pillows and progressing to firmer surfaces.

15. Encourage verbalization regarding loss of the body part, and assist the client to identify coping mechanisms to deal with the loss.

C. Interventions for below-the-knee amputation
1. Prevent edema.
2. Do not allow the residual limb to hang over the edge of the bed.
3. Discourage long periods of sitting to lessen complications of knee flexion.

D. Interventions for above-the-knee amputation
1. Prevent internal or external rotation of the limb.
2. Place a sandbag, rolled towel, or trochanter roll along the outside of the thigh to prevent external rotation.

E. Rehabilitation
1. Instruct the client in crutch walking.
2. Prepare the residual limb for a prosthesis.
3. Prepare the client for fitting of the residual limb for a prosthesis.
4. Instruct the client in exercises to maintain range of motion and upper body strengthening.
5. Provide psychosocial support to the client

XIV. RHEUMATOID ARTHRITIS

A. Description
1. Rheumatoid arthritis is a chronic systemic inflammatory disease (immune complex–disorder); the cause may be related to a combination of environmental and genetic factors.
2. Rheumatoid arthritis leads to destruction of connective tissue and synovial membrane within the joints.
3. Rheumatoid arthritis weakens the joint, leading to dislocation, and permanent deformity of the joint.
4. Formation of pannus occurs at the junction of synovial tissue and articular cartilage and projects into the joint cavity, causing necrosis.
5. Exacerbations of disease manifestations occur during periods of physical or emotional stress and fatigue.

6. Vasculitis can impede blood flow, leading to organ or organ system malfunction and failure because of tissue ischemia.

B. Data collection
1. Inflammation, tenderness, and stiffness of the joints
2. Moderate to severe pain with morning stiffness lasting longer than 30 minutes
3. Joint deformities, muscle atrophy, and decreased range of motion in affected joints
4. Spongy, soft feeling in the joints
5. Low-grade temperature, fatigue, and weakness
6. Anorexia, weight loss, and anemia
7. Elevated sedimentation rate and positive rheumatoid factor
8. Radiographic study showing joint deterioration
9. Synovial tissue biopsy reveals inflammation

C. Rheumatoid factor
1. A blood test used to assist in the diagnosis
2. Values
   a. Nonreactive: 0 to 39 international units/mL
   b. Weakly reactive: 40 to 79 international units/mL
   c. Reactive: greater than 80 international units/mL

D. Pain: A combination of pharmacological therapies including NSAIDs, disease-modifying antirheumatic drugs (DMARDs), and glucocorticoids

E. Physical mobility
1. Preserve joint function.
2. Provide range-of-motion exercises to maintain joint motion and muscle strengthening.
3. Balance rest and activity.
4. Splints may be used during acute inflammation to prevent deformity.
5. Prevent flexion contractures.
6. Apply heat or cold therapy to joints as prescribed.
7. Apply paraffin baths and massage as prescribed.
8. Encourage consistency with exercise program.
9. Use joint-protecting devices.
10. Avoid weight bearing on inflamed joints.

F. Self-care (Box 59-5)
1. Assess the need for assistive devices such as raised toilet seats, self-rising chairs, wheelchairs, and scooters to facilitate mobility.
2. Collaborate with an occupational therapist or HCP to obtain assistive or adaptive devices.
3. Instruct the client in alternative strategies for providing activities of daily living.

G. Fatigue
1. Identify factors that may contribute to fatigue.
2. Monitor for signs of anemia, and administer iron, folic acid, and vitamins as prescribed.
3. Monitor for medication-related blood loss by testing the stool for occult blood.

Box 59-5 Client Education for Rheumatoid Arthritis and Degenerative Joint Disease

Assist the client to identify and correct safety hazards in the home.

Instruct the client on the correct use of assistive or adaptive devices.

Instruct the client in energy conservation measures.

Review the prescribed exercise program.

Instruct the client to sit in a chair with a high, straight back.

Instruct the client to use only a small pillow when lying down.

Instruct the client on measures to protect the joints.

Instruct the client regarding prescribed medications.

Stress the importance of follow-up visits with the HCP.

---

4. Instruct the client in measures to conserve energy, such as pacing activities and obtaining assistance when possible.

H. Disturbed body image
1. Assess the client's reaction to the body change.
2. Encourage the client to verbalize feelings.
3. Assist the client with self-care activities and grooming.
4. Encourage the client to wear street clothes.

I. Surgical interventions: Minimally invasive procedures may be prescribed.
1. Synovectomy: surgical removal of the synovia to help maintain joint function
2. Arthrodesis: bony fusion of a joint to regain some mobility
3. Joint replacement (arthroplasty): surgical replacement of diseased joints with artificial joints, which is performed to restore motion to a joint and function to the muscles, ligaments, and other soft tissue structures that control a joint

XV. OSTEOARTHRITIS (DEGENERATIVE JOINT DISEASE)

A. Description
1. Osteoarthritis is progressive degeneration of the joints as a result of wear and tear.
2. It causes the formation of bony buildup and the loss of articular cartilage in peripheral and axial joints.
3. Osteoarthritis affects the weight-bearing joints and joints that receive the greatest stress, such as the hips, knees, and lower vertebral column and hands.
4. Primary osteoarthritis is usually a result of trauma or another joint insult; there is no known cause for idiopathic osteoarthritis.

B. Data collection
1. Client experiences joint pain that diminishes after rest and intensifies after activity, noted early in the disease process

2. As disease progresses, pain occurs with slight motion or even at rest
3. Symptoms aggravated by temperature change and climate humidity
4. Presence of Heberden's nodes or Bouchard's nodes
5. Joint swelling, crepitus, and limited range of motion
6. Difficulty getting up after prolonged sitting
7. Skeletal muscle disuse atrophy
8. Inability to perform activities of daily living
9. Compression of the spine as manifested by radiating pain, stiffness, and muscle spasms in one or both extremities

C. Pain
1. Administer NSAIDs, muscle relaxants, and other medications as prescribed.
2. Prepare the client for corticosteroid injections into joints as prescribed.
3. Position the joints in function position and avoid flexion of knees and hips.
4. Immobilize the affected joint with a splint or brace until inflammation subsides.
5. Avoid large pillows under the head or knees.
6. Provide a bed or foot cradle to keep linen off the feet.
7. Instruct the client on the importance of moist heat, hot packs or compresses, and paraffin dips as prescribed.
8. Apply cold applications as prescribed when the joint is acutely inflamed.
9. Encourage adequate rest, recommending 10 hours of sleep at night and a 1- to 2-hour nap in the afternoon.

D. Nutrition
1. Encourage a well-balanced diet.
2. Maintain weight within normal range to decrease stress on the joints.

E. Physical mobility
1. Instruct the client to balance activity with rest while participating in an exercise program that limits stressing affected joints.
2. Instruct the client that exercises should be active rather than passive and to stop exercise if pain occurs.
3. Instruct the client to limit exercise when joint inflammation is severe.

F. Surgical management: Minimally invasive procedures may be prescribed.
1. Osteotomy: The bone is resected to correct joint deformity, promote realignment, and reduce joint stress.
2. Total joint replacement or arthroplasty
   a. Total joint replacement is performed when all measures of pain relief have failed.
   b. Hips and knees are replaced most commonly.
   c. Total joint replacement is contraindicated in the presence of infection, advanced osteoporosis, or severe joint inflammation.

Box 59-6 Risk Factors for Osteoporosis

Cigarette smoking
Early menopause
Excessive use of alcohol
Family history
Female gender
Increasing age
Insufficient intake of calcium
Sedentary lifestyle
Thin, small frame
White (European descent) or Asian race

XVI. OSTEOPOROSIS

A. Description
1. Osteoporosis is an age-related metabolic disease.
2. Bone demineralizes, losing calcium and phosphorous salts, leading to fragile bones and subsequent fractures.
3. Bone resorption accelerates as bone formation slows.
4. Osteoporosis occurs most commonly in the wrist, hip, and vertebral column.
5. Osteoporosis can occur postmenopausally or as a result of a metabolic disorder or calcium deficiency.
6. The client may be asymptomatic until the bones become fragile and a minor injury or movement causes a pathological fracture.
7. Primary osteoporosis
   a. Most often occurs in postmenopausal women
   b. Risk factors include decreased calcium intake, deficient estrogen, and limited exercise.
8. Secondary osteoporosis
   a. Causes include prolonged therapy with corticosteroids, thyroid-reducing medications, aluminum-containing antacids, or anticonvulsants
   b. Associated with immobility, alcoholism, malnutrition, or malabsorption
9. Risk factors (Box 59-6)

B. Data collection
1. Possibly asymptomatic
2. Back pain can occur after lifting, bending, or stooping.
3. Back pain that increases with palpation
4. Pelvic or hip pain, especially with weight bearing
5. Problems with balance
6. Decline in height from vertebral compression
7. Kyphosis of the dorsal spine also known as "dowager's hump"
8. Degeneration of lower thorax and lumber vertebrae on radiographic studies

> ⚠ The client with osteoporosis is at risk for pathological fractures.

C. Interventions
1. Assess risk for and prevent injury in the client's personal environment.
   a. Assist the client to identify and correct hazards in his or her environment.
   b. Position household items and furniture for an unobstructed walkway.
   c. Use side rails to prevent falls.
   d. Instruct in the use of assistive devices such as a cane or walker.
   e. Encourage use of a firm mattress.
2. Provide personal care to the client to reduce injuries.
   a. Move the client gently when turning and repositioning.
   b. Assist with ambulation if client is unsteady.
   c. Provide gentle range-of-motion exercises.
   d. Apply a back brace as prescribed during an acute phase to immobilize the spine and provide spinal column support.
3. Provide client instructions to promote optimal level of health and function
   a. Instruct the client in the use of good body mechanics
   b. Instruct the client in exercises to strengthen abdominal and back muscles to improve posture and provide support for the spine.
   c. Instruct the client to avoid activities that can cause vertebral compression.
   d. Instruct the client to eat a diet high in protein, calcium, vitamins C and D, and iron.
   e. Instruct the client to avoid alcohol and coffee.
   f. Instruct the client to maintain an adequate fluid intake to prevent renal calculi.
4. Administer medication to promote bone strength and decrease pain.
   a. Administer calcium, vitamin D, and phosphorus as prescribed for bone metabolism.
   b. Administer calcitonin as prescribed to inhibit bone loss.
   c. Administer estrogen or androgens to decrease the rate of bone resorption as prescribed.
   d. Administer analgesics, muscle relaxants, anti-inflammatory medications and biophosphonates as prescribed.

XVII. GOUT

A. Description
1. Gout is a systemic disease in which urate crystals deposit in joints and other body tissues.
2. Gout leads to abnormal amounts of uric acid in the body.
3. Primary gout results from a disorder of purine metabolism.
4. Secondary gout involves excessive uric acid in the blood that is caused by another disease.

B. Phases
1. Asymptomatic: Client has no symptoms but serum uric acid is elevated
2. Acute: Client has excruciating pain and inflammation of one or more small joints, especially the great toe
3. Intermittent: Client has intermittent periods without symptoms between acute attacks
4. Chronic: Results from repeated episodes of acute gout
   a. Chronic gout results in deposits of urate crystals under the skin.
   b. Chronic gout results in deposits of urate crystals within major organs such as kidneys, leading to organ dysfunction.

 C. Data collection
1. Swelling and inflammation of the joints, leading to excruciating pain
2. Tophi: Hard, irregular-shaped nodules in the skin containing chalky deposits of sodium urate
3. Low-grade fever, malaise, and headache
4. Pruritis from urate crystals in the skin
5. Presence of renal stones from elevated uric acid levels

D. Interventions
1. Provide a low-purine diet as prescribed; foods such as organ meats, wines, and aged cheese should be avoided.
2. Encourage a high fluid intake of 2000 mL to prevent stone formation.
3. Encourage a weight-reduction diet if required.
4. Instruct the client to avoid alcohol and starvation diets, because they may precipitate a gout attack.
5. Increase urinary pH (above 6) by eating alkaline ash foods such as milk and other dairy products.
6. Provide bedrest during the acute attacks with affected extremity elevated.
7. Monitor joint range-of-motion ability and for swelling and inflammation.
8. Position the joint in mild flexion during an acute attack.
9. Protect the affected joint from excessive movement or direct contact with sheets or blankets.
10. Provide heat or cold for local treatments to the affected joint as prescribed.
11. Administer medications such as analgesics, anti-inflammatory medications, and uricosuric agents as prescribed.

MORE QUESTIONS ON EVOLVE!

Practice Questions

621. A nurse is one of several people who witness a vehicle hit a pedestrian at a fairly low speed on a small street. The individual is dazed and tries to get up, and the leg appears fractured. The nurse would plan to:
1. Try to manually reduce the fracture.
2. Assist the person to get up and walk to the sidewalk.
3. Leave the person for a few moments to call an ambulance.
4. Stay with the person and encourage the person to remain still.

622. A nurse witnesses a client sustain a fall and suspects that the client's leg may be fractured. Which action is the priority?
1. Take a set of vital signs.
2. Call the radiology department.
3. Immobilize the leg before moving the client.
4. Reassure the client that everything will be fine.

623. A client with a hip fracture asks the nurse why Buck's extension traction is being applied before surgery. The nurse's response is based on the understanding that Buck's extension traction primarily:
1. Allows bony healing to begin before surgery
2. Provides rigid immobilization of the fracture site
3. Lengthens the fractured leg to prevent severing of blood vessels
4. Provides comfort by reducing muscle spasms and provides fracture immobilization

624. A nurse is evaluating the pin sites of a client in skeletal traction. The nurse would be least concerned with which finding?
1. Inflammation
2. Serous drainage
3. Pain at a pin site
4. Purulent drainage

625. A nurse is caring for the client who has had skeletal traction applied to the left leg. The client is complaining of severe left leg pain. Which action should the nurse take first?
1. Provide pin care.
2. Call the health care provider (HCP).
3. Check the client's alignment in bed.
4. Medicate the client with an analgesic.

626. A nurse has provided instructions regarding specific leg exercises for the client immobilized in right skeletal lower leg traction. The nurse determines that the client needs further instruction if the nurse observes the client:
1. Pulling up on the trapeze
2. Flexing and extending the feet
3. Doing quadriceps-setting and gluteal-setting exercises
4. Performing active range of motion (ROM) to the right ankle and knee

627. A nurse is checking the casted extremity of a client. The nurse would check for which of the following signs and symptoms indicative of infection?
1. Dependent edema
2. Diminished distal pulse
3. Presence of a "hot spot" on the cast
4. Coolness and pallor of the extremity

628. A client has sustained a closed fracture and has just had a cast applied to the affected arm. The client is complaining of intense pain. The nurse has elevated the limb, applied an ice bag, and administered an analgesic, which was ineffective in relieving the pain. The nurse interprets that this pain may be caused by:
1. Infection under the cast
2. The anxiety of the client
3. Impaired tissue perfusion
4. The newness of the fracture

629. A nurse is assigned to care for a client with multiple traumas who is admitted to the hospital. The client has a leg fracture, and a plaster cast has been applied. In positioning the casted leg, the nurse should:
1. Keep the leg in a level position.
2. Elevate the leg for 3 hours, and put it flat for 1 hour.
3. Keep the leg level for 3 hours, and elevate it for 1 hour.
4. Elevate the leg on pillows continuously for 24 to 48 hours.

630. A client is complaining of skin irritation from the edges of a cast applied the previous day. The nurse should plan for which of the following actions?
1. Massaging the skin at the rim of the cast
2. Petaling the cast edges with adhesive tape
3. Using a rough file to smooth the cast edges
4. Applying lotion to the skin at the rim of the cast

631. A client is being discharged home after application of a plaster leg cast. The nurse determines that the client understands proper care of the cast if the client states to:
1. Avoid getting the cast wet.
2. Cover the casted leg with warm blankets.
3. Use the fingertips to lift and move the leg.
4. Use a padded coat hanger end to scratch under the cast.

632. A nurse is planning to provide instructions to the client about how to stand on crutches. In the instructions, the nurse plans to tell the client to place the crutches:
1. 3 inches to the front and side of the client's toes
2. 8 inches to the front and side of the client's toes
3. 20 inches to the front and side of the client's toes
4. 15 inches to the front and side of the client's toes

633. A nurse is evaluating the client's use of a cane for left-sided weakness. The nurse would intervene and correct the client if the nurse observed that the client:
1. Holds the cane on the right side
2. Moves the cane when the right leg is moved
3. Leans on the cane when the right leg swings through
4. Keeps the cane 6 inches out to the side of the right foot

634. A nurse is caring for a client with fresh application of a plaster leg cast. The nurse plans to prevent the development of compartment syndrome by:
1. Elevating the limb and applying ice to the affected leg
2. Elevating the limb and covering the limb with bath blankets
3. Keeping the leg horizontal and applying ice to the affected leg
4. Placing the leg in a slightly dependent position and applying ice

635. A nurse is preparing a list of cast care instructions for a client who just had a plaster cast applied to his right forearm. Which instructions should the nurse include on the list? **Select all that apply.**
☐ 1. Keep the cast and extremity elevated.
☐ 2. The cast needs to be kept clean and dry.
☐ 3. Allow the wet cast 24 to 72 hours to dry.
☐ 4. Expect tingling and numbness in the extremity.
☐ 5. Use a hair dryer set on a warm to hot setting to dry the cast.
☐ 6. Use a soft padded object that will fit under the cast to scratch the skin under the cast.

ANSWERS

621. 4

Rationale: With a suspected fracture, the client is not moved unless it is dangerous to remain in that spot. The nurse should remain with the client and have someone else call for emergency help. A fracture is not reduced at the scene. Before moving the client, the site of the fracture is immobilized to prevent further injury.

Test-Taking Strategy: Use the process of elimination. Eliminate options 1 and 2 first, because these actions could result in further injury to the client. From the remaining options, the most prudent action would be for the nurse to remain with

the client and have someone else call for emergency assistance. Review immediate care of the client with a fracture if you had difficulty with this question.
Level of Cognitive Ability: Applying
Client Needs: Physiological Integrity
Integrated Process: Nursing Process/Implementation
Content Area: Adult Health/Musculoskeletal
Reference: Christensen, Kockrow, p. 758. 2011. *Foundations of nursing.*

622. 3
Rationale: When a fracture is suspected, it is imperative that the area is splinted before the client is moved. Emergency help should be called if the client is not hospitalized; a health care provider is called for the hospitalized client. The nurse should remain with the client and provide realistic reassurance. The nurse does not prescribe radiology tests.
Test-Taking Strategy: Note the strategic word "priority." Eliminate option 2, because the nurse does not prescribe x-rays. Option 4 is eliminated next, because the nurse never tells a client that "everything will be fine." From the remaining options, focus on the data in the question. Immobilizing the limb is imperative for the client's safety, which makes it a better choice than taking vital signs. Review care of the client when a fracture is suspected if you had difficulty with this question.
Level of Cognitive Ability: Applying
Client Needs: Physiological Integrity
Integrated Process: Nursing Process/Implementation
Content Area: Adult Health/Musculoskeletal
References: Christensen, Kockrow, p.758. 2011. *Foundations of nursing.*
deWit, p. 786. 2009.

623. 4
Rationale: Buck's extension traction is a type of skin traction often applied after hip fracture, before the fracture is reduced in surgery. It reduces muscle spasms and helps immobilize the fracture. It does not lengthen the leg for the purpose of preventing blood vessel severance. It also does not allow for bony healing to begin.
Test-Taking Strategy: Use the process of elimination. Recalling the purpose of traction will assist in eliminating options 1 and 3. From the remaining options, eliminate option 2 because of the words "rigid immobilization." Review this type of traction if you had difficulty with this question.
Level of Cognitive Ability: Applying
Client Needs: Physiological Integrity
Integrated Process: Nursing Process/Implementation
Content Area: Adult Health/Musculoskeletal
Reference: Christensen, Kockrow, pp. 156–157. 2011. *Adult health nursing.*

624. 2
Rationale: A small amount of serous drainage is expected at pin insertion sites. Signs of infection such as inflammation, purulent drainage, and pain at the pin site are not expected findings and should be reported.
Test-Taking Strategy: Note the strategic words "least concerned with." Options 1 and 4 indicate infection and are eliminated. To select between options 2 and 3, look at them carefully. The complaint of pain is at "a pin site" only. It gives

no indication that the pain is related to the fracture or muscle spasm. Because serous drainage is an expected finding, you would select this over the complaint of pain. Review care of the client in skeletal traction if you had difficulty with this question.
Level of Cognitive Ability: Evaluating
Client Needs: Physiological Integrity
Integrated Process: Nursing Process/Evaluation
Content Area: Adult Health/Musculoskeletal
References: Christensen, Kockrow, p. 157. 2011. *Adult health nursing.*
Linton, p. 969. 2012.

625. 3
Rationale: A client who complains of severe pain may need realignment or may have had traction weights prescribed that are too heavy. The nurse realigns the client and, if ineffective, calls the HCP. Severe leg pain, once traction has been established, indicates a problem. Medicating the client should be done after trying to determine and treat the cause. Providing pin care is unrelated to the problem as described.
Test-Taking Strategy: Note the strategic word "first." Use the steps of the nursing process. Option 3 is the only option that addresses data collection. Review care of the client in skeletal traction if you had difficulty with this question.
Level of Cognitive Ability: Applying
Client Needs: Physiological Integrity
Integrated Process: Nursing Process/Implementation
Content Area: Adult Health/Musculoskeletal
References: Christensen, Kockrow, p. 157. 2011. *Adult health nursing.*
deWit, p. 793. 2009.
Linton, p. 969. 2012.

626. 4
Rationale: Exercise is indicated within therapeutic limits for the client in skeletal traction to maintain muscle strength and ROM. The client may pull up on the trapeze, perform active ROM with uninvolved joints, and do isometric muscle-setting exercises (e.g., quadriceps- and gluteal-setting exercises). The client may also flex and extend his or her feet.
Test-Taking Strategy: Note the strategic words "needs further instruction." These words indicate a negative event query and the need to select the incorrect client action. Options 1 and 3 are most easily identified as correct actions and are therefore eliminated as possible answers. To select between options 2 and 4, imagine the lines of pull on the fracture site with the movements described. Although flexing and extending the feet does not disrupt the line of pull from the traction, performing active ROM to the affected knee and ankle does. Review care of the client in traction if you had difficulty with this question.
Level of Cognitive Ability: Evaluating
Client Needs: Physiological Integrity
Integrated Process: Teaching and Learning
Content Area: Adult Health/Musculoskeletal
References: Christensen, Kockrow, p. 157. 2011. *Adult health nursing.*
Lewis, Dirksen, Heitkemper, Bucher, Camera, p. 1600. 2011.

627. 3
Rationale: Signs and symptoms of infection under a casted area include odor or purulent drainage from the cast, or the

presence of "hot spots," which are areas of the cast that are warmer than others. The health care provider should be notified if any of these occur. Signs of impaired circulation in the distal limb include coolness and pallor of the skin, diminished arterial pulse, and edema.

Test-Taking Strategy: Begin to answer this question by thinking of what you would expect to find with infection: redness, swelling, heat, and purulent drainage. With these in mind, options 2 and 4 can be eliminated. To select between options 1 and 3, "dependent edema" is not necessarily indicative of infection; swelling would be continuous. The "hot spot" on the cast could signify infection underneath that area. Review the complications of a cast if you had difficulty with this question.

Level of Cognitive Ability: Applying
Client Needs: Physiological Integrity
Integrated Process: Nursing Process/Data Collection
Content Area: Adult Health/Musculoskeletal
References: deWit, p. 791. 2009.
Ignatavicius, Workman, p. 1189. 2010.

628. 3

Rationale: Most pain associated with fractures can be minimized with rest, elevation, application of cold, and administration of analgesics. Pain that is not relieved from these measures should be reported to the health care provider, because it may be the result of impaired tissue perfusion, tissue breakdown, or necrosis. Because this is a new closed fracture and cast, infection would not have had time to set in.

Test-Taking Strategy: Use the process of elimination. Options 2 and 4 can be eliminated first, based on the description in the question. Because the fracture and cast are so new, it is extremely unlikely that infection could have set in. The most likely option is impaired tissue perfusion, because pain from ischemia is not relieved by comfort measures and analgesics. Review the complications of a cast if you had difficulty with this question.

Level of Cognitive Ability: Analyzing
Client Needs: Physiological Integrity
Integrated Process: Nursing Process/Data Collection
Content Area: Adult Health/Musculoskeletal
References: deWit, pp. 790–791. 2009.
Linton, p. 972 . 2012.

629. 4

Rationale: A casted extremity is elevated continuously for the first 24 to 48 hours to minimize swelling and to promote venous drainage. Therefore, the other options are incorrect.

Test-Taking Strategy: Use the process of elimination. Recall that edema sets in after fracture and can be aggravated by casting. For this reason, options 1 and 3 are the least helpful and can be eliminated first. There is no useful purpose for the timing in option 2. Review care of the client with a cast if you had difficulty with this question.

Level of Cognitive Ability: Applying
Client Needs: Physiological Integrity
Integrated Process: Nursing Process/Implementation
Content Area: Adult Health/Musculoskeletal
Reference: Christensen, Kockrow, pp. 154–155. 2011. *Adult health nursing.*

630. 2

Rationale: The edges of the cast can be petaled with tape to minimize skin irritation. If a client has a cast applied and returns home, the client can be taught to do the same. Massaging and applying lotion will not alleviate the skin irritation from the cast edges. Filing the edges will cause cast material to fall into the cast and could lead to skin irritation under the cast.

Test-Taking Strategy: Use the process of elimination. Options 1 and 4 are comparable or alike, and neither helps to get rid of the cause of the irritation, so they are eliminated first. Imagine the use of a "rough file"; it would create plaster chips and dust, which could go underneath the cast. Review cast petaling if you had difficulty with this question.

Level of Cognitive Ability: Applying
Client Needs: Physiological Integrity
Integrated Process: Nursing Process/Planning
Content Area: Adult Health/Musculoskeletal
Reference: deWit, pp. 791, 793. 2009.

631. 1

Rationale: A plaster cast must remain dry to keep its strength. The cast should be handled using the palms of the hands, not the fingertips, until fully dry. Air should circulate freely around the cast to help it dry; the cast also gives off heat as it dries. The client should never scratch under the cast; a cool hair dryer may be used to eliminate itching.

Test-Taking Strategy: Knowledge of cast care is needed to answer this question. Knowing that a wet cast can be dented with the fingertips, causing pressure underneath, helps you eliminate option 3 first. Knowing that the cast needs to dry helps you eliminate option 2 next. Option 4 is dangerous to skin integrity and is also eliminated. Plaster casts, once they have dried after application, should not become wet. Review home care instructions for a client with a cast if you had difficulty with this question.

Level of Cognitive Ability: Evaluating
Client Needs: Physiological Integrity
Integrated Process: Nursing Process/Evaluation
Content Area: Adult Health/Musculoskeletal
Reference: Linton, p. 968. 2012.

632. 2

Rationale: The classic tripod position is taught to the client before giving instructions on gait. The crutches are placed anywhere from 6 to 10 inches in front and to the side of the client, depending on the client's body size. This provides a wide enough base of support to the client and improves balance.

Test-Taking Strategy: Use the process of elimination and visualize each position. Three inches and 20 inches seem excessively short and long, respectively. These options can be eliminated first. Of the remaining options, 8 inches seems more in keeping with the normal length of a stride than 15 inches. Review crutch walking if you had difficulty with this question.

Level of Cognitive Ability: Applying
Client Needs: Safe and Effective Care Environment
Integrated Process: Teaching and Learning
Content Area: Adult Health/Musculoskeletal
Reference: Linton, pp. 969–970. 2012.

633. 2

Rationale: The cane is held on the stronger side to minimize stress on the affected extremity and provide a wide base of support. The cane is held 6 inches lateral to the fifth great toe. The cane is moved forward with the affected leg. The client leans on the cane for added support while the stronger side swings through.

Test-Taking Strategy: Note the strategic word "intervenes." This word indicates a negative event query and the need to select the incorrect client action. Knowing that the cane is held on the stronger side helps you eliminate options 1 and 4 first. To select from the remaining options, recall that the client moves the cane with the weaker leg and leans on it for support when the stronger leg swings through. Review client instructions for cane walking if you had difficulty with this question.

Level of Cognitive Ability: Applying
Client Needs: Safe and Effective Care Environment
Integrated Process: Teaching and Learning
Content Area: Adult Health/Musculoskeletal
References: deWit, p. 779. 2009.
Linton, p. 971. 2012.

634. 1

Rationale: Compartment syndrome is prevented by controlling edema. This is achieved most optimally with elevation and application of ice. Therefore, the other options are incorrect.

Test-Taking Strategy: Use the process of elimination. Recalling that edema is controlled or prevented with limb elevation helps you eliminate options 3 and 4 first. From the remaining options, think about the effects of ice versus bath blankets. Ice will further control edema, but bath blankets will produce heat and prevent air circulation needed for the cast to dry. Review measures to prevent compartment syndrome if you had difficulty with this question.

Level of Cognitive Ability: Applying
Client Needs: Physiological Integrity
Integrated Process: Teaching and Learning
Content Area: Adult Health/Musculoskeletal
Reference: Linton, p. 963. 2012.

635. 1, 2, 3

Rationale: A plaster cast takes 24 to 72 hours to dry (synthetic casts dry in 20 minutes). The cast and extremity may be elevated to reduce edema. A wet cast is handled with the palms of the hand until it is dry, and the extremity is turned (unless contraindicated) so that all sides of the wet cast will dry. A cool setting on the hair dryer can be used to dry a plaster cast. (Heat cannot be used on a plaster cast, because the cast heats up and burns the skin.) The cast needs to be kept clean and dry, and the client is instructed not to stick anything under the cast because of the risk of breaking skin integrity. The client is instructed to monitor the extremity for circulatory impairment such as pain, swelling, discoloration, tingling, numbness, coolness, or diminished pulse. The health care provider is notified immediately if circulatory impairment occurs.

Test-Taking Strategy: Focus on the subject, a plaster cast. Recalling that edema occurs following a fracture and recalling the complications associated with a cast will assist you in answering the question. Review cast care instructions if you had difficulty with this question.

Level of Cognitive Ability: Applying
Client Needs: Physiological Integrity
Integrated Process: Teaching and Learning
Content Area: Adult Health/Musculoskeletal
References: deWit, p. 788. 2009.
Christensen, Kockrow, pp. 154–155. 2011. *Adult health nursing.*

Musculoskeletal Medications

I. SKELETAL MUSCLE RELAXANTS

A. Description

1. Skeletal muscle relaxants (Box 60-1) act directly on the neuromuscular junction or act indirectly on the central nervous system (CNS).
2. Centrally acting muscle relaxants depress neuron activity in the spinal cord or brain.
3. Peripherally acting muscle relaxants act directly on the skeletal muscles, interfering with calcium release from muscle tubules and thus preventing the fibers from contracting.
4. Skeletal muscle relaxants are used to prevent or relieve muscle spasms and treat spasticity associated with spinal cord disease or lesions, acute painful musculoskeletal conditions, and chronic debilitating disorders such as multiple sclerosis, brain attacks (stroke), or cerebral palsy.
5. Skeletal muscle relaxants are contraindicated in clients with severe liver, renal, or heart disease; these medications are often metabolized in the liver or excreted from the kidney.
6. Skeletal muscle relaxants should not be taken with CNS depressants, such as barbiturates, opioids, alcohol, sedatives, hypnotics, or tricyclic antidepressants, unless specifically prescribed.

B. Side effects

1. Dizziness and hypotension
2. Drowsiness and muscle weakness
3. Dry mouth
4. Gastrointestinal upset
5. Photosensitivity
6. Liver toxicity

C. Interventions

1. Obtain a medical history.
2. Monitor vital signs.
3. Monitor for CNS side effects.
4. Determine risk for injury.
5. Monitor involved joints and muscles for pain and mobility.
6. Monitor renal function studies.
7. The client is instructed to take the medication with food to decrease gastrointestinal upset.
8. The client is instructed to report side effects.

9. The client is instructed to avoid alcohol and CNS depressants.
10. The client is instructed to avoid activities requiring alertness such as driving or operating equipment.

⚠ Monitor liver function tests when a client is taking a skeletal muscle relaxant because hepatotoxicity can occur.

D. Nursing considerations

1. Baclofen (Lioresal)
   a. Baclofen causes CNS effects such as drowsiness, dizziness, weakness, and fatigue and nausea, constipation, and urinary retention.
   b. Administered with caution in the client with renal or hepatic dysfunction or a seizure disorder.
   c. Baclofen can be administered by the health care provider through intrathecal infusion using an implantable pump or direct intrathecal administration over 1 minute.
   d. The client with an implantable pump is instructed to maintain medication refill appointments to prevent the pump from emptying and experiencing sudden withdrawal symptoms (which could be life threatening).
2. Carisoprodol (Soma)
   a. The client is advised to take the medication with food to prevent gastrointestinal upset.
   b. The client is instructed to report any rash or hypersensitivity to the health care provider (HCP).
3. Chlorzoxazone (Paraflex, Parafon Forte DSC, Remular-S)
   a. Monitor the client for hypersensitivity reactions such as urticaria, redness or itching, and possibly angioedema.
   b. Chlorzoxazone may cause malaise and may cause the urine to turn orange or red.
   c. Chlorzoxazone can cause hepatitis and hepatic necrosis.
4. Cyclobenzaprine (Flexeril)
   a. Cyclobenzaprine is contraindicated in clients who have received monoamine oxidase inhibitors (MAOIs) within 14 days of initiation of cyclobenzaprine therapy and in clients with cardiac disorders.

859

b. Cyclobenzaprine has significant anticholinergic (atropine-like) effects and should be used with caution in clients with a history of urinary retention, angle-closure glaucoma, or increased intraocular pressure.

c. Cyclobenzaprine should be used only for short-term therapy (2 to 3 weeks).

5. Dantrolene (Dantrium)
   a. Dantrolene acts directly on skeletal muscles to relieve spasticity.
   b. Liver damage is the most serious adverse effect.
   c. Liver function values should be monitored before the initiation of treatment and during treatment.
   d. Dantrolene can cause gastrointestinal bleeding, urinary frequency, impotence, photosensitivity, rash, and muscle weakness.
   e. The client is instructed to wear protective clothing when in the sun.
   f. The client is instructed to notify the HCP if rash, bloody or tarry stools, or yellow discoloration of the skin or eyes occurs.

6. Diazepam (Valium)
   a. Acts in the CNS to suppress spasticity; does not affect skeletal muscle directly
   b. Sedation is a common side effect.

7. Methocarbamol (Robaxin)
   a. The parenteral form is contraindicated in clients with renal impairment.
   b. The parenteral form can cause hypotension, bradycardia, anaphylaxis, and seizures, especially when the medication is given too rapidly.
   c. Monitor site for extravasation, which can result in thrombophlebitis and tissue sloughing.
   d. Methocarbamol may cause the urine to turn brown, black, or green.
   e. The client is informed to notify the HCP if blurred vision, nasal congestion, urticaria, or rash occurs.

8. Tizanidine (Zanaflex) and metaxalone (Skelaxin): Can cause liver damage

9. Orphenadrine (Norflex) has significant anticholinergic (atropine-like) effects and should be used with caution in clients with a history of urinary retention, angle-closure glaucoma, or increased intraocular pressure.

Box 60-1 Skeletal Muscle Relaxants

Baclofen (Lioresal)
Carisoprodol (Soma)
Chlorzoxazone (Paraflex, Parafon Forte, Remular-S)
Cyclobenzaprine (Flexeril)
Dantrolene (Dantrium)
Diazepam (Valium)
Metaxalone (Skelaxin)
Methocarbamol (Robaxin)
Tizanidine (Zanaflex)

⚠ Safety is a primary concern when the client is taking a skeletal muscle relaxant because these medications cause drowsiness.

II. ANTIGOUT MEDICATIONS

A. Description
   1. Antigout medications (Box 60-2) reduce uric acid production and increase uric acid excretion (uricosuric) to prevent or relieve gout or to manage hyperuricemia.
   2. Nonsteroidal anti-inflammatory drugs (NSAIDs) are used for their anti-inflammatory effects and to relieve pain during an acute gouty attack (see Chapter 58 for information on NSAIDs).
   3. Glucocorticoids may be prescribed to reduce inflammation during an acute gouty attack (see Chapter 46 for information on glucocorticoids).
   4. Antigout medications should be used cautiously in clients with gastrointestinal, renal, cardiac, or hepatic disease.

B. Side effects
   1. Headaches
   2. Nausea, vomiting, and diarrhea
   3. Blood dyscrasias, such as bone marrow depression
   4. Flushed skin and rash
   5. Uric acid kidney stones
   6. Sore gums
   7. Metallic taste

C. Interventions
   1. Monitor serum uric acid levels.
   2. Monitor intake and output.
   3. Maintain a fluid intake of at least 2000 to 3000 mL/day to avoid kidney stones.
   4. Monitor complete blood cell count and renal and liver function.
   5. The client is instructed to avoid alcohol and caffeine because these products can increase uric acid levels.
   6. The client is encouraged to comply with therapy to prevent elevated uric acid levels, which can trigger a gout attack.
   7. The client is instructed to avoid foods high in purine as prescribed, such as wine, alcohol, organ meats, sardines, salmon, scallops, and gravy.
   8. The client is instructed to take the medication with food to decrease gastric irritation.

Box 60-2 Antigout Medications

Allopurinol (Zyloprim)
Colchicine
Probenecid
Sulfinpyrazone (Anturane)

9. The client is instructed to report side effects to the HCP.

10. The client is advised to minimize exposure to sunlight and have an annual eye examination because visual changes can occur from prolonged use of allopurinol.

11. The client is instructed not to take aspirin with these medications because this could trigger a gout attack.

D. Nursing considerations

1. Allopurinol (Zyloprim)

   a. Can increase the effect of warfarin (Coumadin) and oral hypoglycemic agents

   b. The client is instructed not to take large doses of vitamin C while taking allopurinol, because kidney stones may occur.

   c. Hypersensitivity syndrome (rare) can occur, characterized by rash, fever, eosinophilia, and dysfunction of the liver and kidneys (medication is stopped and the HCP is notified.

2. Colchicine

   a. Used with caution in older clients, debilitated clients, and clients with cardiac, renal, and/or gastrointestinal disease

   b. If gastrointestinal symptoms occur (nausea, vomiting, diarrhea, and abdominal pain), the medication is stopped and the HCP is notified.

3. Probenecid

   a. Mild gastrointestinal effects can occur and can be reduced by taking the medication with food.

   b. Aspirin and other salicylates interfere with the uricosuric action of the medication.

4. Sulfinpyrazone (Anturane)

   a. Contraindicated in clients with active ulcer disease; used with caution in clients with a history of ulcer disease

   b. Salicylates counteract the uricosuric action of the medication.

c. Inhibits hepatic metabolism of tolbutamide (Orinase), causing hypoglycemia, and warfarin, causing bleeding tendencies

⚠ The concurrent use of antigout medications and aspirin causes elevated uric acid levels; the client should be instructed to take acetaminophen (Tylenol) if prescribed rather than aspirin.

III. ANTIARTHRITIC MEDICATIONS (Box 60-3)

A. Description (Figure 60-1)

1. Rheumatoid arthritis occurs as inflammation progresses into the synovia, cartilage, and bone; if this inflammation is not controlled, it will lead to joint destruction, thus affecting client mobility and comfort.

2. The focus of treatment is early diagnosis and aggressive treatment in order to preserve joint function.

Box 60-3 Antiarthritic Medications

Anakinra (Kineret)
Adalimumab (Humira)
Auranofin (Ridaura)
Aurothioglucose (Solganal)
Azathioprine (Imuran)
Cyclosporine; alcohol (Neoral)
Etanercept (Enbrel)
Gold sodium thiomalate (Aurolate, Myochrysine)
Leflunomide (Arava)
Methotrexate (Rheumatrex, Trexall)
Penicillamine (Cuprimine)
Infliximab (Remicade)
Sulfasalazine (Azulfidine)

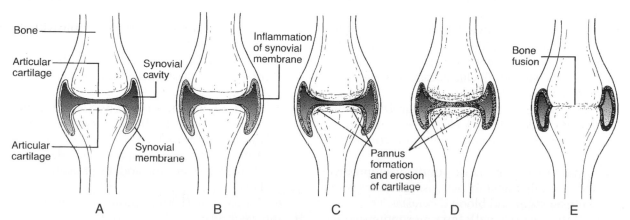

▲ **FIGURE 60-1** Progressive joint degeneration in rheumatoid arthritis. **A,** Healthy joint. **B,** Inflammation of synovial membrane. **C,** Onset of pannus formation and cartilage erosion. **D,** Pannus formation progresses and cartilage deteriorates further. **E,** Complete destruction of joint cavity together with fusion of articulating bones. (From Lehne, R. [2010]. *Pharmacology for nursing care* [7th ed.]. St. Louis: Saunders.)

3. Medication therapy includes NSAIDs, glucocorticoids, and disease-modifying antirheumatic drugs (DMARDs).
4. Gold salts: Use of gold salts has decreased, but their purpose is to reduce the progression of joint damage caused by arthritic processes. Gold toxicity, which includes pruritis, rash, metallic taste, stomatitis, and diarrhea, can occur; if toxicity occurs, dimercaprol (BAL in oil) may be prescribed to enhance gold excretion.

B. DMARDs
1. Description
   a. DMARDs are effective antirheumatic medications that are used to slow the degenerative effects of the disorder.
   b. DMARDs are usually prescribed secondary to NSAIDs but are often the first choice in the treatment of severe arthritis.
2. Common side effects of DMARDs include injection site inflammation and pain, ecchymosis and edema, pancytopenia and infection, fatigue, headache, nausea, vomiting, flu-like symptoms, and allergic response.
3. Interventions
   a. The client is instructed to monitor for signs of infection and report signs to the HCP.
   b. Monitor the injection site for signs of irritation, pain, inflammation, and swelling.
   c. The client is instructed to consult with the HCP before receiving live vaccines and to avoid exposure to infections.
   d. The client is informed about the importance of laboratory tests for neutrophil counts, white blood cell counts, and platelet counts before initiation of treatment and during treatment.
4. Anakinra (Kineret): Injection site reactions are common (pruritus, erythema, rash, pain).
5. Adalimumab (Humira)
   a. Injection site reactions are common.
   b. Has been associated with neurological injury (numbness, tingling, dizziness, disturbed vision, weakness in the legs)
6. Auranofin (Ridaura): Oral gold preparation (not commonly used)
7. Gold sodium thiomalate (Aurolate, Myochrysine), aurothioglucose (Solganal): Intramuscular gold preparations (not commonly used)
8. Azathioprine (Imuran): Immunosuppressive and anti-inflammatory actions; toxic effects include hepatitis and blood dyscrasias.
9. Cyclosporine (Neoral): Immunosuppressive actions; can cause nephrotoxicity
10. Etanercept (Enbrel)
    a. Injection site reactions are common.

b. Poses a risk for heart failure; has been associated with central nervous system demyelinating disorders and hematological disorders
11. Hydroxychloroquine sulfate: Associated with retinal damage; the client is informed to contact the HCP if visual disturbances occur.
12. Leflunomide (Arava): Side effects include diarrhea, respiratory infection, reversible alopecia, rash, and nausea; is hepatotoxic.
13. Methotrexate (Rheumatrex, Trexall): Can cause hepatic fibrosis, bone marrow suppression, gastrointestinal ulceration, and pneumonitis
14. Penicillamine (Cuprimine): Can cause bone marrow suppression and autoimmune disorders
15. Infliximab (Remicade): Can cause infusion reactions (fever, chills, pruritus, urticaria, chest pain); is hepatotoxic
16. Sulfasalazine (Azulfidine): Can cause gastrointestinal and dermatological reactions, bone marrow suppression, hepatitis

C. NSAIDs may be prescribed for their anti-inflammatory and analgesic effects. (See Chapter 58 for information on NSAIDs.)

D. Glucocorticoids may be prescribed for their anti-inflammatory effects. (See Chapter 46 for information on glucocorticoids.)

IV. MEDICATIONS TO PREVENT AND TREAT OSTEOPOROSIS

A. Description
1. Osteoporosis is characterized by low bone mass and increased bone fragility.
2. Calcium and vitamin D supplementation can reduce the risk of osteoporosis; calcium maximizes bone growth early in life and maintains bone integrity later in life, and vitamin D ensures calcium absorption (see Chapter 46 for information on calcium and vitamin D supplements).
3. Treatment is aimed at reducing the occurrence of fractures by maintaining or increasing bone strength.
4. Medications that decrease bone resorption (antiresorptive) and medications that promote bone formation are used.
5. Antiresorptive medications include raloxifene (Evista), calcitonin, and bisphosphonates (see later).
6. Teriparatide (Fortéo) promotes bone growth.

B. Interventions
1. Salmon calcitonin (Miacalcin)
   a. Calcitonin is secreted by the thyroid gland and inhibits osteoclastic bone resorption.

b. Instruct the client how to administer the intranasal or subcutaneous form, depending on the route prescribed.

c. Intranasal route: Examine the nares for irritation; alternate nostrils for doses.

d. When calcitonin is taken, it is important to monitor for hypocalcemia.

2. Bisphosphonates (Box 60-4)

a. Bisphosphonates inhibit osteoclast-mediated bone resorption, thereby increasing total bone mass.

b. Bisphosphonates include alendronate (Fosamax), risedronate (Actonel), and ibandronate (Boniva).

c. Contraindicated for clients with esophageal disorders that can impede swallowing and for clients who cannot sit or stand for at least 30 minutes (60 minutes with ibandronate).

d. After taking the medication the client is instructed to postpone ingesting anything for at least 30 minutes (60 minutes with ibandronate).

e. Adverse effects include esophagitis, muscle pain, and ocular problems; the client is instructed to contact the HCP if adverse effects occur.

⚠ Because of the risk of esophagitis, bisphosphonates must be administered in the morning before eating or drinking with a full glass of water; the client must then remain sitting or standing for at least 30 minutes (60 minutes with ibandronate).

3. Raloxifene (Evista)

a. Antiresorptive medication (nonbisphosphonate)

b. Contraindicated in clients who have a history of venous thrombotic events

c. Needs to be discontinued 72 hours before prolonged immobilization periods (such as with periods of extended bed rest)

d. The client is instructed to avoid extended periods of restricted activity (such as when traveling).

Box 60-4 Medications to Prevent or Treat Osteoporosis

Calcium and vitamin D
Alendronate (Fosamax)
Calcitonin, salmon (Miacalcin)
Ibandronate (Boniva)
Raloxifene (Evista)
Risedronate (Actonel)
Teriparatide (Fortéo)

4. Teriparatide (Fortéo)

a. Teriparatide stimulates new bone formation, thus increasing bone mass.

b. Teriparatide is a portion of the human parathyroid hormone and works by increasing the action of osteoblasts.

c. Reserved for use in clients at high risk for fractures

d. Has been associated with the development of bone cancer

MORE QUESTIONS ON EVOLVE!

Practice Questions

636. The client has been on treatment for rheumatoid arthritis for 3 weeks. During the administration of etanercept (Enbrel), it is most important for the nurse to check:
    1. The injection site for itching and edema
    2. The white blood cell counts and platelet counts
    3. Whether the client is experiencing fatigue and joint pain
    4. A metallic taste in the mouth, with a loss of appetite

637. Baclofen (Lioresal) is prescribed for the client with multiple sclerosis. The nurse assists in planning care, knowing that the primary therapeutic effect of this medication is which of the following?
    1. Increased muscle tone
    2. Decreased muscle spasms
    3. Increased range of motion
    4. Decreased local pain and tenderness

638. A nurse is monitoring a client receiving baclofen (Lioresal) for side effects related to the medication. Which of the following would indicate that the client is experiencing a side effect?
    1. Polyuria
    2. Diarrhea
    3. Drowsiness
    4. Muscular excitability

639. A nurse is reinforcing discharge instructions to a client receiving baclofen (Lioresal). Which of the following would the nurse include in the instructions?
    1. Restrict fluid intake.
    2. Avoid the use of alcohol.
    3. Stop the medication if diarrhea occurs.
    4. Notify the health care provider if fatigue occurs.

640. A client with acute muscle spasms has been taking baclofen (Lioresal). The client calls the clinic nurse because of continuous feelings of weakness and

fatigue and asks the nurse about discontinuing the medication. The nurse should make which appropriate response to the client?

1. "You should never stop the medication."
2. "It is best that you taper the dose if you intend to stop the medication."
3. "It is okay to stop the medication if you think that you can tolerate the muscle spasms."
4. "Weakness and fatigue commonly occur and will diminish with continued medication use."

641. Dantrolene sodium (Dantrium) is prescribed for a client experiencing flexor spasms, and the client asks the nurse about the action of the medication. The nurse responds, knowing that the therapeutic action of this medication is which of the following?

1. Depresses spinal reflexes
2. Acts directly on the skeletal muscle to relieve spasticity
3. Acts within the spinal cord to suppress hyperactive reflexes
4. Acts on the central nervous system (CNS) to suppress spasms

642. A nurse is reviewing the laboratory studies on a client receiving dantrolene sodium (Dantrium). Which laboratory test would identify an adverse effect associated with the administration of this medication?

1. Creatinine
2. Liver function tests
3. Blood urea nitrogen
4. Hematological function tests

643. A nurse is reviewing the record of a client who has been prescribed baclofen (Lioresal). Which of the following disorders, if noted in the client's history, would alert the nurse to contact the health care provider?

1. Seizure disorders
2. Hyperthyroidism
3. Diabetes mellitus
4. Coronary artery disease

644. Cyclobenzaprine (Flexeril) is prescribed for a client to treat muscle spasms, and the nurse is reviewing the client's record. Which of the following disorders, if noted in the client's record, would indicate a need to contact the health care provider regarding the administration of this medication?

1. Glaucoma
2. Emphysema
3. Hyperthyroidism
4. Diabetes mellitus

645. In monitoring a client's response to disease-modifying antirheumatic drugs (DMARDs), which findings would the nurse interpret as acceptable responses? **Select all that apply.**

☐ 1. Symptom control during periods of emotional stress
☐ 2. Normal white blood cell counts, platelet, and neutrophil counts
☐ 3. Radiological findings that show nonprogression of joint degeneration
☐ 4. An increased range of motion in the affected joints 3 months into therapy
☐ 5. Inflammation and irritation at the injection site 3 days after injection is given
☐ 6. A low-grade temperature upon rising in the morning that remains throughout the day

ANSWERS

636. 2

Rationale: Infection and pancytopenia are side effects of etanercept (Enbrel). Laboratory studies are performed before and during drug treatment. The appearance of abnormal white blood cell counts and abnormal platelet counts can alert the nurse to a potentially life-threatening infection. Injection site itching is a common occurrence following administration. A metallic taste with loss of appetite are not common signs of side effects of this medication.

Test-Taking Strategy: Use the process of elimination. Option 4 can be eliminated, because this is not a common side effect. In early treatment, residual fatigue and joint pain may still be apparent. Option 2 monitors for a hematological disorder, which could indicate a reason for discontinuing this medication and should be reported. Review this medication if you had difficulty with this question.

Level of Cognitive Ability: Analyzing

Client Needs: Physiological Integrity
Integrated Process: Nursing Process/Data Collection
Content Area: Pharmacology
References: Hodgson, Kizior, p. 449. 2012. Ignatavicius, Workman, p. 343. 2010.

637. 2

Rationale: Baclofen is a skeletal muscle relaxant and central nervous system depressant and acts at the spinal cord level to decrease the frequency and amplitude of muscle spasms in clients with spinal cord injuries or diseases and in clients with multiple sclerosis. Options 1, 3, and 4 are incorrect.

Test-Taking Strategy: Focus on the client's diagnosis. Recalling the action of this medication will direct you to option 2. Review this medication if you had difficulty with this question.

Level of Cognitive Ability: Understanding
Client Needs: Physiological Integrity
Integrated Process: Nursing Process/Planning

Content Area: Pharmacology
Reference: Lehne, p. 241. 2010.

638. 3

Rationale: Baclofen is a central nervous system (CNS) depressant and frequently causes drowsiness, dizziness, weakness, and fatigue. It can also cause nausea, constipation, and urinary retention. Clients should be warned about the possible reactions. Options 1, 2, and 4 are not side effects.
Test-Taking Strategy: Use the process of elimination. Recalling that baclofen is a CNS depressant used to treat muscle spasticity will direct you to option 3. If you had difficulty with this question, review the side effects of this medication.
Level of Cognitive Ability: Analyzing
Client Needs: Physiological Integrity
Integrated Process: Nursing Process/Data Collection
Content Area: Pharmacology
Reference: Lehne, pp. 241, 244. 2010.

639. 2

Rationale: Baclofen is a central nervous system (CNS) depressant. The client should be cautioned against the use of alcohol and other CNS depressants, because baclofen potentiates the depressant activity of these agents. Constipation rather than diarrhea is an adverse effect of baclofen. It is not necessary to restrict fluids, but the client should be warned that urinary retention can occur. Fatigue is related to a CNS effect that is most intense during the early phase of therapy and diminishes with continued medication use. It is not necessary that the client notify the health care provider if fatigue occurs.
Test-Taking Strategy: Recalling that baclofen is a CNS depressant will direct you to the correct option. If you were unsure of the correct option, use general principles related to medication administration. Alcohol should be avoided with the use of medications. Review this medication if you had difficulty with this question.
Level of Cognitive Ability: Applying
Client Needs: Physiological Integrity
Integrated Process: Teaching and Learning
Content Area: Pharmacology
Reference: Lehne, p. 241. 2010.

640. 4

Rationale: The client should be instructed that symptoms such as drowsiness, weakness, and fatigue are more intense in the early phase of therapy and diminish with continued medication use. The client should be instructed never to withdraw or stop the medication abruptly, because abrupt withdrawal can cause visual hallucinations, paranoid ideation, and seizures. It is best for the nurse to inform the client that these symptoms will subside and encourage the client to continue the use of the medication.
Test Taking Strategy: Use the process of elimination. Eliminate option 1 first because it is a rather extreme nursing response. Next, eliminate options 2 and 3 because these responses do not represent the scope of nursing practice or nursing actions. Review this medication if you had difficulty with this question.
Level of Cognitive Ability: Applying
Client Needs: Physiological Integrity
Integrated Process: Communication and Documentation

Content Area: Pharmacology
Reference: Lehne, p. 241. 2010.

641. 2

Rationale: Dantrium acts directly on skeletal muscle to relieve muscle spasticity. The primary action is the suppression of calcium release from the sarcoplasmic reticulum. This in turn decreases the ability of the skeletal muscle to contract. Options 1, 3, and 4 are not actions of the medication.
Test-Taking Strategy: Use the process of elimination. Options 1, 3, and 4 are all comparable or alike in that they address CNS suppression and the depression of reflexes. Therefore, eliminate these options. Review this medication if you had difficulty with this question.
Level of Cognitive Ability: Applying
Client Needs: Physiological Integrity
Integrated Process: Nursing Process/Implementation
Content Area: Pharmacology
Reference: Hodgson, Kizior, p. 302. 2012.

642. 2

Rationale: Dose-related liver damage is the most serious adverse effect of dantrolene. To reduce the risk of liver damage, liver function tests should be performed before treatment and periodically throughout the treatment course. It is administered in the lowest effective dosage for the shortest time necessary.
Test-Taking Strategy: Use the process of elimination. Eliminate options 1 and 3 because these tests both assess kidney function. From the remaining options, it is necessary to recall that this medication affects liver function. Review this medication if you had difficulty with this question.
Level of Cognitive Ability: Analyzing
Client Needs: Physiological Integrity
Integrated Process: Nursing Process/Data Collection
Content Area: Pharmacology
Reference: Hodgson, Kizior, p. 303–304. 2012.

643. 1

Rationale: Clients with seizure disorders may have a lowered seizure threshold when baclofen is administered. Concurrent therapy may require an increase in the anticonvulsive medication. The disorders in options 2, 3, and 4 are not a concern when the client is taking baclofen.
Test-Taking Strategy: Knowledge regarding the contraindications and the cautions associated with the administration of baclofen is required to answer this question. Remember, a lowered seizure threshold can occur when baclofen is administered. If you are unfamiliar with these contraindications and cautions, review this content.
Level of Cognitive Ability: Analyzing
Client Needs: Safe and Effective Care Environment
Integrated Process: Nursing Process/Data Collection
Content Area: Pharmacology
References: Kee, Hayes, McCuistion, p. 351. 2009. Skidmore-Roth, p. 181. 2010.

644. 1

Rationale: Because this medication has anticholinergic effects, it should be used with caution in clients with a history of urinary retention, angle-closure glaucoma, and increased intraocular pressure. Cyclobenzaprine hydrochloride should be used only for short-term 2- to 3-week therapy.

Test-Taking Strategy: Recalling that this medication has anticholinergic effects will assist in directing you to option 1. If you are unfamiliar with this medication and the contraindications associated with its administration, review this content.

Level of Cognitive Ability: Analyzing
Client Needs: Safe and Effective Care Environment
Integrated Process: Nursing Process/Data Collection
Content Area: Pharmacology
Reference: Hodgson, Kizior, p. 286. 2012.

❖ **645. 1, 2, 3, 4**
Rationale: Because emotional stress frequently exacerbates the symptoms of rheumatoid arthritis, the absence of symptoms is a positive finding. DMARDs are given to slow progression of joint degeneration. In addition, the improvement in the range of motion after 3 months of therapy with normal blood work is a positive finding. Temperature elevation and inflammation and irritation at the medication injection site could indicate signs of infection.

Test-Taking Strategy: Use the process of elimination and focus on the subject—acceptable responses to therapy. Recalling that signs of an infection can indicate an unexpected finding will assist in eliminating options 5 and 6. Review the expected effects of this medication if you had difficulty with this question.

Level of Cognitive Ability: Analyzing
Client Needs: Physiological Integrity
Integrated Process: Nursing Process/Data Collection
Content Area: Pharmacology
References: Kee, Hayes, McCuistion, pp. 365–366. 2009. Lehne, pp. 856–857. 2010.

UNIT 18

The Adult Client with an Immune Disorder

PYRAMID TERMS

acquired immunodeficiency syndrome A chronic illness caused by the human immunodeficiency virus (HIV) and characterized by the breakdown of the immune system

acquired immunity Immunity received passively from the mother's antibodies, animal serum, or production of antibodies in response to a disease; immunization produces active acquired immunity

allergy An abnormal, individual response to certain substances that normally do not trigger such an exaggerated reaction

cellular response A delayed response against slowly developing bacterial infections; also called delayed hypersensitivity

human immunodeficiency virus (HIV) A life-threatening virus that is transmitted from one person to another through blood and body fluids

humoral response An immediate response that provides protection against acute, rapidly developing bacterial and viral infections

immunodeficiency The absence or inadequate production of immune bodies

natural immunity Also called innate immunity; present at birth

Kaposi's sarcoma Skin lesions that occur in individuals with a compromised immune system

Lyme disease An infection acquired from a tick bite; ticks live in wooded areas and survive by attaching to a host

PYRAMID TO SUCCESS

Pyramid points focus on the effects of and complications associated with an immune deficiency. Specific focus relates to the nursing care related to the disorder, the impact of the treatment or disorder, and client adaptation.

Acquired immunodeficiency syndrome is a pyramid focus, along with protecting the client from infection, and preventing the transmission of infection to other individuals. Psychosocial issues relate to social isolation and the body-image disturbances that can occur as a result of the immune disorder.

CLIENT NEEDS

Safe and Effective Care Environment

- Acting as an advocate related to the client's decisions
- Addressing advance directives
- Consulting with members of the health care team
- Establishing priorities
- Handling hazardous and infectious materials safely
- Implementing standard and other precautions
- Maintaining asepsis
- Maintaining confidentiality regarding diagnosis
- Obtaining informed consent for treatments and procedures
- Preventing infection
- Upholding client rights

Health Promotion and Maintenance

- Ensuring that the client receives recommended immunizations
- Implementing health screening measures
- Monitoring for expected body-image changes
- Preventing disease related to infection
- Providing health promotion programs
- Respecting client lifestyle choices

Psychosocial Integrity

- Assisting in mobilizing appropriate support and resource systems
- Assisting the client and family to cope
- Assisting the client to cope, adapt, and problem-solve during illness or stressful events
- Considering religious, spiritual, and cultural preferences
- Discussing grief and loss related to death and the dying process
- Promoting a positive environment to maintain optimal quality of life

Physiological Integrity

- Managing pain
- Managing medical emergencies
- Monitoring for the expected and unexpected responses to treatments
- Promoting nutrition
- Protecting the client from infection
- Providing basic care and comfort
- Reviewing diagnostic test and laboratory test results

Immune Disorders

 I. FUNCTIONS OF THE IMMUNE SYSTEM

A. The immune system provides protection against invasion from microorganisms from outside the body.

B. The immune system protects the body from internal threats and maintains the internal environment by removing dead or damaged cells.

II. IMMUNE RESPONSE

A. T- and B-cells
   1. Lymphocytes migrate to lymphoid tissue where they wait to form sensitized lymphocytes for cellular immunity or antibodies for humoral immunity.
   2. Some B-cells lie dormant until a specific antigen enters the body, at which time they greatly increase in number and are available for defense.
   3. T-cells are responsible for rejection of transplanted tissue.
   4. T- and B-cells are necessary for a normal immune response.

B. Humoral response
   1. **Humoral response** is immediate.
   2. This type of response provides protection against acute, rapidly developing bacterial and viral infections.

C. Cellular response
   1. **Cellular response** is delayed and is called delayed hypersensitivity.
   2. This type of response is active against slowly developing bacterial infections and is involved in autoimmune response, some allergic reactions, and rejection of foreign cells.

III. IMMUNITY

A. Natural immunity
   1. Also called innate or native immunity
   2. Present at birth and includes biochemical, physical, and mechanical barriers of defense as well as the inflammatory response

B. Acquired immunity
   1. **Acquired** or adaptive **immunity** is received passively from the mother's antibodies, animal serum, or from the production of antibodies in response to a disease.
   2. Immunization produces active **acquired immunity**.

IV. IMMUNIZATIONS (refer to Chapter 39 for information about immunizations)

V. LABORATORY STUDIES

A. Antinuclear antibody (ANA) titer
   1. ANA titer is a blood test used in the differential diagnosis of rheumatic diseases and to detect antinucleoprotein factors and patterns associated with certain autoimmune diseases.
   2. The test is positive at a titer of 1:20 or 1:40, depending on the laboratory.
   3. A positive result does not necessarily confirm a disease.
   4. The ANA titer is positive in most individuals diagnosed with systemic lupus erythematosus (SLE).
   5. An ANA titer result can be false positive in a small proportion of the normal population.

B. Anti–double-stranded DNA (dsDNA) antibody test
   1. The anti-dsDNA antibody test is a blood test done specifically to identify or differentiate DNA antibodies found in SLE.
   2. The test supports a diagnosis, monitors disease activity and response to therapy, and establishes a prognosis for SLE.
   3. Values
      a. Negative: Less than 70 units by enzyme-linked immunosorbent assay (ELISA)
      b. Borderline: 70 to 200 units
      c. Positive: Greater than 200 units

C. Refer to Chapter 11 for testing related to **acquired immunodeficiency syndrome (AIDS)**.

D. Skin testing
  1. Description
     a. The administration of an allergen to the surface of the skin or into the dermis
     b. Administered by patch, scratch, or intradermal techniques
  2. Interventions preprocedure
     a. Discontinue systemic corticosteroids or antihistamine therapy 5 days before the test as prescribed.
     b. Obtain informed consent.
  3. Interventions postprocedure
     a. Record the site, date, and time of the test.
     b. Record the date and the time for follow-up site reading.
     c. Inspect the site for erythema, papules, vesicles, edema, and wheal (Figure 61-1).
     d. Measure wheal and document size and other findings.
     e. Provide the client with a list of potential allergens, if identified.

⚠ Have resuscitation equipment available if skin testing is performed, because the allergen may induce an anaphylactic reaction.

VI. IMMUNODEFICIENCY

A. Description
  1. **Immunodeficiency** is the absence or inadequate production of immune bodies.
  2. The disorder can be congenital (primary) or acquired (secondary).

Test Results	Interpretation
	Negative—Wheal less than 0.5 cm in diameter
	Positive—Wheal 0.5 cm in diameter (1+)
	Positive—Wheal 1.0 cm in diameter (2+)
	Positive—Wheal 1.5 cm in diameter (3+)
	Positive—Wheal 2.0 cm in diameter (4+)

▲ **FIGURE 61-1** Interpretation of intradermal allergy test results based on size of wheal after 15 to 30 minutes. (From Monahan, F., Sands, J., Neighbors, M., et al. [2007]. *Phipps' medical surgical nursing: Concepts and clinical practice* [8th ed.]. St. Louis: Mosby.)

  3. Treatment depends on the inadequacy of immune bodies and its primary cause.
B. Data collection
  1. Factors that decrease immune function
  2. Frequent infections
  3. Nutritional status
  4. Medication history, such as use of corticosteroids for long periods
  5. History of alcohol or drug abuse
C. Interventions
  1. Protect the client from infection.
  2. Promote a balanced diet with adequate nutrition.
  3. Use strict aseptic technique for all procedures.
  4. Provide psychosocial care regarding lifestyle changes and role changes.
  5. Instruct the client in measures to prevent infection and to wear a Medic Alert bracelet.

⚠ The priority concern for a client with immunodeficiency is infection.

VII. HYPERSENSITIVITY AND ALLERGY

A. Description
  1. An **allergy** is an abnormal, individual response to certain substances that normally do not trigger such an exaggerated reaction.
  2. In some types of allergies, a reaction occurs on a second and subsequent contact with the allergen.
  3. Skin testing may be done to determine the allergen.
  4. Types of hypersensitivity reactions (Table 61-1).
B. Data collection
  1. History of exposure to allergens
  2. Itching, tearing, and burning of eyes and skin
  3. Rashes
  4. Nose twitching and nasal stuffiness
C. Interventions
  1. Identification of the specific allergen
  2. Management of the symptoms with antihistamines, anti-inflammatory agents, or corticosteroids
  3. Ointments, creams, wet compresses, and soothing baths for local reactions
  4. Desensitization programs may be recommended

VIII. ANAPHYLAXIS

A. Description
  1. Anaphylaxis is a serious and immediate hypersensitivity reaction with the release of histamine from the damaged cells.
  2. Anaphylaxis can be systemic or cutaneous (localized)
B. Data collection (Figure 61-2)
C. Interventions (see Priority Nursing Actions)

IX. LATEX ALLERGY

A. Description

1. Latex **allergy** is a hypersensitivity to latex.
2. The source of the allergic reaction is thought to be the proteins in the natural rubber latex or the various chemicals used in the manufacturing process of latex gloves.
3. Symptoms of the **allergy** can range from mild contact dermatitis to moderately severe symptoms of rhinitis, conjunctivitis, urticaria, and bronchospasm to severe life-threatening anaphylaxis.

B. Common routes of exposure (Box 61-1)

1. Cutaneous: Natural latex gloves and latex balloons
2. Percutaneous and parenteral: IV lines and catheters; hemodialysis equipment

TABLE 61-1 Types of Hypersensitivity Reactions

Type	Causative Component	Pathological Process	Reaction
I: Immediate, anaphylactic	IgE	Mast cell degranulation ↓ Histamine and leukotriene release	Anaphylaxis Atopic diseases Skin reactions
II: Cytolytic, cytotoxic	IgG IgM Complement	Complement fixation ↓ Cell lysis	ABO incompatibility Drug-induced hemolytic anemia
III: Immune complex	Antigen-antibody complexes	Deposition in vessels and tissue walls ↓ Inflammation	Arthus reaction Serum sickness Systemic lupus erythematosus Acute glomerulonephritis
IV: Cell-mediated, delayed	Sensitized T cells	Lymphokine release	Tuberculosis Contact dermatitis Transplant rejection

Ig, Immunoglobulin.
From Black, J., & Hawks, J. (2009). *Medical-surgical nursing: Clinical management for positive outcomes* (8th ed.). St. Louis: Saunders.

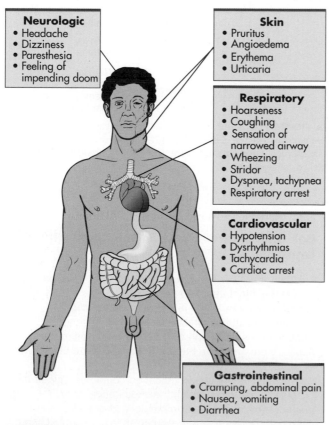

Neurologic
- Headache
- Dizziness
- Paresthesia
- Feeling of impending doom

Skin
- Pruritus
- Angioedema
- Erythema
- Urticaria

Respiratory
- Hoarseness
- Coughing
- Sensation of narrowed airway
- Wheezing
- Stridor
- Dyspnea, tachypnea
- Respiratory arrest

Cardiovascular
- Hypotension
- Dysrhythmias
- Tachycardia
- Cardiac arrest

Gastrointestinal
- Cramping, abdominal pain
- Nausea, vomiting
- Diarrhea

▲ **FIGURE 61-2** Clinical manifestations of a systemic anaphylactic reaction. (From Lewis, S., Heitkemper, M., & Dirksen, S. [2011]. *Medical-surgical nursing: Assessment and management of clinical problems* [8th ed.]. St. Louis: Mosby.)

■■■■ **PRIORITY NURSING ACTIONS!** ■■■■

Actions to Take if a Client Develops Anaphylaxis

1. Quickly assess respiratory status and maintain a patent airway.
2. Call the health care provider (HCP) or Rapid Response Team.
3. Administer oxygen.
4. Prepare to start an IV line and infuse normal saline.
5. Prepare to administer diphenhydramine (Benadryl) and epinephrine (Adrenalin).
6. Document the event, actions taken, and the client's response.

If the client experiences an anaphylactic reaction, the immediate action would be to assess the respiratory status quickly and maintain a patent airway. The HCP or Rapid Response Team is called. In the meantime, the nurse stays with the client and monitors the client's vital signs and for signs of shock. An IV device is inserted if one is not already in place and normal saline is infused. The nurse then prepares for the administration of diphenhydramine and epinephrine and other medications as prescribed. The head of the bed is elevated if the client's blood pressure is normal. The client's feet and legs may be raised. The nurse documents the event, actions taken, and the client's response.

Reference: Black, J., & Hawks, J. (2009). *Medical-surgical nursing: Clinical management for positive outcomes* (8th ed., pp. 2167–2168). St. Louis: Saunders.

Box 61-1 Products That May Contain Natural Rubber Latex

Ace bandages (brown)
Adhesive or elastic bandages
Ambu Bag
Balloons
Blood pressure cuff (tubing and bladder)
Catheter leg bag straps
Catheters
Condoms
Diaphragms
Elastic pressure stockings
Electrocardiogram pads
Feminine hygiene pads
Gloves
Intravenous catheters, tubing, and rubber injection ports
Levin tubes
Pads for crutches
Prepackaged enema kits
Rubber stoppers on medication vials
Stethoscopes
Syringes

Note: Health care agencies use as many non-latex products as possible and have non-latex supplies available for clients with a latex allergy.

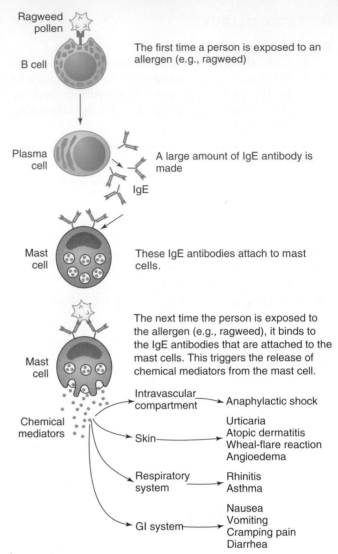

The first time a person is exposed to an allergen (e.g., ragweed)

B cell

Plasma cell — A large amount of IgE antibody is made

IgE

Mast cell — These IgE antibodies attach to mast cells.

Mast cell — The next time the person is exposed to the allergen (e.g., ragweed), it binds to the IgE antibodies that are attached to the mast cells. This triggers the release of chemical mediators from the mast cell.

Chemical mediators
Intravascular compartment → Anaphylactic shock
Skin → Urticaria / Atopic dermatitis / Wheal-flare reaction / Angioedema
Respiratory system → Rhinitis / Asthma
GI system → Nausea / Vomiting / Cramping pain / Diarrhea

▲ **FIGURE 61-3** Steps in a type I allergic reaction. (From Lewis, S., Heitkemper, M., & Dirksen, S. [2011]. *Medical-surgical nursing: Assessment and management of clinical problems* [8th ed.]. St. Louis: Mosby.)

  3. Mucosal: Use of latex condoms, catheters, airways, and nipples
  4. Aerosol: Aerosolization of powder from latex gloves can occur when gloves are dispensed from the box or when gloves are removed from the hands.
C. At-risk individuals
  1. Health care workers
  2. Individuals who work in the rubber industry
  3. Individuals having multiple surgeries
  4. Individuals with spina bifida
  5. Individuals who wear gloves frequently such as food handlers, hairdressers, and auto mechanics
  6. Individuals allergic to kiwis, bananas, pineapples, tropical fruits, grapes, avocados, potatoes, hazelnuts, and water chestnuts

D. Data collection
  1. Anaphylaxis or type I hypersensitivity is a response to natural rubber latex (Figure 61-3; also see Figure 61-2).
  2. A delayed type IV hypersensitivity can occur within 6 to 48 hours. Symptoms of contact dermatitis include pruritus, edema, erythema, vesicles, papules, and crusting and thickening of the skin.

E. Interventions (Box 61-2)

X. AUTOIMMUNE DISEASE

A. Description
  1. The body is unable to recognize its own cells as a part of itself.

  2. Autoimmune disease can affect collagenous tissue.

Box 61-2 Interventions for the Client with a Latex Allergy

Ask the client about a known allergy to latex when performing the initial assessment.
Identify risk factors to a latex allergy in the client.
Use non-latex gloves and all latex-safe supplies.
Keep a latex-safe supply cart near the client's room.
Apply a cloth barrier to the client's arm under a blood pressure cuff.
Use latex-free syringes, medication containers (glass ampules), and latex-safe intravenous equipment.
Instruct the client to wear a Medic-Alert bracelet.
Instruct the client about the importance of informing health care providers and local and paramedic ambulance companies about the allergy.

B. Systemic lupus erythematosus (SLE)
1. Description
   a. A chronic progressive systemic inflammatory disease that can cause major organs and systems to fail
   b. Connective tissue and fibrin deposits collect in blood vessels on collagen fibers and on organs.
   c. The deposits lead to necrosis and inflammation in blood vessels, lymph nodes, gastrointestinal tract, and pleura.
   d. No cure for the disease is known.
2. Causes
   a. The cause of SLE is unknown, and SLE is thought to result from a defect in the immunological mechanisms and have a genetic origin.
   b. Precipitating factors include medications, stress, genetic factors, sunlight or ultraviolet light, and pregnancy.
   c. Discoid lupus erythematosus is possible with some medications but totally disappears after the medication is stopped; the only manifestation is the skin rash that occurs in lupus.
3. Data collection
   a. Assess for precipitating factors.
   b. Erythema or rashes, commonly butterfly rash of the face
   c. Dry, scaly, raised rash on the face or upper body
   d. Fever
   e. Weakness, malaise, and fatigue
   f. Anorexia
   g. Weight loss
   h. Photosensitivity
   i. Joint pain
   j. Erythema of the palms
   k. Anemia
   l. Positive ANA test and lupus erythematosus (LE) preparation
   m. Elevated sedimentation rate and C-reactive protein
4. Interventions
   a. Monitor skin integrity and provide frequent oral care.
   b. Instruct the client to clean the skin with a mild soap, avoiding harsh and perfumed substances.
   c. Assist with the use of ointments and creams for the rash as prescribed.
   d. Identify factors contributing to fatigue.
   e. Administer iron, folic acid, or vitamin supplements as prescribed if anemia occurs.
   f. Provide a high-vitamin and high-iron diet.
   g. Provide a high-protein diet if there is no evidence of kidney disease.
   h. Instruct in measures to conserve energy, such as pacing activities and balancing rest with exercise.
   i. Administer topical or systemic corticosteroids, salicylates, and nonsteroidal anti-inflammatory drugs as prescribed for pain and inflammation.
   j. Administer medications to decrease the inflammatory response as prescribed.
   k. Instruct the client to avoid exposure to sunlight and ultraviolet light.
   l. Monitor for proteinuria and red blood cell casts in the urine.
   m. Monitor for bruising, bleeding, and injury.
   n. Assist with plasmapheresis as prescribed to remove autoantibodies and immune complexes from the blood before organ damage occurs.
   o. Monitor for signs of organ involvement such as pleuritis, nephritis, pericarditis, coronary artery disease, hypertension, neuritis, anemia, and peritonitis.
   p. Note that lupus nephritis occurs early in the disease process.
   q. Provide supportive therapy as major organs become affected.
   r. Provide emotional support and encourage the client to verbalize feelings.
   s. Provide information regarding support groups and encourage the use of community resources.

⚠ For the client with SLE, monitor the blood urea nitrogen and creatinine levels frequently for signs of renal impairment.

C. Scleroderma (systemic sclerosis)
1. Description
   a. Scleroderma is a chronic connective tissue disease similar to SLE that is characterized by inflammation, fibrosis, and sclerosis.
   b. This disorder affects the connective tissue throughout the body.
   c. It causes fibrotic changes involving the skin, synovial membranes, esophagus, heart, lungs, kidneys, and gastrointestinal tract.
   d. Treatment is directed toward forcing the disease into remission and slowing its progress.
2. Data collection
   a. Pain
   b. Stiffness and muscle weakness
   c. Pitting edema of the hands and fingers that progresses to the rest of the body
   d. Taut and shiny skin that is free from wrinkles
   e. Skin tissue is tight, hard, and thick, and it loses its elasticity and adheres to underlying structures.
   f. Dysphagia
   g. Decreased range of motion
   h. Joint contractures
   i. Inability to perform activities of daily living

3. Interventions
   a. Encourage activity as tolerated.
   b. Maintain a constant room temperature.
   c. Provide small frequent meals while eliminating foods that stimulate gastric secretions, such as spicy foods, caffeine, and alcohol.
   d. Advise the client to sit up for 1 to 2 hours after meals if esophageal involvement exists
   e. Provide supportive therapy as the major organs become affected.
   f. Administer corticosteroids as prescribed for inflammation.
   g. Provide emotional support and encourage the use of resources as necessary.

D. Polyarteritis nodosa
   1. Description
      a. Polyarteritis nodosa is a collagen disease and a form of systemic vasculitis that causes inflammation of the arteries in visceral organs, brain, and skin.
      b. Treatment is similar to the treatment for SLE.
      c. Polyarteritis nodosa affects middle-aged men.
      d. The cause is unknown, prognosis is poor.
      e. Renal disorders and cardiac involvement are the most frequent causes of death.
   2. Data collection
      a. Malaise and weakness
      b. Low-grade fever
      c. Severe abdominal pain
      d. Bloody diarrhea
      e. Weight loss
      f. Elevated sedimentation rate
   3. Interventions
      a. Provide supportive care as required.
      b. Provide a well-balanced diet.
      c. Administer corticosteroids, cyclophosphamide, and analgesics to control pain and inflammation.
      d. Provide emotional support and encourage the client to verbalize feelings.
      e. Initiate support services for the client.

E. Pemphigus
   1. Description
      a. A group of related disorders including vulgaris, vegetans, foliaceus, and erythematosus
      b. Pemphigus is a rare autoimmune disease that occurs predominantly between middle and old age.
      c. The cause is unknown, and the disorder is potentially fatal.
      d. Treatment is aimed at suppressing the immune response that causes blister formation.
   2. Data collection
      a. Lesions that appear as fragile flaccid bullae
      b. Partial-thickness wounds that bleed, weep, and form crusts when bullae are disrupted
      c. Debilitation, malaise, and pain

   d. Chewing and swallowing difficulties
   e. Nikolsky's sign: separation of the epidermis caused by rubbing the skin
   f. Leukocytosis, eosinophilia, foul-smelling discharge from skin
   3. Interventions
      a. Provide supportive care.
      b. Provide oral hygiene and increase fluid intake.
      c. Soothe oral lesions with baths as prescribed for relief of symptoms.
      d. Administer topical or systemic antibiotics as prescribed for secondary infections.
      e. Administer corticosteroids and cytotoxic agents as prescribed to bring about remission.

XI. GOODPASTURE'S SYNDROME

A. Description
   1. Goodpasture's syndrome is an autoimmune disorder; autoantibodies are made against the glomerular basement membrane and alveolar basement membrane.
   2. Goodpasture's syndrome is most common in males and young adults who smoke, and the exact cause is unknown.
   3. The lungs and the kidneys are affected primarily, and the disorder is usually not diagnosed until significant pulmonary or renal involvement occurs.

B. Data collection
   1. Clinical manifestations indicating pulmonary and renal involvement
   2. Shortness of breath
   3. Hemoptysis
   4. Decreased urine output
   5. Edema and weight gain
   6. Hypertension and tachycardia

C. Interventions
   1. Focus on suppressing the autoimmune response with medications such as corticosteroids and with plasmapheresis (filtration of the plasma to remove some proteins) to remove the autoantibodies.
   2. Provide supportive therapy for pulmonary and renal involvement.

XII. LYME DISEASE

A. Description
   1. **Lyme disease** is an infection caused by the spirochete *Borrelia burgdorferi*, acquired from a tick bite (ticks live in wooded areas and survive by attaching to a host).
   2. Infection with the spirochete stimulates inflammatory cytokines and autoimmune mechanisms.

B. Data collection (Box 61-3)

 The typical ring shaped rash of Lyme disease does not occur in all clients. Many clients never develop a rash. Additionally, if a rash does occur, it can occur anywhere on the body, not only at the site of the bite.

C. Interventions
1. Gently remove the tick with tweezers, wash skin with antiseptic, and dispose of the tick by flushing it down the toilet; the tick may also be disposed of by placing it in a sealed jar so that the HCP can inspect it and determine its type.
2. Obtain a blood test 4 to 6 weeks after a bite to detect the presence of the disease (testing before this time is not reliable).
3. Instruct the client in the administration of antibiotics as prescribed if the disease is confirmed.
4. Instruct the client to avoid areas that contain ticks, such as wooded grassy areas, especially in the summer months.
5. Instruct the client to wear long-sleeved tops, long pants, closed shoes, and hats while outside.
6. Instruct the client to spray the body with tick repellent before going outside.
7. Instruct the client to examine the body when returning inside for the presence of ticks.

Box 61-3 Data Collection and Stages of Lyme Disease

First Stage
Symptoms can occur several days to months following the bite.
A small red pimple develops that spreads into a ring-shaped rash.
Rash may be large or small or may not occur at all.
Flu-like symptoms occur, such as headaches, stiff neck, muscle aches, and fatigue.

Second Stage
This stage occurs several weeks following the bite.
Joint pain occurs.
Neurological complications occur.
Cardiac complications occur.

Third Stage
Large joints become involved.
Arthritis progresses.

XIII. IMMUNODEFICIENCY SYNDROMES

A. Acquired immunodeficiency syndrome (AIDS)
1. **AIDS** is a viral disease caused by **human immunodeficiency virus (HIV)** that destroys T cells, thereby increasing susceptibility to infection and malignancy (Figure 61-4).
2. The syndrome is manifested clinically by opportunistic infection and unusual neoplasms.
3. **AIDS** is considered a chronic illness.
4. The disease has a long incubation period, sometimes up to 10 years or more.
5. Manifestations may not appear until late in the infection.

▲ **FIGURE 61-4** The life cycle of HIV. (From Ignatavicius, D., & Workman, M. [2010]. *Medical surgical nursing: Patient-centered collaborative care* [6th ed.]. St. Louis: Saunders.)

Box 61-4 Tests Used to Evaluate HIV Progression

Complete Blood Cell Count
WBC count normal to decreased
Lymphopenia (<30% of the normal number of WBCs)
Thrombocytopenia (decreased platelet count)

Lymphocyte Screen
Reduced CD4+/CD8+ T-cell ratio
CD4+ (helper) lymphocytes decreased
CD8+ lymphocytes increased

Quantitative Immunoglobin
IgG increased
IgA frequently increased

Chemistry Panel
Lactate dehydrogenase increased (all fractions)
Serum albumin decreased
Total protein increased
Cholesterol decreased

AST and ALT elevated

Anergy Panel
Nonreactive (anergic) or poorly reactive to infectious agents or environmental materials (e.g., pokeweed, phytohemagglutinin mitogens and antigens, mumps, *Candida*)

Hepatitis B Surface Antigen
To detect the presence of hepatitis C

Blood Cultures
To detect septicemia

Chest Radiograph
To detect *Pneumocystis jiroveci* infection or tuberculosis

ALT, Alanine aminotransferase; *AST*, aspartate aminotransferase; immunoglobulin; *WBC*, white blood cell.
From Copstead, L., & Banasik, J. (2010). *Pathophysiology* (4th ed.). St. Louis: Saunders.

B. Diagnosis and monitoring the client with **AIDS**
  1. Refer to Chapter 11 for diagnostic tests.
  2. Refer to Box 61-4 for tests used to evaluate the progression of **HIV** infection.
C. High-risk groups
  1. Heterosexual or homosexual contact with high-risk individuals
  2. Intravenous drug abusers
  3. Persons receiving blood products
  4. Health care workers
  5. Babies born to infected mothers
D. Data collection
  1. Malaise, fever, anorexia, weight loss, influenza-like symptoms
  2. Lymphadenopathy of at least 3 months
  3. Leukopenia
  4. Diarrhea
  5. Fatigue
  6. Night sweats
  7. Presence of opportunistic infections
  8. Protozoal infections (*P. jiroveci* pneumonia [major source of mortality])
  9. Neoplasms (**Kaposi's sarcoma**: purplish/red lesions of internal organs and skin), B-cell non-Hodgkin's lymphoma, cervical cancer
  10. Fungal infections (candidiasis, histoplasmosis)
  11. Viral infections (cytomegalovirus, herpes simplex)
  12. Bacterial infections
E. Interventions
  1. Provide respiratory support.
  2. Administer oxygen and respiratory treatments as prescribed.
  3. Provide psychosocial support as needed.
  4. Maintain fluid and electrolyte balance.
  5. Monitor for signs of infection.

  6. Prevent the spread of infection.
  7. Initiate standard and other precautions as necessary.
  8. Provide comfort as necessary.
  9. Provide meticulous skin care.
  10. Provide adequate nutritional support as prescribed.
  11. Refer to Chapters 22 and 39 for additional information on **AIDS**.
F. Kaposi's sarcoma
  1. Description: skin lesions that occur primarily in individuals with a compromised immune system
  2. Data collection
     a. **Kaposi's sarcoma** is a slow-growing tumor that appears as a raised, oblong, purplish/reddish-brown lesion, and that may or may not be tender.
     b. Organ involvement includes the lymph nodes, airways, or lungs, or any part of the gastrointestinal tract from the mouth to anus.
  3. Interventions
     a. Maintain standard and other precautions as necessary.
     b. Provide protective isolation if the immune system is depressed.
     c. Prepare the client for radiation therapy or chemotherapy as prescribed.
     d. Administer immunotherapy, as prescribed, to stabilize the immune system.

XIV. POST-TRANSPLANTATION IMMUNODEFICIENCY

A. Description
  1. Secondary **immunodeficiency** is immunosuppression caused by therapeutic agents.

2. The client must take immunosuppression agents for the rest of his or her life posttransplant to decrease rejection of the transplanted organ or tissue.

B. Diagnosis and monitoring of posttransplant clients
1. Check renal and hepatic function.
2. Monitor the complete cell count with differential to monitor for signs of infection.
3. Assess all body secretions periodically for blood.

C. High-risk clients
1. Clients with a history of malignancy or pre-malignancy have an increased susceptibility to malignancy if immunosuppressed.
2. Clients with recent infection or exposure to tuberculosis, herpes zoster, or chickenpox have a high risk for severe generalized disease when on immunosuppressive agents.

D. Data collection
1. Monitor for signs of opportunistic infections.
2. Monitor nutritional status.
3. Monitor for signs of rejection (signs will depend on the organ or tissue transplant).

E. Interventions
1. Strict aseptic technique is necessary.
2. Provide teaching regarding asepsis and the signs of infection and rejection.
3. Provide psychosocial support as needed.
4. Provide client teaching about immunosuppressants.

MORE QUESTIONS ON EVOLVE!

Practice Questions

646. Which of the following individuals is least likely at risk for the development of Kaposi's sarcoma?
1. A kidney transplant client
2. A male with a history of same-sex partners
3. A client receiving antineoplastic medications
4. An individual working in an environment where exposure to asbestos exists

647. The nurse prepares to give a bath and change the bed linens on a client with cutaneous Kaposi's sarcoma lesions. The lesions are open and draining a scant amount of serous fluid. Which of the following would the nurse incorporate in the plan during the bathing of this client?
1. Wearing gloves
2. Wearing a gown and gloves
3. Wearing a gown, gloves, and a mask
4. Wearing a gown and gloves to change the bed linens and gloves only for the bath

648. A client is suspected of having systemic lupus erythematous. The nurse monitors the client, knowing that which of the following is one of the initial characteristic signs of systemic lupus erythematous?
1. Weight gain
2. Subnormal temperature
3. Elevated red blood cell count
4. Rash on the face across the bridge of the nose and on the cheeks

649. A client with pemphigus is being seen in the clinic regularly. The nurse plans care based on which of the following descriptions of this condition?
1. The presence of tiny red vesicles
2. An autoimmune disease that causes blistering in the epidermis
3. The presence of skin vesicles found along the nerve caused by a virus
4. The presence of red, raised papules and large plaques covered by silvery scales

650. The client is brought to the emergency department and is experiencing an anaphylactic reaction from eating shellfish. The nurse implements which immediate action?
1. Maintaining a patent airway
2. Administering a corticosteroid
3. Administering epinephrine (Adrenalin)
4. Instructing the client on the importance of obtaining a Medic-Alert bracelet

651. The nurse is assisting in planning care for a client with a diagnosis of immune deficiency. The nurse would incorporate which of the following as a priority in the plan of care?
1. Protecting the client from infection
2. Providing emotional support to decrease fear
3. Encouraging discussion about lifestyle changes
4. Identifying factors that decreased the immune function

652. A client calls the office of his primary care health care provider and tells the nurse that he was just stung by a bumblebee while gardening. The client is afraid of a severe reaction, because the client's neighbor experienced such a reaction just 1 week ago. The appropriate nursing action is to:
1. Advise the client to soak the site in hydrogen peroxide.
2. Ask the client if he ever sustained a bee sting in the past.
3. Tell the client to call an ambulance for transport to the emergency room.
4. Tell the client not to worry about the sting unless difficulty with breathing occurs.

653. The nurse is assisting in administering immunizations at a health care clinic. The nurse understands that immunization provides which of the following?

1. Protection from all diseases
2. Innate immunity from disease
3. Natural immunity from disease
4. Acquired immunity from disease

654. The nurse is assigned to care for a client with systemic lupus erythematosus (SLE). The nurse plans care knowing that this disorder is:
1. A local rash that occurs as a result of allergy
2. A disease caused by overexposure to sunlight
3. An inflammatory disease of collagen contained in connective tissue
4. A disease caused by the continuous release of histamine in the body

655. The camp nurse prepares to instruct a group of children about Lyme disease. Which of the following information would the nurse include in the instructions?
1. Lyme disease is caused by a tick carried by deer.
2. Lyme disease is caused by contamination from cat feces.
3. Lyme disease can be contagious by skin contact with an infected individual.
4. Lyme disease can be caused by the inhalation of spores from bird droppings.

656. The client is diagnosed with stage I of Lyme disease. The nurse assesses the client for which characteristic of this stage?
1. Arthralgias
2. Flu-like symptoms
3. Enlarged and inflamed joints
4. Signs of neurological disorders

657. A female client arrives at the health care clinic and tells the nurse that she was just bitten by a tick and would like to be tested for Lyme disease. The client tells the nurse that she removed the tick and flushed it down the toilet. Which of the following nursing actions is appropriate?
1. Refer the client for a blood test immediately.

2. Inform the client that there is not a test available for Lyme disease.
3. Tell the client that testing is not necessary unless arthralgia develops.
4. Instruct the client to return in 4 to 6 weeks to be tested, because testing before this time is not reliable.

658. A Cub Scout leader who is a nurse is preparing a group of Cub Scouts for an overnight camping trip and instructs the scouts about the methods to prevent Lyme disease. Which statement by one of the Cub Scouts indicates a need for further instructions?
1. "I need to bring a hat to wear during the trip."
2. "I should wear long-sleeved tops and long pants."
3. "I should not use insect repellent because it will attract the ticks."
4. "I need to wear closed shoes and socks that can be pulled up over my pants."

659. The client with acquired immunodeficiency syndrome is diagnosed with cutaneous Kaposi's sarcoma. Based on this diagnosis, the nurse understands that this has been confirmed by which of the following?
1. Swelling in the genital area
2. Swelling in the lower extremities
3. Punch biopsy of the cutaneous lesions
4. Appearance of reddish-blue lesions on the skin

660. Which interventions would apply in the care of a client at high risk for an allergic response to a latex allergy. **Select all that apply**.
 ❑ 1. Use non-latex gloves.
 ❑ 2. Use medications from glass ampules.
 ❑ 3. Place the client in a private room only.
 ❑ 4. Do not puncture rubber stoppers with needles.
 ❑ 5. Keep a latex-safe supply cart available in the client's area.
 ❑ 6. Use a blood pressure cuff from an electronic device only to measure the blood pressure.

ANSWERS

646. 4

Rationale: Kaposi's sarcoma is a vascular malignancy that presents as a skin disorder and is a common acquired immunodeficiency syndrome indicator. It is seen frequently in men with a history of same-sex partners. Although the cause of Kaposi's sarcoma is not known, it is considered to be the result of an alteration or failure in the immune system. The renal transplant client and the client receiving antineoplastic medications are at risk for immunosuppression. Exposure to asbestos is not related to the development of Kaposi's sarcoma.

Test-Taking Strategy: Use the process of elimination. Note the strategic words "least likely at risk." Option 2 can be eliminated easily. Note that options 1 and 3 are comparable or alike. These clients are at risk for immunosuppression. With this in mind, these options can be eliminated. If you had difficulty with this question, review the risk factors associated with Kaposi's sarcoma.
Level of Cognitive Ability: Analyzing
Client Needs: Physiological Integrity
Integrated Process: Nursing Process/Data Collection
Content Area: Adult Health/Immune
References: Christensen, Kockrow, p. 734. 2011. *Adult health nursing.* Linton, p. 1196. 2012.

647. 2

Rationale: Gowns and gloves are required if the nurse anticipates contact with soiled items, such as wound drainage, or while caring for a client who is incontinent with diarrhea or a client who has an ileostomy or colostomy. Masks are not required unless droplet or airborne precautions are necessary. Regardless of the amount of wound drainage, a gown and gloves must be worn.

Test-Taking Strategy: Use the process of elimination and think about the method of transmission of infection when answering a question of this type. Read the question, noting the task that is presented in this case is bathing and changing linens. Eliminate option 3, because the method of transmission is not respiratory. Eliminate options 1 and 4, because neither provides adequate protection based on the method of transmission. If you had difficulty with this question, review standard and transmission-based precautions.

Level of Cognitive Ability: Applying
Client Needs: Safe and Effective Care Environment
Integrated Process: Nursing Process/Planning
Content Area: Adult Health/Immune
Reference: deWit, pp. 120, 1189–1190. 2009.

648. 4

Rationale: Skin lesions or rash on the face across the bridge of the nose and on the cheeks is an initial characteristic sign of systemic lupus erythematosus (SLE). Fever and weight loss may also occur. Anemia is most likely to occur later in SLE.

Test-Taking Strategy: Use the process of elimination and note the strategic words "characteristic sign." Recalling the characteristic butterfly rash associated with SLE will direct you to the correct option. If you are unfamiliar with this disorder, review this content.

Level of Cognitive Ability: Analyzing
Client Needs: Physiological Integrity
Integrated Process: Nursing Process/Data Collection
Content Area: Adult Health/Immune
Reference: Christensen, Kockrow, pp. 85–86. 2011. *Adult health nursing.*

649. 2

Rationale: Pemphigus is an autoimmune disease that causes blistering in the epidermis. The client has large flaccid blisters (bullae). Because the blisters are in the epidermis, they have a thin covering of skin and break easily, leaving large denuded areas of skin. On initial examination, clients may have crusting areas instead of intact blisters. Option 1 describes eczema, option 3 describes herpes zoster, and option 4 describes psoriasis.

Test-Taking Strategy: Use the process of elimination. Recalling that pemphigus vulgaris is an autoimmune disorder will direct you to the correct option. If you had difficulty with this question, review the characteristics of this disorder.

Level of Cognitive Ability: Understanding
Client Needs: Physiological Integrity
Integrated Process: Nursing Process/Planning
Content Area: Adult Health/Immune
Reference: Linton, p. 1193. 2012.

650. 1

Rationale: If the client experiences an anaphylactic reaction, the immediate action would be to maintain a patent airway.

The client then would receive epinephrine. Corticosteroids may also be prescribed. The client will need to be instructed about obtaining and wearing a Medic-Alert bracelet, but this is not the immediate action.

Test-Taking Strategy: Focus on the strategic word "immediate." This strategic word tells you that you need to prioritize your nursing actions. Use the ABCs—airway, breathing, and circulation—to answer the question. Airway is always the priority. Review care to the client experiencing an anaphylactic reaction if you had difficulty with this question.

Level of Cognitive Ability: Applying
Client Needs: Physiological Integrity
Integrated Process: Nursing Process/Implementation
Content Area: Critical Care
Reference: Christensen, Kockrow, p. 728. 2011. *Adult health nursing.*

651. 1

Rationale: The client with immune deficiency has inadequate or absent immune bodies and is at risk for infection. The priority nursing intervention would be to protect the client from infection. Options 2, 3, and 4 may be components of care but are not the priority.

Test-Taking Strategy: Use Maslow's hierarchy of needs theory to answer the question. Remember that physiological needs are the priority. This will direct you to the correct option. Review the care of a client with immune deficiency if you had difficulty with this question.

Level of Cognitive Ability: Applying
Client Needs: Physiological Integrity
Integrated Process: Nursing Process/Planning
Content Area: Adult Health/Immune
Reference: deWit, pp. 234–236. 2009.

652. 2

Rationale: In some types of allergies, a reaction occurs only on second and subsequent contacts with the allergen. Therefore, the appropriate action would be to ask the client if he ever received a bee sting in the past. Option 1 is not appropriate advice. Option 3 is unnecessary. The client should not be told "not to worry."

Test-Taking Strategy: Use the steps of the nursing process to answer the question. Option 2 is the only option that addresses data collection. Review information related to allergic reactions if you had difficulty with this question.

Level of Cognitive Ability: Applying
Client Needs: Physiological Integrity
Integrated Process: Nursing Process/Implementation
Content Area: Adult Health/Immune
References: deWit, p. 258. 2009.
Linton, p. 253. 2012.

653. 4

Rationale: Acquired immunity can occur by receiving an immunization that causes antibodies to a specific pathogen to form. Natural (innate) immunity is present at birth. No immunization protects the client from all diseases.

Test-Taking Strategy: Use the process of elimination and knowledge regarding immunity to disease to answer the question. Eliminate option 1 first because of the closed-ended word

"all." Next eliminate options 2 and 3 because they are comparable or alike. Review natural and acquired immunity if you had difficulty with this question.
Level of Cognitive Ability: Understanding
Client Needs: Health Promotion and Maintenance
Integrated Process: Nursing Process/Implementation
Content Area: Adult Health/Immune
Reference: Christensen, Kockrow, p. 720. 2011. *Adult health nursing.*

654. 3
Rationale: SLE is an inflammatory disease of collagen contained in connective tissue. Options 1, 2, and 4 are not associated with this disease.
Test-Taking Strategy: Use the process of elimination. Eliminate option 1 because SLE is a systemic disorder, not a local one. Next eliminate option 2 because of its similarity to option 1. From the remaining options, select option 3 because of its systemic characteristic. If you are unfamiliar with this disorder, review its characteristics.
Level of Cognitive Ability: Understanding
Client Needs: Physiological Integrity
Integrated Process: Nursing Process/Planning
Content Area: Adult Health/Immune
Reference: Christensen, Kockrow, pp. 85–87. 2011. *Adult health nursing.*

655. 1
Rationale: Lyme disease is a multisystem infection that results from a bite by a tick carried by several species of deer. Persons bitten by *Ixodes* ticks can be infected with the spirochete *Borrelia burgdorferi.* Lyme disease cannot be transmitted from one person to another. Toxoplasmosis is caused from the ingestion of cysts from contaminated cat feces. Histoplasmosis is caused by the inhalation of spores from bat or bird droppings.
Test-Taking Strategy: Use the process of elimination. Recalling that this disease is caused by a bite will assist in eliminating the incorrect options. If you had difficulty with this question, review the cause of Lyme disease.
Level of Cognitive Ability: Applying
Client Needs: Health Promotion and Maintenance
Integrated Process: Teaching and Learning
Content Area: Adult Health/Immune
Reference: Linton, p. 254. 2012.

656. 2
Rationale: The hallmark of stage I is the development of a skin rash within 2 to 30 days of infection, generally at the site of the tick bite. The rash develops into a concentric ring, giving it a bull's-eye appearance. The lesion enlarges up to 50 to 60 cm, and smaller lesions develop farther away from the original tick bite. In stage I, most infected persons develop flu-like symptoms that last 7 to 10 days; these symptoms may reoccur later. Neurological deficits occur in stage II. Arthralgias and joint enlargements are most likely to occur in stage III.
Test-Taking Strategy: Use the process of elimination and eliminate options 1 and 3 first, because they are comparable or alike. Next, note that the question asks for the characteristic of stage I. From the remaining two options, select the least serious one because the subject of the question relates to stage I.

Expect neurological disorders to occur with progression of the disease. If you had difficulty with this question, review the stages of Lyme disease.
Level of Cognitive Ability: Understanding
Client Needs: Physiological Integrity
Integrated Process: Nursing Process/Data Collection
Content Area: Adult Health/Immune
Reference: Linton, p. 254. 2012.

657. 4
Rationale: A blood test is available to detect Lyme disease; however, the test is not reliable if performed before 4 to 6 weeks following the tick bite. Antibody formation takes place in the following manner: immunoglobulin M is detected 3 to 4 weeks after Lyme disease onset, peaks at 6 to 8 weeks, and then gradually disappears; immunoglobulin G is detected 2 to 3 months after infection and may remain elevated for years. Options 1, 2, and 3 are incorrect.
Test-Taking Strategy: Use the process of elimination. Eliminate option 1 first. The word "immediately" should indicate that this is potentially an incorrect option. A blood test is available; therefore, eliminate option 2. Eliminate option 3, because treatment should begin before the arthralgia develops. If you had difficulty with this question, review the method of diagnosing Lyme disease.
Level of Cognitive Ability: Applying
Client Needs: Physiological Integrity
Integrated Process: Nursing Process/Implementation
Content Area: Adult Health/Immune
Reference: Linton, p. 254. 2012.

658. 3
Rationale: In the prevention of Lyme disease, individuals need to be instructed to use an insect repellent on the skin and clothes when in an area where ticks are likely to be found. Long-sleeved tops and long pants, closed shoes, and a hat or cap should be worn. If possible, one should avoid heavily wooded areas or areas with thick underbrush. Socks can be pulled up and over the pant legs to prevent ticks from entering under clothing.
Test-Taking Strategy: Use the process of elimination and note the strategic words "need for further instructions." These words indicate a negative event query and ask you to select an option that is an incorrect statement. Note that option 3 uses the words "should not." Reading carefully will assist in directing you to this option. If you had difficulty with this question, review the measures to prevent contact with ticks.
Level of Cognitive Ability: Evaluating
Client Needs: Safe and Effective Care Environment
Integrated Process: Teaching and Learning
Content Area: Adult Health/Immune
Reference: Ignatavicius, Workman, p. 356. 2010.

659. 3
Rationale: Kaposi's sarcoma lesions begin as red, dark blue, or purple macules on the lower legs that change into plaques. These large plaques ulcerate or open and drain. The lesions spread by metastasis through the upper body and then to the face and oral mucosa. They can move to the lymphatic system, lungs, and gastrointestinal tract. Late disease results in swelling and pain in the lower extremities, penis, scrotum, or

face. Diagnosis is made by punch biopsy of cutaneous lesions and biopsy of pulmonary and gastrointestinal lesions.

Test-Taking Strategy: Use the process of elimination. Eliminate options 1 and 2 first, because these symptoms occur late in the development of Kaposi's sarcoma. From the remaining options, note the strategic word "confirmed." This strategic word will assist in directing you to the option that will confirm the diagnosis: the biopsy of the lesions. Review diagnostic measures for Kaposi's sarcoma if you had difficulty with this question.

Level of Cognitive Ability: Analyzing
Client Needs: Physiological Integrity
Integrated Process: Nursing Process/Data Collection
Content Area: Adult Health/Immune
Reference: Christensen, Kockrow, p. 750. 2011. *Adult health nursing.*

❖ **660. 1, 2, 4, 5**
Rationale: If a client is allergic to latex and is at high risk for an allergic response, the nurse would use non-latex gloves and latex-safe supplies and would keep a latex-safe supply cart available in the client's area. Any supplies or materials that contain latex would be avoided. These include blood pressure cuffs and medication bottles with a rubber stopper that requires puncture with a needle. It is not necessary to place the client in a private room.

Test-Taking Strategy: Focus on the subject, the client is at high risk for an allergic response to a latex allergy. Recalling that items that contain rubber are likely to contain latex will direct you to the correct interventions. Also noting the closed-ended word "only" in options 3 and 6 will assist in eliminating these options. Review care to the client with a latex allergy if you had difficulty with this question.

Level of Cognitive Ability: Applying
Client Needs: Safe and Effective Care Environment
Integrated Process: Nursing Process/Implementation
Content Area: Adult Health/Immune
Reference: Christensen, Kockrow, pp. 26–28. 2011. *Adult health nursing.*

62

Immunological Medications

I. HUMAN IMMUNODEFICIENCY VIRUS (HIV) AND ACQUIRED IMMUNODEFICIENCY SYNDROME (AIDS)

A. Medications include nucleoside-nucleotide reverse transcriptase inhibitors, non-nucleoside reverse transcriptase inhibitors, protease inhibitors, and fusion inhibitors (Box 62-1 and Figure 62-1).

B. Nucleoside-nucleotide reverse transcriptase inhibitors and non-nucleoside reverse transcriptase inhibitors work by inhibiting the activity of reverse transcriptase.

C. Protease inhibitors work by interfering with the activity of the enzyme protease.

D. Fusion inhibitors work by inhibiting the binding of human **immunodeficiency** virus to cells.

E. Standard treatment consists of using three or four medications in regimens known as highly active antiretroviral therapy (HAART); this therapy is not curative but can delay or reverse loss of immune function, preserve health, and prolong life.

F. Other medications include those that are used to treat complications or opportunistic infections that develop (see Box 62-1).

G. Nucleoside-nucleotide reverse transcriptase inhibitors (NNRTIs)

1. Abacavir (Ziagen): Can cause nausea; monitor for hypersensitivity reaction, including fever, nausea, vomiting, diarrhea, lethargy, malaise, sore throat, shortness of breath, cough, and rash

2. Abacavir; Lamivudine (Epzicom): In addition to the effects that can occur from abacavir and lamivudine, hypersensitivity reactions, lactic acidosis, and severe hepatomegaly can occur.

3. Didanosine (Videx): Can cause nausea, diarrhea, peripheral neuropathy, hepatotoxicity, and pancreatitis

4. Emtricitabine (Emtriva): Can cause headache, diarrhea, nausea, rash, hyperpigmentation of the palms and soles, lactic acidosis, and severe hepatomegaly

5. Emtricitabine; tenofovir (Truvada): In addition to the effects that can occur from emtricitabine and tenofovir, lactic acidosis and severe hepatomegaly can occur.

6. Lamivudine (Epivir): Causes nausea and nasal congestion

7. Lamivudine; zidovudine (Combivir): Can cause anemia and neutropenia and lactic acidosis with hepatomegaly

8. Lamivudine; zidovudine; abacavir (Trizivir): In addition to the effects that can occur from lamivudine, zidovudine, and abacavir, hypersensitivity reactions, anemia, neutropenia, lactic acidosis, and severe hepatomegaly can occur.

9. Stavudine (d4t, Zerit): Can cause peripheral neuropathy and pancreatitis

10. Tenofovir (Viread): Can cause nausea and vomiting

11. Zalcitabine (ddC, Hivid): Can cause oral ulcers, peripheral neuropathy, hepatotoxicity, and pancreatitis

12. Zidovudine (Retrovir, azidothymidine, AZT, ZDV): Can cause nausea, vomiting, anemia, leukopenia, myopathy, fatigue, and headache

H. Non-nucleoside reverse transcriptase inhibitors (NRTIs)

1. Delavirdine (Rescriptor): Can cause rash, liver function changes, and pruritis

2. Efavirenz (Sustiva): Can cause rash, dizziness, confusion, difficulty concentrating, dreams, and encephalopathy

3. Nevirapine (Viramune): Can cause rash, Stevens-Johnson syndrome, hepatitis, and increased transaminase levels

I. Protease inhibitors (PIs)

1. Amprenavir; vitamin E (Agenerase)
   a. Can cause nausea, vomiting, headache, altered taste sensations, perioral paresthesia, rashes, and increased results of liver function studies
   b. Oral solution contains an alcohol that can interact with metronidazole (Flagyl); can cause feelings of inebriation

2. Atazanavir (Reyataz): Can cause nausea, headache, infection, vomiting, diarrhea, drowsiness, insomnia, fever, hyperglycemia, hyperlipidemia, and increased bleeding in clients with hemophilia

Box 62-1 Medications for HIV and AIDS

Nucleoside-Nucleotide Reverse Transcriptase Inhibitors (NNRTIs)
Abacavir (Ziagen)
Abacavir; lamivudine (Epzicom)
Didanosine (Videx)
Emtricitabine (Emtriva)
Emtricitabine; tenofovir (Truvada)
Emtricitabine; tenofovir; efavirenz (Atripla)
Lamivudine (Epivir)
Lamivudine; zidovudine (Combivir)
Lamivudine; zidovudine; abacavir (Trizivir)
Stavudine (d4t, Zerit XR)
Tenofovir (Viread)
Zidovudine (Retrovir, azidothymidine, AZT, ZDV)

Non-Nucleoside Reverse Transcriptase Inhibitors (NRTIs)
Delavirdine (Rescriptor)
Efavirenz (Sustiva)
Etravirine (Intelence)
Nevirapine (Viramune)

Protease Inhibitors (PIs)
Amprenavir; vitamin E (Agenerase)
Atazanavir (Reyataz)
Danunavir (Prezista)
Fosamprenavir (Lexiva)
Indinavir (Crixivan)
Lopinavir; ritonavir (Kaletra)
Nelfinavir (Viracept)

Ritonavir (Norvir)
Saquinavir (Invirase)
Tipranavir (Aptivus)

Integrase Inhibitor
Raltegravir (Isentress)

Fusion Inhibitor
Enfuvirtide (Fuzeon)

CCR5 Antagonist
Maraviroc (Selzentry)

Anti-Inflammatory Medication
Sulfasalazine (Azulfidine)

Anti-Infective Medications
Atovaquone (Mepron)
Metronidazole (Flagyl)
Pentamidine isethionate (Pentam 300)
Sulfamethoxazole; trimethoprim (Bactrim)

Antifungal Medications
Amphotericin B (Fungizone)
Fluconazole (Diflucan)
Ketoconazole

Antiviral Medications
Acyclovir (Zovirax)
Foscarnet
Ganciclovir (Cytovene)

3. Fosamprenavir (Lexiva): Similar to amprenavir; can cause nausea, vomiting, headache, altered taste sensations, perioral paresthesia, rashes, and increased results of liver function studies
4. Indinavir (Crixivan): Can cause nausea, diarrhea, hyperbilirubinemia, nephritis, and kidney stones
5. Lopinavir-ritonavir combination (Kaletra): Can cause nausea, diarrhea, altered taste sensations, circumoral paresthesia, and hepatitis
6. Nelfinavir (Viracept): Can cause nausea, flatulence, and diarrhea
7. Ritonavir (Norvir): Can cause nausea, vomiting, diarrhea, altered taste sensations, circumoral paresthesia, hepatitis, and increased triglyceride levels
8. Saquinavir (Invirase): Can cause nausea, diarrhea, photosensitivity, and headache
9. Tipranavir (Aptivus): Hepatotoxicity (liver damage); can also cause nausea, vomiting, diarrhea, headache, and fatigue
J. Integrase inhibitor: Raltegravor (Isentress)
1. Stops HIV replication and is used in combination with other antiretroviral medications
2. Common side effects include nausea, diarrhea, fatigue, headache, and itching
K. Chemokine receptor 5 (CCR5) antagonist: Maraviroc (Selzentry)

1. Binds with CCR5 and blocks viral entry
2. Most common side effects are cough, dizziness, pyrexia, rash, abdominal pain, musculoskeletal symptoms, and upper respiratory tract infections; liver injury, and cardiovascular events have occurred in some clients
L. Fusion inhibitor: Enfuvirtide (Fuzeon) can cause skin irritation at injection site, fatigue, nausea, insomnia, and peripheral neuropathy.
M. Anti-infective medications: Used to treat opportunistic infections such as *Pneumocystis jiroveci* pneumonia; *Toxoplasma* encephalitis is treated with sulfamethoxazole-trimethoprim (Bactrim; see Box 62-1)
N. Antifungal medications: Used to treat candidiasis, cryptococcal meningitis (see Box 62-1)
O. Antiviral medications: Used to treat cytomegalovirus retinitis, herpes simplex, varicella zoster virus (see Box 62-1)

 The client with HIV or AIDS is at high risk for the development of opportunistic infections.

II. **IMMUNOSUPPRESSANTS** (Box 62-2 and Figure 62-2)

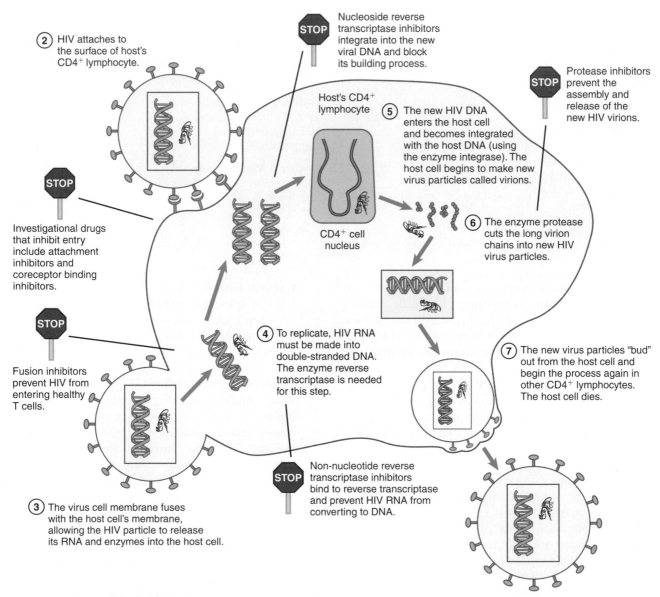

1. HIV virus: HIV genetic material encoated by a protein shell. GP120 proteins are able to attach to CD₄ receptors on the surface of the host's CD4⁺ T cells.

2. HIV attaches to the surface of host's CD4⁺ lymphocyte.

STOP Nucleoside reverse transcriptase inhibitors integrate into the new viral DNA and block its building process.

STOP Protease inhibitors prevent the assembly and release of the new HIV virions.

5. The new HIV DNA enters the host cell and becomes integrated with the host DNA (using the enzyme integrase). The host cell begins to make new virus particles called virions.

Host's CD4⁺ lymphocyte

STOP Investigational drugs that inhibit entry include attachment inhibitors and coreceptor binding inhibitors.

CD4⁺ cell nucleus

6. The enzyme protease cuts the long virion chains into new HIV virus particles.

STOP Fusion inhibitors prevent HIV from entering healthy T cells.

4. To replicate, HIV RNA must be made into double-stranded DNA. The enzyme reverse transcriptase is needed for this step.

7. The new virus particles "bud" out from the host cell and begin the process again in other CD4⁺ lymphocytes. The host cell dies.

3. The virus cell membrane fuses with the host cell's membrane, allowing the HIV particle to release its RNA and enzymes into the host cell.

STOP Non-nucleotide reverse transcriptase inhibitors bind to reverse transcriptase and prevent HIV RNA from converting to DNA.

▲ **FIGURE 62-1** Steps in the life cycle of the human immunodeficiency virus (HIV), with correlation to medications. (From Black, J., & Hawks, J. [2009]. *Medical-surgical nursing: Clinical management for positive outcomes* [8th ed.]. St. Louis: Saunders.)

Box 62-2 Immunosuppressants

Calcineurin Inhibitors
Cyclosporine (Sandimmune, Gengraf, Neoral)
Tacrolimus (Prograf)

Cytotoxic Medications
Azathioprine (Imuran)
Cyclophosphamide (Neosar)
Methotrexate (Rheumatrex, Trexall)
Mycophenolate mofetil (CellCept)
Mycophenolic acid (Myfortic)

Antibodies
Basiliximab (Simulect)
Daclizumab (Zenapax)
Lymphocyte immune globulin, antithymocyte globulin (equine)
Muromonab-CD3 (Orthoclone OKT3)
$Rh_o(D)$ immune globulin (RhoGAM)

Other
Sirolimus (Rapamune)

Glucocorticoids
See Chapter 46

A. Description: Immunosuppressants are used for transplant clients to prevent organ or tissue rejection and to treat autoimmune disorders such as systemic lupus erythematosus.
B. Cyclosporine (Sandimmune, Gengraf, Neoral)
  1. Used for prevention of rejection following allogenic organ transplantation
  2. Usually administered with a glucocorticoid and another immunosuppressant
  3. Most common adverse effects are nephrotoxicity, infection, hypertension, and hirsutism
C. Tacrolimus (Prograf)
  1. Used for prevention of rejection following liver or kidney transplantation
  2. Adverse effects include nephrotoxicity, neurotoxicity, gastrointestinal effects, hypertension, hyperkalemia, hyperglycemia, hirsutism, and gum hyperplasia.
D. Azathioprine (Imuran)
  1. Generally used with renal transplant clients
  2. Can cause neutropenia and thrombocytopenia
E. Cyclophosphamide (Neosar)
  1. Used for its immunosuppressant action to treat autoimmune disorders
  2. Can cause neutropenia and hemorrhagic cystitis
F. Methotrexate (Rheumatrex, Trexall)
  1. Used for its immunosuppressant action to treat autoimmune disorders
  2. Can cause hepatic fibrosis and cirrhosis, bone marrow suppression, ulcerative stomatitis, and renal damage
G. Mycophenolate mofetil (CellCept) and mycophenlic acid (Myfortic)
  1. Used to prevent rejection following kidney, heart, and liver transplantation

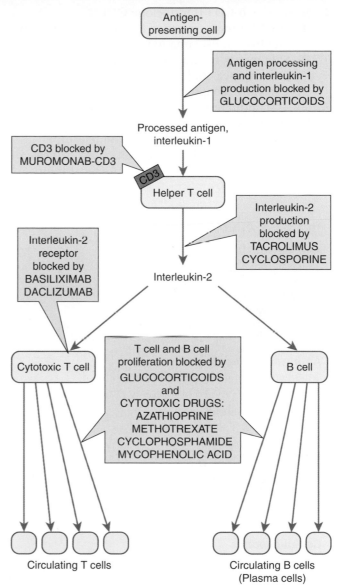

▲ **FIGURE 62-2** Sites of action of immunosuppressant drugs. (From Lehne, R. [2010]. *Pharmacology for nursing care* [7th ed.]. St. Louis: Saunders.)

  2. Can cause diarrhea, vomiting, neutropenia, sepsis; increased risk of infection and malignancies, especially lymphomas
H. Basiliximab (Simulect); daclizumab (Zenapax)
  1. Used to prevent rejection following kidney transplantation
  2. Can cause severe acute hypersensitivity reactions including anaphylaxis
I. Lymphocyte immune globulin, antithymocyte globulin (equine)
  1. Used to prevent rejection following kidney, heart, liver, and bone marrow transplantation
  2. Side effects include fever, chills, leukopenia, and skin reactions
  3. Can cause anaphylactoid reactions

J. Muromonab-CD3 (Orthoclone OKT3)
  1. Used to prevent rejection following kidney, heart, and liver transplantation
  2. Side effects include fever, chills, dyspnea, chest pain, nausea, and vomiting
  3. Can cause anaphylactoid reactions
K. $Rh_o(D)$ immune globulin (RhoGAM; see Chapter 27)
L. Sirolimus (Rapamune)
  1. Used to prevent renal transplant rejection
  2. Increases the risk of infection; raises cholesterol and triglyceride levels; can cause renal injury

  3. Other side effects include rash, acne, anemia, thrombocytopenia, joint pain, diarrhea, and hypokalemia.

⚠ Monitor the client taking an immunosuppressant closely for signs of infection.

III. IMMUNIZATIONS (see Chapter 39)

Box 62-3 Antibiotics

Aminoglycosides
Amikacin (Amikin)
Gentamicin
Kanamycin (Kantrex)
Neomycin (Neo-Fradin)
Streptomycin
Tobramycin (Nebcin)

Antimycobacterials
Antituberculosis agents (see Chapter 50)
Leprostatics: Clofazimine (Lamprene) and dapsone

Antifungal Medications
Amphotericin B (Fungizone)
Fluconazole (Diflucan)
Ketoconazole

Antiviral Medications
Acyclovir (Zovirax)
Foscarnet
Ganciclovir (Cytovene)

Cephalosporins
Cefaclor (Ceclor)
Cefadroxil (Duricef)
Cefazolin (Ancef, Kefzol)
Cefdinir (Omnicef)
Cefditoren (Spectracef)
Cefepime (Maxipime)
Cefotaxime (Claforan)
Cefotetan (Cefotan)
Cefoxitin (Mefoxin)
Cefopodoxime (Vantin)
Cefprozil (Cefzil)
Ceftazidime (Ceptaz, Fortaz, Tazicef)
Ceftibuten (Cedax)
Ceftizoxime (Cefizox)
Ceftriaxone (Rocephin)
Cefuroxime (Ceftin)
Cephalexin (Keflex)
Loracarbef (Lorabid)

Fluoroquinolones
Ciprofloxacin (Cipro)
Gatifloxacin (Tequin)
Gemifloxacin (Factive)
Levofloxacin (Levaquin)

Lomefloxacin (Maxaquin)
Moxifloxacin (Avelox)
Norfloxacin (Noroxin)
Ofloxacin (Floxin)
Trovafloxacin (Trovan)

Lincosamides
Clindamycin (Cleocin)
Lincomycin (Lincocin)

Macrolides
Azithromycin (Zithromax)
Clarithromycin (Biaxin)
Dirithromycin (Dynabac)
Erythromycin

Monobactam
Aztreonam (Azactam)

Penicillins
Amoxicillin (Amoxil)
Ampicillin (Principen)
Carbenicillin (Geocillin)
Penicillin G (Bicillin L-A, Permapen, Pfizerpen, Wycillin)
Penicillin V (Veetids)
Piperacillin
Ticarcillin (Ticar)

Penicillinase-Resistant Penicillins
Dicloxacillin
Nafcillin
Oxacillin

Sulfonamides
Sulfamethoxazole
Sulfadiazine
Sulfasalizine
Sulfisoxazole
Trimethoprim; sulfamethoxazole (TMP-SMZ; Bactrim, Cotrim, Septra)

Tetracyclines
Demeclocycline (Declomycin)
Doxycycline (Vibramycin)
Minocycline (Minocin)
Oxytetracycline (Terramycin)
Tetracycline (Sumycin)

IV. ANTIBIOTICS (Box 62-3)

A. Inhibit the growth of bacteria

B. Include medication classifications of aminoglycosides, cephalosporins, fluoroquinolones, macrolides, lincosamides, monobactams, penicillins and penicillinase-resistant penicillins, sulfonamides, tetracyclines, antimycobacterials, antifungals (see Box 62-3)

C. Adverse effects (Table 62-1)

D. Nursing considerations

1. Check for allergies.
2. Monitor appropriate laboratory values before therapy as appropriate and during therapy to assess for adverse effects.
3. Monitor for adverse effects and report to the health care provider if any occur.
4. The appropriate method of administration is determined and instructions are provided to the client.

TABLE 62-1 Antibiotics and their Adverse Effects

Classification	Adverse Effects
Aminoglycosides	Ototoxicity Confusion, disorientation Renal toxicity Gastrointestinal irritation Palpitations, blood pressure changes Hypersensitivity reactions
Cephalosporins	Gastrointestinal disturbances Pseudomembranous colitis Headache, dizziness, lethargy, paresthesias Nephrotoxicity Superinfections
Fluoroquinolones	Headache, dizziness, insomnia, depression Gastrointestinal effects Bone marrow depression Fever, rash, photosensitivity
Macrolides	Gastrointestinal effects Pseudomembranous colitis Confusion, abnormal thinking Superinfections Hypersensitivity reactions
Lincosamides	Gastrointestinal effects Pseudomembranous colitis Bone marrow depression
Monobactams	Gastrointestinal effects Hepatotoxicity Allergic reactions
Penicillins and penicillinase-resistant penicillins	Gastrointestinal effects, including sore mouth and furry tongue Superinfections Hypersensitivity reactions, including anaphylaxis
Sulfonamides	Gastrointestinal effects Hepatotoxicity Nephrotoxicity Bone marrow depression Dermatological effects, including hypersensitivity and photosensitivity Headache, dizziness, vertigo, ataxia, depression, seizures
Tetracyclines	Gastrointestinal effects Hepatotoxicity Teeth (staining) and bone damage Superinfections Dermatological reactions, including rash and photosensitivity Hypersensitivity reactions
Antimycobacterials, leprostatics	Gastrointestinal effects Neuritis, dizziness, headache, malaise, drowsiness, hallucinations
Antifungals	Gastrointestinal effects Headache, rash, anemia, hepatotoxicity, hearing loss, peripheral neuritis

5. Monitor intake and output.
6. Encourage fluid intake (unless contraindicated).
7. Initiate safety precautions because of possible central nervous system effects.
8. The client is taught about the medication and how to take the medication; the importance of completing the full prescribed course is emphasized.

MORE QUESTION ON EVOLVE!

Practice Questions

661. The client who is human immunodeficiency virus seropositive has been taking stavudine (d4t, Zerit). The nurse monitors which of the following most closely while the client is taking this medication?
1. Gait
2. Appetite
3. Level of consciousness
4. Hemoglobin and hematocrit blood levels

662. The client with acquired immunodeficiency syndrome has begun therapy with zidovudine (Retrovir, Azidothymidine, AZT, ZDV). The nurse carefully monitors which of the following laboratory results during treatment with this medication?
1. Blood culture
2. Blood glucose level
3. Blood urea nitrogen
4. Complete blood count

663. The nurse is reviewing the results of serum laboratory studies drawn on a client with acquired immunodeficiency syndrome who is receiving didanosine (Videx). The nurse interprets that the client may have the medication discontinued by the health care provider if which of the following significantly elevated results is noted?
1. Serum protein
2. Blood glucose
3. Serum amylase
4. Serum creatinine

664. The nurse is caring for a postrenal transplant client taking cyclosporine (Sandimmune, Gengraf, Neoral). The nurse notes an increase in one of the client's vital signs, and the client is complaining of a headache. What is the vital sign that is most likely increased?
1. Pulse
2. Respirations
3. Blood pressure
4. Pulse oximetry

665. Amikacin (Amikin) is prescribed for a client with a bacterial infection. The client is instructed to contact the health care provider (HCP) immediately if which of the following occurs?
1. Nausea
2. Lethargy
3. Hearing loss
4. Muscle aches

666. The nurse is assigned to care for a client with cytomegalovirus retinitis and acquired immunodeficiency syndrome who is receiving foscarnet. The nurse should check the latest results of which of the following laboratory studies while the client is taking this medication?
1. CD4 cell count
2. Serum albumin
3. Serum creatinine
4. Lymphocyte count

667. The client with acquired immunodeficiency syndrome and *Pneumocystis jiroveci* infection has been receiving pentamidine isethionate (Pentam 300). The client develops a temperature of 101 ° F. The nurse does further monitoring of the client, knowing that this sign would most likely indicate:
1. The dose of the medication is too low.
2. The client is experiencing toxic effects of the medication.
3. The client has developed inadequacy of thermoregulation.
4. The result of another infection caused by leukopenic effects of the medication.

668. Saquinavir (Invirase) is prescribed for the client who is human immunodeficiency virus seropositive. The nurse reinforces medication instructions and tells the client to:
1. Avoid sun exposure.
2. Eat low-calorie foods.
3. Eat foods that are low in fat.
4. Take the medication on an empty stomach.

669. Ketoconazole is prescribed for a client with a diagnosis of candidiasis. Select the interventions that the nurse includes when administering this medication. **Select all that apply**.
- ❏ 1. Restrict fluid intake.
- ❏ 2. Instruct the client to avoid alcohol.
- ❏ 3. Monitor hepatic and liver function studies.
- ❏ 4. Administer the medication with an antacid.
- ❏ 5. Instruct the client to avoid exposure to the sun.
- ❏ 6. Administer the medication on an empty stomach.

❖ **670.** A client with human immunodeficiency virus is taking nevirapine (Viramune). The nurse should monitor for which adverse effects of the medication? **Select all that apply.**

❏ 1. Rash
❏ 2. Hepatotoxicity
❏ 3. Hyperglycemia
❏ 4. Peripheral neuropathy
❏ 5. Reduced bone mineral density

ANSWERS

661. 1

Rationale: Stavudine (d4t, Zerit) is an antiretroviral used to manage human immunodeficiency virus infection in clients who do not respond to or who cannot tolerate conventional therapy. The medication can cause peripheral neuropathy, and the nurse should monitor the client's gait closely and ask the client about paresthesia. Options 2, 3, and 4 are unrelated to the use of the medication.
Test-Taking Strategy: Focus on the name of the medication. Recalling that this medication causes peripheral neuropathy will direct you to the correct option. If you are not familiar with this medication and the important data collection measures, review this content.
Level of Cognitive Ability: Analyzing
Client Needs: Physiological Integrity
Integrated Process: Nursing Process/Data Collection
Content Area: Pharmacology
Reference: Hodgson, Kizior, pp. 1081–1082. 2012.

662. 4

Rationale: A common side effect of therapy with zidovudine is leukopenia and anemia. The nurse monitors the complete blood count results for these changes. Options 1, 2, and 3 are unrelated to the use of this medication.
Test-Taking Strategy: Focus on the name of the medication. Recalling that zidovudine causes leukopenia and anemia will direct you to the correct option. Review this medication if you had difficulty with this question.
Level of Cognitive Ability: Analyzing
Client Needs: Physiological Integrity
Integrated Process: Nursing Process/Data Collection
Content Area: Pharmacology
Reference: Hodgson, Kizior, p. 1229. 2012.

663. 3

Rationale: Didanosine (Videx) can cause pancreatitis. A serum amylase level that is increased 1.5 to 2 times normal may signify pancreatitis in the client with acquired immunodeficiency syndrome and is potentially fatal. The medication may have to be discontinued. The medication is also hepatotoxic and can result in liver failure.
Test-Taking Strategy: Focus on the name of the medication. Recalling that this medication can cause damage to the pancreas and is hepatotoxic will direct you to the correct option. Review this medication if you had difficulty with this question.
Level of Cognitive Ability: Analyzing
Client Needs: Physiological Integrity
Integrated Process: Nursing Process/Data Collection
Content Area: Pharmacology
Reference: Hodgson, Kizior, p. 349–351. 2012.

664. 3

Rationale: Hypertension can occur in a client taking cyclosporine (Sandimmune, Gengraf, Neoral), and because this client is also complaining of a headache, the blood pressure is the vital sign to be monitoring most closely. Other adverse effects include infection, nephrotoxicity, and hirsutism. Options 1, 2, and 4 are unrelated to the use of this medication.
Test-Taking Strategy: Focus on the name of the medication and the data in the question, and recall that this medication can cause hypertension. Review the adverse effects of this medication if you had difficulty with this question.
Level of Cognitive Ability: Analyzing
Client Needs: Physiological Integrity
Integrated Process: Nursing Process/Data Collection
Content Area: Pharmacology
Reference: Hodgson, Kizior, pp. 289–291. 2012.

665. 3

Rationale: Amikacin (Amikin) is an aminoglycoside. Adverse effects of aminoglycosides include ototoxicity (hearing problems), confusion, disorientation, gastrointestinal irritation, palpitations, blood pressure changes, nephrotoxicity, and hypersensitivity. The nurse instructs the client to report hearing loss to the HCP immediately. Lethargy and muscle aches are not associated with the use of this medication. It is not necessary to contact the HCP immediately if nausea occurs. If nausea persists or results in vomiting, the HCP should be notified.
Test-Taking Strategy: Note the strategic words "contact the HCP immediately." Recalling that this medication is an aminoglycoside (most aminoglycoside medication names end in the letters -*cin*) and that aminogylcosides are ototoxic will direct you to the correct option. Review the adverse effects of aminoglycosides if you had difficulty with this question.
Level of Cognitive Ability: Applying
Client Needs: Physiological Integrity
Integrated Process: Teaching and Learning
Content Area: Pharmacology
Reference: Hodgson, Kizior, pp. 48–50. 2012.

666. 3

Rationale: Foscarnet is toxic to the kidneys. Serum creatinine is monitored before therapy, two to three times per week during induction therapy, and at least weekly during maintenance therapy. Foscarnet may also cause decreased levels of calcium, magnesium, phosphorus, and potassium. Thus these levels are also measured with the same frequency.
Test-Taking Strategy: Use the process of elimination. Recalling that this medication is nephrotoxic will direct you to the correct option. Review this medication if you are unfamiliar with it.

Level of Cognitive Ability: Analyzing
Client Needs: Physiological Integrity
Integrated Process: Nursing Process/Data Collection
Content Area: Pharmacology
Reference: Hodgson, Kizior, p. 518. 2012.

667. 4

Rationale: Frequent side effects of this medication include leukopenia, thrombocytopenia, and anemia. The client should be monitored routinely for signs and symptoms of infection. Options 1, 2, and 3 are inaccurate interpretations.
Test-Taking Strategy: Use the process of elimination focusing on the strategic words "develops a temperature." Note the relationship between these strategic words and the correct option. Review the side effects of this medication if you had difficulty with this question.
Level of Cognitive Ability: Analyzing
Client Needs: Physiological Integrity
Integrated Process: Nursing Process/Data Collection
Content Area: Pharmacology
References: Hodgson, Kizior, pp. 917–919. 2012.
Lehne, p. 1161. 2010.

668. 1

Rationale: Saquinavir (Invirase) is an antiretroviral (protease inhibitor) used with other antiretroviral medications to manage human immunodeficiency virus infection. Saquinavir is administered with meals and is best absorbed if the client consumes high-calorie, high-fat meals. Saquinavir can cause photosensitivity, and the nurse should instruct the client to avoid sun exposure.
Test-Taking Strategy: Use the process of elimination. Options 2 and 3 can be eliminated first, knowing that these dietary measures would not likely be prescribed for this client. From the remaining options, you must know that this medication can cause photosensitivity. Review this medication if you had difficulty with this question.
Level of Cognitive Ability: Applying
Client Needs: Physiological Integrity
Integrated Process: Teaching and Learning
Content Area: Pharmacology
Reference: Hodgson, Kizior, pp. 1042–1043. 2012.

669. 2, 3, 5

Rationale: Ketoconazole is an antifungal medication. It is administered with food (not on an empty stomach) and antacids are avoided for 2 hours after taking the medication to ensure absorption. The medication is hepatotoxic and the nurse monitors liver function studies. The client is instructed to avoid exposure to the sun because the medication increases photosensitivity. The client is also instructed to avoid alcohol. There is no reason for the client to restrict fluid intake. In fact, this could be harmful to the client.
Test-Taking Strategy: Use general medication guidelines to assist in selecting the correct interventions. Also remember that this medication is administered with food and that it is hepatotoxic. Review this medication if you had difficulty with this question.
Level of Cognitive Ability: Analyzing
Client Needs: Physiological Integrity
Integrated Process: Nursing Process/Implementation
Content Area: Pharmacology
Reference: Hodgson, Kizior, pp. 648–650. 2012.

670. 1, 2

Rationale: Nevirapine (Viramune) is a non-nucleoside reverse transcriptase inhibitors (NRTI) that is used to treat HIV infection. It is used in combination with other antiretroviral medications to treat HIV. Adverse effects include rash, Stevens-Johnson syndrome, hepatitis, and increased transaminase levels. Hyperglycemia, peripheral neuropathy, and reduced bone density are not adverse effects of this medication.
Test-Taking Strategy: Specific knowledge regarding the adverse effects of this medication is needed to answer this question correctly. Remember that rash, Stevens-Johnson syndrome, hepatitis, and increased transaminase levels are adverse effects of nevirapine. Review this medication if you had difficulty with this question.
Level of Cognitive Ability: Analyzing
Client Needs: Physiological Integrity
Integrated Process: Nursing Process/Implementation
Content Area: Pharmacology
Reference: Lehne, p. 1099. 2010.

UNIT 19

The Adult Client with a Mental Health Disorder

PYRAMID TERMS

abuse An act of misuse, deceit, or exploitation toward another individual that results in injury, damage, maltreatment, or corruption; can also refer to misuse of a chemical substance such as a controlled drug

addiction Also known as drug dependence; incorporates the concepts of loss of control with respect to the use of a drug, taking the drug despite related problems and complications, and a tendency to relapse

coping mechanisms Methods of adjusting to environmental stress without altering one's own goals or purposes; can include both conscious and unconscious mechanisms

crisis A temporary state of disequilibrium in which an individual's usual coping mechanisms or problem-solving methods fail. It can result in personality growth or personality disorganization.

defense mechanisms A coping mechanism (protective defense) of the ego that attempts to protect the individual from feelings of inadequacy and worthlessness and prevent awareness of anxiety. When anxiety is too painful, the individual copes by using defense mechanisms to protect the ego and decrease anxiety.

milieu The physical and social environment in which an individual lives. Milieu therapy focuses on positive physical and social environmental manipulation to produce positive change.

rape-trauma syndrome A syndrome characterized by an acute phase and a long-term reorganization process that occurs after an actual or attempted sexual assault. Each phase has separate symptoms.

restraints (security devices) Physical restraints include any manual method or mechanical device, material, or equipment that inhibits free movement. Chemical restraints include the administration of medications for the specific purpose of inhibiting a specific behavior or movement.

seclusion Placing a client alone in a specially designed room for protection and close supervision. It is the last measure in a process to maximize safety to the client and others.

suicide The ultimate act of self-destruction in which an individual purposefully ends his or her own life

suicide attempt Any willful, self-inflicted, or life-threatening attempt by an individual that has not led to death

PYRAMID TO SUCCESS

The Pyramid to Success focuses on the therapeutic nurse-client relationship, client rights, hospital admission procedures, ethical and legal issues related to the care of the client with a mental health disorder, grief and loss, and end-of-life issues. Pyramid points focus on the use of restraints, seclusion, and electroconvulsive therapy (ECT). Focus on care of the client with an addiction, such as an eating disorder or drug or alcohol disorder. Additional focus areas include anxiety, depression, suicide, abuse and violence, rape crisis interventions, posttraumatic stress disorders, obsessive-compulsive disorders, schizophrenia, and bipolar disorders. Pyramid points address the use of medications prescribed for the client with a mental health disorder, particularly lithium and the benzodiazepines.

CLIENT NEEDS

Safe and Effective Care Environment

- Ensuring client advocacy
- Implementing legal responsibilities related to reporting incidences of violence and abuse

- Maintaining confidentiality
- Obtaining informed consent related to treatments, such as restraints, seclusion, and electroconvulsive therapy (ECT)
- Providing psychiatric consultations and referrals
- Providing safety to client and others
- Upholding client rights
- Using restraints and seclusion appropriately and safely

Health Promotion and Maintenance

- Identifying individual lifestyle choices
- Performing psychosocial assessment techniques
- Providing health promotion programs related to addictions
- Identifying community resources for the client

Psychosocial Integrity

- Monitoring for abuse/neglect situations
- Monitoring for chemical dependency
- Monitoring for domestic violence
- Addressing grief and loss and end-of-life issues
- Caring for the client who has been sexually abused or raped

- Considering religious, cultural, and spiritual influences on health
- Developing a therapeutic nurse-client relationship
- Identifying appropriate counseling techniques
- Identifying coping mechanisms
- Identifying support systems
- Implementing behavioral interventions
- Providing crisis intervention
- Providing a therapeutic milieu
- Teaching stress management techniques

Physiological Integrity

- Administering medications as prescribed
- Assessing for abusive and self-destructive behavior
- Monitoring elimination patterns
- Monitoring for alterations in body systems related to addictions
- Monitoring for expected and untoward effects of medications
- Monitoring for potential complications related to medications and electroconvulsive therapy
- Monitoring laboratory values related to medication therapy
- Monitoring rest and sleep patterns
- Providing adequate nutrition
- Providing personal hygiene measures

Foundations of Psychiatric Mental Health Nursing

 I. THE NURSE-CLIENT RELATIONSHIP

A. Principles
1. Genuineness, respect, and empathic understanding are characteristics important to the development of a therapeutic nurse-client relationship.
2. The client should be cared for in a holistic manner.
3. The nurse considers the client's cultural beliefs and values in assessing the client's response to the nurse-client relationship and his or her adaptation to stressors.
4. Appropriate limits and boundaries define and facilitate a therapeutic nurse-client relationship.
5. Honest and open communication is an important cornerstone for the development of trust—an underpinning of the therapeutic nurse-client relationship.
6. The nurse uses therapeutic communication techniques to encourage the client to express thoughts and feelings as they address identified problem areas.
7. The nurse respects the client's confidentiality and limits discussion of the client to members of the treatment team.
8. The goal of the nurse-client relationship is to assist the client to develop problem-solving and **coping mechanisms**.

 The nurse needs to consider the religious and spiritual practices of the client and whether these practices may give the client hope, comfort, and support while healing.

B. Phases of a therapeutic nurse-client relationship
1. Preinteraction phase
   a. The preinteraction phase begins before the nurse's first contact with the client.
   b. The nurse's task in the preinteraction phase is to explore any preconceived ideas, stereotypes, biases, and values that may impinge on the nurse-client relationship.
2. Orientation or introductory phase
   a. Acceptance, trust, and boundaries are established.

   b. Expectations and the time frame of the relationship are identified (establishing a contract).
   c. Client-centered goals are defined.
   d. Termination and separation of the relationship are discussed in anticipation of the time-limited nature of the relationship.
3. Working phase
   a. Exploring, focusing on, and evaluating the client's concerns and problems occurs; an attitude of acceptance and active listening assists the client to express thoughts and feelings.
   b. Encouraging independence in the client facilitates recovery and leads to readiness for termination.
4. Termination or separation phase
   a. Prepare the client for termination and separation on initial contact.
   b. Evaluate progress and achievement of goals.
   c. Identify responses related to termination and separation, such as anger, distancing from the relationship, a return of symptoms, and dependency.
   d. Encourage the client to express feelings about termination.
   e. Identify the client's strengths and anticipated needs for follow-up care.
   f. Refer the client to community resources and/or other support systems.

II. THERAPEUTIC COMMUNICATION PROCESS

A. Principles
1. Communication includes verbal and nonverbal expression (Figure 63-1).
2. Successful communication includes appropriateness, efficiency, flexibility, and feedback.
3. Anxiety in the nurse or client impedes communication.
4. Communication needs to be goal directed within a professional framework.

▲ **FIGURE 63-1** Operational definition of communication. (From Varcarolis, E., & Halter, M. [2010]. *Foundations of psychiatric mental health nursing* [6th ed.]. St. Louis: Saunders.)

B. Therapeutic and nontherapeutic communication techniques (Box 63-1)

III. MENTAL HEALTH

A. Mental health is a lifelong process of successful adaptation to a changing internal and external environment.

B. The mentally healthy individual is *in contact with reality,* is able to relate to people and situations in their environment, and can resolve conflicts within a problem-solving framework.

C. The mentally healthy individual has psychobiological resilience.

IV. PSYCHIATRIC/MENTAL HEALTH ILLNESS

A. Description

1. Psychiatric illness is the loss of ability to respond to the environment in ways that are in harmony with oneself or the expectations of society.

2. It is characterized by thought or behavior patterns that impair functioning and cause distress.

B. Personality characteristics

1. Self-concept is distorted.

2. Perception of strengths and weaknesses is not realistic.

3. Thoughts and perceptions may not be reality-based.

Box 63-1 Therapeutic and Nontherapeutic Communication Techniques

Therapeutic Techniques	**Nontherapeutic Techniques**
Clarifying and validating	Asking the client, "Why?"
Encouraging formulation of a plan of action	Being defensive or challenging the client
Focusing and refocusing	Changing the subject
Giving information and presenting reality	Giving advice or approval or disapproval
Listening	Making stereotypical comments
Maintaining neutral responses	Making value judgments
Maintaining silence	Placing the client's feelings on hold
Providing acknowledgment and feedback	Providing false reassurance
Providing nonverbal encouragement	
Reflecting	
Restating	
Sharing perceptions	
Summarizing	
Using broad openings and open ended questions	

---

4. The ability to find meaning and purpose in life may be impaired.
5. Life direction and productivity may be disturbed.
6. Meeting one's own needs may be problematic.
7. Excessive reliance or preoccupation on the thoughts, opinions, and actions of self or others may be present.

C. Adaptations to stress
  1. The individual's sense of self-control and environmental mastery may be affected.
  2. Perception of the environment may be distorted.
  3. **Coping mechanisms** may be ineffective or nonexistent.

D. Interpersonal relationships
  1. Interpersonal relationships may suffer or even be minimally existent.
  2. The ability to enjoy sustained intimacy in relationships is impaired.

 V. COPING AND DEFENSE MECHANISMS

A. Coping mechanisms
  1. Coping involves any effort to decrease anxiety.
  2. **Coping mechanisms** can be constructive or destructive, task oriented in relation to direct problem-solving, or defense oriented and regulating the response to protect oneself.

B. Defense mechanisms
  1. As anxiety increases, the individual copes by using **defense mechanisms**.
  2. A **defense mechanism** is a **coping mechanism** used in an effort to protect the individual from feelings of anxiety; as anxiety increases and becomes overwhelming, the individual copes by using **defense mechanisms** to protect the ego and decrease anxiety (Box 63-2).

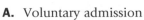 Coping mechanisms and defense mechanisms are used by the client to decrease anxiety.

C. Interventions
  1. Assist the client to identify the source of anxiety and to explore methods to reduce anxiety.
  2. Assess the client's use of **defense mechanisms**.
  3. Facilitate appropriate use of **defense mechanisms**.
  4. Determine whether the **defense mechanisms** used by the client are effective for him or her or create additional distress.
  5. Avoid criticizing the client's behavior and use of **defense mechanisms**.

VI. DIAGNOSTIC AND STATISTICAL MANUAL OF MENTAL HEALTH DISORDERS

A. The *Diagnostic and Statistical Manual of Mental Health Disorders*, from the American Psychiatric Association, provides guidelines for health care personnel for identifying and categorizing mental illness.

B. The manual is a system used in clinical, research, and educational settings, in which diagnostic criteria are included for each mental health disorder.

C. The manual addresses culturally diverse populations and illness that may be associated with a particular culture.

D. The guidelines in the manual assist the health care team to plan and evaluate the treatment plan.

VII. TYPES OF MENTAL HEALTH ADMISSIONS AND DISCHARGES

A. Voluntary admission
  1. The client (or the client's guardian) seeks admission for care.
  2. The voluntary client is free to sign out of the hospital with health care provider (HCP) notification and prescription.
  3. Detaining a voluntary client against his or her will is termed false imprisonment.
  4. Civil rights are retained fully by the client (Box 63-3).

Box 63-2 Types of Defense Mechanisms

Compensation: Putting forth extra effort to achieve in areas where one has a real or imagined deficiency

Conversion: The expression of emotional conflicts through physical symptoms

Denial: Disowning consciously intolerable thoughts and impulses

Displacement: Feelings toward one person are directed to another who is less threatening, thereby satisfying an impulse with a substitute object

Dissociation: The blocking off of an anxiety-provoking event or period of time from the conscious mind

Fantasy: Gratification by imaginary achievements and wishful thinking

Fixation: Never advancing to the next level of emotional development and organization; the persistence in later life of interests and behavior patterns appropriate to an earlier age

Identification: The unconscious attempt to change oneself to resemble an admired person

Insulation: Withdrawing into passivity and becoming inaccessible to avoid further threatening situations

Intellectualization: Excessive reasoning to avoid feelings; the thinking is disconnected from feelings, and situations are dealt with at a cognitive level

Introjection: A type of identification in which the individual incorporates the traits or values of another into self

Isolation: Response in which a person blocks feelings associated with an unpleasant experience

Projection: Transferring one's internal feelings, thoughts, and unacceptable ideas and traits to someone else

Rationalization: An attempt to make unacceptable feelings and behaviors acceptable by justifying the behavior

Reaction formation: Developing conscious attitudes and behaviors and acting out behaviors opposite to what one really feels

Regression: Returning to an earlier developmental stage to express an impulse to deal with anxiety

Repression: An unconscious process in which the client blocks undesirable and unacceptable thoughts from conscious expression

Splitting: Tendency to view others or events as either all good or all bad. This allows the individual to hold opposite and nonintegrated views.

Sublimation: Replacement of an unacceptable need, attitude, or emotion with one more socially acceptable

Substitution: The replacement of a valued unacceptable object with an object that is more acceptable to the ego

Suppression: The conscious, deliberate forgetting of unacceptable or painful thoughts, ideas, and feelings

Symbolization: The conscious use of an idea or object to represent another actual event or object; many times the meaning is not clear because the symbol may be representative of something unconscious

Undoing: Engaging in behavior that is considered to be opposite of a previous unacceptable behavior, thought, or feeling

Box 63-3 Client Rights

Right to accessible health care

Right to coordination and continuity of health care

Right to courteous and individualized health care

Right to information about the qualifications, names, and titles of personnel delivering care

Right to refuse observation by those not directly involved in care

Right to privacy and confidentiality

Right to informed consent

Right to treatment and to refuse treatment

Right to treatment in the least restrictive setting

Right not to be subjected to unnecessary restraints

Right to habeas corpus; may request a hearing at any time to be released from the hospital

Right to information about diagnosis, prognosis, and treatment

Right to information on the charges of service

Right to communicate with people outside the hospital through written correspondence, telephone, and personal visits

Right to keep clothing and personal effects

Right to be employed

Right to religious freedom

Right to execute wills

Right to retain licenses, privileges, or permits established by the law, such as a driver's or professional license

Adapted from Stuart, G. (2009). *Principles and practice of psychiatric nursing* (9th ed.). St. Louis: Mosby.

B. Right to confidentiality

1. A client has a right to confidentiality of their medical information. The Health Insurance Portability and Accountability Act (HIPAA) of 1996 ensures client confidentiality with regard to release and electronic transmission of data.

2. Information sometimes must be released in life-threatening situations without the client's consent.

3. In the event of a specific threat against an identified individual, the HCP has a legal obligation to warn intended victim(s) of a client's threats of harm

! Except in an emergency situation, client information can be released only with the client's informed consent, which specifies the information that can be released and the timeframe for which the release is valid.

C. Involuntary admission
1. Involuntary admission may be necessary when a person is mentally ill, is a danger to self or others, or is in need of psychiatric treatment or physical care.
2. Involuntary admission occurs when a client is admitted or detained involuntarily for mental health treatment because of actual or imminent danger to self or others.
3. The client who is admitted involuntarily retains his or her right for informed consent.
4. The client retains the right to refuse treatments, including medications, unless a separate and specific treatment order is obtained from the court.
5. The client loses the right to refuse treatment when the client poses an immediate danger to self or others, requiring immediate action by the health care team.
6. An order from a judge is required for involuntary admissions except in the case of emergency, which allows time to obtain the necessary order from a judge. In the case of all involuntary admissions, legal counsel must be provided for the client.
7. A court hearing is held by a judge within a specified time for clients admitted involuntarily. The specific time varies by state.
8. In most states, the client can institute a court hearing to seek an expedient judicial discharge (a writ of habeas corpus).
9. At the court hearing, a determination is made as to whether the client may be released from the hospital or detained for further treatment and evaluation or committed to a mental health facility for an undetermined time period.
10. The client has the right to treatment in the least restrictive treatment environment. If treatment objectives can be achieved, for example, by court-ordered treatment to an outpatient facility as opposed to an inpatient facility, the client has the right to be treated in the former setting.
11. The client is considered legally competent unless he or she has been declared incompetent through a legal hearing separate from the involuntary commitment hearing.
12. In the course of providing nursing care and carrying out medical presriptions, if the nurse believes that a client lacks competency to make informed decisions, action should be initiated to determine if a legal guardian needs to be appointed by the court.

D. Release from the hospital
1. Description
   a. A client may be released voluntarily, against medical advice, or with conditions (conditional release).
   b. The client who sought voluntary admission has the right to demand to be released.
2. Voluntary release
   a. In the absence of an act of self-harm or danger to others, a voluntary client should never be detained.
   b. If a voluntary client wishes to be discharged from treatment but is considered potentially dangerous to self or others, the HCP can prescribe the client to be detained while legal proceedings for involuntary status are sought.
   c. Some states provide for conditional release of involuntarily hospitalized clients. This enables the treating HCP to prescribe continued treatment on an outpatient basis as opposed to discharging the client to follow up on his or her own initiative.
   d. Conditional release usually involves outpatient treatment for a specified period to determine the client's compliance with medication protocol, ability to meet basic needs, and ability to reintegrate into the community.
   e. An involuntary client who is released conditionally may be reinstitutionalized while the commitment is still in effect without recommencement of formal admission procedures.
3. Discharge planning and follow-up care
   a. Discharge (unconditional release) is the termination of the client-institution relationship.
   b. This release may be prescribed by the psychiatrist, court, or administration for involuntarily admitted clients and may be requested by voluntary clients at any time.
   c. In most states, the client can institute a court hearing to seek an expedient judicial discharge (writ of habeas corpus).
   d. Discharge planning and follow-up care are important for the continued well-being of the client with a mental health disorder.
   e. After-care case managers are used to facilitate the client's adaptation back into the community and provide early referral if the treatment plan is not successful.

VIII. MILIEU THERAPY

A. Description
1. The **milieu** refers to the physical and social environment in which an individual is receiving treatment.

2. **Milieu** therapy uses a safe environment to meet the individual client's treatment needs.

3. Safety is the number one priority in managing the **milieu**.

4. **Milieu** therapy is staffed by persons educated to provide support, understanding, and individual attention. All encounters with the client have the goal of being "therapeutic."

5. All members of the treatment team contribute to the planning and functioning of the **milieu**. The team generally includes the registered nurse, social worker, exercise therapist, recreational therapist, psychologist, psychiatrist, occupational therapist, clinical nurse specialist, or nurse practitioner.

6. All treatment team members are viewed as significant and valuable to the client's successful treatment outcomes.

B. Focus of **milieu** therapy

1. To use the physical and social environment to effect a positive change directed toward accomplishing the client's treatment goals.

2. To use community meetings, activity groups, social skills groups, and physical exercise programs to accomplish treatment goals.

3. To have one-to-one relationships with staff to examine client behaviors, feelings, and interactions within the context of the therapeutic group activities.

⚠ The focus of milieu therapy is to empower the client through involvement in setting his or her own goals and to develop purposeful relationships with the staff to assist in meeting these goals.

IX. INTERPERSONAL PSYCHOTHERAPY

A. Description

1. A treatment modality that uses a therapeutic relationship to modify the client's feelings, attitudes, and behaviors

2. Therapeutic communication forms the foundation of the therapist-client relationship

B. Focus of interpersonal psychotherapy.

1. To establish a contract, clarify roles, and work within an agreed-upon time frame toward meeting the client's goals.

2. Focusing on the therapist-client relationship is used as a way for clients to examine other relationships in his or her life.

C. Levels of psychotherapy

1. Supportive therapy

a. Allows the client to express feelings, explore alternatives, and make decisions in a safe, caring environment

b. May be needed briefly or over a period of years

c. No plan exists to introduce new methods of coping; instead, the therapist reinforces the client's existing **coping mechanisms**

2. Re-educative therapy

a. Involves learning new ways of perceiving and behaving

b. The client explores alternatives in a planned, systematic way and requires a longer period of therapy than supportive therapy.

c. The client enters into a contract that specifies desired changes of behavior.

d. May include short-term psychotherapy, reality therapy, cognitive restructuring, behavior modification, and the development of coping skills.

3. Reconstructive therapy

a. Involves the use of psychotherapy or psychoanalysis to make major changes in the client's life

b. May require several years of therapy and focuses on all aspects of the client's life

c. Emotional and cognitive restructuring of self takes place.

d. Positive outcomes include a greater understanding of self and others, more emotional freedom, and the development of potential abilities.

X. BEHAVIOR THERAPY

A. A treatment approach that uses the principles of Skinnerian (operant conditioning) or Pavlovian (classical conditioning) behavior theory to bring about behavioral change

B. The belief is that most behaviors are learned.

C. Operant conditioning refers to the manipulation of selected reinforcers to elicit and strengthen desired behavioral responses. The reinforcer refers to the consequence of the behavior, which is defined as anything that increases the occurrence of a behavior (Figure 63-2).

D. In classical conditioning (respondent conditioning) the individual responds to a stimulus but is basically a passive agent (see Figure 63-2).

E. Desensitization is a form of behavior therapy by which exposure to increasing increments of a feared

▲ FIGURE 63-2 Respondent versus operant conditioning. (From Varcarolis, E., & Halter, M. [2010]. *Foundations of psychiatric mental health nursing* [6th ed.]. St. Louis: Saunders.)

stimulus paired with increasing levels of relaxation helps to reduce the intensity of fear to a more tolerable level.

F. Aversion therapy is a form of behavior therapy by which negative reinforcement is used to change behavior; for example, a stimulus *attractive* to the client is paired with an *unpleasant* event in hopes of endowing the stimulus with negative properties, thereby dissuading the behavior.

G. Modeling is behavioral therapy in which the therapist acts as a role model for specific identified behaviors so that the client learns through imitation.

XI. COGNITIVE THERAPY

A. An active, directive, time-limited, structured approach used to treat a variety of disorders including anxiety, depression, and phobias

B. Based on the principle that how an individual feels and behaves is determined by how they think about the world and his or her place in it. The individual's cognitions are based on the attitudes or assumptions developed from previous experiences.

C. Therapeutic techniques are designed to identify, reality test, and correct distorted conceptualizations and the dysfunctional beliefs underlying these cognitions.

D. The therapist helps the individual to change the way he or she thinks, thereby reducing symptoms.

XII. GROUP DEVELOPMENT AND GROUP THERAPY

A. Description: Group therapy involves a therapist and ideally five to eight members working on his or her individual goals within the context of a group, which presumably increases the opportunity for feedback and support.

B. Stages of group development
  1. Initial stage
     a. During this stage, group development involves superficial rather than open and trusting communication.
     b. Members become acquainted with each other and search for similarity between themselves and other group members.
     c. Members may be unclear about the purpose or goals of the group.
     d. Group norms, roles, and responsibilities are established.
  2. Working stage
     a. During this stage, the real work of the group is accomplished.
     b. Members are familiar with each other, the group leader, and the group roles, and they feel free to address and attempt to solve their problem.
     c. Both conflict and cooperation surface during the group's work as the members learn to work with each other.

  3. Termination stage
     a. Members' feelings are explored regarding their accomplishments and the impending termination of the group.
     b. The termination stage provides an opportunity for members to learn to deal more realistically and comfortably with this normal part of human experience.

C. Group therapy models (*Note:* These models apply to individual or group psychotherapy.)
  1. Psychoanalytical group psychotherapy
     a. The therapist holds a main position.
     b. Each client in the group has a relationship with the therapist.
     c. Communication is focused on three levels: unconscious, semiconscious, and conscious information.
  2. Transactional analysis
     a. The three ego states of the individual are examined.
     b. The goal is for individuals in the group to communicate from the proper ego states for the situation and responses of others, thereby lessening conflict and promoting mature relationships.
  3. Rational emotive therapy is a kind of cognitive therapy in which the therapist focuses on how irrational beliefs and thoughts contribute to psychological distress.
  4. Rogerian therapy
     a. The therapist's goal is to help the members express their feelings toward one another during group sessions.
     b. The therapist's role is one of encouraging the expression of feelings, clarifying these feelings with clients, and accepting clients and their feelings nonjudgmentally.
  5. Gestalt therapy
     a. Emphasis is on the "here and now."
     b. Emphasizes self-expression, self-exploration, and self-awareness in the present.
     c. The client and therapist focus on everyday problems and try to solve them.
     d. The individual becomes aware of the total self and the surrounding environment.
     e. Awareness of the problem renders the client capable of change.
     f. The therapist's role is to help the members express their feelings and grow from their experiences.
  6. Interpersonal group therapy: promotes the individual's comfort with others in the group, which then transfers to other relationships.
  7. Self-help or support groups (Box 63-4)

⚠ Support groups are based on the premise that individuals who have experienced a problem are able to help others who have a similar problem.

Box 63-4 Examples of Self-Help or Support Groups

Adult Children of Alcoholics
Al-Anon
Alcoholics Anonymous
Co-dependents Anonymous
Gamblers Anonymous
Narcotics Anonymous
Overeaters Anonymous
Cancer Support
Mental Illness support groups
Bereavement groups
Parents Without Partners
Recovery groups, such as for those who have experienced trauma
Smoking cessation
Unexpected body-image changes, such as mastectomy or colostomy

XIII. FAMILY THERAPY

A. Family therapy is a specific intervention mode based on the premise that the member who has the presenting symptoms will signal the presence of problems in the entire family. This premise also assumes that a change in one member will bring about changes in other members.

B. The therapist works to assist family members to identify and express their thoughts and feelings; define family roles and rules; try new, more productive styles of relating; and restore strength to the family.

MORE QUESTIONS ON EVOLVE!

Practice Questions

671. A nurse is assigned to care for a client who is experiencing disturbed thought processes. The nurse is told that the client believes that the food is being poisoned. Which communication technique does the nurse plan to use to encourage the client to eat?

1. Open-ended questions and silence
2. Focusing on self-disclosure regarding food preferences
3. Stating the reasons that the client may not want to eat
4. Offering opinions about the necessity of adequate nutrition

672. A nurse is assigned to care for a client admitted to the hospital after sustaining an injury from a house fire. The client attempted to save a neighbor involved in the fire but, in spite of the client's efforts, the neighbor died. Which action would the nurse take to enable the client to work through the meaning of the crisis?

1. Identifying the client's ability to function
2. Identifying the client's potential for self-harm
3. Inquiring about the client's feelings that may affect coping
4. Inquiring about the client's perception of the cause of the neighbor's death

673. A nurse is assisting with the data collection on a client admitted to the psychiatric unit. The nurse reviews the data obtained and identifies which of the following as a priority concern?

1. The client's report of suicidal thoughts
2. The client's report of not eating or sleeping
3. The presence of bruises on the client's body
4. The family member is disapproving of the treatment

674. Laboratory work is prescribed for a client who has been experiencing delusions. When the laboratory technician approaches the client to obtain a specimen of the client's blood, the client begins to shout, "You're all vampires. Let me out of here!" The nurse who is present at the time should respond by stating which of the following?

1. "The technician will leave and come back later for your blood."
2. "What makes you think that the technician wants to hurt you?"
3. "Are you fearful and think that others may want to hurt you?"
4. "The technician is not going to hurt you, but is going to help you!"

675. An intoxicated client is brought to the emergency department by local police. The client is told that the health care provider (HCP) will be in to see the client in about 30 minutes. The client becomes very loud and offensive and wants to be seen by the HCP immediately. The nurse assisting to care for the client would plan for which appropriate nursing intervention?

1. Watch the behavior escalate before intervening.
2. Attempt to talk with the client to de-escalate the behavior.
3. Offer to take the client to an examination room until he or she can be treated.
4. Inform the client that he or she will be asked to leave if the behavior continues.

676. A client is admitted to a psychiatric unit for treatment of psychotic behavior. The client is at the locked exit door and is shouting, "Let me out! There's nothing wrong with me! I don't belong here!" The nurse identifies this behavior as:

1. Denial
2. Projection
3. Regression
4. Rationalization

677. A client says to the nurse, "I'm going to die, and I wish my family would stop hoping for a 'cure'! I get so angry when they carry on like this! After all, I'm the one who's dying." The therapeutic response by the nurse is:
1. "Have you shared your feelings with your family?"
2. "I think we should talk more about your anger with your family."
3. "You're feeling angry that your family continues to hope for you to be 'cured'?"
4. "Well, it sounds like you're being pretty pessimistic. After all, years ago people died of pneumonia."

678. A nurse in a psychiatric unit is assigned to care for a client admitted to the unit 2 days ago. On review of the client's record, the nurse notes that the admission was a voluntary admission. Based on this type of admission, the nurse would expect which of the following?
1. The client will be angry and will refuse care.
2. The client will participate in the treatment plan.
3. The client will be very resistant to treatment measures.
4. The client's family will be very resistant to treatment measures.

679. A licensed practical nurse (LPN) enters a client's room, and the client is demanding release from the hospital. The LPN reviews the client's record and notes that the client was admitted 2 days ago for treatment of an anxiety disorder, and that the admission was a voluntary admission. The LPN reports the findings to the registered nurse (RN) and expects that the RN will take which of the following actions?
1. Contact the health care provider (HCP).
2. Call the client's family.
3. Persuade the client to stay a few more days.
4. Tell the client that discharge is not possible at this time.

680. A client is admitted to the psychiatric nursing unit. When collecting data from the client, the nurse notes that the client was admitted on an involuntary status. Based on this type of admission, the nurse likely expects that the client:
1. Presents a harm to self
2. Requested the admission

3. Consented to the admission
4. Provided written application to the facility for admission

681. Following a group therapy session, a client approaches the licensed practical nurse (LPN) and verbalizes a need for seclusion because of uncontrollable feelings. The LPN reports the findings to the registered nurse (RN) and expects that the RN will take which of the following actions?
1. Call the client's family.
2. Place the client in seclusion immediately.
3. Inform the client that seclusion has not been prescribed.
4. Get a written prescription from the health care provider (HCP) and obtain an informed consent.

682. A nurse is providing care to a client admitted to the hospital with a diagnosis of anxiety disorder. The nurse is talking with the client and the client says, "I have a secret that I want to tell you. You won't tell anyone about it, will you?" The appropriate nursing response is which of the following?
1. "No, I won't tell anyone."
2. "I cannot promise to keep a secret."
3. "If you tell me the secret, I will tell it to your doctor."
4. "If you tell me the secret, I will need to document it in your record."

683. A psychiatric nurse is greeted by a neighbor in a local grocery store. The neighbor says to the nurse, "How is Carol doing? She is my best friend and is seen at your clinic every week." The appropriate nursing response is which of the following?
1. "I cannot discuss any client situation with you."
2. "I'm not supposed to discuss this, but since you are my neighbor, I can tell you that she is doing great!"
3. "You may want to know about Carol, so you need to ask her yourself so you can get the story firsthand."
4. "I'm not supposed to discuss this, but since you are my neighbor, I can tell you that she really has some problems!"

684. A nurse is preparing a client for the termination phase of the nurse-client relationship. Which nursing task would the nurse appropriately plan for this phase?
1. Plan short-term goals.
2. Identify expected outcomes.
3. Assist in making appropriate referrals.
4. Assist in developing realistic solutions.

❖ **685.** The nurse in the mental health unit reviews the therapeutic and nontherapeutic communication techniques with a nursing student. Which of the following are therapeutic communication techniques? **Select all that apply.**

☐ 1. Restating
☐ 2. Listening
☐ 3. Asking the client, "Why?"
☐ 4. Maintaining neutral responses
☐ 5. Giving advice or approval or disapproval
☐ 6. Providing acknowledgment and feedback

ANSWERS

671. 1

Rationale: Open-ended questions and silence are strategies used to encourage clients to discuss their problem. Options 3 and 4 do not encourage the client to express feelings. The nurse should not offer opinions and should not state the reasons, but should encourage the client to identify the reasons for the behavior. Option 2 is not a client-centered intervention.

Test-Taking Strategy: Use the process of elimination. Eliminate options 3 and 4 first, because they do not support client expression of feelings. Eliminate option 2 next, because it is not a client-centered intervention. Focusing on the client's feelings will direct you to option 1. Review therapeutic communication techniques if you had difficulty with this question.

Level of Cognitive Ability: Applying
Client Needs: Psychosocial Integrity
Integrated Process: Caring
Content Area: Mental Health
Reference: Morrison-Valfre, pp. 104–105. 2009.

672. 3

Rationale: The client must first deal with feelings and negative responses before the client is able to work through the meaning of the crisis. Option 3 pertains directly to the client's feelings. Options 1, 2, and 4 do not directly address the client's feelings.

Test-Taking Strategy: Use the process of elimination. Focusing on the feelings of the client will direct you to the correct option. Review the nurse's actions in a crisis situation if you had difficulty with this question.

Level of Cognitive Ability: Applying
Client Needs: Psychosocial Integrity
Integrated Process: Nursing Process/Implementation
Content Area: Mental Health
References: Christensen, Kockrow, pp. 1131–1132. 2011. *Foundations of nursing.*
Morrison-Valfre, p. 77. 2009.

673. 1

Rationale: The client's thoughts are extremely important when verbalized. Suicidal thoughts are the highest priority. Options 2, 3, and 4 will all affect the treatment of the client but are not of greatest importance at this time.

Test-Taking Strategy: The client is the focus of the question; therefore, eliminate option 4. Focus on the strategic words "priority concern" and use prioritizing skills. Remember, if the client verbalizes suicidal thoughts, it is a priority concern. Review data collection techniques related to the suicidal client if you had difficulty with this question.

Level of Cognitive Ability: Analyzing
Client Needs: Psychosocial Integrity
Integrated Process: Nursing Process/Data Collection

Content Area: Mental Health
Reference: Morrison-Valfre, pp. 87–88, 303–304. 2009.

674. 3

Rationale: Option 3 is the only option that recognizes the client's need. This response helps the client focus on the emotion underlying the delusion but does not argue with it. If the nurse attempts to change the client's mind, the delusion may, in fact, be even more strongly held. Options 1, 2, and 4 do not focus on the client's feelings.

Test-Taking Strategy: Use therapeutic communication techniques and knowledge regarding the dynamics of delusions and how delusions meet the client's underlying needs. This will direct you to option 3. In addition, option 3 focuses on the client's feelings. Review therapeutic communication techniques if you had difficulty with this question.

Level of Cognitive Ability: Applying
Client Needs: Psychosocial Integrity
Integrated Process: Communication and Documentation
Content Area: Mental Health
Reference: Morrison-Valfre, pp. 35, 104–105. 2009.

675. 3

Rationale: Safety of the client, other clients, and staff is of prime concern. When dealing with an impaired individual, trying to talk may be out of the question. Waiting to intervene could cause the client to become even more agitated and a threat to others. Option 4 would only further aggravate an already agitated individual. Option 3 is in effect an isolation technique that allows for separation from others and provides a less stimulating environment, where the client can maintain dignity.

Test-Taking Strategy: Focus on the subject of the question and use the process of elimination. Noting that the client is inebriated will assist in directing you to option 3. Option 3 most directly addresses the situation and the behavior and feelings of the client. Review nursing interventions for a client who is inebriated if you had difficulty with this question.

Level of Cognitive Ability: Applying
Client Needs: Psychosocial Integrity
Integrated Process: Nursing Process/Planning
Content Area: Mental Health
Reference: Varcarolis, Halter, pp. 429–431. 2009.

676. 1

Rationale: Denial is refusal to admit to a painful reality and is treated as if it does not exist. In projection, a person unconsciously rejects emotionally unacceptable features and attributes them to other people, objects, or situations. In regression, the client returns to an earlier, more comforting, although less mature way of behaving. Rationalization is justifying the unacceptable attributes about oneself.

Test-Taking Strategy: Use the process of elimination. Note the strategic words, "There's nothing wrong with me!" Select the option that recognizes the client's attempt to avoid looking at the reality of the situation. If you had difficulty with this question, review defense mechanisms.
Level of Cognitive Ability: Understanding
Client Needs: Psychosocial Integrity
Integrated Process: Nursing Process/Data Collection
Content Area: Mental Health
Reference: Morrison-Valfre, pp. 39, 193. 2009.

677. 3

Rationale: Reflection is the therapeutic communication technique that redirects the client's feelings back to validate what the client is saying. In option 2, the nurse attempts to use focusing, but the attempt to discuss central issues is premature. In option 4, the nurse makes a judgment and is nontherapeutic in the one-on-one relationship. In option 1, the nurse is attempting to assess the client's ability to openly discuss feelings with family members. Although this may be appropriate, the timing is somewhat premature and closes off facilitation of the client's feelings.
Test-Taking Strategy: Use therapeutic communication techniques. Note that option 3 uses the therapeutic technique of reflection and focuses on the client's feelings. Options 1, 2, and 4 are nontherapeutic at this time. Review therapeutic communication techniques if you had difficulty with this question.
Level of Cognitive Ability: Applying
Client Needs: Psychosocial Integrity
Integrated Process: Communication and Documentation
Content Area: Mental Health
References: Christensen, Kockrow, p. 1130. 2011. *Foundations of nursing.*
Morrison-Valfre, pp. 104–105. 2009.

678. 2

Rationale: Generally, voluntary admission is sought by the client or client's guardian. If the client seeks voluntary admission, the most likely expectation is that the client will participate in the treatment program.
Test-Taking Strategy: Use the process of elimination. Note the strategic words "voluntary admission." This will direct you to option 2. In addition, note that options 1, 3, and 4 are comparable or alike. Review the various types of hospital admission processes if you had difficulty with this question.
Level of Cognitive Ability: Understanding
Client Needs: Psychosocial Integrity
Integrated Process: Nursing Process/Planning
Content Area: Mental Health
Reference: Morrison-Valfre, pp. 24–25. 2009.

679. 1

Rationale: Generally, voluntary admission is sought by the client or client's guardian. Voluntary clients have the right to demand and obtain release. The best nursing action is to contact the HCP.
Test-Taking Strategy: Use the process of elimination. Noting the type of hospital admission will assist in eliminating option 4. It is inappropriate to "persuade" a client to stay in the hospital. Option 2 should be eliminated simply based on the issue

of client rights and the issue of confidentiality. Review the various types of hospital admission and discharge processes if you had difficulty with this question.
Level of Cognitive Ability: Applying
Client Needs: Safe and Effective Care Environment
Integrated Process: Nursing Process/Implementation
Content Area: Mental Health
References: Morrison-Valfre, p. 24. 2009.
Varcarolis, Halter, pp. 520, 522–523. 2009.

680. 1

Rationale: Involuntary admission is made without the client's consent. Involuntary admission is necessary when a person is a danger to self or others or is in need of psychiatric treatment or physical care. Options 2, 3, and 4 describe the process of voluntary admission.
Test-Taking Strategy: Use the process of elimination. Note the strategic words "involuntary status." This should direct you to option 1. Also, note that options 2, 3, and 4 are comparable or alike. Review the process of involuntary admission if you had difficulty with this question.
Level of Cognitive Ability: Understanding
Client Needs: Psychosocial Integrity
Integrated Process: Nursing Process/Planning
Content Area: Mental Health
Reference: Morrison-Valfre, p. 24. 2009.

681. 4

Rationale: A client may request to be secluded or restrained. Federal laws require the consent of the client, unless an emergency situation exists in which an immediate risk to the client or others can be documented. The use of seclusion and restraint is permitted only on the written prescription of the health care provider (HCP), which must be reviewed and renewed every 24 hours. It must also specify the type of restraint to be used.
Test-Taking Strategy: Use the process of elimination. There is no reason to call the family at this time; therefore, eliminate option 1. Knowing that a HCP's written prescription is necessary in this situation will assist in eliminating option 2. Option 3 is not the best choice because this information, if given to a client experiencing uncontrollable feelings, may cause escalation of the feelings. Review the procedures for seclusion if you had difficulty with this question.
Level of Cognitive Ability: Applying
Client Needs: Safe and Effective Care Environment
Integrated Process: Nursing Process/Implementation
Content Area: Mental Health
References: Varcarolis, Halter, pp. 522–524. 2009.

682. 2

Rationale: The nurse should never promise to keep a secret. Secrets are appropriate in a social relationship, but not in a therapeutic one. The nurse needs to be honest with the client and tell the client that a promise cannot be made to keep the secret.
Test-Taking Strategy: Use the process of elimination and knowledge of therapeutic communication techniques. Option 1 can be eliminated because it is inappropriate. Also, options 3 and 4 are not only inappropriate, but are threatening to an

extent and may even block further communication. Review the principles related to a therapeutic nurse-client relationship if you had difficulty with this question.

Level of Cognitive Ability: Applying
Client Needs: Psychosocial Integrity
Integrated Process: Communication and Documentation
Content Area: Mental Health
References: Morrison-Valfre, pp. 104-105, 110. 2009.

683. 1

Rationale: A nurse is required to maintain confidentiality regarding clients and their care. Confidentiality is basic to the therapeutic relationship and is a client's right. Option 3 is correct in a sense; however, it is a rather blunt statement. Both options 2 and 4 identify statements that do not maintain client confidentiality.

Test-Taking Strategy: Use the process of elimination. Focus on the subject of the question, maintaining confidentiality. This should assist in eliminating options 2 and 4. From the remaining options, select option 1 over option 3 because it is most direct and correct. Option 3 is a rather blunt and somewhat rude statement. Review confidentiality issues if you had difficulty with this question.

Level of Cognitive Ability: Applying
Client Needs: Safe and Effective Care Environment
Integrated Process: Communication and Documentation
Content Area: Mental Health
References: Morrison-Valfre, p. 25. 2009.

684. 3

Rationale: Tasks of the termination phase include evaluating client performance, evaluating achievement of expected outcomes, evaluating future needs, making appropriate referrals, and dealing with the common behaviors associated with termination. Options 1, 2, and 4 identify the tasks of the working phase of the relationship.

Test-Taking Strategy: Noting the strategic words "termination phase" should direct you to the correct option. If you are unfamiliar with the appropriate tasks of the phases of the nurse-client relationship, review this content.

Level of Cognitive Ability: Applying
Client Needs: Psychosocial Integrity
Integrated Process: Nursing Process/Planning
Content Area: Mental Health
Reference: Morrison-Valfre, p. 115. 2009.

685. 1, 2, 4, 6 ❖

Rationale: Some of the therapeutic communication techniques include listening, maintaining silence, maintaining neutral responses, using broad openings and open-ended questions, focusing and refocusing, restating, clarifying and validating, sharing perceptions, reflecting, providing acknowledgment and feedback, giving information and presenting reality, encouraging formulation of a plan of action, providing nonverbal encouragement, and summarizing.

Test-Taking Strategy: Focus on the subject, therapeutic communication techniques. This will assist you in selecting the correct answers. Review therapeutic and nontherapeutic techniques if you had difficulty with this question.

Level of Cognitive Ability: Understanding
Client Needs: Psychosocial Integrity
Integrated Process: Teaching and Learning
Content Area: Mental Health
Reference: Morrison-Valfre, pp. 104–105. 2009.

Mental Health Disorders

I. ANXIETY

A. Description
1. Anxiety is a normal response to stress.
2. A subjective experience that includes feelings of apprehension, uneasiness, uncertainty, or dread
3. Occurs as a result of threats that may be misperceived or misinterpreted or as a result of a threat to identity or self-esteem
4. May result when values are threatened or preceding new experiences

B. Types of anxiety
1. Normal: A healthy type of anxiety
2. Acute: Precipitated by imminent loss or change that threatens one's sense of security
3. Chronic: Anxiety that persists as a characteristic response to daily activities

C. Levels of anxiety
1. Mild
   a. Associated with the tension of everyday life
   b. The individual is alert.
   c. The perceptual field is increased.
   d. Mild anxiety can be motivating, produce growth, enhance creativity, and increase learning.
2. Moderate
   a. The focus is on immediate concerns.
   b. Moderate anxiety narrows the perceptual field.
   c. Selective inattentiveness occurs.
   d. Learning and problem solving still occur.
3. Severe
   a. Severe anxiety is a feeling that something bad is about to happen.
   b. A significant narrowing in the perceptual field occurs.
   c. Focus is on minute or scattered details.
   d. All behavior is directed at relieving the anxiety.
   e. Learning and problem solving are not possible.
   f. The individual needs direction to focus.
4. Panic
   a. Panic is associated with dread and terror and a sense of impending doom.
   b. The personality is disorganized.
   c. The individual is unable to communicate or function effectively.
   d. Increased motor activity occurs.
   e. Loss of rational thoughts with distorted perception occurs.
   f. Inability to concentrate occurs.
   g. If prolonged, panic can lead to exhaustion and death.

D. Interventions: General nursing measures (see Priority Nursing Actions)

■■■ PRIORITY NURSING ACTIONS! ■■■

Actions to Take for a Client Experiencing Anxiety
1. Provide a calm environment, decrease environmental stimuli, and stay with the client.
2. Ask the client to identify what and how he or she feels.
3. Encourage the client to describe and discuss his or her feelings.
4. Help the client to identify the causes of the feelings if he or she is having difficulty doing so.
5. Listen to the client for expressions of helplessness and hopelessness.
6. Document the event, significant information, actions taken and follow-up actions, and the client's response.

If a client experiences anxiety, immediate actions are to provide a calm environment, decrease environmental stimuli, and stay with the client. Excess stimulation would escalate the anxiety. Next, asking the client to identify what and how he or she feels and helping the client to identify the causes of the feelings help to increase his or her awareness of the connection between behaviors and feelings. This awareness helps to decrease the anxiety. While listening to the client, the nurse observes for expressions of helplessness and hopelessness that could indicate self-harm intentions. The nurse provides follow-up care as needed based on observations and assessments. Finally, the nurse documents the event, significant information, actions taken and follow-up actions, and the client's response.

Reference: *Varcarolis, E., & Halter, M. (2009). Essentials of psychiatric mental health nursing: A communication approach to evidence-based care (p. 132). St. Louis: Saunders.*

1. Recognize the anxiety.
2. Establish trust.
3. Protect the client.
4. Do not criticize **coping mechanisms**.
5. Do not force the client into situations that provoke anxiety.
6. Modify the environment by setting limits or limiting interaction with others.
7. Provide creative outlets.
8. Provide activities that limit the amount of time for destructive behavior.
9. Promote relaxation techniques such as breathing exercises or guided imagery.
10. Monitor vital signs and administer antianxiety medications as prescribed.

⚠ The immediate nursing action for a client with anxiety is to decrease stimuli in the environment and provide a calm and quiet environment.

E. Interventions: Mild to moderate levels
1. Help the client identify the anxiety.
2. Encourage the client to talk about feelings and concerns.
3. Help the client identify thoughts and feelings that occurred before the onset of anxiety.
4. Encourage problem-solving.
5. Encourage gross motor exercise.

F. Interventions: Severe to panic levels
1. Reduce the anxiety quickly.
2. Use a calm manner.
3. Always remain with the client.
4. Provide clear, simple statements.
5. Use a low-pitched voice.
6. Attend to the physical needs of the client.
7. Provide gross motor activity.
8. Administer antianxiety medications as prescribed.

II. GENERALIZED ANXIETY DISORDER

A. Description
1. Generalized anxiety disorder is an unrealistic anxiety about everyday worries that persists over time and is not associated with another psychiatric or medical disorder.
2. Physical symptoms occur.

B. Data collection
1. Restlessness and inability to relax
2. Episodes of trembling and shakiness
3. Chronic muscular tension
4. Dizziness
5. Inability to concentrate
6. Chronic fatigue and sleep problems
7. Inability to recognize the connection between the anxiety and physical symptoms
8. Client is focused on the physical discomfort

C. Panic disorder
1. Description
   a. Panic disorder produces a sudden onset of feelings of intense apprehension and dread.
   b. The cause usually cannot be identified.
   c. Severe, recurrent, intermittent anxiety attacks lasting 5 to 30 minutes occur.
2. Data collection
   a. Choking sensation
   b. Labored breathing
   c. Pounding heart
   d. Chest pain
   e. Dizziness
   f. Nausea
   g. Blurred vision
   h. Numbness or tingling of the extremities
   i. A sense of unreality and helplessness
   j. A fear of being trapped
   k. A fear of dying
3. Interventions
   a. Remain with the client.
   b. Attend to the physical symptoms.
   c. Assist the client to identify the thoughts that aroused the anxiety and identify the basis for these thoughts.
   d. Assist the client to change the unrealistic thoughts to more realistic thoughts.
   e. Use cognitive restructuring to replace distorted thinking.
   f. Administer antianxiety medications if prescribed.

III. POSTTRAUMATIC STRESS DISORDER

A. Description: After experiencing a psychologically traumatic event, the individual is prone to re-experience the event and have recurrent and intrusive dreams or flashbacks.

B. Stressors
1. Natural disaster
2. Terrorist attack
3. Combat experiences
4. Accidents
5. Rape
6. Crime or violence
7. Sexual, physical, or emotional **abuse**
8. Re-experiencing the event as flashbacks

C. Data collection
1. Emotional numbness
2. Detachment
3. Depression
4. Anxiety
5. Sleep disturbances and nightmares
6. Flashbacks of the event
7. Hypervigilance
8. Guilt about surviving the event

9. Poor concentration and avoidance of activities that trigger the memory of the event

D. Interventions (Box 64-1)

IV. PHOBIAS

A. Description
1. An irrational fear of an object or situation that persists, although the person may recognize it as unreasonable
2. Associated with panic level anxiety if the object, situation, or activity cannot be avoided
3. **Defense mechanisms** commonly used include repression and displacement.

B. Types (Box 64-2)

C. Interventions
1. Identify the basis of the anxiety.

Box 64-1 Interventions for Posttraumatic Stress Disorder

Be nonjudgmental and supportive.

Assure the client that his or her feelings and behaviors are normal reactions.

Assist the client to recognize the association between his or her feelings and behaviors and the trauma experience.

Encourage the client to express his or her feelings. Provide individual therapy that addresses loss of control or anger issues.

Assist the client to develop adaptive coping mechanisms and use relaxation techniques.

Encourage the use of support groups.

Facilitate a progressive review of the trauma experience.

Encourage the client to establish and reestablish relationships.

Inform the client that hypnotherapy or systematic desensitization may be used as a form of treatment.

Box 64-2 Types of Phobias

Acrophobia: Fear of heights
Agoraphobia: Fear of open spaces
Astraphobia: Fear of electrical storms
Claustrophobia: Fear of closed spaces
Hematophobia: Fear of blood
Hydrophobia: Fear of water
Monophobia: Fear of being alone
Mysophobia: Fear of dirt or germs
Nyctophobia: Fear of darkness
Pyrophobia: Fear of fires
Social phobia: Fear of situations in which one might be embarrassed or criticized and the fear of making a fool of oneself
Xenophobia: Fear of strangers
Zoophobia: Fear of animals

---

2. Allow the client to verbalize feelings about the anxiety-producing object or situation. Frequently talking about the feared object is the first step in the desensitization process.
3. Teach relaxation techniques such as breathing exercises, muscle relaxation exercises, and visualization of pleasant situations.
4. Promote desensitization by gradually introducing the individual to the feared object or situation in small doses.

⚠️ Always stay with the client experiencing anxiety to promote safety and security. Never force the client to have contact with the phobic object or situation.

V. OBSESSIVE-COMPULSIVE DISORDER

A. Obsessions: Preoccupation with persistent intrusive thoughts and ideas

B. Compulsion
1. A compulsion is the performance of rituals or repetitive behaviors designed to prevent some event, divert unacceptable thoughts, and decrease anxiety.
2. Obsessions and compulsions often occur together and can disrupt normal daily activities.
3. Anxiety occurs when one resists obsessions or compulsions, and from being powerless to resist the thoughts or rituals.
4. Obsessive thoughts can involve issues of violence, aggression, sexual behavior, orderliness, or religion and can uncontrollably interrupt conscious thoughts and the ability to function.

C. Compulsive behavior patterns (behaviors or rituals)
1. Compulsive behavior patterns decrease the anxiety.
2. The patterns are associated with the obsessive thoughts.
3. The patterns neutralize the thought.
4. During stressful times, the ritualistic behavior increases.
5. **Defense mechanisms** include repression, displacement, and undoing.

D. Interventions (Box 64-3)

VI. SOMATOFORM DISORDERS

A. Description
1. Somatoform disorders are characterized by persistent worry or complaints regarding physical illness without supporting physical findings.
2. The client focuses on the physical signs and symptoms and is unable to control the signs and symptoms.
3. The physical signs and symptoms increase with psychosocial stressors.
4. The anxiety is redirected into a somatic concern.

Box 64-3 Interventions for Obsessive-Compulsive Disorder

Ensure that basic needs (food, rest, grooming) are met.

Identify the situations that precipitate the compulsive behavior; encourage the client to verbalize concerns and feelings.

Be empathetic toward the client, and be aware of his or her need to perform the compulsive behavior.

Do not interrupt the compulsive behaviors unless they jeopardize the safety of the client or others (provide for client safety related to the behavior).

Allow time for the client to perform the compulsive behavior but set limits on behaviors that may interfere with the client's physical well-being to protect the client from physical harm.

Implement a schedule for the client that distracts from the behaviors (structure simple activities, games, or tasks for the client).

Establish a written contract that will assist the client to decrease the frequency of compulsive behaviors gradually.

Recognize and reinforce positive nonritualistic behaviors.

---

5. The client may unconsciously use somatization for secondary gains such as increased attention and decreased responsibilities.

B. Conversion disorder
  1. Description
     a. A physical symptom or a deficit suggesting loss or altered body function related to psychological conflict or a neurological disorder.
     b. Conversion disorder is an expression of a psychological conflict or need.
     c. The most common conversion symptoms are blindness, deafness, paralysis, and the inability to talk.
     d. Conversion disorder has no organic cause.
     e. Symptoms are beyond the conscious control of the client and are directly related to conflict.
     f. The development of physical symptoms reduces anxiety.
  2. Data collection
     a. "La belle indifference": unconcerned with symptoms
     b. Physical limitation or disability
     c. Feelings of guilt, anxiety, or frustration
     d. Low self-esteem and feelings of inadequacy
     e. Unexpressed anger or conflict
     f. Secondary gain

C. Hypochondriasis
  1. Description
     a. The preoccupation with fears of having a serious disease

  b. No evidence of physical illness exists
  c. Hypochondriasis significantly impairs social and occupational functioning
  2. Data collection
     a. Preoccupation with physical functioning
     b. Frequent somatic complaints
     c. Complaints of fatigue and insomnia
     d. Anxiety
     e. Difficulty expressing feelings
     f. Extensive use of home remedies or non-prescription medications
     g. Repeatedly visiting the doctor in spite of repeated reassurance and normal test results
     h. Secondary gain

D. Somatization disorder
  1. Description
     a. The client has multiple physical complaints involving multiple body systems.
     b. The etiology of these complaints is presumed to be psychological.
  2. Data collection
     a. Physical complaints of pain, denial of emotional problems, and signs of anxiety, fear, and low self-esteem may be present.
     b. Secondary gain: The client may unconsciously use somatization for secondary gains such as increased attention and decreased responsibilities.

E. Interventions
  1. Obtain a nursing history and assess for physical problems.
  2. Explore with the client the needs being met by the physical symptoms.
  3. Assist the client to identify alternative ways of meeting needs.
  4. Assist the client to relate feelings and conflicts to the physical symptoms.
  5. Convey understanding that the physical symptoms are real to the client.
  6. Assure the client that physical illness has been ruled out.
  7. Explore the source of anxiety and stimulate verbalization of anxiety.
  8. Encourage the use of relaxation techniques as the anxiety increases.
  9. Use a pain assessment scale if the client complains of pain, and implement pain-reduction measures as required.
  10. Report and assess any new physical complaint.
  11. Encourage diversional activities.
  12. Provide positive feedback.
  13. Assist the client in recognizing his or her own feelings and emotions.
  14. Administer antianxiety medications if prescribed.

⚠ For a client with a somatoform disorder, allow a specific time period for the client to discuss physical complaints because the client will feel less threatened if this behavior is limited rather than stopped completely. However, avoid responding with positive reinforcement about the physical complaints.

VII. DISSOCIATIVE DISORDER

A. Description
1. Dissociative disorder is a disruption in integrative functions of memory, consciousness, or identity.
2. Dissociative disorder is associated with exposure to an extremely traumatic event.

B. Dissociative identity disorder (multiple personality)
1. Description
   a. Two or more fully developed distinct and unique personalities exist within the person.
   b. The host is the primary personality and the other personalities are referred to as *alters*.
   c. Alter personalities may take full control of the client, one at a time, and may or may not be aware of each other.
   d. The alters may be aware of the host but the host is not usually aware of the alter(s).
2. Data collection
   a. The client may have an inability to recall important information (unrelated to ordinary forgetfulness).
   b. Transition from one personality to the other is related to stress or a traumatic event and is sudden.
   c. Dissociation is used as a method of distancing and defending one's self from anxiety and traumatizing experiences.

C. Dissociative amnesia
1. Description
   a. The inability to remember important personal information because it provokes anxiety.
   b. Memory impairment may range from partial to almost complete.
2. Data collection
   a. Localized: The client blocks out all memories about a specified period.
   b. Selective: The client recalls some but not all memories about a specified period.
   c. Generalized: The client has a loss of all memory about past life.

D. Dissociative fugue
1. Description
   a. The client assumes a new identity in a new environment.
   b. The disorder may occur suddenly.
2. Data collection
   a. The client may drift from place to place.
   b. The client develops few social relationships.
   c. When the fugue lifts, the client returns home and is unable to recall the fugue state.

E. Depersonalization disorder
1. Description: An altered self-perception in which one's own reality is temporarily lost or changed
2. Data collection
   a. Feelings of detachment
   b. Intact reality testing

F. Interventions
1. Develop a trusting relationship with the client.
2. Encourage verbal expression of painful experiences, anxieties, and concerns.
3. Explore methods of coping.
4. Identify sources of conflict.
5. Focus on the client's strengths and skills.
6. Orient the client.
7. Provide nondemanding simple routines.
8. Allow the client to progress at his or her own pace.
9. Implement stress-reduction techniques.
10. Plan for individual, group, and/or family psychotherapy to integrate dissociated aspects of personality or memory and expand self-awareness.

VIII. MOOD DISORDERS

A. Bipolar disorder
1. Description (Box 64-4)
   a. Bipolar disorder is characterized by episodes of mania and depression with periods of normal mood and activity in between.
   b. The medication of choice has traditionally been lithium carbonate, which can be toxic and therefore requires the regular monitoring of serum lithium levels.
   c. Other medications such as divalproex (Valproate), olanzapine (Zyprexa), and carbamazepine (Tegretol) may also be prescribed to reduce the symptoms of acute bipolar manic episodes.
2. Interventions for mania (Box 64-5)
   a. Remove hazardous objects from the environment (this should be done for all clients).
   b. Assess the client closely for fatigue.
   c. Use comfort measures to promote sleep.
   d. Provide frequent rest periods.
   e. Monitor the client's sleep patterns.
   f. Provide a private room if possible.
   g. Administer a hypnotic or sedative medication as prescribed.
   h. Encourage the client to ventilate feelings.
   i. Use calm, slow interactions.
   j. Help the client focus on one topic during the conversation.
   k. Ignore or distract the client from grandiose thinking.

l. Present reality to the client.
m. Do not argue with the client.
n. Limit group activities and assess the client's tolerance level.
o. Provide high-calorie finger foods and fluids.
p. Supervise the client's choice of clothing.
q. Reduce environmental stimuli.
r. Set limits on inappropriate behaviors.
s. Provide physical activities and outlets for tension.
t. Avoid competitive games.
u. Provide gross motor activities such as walking and writing.
v. Provide structured activities or one-to-one activities with the nurse.
w. Provide simple and direct explanations for routine procedures.
x. Supervise the administration of medication.
3. Major depressive disorder.
   a. Data collection (see Box 64-4).
   b. Interventions for depressed clients (Box 64-6).

Box 64-4 Data Collection: Bipolar Disorder

Mania
Becomes angry quickly
Delusional self-confidence
Distracted by environmental stimuli
Extroverted personality
Flight of ideas
Grandiose and persecutory delusions
High and unstable affect
Inability to eat or sleep because of involvement in more important things
Inability to sleep yet still active
Inappropriate affect
Inappropriate dress
Initiation of activity
Pressured speech
Restlessness
Sexually promiscuous
Significant decrease in appetite
Unlimited energy
Urgent motor activity

Depression
Increased or decreased appetite
Decrease in activities of daily living
Decreased emotion and physical activity
Easily fatigued
Inability to make decisions
Poor concentration
Internalizing hostility
Introverted personality
Social isolation and withdrawn from groups
Lack of energy
Lack of initiative
Lack of self-confidence and low self-esteem
Lack of sexual interest
Psychomotor retardation
Suicidal thinking

Box 64-5 Dealing with Inappropriate Behaviors Associated with Bipolar Disorder

Aggressive Behavior
Assist the client in identifying feelings of frustration and aggression.
Encourage the client to talk out instead of acting out feelings of frustration.
Assist the client in identifying precipitating events or situations that lead to aggressive behavior.
Describe the consequences of the behavior on self and others.
Assist in identifying previous coping mechanisms.
Assist the client in problem-solving techniques to cope with frustration or aggression.

De-Escalation Techniques
Maintain safety for the client, other clients, and self.
Maintain a large personal space and use a nonaggressive posture.
Use a calm approach and communicate with a calm, clear tone of voice (be assertive, not aggressive).
Determine what the client considers to be his or her need.

Avoid verbal struggles.
Provide the client with clear options that deal with the client's behavior.
Assist the client with problem-solving and decision-making regarding the options.

Manipulative Behavior
Set clear, consistent, realistic, and enforceable limits, and communicate expected behaviors.
Be clear about the consequences associated with exceeding set limits and follow through with the consequences in a nonpunitive manner if necessary.
Discuss the client's behavior in a nonjudgmental and nonthreatening manner.
Avoid power struggles with the client (avoid arguing with the client).
Assist the client in developing means of setting limits on personal behavior.

⚠️ Monitor a depressed client closely for signs of suicidal ideation. If the client presents with increased energy, monitor closely because it could mean that he or she now has the energy to perform the suicide act.

IX. SCHIZOPHRENIA

A. Description

1. Schizophrenia is a group of mental disorders characterized by psychotic features (hallucinations and delusions), disordered thought processes, and disrupted interpersonal relationships.

2. Disturbances in affect, mood, behavior, and thought processes occur.

B. Data collection (Figure 64-1)

1. Physical characteristics
   a. Unkempt appearance
   b. Body image distortions
   c. May be preoccupied with somatic complaints
   d. May neglect hygiene, eating, sleeping, and elimination

2. Motor activity (Box 64-7)
   a. Catatonic posturing: Holding bizarre postures for long periods
   b. Catatonic excitement: Moving excitedly with no environmental stimuli present

---

Box 64-6 Interventions for Depressed Clients

Assess for suicidal ideation.

Provide safety from suicidal actions (be certain that there are no harmful objects in the environment).

Assist with activities of daily living.

Use gentle encouragement to participate in activities of daily living and unit therapies.

Do not push decision-making or making complex choices. Make decisions that the client is not ready to make.

Monitor sleep patterns.

Monitor nutritional intake and weight.

Provide achievable activities in which the client can achieve success (focus on strengths).

Remind the client of times when he or she felt better and was successful.

Spend time with the client to convey the client's value.

Respond to anger therapeutically.

Box 64-7 Abnormal Motor Behaviors

Description

Abnormal motor behavior or activity displayed by the mentally ill client and occurring as a result of a psychiatric disorder

Types of Abnormal Motor Behaviors

Echolalia

Repeating the speech of another person

Echopraxia

Repeating the movements of another person

Waxy Flexibility

Having one's arms or legs placed in a certain position and holding that same position for hours

---

▲ **FIGURE 64-1** Treatment-relevant dimensions of schizophrenia. (From Varcarolis, E., & Halter, M. [2010]. *Foundations of psychiatric mental health nursing* [6th ed.]. St. Louis: Saunders.)

  c. Possible total immobilization
  d. Inability to respond to commands or responding only to commands
  e. Waxy flexibility
  f. Repetitive or stereotyped movements
  g. Motor activity that may be increased as evidenced by agitation, pacing, inability to sleep, loss of appetite and weight, and impulsiveness
  h. Possible inability to initiate activity (anergia)
3. Emotional characteristics
  a. Mistrust may be present.
  b. View of the world as threatening and unsafe
  c. Affect may be blunted, flat, or inappropriate.
  d. May display feelings of ambivalence, helplessness, anxiety, anger, guilt, or depression in response to hallucinations, delusions, or as a result of the grief related to losses imposed by this illness.
4. Compulsive rituals: performed as an attempt to solve conflicting feelings by constant, repetitive activity
5. Overcompliance: attempt to deny responsibility for any action by doing only what another instructs exactly
6. Affective disturbances
  a. Flat or incongruent affect or inappropriate affect
  b. Altered thought processes
7. Abnormal thought processes (Box 64-8)
  a. Impaired reality testing
  b. Fragmentation of thoughts
  c. Thought blocking
  d. Loose associations
  e. Echolalia
  f. Distorted perception of the environment
  g. Neologisms
  h. Magical thinking

  i. Inability to conceptualize meaning in words or thoughts
  j. Inability to organize facts logically
  k. Delusions associated with thought processes or content
8. Types of delusions (Box 64-9)
  a. Loss of reference in which the client believes that certain events, situations, or interactions are related directly to self

Box 64-9 Delusions

Description
A false belief held to be true even when there is evidence to the contrary

Types

Grandeur
The false belief that one is a powerful and important person

Jealousy
The false belief that one's partner or mate is going out with other persons

Persecution
The thought that one is being singled out for harm by others

Interventions
Ask the client to describe the delusion.
Be open and honest in interactions to reduce suspiciousness.
Focus the conversation on reality-based topics rather than the delusion.
Encourage the client to express feelings and focus on the feelings that the delusions generate.
If the client obsesses on the delusion, set firm limits on the amount of time for talking about the delusion.
Do not dispute with the client or try to convince him or her that the delusions are false.
Validate if part of the delusion is real.

Box 64-8 Abnormal Thought Processes

Description
Abnormal thought processes displayed by the mentally ill client and occurring as a result of a psychiatric disorder

Circumstantiality
Before getting to the point or answering a question, the individual gets caught up in countless details and explanations

Confabulation
Filling a memory gap with detailed fantasy believed by the teller. The purpose of confabulation is to maintain self-esteem. This is seen in organic conditions such as Korsakoff's psychosis.

Flight of Ideas
A constant flow of speech in which the individual jumps from one topic to another in rapid succession. A connection

between topics exists, although it is sometimes difficult to identify. This is seen in manic states.

Looseness of Association
Haphazard, illogical, and confused thinking and interrupted connections in thought. This is seen mostly in schizophrenic disorders.

Neologisms
Words that an individual makes up that only have meaning for the individual. This is often part of a delusional system.

Thought Blocking
A sudden cessation of a thought in the middle of a sentence; the client is unable to continue the train of thought. Often sudden new thoughts come up unrelated to the topic.

Word Salad
A mixture of words and phrases that have no meaning

b. Delusions of persecution in which the client believes that he or she is being harassed, threatened, or persecuted by some powerful force

c. Delusions of grandeur in which the client attaches special significance to self in relation to others or the universe and has an exaggerated sense of self that has no basis in reality

d. Somatic delusions in which the client believes that his or her body is changing or responding in an unusual way, which has no basis in reality

9. Perceptual distortions
   a. Illusions that may be brief experiences with a misinterpretation or misperception of reality
   b. Hallucinations (five senses) such as perceiving objects, sensations, or images with no basis in reality (Box 64-10)

10. Language and communication disturbances (Box 64-11)
    a. Related to disorders in thought process
    b. Inability to organize language

c. Difficulty communicating clearly

d. Inappropriate responses to a situation

e. A single word or phrase that may represent the whole meaning of the conversation such that the client may feel that he or she has communicated adequately

f. Development of a private language

C. Subtypes of schizophrenia: Note that the updated *Diagnostic and Statistical Manual of Mental Disorders* (DSM-5) no longer uses subtypes as diagnostic criteria.

1. Paranoid schizophrenia
   a. Suspiciousness and aloofness
   b. Hostility
   c. Delusions
   d. Auditory hallucinations
   e. Anxiety and anger
   f. Persecutory themes
   g. Violence

2. Disorganized schizophrenia
   a. Extreme social withdrawal
   b. Disorganized speech or behavior
   c. Flat or inappropriate affect
   d. Silliness unrelated to speech
   e. Stereotyped behaviors
   f. Grimacing mannerisms
   g. Inability to perform activities of daily living

3. Catatonic schizophrenia
   a. Psychomotor disturbances
   b. Immobility
   c. Stupor
   d. Waxy flexibility
   e. Excessive purposeless motor activity
   f. Echolalia
   g. Automatic obedience
   h. Stereotyped or repetitive behavior

4. Undifferentiated schizophrenia
   a. Delusions and hallucinations
   b. Disorganized speech

Box 64-10 Hallucinations

Description

A sense (occurs with one of the five senses) perception for which no external stimuli exist. This can have an organic or functional cause.

Types

Auditory

Hearing voices when none are present

Gustatory

Experiencing taste in the absence of stimuli

Olfactory

Smelling smells that do not exist

Tactile

Feeling touch sensations in the absence of stimuli

Visual

Seeing things that are not there

Command

"Voices" that direct a person to take action that is often harmful

Interventions

Ask the client directly about the hallucination.

Avoid reacting to the hallucination as if it were real.

Decrease stimuli or move the client to another area.

Do not negate the client's experience.

Focus on reality-based topics.

Attempt to engage the client's attention through a concrete activity.

Respond verbally to anything real that the client talks about.

Avoid touching the client.

Monitor for signs of increasing anxiety or agitation, which may indicate that the hallucinations are increasing.

Box 64-11 Language and Communication Disturbances

Clang association: Repetition of words or phrases that are similar in sound but in no other way

Echolalia: Repetition of words or phrases heard from another person

Mutism: Absence of verbal speech

Neologism: A new word devised that has special meaning only to the client

Pressured speech: Speaking as if the words are being forced out quickly

Verbigeration: Purposeless repetition of words or phrases

Word salad: Form of speech in which words or phrases are connected meaninglessly

c. Disorganized or catatonic behavior

d. Flat affect

e. Social withdrawal

5. Residual schizophrenia

a. Diagnosed as schizophrenic in the past

b. Time limited between attacks but may last for many years

c. The client exhibits considerable social isolation and withdrawal and impaired role functioning.

D. Interventions (Box 64-12)

E. Interventions: active hallucinations

1. Monitor for hallucination cues and assess content of hallucinations.

2. Intervene with one-on-one contact.

3. Decrease stimuli or move the client to another area.

4. Avoid conveying to the client that others are also experiencing the hallucination.

5. Respond verbally to anything real that the client talks about.

6. Avoid touching the client.

7. Encourage the client to express feelings.

8. During a hallucination, attempt to engage the client's attention through a concrete activity.

9. Accept and do not joke about or judge the client's behavior.

10. Provide easy activities and a structured environment with routine activities of daily living.

11. Monitor for signs of increasing fear, anxiety, or agitation.

12. Decrease stimuli as needed.

13. Administer medications as prescribed.

⚠ For a client with hallucinations, safety is the first priority. Ensure that the client does not have an auditory command telling him or her to harm self or others.

F. Interventions: Delusions

1. Interact based on reality.

2. Encourage the client to express feelings.

3. Do not dispute the client or try to convince the client that delusions are false.

4. Initially, initiate activities on a one-on-one basis.

5. Alter hospital routines as necessary, such as using canned or packaged food or food from home.

6. Recognize accomplishments and provide positive feedback for successes.

X. PARANOID DISORDERS

A. Description

1. Paranoid disorder is a concrete, pervasive delusional system characterized by persecutory and grandiose beliefs.

2. The client demonstrates suspicion and mistrust of others.

3. The client is often viewed by others as hostile, stubborn, and defensive.

B. Behaviors

1. Suspicious and mistrustful

2. Emotionally distant

3. Distortion of reality

Box 64-12 Interventions for Schizophrenia

Assess the client's physical needs.

Set limits on the client's behaviors when it interferes with others and becomes disruptive.

Maintain a safe environment.

Initiate one-on-one interaction and progress to small groups as tolerated.

Spend time with the client even if he or she is unable to respond.

Monitor for altered thought processes.

Maintain ego boundaries and avoid touching the client.

Limit the time of interaction with the client.

Avoid an overly warm approach. A neutral approach is less threatening.

Do not make promises to the client that cannot be kept.

Establish daily routines.

Assist the client to improve grooming and accept responsibility for personal care.

Sit with the client in silence if necessary.

Provide brief and frequent contact with the client.

Tell the client when you are leaving.

Tell the client when you do not understand.

Do not "go along" with the client's delusions or hallucinations.

Provide simple, concrete activities, such as puzzles or word games.

Reorient the client as necessary.

Help the client establish what is real and unreal.

Stay with the client if he or she is frightened.

Speak to the client in a simple, direct, and concise manner.

Reassure the client that the environment is safe.

Remove the client from group situations if the client's behavior is too bizarre, disturbing, or dangerous to others.

Set realistic goals.

Initially, do not offer choices to the client, and gradually assist him or her in making decisions.

Use canned or packaged food, especially with the paranoid schizophrenic client.

Provide a radio or tape player at night for insomnia.

Explain to the client everything that is being done.

Set limits on the client's behavior if he or she cannot.

Decrease excessive stimuli in the environment.

Monitor for suicide risk.

Assist the client to use alternative means to express feelings through music or art therapy or writing.

4. Poor insight and poor judgments
5. Hypervigilant
6. Low self-esteem
7. Highly sensitive, difficulty in admitting own error, and taking pride in being correct
8. Hypercritical and intolerant of others
9. Hostile, aggressive, and quarrelsome
10. Evasive
11. Exhibits concrete thinking

C. Delusions
1. Delusions serve a purpose in establishing identity and self-esteem.
2. Client may have grandiose and persecutory delusions.
3. Process of delusion includes denial, projection, and rationalization.
4. As trust in others increases, the need for delusions decreases.

D. Types of paranoid disorders
1. Paranoid personality disorder
   a. Suspicious
   b. Nonpsychotic
   c. No hallucinations or delusions
   d. No symptoms of schizophrenia
2. Paranoid-induced state
   a. Abrupt onset in response to stress and subsides when stress decreases
   b. No hallucinations but experiences paranoid delusions
   c. May be sensitive and suspicious before the development of delusions
   d. No symptoms of schizophrenia
3. Paranoia
   a. Exhibits an organized delusional system
   b. No hallucinations
   c. Reserved and sensitive before onset
   d. Psychotic state
   e. No symptoms of schizophrenia
4. Paranoid schizophrenia
   a. Before onset, the client becomes cold, withdrawn, distrustful, resentful, argumentative, sarcastic, and defiant.
   b. Bizarre, numerous, and changeable delusions occur.
   c. Delusions become less logical as the client becomes more disorganized.
   d. Persecutory hallucinations occur.
   e. Psychotic state ensues.
   f. All symptoms of schizophrenia are present.

E. Interventions (Box 64-13)

⚠ Do not whisper or laugh in front of a client with a paranoid disorder because the client will think that you are talking about or laughing at him or her. This increases the paranoia.

XI. PERSONALITY DISORDERS

A. Description
1. Personality disorders include various inflexible maladaptive behavior patterns or traits that may impair functioning and relationships.
2. The individual usually remains in touch with reality and typically has a lack of insight into his or her behavior.
3. Stress exacerbates manifestations of the personality disorder.
4. In severe cases the personality disorder may deteriorate to a psychotic state.

B. Characteristics
1. Poor impulse control
   a. Acting out to manage internal pain
   b. Forms of acting out include physical and verbal attacks, such as yelling and swearing, and self-injurious behaviors such as cutting own skin, banging the head, punching self, manipulation, substance **abuse**, promiscuous sexual behaviors, and **suicide attempts**.

Box 64-13 Interventions for Paranoid Disorders

Assess for suicide risk.
Diminish suspicious behavior.
Avoid direct eye contact.
Establish a trusting relationship.
Promote increased self-esteem.
Remain calm, nonthreatening, and nonjudgmental.
Provide continuity of care.
Respond honestly to the client.
Follow through on commitments made to the client.
Acknowledge the client's feelings, but tell him or her that you do not share his or her interpretation of an event.
Provide a daily schedule of activities.
Assist the client to identify diversionary activities.
Gradually introduce the client to groups.

Refocus conversation to reality-based topics.
Use role playing to help the client identify thoughts and feelings.
Provide positive reinforcement for successes.
Do not argue with delusions.
Use concrete, specific words.
Do not be secretive with the client.
Do not whisper in the client's presence.
Assure the client that he or she will be safe.
Involve the client in noncompetitive tasks.
Provide the client opportunity to complete small tasks.
Monitor eating, drinking, sleeping, and elimination patterns.
Limit physical contact.
Monitor for agitation and decrease stimuli as needed.

    c. Client may be preoccupied with self, religion, or sex.

  2. Mood characteristics

    a. May experience abandonment and depression

    b. Moods may include rage, guilt, fear, and emptiness

  3. Impaired judgment

    a. Difficulty with problem solving

    b. Inability to perceive the consequences of behavior

  4. Impaired reality testing: distortion of reality and often projection of own feelings onto others

  5. Impaired object relations: rigid and inflexible, with difficulty in intimate relationships

  6. Impaired self-perception: distorted self-perception and experience of self-hate or self-idealization

  7. Impaired thought processes

    a. Concrete or diffuse thinking

    b. Difficulty concentrating

    c. Impaired memory

  8. Impaired stimulus barrier

    a. Inability to regulate incoming sensory stimuli

    b. Increased excitability

    c. Excessive response to noise and light

    d. Poor attention span

    e. Agitated

    f. Insomnia

C. Cluster A Personality Disorders include the odd/eccentric types: schizoid, schizotypal, and paranoid

  1. Schizoid personality disorder is characterized by an inability to form warm, close social relationships.

    a. Social detachment and lack of close relationships

    b. Interest in solitary activities

    c. Aloof and indifferent

    d. Restricted expression of emotions

    e. Lack of interest in others

  2. Schizotypal personality disorder is characterized by the display of abnormal or highly unusual thoughts, perceptions, speech, and behavior patterns.

    a. Suspicious

    b. Paranoia

    c. Magical thinking

    d. Odd thinking and speech

    e. Relationship deficits

  3. Paranoid personality disorder is characterized by suspiciousness and mistrust of others.

    a. May be argumentative

    b. May be hostile, aloof

    c. May be rigid, critical, and controlling of others

    d. May have thoughts of grandiosity

D. Cluster B Personality Disorders include the overemotional, erratic types: histrionic, narcissistic, borderline, and antisocial

  1. Histrionic personality disorder is characterized by overly dramatic and intensely expressive behavior.

    a. Lively and dramatic and enjoys being the center of attention

    b. Has poor and shallow interpersonal relations

    c. May be sexually seductive or provocative

    d. Dramatizes their life and may appear theatrical

    e. Overly concerned with appearance

    f. Easily bored

  2. Narcissistic personality disorder is characterized by an increased sense of self-importance, preoccupation with fantasies and a sense of unlimited success.

    a. Need for admiration and inflation of accomplishments

    b. Overestimation of abilities and underestimation of contributions of others

    c. Lack of empathy and sensitivity to the needs of others

  3. Antisocial personality disorder is comprised of a pattern of irresponsible and antisocial behavior, selfishness, an inability to maintain lasting relationships, poor sexual adjustment, a failure to accept social norms, and a tendency toward irritability and aggressiveness.

    a. Perceives the world as hostile

    b. Superficial charm and hostility

    c. No shame or guilt

    d. Self-centered

    e. Unreliable

    f. Easily bored

    g. Poor work history

    h. Inability to tolerate frustration

    i. Views others as objects to be manipulated

    j. Poor judgment

    k. Impulsive

  4. Borderline personality disorder is characterized by instability in interpersonal relationships, unstable mood and self-image, and impulsive and unpredictable behavior.

    a. Unclear identity

    b. Unstable and intense

    c. Extreme shifts in mood

    d. Easily angered

    e. Easily bored

    f. Argumentative

    g. Depression

    h. Self-destructive behavior

    i. Manipulation

    j. Inability to tolerate anxiety

    k. Chronic feelings of emptiness and fear of being alone

    l. Splitting (sees others as all good or all bad; creates conflict between individuals by playing one person against another)

E. Cluster C Personality Disorders include the anxious, fearful types of personality disorders: obsessive-compulsive personality, avoidant, and dependent.

1. Obsessive-compulsive personality disorder is characterized by difficulty expressing warm and tender emotions, perfectionism, stubbornness, the need to control others, and a devotion to work.
   a. Overly conscientious
   b. Inflexible and preoccupied with details and rules
   c. Extreme devotion to work to the exclusion of leisure activities and friendships
   d. Miserly and stubborn
   e. Hoarding behavior
   f. Engages in rituals
2. Avoidant personality disorder is characterized by social withdrawal and extreme sensitivity to potential rejection
   a. Feelings of inadequacy
   b. Hypersensitive to reactions of others and poor reaction to criticism
   c. Social isolation
   d. Lack of support system
3. Dependent personality disorder is characterized by intense lack of self-confidence and low self-esteem, and lack of ability to function independently, such that the individual passively allows others to make decisions and assume responsibility for major areas in the person's life. The dependent client has great difficulty making decisions.

F. General interventions for the client with a personality disorder
1. Maintain safety against self-destructive behaviors.
2. Allow the client to make choices and be as independent as possible.
3. Encourage the client to discuss feelings rather than act them out.
4. Provide consistency in response to the client's acting-out behaviors.
5. Discuss expectations and responsibilities with the client.
6. Discuss the consequences that follow certain behaviors.
7. Inform the client that harm to self, others, and property is unacceptable.
8. Identify splitting behavior.
9. Assist the client to deal directly with anger.
10. Develop a written safety and/or behavioral contract with the client.
11. Encourage the client to keep a journal recording daily feelings.
12. Encourage the client to participate in group activities, and praise nonmanipulative behavior.
13. Set and maintain limits to decrease manipulative behavior.
14. Remove the client from group situations in which attention-seeking behaviors occur.
15. Provide realistic praise for positive behaviors in social situations.

XII. COGNITIVE IMPAIRMENT DISORDERS

A. Autism: Refer to Chapter 31
B. Attention deficit hyperactivity disorder: refer to Chapter 31
C. Dementia and Alzheimer's disease
1. Dementia
   a. Dementia is a syndrome with progressive deterioration in intellectual functioning; secondary to structural or functional changes.
   b. Long- and short-term memory loss occurs with impairment in judgment, abstract thinking, problem-solving ability, and behavior.
   c. Dementia results in a self-care deficit.
   d. The most common type of dementia is Alzheimer's disease.
2. Alzheimer's disease (Box 64-14)
   a. Alzheimer's disease is an irreversible form of senile dementia from nerve cell deterioration.
   b. Individuals with Alzheimer's disease experience cognitive deterioration and progressive loss of ability to carry out activities of daily living.
   c. The client experiences a steady decline in physical and mental functioning and usually requires long-term care facility placement in the final stages of the illness.
3. Interventions
   a. Identify and reinforce retained skills.
   b. Provide continuity of care.
   c. Orient the client to the environment.
   d. Furnish the environment with familiar possessions.
   e. Acknowledge the client's feelings.
   f. Help the client and family members manage memory deficits and behavior changes.
   g. Encourage the family members to express feelings about caregiving.
   h. Provide the caregiver support and identify the resources and support groups available.
   i. Monitor activities of daily living.

Box 64-14 Alzheimer's Disease

Agnosia: Failure to recognize or identify objects despite intact sensory function
Amnesia: Loss of memory caused by brain degeneration
Aphasia: Language disturbance in understanding and expressing the spoken word
Apraxia: Inability to perform motor activities despite intact motor function

j. Remind the client how to perform self-care activities.

k. Help the client maintain independence.

l. Provide the client with consistent routines.

m. Provide exercise such as walking with an escort.

n. Avoid activities that tax the memory.

o. Allow the client plenty of time to complete a task.

p. Use constant encouragement in a simple step-by-step approach.

q. Provide activities that distract and occupy time, such as listening to music, coloring, and watching television.

r. Provide the client with mental stimulation with simple games or activities.

4. Wandering
   a. Provide a safe environment.
   b. Prevent unsafe wandering.
   c. Provide close supervision.
   d. Close and secure doors.
   e. Use identification bracelets and electronic surveillance.

⚠ Providing a safe environment is a priority in the care of a client with Alzheimer's disease.

5. Communication
   a. Adapt to the communication level of the client.
   b. Use a firm volume and a low-pitched voice to communicate.
   c. Stand directly in front of the client and maintain eye contact.
   d. Call the client by name and identify self. Wait for a response.
   e. Use a calm and reassuring voice.
   f. Use pantomime gestures if the client is unable to understand spoken words.
   g. Speak slowly and clearly, using short words and simple sentences.
   h. Ask only one question at a time and give one direction at a time.
   i. Repeat questions if necessary but do not rephrase.

6. Impaired judgment
   a. Remove throw rugs, toxic substances, and dangerous electrical appliances from the environment.
   b. Reduce hot water heater temperature.

7. Altered thought processes
   a. Call the client by name.
   b. Orient the client frequently.
   c. Use familiar objects in the room.
   d. Place a calendar and clock in a visible place.
   e. Maintain familiar routines.
   f. Allow the client to reminisce.

g. Make tasks simple.

h. Allow time for the client to complete a task.

i. Provide positive reinforcement for positive behaviors.

8. Altered sleep patterns
   a. Allow the client to wander in a safe place until he or she becomes tired.
   b. Prevent shadows in the room by using indirect light.
   c. Avoid the use of hypnotics because they cause confusion and aggravate the sundown effect.

9. Agitation
   a. Assess the precipitant of the agitation.
   b. Reassure the client.
   c. Remove items that can be hazardous during the time of agitation.
   d. Approach the client slowly and calmly from the front, and then speak, gesture, and move slowly.
   e. Remove client to a less stressful environment; decrease excess stimuli.
   f. Use touch gently.
   g. Do not argue with or force the client.

XIII. PSYCHOSEXUAL ALTERATIONS

A. Sexuality
   1. One's sense of being a sexual individual
   2. Includes how one looks, behaves, and relates to others

B. Sexual expression (Box 64-15)

C. Alterations in sexual behavior
   1. Transsexualism: Feeling that one's gender is inappropriate and desiring to acquire sexual characteristics of the opposite gender
   2. Exhibitionism: Sexual urges and fantasies and exposure of genitals to strangers to bring sexual gratification and/or arousal
   3. Fetishism: Using nonliving objects for sexual gratification
   4. Pedophilia: Desiring sexual activity with a child under age 13
   5. Sexual masochism: Sexual gratification that involves receiving pain
   6. Sexual sadism: Sexual gratification that involves inflicting pain

Box 64-15 Sexual Expression

Bisexuality: Sexual attraction to and activity with both genders

Heterosexuality: Male-female sexual relationships

Homosexuality: Sexual attraction to a member of the same gender

Transvestism: Obsession with wearing clothing of the opposite gender

7. Voyeurism: Sexual gratification through observing others disrobing or engaging in sexual activity
8. Zoophilia: Intense sexual arousal or desire for sexual contact with animals
9. Frotteurism: Intense sexual arousal or desire when rubbing against a nonconsenting person

D. Interventions
1. Assess sexual history, history of trauma or **abuse**, and precipitating event for the sexual disorder.
2. Encourage the client to explore personal beliefs.
3. Provide a nonjudgmental attitude.
4. Provide supportive psychotherapy.

MORE QUESTIONS ON EVOLVE!

Practice Questions

686. A client with delirium becomes agitated and confused at night. The best initial intervention by the nurse is to:
1. Move the client next to the nurse's station.
2. Use a night light and turn off the television.
3. Keep the television and a soft light on during the night.
4. Play soft music during the night and maintain a well-lit room.

687. A nurse is collecting data on a client who is actively hallucinating. Which nursing statement would be therapeutic at this time?
1. "I know you feel 'they are out to get you,' but it's not true."
2. "I can hear the voice and she wants you to come to dinner."
3. "Sometimes people hear things or voices others can't hear."
4. "I talked to the voices you're hearing and they won't hurt you now."

688. A nurse is caring for a client with a diagnosis of depression. The nurse monitors for signs of constipation and urinary retention, knowing that these problems are likely caused by:
1. Poor dietary choices
2. Lack of exercise and poor diet
3. Inadequate dietary intake and dehydration
4. Psychomotor retardation and side effects of medication

689. A client is admitted to the in-patient unit and is being considered for electroconvulsive therapy (ECT). The client appears calm, but the family is hypervigilant and anxious. The client's mother begins to cry and states, "My child's brain will be destroyed. How can the doctor do this?" The nurse makes which therapeutic response?
1. "It sounds as though you need to speak to the psychiatrist."
2. "Perhaps you'd like to see the ECT room and speak to the staff."
3. "Your child has decided to have this treatment. You should be supportive of the decision."
4. "It sounds as though you have some concerns about the ECT procedure. Why don't we sit down together and discuss any concerns you may have?"

690. A client who is diagnosed with pedophilia and has been recently paroled as a sex offender says, "I'm in treatment and I have served my time. Now this group has posters of me all over the neighborhood telling about me with my picture on it." Which of the following is an appropriate response by the nurse?
1. "When children are hurt as you hurt them, people want you isolated."
2. "You're lucky it doesn't escalate into something pretty scary after your crime."
3. "You understand that people fear for their children, but you're feeling unfairly treated?"
4. "You seem angry, but you have committed serious crimes against several children, so your neighbors are frightened."

691. A nurse is preparing for the hospital discharge of a client with a history of command hallucinations to harm self or others. The nurse instructs the client about interventions for hallucinations and anxiety and determines that the client understands the interventions when the client states:
1. "My medications won't make me anxious."
2. "I'll go to a support group and talk so that I won't hurt anyone."
3. "I won't get anxious or hear things if I get enough sleep and eat well."
4. "I can call my therapist when I'm hallucinating so that I can talk about my feelings and plans and not hurt anyone."

692. A nurse observes that a client is psychotic, pacing, and agitated and is making aggressive gestures. The client's speech pattern is rapid and the client's affect is belligerent. Based on these observations, the nurse's immediate priority of care is to:
1. Provide safety for the client and other clients on the unit.
2. Provide the clients on the unit with a sense of comfort and safety.
3. Assist the staff in caring for the client in a controlled environment.
4. Offer the client a less-stimulating area to calm down and gain control.

693. A nurse is caring for a client diagnosed with catatonic stupor. The client is lying on the bed, with the body pulled into a fetal position. The appropriate nursing intervention is which of the following?
1. Ask direct questions to encourage talking.
2. Leave the client alone and intermittently check on him.
3. Sit beside the client in silence and verbalize occasional open-ended questions.
4. Take the client into the dayroom with other clients so they can help watch him.

694. A mother of a teenage client with an anxiety disorder is concerned about her daughter's progress on discharge. She states that her daughter "stashes food, eats all the wrong things that make her hyperactive," and "hangs out with the wrong crowd." In helping the mother prepare for her daughter's discharge, the nurse suggests that the mother:
1. Restrict the daughter's socializing time with her friends.
2. Restrict the amount of chocolate and caffeine products in the home.
3. Keep her daughter out of school until she can adjust to the school environment.
4. Consider taking time from work to help her daughter readjust to the home environment.

695. A client is unwilling to go out of the house for fear of "doing something crazy in public." Because of this fear, the client remains homebound except when accompanied outside by the spouse. The nurse determines that the client has:
1. Agoraphobia
2. Hematophobia
3. Claustrophobia
4. Hypochondriasis

696. A client has reported that crying spells have been a major problem over the past several weeks, and that the doctor said that depression is probably the reason. The nurse observes that the client is sitting slumped in the chair and the clothes that the client is wearing do not fit well. The nurse interprets that further data collection should focus on:
1. Weight loss
2. Sleep patterns
3. Medication compliance
4. Onset of the crying spells

697. A client was admitted to a medical unit with acute blindness. Many tests are performed and there seems to be no organic reason why this client cannot see. The nurse later learns that the client became blind after witnessing a hit-and-run car crash, in which a family of three was killed. The nurse suspects that the client may be experiencing a:
1. Psychosis
2. Repression
3. Conversion disorder
4. Dissociative disorder

698. A manic client announces to everyone in the dayroom that a stripper is coming to perform that evening. When the psychiatric nurse's aide firmly states that the client's behavior is not appropriate, the manic client becomes verbally abusive and threatens physical violence to the nurse's aide. Based on the analysis of this situation, the nurse determines that the appropriate action would be to:
1. Escort the manic client to his or her room.
2. Orient the client to time, person, and place.
3. Tell the client that the behavior is not appropriate.
4. Tell the client that smoking privileges are revoked for 24 hours.

699. A nurse notes documentation in a client's record that the client is experiencing delusions of persecution. The nurse understands that these types of delusions are characteristic of which of the following?
1. The false belief that one is a very powerful person
2. The false belief that one is a very important person
3. The false belief that one is being singled out for harm by others
4. The false belief that one's partner is going out with other people

700. Which nursing interventions are appropriate for a hospitalized client with mania who is exhibiting manipulative behavior? **Select all that apply.** ❖
☐ 1. Communicate expected behaviors to the client.
☐ 2. Ensure that the client knows that he or she is not in charge of the nursing unit.
☐ 3. Assist the client in developing means of setting limits on personal behavior.
☐ 4. Follow through about the consequences of behavior in a nonpunitive manner.
☐ 5. Enforce rules and inform the client that he or she will not be allowed to attend therapy groups.
☐ 6. Be clear with the client regarding the consequences of exceeding limits set regarding behavior.

ANSWERS

686. 2

Rationale: It is important to provide a consistent daily routine and a low-stimulation environment when the client is agitated and confused. Noise levels including a radio and television may add to the confusion and disorientation. Moving the client next to the nurses' station is not the initial intervention.
Test-Taking Strategy: Use the process of elimination and note the strategic word "initial" in the question. Eliminate options 3 and 4 first because they are comparable or alike. From the remaining options, recalling that a low-stimulation environment is best will direct you to option 2. Review measures related to the client with agitation and confusion if you had difficulty with this question.
Level of Cognitive Ability: Applying
Client Needs: Psychosocial Integrity
Integrated Process: Nursing Process/Implementation
Content Area: Mental Health
References: Stuart, p. 404. 2009.

687. 3

Rationale: It is important for the nurse to reinforce reality with the client. Options 1, 2, and 4 do not reinforce reality but reinforce the hallucination that the voices are real.
Test-Taking Strategy: Use the process of elimination. Note that options 1, 2, and 4 all indicate reinforcement to the client that the voices are real. Option 3 is the only statement that indicates reality. Review nursing interventions related to the client who is hallucinating if you had difficulty with this question.
Level of Cognitive Ability: Applying
Client Needs: Psychosocial Integrity
Integrated Process: Communication and Documentation
Content Area: Mental Health
Reference: Morrison-Valfre, pp. 92, 104–105. 2009.

688. 4

Rationale: Constipation can be related to inadequate food intake, lack of exercise, and poor diet. In this situation, urinary retention is most likely caused by medications. Option 4 is the only option that addresses both constipation and urinary retention.
Test-Taking Strategy: Use the process of elimination and focus on the data in the question. Options 1, 2, and 3 are all comparable or alike and address diet. Option 4 addresses both concerns of constipation and urinary retention. If you had difficulty with this question, review the interventions for a client with depression and the effects of medications prescribed for this disorder.
Level of Cognitive Ability: Analyzing
Client Needs: Physiological Integrity
Integrated Process: Nursing Process/Data Collection
Content Area: Mental Health
Reference: Morrison-Valfre, p. 228. 2009.

689. 4

Rationale: The nurse needs to encourage the family and client to verbalize their fears and concerns. Option 4 is the only option that encourages verbalization. Options 1, 2, and 3 avoid dealing with the client or family concerns.

Test-Taking Strategy: Use therapeutic communication techniques and focus on the client's and family's feelings and concerns. This will direct you to option 4. Review these techniques if you had difficulty with this question.
Level of Cognitive Ability: Applying
Client Needs: Psychosocial Integrity
Integrated Process: Nursing Process/Implementation
Content Area: Mental Health
References: Christensen, Kockrow, pp. 1143, 1150. 2011. *Foundations of nursing.*
Stuart, pp. 537–538. 2009.

690. 3

Rationale: Focusing and verbalizing the implied concern is the therapeutic response because it assists the client to clarify thinking and re-examine what the client is really saying. Option 3 is the only option that reflects the use of this therapeutic communication technique. Option 1 is insensitive and anxiety-provoking. Option 4 does not facilitate the client's expression of feelings. Option 2 gives advice and does not facilitate the client's expression of feelings.
Test-Taking Strategy: Use therapeutic communication techniques to answer the question. Remembering to focus on the client's feelings and concerns will direct you to the correct option. Review these techniques if you had difficulty with this question.
Level of Cognitive Ability: Applying
Client Needs: Psychosocial Integrity
Integrated Process: Communication and Documentation
Content Area: Mental Health
References: Morrison-Valfre, pp. 104–105. 2009.
Stuart, p. 494. 2009.

691. 4

Rationale: There may be an increased risk for impulsive and/or aggressive behavior if a client is receiving command hallucinations to harm self or others. Talking about the auditory hallucinations can interfere with the subvocal muscular activity associated with a hallucination. Option 4 is a specific agreement to seek help and evidences self-responsible commitment and control over his or her own behavior.
Test-Taking Strategy: Use the process of elimination. Note the relation between the word "hallucinations" in the question and the correct option. Review care of the client with command hallucinations if you had difficulty with this question.
Level of Cognitive Ability: Evaluating
Client Needs: Psychosocial Integrity
Integrated Process: Nursing Process/Evaluation
Content Area: Mental Health
Reference: Swearingen, pp. 708–709. 2012.

692. 1

Rationale: Safety of the client and other clients is the priority. Option 1 is the only option that addresses the client and other clients' safety needs. Option 4 addresses the client's needs. Option 2 addresses other clients' needs. Option 3 is not client centered.
Test-Taking Strategy: Use the process of elimination and focus on the subject, safety. Option 1 is the umbrella option and addresses the safety of all. Review care of the psychotic client if you had difficulty with this question.

Level of Cognitive Ability: Applying
Client Needs: Safe and Effective Care Environment
Integrated Process: Nursing Process/Implementation
Content Area: Mental Health
Reference: Morrison-Valfre, p. 351. 2009.

693. 3

Rationale: Clients with catatonic stupor may be immobile and mute and may require consistent, repeated approaches. The nurse facilitates communication with the client by sitting in silence, asking open-ended questions, and pausing to provide opportunities for the client to respond. The nurse would not leave the client alone. Fortunately, with pharmacotherapy and improved individual management, severe catatonic symptoms rarely occur. Option 4 relies on other clients to care for this one, which is an inappropriate expectation. Asking direct questions of this client is not therapeutic. Option 3 is the best action because it provides for client supervision and communication as appropriate.
Test-Taking Strategy: Use the process of elimination. Eliminate option 2 because the nurse would not leave the client alone. Eliminate option 4 next because this action relies on other clients to care for this one. Eliminate option 1 because asking direct questions of this client is not therapeutic. Review care of the client with catatonic stupor if you had difficulty with this question.
Level of Cognitive Ability: Applying
Client Needs: Psychosocial Integrity
Integrated Process: Nursing Process/Implementation
Content Area: Mental Health
Reference: Varcarolis, Halter, pp. 275. 277. 2009.

694. 2

Rationale: Clients with anxiety disorder should abstain from or limit their intake of caffeine, chocolate, and alcohol. These products have the potential of increasing anxiety. Options 1 and 3 are unreasonable and are an unhealthy approach. It may not be realistic for a family member to take time away from work.
Test-Taking Strategy: Use the process of elimination. Options 1, 3, and 4 are comparable or alike and are concerned with monitoring or curtailing the client's physical activities. Option 2 addresses preparation of the client's environment and focuses on the concern or subject expressed in the question. Review discharge planning for the client with anxiety disorder if you had difficulty with this question.
Level of Cognitive Ability: Applying
Client Needs: Psychosocial Integrity
Integrated Process: Teaching and Learning
Content Area: Mental Health
References: Stuart, p. 223. 2009.
Swearingen, p. 677. 2012.

695. 1

Rationale: Agoraphobia is a fear of being alone in open or public places where escape might be difficult. Agoraphobia includes experiencing fear or a sense of helplessness or embarrassment if a phobic attack occurs. Avoidance of such situations usually results in the reduction of social and professional interactions. Hematophobia is the fear of blood.

Claustrophobia is a fear of closed-in places. Clients with hypochondriacal symptoms focus their anxiety on physical complaints and are preoccupied with their health.
Test-Taking Strategy: Use the process of elimination and focus on the data in the question. Recalling the specific types of phobias and associated client behaviors will direct you to the correct option. If you had difficulty with this question, review phobia types and associated client behaviors.
Level of Cognitive Ability: Understanding
Client Needs: Psychosocial Integrity
Integrated Process: Nursing Process/Data Collection
Content Area: Mental Health
References: Morrison-Valfre, p. 197. 2009.
Swearingen, p. 678. 2012.

696. 1

Rationale: All the options are possible issues to address; however, the weight loss is the first item that needs further data collection because ill-fitting clothing could indicate a problem with nutrition. The client has already told the nurse that the crying spells have been a problem. Medication or sleep patterns are not mentioned or addressed in the question.
Test-Taking Strategy: Use the process of elimination and Maslow's Hierarchy of Needs theory to answer the question. Focusing on the data in the question will assist in eliminating the incorrect options. Review the priorities of care for a client with depression if you had difficulty with this question.
Level of Cognitive Ability: Analyzing
Client Needs: Physiological Integrity
Integrated Process: Nursing Process/Data Collection
Content Area: Mental Health
References: Christensen, Kockrow, p. 1145. 2011. *Foundations of nursing.*
Morrison-Valfre, p. 228. 2009.

697. 3

Rationale: A conversion disorder is the alteration or loss of a physical function that cannot be explained by any known pathophysiological mechanism. It is thought to be an expression of a psychological need or conflict. In this situation, the client witnessed an accident that was so psychologically painful that the client became blind. A dissociative disorder is a disturbance or alteration in the normally integrative functions of identity, memory, or consciousness. Psychosis is a state in which a person's mental capacity to recognize reality, communicate, and relate to others is impaired, thus interfering with the person's capacity to deal with life's demands. Repression is a coping mechanism in which unacceptable feelings are kept out of awareness.
Test-Taking Strategy: Use the process of elimination. Noting that the client evidences no organic reason to account for the blindness will direct you to the correct option. If you had difficulty with this question, review conversion disorders and defense mechanisms.
Level of Cognitive Ability: Understanding
Client Needs: Psychosocial Integrity
Integrated Process: Nursing Process/Data Collection
Content Area: Mental Health
References: Morrison-Valfre, pp. 242. 243. 2009.

698. 1

Rationale: The client is at risk for injury to self and others and therefore should be escorted out of the dayroom. Option 4 may increase the agitation that already exists in this client. Orientation will not halt the behavior. Telling the client that the behavior is not appropriate has already been attempted by the psychiatric nurse's aide.

Test-Taking Strategy: Use the process of elimination and therapeutic interventions for the manic client. Options 2, 3, and 4 will not de-escalate the client's agitation. If you had difficulty with this question, review the appropriate interventions in dealing with a manic client.

Level of Cognitive Ability: Applying
Client Needs: Psychosocial Integrity
Integrated Process: Nursing Process/Implementation
Content Area: Mental Health
References: Swearingen, p. 684. 2012.
Varcarolis, Halter, pp. 254–255. 2009.

699. 3

Rationale: A delusion is a false belief held to be true even when there is evidence to the contrary. A delusion of persecution is the thought that one is being singled out for harm by others. A delusion of grandeur is the false belief that he or she is a very powerful and important person. A delusion of jealousy is the false belief that one's partner is going out with other people.

Test-Taking Strategy: Use the process of elimination. Eliminate options 1 and 2 first since they are comparable or alike. From the remaining options, note the relationship between the word "persecution" in the question and the description in option 3. Review the description of the types of delusions if you had difficulty with this question.

Level of Cognitive Ability: Understanding
Client Needs: Psychosocial Integrity
Integrated Process: Nursing Process/Data Collection
Content Area: Mental Health
Reference: Morrison-Valfre, pp. 180, 348. 2009.

700. 1, 3, 4, 6

Rationale: Interventions for dealing with the client exhibiting manipulative behavior include setting clear, consistent, and enforceable limits on manipulative behaviors; being clear with the client regarding the consequences of exceeding limits set; following through with the consequences in a nonpunitive manner; and assisting the client in developing means of setting limits on personal behaviors. Enforcing rules and informing the client that he or she will not be allowed to attend therapy groups is a violation of a client's rights. Ensuring that the client knows that he or she is not in charge of the nursing unit is inappropriate; power struggles need to be avoided.

Test-Taking Strategy: Focus on the subject, manipulative behavior. Recalling clients' rights and that power struggles need to be avoided will assist in selecting the correct interventions. Review care to the client with manipulative behavior if you had difficulty with this question.

Level of Cognitive Ability: Applying
Client Needs: Psychosocial Integrity
Integrated Process: Nursing Process/Implementation
Content Area: Mental Health
Reference: Varcarolis, Halter, p. 259. 2009.

65

Addictions

I. EATING DISORDERS

A. Description: Eating disorders are characterized by uncertain self-identification and grossly disturbed eating habits (Figure 65-1).

B. Compulsive overeating
1. Compulsive overeating is binge-like overeating without purging.
2. Food consumption is out of the individual's control and occurs in a stereotyped fashion.
3. The client may be repulsed by eating, and the eating relieves tension but does not produce pleasure.
4. The client is aware that eating patterns are abnormal and feels depressed after eating.
5. The client eats secretly during a binge and consumes high-calorie and easily digestible food.
6. The client repeatedly tries to diet but without success.
7. The client feels helpless and hopeless about weight.
8. When experiencing guilt, anger, depression, boredom, loneliness, inadequacy, or ambivalence, the client responds by eating.

C. Anorexia nervosa
1. Description
   a. The onset often is associated with a stressful life event.
   b. The client intensely fears obesity.
   c. Body image is distorted, and the client has a disturbed self-concept.
   d. The client is preoccupied with foods that prevent weight gain and has a phobia against foods that produce weight gain.
   e. The eating disorder can be life threatening.
   f. Death can occur from starvation, **suicide,** cardiomyopathies, or electrolyte imbalance.
2. Data collection
   a. Refusal to eat and appetite loss
   b. Appetite denial
   c. Feelings of lack of control
   d. Self-induced vomiting and self-administered enemas
   e. Compulsive exercising

   f. Overachiever and perfectionist
   g. Decreased temperature, pulse, and blood pressure
   h. Weight loss
   i. Gastrointestinal disturbances
   j. Constipation
   k. Electrolyte imbalances
   l. Scaly, dry skin
   m. Presence of lanugo on extremities
   n. Sleep disturbances
   o. Hormone deficiencies
   p. Amenorrhea for at least three consecutive menstrual periods
   q. Teeth and gum deterioration
   r. Cyanosis and numbness of extremities
   s. Esophageal varices from vomiting
   t. Bone degeneration

The client with an eating disorder experiences an altered body image.

D. Bulimia nervosa
1. Description
   a. The client indulges in eating binges followed by purging behaviors.
   b. Most clients remain within a normal weight range but feel that their lives are dominated by the eating-related conflict.
2. Data collection
   a. Preoccupied with body shape and weight
   b. Consumption of high-calorie food in secret; guilt about secretive eating
   c. Binge-purge syndrome
   d. Attempts to lose weight through diets, vomiting, enemas, cathartics, and amphetamines or diuretics
   e. Has need for control yet experiences feelings of powerlessness or loss of control
   f. Low self-esteem
   g. Poor interpersonal relationships
   h. Decreased or absent interest in sex
   i. Mood swings
   j. Electrolyte imbalances

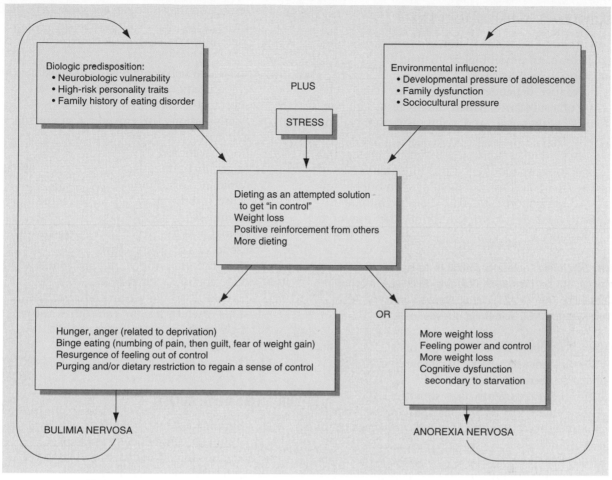

▲ **FIGURE 65-1** Cycle of eating disorders. (From Fortinash, K., & Worret, P. [2012]. *Psychiatric mental health nursing* [5th ed.]. St. Louis: Mosby.)

k. Loss of tooth enamel and dental decay
l. Stomach ulcers and rectal bleeding
m. Esophageal varices from vomiting
n. Cardiac disease and hypertension

E. Interventions: Clients with an eating disorder

1. Assess the client's nutritional status and the severity of any medical problems.
2. Establish a one-to-one therapeutic relationship with the client. The nurse must establish trust and recognize any client reluctance to establish a relationship.
3. Establish a contract with the client concerning the nutritional plan for the day.
4. Assist the client to identify precipitants to the eating disorder.
5. Encourage the client to express feelings about the eating behavior and about how he or she feels about their body.
6. Be accepting and nonjudgmental.
7. Work with the client on exploring self-concept and establishing identity.
8. Implement behavior modification techniques.

9. Supervise the client during mealtimes and for a specified period after meals.
10. Set a time limit for each meal.
11. Provide a pleasant, relaxed environment for eating.
12. Monitor for signs of physical complications related to the eating disorder.
13. Record intake and output.
14. Weigh the client daily at the same time, using the same scale, after the client voids.
15. When weighing the client, ensure that the client is wearing the same clothing as when the previous weight was taken.
16. Monitor and restore fluid and electrolyte balance.
17. Monitor elimination patterns.
18. Assess and limit the client's activity level.
19. Encourage the client to participate in diversional activities.
20. Assess the client's suicidal potential.
21. Administer antidepressant medication if prescribed.
22. Encourage psychotherapy.
23. Refer the client to support groups.

II.   SUBSTANCE ABUSE DISORDERS

A. Description: Substance **abuse** disorders cause behavioral and physiological changes (Box 65-1).

B. Substance dependence
1. Substance dependence is a pattern of repeated use of a substance, which usually results in tolerance, withdrawal, and compulsive drug-taking behavior.
2. The client takes substances in larger amounts and over longer periods than was intended.
3. The client has the desire to cut down but has unsuccessful efforts to decrease or discontinue use.
4. Daily activities revolve around the use of a substance.

 Screening tools are available to assess a substance abuse disorder, including Michigan Alcohol Screening Test (MAST), Drug Abuse Screening Test (DAST), and CAGE screening questionnaire.

C. Substance tolerance is the need for increased amounts of the substance to achieve the desired effect.

D. Substance **abuse**
1. The client recurrently uses substances.
2. The client experiences recurrent, significant harmful consequences related to the use of substances.
3. The client may have legal issues to resolve, and involvement with the legal system is not uncommon.

E. Substance withdrawal
1. Physiological and substance-specific cognitive symptoms occur.
2. Substance withdrawal occurs when an individual experiences a decrease in blood levels of a substance to which they are physiologically dependent.

F. Other factors to consider in the client with a substance-related disorder
1. Rebellion and peer group pressure in adolescence may contribute to the onset of substance use.
2. Substance use may become a coping mechanism for decreasing physical and emotional pain.

Box 65-1 CAGE Screening Test

C: Have you ever felt the need to cut down on your drinking/drug use?

A: Have you ever been annoyed at criticism of your drinking/drug use?

G: Have you ever felt guilty about something you have done when you have been drinking or taking drugs?

E: Have you ever had an eye opener: drinking or taking drugs first thing in the morning to get going or to avoid withdrawal symptoms?

---

3. Depression may precede or occur as a result of or in association with substance use.
4. Grief and loss may be associated with substance use.

G. Dysfunctional behaviors related to substance **abuse**
1. Preoccupation with obtaining and using substance
2. Manipulation to avoid consequences of behavior
3. Impulsiveness
4. Anger, including physical and verbal **abuse**
5. Avoidance of relationships
6. Sense of self-importance and requiring special treatment
7. Denial; blaming everything but the substance use for his or her problems
8. Uses rationalization and projection to justify unacceptable behavior
9. Likely to be involved in codependent relationships whereby a significant other also unknowingly serves as a significant enabler
10. Low self-esteem
11. Depression

III.   ALCOHOL ABUSE

A. Description
1. Alcohol is a central nervous system (CNS) depressant affecting all body tissues.
2. Physical dependence is a biological need for alcohol to avoid physical withdrawal symptoms, whereas psychological dependence refers to craving for the subjective effect of alcohol.

B. Risk factors
1. Biological predisposition. Genetic and familial predisposition may be a risk factor.
2. Depressed and highly anxious characteristics
3. Low self-esteem
4. Poor self-control
5. History of rebelliousness, poor school performance, or delinquency
6. Poor parental relationships

C. Data collection
1. Slurred speech
2. Uncoordinated movements
3. Unsteady gait
4. Restlessness
5. Belligerence
6. Confusion
7. Sneaking drinks, drinking in the morning, and experiencing blackouts
8. Binge drinking
9. Arguments about drinking
10. Missing work
11. Increased tolerance to alcohol
12. Intoxication, with blood alcohol levels of 0.1% (100 mg alcohol per deciliter of blood) or higher

⚠ Part of the assessment should include the type of alcohol, how much consumed, and for how many years.

D. Psychological symptoms
1. Depression
2. Hostility
3. Suspiciousness
4. Rationalization
5. Irritability
6. Isolation
7. Decrease in inhibitions
8. Decrease in self-esteem
9. Denial that a problem exists

E. Complications associated with chronic alcohol use
1. Vitamin deficiencies
   a. Vitamin B deficiency causing peripheral neuropathies
   b. Thiamine deficiency causing Korsakoff's syndrome (a form of amnesia)
2. Alcohol-induced persistent amnesic disorder causing severe memory problems
3. Wernicke's encephalopathy (degenerative condition of the brain) causing confusion, ataxia, and abnormal eye movements
4. Hepatitis; cirrhosis of the liver
5. Esophagitis and gastritis
6. Pancreatitis
7. Anemias
8. Immune system dysfunctions
9. Brain damage
10. Peripheral neuropathy
11. Cardiac disorders

IV. ALCOHOL WITHDRAWAL

A. Description
1. Early signs develop within a few hours after cessation of alcohol intake.
2. These signs peak after 24 to 48 hours and then rapidly disappear, unless the withdrawal progresses to alcohol withdrawal delirium.
3. At the onset of withdrawal (Box 65-2), follow agency protocol using specified withdrawal assessment scales as indicated by unit or agency policy.
4. Chlordiazepoxide (Librium) is the most commonly prescribed medication for acute alcohol withdrawal and is usually given orally unless a more immediate onset is required. Any benzodiazepine will decrease the withdrawal symptoms because of cross tolerance (see Chapter 67 for a list of benzodiazepines).
5. An intramuscular injection of vitamin B_1 (thiamine) followed by several days of oral administration is administered to prevent Wernicke-Korsakoff's syndrome.

B. Withdrawal (see Box 65-2)
C. Withdrawal delirium: The state of delirium usually peaks 48 to 72 hours after cessation or reduction of intake (although can occur later) and lasts 2 to 3 days (Box 65-3).

⚠ Withdrawal delirium is a medical emergency. Death can occur from myocardial infarction, fat emboli, peripheral vascular collapse, electrolyte imbalance, aspiration pneumonia, or suicide.

D. Interventions
1. Provide care in a nonjudgmental manner.
2. Check the client frequently.
3. Monitor vital signs and neurological signs (as often as every 15 minutes) and provide one-to-one supervision.
4. Provide a quiet, nonstimulating environment. Encourage family members (one at a time) to stay with the client to minimize anxiety.
5. Orient the client frequently.
6. Explain all treatments and procedures in a quiet and simple manner.

Box 65-2 Early Signs of Alcohol Withdrawal

Anorexia (nausea and vomiting may occur)
Anxiety
Being easily startled
Hyperalertness
Hypertension
Insomnia
Irritability
Jerky movements
Possibly experiences hallucinations, illusions, or vivid nightmares
Possibly reports a feeling of "shaking inside"
Seizures (usually appear 7–48 hours after cessation of alcohol)
Tachycardia
Tremors

Box 65-3 Manifestations of Alcohol Withdrawal Delirium

Agitation
Anorexia
Anxiety
Delirium
Diaphoresis
Disorientation with fluctuating levels of consciousness
Fever (temperature of 100° to 103° F)
Hallucinations and delusions
Insomnia
Tachycardia and hypertension

7. Initiate seizure precautions.
8. Administer sedating or anticonvulsant medication as prescribed.
9. Provide small, frequent, high-carbohydrate foods (administer antiemetic before meals as needed).
10. Monitor intake and output.
11. Administer vitamins (multivitamin, vitamin B complex [including thiamine], and vitamin C).
12. Assist the client with activities of daily living and assist with ambulation if stable.
13. Allow the client to express fears.

E. Disulfiram (Antabuse) therapy
   1. Description
      a. Disulfiram is an alcohol deterrent used for alcoholic dependence.
      b. The medication sensitizes the client to alcohol, so a disulfiram-alcohol reaction occurs if alcohol is ingested.
      c. The client must abstain from alcohol for at least 12 hours before the initial dose is administered.
      d. Adverse effects usually begin within minutes to a half hour after consuming alcohol and may last ½ to 2 hours.
      e. Avoid alcohol consumption for up to 14 days after disulfiram therapy has been discontinued because it places the client at risk for a disulfiram-alcohol reaction.
   2. Adverse reactions
      a. Facial flushing
      b. Sweating
      c. Throbbing headache
      d. Neck pain
      e. Nausea and vomiting
      f. Hypotension
      g. Tachycardia
      h. Respiratory distress
   3. Client education
      a. Educate as to the effects of the medication
      b. Ensure that the client agrees to abstain from alcohol and any substances that contain alcohol.
      c. Instruct the client that the effects of the medication may occur for several days after discontinuance.
      d. Other medications used to assist with cravings include acamprosate calcium (Campral), naltrexone (ReVia), and nalmefene (Revex).

F. Dealing with the client who **abuses** alcohol (Boxes 65-4 and 65-5).

⚠ Instruct the client who is on disulfiram (Antabuse) therapy to avoid the use of substances that contain alcohol, such as cough medicines, rubbing compounds, vinegar, mouthwashes, and aftershave lotions. The client needs to read the labels of all products.

V. DRUG DEPENDENCY

A. Central nervous system (CNS) depressants
   1. CNS depressants can include alcohol, benzodiazepines, and barbiturates, and they act as a depressant, sedative, and/or hypnotic.
   2. Intoxication (Box 65-6)
   3. Overdose can produce cardiovascular or respiratory depression, coma, shock, convulsions, and death.

Box 65-4 Dealing with the Client Who Abuses Alcohol

Direct the client's focus to the substance abuse problem.
Identify with the client those situations that precipitate angry feelings.
Set limits on manipulative behavior and verbal and physical abuse.
Hold the client firmly to reasonable limits, consistently reinforcing rules, with equitable consequences for breaking rules.
Hold the client accountable for all behaviors.
Assist the client to explore strengths and weaknesses.
Encourage focusing on strengths if the client is losing control.
Encourage the client to participate in group therapy and support groups.

Box 65-5 Therapies for Substance Abuse Clients and Their Families

Behavior therapy, aversion conditioning with disulfiram (Antabuse) or another medication
Hospitalization
Psychotherapy (individual, group, family)
Support groups such as Alcoholics Anonymous; Narcotics Anonymous; Pills Anonymous; Al-Anon, Al-a-Teen, or Narc-Anon (for family members and friends of alcoholics or addicts); and Adult Children of Alcoholics
Transitional living programs (halfway houses)

Box 65-6 Intoxication: Central Nervous System Depressants

Drowsiness
Hypotension
Impairment of memory, attention, judgment, and social or occupational functioning
Incoordination and unsteady gait
Irritability
Slurred speech

4. Overdose: If the client is awake, vomiting is induced and activated charcoal is administered. If the client is comatose, airway establishment and maintenance and gastric lavage with activated charcoal are the priorities. Seizure precautions are indicated.
5. Flumazenil (Romazicon) intravenously may be used in benzodiazepine overdose to reverse the effects.
6. Withdrawal effects include nausea, vomiting, tachycardia, diaphoresis, irritability, tremors, insomnia, and seizures. Withdrawal must be treated with a carefully titrated similar drug (abrupt withdrawal can lead to death).
7. Withdrawal from CNS depressants such as barbiturates is generally treated with a barbiturate such as phenobarbital or a long-acting benzodiazepine.

B. CNS stimulants
1. CNS stimulants can include amphetamines, cocaine, and crack.
2. Intoxication (Box 65-7)
3. Overdose can produce respiratory distress, ataxia, hyperpyrexia, seizures, coma, brain attack (stroke), myocardial infarction, and death.
4. Overdose is treated with antipsychotics and management of associated effects.
5. Withdrawal effects include fatigue, depression, agitation, apathy, anxiety, insomnia, disorientation, lethargy, and craving.
6. Withdrawal is treated with antidepressants, a dopamine agonist, or bromocriptine (Parlodel). Withdrawal is primarily supportive, particularly when dealing with the severe depression and suicidal ideation that accompanies stimulant withdrawal.

C. Opioids
1. Opioids can include opium, heroin, meperidine (Demerol), morphine sulfate, codeine sulfate, methadone (Dolophine), hydromorphone (Dilaudid), and fentanyl (Sublimaze).
2. Intoxication (Box 65-8)
3. Overdose can produce respiratory depression, coma, shock, seizures, and death.
4. Overdose is treated with an opioid antagonist such as naloxone (Narcan).

5. Withdrawal effects include yawning, insomnia, irritability, rhinorrhea, diaphoresis, cramps, nausea and vomiting, muscle aches, chills, fever, lacrimation, and diarrhea.
6. Withdrawal may be treated by methadone detoxification or tapering dosage with other opioids.
7. Clonidine (Catapres) as an α-adrenergic blocker assists in reducing the severity of sympathetic nervous system–generated withdrawal discomfort.
8. Specific symptom management measures may also be used (e.g., bismuth subsalicylate [Kaopectate] for diarrhea, acetaminophen [Tylenol] for muscle aches).

D. Hallucinogens
1. Hallucinogens can include lysergic acid diethylamide (LSD), mescaline (peyote), psilocybin (mushrooms), or phencyclidine (PCP).
2. Intoxication (Box 65-9)
3. Overdose effects of LSD, peyote, and psilocybin include psychosis, brain damage, and death. Effects of PCP include psychosis, hypertensive crisis, hyperthermia, seizures, and respiratory arrest.
4. Treatment (LSD, peyote, psilocybin) involves low environmental stimuli (speak slowly, clearly, and in a low voice) and medications to treat anxiety.

Box 65-8 Intoxication: Opioids

Constricted pupils
Decreased respirations
Drowsiness
Euphoria
Hypotension
Impaired memory, attention, and judgment
Psychomotor retardation
Slurred speech

Box 65-7 Intoxication: Central Nervous System Stimulants

Dilated pupils
Euphoria
Hypertension
Impaired judgment and social or occupational functioning
Insomnia
Nausea and vomiting
Paranoia, delusions, or hallucinations
Potential for violence
Tachycardia

Box 65-9 Intoxication: Hallucinogens

Agitation and belligerence
Anxiety and depression
Bizarre, regressive, or violent behavior
Blank stare
Diaphoresis
Dilated pupils
Elevated vital signs including blood pressure
Hallucinations
Impaired judgment and social and occupational functioning
Incoordination
Muscular rigidity and chronic jerking
Paranoia
Seizures
Tachycardia
Tremors

5. Treatment (PCP) involves possible gastric lavage (if alert), acidifying urine to assist in excreting drug, and interventions to treat behavioral disturbances, hyperthermia, hypertension, and respiratory distress.

6. Withdrawal is primarily supportive and may include medications to target particular problem behaviors, such as agitation.

E. Inhalants

1. Inhalants can include gases or liquids such as butane, paint thinner, paint and wax removers, airplane glue, nail polish remover, and nitrous oxide.
2. Intoxication (Box 65-10)
3. Overdose can cause damage to the nervous system and death.
4. Withdrawal management is mainly supportive, including treating affected body systems.

F. Marijuana (*Cannabis sativa*)

1. Marijuana generally is smoked but can be ingested.
2. Marijuana causes euphoria, detachment, relaxation, talkativeness, slowed perception of time, anxiety, or paranoia.
3. Long-term dependence can result in lethargy, difficulty concentrating, memory loss, and possibly chronic respiratory disorders.
4. Withdrawal management is mainly supportive.

G. Other recreational and club drugs

1. Other recreational drugs include ecstasy (methylenedioxymethamphetamine) GHB (gamma-hydroxybutyrate), methamphetamine (crank, meth, and other slang names), and ketamine.
2. Effects include euphoria, increased energy, increased self-confidence, and increased sociability.
3. Adverse effects include hyperthermia, rhabdomyolysis, renal failure, hepatotoxicity, depression, panic attacks, psychosis, cardiovascular collapse, and death.
4. The use of over-the-counter medications containing ephedrine or pseudoephedrine to manufacture illegal supplies of methamphetamine has led many states to adopt laws requiring limited sales and signatures for the purchase of these medications.
5. Programs for **addiction** also address nicotine withdrawal and the pharmacologic and psychotherapeutic interventions for this problem, such as nicotine patches, nicotine inhalers, and bupropion (Zyban) for the reduction of withdrawal and cravings.

6. Anabolic steroids have also gained increased attention as increasing adverse events including death have become more present in the public media.

H. Interventions: Withdrawal

1. Initiate seizure precautions.
2. Hydrate the client.
3. Monitor vital signs every hour.
4. Monitor intake and output.
5. Orient client frequently.
6. Maintain minimal stimuli.
7. Approach the client in an accepting and nonjudgmental manner.
8. Direct the client's focus to the substance **abuse** problem.
9. Assist the client with identifying situations that precipitate angry feelings.
10. Assist the client to deal with emotions.
11. Limit the client's blame-placing or rationalizing to explain the substance **abuse** problem.
12. Assist the client to use assertive techniques rather than manipulation to meet needs.
13. Set limits on manipulative behavior and verbal and physical **abuse**.
14. Maintain firm and reasonable limits, consistently reinforcing rules, with reasonable consequences for breaking rules.
15. Hold the client accountable for all behaviors.
16. Assist the client to explore strengths and weaknesses.
17. Encourage focusing on strengths if the client is losing control.
18. Encourage the client to participate in unit activities.
19. Encourage the client to participate in group therapy and support groups.
20. Box 65-11 delineates nursing care for clients.

Box 65-10 Intoxication: Inhalants

Enhancement of sexual pleasure
Euphoria
Excitation followed by drowsiness, lightheadedness, disinhibition, and agitation
Giggling and laughter

Box 65-11 Withdrawal: Nursing Care

Obtain information regarding the drug type and amount consumed.
Assess vital signs.
Remove unnecessary objects from the environment.
Provide one-to-one supervision if necessary.
Provide a quiet, calm environment with minimal stimuli.
Maintain client orientation.
Ensure the client's safety by implementing seizure precautions.
Use restraints, if necessary and prescribed, to prevent the client from harming self and others.
Provide for physical needs.
Provide food and fluids as tolerated.
Administer medications as prescribed to decrease withdrawal symptoms.
Collect blood and urine samples for drug screening.

I. Dual diagnoses
   1. Sometimes the use of alcohol and drugs masks underlying psychiatric pathology.
   2. Psychiatric pathology may also be precipitated by substance use and **abuse**.
   3. When psychiatric disorders and substance **abuse** are both present, it is often referred to as dual diagnosis.
   4. Separating out psychiatric diagnosis and substance dependence can only be done over time after a sustained period of abstinence.
J. **Addiction** and **abuse** in health care professionals: Suspicious signs
   1. Frequently reporting that drugs have been wasted without being witnessed by another nurse
   2. Administering maximum dosages of controlled substances when other nurses do not
   3. A variance in usual pain relief in the absence of a change in dosage or frequency in their clients
   4. Work patterns include the following: always volunteering to carry opioid (narcotic) drug cabinet or drawer keys, choosing shifts in which less supervision is present, choosing work areas in which the use of controlled substances is high, such as critical care units, operating room, anesthesia, and trauma units.
   5. Nurses have a professional and ethical obligation to report impaired co-workers.
   6. The majority of impaired nurses are able to return to work through the State Board of Nursing assistance and monitoring programs. Such programs usually require strict adherence to clearly stated rules and regular reports and drug screens.
K. Codependency issues
   1. Codependency refers to the presence of coexisting behaviors present in a significant other, which serves to enable the addict or alcoholic to continue the irresponsible patterns of use without experiencing consequences.
   2. Examples of codependency: paying bills the addict or alcoholic is responsible for; bailing the addict or alcoholic out of jail, helping the addict or alcoholic to call in sick
   3. It is important to address codependency issues with the family to maximize the chance for recovery of both the client with the **addiction** and the person with codependent behaviors.

MORE QUESTIONS ON EVOLVE!

Practice Questions

701. A nurse is caring for a female client who was recently admitted to the hospital for anorexia nervosa. The nurse enters the client's room and notes that the client is doing vigorous push-ups. Which nursing action is appropriate?

   1. Interrupt the client and weigh her immediately.
   2. Interrupt the client and offer to take her for a walk.
   3. Allow the client to complete her exercise program.
   4. Tell the client that she is not allowed to exercise vigorously.

702. A nurse is caring for a client with anorexia nervosa. The nurse is monitoring the behavior of the client and understands that the client with anorexia nervosa manages anxiety by:
   1. Engaging in immoral acts
   2. Always reinforcing self-approval
   3. Observing rigid rules and regulations
   4. Having the need to always make the right decision

703. A nursing student is developing a plan of care for the hospitalized client with bulimia nervosa. The nursing instructor intervenes if the student documents which incorrect intervention in the plan?
   1. Monitor intake and output.
   2. Monitor electrolyte levels.
   3. Observe for excessive exercise.
   4. Monitor for the use of laxatives and diuretics.

704. A nurse is monitoring a client who abuses alcohol for signs of alcohol withdrawal delirium. The nurse monitors for which of the following?
   1. Hypotension, ataxia, vomiting
   2. Stupor, agitation, muscular rigidity
   3. Hypotension, bradycardia, agitation
   4. Hypertension, disorientation, hallucinations

705. The spouse of a client admitted to the hospital for alcohol withdrawal says to the nurse, "I should get out of this bad situation." The most helpful response by the nurse would be:
   1. "Why don't you tell your husband about this?"
   2. "This is not the best time to make that decision."
   3. "What do you find difficult about this situation?"
   4. "I agree with you. You should get out of this situation."

706. A nurse is caring for a client who is suspected of being dependent on drugs. Which question would be appropriate for the nurse to ask when collecting data from the client regarding drug abuse?
   1. "Why did you get started on these drugs?"
   2. "How much do you use and what effect does it have on you?"
   3. "How long did you think you could take these drugs without someone finding out?"
   4. The nurse does not ask any questions because of fear that the client is in denial and will throw the nurse out of the room.

707. A client who has been drinking alcohol on a regular basis admits to having "a problem" and is asking for assistance with the problem. The nurse would encourage the client to attend which of the following community groups?
1. Al-Anon
2. Fresh Start
3. Families Anonymous
4. Alcoholics Anonymous

708. A client with a diagnosis of anorexia nervosa, who is in a state of starvation, is in a two-bed hospital room. A newly admitted client will be assigned to this client's room. Which client would be an appropriate choice as this client's roommate?
1. A client with pneumonia
2. A client receiving diagnostic tests
3. A client who thrives on managing others
4. A client who could benefit from the client's assistance at mealtime

709. A nurse is assigned to care for a client at risk for alcohol withdrawal. The nurse monitors the client, knowing that the early signs of withdrawal will usually develop within how much time after cessation or reduction of alcohol intake?
1. In 7 days
2. In 14 days
3. In 21 days
4. Within a few hours

710. A nurse determines that the wife of an alcoholic client is benefiting from attending an Al-Anon group when the nurse hears the wife say:
1. "I no longer feel that I deserve the beatings my husband inflicts on me."
2. "My attendance at the meetings has helped me to see that I provoke my husband's violence."
3. "I enjoy attending the meetings because they get me out of the house and away from my husband."
4. "I can tolerate my husband's destructive behaviors now that I know they are common in alcoholics."

711. A female client with anorexia nervosa is a member of a support group. The client has verbalized that she would like to buy some new clothes but her finances are limited. Group members have brought some used clothes for the client to replace her old clothes. The client believes that the new clothes were much too tight, so she has reduced

her calorie intake to 800 calories daily. The nurse identifies this behavior as:
1. Normal
2. Regression
3. Indicative of the client's ambivalence
4. Evidence of the client's altered and distorted body image

712. A hospitalized client with a history of alcohol abuse tells the nurse, "I am leaving now. I have to go. I don't want any more treatment. I have things that I have to do right away." The client has not been discharged. In fact, the client is scheduled for an important diagnostic test to be performed in 1 hour. After the nurse discusses the client's concerns with the client, the client dresses and begins to walk out of the hospital room. The appropriate nursing action is to:
1. Call the nursing supervisor
2. Call security to block all exit areas
3. Restrain the client until the health care provider (HCP) can be reached
4. Tell the client that she cannot return to this hospital again if she leaves now

713. A nursing student is asked to identify the characteristics of bulimia nervosa. Which response by the student indicates a need to further research the disorder?
1. Dental erosion
2. Electrolyte imbalances
3. Enlarged parotid glands
4. Body weight well below ideal range

714. A nurse is caring for a client who has a history of opioid abuse and is monitoring the client for signs of withdrawal. Which clinical manifestations are specifically associated with withdrawal from opioids?
1. Dilated pupils, tachycardia, and diaphoresis
2. Yawning, irritability, diaphoresis, cramps, and diarrhea
3. Tachycardia, hypertension, sweating, and marked tremors
4. Depressed feelings, high drug craving, fatigue, and agitation

715. Which of the following are appropriate interventions for caring for the client in alcohol withdrawal? **Select all that apply.**
❏ 1. Monitor vital signs.
❏ 2. Maintain an NPO status.
❏ 3. Provide a safe environment.
❏ 4. Address hallucinations therapeutically.
❏ 5. Provide stimulation in the environment.
❏ 6. Provide reality orientation as appropriate.

ANSWERS

701. 2

Rationale: Clients with anorexia nervosa are frequently preoccupied with vigorous exercise and push themselves beyond normal limits to work off caloric intake. The nurse must provide for appropriate exercise as well as place limits on vigorous activities. Options 1, 3, and 4 are inappropriate nursing actions.

Test-Taking Strategy: Use the process of elimination. Recalling that the nurse needs to set firm limits with clients who have this disorder will direct you to option 2. If you had difficulty with this question, review interventions for the client with anorexia nervosa.

Level of Cognitive Ability: Applying
Client Needs: Physiological Integrity
Integrated Process: Nursing Process/Implementation
Content Area: Mental Health
Reference: Stuart, p. 470. 2009.

702. 3

Rationale: Clients with anorexia nervosa have the desire to please others. Their need to be correct or perfect interferes with rational decision-making processes. These clients are moralistic. Rules and rituals help the clients manage their anxiety. Options 1, 2, and 4 are incorrect.

Test-Taking Strategy: Use the process of elimination and focus on the subject—managing anxiety. Eliminate options 2 and 4 because of the closed-ended word "always." Eliminate option 1 because it is not characteristic of the client with anorexia. Review the characteristics associated with this disorder if you had difficulty with this question.

Level of Cognitive Ability: Understanding
Client Needs: Psychosocial Integrity
Integrated Process: Nursing Process/Data Collection
Content Area: Mental Health
References: Stuart, pp. 463, 469–470. 2009.
Varcarolis, Halter, p. 202. 2009.

703. 3

Rationale: Excessive exercise is a characteristic of anorexia nervosa, not bulimia nervosa. Frequent vomiting, in addition to laxative and diuretic abuse, may lead to dehydration and electrolyte imbalance. Monitoring for dehydration and electrolyte imbalance are important nursing actions. Option 3 is the only option that is not associated with care of the client with bulimia.

Test-Taking Strategy: Note the strategic word "incorrect" in the question. This word indicates a negative event query and the need to select the incorrect intervention. Options 1, 2, and 4 are comparable or alike and directly or indirectly infer concern about fluid and electrolyte balance. Option 3 is different from the other options. Review the characteristics associated with bulimia nervosa if you had difficulty with this question.

Level of Cognitive Ability: Analyzing
Client Needs: Physiological Integrity
Integrated Process: Nursing Process/Planning
Content Area: Mental Health
References: Christensen, Kockrow, p. 1148. 2011. *Foundations of nursing.*
Morrison-Valfre, pp. 153, 250–251. 2009.

704. 4

Rationale: The symptoms associated with alcohol withdrawal delirium typically are anxiety, insomnia, anorexia, hypertension, disorientation, visual or tactile hallucinations, agitation, fever, and delusions.

Test-Taking Strategy: Use the process of elimination. Review each option carefully to ensure that all the symptoms are contained in the correct option. Eliminate options 1 and 3 first, knowing that hypertension rather than hypotension occurs. From the remaining options, recalling that the client who is stuporous is not likely to exhibit agitation will direct you to option 4. Review the symptoms associated with alcohol withdrawal if you had difficulty with this question.

Level of Cognitive Ability: Analyzing
Client Needs: Physiological Integrity
Integrated Process: Nursing Process/Data Collection
Content Area: Mental Health
Reference: Stuart, pp. 434–435. 2009.

705. 3

Rationale: The most helpful response is the one that encourages the client to problem solve. Giving advice implies that the nurse knows what is best and can also foster dependency. The nurse should not agree with the client nor should the nurse request that the client provide explanations.

Test-Taking Strategy: Use therapeutic communication techniques. Eliminate option 1 because of the word "why," which should be avoided in communication. Eliminate option 4 because the nurse is agreeing with the client. Eliminate option 2 because this option places the client's feelings on hold. Option 3 is the only option that addresses the client's feelings. Review therapeutic communication techniques if you had difficulty with this question.

Level of Cognitive Ability: Applying
Client Needs: Psychosocial Integrity
Integrated Process: Communication and Documentation
Content Area: Mental Health
References: Morrison-Valfre, pp. 104–105. 2009.
Stuart, pp. 435–436. 2009.

706. 2

Rationale: Whenever the nurse collects data from a client who is dependent on drugs, it is best for the nurse to attempt to elicit information by being nonjudgmental and direct. Option 1 is incorrect because it is judgmental, off focus, and reflects the nurse's bias. Option 3 is incorrect because it is judgmental, insensitive, and aggressive, which is nontherapeutic. Option 4 is incorrect because it indicates passivity on the nurse's part and uses rationalization to avoid the therapeutic nursing intervention.

Test-Taking Strategy: Use the process of elimination and therapeutic communication techniques to answer the question. Option 2 is the statement that is nonjudgmental and direct. Review data collection of a client who is a drug abuser if you had difficulty with this question.

Level of Cognitive Ability: Applying
Client Needs: Psychosocial Integrity
Integrated Process: Nursing Process/Data Collection
Content Area: Mental Health
Reference: Morrison-Valfre, p. 318. 2009.

707. 4

Rationale: Alcoholics Anonymous is a major self-help organization for the treatment of alcoholism. Option 1 is a group for families of alcoholics. Option 3 is for parents of children who abuse substances. Option 2 is for nicotine addicts.

Test-Taking Strategy: Use the process of elimination. If you are unfamiliar with these support groups, note the relation between "drinking" in the question and "Alcoholics" in the correct option. Familiarize yourself with the purposes of specific support groups if you had difficulty with this question.

Level of Cognitive Ability: Applying
Client Needs: Safe and Effective Care Environment
Integrated Process: Nursing Process/Implementation
Content Area: Mental Health
Reference: Morrison-Valfre, p. 316. 2009.

708. 2

Rationale: The client receiving diagnostic tests is an appropriate roommate. The client with anorexia is most likely experiencing hematological complications, such as leukopenia. Having a roommate with pneumonia would place the client with anorexia nervosa at risk for infection. The client with anorexia nervosa should not be put in a situation in which he or she can focus on the nutritional needs of others or be managed by others, because this may contribute to sublimation and suppression of his or her own hunger.

Test-Taking Strategy: Use the process of elimination and note the strategic words "in a state of starvation." Recalling the characteristics and complications associated with anorexia nervosa will direct you to othe correct option. Review care of the client with anorexia nervosa if you have difficulty with this question.

Level of Cognitive Ability: Analyzing
Client Needs: Safe and Effective Care Environment
Integrated Process: Nursing Process/Planning
Content Area: Mental Health
Reference: Stuart, pp. 461–462. 2009.

709. 4

Rationale: Early signs of alcohol withdrawal develop within a few hours after cessation or reduction of alcohol and peak after 24 to 48 hours.

Test-Taking Strategy: Use the process of elimination and note the strategic words "early" and "usually develop." This will assist in directing you to option 4. If you are unfamiliar with the manifestations associated with alcohol withdrawal, review this content.

Level of Cognitive Ability: Understanding
Client Needs: Physiological Integrity
Integrated Process: Nursing Process/Data Collection
Content Area: Mental Health
Reference: Stuart, pp. 434–435. 2009.
Varcarolis, Halter, p. 342. 2009.

710. 1

Rationale: Al-Anon support groups are a protected, supportive opportunity for spouses and significant others to learn what to expect and to obtain suggestions about successful behavioral changes. Option 1 is the healthiest response, because it exemplifies an understanding that the alcoholic partner is responsible for his behavior and cannot be allowed to blame family members for loss of control. The nonalcoholic partner should

not feel responsible when the spouse loses control (option 2). Option 4 indicates that the wife remains codependent. Option 3 indicates that the group is being seen as an escape, not a place to work on issues.

Test-Taking Strategy: Use the process of elimination and focus on the subject of the question—benefiting from attending an Al-Anon group. This will direct you to the correct option. Review the purpose of this type of support group if you had difficulty with this question.

Level of Cognitive Ability: Evaluating
Client Needs: Psychosocial Integrity
Integrated Process: Nursing Process/Evaluation
Content Area: Mental Health
Reference: Varcarolis, Halter, p. 353. 2009.

711. 4

Rationale: Altered or distorted body image is a concern with clients with anorexia nervosa. Although the client may struggle with ambivalence and present with regressed behavior, the client's coping pattern relates to the basic issue of distorted body image. The client's behavior is not normal.

Test-Taking Strategy: Use the process of elimination. Focus on the information provided in the question to determine that the subject relates to a distorted body image. This will direct you to the correct option. If you had difficulty with this question, review the characteristics associated with the client with anorexia nervosa.

Level of Cognitive Ability: Understanding
Client Needs: Psychosocial Integrity
Integrated Process: Nursing Process/Data Collection
Content Area: Mental Health
Reference: Stuart, p. 472. 2009.

712. 1

Rationale: A nurse can be charged with false imprisonment if a client is made to wrongfully believe that he or she cannot leave the hospital. Most health care facilities have documents that the client is asked to sign, which relate to the client's responsibilities when he or she leaves against medical advice (AMA). The client should be asked to sign this document before leaving. The nurse should request that the client wait to speak to the HCP before leaving, but, if the client refuses to do so, the nurse cannot hold the client against his or her will. Restraining the client and calling security to block exits constitutes false imprisonment. Any client has a right to health care (option 4) and cannot be told otherwise.

Test-Taking Strategy: Use the process of elimination. Keeping the concept of false imprisonment in mind, eliminate options 2 and 3 because they are comparable or alike. Eliminate option 4, knowing that any client has a right to health care. Review the points related to false imprisonment if you had difficulty with this question.

Level of Cognitive Ability: Applying
Client Needs: Safe and Effective Care Environment
Integrated Process: Nursing Process/Implementation
Content Area: Mental Health
Reference: Varcarolis, Halter, p. 528. 2009.

713. 4

Rationale: Clients with bulimia nervosa may not initially appear to be physically or emotionally ill. They are often at or slightly below ideal body weight. On further inspection, the client demonstrates enlargement of the parotid glands with dental erosion and caries if he or she has been inducing vomiting. Electrolyte imbalances are present.

Test-Taking Strategy: Use the process of elimination and note the strategic words "need to further research." Focusing on the client's diagnosis will direct you to option 4. Option 4 is a characteristic sign of anorexia nervosa, not bulimia nervosa. Review the characteristics of these disorders if you had difficulty with this question.

Level of Cognitive Ability: Evaluating
Client Needs: Physiological Integrity
Integrated Process: Teaching and Learning
Content Area: Mental Health
Reference: Stuart, p. 459. 2009.

714. 2

Rationale: Opioids are central nervous system (CNS) depressants. Withdrawal effects include yawning, insomnia, irritability, rhinorrhea, diaphoresis, cramps, nausea and vomiting, muscle aches, chills, fever, lacrimation, and diarrhea. Withdrawal is treated by methadone tapering or medication detoxification. Option 2 identifies the clinical manifestations associated with withdrawal from opioids. Option 3 describes withdrawal from alcohol. Option 1 describes intoxication from hallucinogens. Option 4 describes withdrawal from cocaine.

Test-Taking Strategy: Focus on the subject of the question—the clinical manifestations associated with withdrawal from opioids. Recalling that opioids are CNS depressants will direct

you to option 2. If you had difficulty with this question, review the manifestations associated with opioid withdrawal.

Level of Cognitive Ability: Analyzing
Client Needs: Physiological Integrity
Integrated Process: Nursing Process/Data Collection
Content Area: Mental Health
Reference: Stuart, pp. 434–435. 2009.

715. 1, 3, 4, 6   ❖

Rationale: When the client is experiencing withdrawal from alcohol, the priority for care is to prevent the client from harming himself or herself or others. The nurse would provide a low stimulating environment to maintain the client in as calm a state as possible. The nurse would monitor the vital signs closely and report abnormal findings. The nurse would frequently reorient the client to reality and would address hallucinations therapeutically. Adequate nutritional and fluid intake needs to be maintained.

Test-Taking Strategy: Use therapeutic communication techniques to assist in selecting the correct interventions. Also, recalling the characteristics associated with alcohol withdrawal will assist in answering correctly. Review these interventions if you had difficulty with this question.

Level of Cognitive Ability: Applying
Client Needs: Psychosocial Integrity
Integrated Process: Nursing Process/Implementation
Content Area: Mental Health
Reference: Stuart, pp. 434–435. 2009.

Crisis Theory and Intervention

66

I. CRISIS INTERVENTION

A. Description
1. **Crisis** is a temporary state of severe emotional disorganization caused by failure of **coping mechanisms** and lack of support.
2. Decision making and problem solving are inadequate.
3. Treatment is aimed at assisting the client and the family through the stressful situation.

B. Phases of a **crisis**
1. Phase 1: external precipitating event
2. Phase 2
   a. Perception of the threat
   b. Increase in anxiety
   c. Client may cope or resolve the **crisis**.
3. Phase 3
   a. Failure of coping
   b. Increasing disorganization
   c. Emergence of physical symptoms
   d. Relationship problems
4. Phase 4
   a. Mobilization of internal and external resources
   b. Goal is to return the individual to at least a pre-crisis level of functioning

C. Types of crises (Box 66-1)

D. **Crisis** intervention
1. Treatment is immediate, supportive, and directly responsive to the immediate **crisis**.
2. Interventions are goal directed.
3. Feelings of the client are acknowledged.
4. Intervention provides opportunities for expression and validation of feelings.
5. Connections are made between the meaning of the event and the **crisis**.
6. Client explores alternative **coping mechanisms** and tries out new behaviors.

II. GRIEF

A. Grief is a natural emotional response to loss that individuals must experience as they attempt to accept the loss.

B. Grief usually involves moving through a series of stages or tasks to help resolve the grief (Box 66-2).

C. Feelings associated with grief can include anger, frustration, loneliness, sadness, guilt, regret, or peace.

D. Healing can occur when the pain of the loss has lessened and the survivor has adapted to life without the deceased. The survivor will continue to experience memories of the deceased.

E. Types of grief
1. Normal grief: Physical, emotional, cognitive, or behavioral reactions can occur. The process of resolution can take months to years.
2. Anticipatory grief occurs before the loss and is associated with an acute, chronic, or terminal illness.
3. Disenfranchised grief occurs when a loss is experienced and cannot be acknowledged openly. (Societal norms do not define the loss as a loss within its traditional definition.)
4. Dysfunctional grief occurs with prolonged emotional instability and a lack of progression to successful coping with the loss.
5. Children's grief is based on their developmental level (Box 66-3).

III. LOSS

A. Loss is the absence of something desired or previously thought to be available.

B. Actual loss can be identified by others and can arise in response to or in anticipation of a situation.

C. Perceived loss is experienced by one person and cannot be verified by others.

D. Anticipatory loss is experienced before the loss occurs.

E. Mourning
1. The outward and social expression of loss.
2. May be dictated by cultural and religious beliefs

F. Bereavement
1. Includes the inner feelings and the outward reactions of the survivor.
2. Includes grief and mourning.

IV. NURSE'S ROLE: GRIEF AND LOSS (Box 66-4)

A. Allow ongoing opportunities for fully informed choices.

Box 66-1 Types of Crises

Maturational Crisis

Relates to developmental stages and associated role changes; examples include marriage, birth of a child, and retirement

Situational Crisis

Arises from an external source, is often unanticipated, and is associated with a life event that upsets an individual or a group's psychological equilibrium; examples include loss of a job or a change in job, a change in financial status, death of a loved one, divorce, abortion, and severe physical or mental illness

Adventitious Crisis

Relates to a crisis of disaster or an event that is not a part of everyday life and is unplanned and accidental. This type of crisis may result from a natural disaster such as a flood, earthquake, hurricane, fire, or tornado; a national disaster such as war, riots, acts of terrorism; or a crime of violence such as rape, assault, murder, spousal or child abuse.

Box 66-2 The Grief Response

Stage 1: Shock and Disbelief

The survivor may have feelings of numbness, difficulties with decision making, emotional outbursts, denial, and isolation.

Stage 2: Experiencing the Loss

The survivor may feel angry at the loved one who died or may feel guilt about the death.

Bargaining and/or depression may also occur in this stage.

Stage 3: Reintegration

The survivor begins to reorganize his or her life and accepts the reality of the loss.

B. Facilitate the grief process. Assess grief and assist the survivor to feel the loss and complete the tasks of the grief process.

C. Grief affects survivors physically, psychologically, socially, and spiritually; therefore, a multidisciplinary team approach including a bereavement specialist facilitates the grief process.

⚠ The nurse's role in the grief and loss process includes communicating with the client, family members, and significant other. The nurse must consider the survivor's culture, religion, family structure, individual life experiences, coping skills, and support systems.

V. END OF LIFE

A. Description: End of life refers to issues related to death and dying.

B. Cultural and religious issues (see Chapter 6 and Box 6-4 for information regarding cultural and religious issues)

Box 66-3 Children's Grief

Birth to 1 Year

The infant has no concept of death.

The infant reacts to the loss of mother or caregiver.

1 to 2 Years

The child may see death as reversible.

The grief response occurs only to the death of the significant person in the child's life.

The child may scream, withdraw, or become disinterested in the environment.

2 to 5 Years

The child may see death as reversible.

The child has a sense of loss and is concerned about who will provide care.

Regression or aggressive behavior may occur.

5 to 9 Years

The child begins to see death as permanent.

The child may feel responsible for the occurrence.

The child has difficulty concentrating.

Preadolescent Through Adolescence

The adolescent sees death as permanent.

The adolescent experiences a strong emotional reaction.

The adolescent may regress.

Box 66-4 Communication Process

Determine how much the client and family want to know.

Determine whether there is a spokesperson for the family.

Be aware of cultural and religious beliefs and how they may affect the communication process. Consider personal space issues, eye contact, and touch.

Obtain an interpreter if necessary.

Allow opportunity for informed choices.

Assist with the decision-making process if asked. Use problem solving to assist in decision-making, and avoid interjecting personal views or opinions.

Encourage expression of feelings, concerns, and fears.

Be honest and truthful, and let the client and family know that you will not abandon them.

Ask the client and family about their expectations and needs.

Be a sensitive listener. Sit in silence if necessary and appropriate.

Extend touch and hold the client's or family member's hand if appropriate.

Encourage reminiscing.

If you do not know what to do in a particular situation, seek assistance.

If you do not know what to say to a client or family who is talking about death, listen attentively and use therapeutic communication techniques such as open-ended questions or reflection.

Acknowledge your own feelings. Let the client and family know that the topic of conversation is a difficult one and that you do not know what to say.

Realize that it is acceptable to cry with the client and family during the grief process.

C. Legal and ethical issues
1. Outcomes related to care during illness and the dying experience should be based on the client's wishes.
2. Issues for consideration may include organ and tissue donations, advance directives or other legal documents, withholding or withdrawing treatment, and cardiopulmonary resuscitation.

D. Palliative care
1. Palliative care focuses on caring interventions and symptom management rather than cure for diseases that no longer respond to treatment.
2. A pain- and symptom-controlled environment is established. (The dying client should be as pain free and as comfortable as possible.)
3. Hospice care provides support and care for clients in the last phases of incurable diseases so that they might live as fully and as comfortably as possible. The client and family needs are the focus of any intervention.

E. Near-death physiological manifestations
1. As death approaches, metabolism is reduced and the body gradually slows down until all function ends.
2. Sensory: The client experiences blurred vision, decreased sense of taste and smell, decreased pain and touch perception, and loss of blink reflex. The client also appears to stare. (Hearing is believed to be the last sense lost.)
3. Respirations
   a. Respirations may be rapid, slow, shallow, and irregular.
   b. Respirations may be noisy and wet sounding (death rattle).
   c. Cheyne-Stokes respiration is alternating periods of apnea and deep, rapid breathing.
4. Circulation
   a. Heart rate slows, and blood pressure falls progressively.
   b. Skin is cool to touch, and the extremities become pale, mottled, and cyanotic.
   c. Skin is wax-like very near death.
5. Urinary output gradually decreases. Incontinence may occur.
6. Gastrointestinal motility and peristalsis diminish, leading to constipation, gas accumulation, and distention. A bowel movement may occur before death or at the time of death.
7. Musculoskeletal system: The client gradually loses ability to move, has difficulty speaking and swallowing, and loses the gag reflex.

F. Death
1. Death occurs when all vital organs and body systems cease to function.
2. Generally respirations cease first, and then the heart beat stops a few minutes thereafter.

G. Brain death occurs when the cerebral cortex stops functioning or is irreversibly damaged.

H. Nursing care
1. Frequency of assessment depends on the client's stability (at least every 8 hours). As changes occur, assessment needs to be done more frequently.
2. Physical care (Box 66-5)

⚠ Avoid repeated, unnecessary assessments on a dying client. Assessment should be limited to obtaining essential data.

Box 66-5 Physical Care to the Dying Client

Pain
Administer pain medication.
Do not delay or deny pain medication.

Dyspnea
Elevate the head of the bed or position on the side.
Administer supplemental oxygen.
Suction fluids from the airway as needed.

Skin
Assess color and temperature.
Assess for breakdown.
Implement measures to prevent breakdown.

Dehydration
Maintain regular oral care.
Encourage taking ice chips and sips of fluid.
Do not force the client to eat or drink.
Use moist cloths to provide moisture to the mouth.
Apply lubricant to the lips and oral mucous membranes.

Anorexia, Nausea, and Vomiting
Provide antiemetics before meals.
Have family members provide the client's favorite foods.
Provide frequent small portions of favorite foods.

Elimination
Monitor urinary and bowel elimination.
Place absorbent pads under the client and check frequently.

Weakness and Fatigue
Provide rest periods.
Assess tolerance for activities.
Provide assistance and support as needed for maintaining bed or chair positions.

Restlessness
Maintain a calm soothing environment.
Do not restrain.
Limit the number of visitors at the client's bedside.
Allow a family member to stay with the client.

3. Psychosocial care
   a. Monitor for anxiety and depression.
   b. Monitor for fear (Box 66-6).
   c. Encourage the client and family to express feelings.
   d. Provide support and advocacy for the client and family.
   e. Provide privacy for the client and family.
   f. Provide a private room for the client.
4. Postmortem care (Box 66-7)
   a. Maintain respect and dignity for the client.
   b. Determine whether the client is an organ donor. If so, follow appropriate procedures related to the donation.
   c. Consider cultural rituals, state laws, and agency procedures when performing postmortem care.
   d. Prepare the body for immediate viewing by the family.
   e. Provide privacy and time for the family to be with the deceased person.

VI. DEPRESSION

A. Description (refer to Chapter 64)
   1. Depression affects feelings, thoughts, and behaviors.

Box 66-6 Fear Associated with Dying

Fear of Pain
Fear of pain may occur based on anxieties related to dying.
Do not delay or deny pain relief measures to a terminally ill client.

Fear of Loneliness and Abandonment
Allow family members to stay with the client.
Holding hands and touching (if culturally acceptable) and listening to the client are important.

Fear of Being Meaningless
Client may feel hopeless and powerless.
Encourage life reviews and focus on the positive aspects of the client's life.

Adapted from Lewis, S., Heitkemper, M., & Dirksen, S. (2011). Medical-surgical nursing: Assessment and management of clinical problems (8th ed.). St. Louis: Mosby.

Box 66-7 General Postmortem Procedures

Close the client's eyes.
Replace dentures.
Wash the body.
Place pads under the perineum.
Remove tubes and dressings.
Straighten the body and place a pillow under the head in preparation for family viewing.

---

2. It can occur after a loss, including loss of self-esteem, the end of a significant relationship, the death of a loved one, or a traumatic event.
3. The loss is followed by grief and mourning. If this process does not resolve, depression results.
4. Depression may be mild, moderate, or severe.
5. Treatment includes counseling, antidepressant medication, alternative medications, light therapy, and electroconvulsive therapy (ECT).

B. Mild depression
   1. Triggered by an external event, and the experience follows the normal grief reaction.
   2. Lasts less than 2 weeks
   3. Feeling sad
   4. Feeling let down or disappointed
   5. Mild alterations in sleep patterns
   6. Feeling less alert
   7. Irritability
   8. Disinterested in spending time with others
   9. Increased use of alcohol or drugs

C. Moderate depression
   1. Persists over time
   2. The person experiences a sense of change and often seeks help.
   3. Despondent and gloomy
   4. Dejected
   5. Low self-esteem
   6. Helplessness and powerlessness
   7. May experience intense anxiety and anger
   8. Diurnal variation: The person may feel better at a certain time of the day, such as in the morning.
   9. Slow thought processes and difficulty in concentrating
   10. Rumination: Persistent thinking about and discussion of a particular subject
   11. Negative thinking and suicidal thoughts
   12. Sleep disturbances
   13. Social withdrawal
   14. Anorexia, weight loss, and fatigue
   15. Somatic complaints
   16. Menstrual changes
   17. Increased use of alcohol or drugs

D. Severe depression
   1. Intense and pervasive
   2. Despair and hopelessness
   3. Guilt and worthlessness
   4. Flat affect
   5. May show agitation and pace about
   6. Poor posture and unkempt appearance
   7. Decreased speech
   8. Self-destructive thoughts (suicidal ideations); however, the client may lack energy to act on the thought
   9. Social withdrawal
   10. Poor concentration and overwhelmed by simple tasks
   11. Severe psychomotor retardation

12. Anorexia and considerable weight loss
13. Constipation and urinary retention
14. Lack of sexual interest
15. Terminal insomnia
16. Diurnal variation: The person feels worse in the morning and better as the day goes on.
17. Delusions and hallucinations

E. Interventions
1. Altered thought processes
   a. Encourage the client to discuss losses or changes in the life situation.
   b. Encourage the client to express sadness or anger and allow adequate time for verbal responses.
   c. Assist the client in developing short-term goals.
   d. Encourage the use of problem solving and positive thinking.
   e. Limit decision making.
   f. Spend short periods throughout the day with the client.
   g. Be on time when a schedule is planned with the client.
   h. Sit in silence with the client who is not verbalizing.
   i. Use simple, concrete words when communicating.
   j. Avoid a cheerful attitude.
2. Risk for self-harm
   a. Assess for **suicide** clues and intervene to provide safety precautions as necessary.
   b. Ask the client directly, "Have you thought of hurting yourself?"
   c. Assess lethality of plans.
   d. Do not leave the client alone for extended periods.
   e. If the client has a suicidal plan, place on a one-to-one supervision.
   f. Form a suicidal contract with the client.

⚠ For a client at risk for self-harm, ask the client directly, "Have you thought of hurting yourself?"

3. Activity intolerance
   a. Encourage daily exercise.
   b. Assist with activities of daily living if the client is unable to perform them.
   c. Begin with one-to-one activities.
   d. Provide activities for easy mastery to increase self-esteem and assist to alleviate guilt feelings.
   e. Provide activities that do not require a great deal of concentration (simple card games, drawing).
   f. Engage in gross motor activities (walking).
   g. Eventually bring the client into small group activities and then large groups.

4. Altered nutrition
   a. Ensure adequate nutrition.
   b. Offer small, high-calorie, high-protein snacks, and fluids throughout the day.
   c. Stay with the client during meals.
   d. Weigh the client weekly.
   e. Assess bowel patterns for constipation.
5. Sleep pattern disturbance
   a. Ensure adequate sleep.
   b. Provide rest periods after activities.
   c. Encourage the client to dress and stay out of bed during the day.
   d. Provide relaxation measures at bedtime.
   e. Decrease environmental stimuli at bedtime.
   f. Spend time with the client before bedtime.

VII. ELECTROCONVULSIVE THERAPY (ECT)

A. Description
1. An effective treatment for depression that consists of inducing a grand mal (tonic-clonic) seizure by passing an electrical current through electrodes that are attached to the temples.
2. The administration of a muscle relaxant minimizes seizure activity, preventing damage to long bones and cervical vertebrae.
3. The usual course is 6 to 12 treatments given two to three times per week.
4. Maintenance ECT once a month may help to decrease the relapse rate for the client with recurrent depression.
5. ECT is not a permanent cure.
6. Not necessarily effective in the client with dysthymic depression or the client with depression and personality disorders, those with drug dependence, or those with depression as a result of situational or social difficulties.
7. At-risk clients include those with recent myocardial infarction, brain attack (stroke) or cerebral vascular malformation, or clients with intracranial mass lesions.

B. Uses
1. Clients with major depressive and bipolar-depressive disorders, especially when psychotic symptoms are present, such as delusions of guilt, somatic delusions, and delusions of infidelity
2. Clients who have depression with marked psychomotor retardation and stupor
3. Manic clients whose conditions are resistant to lithium and antipsychotic medications and in clients who are rapid cyclers. (A client with a bipolar disorder who has many episodes of mood swings close together.)
4. Clients with schizophrenia (especially catatonia), those with schizoaffective syndromes, and psychotic clients

Box 66-8 Electroconvulsive Therapy (ECT): Indications for Use

When antidepressant medications have no effect
When there is a need for a rapid definitive response such as when a client is suicidal or homicidal
The client is in extreme agitation or stupor.
The risks of other treatments outweigh the risk of ECT
The client has a history of poor medication response, a history of good ECT response, or both.
The client prefers ECT as a treatment.

 C. Indications for use (Box 66-8)

 D. Preprocedure
1. Explain the procedure to the client.
2. Encourage the client to discuss feelings, including myths regarding ECT.
3. Teach the client and family what to expect.
4. Informed consent must be obtained when voluntary clients are being treated.
5. For involuntary clients, when informed consent cannot be obtained, permission may be obtained from the next of kin, although in some states the permission for ECT must be obtained from the court.
6. NPO after midnight or at least 4 hours before treatment.
7. Take baseline vital signs.
8. Ask the client to void.
9. Remove hairpins, contact lenses, and dentures.
10. Administer preoperative medication if prescribed. Glycopyrrolate (Robinul) or atropine sulfate may be prescribed to prevent the potential for aspiration and minimize bradydysrhythmia in response to electrical stimulus.

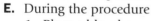 **E.** During the procedure
1. Place a blood pressure cuff on one of the client's arms.
2. An IV line is inserted and EEG and ECG electrodes are attached.
3. A pulse oximeter is placed onto the client's finger.
4. Blood pressure is monitored throughout the treatment.
5. Medications administered may include a short-acting anesthetic such as methohexital sodium (Brevital Sodium), thiopental sodium (Pentothal), and a muscle relaxant such as succinylcholine (Anectine).
6. 100% oxygen by mask via positive pressure is administered throughout the procedure.
7. An airway or bite block is placed to prevent biting the tongue.
8. Electrical stimulus is administered and the seizure should last 30 to 60 seconds.

 F. Postprocedure
1. The client will be transported to a recovery room with the blood pressure cuff and oximeter in place, where oxygen, suction, and other emergency equipment is available.
2. Once the client is awake, talk to the client and take vital signs.
3. The client may be confused. Provide frequent orientation (brief, distinct, and simple) and reassurance.
4. The client returns to the nursing unit when at least a 90% oxygen saturation level is maintained, vital signs are stable, and mental status is satisfactory.
5. Assess the gag reflex before giving the client fluids, food, or medication.

G. Potential side effects
1. Major side effects include confusion, disorientation, and short-term memory loss.
2. The client may be confused and disoriented upon awakening.
3. Memory deficits may occur, but memory usually recovers completely, although some clients have memory loss lasting up to 6 months.

VIII. SUICIDAL BEHAVIOR

A. Description
1. Suicidal clients characteristically have feelings of worthlessness, guilt, and hopelessness that are so overwhelming that they feel unable to go on with life and feel unfit to live.
2. The nurse caring for a depressed client always considers the possibility of **suicide**.

B. High-risk groups
1. Those with a history of previous **suicide attempts**
2. Family history of **suicide attempts**
3. Adolescents
4. Older clients
5. Disabled or terminally ill adults
6. Clients with personality disorders
7. Clients with organic brain syndrome or dementia
8. Depressed or psychotic clients
9. Substance abusers

C. Clues (Box 66-9)

D. Data collection (Box 66-10)

E. Interventions
1. Initiate **suicide** precautions.
2. Remove harmful objects.
3. Do not leave the client alone.
4. Provide a nonjudgmental, caring attitude.
5. Develop a contract that is written, dated, and signed and that indicates alternative behavior at times of suicidal thoughts.
6. Encourage the client to talk about feelings and identify positive aspects about self.
7. Encourage active participation in own care.
8. Keep the client active by assigning achievable tasks.
9. Check that visitors do not leave harmful objects in the client's room.

10. Identify support systems.
11. Do not allow the client to leave the unit unless accompanied by a staff member.
12. Continue to assess the client's **suicide** potential.

⚠ Provide one-to-one supervision at all times for the client at risk for suicide.

IX. ABUSIVE BEHAVIORS

A. Anger
  1. A feeling of annoyance that may be displaced onto an object or person.
  2. Used to avoid anxiety and gives a feeling of power in situations in which the person feels out of control.

Box 66-9 Suicidal Clues

Giving away personal, special, and prized possessions
Canceling social engagements
Making out or changing a will
Taking out or changing insurance policies
Positive or negative changes in behavior
Poor appetite
Sleeping difficulties
Feelings of hopelessness
Difficulty in concentrating
Loss of interest in activities
Client statements that indicate intent to attempt suicide
Sudden calmness or improvement in a depressed client
Client questions about poisons, guns, or other lethal objects

---

Box 66-10 Suicidal Client: Data Collection

The Plan
Does the client have a plan?
What is the plan, how lethal is the plan, and how likely is death to occur?
Does the client have the means to carry out the plan?

Client History of Attempts
What suicide attempts occurred in the past and what were the outcomes (i.e., physiological injuries)?
Was the client accidentally rescued?
Have the past attempts and methods been the same, or have methods increased in lethality?

Psychosocial
Is the client alone or alienated from others?
Is hostility or depression present?
Do hallucinations exist?
Is substance abuse present?
Has the client had any recent losses or physical illness?
Has the client had any environmental or lifestyle changes?

B. Aggression can be harmful and destructive when not controlled.
C. Violence is the physical force that is threatening to the safety of self and others.
D. Data collection
  1. History of violence or self-harm
  2. Poor impulse control and low tolerance of frustration
  3. Defiance and argumentativeness
  4. Raising of voice
  5. Making verbal threats
  6. Pacing and agitation
  7. Muscle rigidity
  8. Flushed face
  9. Glaring at others
E. Interventions
  1. Maintain safety.
  2. Use a calm approach and communicate with a calm, clear tone of voice. (Be assertive but not aggressive, and avoid verbal struggles.)
  3. Maintain a large personal space and use a nonaggressive posture.
  4. Listen actively and acknowledge the client's anger.
  5. Determine what the client considers to be his or her need.
  6. Provide the client with clear options that deal with the client's behavior, set limits on behavior, and make the client aware of the consequences of anger and violence.
  7. Discuss the use of **restraints** or **seclusion** if the client is unable to control angry behavior that may lead to violence.
  8. Assist the client with problem solving and decision making regarding the options.
F. **Restraints and seclusion**
  1. Description
     a. Physical **restraints**: Any manual method or mechanical device, material, or equipment that inhibits free movement
     b. **Seclusion**: A process in which a client is placed alone in a specially designed room for protection and close supervision
     c. Chemical **restraints**: Medications given for a specific purpose of inhibiting a specific behavior or movement and that have an impact on the client's ability to relate to the environment
  2. Use of **restraints** and **seclusion**

⚠ Restraints require a written prescription by the health care provider, which must be reviewed and renewed every 24 hours. The prescription must specify the type of restraint or seclusion, and the criteria for release. (Agency policy and procedures must be followed.)

     a. **Restraints** and **seclusion** should never be used as punishment or for the convenience of the health care staff.

b. **Restraints** and **seclusion** are used when behavior is physically harmful to the client or others and when alternative or less restrictive measures are insufficient in protecting the client or others from harm.

c. The nurse must document the behavior leading to the use of **restraints** or **seclusion**.

d. **Restraints** and **seclusion** are used when the client anticipates that a controlled environment would be helpful and requests **seclusion**.

e. In an emergency, the qualified nurse may place a client in **restraints** or **seclusion** and obtain a written or verbal prescription as soon as possible thereafter.

f. Within 1 hour of the initiation of **restraints** or **seclusion**, the psychiatrist must make a face-to-face assessment and evaluation of the client and must continuously reevaluate the need for continued restraint or **seclusion**.

g. While in **restraints** or **seclusion**, the client must be protected from all sources of harm by having one-to-one supervision with a staff member within an arm's length of the client.

h. The client in **restraints** or **seclusion** needs constant one-to-one supervision. Physical, safety, and comfort needs must be assessed every 15 to 30 minutes, and these observations are also documented (such as food, fluids, bathroom needs, range-of-motion exercise, and ambulation).

X. FAMILY VIOLENCE

A. Description (Figure 66-1)
 1. The violence begins with threats or verbal or physical minor assaults (tension building), and the victim attempts to comply with the requests of the abuser.
 2. The abuser loses control and becomes destructive and harmful (acute battering) while the victim attempts to protect himself or herself.
 3. After the battering, the abuser then becomes loving and attempts to make peace (calmness and a diffusion of tension).
 4. The abuser justifies that violence is normal and the victim is responsible for the **abuse**.
 5. Outsiders are usually not aware of what is happening in the family.
 6. Family members are isolated socially and lack autonomy and trust among each other. Caring and intimacy in the family are absent.
 7. Family members expect other members of the family to meet their needs, but none are able to do so.
 8. The abuser threatens to abandon the family.

B. Types of violence (Box 66-11)

C. The vulnerable person
 1. The vulnerable person is the one in the family unit against whom violence is perpetrated.
 2. Those most vulnerable are children and older adults.
 3. The perpetrator of violence and the person targeted by the violence can be male or female.
 4. Battering is a crime.

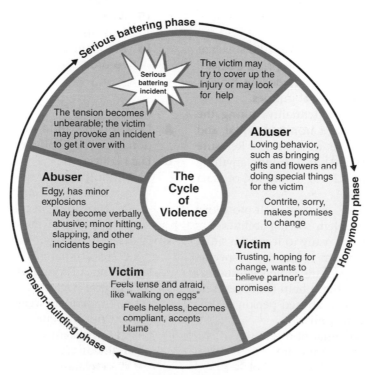

▲ **FIGURE 66-1** The cycle of violence. (Redrawn from YWCA of Annapolis and Anne Arundel County, 1517 Ritchie Highway, Arnold, MD 21012.)

Box 66-11 Types of Violence

Physical violence: Infliction of physical pain or bodily harm
Sexual violence: Any form of sexual contact without consent
Emotional violence: Infliction of mental anguish
Physical neglect: Failure to provide health care to prevent or treat physical or emotional illnesses
Developmental neglect: Failure to provide physical and cognitive stimulation needed to prevent developmental deficits
Educational neglect: Depriving a child of education
Economic exploitation: Illegal or improper exploitation of money, funds, or other resources for one's personal gain

Box 66-12 Data Collection Questions for Violence and Abuse

"Has anyone ever touched you in a way that made you uncomfortable?"
"Is anyone hurting you now?"
"How do you and your partner deal with anger (or disagreement)?"
"Has your partner ever hit you?"
"Have you ever been threatened by _____?"
"Does your partner prevent you from seeing family or friends?"
"Does your partner ever use the children to manipulate you?"
"Did (or does) anyone in your family deal with anger by hitting?"
"Who do you play with most often? Is there anyone you do not like playing with? Are there games you don't like playing?"

D. Characteristics of abusers
1. Impaired self-esteem
2. Strong dependency needs
3. Narcissistic and suspicious
4. History of **abuse** during childhood
5. Perceive victims as their property and believe that they are entitled to **abuse** them

E. Characteristics of victims
1. Victims feel trapped, dependent, helpless, and powerless.
2. Victims of **abuse** may become depressed as they are trapped in the abuser's power and control cycle (see Figure 66-1).
3. As victims' self-esteem becomes diminished with chronic **abuse**, they may blame themselves for the violence and be unable to see a way out of the situation.

F. Interventions
1. Report suspected or actual cases of child **abuse** or **abuse** to the older adult to appropriate authorities. (Follow state and agency guidelines.)
2. Assess for evidence of physical injuries.
3. Ensure privacy and confidentiality during the assessment and provide a nonjudgmental and empathetic approach to foster trust. Reassure the victim that he or she has not done anything wrong. (See Box 66-12 for examples of data collection questions.)
4. Assist the victim to develop self-protective abilities and other problem-solving abilities.
5. Even if the victim is not ready to leave the situation, encourage the victim to develop a specific safety plan (a fast escape if the violence resumes) and the best place to obtain help (hotlines, safe houses, and shelters). An abused person is usually reluctant to call the police.
6. Assess the suicidal potential of the victim.
7. Assess the potential for homicide.
8. Assess for the use of drugs and alcohol.
9. Determine family coping patterns and support systems.

10. Provide support and assistance in coping with contacting the legal system.
11. Assist in resolving family dysfunction with prescribed therapies.
12. Encourage individual therapy for the victim that promotes coping with the trauma and prevents further psychological conflict.
13. Individual therapy that focuses on preventing violent behavior and repairing relationships is encouraged for abusers.
14. Encourage psychotherapy, counseling, group therapy, and support groups to assist family members to develop coping strategies.
15. Assist the family to access community and personal resources.
16. Maintain accurate and thorough medical health records.

XI. CHILD ABUSE (see Chapter 31)

A. Description: Child **abuse** involves physical, emotional, or sexual **abuse** and can involve neglect.
B. Data collection
1. Physical **abuse**
   a. Unexplained bruises, burns, or fractures
   b. Bald spots on the scalp
   c. Apprehensiveness in the child
   d. Extreme aggressiveness or withdrawal
   e. Fear of parents
   f. Lack of crying when approached by a stranger
2. Physical neglect
   a. Inadequate weight gain
   b. Poor hygiene
   c. Consistent hunger (begs or steals food)
   d. Inconsistent school attendance
   e. Constant fatigue
   f. Reports of lack of child supervision
   g. Delinquency

3. Emotional **abuse**
    a. Speech disorders
    b. Habit disorders, such as sucking, biting, and rocking
    c. Learning disorders
    d. Self-harm behaviors
4. Sexual **abuse**
    a. Difficulty walking or sitting
    b. Torn, stained, or bloody underclothing
    c. Pain, swelling, or itching of the genitals
    d. Bruises, bleeding, or lacerations in the genital or anal area
    e. Poor peer relations
    f. Delinquency
    g. Changes in sleep patterns
    h. Self-harm behaviors
5. Shaken baby syndrome
    a. **Abuse** can cause intracranial hemorrhage, leading to cerebral edema and death
    b. Baby often has respiratory problems
    c. Nurse would note full bulging fontanels and a head circumference greater than expected
6. Child abduction
    a. Many cases involve abduction by a family member (usually a parent) who takes or keeps the child and violates a custody order.
    b. The most vulnerable age for children abduction is less than 6 years of age.
    c. Parents at risk for abducting their child include those who have made a prior threat of intent, cases in which there is a suspicion of **abuse** of the child, those wanting the child to grow up in their country of origin, or a parent with a mental illness, especially a sociopathic parent.
C. Interventions
    1. Assess injuries. Support the child during a thorough physical assessment.
    2. The child will likely be removed from the abusive environment to a safe place to prevent further injury while the case is investigated.
    3. Move slowly and avoid any loud noises when near the child.
    4. Communicate with the child at the child's eye level.
    5. Reassure the child that he or she is not "bad" and is not responsible for the abuser's behavior.
    6. Document accurately and completely all information related to the suspected **abuse**.
    7. When working with parents in follow-up care or counseling, assist the parents in identifying stressors and alternative ways to express feelings.
    8. Provide education to the parents, and refer parents to **crisis** hotlines and community support systems such as Parents Anonymous (a group for parents who have abused or fear that they may **abuse** their child physically) or Parents

United International, Inc. (a group devoted to helping sexually abused families).

⚠ Report cases of suspected abuse of a child or older adult to appropriate authorities (follow state and agency guidelines). Reporting is mandated by federal law.

XII. ABUSE TO THE OLDER ADULT

A. Description
    1. **Abuse** to an older adult involves physical, emotional, or sexual **abuse** and can involve neglect or economic exploitation.
    2. Individuals at most risk include those who are dependent because of illness, immobility, or altered mental status.
    3. Factors that contribute to **abuse** and neglect include long-standing family violence, caregiver stress, and the individual's increasing dependence on others.
    4. Victims may attempt to dismiss injuries as accidental, and abusers may prevent victims from receiving proper medical care to avoid discovery.
    5. Victims are often isolated socially by their abusers.
B. Data collection
    1. Physical **abuse**
        a. Sprains, dislocations, or fractures
        b. Abrasions, bruises, or lacerations
        c. Pressure sores
        d. Puncture wounds
        e. Burns
        f. Skin tears
    2. Sexual **abuse**
        a. Torn or stained underclothing
        b. Discomfort or bleeding in the genital area
        c. Difficulty in walking or sitting
        d. Unexplained genital infections or disease
    3. Emotional **abuse**
        a. Confusion
        b. Fearful and agitated
        c. Changes in appetite and weight
        d. Withdrawn and loss of interest in self and social activities
    4. Neglect
        a. Disheveled appearance
        b. Dressed inadequately or inappropriately
        c. Dehydration and malnutrition
        d. Lacking physical needs, such as glasses, hearing aids, and dentures
    5. Signs of medication overdose
    6. Economic exploitation
        a. Inability to pay bills and fearful when discussing finances
        b. Confused, inaccurate, or no knowledge of finances

C. Interventions (see Priority Nursing Actions)
1. Assess for and treat physical injuries.
2. Report cases of suspected **abuse** to appropriate authorities (follow state and agency guidelines).
3. Separate the older adult from the abusive environment if possible and contact adult protective services for assistance in placement while the **abuse** is investigated.
4. Explore alternative living arrangements that are the least restrictive and disruptive to the victim.
5. The older adult who has been abused may need assistance for financial or legal matters.
6. Provide referrals to emergency community resources.
7. When working with caregivers, assess the need for respite care or counseling if needed to deal with caregiver stress.

▬▬▬ PRIORITY NURSING ACTIONS! ▬▬▬

Actions to Take When an Older Client Is Physically Abused
1. Assess and treat the wounds.
2. Remove the victim from immediate danger.
3. Adhere to mandatory abuse reporting laws.
4. Notify the caseworker of the family situation.
5. Document the occurrence, findings, actions taken, and the victim's response.

When a victim is abused, the priority is to assess and treat any physical injuries. The nurse stays with the victim and provides comfort and support. After physical injuries are treated, the nurse ensures that the client is safe and is removed from the threatening environment. Elder abuse needs to be reported, so the nurse would adhere to the mandatory abuse reporting laws of the state. The nurse also contacts the caseworker of the family situation so that the incident is reported and follow-up with the family can occur. If there is no caseworker, the nurse contacts social services or the appropriate service to initiate this process. Finally, the nurse documents the occurrence, findings, actions taken, and the victim's response.

References: Fortinash, K., & Holoday-Worret, P. (2008). *Psychiatric mental health nursing* (4th ed., pp. 491–492). St. Louis: Mosby; and Stuart, G. (2009). *Principles and practice of psychiatric nursing* (9th ed., p. 328). St. Louis: Mosby.

XIII.   RAPE AND SEXUAL ASSAULT

A. Description
1. Rape (sexual assault) is engaging another person in a sexual act and/or sexual intercourse through the use of force and without the consent of the sexual partner.
2. The victim is not required by law to report the rape or assault.
3. Often, the victim is blamed by others and receives no support from significant others.

4. Acquaintance rapes involve someone known to the victim.
5. Statutory rape is the act of sexual intercourse with a person under the age of legal consent, even if the minor consents.
6. Marital rape
    a. The belief that marriage bestows rights to sex whenever wanted and without consent of the partner contributes to the occurrence of marital rape.
    b. Victims of marital rape describe being forced to perform acts they did not wish to perform and being physically abused during sex.

B. Data collection
1. Female client
    a. Obtain the date of the last menstrual period.
    b. Determine the form of birth control used and the last act of intercourse before rape.
    c. Determine the duration of intercourse, orifices violated, and whether penile penetration occurred.
    d. Determine the use of a condom by the perpetrator.
2. Shame, embarrassment, and humiliation
3. Anger and revenge
4. Fear of telling others for fear of not being believed

C. It is important to note that males may be sexually abused both as children and as adults and are the usual targeted victim of pedophiles. Males may have more difficulty with disclosing their **abuse**.

D. Rape trauma syndrome
1. Sleep disturbances and nightmares
2. Loss of appetite
3. Fears, anxiety, phobias, and suspicion
4. Decrease in activities and motivation
5. Disruptions in relationships with partner, family, and friends
6. Self-blame, guilt, and shame
7. Lowered self-esteem and feelings of worthlessness
8. Somatic complaints

E. Interventions
1. Perform data collection in a quiet, private area.
2. Stay with the victim.
3. Assess the victim's stress level before performing treatments and procedures.
4. Victim should not shower, bathe, douche (female), or change clothing until an examination is performed.
5. Obtain written consent for the examination, photographs, laboratory tests, release of information, and laboratory samples.
6. Assist with the female pelvic examination and obtain specimens to detect semen (the pelvic examination may trigger a flashback of the attack). A shower and fresh clothing should be made available to the client after the examination.

7. Preserve any evidence.
8. Treat physical injuries and provide client safety.
9. Document all events in the care of the victim.
10. Reinforce to the victim that surviving the assault is most important. If the victim survived the rape, he or she did exactly what was necessary to stay alive.
11. Refer the victim to **crisis** intervention and support groups.

MORE QUESTIONS ON EVOLVE!

Practice Questions

716. A nurse is caring for an older adult client who has recently lost her husband. The client says, "No one cares about me anymore. All the people I loved are dead." Which response by the nurse is therapeutic?
1. "Right! Why not just 'pack it in'?"
2. "That seems rather unlikely to me."
3. "I don't believe that, and neither do you."
4. "You must be feeling all alone at this point."

717. A nurse is planning care for a client who is being hospitalized because the client has been displaying violent behavior and is at risk for potential harm to others. The nurse avoids which intervention in the plan of care?
1. Facing the client when providing care
2. Ensuring that a security officer is within the immediate area
3. Keeping the door to the client's room open when with the client
4. Assigning the client to a room at the end of the hall to prevent disturbing the other clients

718. Which behaviors observed by the nurse might lead to the suspicion that a depressed adolescent client could be suicidal?
1. The client gives away a prized CD and a cherished autographed picture of the performer.
2. The client runs out of the therapy group swearing at the group leader and then runs to her room.
3. The client gets angry with her roommate when the roommate borrows her clothes without asking.
4. The client becomes angry while speaking on the telephone and slams the receiver down on the hook.

719. A client is admitted to the psychiatric unit after a serious suicidal attempt by hanging. The nurse's most important aspect of care is to maintain client safety and plans to:
1. Request that a peer remain with the client at all times.

2. Remove the client's clothing and place the client in a hospital gown.
3. Assign a staff member to the client who will remain with him or her at all times.
4. Admit the client to a seclusion room where all potentially dangerous articles are removed.

720. The police arrive at the emergency room with a client who has seriously lacerated both wrists. The initial nursing action is to:
1. Administer an antianxiety agent.
2. Examine and treat the wound sites.
3. Secure and record a detailed history.
4. Encourage and assist the client to vent feelings.

721. A nurse is caring for a client with severe depression. Which of the following activities would be appropriate for this client?
1. A puzzle
2. Drawing
3. Checkers
4. Paint by number

722. A client experiencing a severe major depressive episode is unable to address activities of daily living. The appropriate nursing intervention is to:
1. Feed, bathe, and dress the client as needed until the client can perform these activities independently.
2. Offer the client choices and consequences to the failure to comply with the expectation of maintaining activities of daily living.
3. Structure the client's day so that adequate time can be devoted to the client's assuming responsibility for the activities of daily living.
4. Have the client's peers confront the client about how the noncompliance in addressing activities of daily living affects the milieu.

723. An older client is a victim of elder abuse, and the client's family has been attending weekly counseling sessions. Which statement by the abusive family member would indicate the client has learned positive coping skills?
1. "I will be more careful to make sure that my father's needs are met."
2. "Now that my father is moving into my home, I will need to change my ways."
3. "I feel better able to care for my father now that I know where to obtain assistance."
4. "I am so sorry and embarrassed that the abusive event occurred. It won't happen again."

724. A nurse is assisting in planning care for a client being admitted to the nursing unit who has

attempted suicide. Which priority nursing intervention will the nurse include in the plan of care?
1. One-to-one suicide precautions
2. Suicide precautions, with 30-minute checks
3. Checking the whereabouts of the client every 15 minutes
4. Asking that the client report suicidal thoughts immediately

725. A nurse is reviewing the health care record of a client admitted to the psychiatric unit. The nurse notes that the admission nurse has documented that the client is experiencing anxiety as a result of a situational crisis. The nurse would determine that this type of crisis could be caused by:
1. Witnessing a murder
2. The death of a loved one
3. A fire that destroyed the client's home
4. A recent rape episode experienced by the client

726. A nurse is gathering data from a client in crisis. When determining the client's perception of the precipitating event that led to the crisis, the most appropriate question to ask is:
1. "With whom do you live?"
2. "Who is available to help you?"
3. "What leads you to seek help now?"
4. "What do you usually do to feel better?"

727. A nurse is assisting in developing a plan of care for the client in a crisis state. When developing the plan, the nurse will consider which of the following?
1. A crisis state indicates that the individual is suffering from a mental illness.
2. A crisis state indicates that the individual is suffering from an emotional illness.
3. Presenting symptoms in a crisis situation are similar for all individuals experiencing a crisis.
4. A client's response to a crisis is individualized, and what constitutes a crisis for one person may not constitute a crisis for another person.

728. A nurse observes that a client with a potential for violence is agitated, pacing up and down in the hallway, and making aggressive and belligerent gestures at other clients. Which statement would be appropriate to make to this client?
1. "You need to stop that behavior now!"
2. "You will need to be placed in seclusion!"
3. "What is causing you to become agitated?"
4. "You will need to be restrained if you do not change your behavior."

729. During a conversation with a depressed client on a psychiatric unit, the client says to the nurse, "My family would be better off without me." The nurse should make which therapeutic response to the client?
1. "Have you talked to your family about this?"
2. "Everyone feels this way when they are depressed."
3. "You will feel better once your medication begins to work."
4. "You sound very upset. Are you thinking of hurting yourself?"

730. A nurse is preparing to care for a dying client, and several family members are at the client's bedside. Which therapeutic techniques should the nurse use when communicating with the family? **Select all that apply.**
❏ 1. Discourage reminiscing.
❏ 2. Make the decisions for the family.
❏ 3. Encourage expression of feelings, concerns, and fears.
❏ 4. Explain everything that is happening to all family members.
❏ 5. Extend touch and hold the client's or family member's hand if appropriate.
❏ 6. Be honest and truthful and let the client and family know that you will not abandon them.

ANSWERS

716. 4
Rationale: The client is experiencing loss and is feeling hopeless. The therapeutic response by the nurse is the one that attempts to translate words into feelings. In option 2, the nurse is voicing doubt, which is often used when a client verbalizes delusional ideas. In option 3, the nurse is disagreeing with the client, which implies that the nurse has passed judgment on the client's ideas or opinions. In option 1, the nurse uses sarcasm, which gives advice and is nontherapeutic as a nursing response.
Test-Taking Strategy: Use therapeutic communication techniques. Option 4 is the only option that focuses on the client's feelings. Review therapeutic communication techniques if you had difficulty with this question.

Level of Cognitive Ability: Applying
Client Needs: Psychosocial Integrity
Integrated Process: Communication and Documentation
Content Area: Mental Health
Reference: Morrison-Valfre, pp. 104–105, 216-217. 2009.

717. 4
Rationale: The client should be placed in a room near the nurses' station and not at the end of a long, relatively unprotected corridor. The nurse should not isolate himself or herself with a potentially violent client. The door to the client's room should be kept open, and the nurse should never turn away from the client. A security officer or male aide should be within immediate call in case the possibility of violence is suspected.

Test-Taking Strategy: Use the process of elimination and note the strategic word "avoids." This word indicates a negative event query and the need to select the incorrect intervention. Keeping in mind that safety is the subject will direct you to the correct option. If you had difficulty with this question, review guidelines for caring for the violent client.
Level of Cognitive Ability: Applying
Client Needs: Safe and Effective Care Environment
Integrated Process: Nursing Process/Planning
Content Area: Mental Health
Reference: Varcarolis, Halter, p. 431. 2009.

718. 1

Rationale: A depressed, suicidal client often gives away that which is of value as a way of saying "goodbye" and wanting to be remembered. Options 2, 3, and 4 identify acting-out behaviors.
Test-Taking Strategy: Use the process of elimination. Options 2, 3, and 4 are comparable or alike in that they deal with anger and "acting-out behaviors," which are often typical of some adolescents. Option 1 is different in nature and could indicate that the client may be saying goodbye. Review the clues that indicate suicide if you had difficulty with this question.
Level of Cognitive Ability: Analyzing
Client Needs: Psychosocial Integrity
Integrated Process: Nursing Process/Data Collection
Content Area: Mental Health
Reference: Morrison-Valfre, p. 297. 2009.

719. 3

Rationale: Hanging is a serious suicide attempt. The plan of care must reflect action that will promote the client's safety. Constant observation status (one on one) with a staff member who is never less than an arm's length away is the safest intervention.
Test-Taking Strategy: Use the process of elimination. Eliminate option 4 because seclusion should not be the initial intervention. Eliminate option 1 next since the responsibility to safeguard a client is not the peer's responsibility. Eliminate option 2 because removing one's clothing will not maximize all possible safety strategies. Review nursing interventions for the client at risk for suicide if you had difficulty with this question.
Level of Cognitive Ability: Applying
Client Needs: Safe and Effective Care Environment
Integrated Process: Nursing Process/Implementation
Content Area: Mental Health
Reference: Varcarolis, Halter, p. 417. 2009.

720. 2

Rationale: The initial nursing action is to examine and treat the self-inflicted injuries. Injuries from lacerated wrists can lead to a life-threatening situation. Other interventions may follow after the client has been treated medically.
Test-Taking Strategy: Use Maslow's Hierarchy of Needs theory to prioritize. Physiological needs come first. Option 2 addresses the physiological need. Review care of the client who has attempted suicide if you had difficulty with this question.
Level of Cognitive Ability: Applying
Client Needs: Physiological Integrity

Integrated Process: Nursing Process/Implementation
Content Area: Mental Health
References: Stuart, p. 317. 2009.
Varcarolis, Halter, p. 416. 2009.

721. 2

Rationale: Concentration and memory are poor in a client with severe depression. When a client has a diagnosis of severe depression, the nurse needs to provide activities that require little concentration. Activities that have no right or wrong choices or decisions minimize opportunities for the client to put down himself or herself. The nurse can also process the client's feelings by sitting with the client and talking or encouraging the client to write in a journal.
Test-Taking Strategy: Use the process of elimination. Note that options 1, 3, and 4 are comparable or alike in that they all require concentration. It is important to remember that clients with depression have difficulty concentrating and need activities that require little concentration. Review care of the client with severe depression if you had difficulty with this question.
Level of Cognitive Ability: Applying
Client Needs: Psychosocial Integrity
Integrated Process: Nursing Process/Implementation
Content Area: Mental Health
Reference: Stuart, pp. 306, 327. 2009.

722. 1

Rationale: The client with depression may not have the energy or interest to complete activities of daily living. Often, severely depressed clients are unable to perform even the simplest activities of daily living. The nurse assumes this role and completes these tasks with the client. Options 2 and 3 are incorrect because the client lacks the energy and motivation to perform these tasks independently. Option 4 will increase the client's feelings of poor self-esteem and unworthiness.
Test-Taking Strategy: Use the process of elimination and note the strategic words "severe major depressive episode." Eliminate options 2 and 3 because the client lacks the energy and motivation to do these independently. In addition, option 2 may lead to increased feelings of worthlessness as the client fails to meet expectations. Option 4 will increase the client's feelings of poor self-esteem and unworthiness. Review care of the client with severe depression if you had difficulty with this question.
Level of Cognitive Ability: Applying
Client Needs: Physiological Integrity
Integrated Process: Nursing Process/Implementation
Content Area: Mental Health
Reference: Stuart, pp. 301–302. 2009.

723. 3

Rationale: Elder abuse sometimes occurs with family members who are being expected to care for their aging parents. This can cause family members to become overextended, frustrated, or financially depleted. Knowing where in the community to turn for assistance in caring for aging family members can bring much-needed relief. Using these alternatives is a positive alternative coping strategy, which many families use.

Test-Taking Strategy: Use the process of elimination and focus on the subject, a coping strategy. Only option 3 identifies a means of coping with the subjects. The other options are statements of good faith or promises, which may or may not be kept in the future. Option 3 outlines a definitive plan for how to handle the pressure associated with the father's care. Review effective coping strategies if you had difficulty with this question.
Level of Cognitive Ability: Evaluating
Client Needs: Psychosocial Integrity
Integrated Process: Nursing Process/Evaluation
Content Area: Mental Health
References: Morrison-Valfre, pp. 287–288. 2009.
Stuart, pp. 720–721. 2009.

724. 1
Rationale: One-to-one suicide precautions are required for the client who has attempted suicide. Options 2 and 3 are not appropriate, considering the situation. Option 4 may be an appropriate nursing intervention, but the priority is stated in option 1. The best option is constant supervision so that the nurse may intervene as needed if the client attempts to cause harm to him or herself.
Test-Taking Strategy: Use the process of elimination and note the strategic word "priority." Recalling that one-to-one suicide precautions are the priority in caring for a suicidal client will direct you to the correct option. Review interventions for the suicidal client if you had difficulty with this question.
Level of Cognitive Ability: Applying
Client Needs: Safe and Effective Care Environment
Integrated Process: Nursing Process/Implementation
Content Area: Mental Health
References: Stuart, p. 327. 2009.
Varcarolis, Halter, p. 417. 2009.

725. 2
Rationale: A situational crisis is associated with a life event. External situations that could precipitate a situational crisis include loss or change of a job, the death of a loved one, abortion, change in financial status, divorce, and severe illness. Options 1, 3, and 4 identify adventitious crises. An adventitious crisis relates to a crisis, disaster, or event that is not a part of everyday life, is unplanned, and is accidental.
Test-Taking Strategy: Use the process of elimination and focus on the strategic words "situational crisis." This will assist in eliminating options 1, 3, and 4 because they are comparable or alike. If you had difficulty with this question, review the types of crisis.
Level of Cognitive Ability: Understanding
Client Needs: Psychosocial Integrity
Integrated Process: Nursing Process/Data Collection
Content Area: Mental Health
Reference: Morrison-Valfre, p. 206. 2009.

726. 3
Rationale: A nurse's initial task when gathering data from a client in crisis is to assess the individual or family and the problem. The more clearly the problem can be defined, the better the chance a solution can be found. Option 3 will assist in determining data related to the precipitating event that led to the

crisis. Options 1 and 2 identify situational supports. Option 4 identifies personal coping skills.
Test-Taking Strategy: Use the process of elimination and note the strategic words "precipitating event." Focus on these strategic words when selecting the correct option. Eliminate options 1 and 2, because these data will determine support systems. Eliminate option 4, because this question would be asked when determining coping skills. Review data collection methods for a client in crisis if you had difficulty with this question.
Level of Cognitive Ability: Applying
Client Needs: Psychosocial Integrity
Integrated Process: Nursing Process/Data Collection
Content Area: Mental Health
References: Morrison-Valfre, pp. 76–78. 2009.
Varcarolis, & Halter, p. 368. 2009.

727. 4
Rationale: Although each crisis response can be described in similar terms as far as presenting symptoms are concerned, what constitutes a crisis for one person may not constitute a crisis for another person, because each is a unique individual. Being in a crisis state does not mean that the client is suffering from an emotional or mental illness.
Test-Taking Strategy: Use the process of elimination. Eliminate option 3 because of the closed-ended word "all." Next, eliminate options 1 and 2 because a crisis does not indicate "illness." Review the characteristics of a crisis state if you had difficulty with this question.
Level of Cognitive Ability: Understanding
Client Needs: Psychosocial Integrity
Integrated Process: Nursing Process/Data Collection
Content Area: Mental Health
Reference: Varcarolis, Halter, pp. 370–371. 2009.

728. 3
Rationale: The best statement is to ask the client what is causing the agitation. This will assist the client to become aware of the behavior and will assist the nurse in planning appropriate interventions for the client. Option 1 is demanding behavior, which could cause increased agitation in the client. Options 2 and 4 are threats to the client and are inappropriate.
Test-Taking Strategy: Use the process of elimination. Eliminate option 1 because of the demand that it places on the client. Eliminate options 2 and 4 because they indicate threats to the client. Review appropriate nursing interventions for the agitated client if you had difficulty with this question.
Level of Cognitive Ability: Applying
Client Needs: Psychosocial Integrity
Integrated Process: Communication and Documentation
Content Area: Mental Health
Reference: Morrison-Valfre, pp. 104–105, 277. 2009.

729. 4
Rationale: Clients who are depressed may be at risk for suicide. It is critical for the nurse to assess suicidal ideation and plan. The client should be directly asked if a plan for self-harm exists. Options 1, 2, and 3 are not therapeutic responses.
Test-Taking Strategy: Use therapeutic communication techniques. Option 4 is the only option that deals directly with

the client's feelings. Additionally, clients at risk for suicide need to be directly assessed regarding the potential for self-harm. Review data collection techniques for the depressed client if you had difficulty with this question.

Level of Cognitive Ability: Applying
Client Needs: Psychosocial Integrity
Integrated Process: Nursing Process/Data Collection
Content Area: Mental Health
Reference: Morrison-Valfre, p. 228. 2009.

❖ **730. 3, 5, 6**
Rationale: The nurse must determine whether there is a spokesperson for the family and how much the client and family want to know. The nurse needs to allow the family and client the opportunity for informed choices and assist with the decision-making process if asked. The nurse should encourage expression of feelings, concerns, and fears, as well as reminiscing. The nurse needs to be honest and truthful and let the client and family know that they will not be abandoned. It is important to extend touch and hold the client's or family member's hand if appropriate.

Test-Taking Strategy: Recalling therapeutic communication techniques and client and family rights will assist you in answering this question. Review these techniques and care to the dying client if you had difficulty with this question.

Level of Cognitive Ability: Applying
Client Needs: Psychosocial Integrity
Integrated Process: Caring
Content Area: Mental Health
References: Morrison-Valfre, pp. 219–220, 222. 2009.

Psychiatric Medications

I. SELECTIVE SEROTONIN REUPTAKE INHIBITORS (SSRIs) (Box 67-1)

A. Description
1. Inhibit serotonin uptake and elicit an antidepressant response.
2. The potential for medication interactions is high and complete medication assessments must be obtained and evaluated. Inquire about the use of herbal therapies, especially St. John's wort.

B. Side effects
1. Nausea, vomiting, cramping, and diarrhea
2. Dry mouth
3. Central nervous system (CNS) stimulation, including akathisia (restlessness, agitation)
4. Photosensitivity
5. Insomnia, somnolence (sleepy, drowsy)
6. Nervousness
7. Headache, dizziness
8. Seizure activity
9. Weight loss or gain
10. Decreased libido
11. Apathy
12. Tremors
13. Increased sweating

C. Interventions
1. SSRIs interact with a number of medications.
2. Monitor the vital signs, because SSRIs can potentially lower or elevate blood pressure.
3. Monitor weight.
4. Initiate safety precautions, particularly if dizziness occurs.
5. The client is instructed to avoid alcohol.
6. Administered with a snack or meal to reduce the risk of dizziness and lightheadedness.
7. Monitor the suicidal client, especially during improved mood and increased energy levels.
8. The client taking fluoxetine (Prozac) and bupropion (Wellbutrin) is instructed to take the medication early in the day to prevent interference with sleep.
9. For the client on long-term therapy, monitor liver and renal function test results. Altered values may occur requiring dosage adjustments.
10. Monitor white blood cell and neutrophil counts. The medication may be discontinued if levels fall below normal.
11. If priapism (painful, prolonged penile erection) occurs, the medication is withheld and the health care provider (HCP) is notified.
12. The client is informed about the possibility of decreased libido.
13. The client is instructed to change positions slowly to avoid a hypotensive effect.
14. The client is instructed to report any visual changes to the HCP.
15. The client is educated about the potential for discontinuation syndrome if medication is stopped abruptly rather than tapered. The syndrome is characterized by gastrointestinal (GI) distress, behavioral or perceptual oddities, movement problems, and sleep disturbances.
16. Be aware of the potential for serotonin syndrome characterized by elevated temperature, muscle rigidity, elevated creatine phosphokinase (CPK) levels. This risk is greatly increased when SSRIs are given with monoamine oxidase inhibitors (MAOIs). Thus, this medication combination needs to be avoided.
17. The client is instructed that over-the-counter (OTC) cold medicines can increase the likelihood of serotonin syndrome.
18. In pregnancy, consultation with an obstetrician is recommended regarding taking these medications.
19. Monitor the medication response in children, adolescents, and the older client because the response may be different than in an adult client.
20. Psychotherapy is encouraged.

II. TRICYCLIC ANTIDEPRESSANTS (Box 67-2)

A. Description
1. Block the reuptake of norepinephrine (and serotonin) at the presynaptic neuron. It is used to treat depression.
2. May reduce seizure threshold.

Box 67-1 Reuptake Inhibitors

Selective Serotonin Reuptake Inhibitors
Citalopram (Celexa)
Escitalopram (Lexapro)
Fluoxetine (Prozac)
Fluvoxamine (Luvox)
Paroxetine hydrochloride (Paxil, Pexeva)
Sertraline hydrochloride (Zoloft)

Serotonin-Norepinephrine Reuptake Inhibitors
Venlafaxine (Effexor)
Duloxetine (Cymbalta)
Desvenlafaxine (Pristiq)

Atypical Antidepressants
Amoxapine
Bupropion hydrochloride (Wellbutrin)
Mirtazapine (Remeron)
Nefazodone
Trazodone (Desyrel)

Box 67-2 Tricyclic Antidepressants

Amitriptyline hydrochloride
Clomipramine (Anafranil)
Desipramine hydrochloride (Norpramin)
Doxepin hydrochloride (Sinequan)
Imipramine hydrochloride (Tofranil)
Nortriptyline hydrochloride (Aventyl, Pamelor)
Protriptyline hydrochloride (Vivactil)
Trimipramine maleate (Surmontil)

■ PRIORITY NURSING ACTIONS! ■

Actions to Take for a Tricyclic Antidepressant Overdose

1. Check airway and maintain a patent airway.
2. Administer oxygen.
3. Check vital signs.
4. Obtain an electrocardiogram (ECG).
5. Prepare for gastric lavage with activated charcoal.
6. Prepare for the administration of physostigmine (a cholinesterase inhibitor) and antidysrhythmic medications.
7. Document the event, actions taken, and the client's response.

A tricyclic antidepressant overdose can be life threatening. Signs and symptoms include dysrhythmias, including tachycardia, intraventricular blocks, complete atrioventricular block, ventricular fibrillation; hypothermia; flushing; dry mouth; dilation of the pupils; confusion, agitation, hallucinations; and seizures followed by coma. The immediate action is to check the airway and institute measures such as oxygen to maintain a patent airway. Vital signs are checked and monitored and an ECG is obtained to check for dysrhythmias. Gastric lavage with activated charcoal is done to prevent further medication absorption. Physostigmine (a cholinesterase inhibitor) is given to counteract anticholinergic effects and antidysrhythmics are administered as needed. The nurse documents the event, actions taken, and the client's response.

Reference: Lehne, R. (2010). *Pharmacology for nursing care* (7th ed., p. 342). St. Louis: Saunders.

3. May reduce effectiveness of antihypertensive agents.
4. Concurrent use with alcohol or antihistamines can cause CNS depression.
5. Concurrent use with MAOIs can cause hypertensive **crisis**.
6. Cardiac toxicity can occur and all clients should undergo electrocardiographic evaluation before treatment and periodically thereafter.
7. Overdose is life threatening, necessitating immediate treatment (see Priority Nursing Actions!).
8. The tricyclic antidepressant clomipramine (Anafranil) may be used to treat obsessive-compulsive disorder.

B. Side effects
1. Anticholinergic effects: dry mouth, difficulty voiding, dilated pupils and blurred vision, decreased gastrointestinal motility, constipation
2. Photosensitivity
3. Cardiovascular disturbances such as tachycardia, dysrhythmias
4. Orthostatic hypotension
5. Sedation
6. Weight gain

7. Anxiety, restlessness, irritability
8. Decreased or increased libido with ejaculatory and erection disturbances

C. Interventions
1. Monitor the suicidal client, especially during improved mood and increased energy levels.
2. The client is instructed to change positions slowly to avoid a hypotensive effect.
3. Monitor pattern of daily bowel activity.
4. Monitor for urinary retention.
5. For the client on long-term therapy, monitor liver, and renal function test results.
6. Administer with food or milk if gastrointestinal distress occurs.
7. Administer the entire daily oral dose at one time, preferably at bedtime.
8. The client is instructed to avoid alcohol and nonprescription medications to prevent adverse medication interactions.
9. The client is instructed to avoid driving and other activities requiring alertness until the response is known. Sedation is expected in early therapy and may subside with time.
10. When the medication is discontinued by the health care provider, it should be tapered gradually.

11. The potential for medication interactions with OTC cold medication exists.
12. The client is cautioned about photosensitivity and to take measures to prevent exposure to sunlight.
13. Oral hygiene and the use of hard candies and mouth rinses to relieve dry mouth is encouraged.
14. Psychotherapy is encouraged.

⚠ The client is informed that antidepressant medication may take several weeks to produce the desired effect. (The client response may not occur until 2 to 4 weeks after the first dose.)

III. MONOAMINE OXIDASE INHIBITORS (MAOIs) (Box 67-3)

A. Description
1. Inhibit the enzyme monoamine oxidase, which is present in the brain, blood platelets, liver, spleen, and kidneys.
2. Monoamine oxidase metabolizes amines, norepinephrine, and serotonin, so the concentration of these amines increases with MAOI.
3. Used for depression in the client who has not responded to other antidepressant therapies, including electroconvulsive therapy.
4. Concurrent use with amphetamines, antidepressants, dopamine, epinephrine, guanethidine, levodopa, methyldopa, nasal decongestants, norepinephrine, reserpine, tyramine-containing foods, or vasoconstrictors may cause hypertensive **crisis**.
5. Concurrent use with opioid analgesics may cause hypertension, hypotension, coma, or seizures.

B. Side effects
1. Orthostatic hypotension
2. Restlessness
3. Insomnia
4. Dizziness
5. Weakness, lethargy
6. Gastrointestinal upset
7. Dry mouth
8. Weight gain
9. Peripheral edema
10. Anticholinergic effects
11. CNS stimulation, including anxiety, agitation, mania
12. Delay in ejaculation

C. Hypertensive **crisis**
1. Hypertension
2. Occipital headache radiating frontally
3. Neck stiffness and soreness
4. Nausea and vomiting
5. Sweating
6. Fever and chills
7. Clammy skin
8. Dilated pupils

Box 67-3 Monoamine Oxidase Inhibitors

Isocarboxazid (Marplan)
Phenelzine sulfate (Nardil)
Tranylcypromine sulfate (Parnate)
Selegiline (Emsam)

---

9. Palpitations, tachycardia, or bradycardia
10. Constricting chest pain
11. Antidote for hypertensive **crisis**: phentolamine by intravenous injection

D. Interventions
1. Monitor blood pressure frequently for hypertension.
2. Monitor for signs of hypertensive **crisis**.
3. If palpitations or frequent headaches occur, withhold the medication and notify the HCP.
4. Administered with food if gastrointestinal distress occurs.
5. The client is instructed that the medication effect may be noted during the first week of therapy, but maximum benefit may take up to 3 weeks.
6. The client is instructed to report headache, neck stiffness, or neck soreness immediately.
7. The client is instructed to change positions slowly to prevent orthostatic hypotension.
8. The client is instructed to avoid caffeine or OTC preparations such as weight-reducing pills or medications for hay fever and colds.
9. Monitor for client compliance with medication administration.
10. The client is instructed to carry a Medic-Alert card indicating that an MAOI medication is being taken.
11. Administering the medication in the evening is avoided because insomnia may result.
12. When the medication is discontinued by the HCP, it should be discontinued gradually.
13. The client is instructed to avoid foods that require bacteria or molds for their preparation or preservation, and those that contain tyramine (Figure 67-1 and Box 67-4).

⚠ The client is taught about the foods that contain tyramine. Consuming tyramine-containing foods when taking an MAOI can cause hypertensive crisis.

IV. MOOD STABILIZERS (Box 67-5)

A. Description: Affect cellular transport mechanism and enhance serotonin and/or gamma-aminobutyric acid (GABA) function, which are associated with mood.

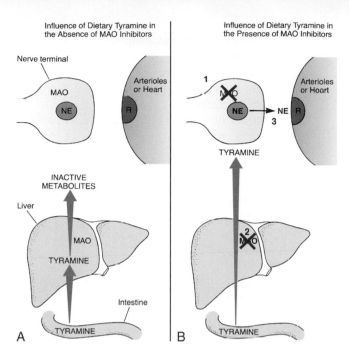

▲ FIGURE 67-1 Interaction between dietary tyramine and monoamine oxidase inhibitors (MAOIs). **A,** In the absence of MAOIs, dietary tyramine is absorbed from the intestine, transported to the liver, and then immediately activated by MAO. No tyramine reaches the general circulation. **B,** Three events occur in the presence of MAOIs: (1) inhibition of neuronal MAO raises levels of norepinephrine (NE) in sympathetic nerve terminals; (2) inhibition of hepatic MAO allows dietary tyramine to pass through the liver and enter systemic circulation intact; (3) on reaching peripheral sympathetic nerve terminals, tyramine promotes the release of accumulated NE stores, thereby causing massive vasoconstriction and excessive stimulation of the heart. *MAO*, Monoamine oxidase; *R*, receptor for NE. (From Lehne, R. [2010]. *Pharmacology for nursing care* [7th ed.]. St. Louis: Saunders.)

Box 67-4 Foods to Avoid That Contain Tyramine

Avocados
Bananas
Beef or chicken liver
Brewer's yeast
Broad beans
Caffeine, such as in coffee, tea, or chocolate
Cheese, especially aged, except cottage cheese
Figs
Meat extracts and tenderizers
Overripe fruit
Papaya
Pickled herring
Raisins
Red wine, beer, sherry
Sausage, bologna, pepperoni, salami
Sour cream
Soy sauce
Yogurt

Box 67-5 Mood Stabilizers

Lithium Preparations
Lithium carbonate (Lithobid)
Lithium citrate

Other Mood Stabilizers
Aripiprazole (Abilify)
Carbamazepine (Tegretol)
Gabapentin (Neurontin)
Lamotrigine (Lamictal)
Olanzapine (Zyprexa)
Olanzapine/fluoxetine (Symbyax)
Oxcarbazepine (Trileptal)
Quetiapine (Seroquel)
Risperidone (Risperdal)
Valproate sodium (Depakene, Depakote, Depacon)
Ziprasidone (Geodon)

B. Lithium
1. Concurrent use with diuretics, fluoxetine (Prozac), methyldopa, or nonsteroidal anti-inflammatory drugs (NSAIDs) increases lithium reabsorption by the kidney or inhibits lithium excretion, either of which increases the risk of lithium toxicity.
2. Acetazolamide (Diamox), theophylline, phenothiazines, or sodium bicarbonate may increase renal excretion of lithium, reducing its effectiveness.
3. The therapeutic dose is only slightly less than the amount producing toxicity.
4. The therapeutic drug serum level of lithium is 0.6 to 1.2 mEq/L. The actual dose at which the therapeutic effect is achieved and the levels at which toxicity appears is highly variable among individuals.
5. The causes of an increase in the lithium level include decreased sodium intake, fluid and electrolyte loss associated with severe sweating, dehydration, diarrhea, or diuretic therapy, and illness or overdose.
6. Serum lithium levels should be checked every 1 to 2 months or whenever any behavioral change suggests an altered serum level.
7. Blood samples to check serum lithium levels should be drawn in the morning, 12 hours after the last dose was taken.

C. Side effects
1. Polyuria
2. Polydipsia
3. Anorexia, nausea
4. Dry mouth
5. Mild thirst
6. Weight gain
7. Abdominal bloating
8. Soft stools or diarrhea
9. Fine hand tremors
10. Inability to concentrate

11. Muscle weakness
12. Lethargy
13. Fatigue
14. Headache
15. Hair loss
16. Hypothyroidism

D. Interventions
1. Monitor the suicidal client, especially during improved mood and increased energy levels.
2. The medication is administered with food to minimize gastrointestinal irritation.
3. The client is instructed to avoid excessive amounts of coffee, tea, or cola, which have a diuretic effect.
4. Diuretics are not administered while the client is taking lithium.
5. The client is instructed to avoid alcohol.
6. The client is instructed to avoid OTC medications.
7. The client is instructed that he or she may take a missed dose within 2 hours of the scheduled time. Otherwise, the client should skip the missed dose and take the next dose at the scheduled time.
8. The client is instructed not to adjust the dosage without consulting the HCP because lithium should be tapered and not discontinued abruptly.
9. The client is instructed in the signs and symptoms of lithium toxicity.
10. The client is instructed to notify the HCP if polyuria, prolonged vomiting, diarrhea, or fever occurs.
11. The client is instructed that the therapeutic response to the medication will be noted in 1 to 3 weeks.
12. Monitor the electrocardiogram (ECG), renal function tests, and thyroid tests (ensure that these tests are performed before the start of therapy).
13. The client is instructed to take the medication with food or milk to decrease GI upset.
14. Monitor weight.

⚠ The client taking lithium (Lithobid) is instructed to maintain a fluid intake of six to eight glasses of water a day and an adequate salt intake to prevent lithium toxicity.

E. Lithium toxicity
1. Description
   a. Occurs when ingested lithium cannot be detoxified and excreted by the kidneys
   b. Symptoms of toxicity begin to appear when the serum lithium level is 1.5 to 2 mEq/L.
2. Mild toxicity
   a. Serum lithium level is 1.5 mEq/L
   b. Apathy

c. Lethargy
d. Diminished concentration
e. Mild ataxia
f. Coarse hand tremors
g. Slight muscle weakness

3. Moderate toxicity
   a. Serum lithium level between 1.5 to 2.5 mEq/L
   b. Nausea, vomiting
   c. Severe diarrhea
   d. Mild to moderate ataxia and incoordination
   e. Slurred speech
   f. Tinnitus
   g. Blurred vision
   h. Muscle twitching
   i. Irregular tremor
4. Severe toxicity
   a. Serum lithium level is higher than 2.5 mEq/L
   b. Nystagmus
   c. Muscle fasciculations
   d. Deep tendon hyperreflexia
   e. Visual or tactile hallucinations
   f. Oliguria or anuria
   g. Impaired level of consciousness
   h. Tonic-clonic seizures or coma, leading to death
5. Interventions for lithium toxicity
   a. Lithium is withheld and the HCP is notified.
   b. Monitor vital signs and level of consciousness.
   c. Monitor cardiac status.
   d. Prepare to obtain samples monitoring lithium, electrolyte, blood urea nitrogen, and creatinine levels and complete blood cell count.
   e. Monitor for suicidal tendencies and institute suicide precautions.

V. ANTIANXIETY OR ANXIOLYTIC MEDICATIONS

A. Description
1. Antianxiety medications depress the CNS, thereby increasing the effects of GABA, which produces relaxation and may depress the limbic system.
2. Benzodiazepines have anxiety-reducing (anxiolytic), sedative-hypnotic, muscle-relaxing, and anticonvulsant actions (Box 67-6).
3. Benzodiazepines are contraindicated in clients with acute narrow-angle glaucoma and should be used cautiously in children and older clients.
4. Benzodiazepines interact with other CNS medications, producing an additive effect.
5. Abrupt withdrawal of benzodiazepines can be potentially life threatening and withdrawal should only be done under medical supervision.

B. Side effects
1. Daytime sedation
2. Ataxia
3. Dizziness

4. Headaches
5. Blurred or double vision
6. Hypotension
7. Tremor
8. Amnesia
9. Slurred speech
10. Urinary incontinence
11. Constipation
12. Paradoxical CNS excitement
13. Lethargy
14. Behavioral change

C. Acute toxicity
1. Somnolence
2. Confusion
3. Diminished reflexes and coma
4. Flumazenil (Romazicon), a benzodiazepine antagonist administered intravenously, will reverse benzodiazepine intoxication in 5 minutes.
5. The client being treated for an overdose of a benzodiazepine may experience agitation, restlessness, discomfort, and anxiety.

D. Interventions
1. Monitor for motor responses such as agitation, trembling, and tension.
2. Monitor for autonomic responses such as cold clammy hands and sweating.
3. Monitor for paradoxical CNS excitement during early therapy, particularly in older and debilitated individuals.
4. Monitor for visual disturbances because the medications can worsen glaucoma.
5. Monitor liver and renal function test results and complete blood cell counts.
6. Reduce the medication dose as prescribed for the older adult client and for the client with impaired liver function.
7. Initiate safety precautions, because the older adult client is at risk for falling when taking the medication for sleep or anxiety.

8. Assist with ambulation if drowsiness or lightheadedness occurs.
9. The client is instructed that drowsiness usually disappears during continued therapy.
10. The client is instructed to avoid tasks that require alertness until the response to the medication is established.
11. The client is instructed to avoid alcohol.
12. The client is instructed not to take other medications without consulting the HCP.
13. The client is instructed not to stop the medication abruptly (can result in seizure activity).

E. Withdrawal
1. To lessen withdrawal symptoms, the dosage of a benzodiazepine should be tapered gradually over 2 to 6 weeks.
2. Abrupt or too-rapid withdrawal results in the following:
   a. Restlessness
   b. Irritability
   c. Insomnia
   d. Hand tremors
   e. Abdominal or muscle cramps
   f. Sweating
   g. Vomiting
   h. Seizures

VI. BARBITURATES AND SEDATIVE-HYPNOTICS (Box 67-7)

A. Description
1. These medications depress the reticular activating system by promoting the inhibitory synaptic action of the neurotransmitter GABA.
2. These medications are used for short-term treatment of insomnia or for sedation to relieve anxiety, tension, and apprehension.

B. Side effects
1. Dizziness and drowsiness

Box 67-6 Benzodiazepines

Alprazolam (Xanax, Niravam)
Chlordiazepoxide (Librium)
Clonazepam (Klonopin)
Clorazepate (Tranxene)
Diazepam (Valium)
Flurazepam (Dalmane)
Lorazepam (Ativan)
Midazolam (Versed)
Oxazepam (Serax)
Quazepam (Doral)
Temazepam (Restoril)
Triazolam (Halcion)

Nonbenzodiazepine Anxiolytics
Buspirone (BuSpar)

Box 67-7 Barbiturates and Sedative-Hypnotics

Barbiturates
Amobarbital (Amytal)
Butabarbital (Butisol)
Pentobarbital (Nembutal)
Phenobarbital (Luminal)
Secobarbital (Seconal)

Sedative-Hypnotics
Chloral hydrate (Aquachloral Supprettes, Somnote)
Eszopiclone (Lunesta)
Meprobamate (Miltown)
Ramelteon (Rozerem)
Zaleplon (Sonata)
Zolpidem (Ambien)

2. Confusion
3. Irritability
4. Allergic reactions
5. Agranulocytosis
6. Thrombocytopenic purpura
7. Megaloblastic anemia

C. Overdose
1. Tachycardia
2. Hypotension
3. Cold and clammy skin
4. Dilated pupils
5. Weak and rapid pulse
6. Signs of shock
7. Depressed respirations
8. Absent reflexes
9. Coma and death may result from respiratory and cardiovascular collapse.

D. Withdrawal
1. Severe withdrawal symptoms begin within 24 hours after the medication is discontinued in an individual with severe medication dependence.
2. Gradual withdrawal is used to detoxify a dependent client.
3. Anxiety
4. Insomnia
5. Nightmares
6. Daytime agitation
7. Tremors
8. Delirium
9. Seizures
10. Behavioral changes

E. Interventions
1. Lower doses are administered as prescribed for the older client.
2. Medications should be used with caution in the client who has suicidal tendencies or has a history of drug **addiction**.
3. Maintain safety by supervising ambulation and using side rails at night.
4. The client is instructed to take the medication as directed.
5. The client is instructed to avoid driving or operating hazardous equipment if drowsiness, dizziness, or unsteadiness occurs.
6. The client is instructed to avoid alcohol.
7. For insomnia, the client is instructed to take the medication 30 minutes before bedtime. The client is instructed avoid taking with a heavy meal to help absorption.
8. The client is instructed that a hangover effect may occur in the morning.
9. The client is instructed not to discontinue the medication abruptly.
10. The client taking chloral hydrate is instructed to take the medication with food and a full glass of water, fruit juice, or ginger ale to prevent gastric irritation.

VII. ANTIPSYCHOTIC MEDICATIONS (Box 67-8)

A. Description
1. Improve the thought processes and the behavior of the client with psychotic symptoms, especially the client with schizophrenia.
2. Affect dopamine receptors in the brain, thereby reducing the psychotic symptoms.
3. Typical antipsychotics are more effective for positive symptoms of schizophrenia such as hallucinations, aggression, and delusions. Typical antipsychotic medications also block the chemoreceptor trigger zone and vomiting center in the brain, producing an antiemetic effect.
4. Atypical antipsychotics are more effective for the negative symptoms of schizophrenia, such as avolition, apathy, and alogia.
5. The effects of antipsychotic medications will be potentiated when given with other medications acting on the CNS.

B. Side effects (Box 67-9)

C. Interventions
1. Monitor vital signs.
2. Monitor for symptoms of neuroleptic malignant syndrome.
3. Monitor urine output.
4. Monitor serum glucose level.
5. Note that the client taking an antipsychotic medication may require long-term medication for parkinsonian symptoms.
6. Administer the medication with food or milk to decrease gastric irritation.
7. For oral use, the liquid form might be preferred, because some clients hide tablets to avoid taking them.
8. Note that the absorption rate is faster with the liquid form of oral medication.

Box 67-8 Antipsychotic Medications

Typical Antipsychotics
Chlorpromazine hydrochloride (Thorazine)
Fluphenazine decanoate (Prolixin Decanoate)
Haloperidol
Loxapine (Loxitane)
Molindone hydrochloride (Moban)
Pimozide (Orap)
Thiothixene hydrochloride (Navane)
Trifluoperazine

Atypical Antipsychotics
Aripiprazole (Abilify)
Clozapine (Clozaril)
Olanzapine (Zyprexa)
Quetiapine (Seroquel)
Risperidone (Risperdal)
Ziprasidone (Geodon)

9. Skin contact with the liquid concentrate is avoided to prevent contact dermatitis.
10. Protect the liquid concentrate from light.
11. Dilute the liquid concentrate with fruit juice.
12. The client is informed that a full therapeutic effect of the medication may not be evident for 3 to 6 weeks after initiation of therapy. However, an observable therapeutic response may be apparent after 7 to 10 days.
13. The client is informed that some medications may cause a harmless change in urine color to pinkish to red-brown.
14. The client is instructed to use sunscreen, hats, and protective clothing when outdoors.
15. The client is instructed to avoid alcohol or other CNS depressants.

Box 67-9 Side Effects of Antipsychotic Medications

Anticholinergic Effects
Dry mouth
Increased heart rate
Urinary retention
Constipation
Hypotension

Extrapyramidal Side Effects
Parkinsonism
Tremors
Mask-like facies
Rigidity
Shuffling gait
Dysphagia
Drooling
Dystonias
Abnormal or involuntary eye movements, including oculogyric crisis
Facial grimacing
Twisting of the torso or other muscle groups
Akathisia
Restlessness
Constant moving about
Tardive Dyskinesia
Protrusion of the tongue
Chewing motion
Involuntary movements of the body and extremities

Other Side Effects
Drowsiness
Blood dyscrasias
Pruritus
Photosensitivity
Elevated blood glucose level
Increased weight
Impaired body temperature regulation
Gynecomastia
Lactation

---

16. The client is instructed to change positions slowly to avoid orthostatic hypotension.
17. The client is instructed to report signs of agranulocytosis, including sore throat, fever, and malaise.
18. The client is instructed to report signs of liver dysfunction, including jaundice, malaise, fever, right upper abdominal pain.
19. When discontinuing antipsychotics, the medication dosage should be reduced gradually to avoid sudden recurrence of psychotic symptoms.

 Monitor for extrapyramidal side effects in the client taking an antipsychotic medication.

VIII. NEUROLEPTIC MALIGNANT SYNDROME

A. Description
1. A potentially fatal syndrome that may occur at any time during therapy with neuroleptic (antipsychotic) medications
2. Although rare, neuroleptic malignant syndrome more commonly occurs at the initiation of therapy, after the client has changed from one medication to another, after a dosage increase, or when a combination of medications is used.

B. Data collection
1. Dyspnea or tachypnea
2. Tachycardia or irregular pulse rate
3. Fever
4. High or low blood pressure
5. Increased sweating
6. Loss of bladder control
7. Skeletal muscle rigidity
8. Pale skin
9. Excessive weakness or fatigue
10. Altered level of consciousness
11. Seizures
12. Severe extrapyramidal side effects
13. Difficulty swallowing
14. Excessive salivation
15. Oculogyric crisis
16. Dyskinesia
17. Elevated white blood cell count, liver function results, and creatinine phosphokinase level

C. Interventions
1. Notify the registered nurse who will then notify the HCP.
2. Monitor the vital signs.
3. Initiate safety and seizure precautions.
4. Prepare to discontinue the medication.
5. Monitor the level of consciousness.
6. Administer antipyretics as prescribed.
7. Use a cooling blanket to lower the body temperature.
8. Monitor electrolyte levels and administer fluids intravenously as prescribed.

IX. MEDICATIONS TO TREAT ATTENTION-DEFICIT/ HYPERACTIVITY DISORDER (Box 67-10)

A. Children with attention-deficit/hyperactivity disorder may require medication to reduce hyperactive behavior and lengthen attention span.

B. Medications that are most effective in controlling this disorder are CNS stimulants.

C. CNS stimulants, which increase agitation and activity in adults, have a calming effect on children with attention-deficit/hyperactivity disorder and increase alertness and sensitivity to stimuli.

D. Side effects
1. Tachycardia
2. Anorexia and weight loss
3. Elevated blood pressure
4. Dizziness
5. Agitation

E. Interventions
1. Monitor for CNS side effects.
2. Obtain a baseline ECG.
3. Monitor the blood pressure.
4. The child and parents are instructed that OTC medications need to be avoided.
5. The child and parents are instructed that the last dose of the day should be taken at least 6 hours before bedtime (14 hours for extended-released forms) to prevent insomnia.
6. Monitor height and weight (particularly in children).
7. Reinforce that several weeks of therapy may be necessary before the therapeutic effect is noted.
8. The client and parents are instructed that a drug-free period may be prescribed to allow growth of the child if the medication has caused growth retardation.

X. MEDICATIONS TO TREAT ALZHEIMER'S DISEASE (Box 67-11)

A. Acetylcholinesterase inhibitors may be used to treat Alzheimer's disease to improve cognitive functions in the early stages.

B. Donepezil (Aricept)
1. An inhibitor of acetylcholinesterase used to treat mild to moderate dementia of Alzheimer's disease.
2. Side effects include nausea and diarrhea.
3. Donepezil can slow the heart rate through its vagotonic effect.

C. Galantamine (Razadyne)
1. An inhibitor of cholinesterase used to treat mild to moderate dementia of Alzheimer's disease.
2. Side effects include nausea, vomiting, diarrhea, anorexia, and weight loss.
3. Can cause bronchoconstriction. Used with caution in clients with asthma and chronic obstructive pulmonary disease.

D. Memantine (Namenda)
1. An NMDA (N-methyl-D-aspartate) receptor antagonist is indicated for moderate to severe Alzheimer's disease.
2. Side effects include dizziness, headache, confusion, and constipation.
3. Should not be used in combination with other NMDA antagonists such as amantadine (Symmetrel) or ketamine (Ketalar). Such combinations produce undesirable additive effects.
4. Sodium bicarbonate and other medications that alkalinize the urine can decrease renal excretion of memantine. Accumulation to toxic levels can result.

E. Rivastigmine (Exelon)
1. Cholinesterase inhibitor used to treat mild to moderate dementia of Alzheimer's disease.
2. Side effects include nausea, vomiting, diarrhea, abdominal pain, and anorexia.
3. Used with caution in clients with peptic ulcer disease, bradycardia, sick sinus syndrome, urinary obstruction, and lung disease because it enhances cholinergic transmission, thus intensifying symptoms of these disorders.

F. Tacrine (Cognex)
1. A centrally acting cholinesterase inhibitor used to treat mild to moderate dementia of Alzheimer's disease.
2. Side effects include ataxia, loss of appetite, nausea, vomiting, and diarrhea.
3. An adverse effect is hepatotoxicity. Liver function studies need to be monitored.

Box 67-10 Medications to Treat Attention-Deficit/Hyperactivity Disorder

Amphetamine
Atomoxetine (Strattera)
Dexmethylphenidate (Focalin)
Dextroamphetamine (Dexedrine)
Dextroamphetamine and amphetamine (Adderall XR)
Methamphetamine (Desoxyn)
Methylphenidate (Ritalin, Concerta, Metadate CD, Methylin)

Box 67-11 Medications to Treat Alzheimer's Disease

Donepezil (Aricept)
Galantamine (Razadyne)
Memantine (Namenda)
Rivastigmine (Exelon)
Tacrine (Cognex)

MORE QUESTIONS ON EVOLVE!

Practice Questions

731. A nurse is caring for a hospitalized client who has been taking clozapine (Clozaril) for the treatment of a schizophrenic disorder. Which laboratory study prescribed for the client will the nurse specifically review to monitor for an adverse effect associated with the use of this medication?
1. Platelet count
2. Cholesterol level
3. White blood cell count
4. Blood urea nitrogen level

732. Disulfiram (Antabuse) is prescribed for a client who is seen in the psychiatric health care clinic. The nurse is collecting data on the client and is providing instructions regarding the use of this medication. Which is most important for the nurse to determine before administration of this medication?
1. A history of hyperthyroidism
2. A history of diabetes insipidus
3. When the last full meal was consumed
4. When the last alcoholic drink was consumed

733. A nurse is collecting data from a client and the client's spouse reports that the client is taking donepezil hydrochloride (Aricept). Which disorder would the nurse suspect that this client may have based on the use of this medication?
1. Dementia
2. Schizophrenia
3. Seizure disorder
4. Obsessive-compulsive disorder

734. Fluoxetine (Prozac)is prescribed for the client. The nurse reinforces instructions to the client regarding the administration of the medication. Which statement by the client indicates an understanding about administration of the medication?
1. "I should take the medication with my evening meal."
2. "I should take the medication at noon with an antacid."
3. "I should take the medication in the morning when I first arise."
4. "I should take the medication right before bedtime with a snack."

735. A client receiving a tricyclic antidepressant arrives at the mental health clinic. Which observation indicates that the client is correctly following the medication plan?
1. Reports not going to work for this past week
2. Complains of not being able to "do anything" anymore

3. Arrives at the clinic neat and appropriate in appearance
4. Reports sleeping 12 hours per night and 3 to 4 hours during the day

736. A nurse is performing a follow-up teaching session with a client discharged 1 month ago who is taking fluoxetine (Prozac). What information would be important for the nurse to gather regarding the adverse effects related to the medication?
1. Cardiovascular symptoms
2. Gastrointestinal dysfunctions
3. Problems with mouth dryness
4. Problems with excessive sweating

737. A client taking buspirone (BuSpar) for 1 month returns to the clinic for a follow-up visit. Which of the following would indicate medication effectiveness?
1. No rapid heartbeats or anxiety
2. No paranoid thought processes
3. No thought broadcasting or delusions
4. No reports of alcohol withdrawal symptoms

738. A client taking lithium carbonate (Lithobid) reports vomiting, abdominal pain, diarrhea, blurred vision, tinnitus, and tremors. The lithium level is checked as a part of the routine follow-up and the level is 3.0 mEq/L. The nurse knows that this level is:
1. Toxic
2. Normal
3. Slightly above normal
4. Excessively below normal

739. A client arrives at the health care clinic and tells the nurse that he has been doubling his daily dosage of bupropion hydrochloride (Wellbutrin) to help him get better faster. The nurse understands that the client is now at risk for which of the following?
1. Insomnia
2. Weight gain
3. Seizure activity
4. Orthostatic hypotension

740. A hospitalized client is started on phenelzine sulfate (Nardil) for the treatment of depression. The nurse instructs the client to avoid consuming which foods while taking this medication? **Select all that apply**.
☐ 1. Figs
☐ 2. Yogurt
☐ 3. Crackers
☐ 4. Aged cheese
☐ 5. Tossed salad
☐ 6. Oatmeal cookies

ANSWERS

731. 3
Rationale: Hematological reactions can occur in the client taking clozapine and include agranulocytosis and mild leukopenia. The white blood cell count should be checked before initiating treatment and should be monitored closely during the use of this medication. The client should also be monitored for signs indicating agranulocytosis, which may include sore throat, malaise, and fever. Options 1, 2, and 4 are unrelated to this medication.
Test-Taking Strategy: Knowledge regarding the adverse effects that can occur in association with the use of clozapine is required to answer this question. Remember, clozapine can cause agranulocytosis and mild leukopenia. If you are unfamiliar with these adverse effects and the laboratory studies that need to be monitored, review this content.
Level of Cognitive Ability: Analyzing
Client Needs: Physiological Integrity
Integrated Process: Nursing Process/Data Collection
Content Area: Pharmacology
Reference: Hodgson, Kizior, pp. 268–269. 2012.

732. 4
Rationale: Disulfiram is used as an adjunct treatment for selected clients with chronic alcoholism who want to remain in a state of enforced sobriety. Clients must abstain from alcohol intake for at least 12 hours before the initial dose of the medication is administered. The most important data are to determine when the last alcoholic drink was consumed. The medication is used with caution in clients with diabetes mellitus, hypothyroidism, epilepsy, cerebral damage, nephritis, and hepatic disease. It is also contraindicated in severe heart disease, psychosis, or hypersensitivity related to the medication.
Test-Taking Strategy: Use the process of elimination, recalling that the medication is used as an adjunct treatment for selected clients with chronic alcoholism. This will assist in directing you to the correct option. Review this medication if you had difficulty with this question.
Level of Cognitive Ability: Analyzing
Client Needs: Physiological Integrity
Integrated Process: Nursing Process/Data Collection
Content Area: Pharmacology
Reference: Lehne, pp. 417–418, 420. 2010.

733. 1
Rationale: Donepezil hydrochloride is a cholinergic agent used in the treatment of mild to moderate dementia of the Alzheimer type. It enhances cholinergic functions by increasing the concentration of acetylcholine. It slows the progression of Alzheimer's disease. Options 2, 3, and 4 are incorrect.
Test-Taking Strategy: Knowledge regarding the use of donepezil hydrochloride is needed to answer this question. Remember, this medication is used to treat mild to moderate dementia. Review this medication if you had difficulty with this question.
Level of Cognitive Ability: Analyzing
Client Needs: Physiological Integrity
Integrated Process: Nursing Process/Data Collection
Content Area: Pharmacology
Reference: Hodgson, Kizior, pp. 374–376. 2012.

734. 3
Rationale: Fluoxetine hydrochloride is administered in the early morning without consideration to meals. Options 1, 2, and 4 are incorrect.
Test-Taking Strategy: Use the process of elimination. Eliminate options 1, 2, and 4 because they are comparable or alike and indicate taking the medication with an antacid or food. If you are unfamiliar with the use of this medication and the client-teaching points, review this content.
Level of Cognitive Ability: Evaluating
Client Needs: Physiological Integrity
Integrated Process: Nursing Process/Evaluation
Content Area: Pharmacology
Reference: Lehne, p. 356. 2010.

735. 3
Rationale: Depressed individuals will sleep for long periods, are not able to go to work, and feel as if they cannot "do anything." Once they have had some therapeutic effect from their medication, they will report resolution of many of these complaints as well as demonstrate an improvement in their appearance.
Test-Taking Strategy: Use the process of elimination. The observations identified in options 1, 2, and 4 are all symptoms of depression. The improvement in appearance indicates a therapeutic response to the medication, thus indicating compliance with the medication regimen. Review the expected effects of tricyclic antidepressants if you had difficulty with this question.
Level of Cognitive Ability: Evaluating
Client Needs: Physiological Integrity
Integrated Process: Nursing Process/Evaluation
Content Area: Pharmacology
Reference: Kee, Hayes, McCuistion, p. 410. 2009.

736. 2
Rationale: The most common adverse effects related to fluoxetine include central nervous system (CNS) and gastrointestinal (GI) system dysfunction. This medication affects the GI system by causing nausea and vomiting, cramping, and diarrhea. Options 1, 3, and 4 are not adverse effects of this medication.
Test-Taking Strategy: Knowledge regarding the adverse effects related to fluoxetine is required to answer this question. Remember that this medication causes CNS and GI system dysfunction. Review these side effects and adverse reactions if you had difficulty with this question.
Level of Cognitive Ability: Analyzing
Client Needs: Physiological Integrity
Integrated Process: Nursing Process/Data Collection
Content Area: Pharmacology
Reference: Hodgson, Kizior, pp. 497–499. 2012.

737. 1
Rationale: Buspirone hydrochloride is not recommended for the treatment of drug or alcohol withdrawal, paranoid thought disorders, or schizophrenia (thought broadcasting or delusions). Buspirone hydrochloride is most often indicated for the treatment of anxiety and aggression.
Test-Taking Strategy: Knowledge regarding the use of buspirone hydrochloride will direct you to the correct option.

Recalling that this medication is an antianxiety drug will direct you to the correct option. Review this medication if you had difficulty with this question.
Level of Cognitive Ability: Evaluating
Client Needs: Physiological Integrity
Integrated Process: Nursing Process/Evaluation
Content Area: Pharmacology
References: Hodgson, Kizior, pp. 154–155. 2012.
Kee, Hayes, McCuistion, p. 407. 2009.

738. 1
Rationale: The therapeutic serum level of lithium is 0.6 to 1.2 mEq/L. A level of 3 mEq/L indicates toxicity.
Test-Taking Strategy: Knowledge regarding the therapeutic serum level of lithium will direct you to the correct option. Remember the therapeutic level is 0.6 to 1.2 mEq/L. Review this level if you had difficulty with this question.
Level of Cognitive Ability: Understanding
Client Needs: Physiological Integrity
Integrated Process: Nursing Process/Data Collection
Content Area: Pharmacology
Reference: Kee, Hayes, McCuistion, pp. 418–419. 2009.

739. 3
Rationale: Bupropion does not cause significant orthostatic blood pressure changes. Seizure activity is common in dosages greater than 450 mg daily. Bupropion frequently causes a drop in body weight. Insomnia is a side effect, but seizure activity causes a greater client risk.

Test-Taking Strategy: Use the process of elimination. Noting that the client has been doubling the medication dose and recalling that seizure activity can occur with higher-than-recommended doses will direct you to option 3. Review this medication if you had difficulty with this question.
Level of Cognitive Ability: Analyzing
Client Needs: Physiological Integrity
Integrated Process: Nursing Process/Data Collection
Content Area: Pharmacology
Reference: Hodgson, Kizior, pp. 154–155. 2012.

740. 1, 2, 4

Rationale: Phenelzine sulfate (Nardil) is a monoamine oxidase inhibitor. The client should avoid taking in foods that are high in tyramine. Use of these foods could trigger a potentially fatal hypertensive crisis. Some foods to avoid include yogurt, aged cheeses, smoked or processed meats, red wines, and fruits such as avocados, raisins, and figs.
Test-Taking Strategy: Recall that phenelzine sulfate is a monoamine oxidase inhibitor and foods high in tyramine must be avoided. Next, from the food items listed in the question, identify the food that contains tyramine. Review the food items to avoid with monoamine oxidase inhibitors if you had difficulty with this question.
Level of Cognitive Ability: Applying
Client Needs: Physiological Integrity
Integrated Process: Nursing Process/Implementation
Content Area: Pharmacology
Reference: Hodgson, Kizior, pp. 922–923. 2012.

UNIT 20

Comprehensive Test

MORE QUESTIONS ON EVOLVE!

Questions

741. A nurse reinforces home care instructions to the parents of a child hospitalized with pertussis. The child is in the convalescent stage and is being prepared for discharge. Which statement by the parents indicates a need for further instructions?
1. "We need to encourage adequate fluid intake."
2. "Coughing spells may be triggered by dust or smoke."
3. "We need to maintain respiratory precautions and a quiet environment for at least 2 weeks."
4. "Good hand-washing techniques need to be instituted to prevent spreading the disease to others."

❖ **742.** A client enters the emergency room confused, twitching, and having seizures. His family states he recently was placed on corticosteroids for arthritis and was feeling better and exercising daily. Upon assessment, he has flushed skin, dry mucous membranes, an elevated temperature, and poor skin turgor. His serum sodium level is 172 mEq/L. Choose the interventions that the health care provider would likely prescribe. **Select all that apply.**
☐ 1. Monitor intake and output.
☐ 2. Monitor the vital signs.
☐ 3. Monitor the electrolyte levels.
☐ 4. Increase water intake orally.
☐ 5. Provide a sodium-reduced diet.
☐ 6. Administer sodium replacements.

743. A nurse is monitoring a client receiving glipizide (Glucotrol). Which outcome indicates an ineffective response from the medication?
1. A decrease in polyuria
2. A decrease in polyphagia
3. A fasting plasma glucose of 100 mg/dL
4. A glycosylated hemoglobin level of 12%

744. A nurse is reinforcing discharge instructions to a client receiving sulfisoxazole. Which of the following would be included in the plan of care for instructions?
1. Maintain a high fluid intake.
2. Discontinue the medication when feeling better.
3. If the urine turns dark brown, call the health care provider immediately.
4. Decrease the dosage when symptoms are improving to prevent an allergic response.

745. Before administering an intermittent tube feeding through a nasogastric tube, the nurse checks for gastric residual volume. The nurse understands that the rationale for checking gastric residual volume before administering the tube feeding is to:
1. Observe the digestion of formula.
2. Check fluid and electrolyte status.
3. Evaluate absorption of the last feeding.
4. Confirm proper nasogastric tube placement.

746. A postoperative client requests medication for flatulence (gas pains). Which medication from the following PRN list should the nurse administer to this client?
1. Ondansetron (Zofran)

    2. Simethicone (Mylicon)
    3. Acetaminophen (Tylenol)
    4. Magnesium hydroxide (milk of magnesia, MOM)

747. A client is admitted to the hospital with a diagnosis of major depression. During the admission interview, the nurse determines that a major concern is the client's altered nutrition related to poor nutritional intake. The appropriate initial nursing intervention related to this concern is:
1. Weigh the client three times per week, before breakfast.
2. Explain to the client the importance of a good nutritional intake.
3. Report the nutritional concern to the psychiatrist and obtain a nutritional consult as soon as possible.
4. Offer the client several small, frequent meals daily, and schedule brief nursing interactions with the client during these times.

748. A client received 20 units of NPH insulin subcutaneously at 8:00 AM. The nurse should check the client for a potential hypoglycemic reaction at what time?
1. 5:00 PM
2. 10:00 AM
3. 11:00 AM
4. 11:00 PM

749. A nurse assists in developing a plan of care for a client with hyperparathyroidism receiving calcitonin-human (Cibacalcin). Which outcome has the highest priority regarding this medication?
1. Relief of pain
2. Absence of side effects
3. Reaching normal serum calcium levels
4. Verbalization of appropriate medication knowledge

750. A nursing instructor asks a nursing student about the cause of hemophilia. The student correctly responds by telling the instructor that:
1. Hemophilia is a Y-linked hereditary disorder.
2. A splenectomy resolves the bleeding disorders.
3. Hemophilia A results from deficiency of factor VIII.
4. A bone marrow transplant is the treatment of choice.

751. A 4-year-old child is admitted to the hospital with suspected acute lymphocytic leukemia (ALL). The nurse understands that which diagnostic study will confirm this diagnosis?
1. A platelet count
2. A lumbar puncture
3. Bone marrow biopsy
4. White blood cell (WBC) count

752. A child with leukemia is experiencing nausea related to medication therapy. The nurse, concerned about the child's nutritional status, should offer which of the following during this episode of nausea?
1. Low-calorie foods
2. Cool, clear liquids
3. Low-protein foods
4. The child's favorite foods

753. To ensure a safe environment for a child admitted to the hospital for a craniotomy to remove a brain tumor, the nurse should include which of the following in the plan of care?
1. Initiating seizure precautions
2. Using a wheelchair for out-of-bed activities
3. Assisting the child with ambulation at all times
4. Avoiding contact with other children on the nursing unit

754. A nurse is preparing to suction an adult client ❖ through the client's tracheostomy tube. Which intervention(s) would the nurse perform for this procedure? **Select all that apply.**
☐ 1. Apply suction for up to 10 to 15 seconds.
☐ 2. Hyperoxygenate the client before suctioning.
☐ 3. Set the wall suction unit pressure at 160 mm Hg.
☐ 4. Apply suction while gently inserting the catheter.
☐ 5. Apply intermittent suction while rotating and withdrawing the catheter.
☐ 6. Advance the catheter until resistance is met and then pull the catheter back 1 cm.

755. A nurse is assisting in caring for a client who has a placenta previa. The nurse understands that a cervical examination will not be performed on the client primarily because it could do which of the following?
1. Initiate premature labor
2. Cause profound hemorrhage
3. Rupture the fetal membranes
4. Increase the chance of infection

756. A mother is breast-feeding her newborn infant. The mother complains to the nurse that she is experiencing severe nipple soreness. The nurse should provide which of the following suggestions to the client?
1. Avoid rotating breast-feeding positions so that the nipple will toughen.
2. Stop nursing during the period of nipple soreness to allow the nipples to heal.
3. Nurse the newborn infant less frequently and substitute a bottle-feeding until the nipples become less sore.

4. Position the newborn infant with the ear, shoulder, and hip in straight alignment and with the baby's stomach against the mother's.

757. Which behavior should the nurse expect a client diagnosed with agoraphobia to describe when discussing the disorder?
    1. A fear of leaving the house
    2. A fear of riding in elevators
    3. A fear of speaking in public
    4. A need to wash hands several times before eating a meal

758. A nurse checks the food on a tray delivered for an Orthodox Jewish client and notes that the client has received a roast beef dinner with whole milk as a beverage. Which action should the nurse take?
    1. Deliver the food tray to the client.
    2. Replace the whole milk with fat-free milk.
    3. Call the dietary department and ask for a different meal.
    4. Ask the dietary department to replace the roast beef with pork.

759. A client is brought to the emergency department by the ambulance team after collapse at home. Cardiopulmonary resuscitation is attempted but is unsuccessful. The wife of the client tells the nurse that the client is an organ donor and that his eyes are to be donated. Which action should the nurse take next?
    1. Place dry, sterile dressings over the eyes of the deceased.
    2. Call the National Donor Association to confirm that the client is a donor.
    3. Close the eyes, elevate the head of the bed, and place a small ice pack on the eyes.
    4. Ask the wife to obtain the legal documents regarding organ donation from the lawyer.

760. A nurse administers a dose of scopolamine (Transderm-Scop) to a postoperative client. The nurse tells the client to expect which of the following side effects of this medication?
    1. Dry mouth
    2. Diaphoresis
    3. Excessive urination
    4. Pupillary constriction

761. A nurse is caring for a child diagnosed with Down syndrome. In describing the disorder to the parents, the nurse bases the explanation on the fact that Down syndrome is a:
    1. Condition characterized by above-average intellectual functioning with deficits in adaptive behavior

    2. Condition characterized by average intellectual functioning and the absence of deficits in adaptive behavior
    3. Condition characterized by subaverage intellectual functioning with the absence of deficits in adaptive behavior
    4. Congenital condition that results in moderate to severe retardation and has been linked to an extra chromosome 21 (group G)

762. A client with a diagnosis of major depression becomes more anxious, reports sleeping poorly, and seems to display increased anger. The nurse interprets the client's behavior as:
    1. The client is at increased risk for suicide.
    2. The client is dealing with pertinent issues.
    3. The client may need some time off the unit.
    4. The client is responding normally to hospitalization.

763. Which of the following electrocardiogram changes should the nurse note on the cardiac monitor with a client whose potassium (K^+) level is 3.2 mEq/L?
    1. U waves
    2. Flat P waves
    3. Elevated T waves
    4. Prolonged PR interval

764. An adult client with hepatic encephalopathy has a serum ammonia level of 120 mcg/dL and receives treatment with lactulose (Chronulac) syrup. The nurse determines that the client has the best and most optimal response if the level changes to which of the following after medication administration?
    1. 2 mcg/dL
    2. 5 mcg/dL
    3. 70 mcg/dL
    4. 100 mcg/dL

765. A nurse assists in developing a plan of care for the child with meningitis. What is the priority nursing diagnosis for this child?
    1. Acute pain
    2. Deficient knowledge related to parenting
    3. Dysfunctional family process
    4. Risk for ineffective cerebral tissue perfusion

766. A nurse is caring for a postoperative client who has been NPO, and the health care provider has prescribed a clear liquid diet. In planning to initiate this diet, which priority item should the nurse place at the client's bedside?
    1. A straw
    2. Code cart
    3. Cardiac monitor
    4. Suction equipment

767. A nurse has given the client taking ethambutol (Myambutol) information about the medication. The nurse determines that the client understands the instructions if the client immediately reports:
1. Impaired sense of hearing
2. Distressing gastrointestinal side effects
3. Orange-red discoloration of body secretions
4. Difficulty discriminating the color red from green

768. A nurse is caring for an older client with a diagnosis of myasthenia gravis and has reinforced self-care instructions. Which statement by the client indicates that further teaching is necessary?
1. "I rest each afternoon after my walk."
2. "I cough and deep breathe many times during the day."
3. "If I get abdominal cramps and diarrhea, I should call my doctor."
4. "I can change the time of my medication on the mornings that I feel strong."

❖ **769.** The nurse should implement which of the following in the care of a child who is having a seizure? **Select all that apply.**
☐ 1. Time the seizure.
☐ 2. Restrain the child.
☐ 3. Stay with the child.
☐ 4. Insert an oral airway.
☐ 5. Place the child in a supine position.
☐ 6. Loosen clothing around the child's neck.

❖ **770.** A nurse is preparing to administer a prescribed intramuscular (IM) dose of meperidine hydrochloride (Demerol), 35 mg, to a client. The medication label reads meperidine hydrochloride, 50 mg/mL. How many milliliters will the nurse administer to the client? **Fill in the blank.**

_____ mL

❖ **771.** A nurse is calculating a client's 24-hour fluid intake. The client consumed coffee (8 oz), water (8 oz), and orange juice (6 oz) for breakfast; soup (4 oz) and iced tea (8 oz) for lunch; and milk (10 oz), tea (8 oz), and water (8 oz) for dinner. The client also consumed 24 oz of water during the day. How many milliliters of fluid did the client consume in the 24-hour period? **Fill in the blank.**

_____mL

772. A client with diabetes mellitus who has been controlled with daily insulin has been placed on atenolol (Tenormin) for the control of angina pectoris. Because of the effects of atenolol, the nurse determines that which of the following is the most reliable indicator of hypoglycemia?
1. Sweating
2. Tachycardia
3. Nervousness
4. Low blood glucose level

❖ **773.** A nurse is asked to regulate the flow rate of an intravenous (IV) solution being administered to a client. The IV bag contains 50 mL of solution and the solution is to be administered over 30 minutes. The administration set has a drop factor of 10 drops (gtt)/mL. The nurse should regulate the roller clamp on the infusion set to deliver how many drops per minute? **Fill in the blank. Round to the nearest whole number.**

_____ gtt/minute

774. Which data would indicate a potential complication associated with age-related changes in the musculoskeletal system?
1. Decrease in height
2. Overall sclerotic lesions
3. Diminished lean body mass
4. Changes in structural bone tissue

775. A nurse provides home care instructions to the mother of a child recovering from Reye's syndrome. Which statement by the mother indicates a need for further instruction?
1. "I need to check for jaundiced skin and eyes every day."
2. "I need to have my child nap during the day to provide rest."
3. "I need to decrease the stimuli at home to prevent intracranial pressure."
4. "I need to give frequent, small, nutritious meals if my child starts to vomit."

❖ **776.** A health care provider prescribes potassium chloride (KCl) elixir, 20 mEq orally twice daily. The medication label states potassium chloride (KCl), 30 mEq/15 mL. The nurse prepares to administer the morning dose. How many milliliters will the nurse prepare to administer one dose? **Fill in the blank.**

_____ mL

777. A nurse provides medication instructions to a client with peptic ulcer disease. Which statement by the client indicates the best understanding of the medication therapy?
1. "Antacids will coat my stomach."
2. "Omeprazole (Prilosec) will coat the ulcer and help it heal."
3. "Sucralfate (Carafate) will change the fluid in my stomach."
4. "The nizatidine (Axid) will cause me to produce less stomach acid."

778. In planning activities for the depressed client, especially during the early stages of hospitalization, which of the following is best?
1. Plan nothing until the client asks to participate in the milieu.
2. Encourage the client to participate in a structured daily program of activities.
3. Give the client a menu of daily activities and insist that the client participate in all activities offered.
4. Provide an activity that is quiet and solitary in nature to avoid increased fatigue, such as working on a puzzle or reading a book.

779. A nurse is assisting in preparing a plan of care for a 4-year-old child hospitalized with nephrotic syndrome. Which dietary intervention is most appropriate for this child?
1. Provide a high-salt diet.
2. Provide a high-protein diet.
3. Discourage visitors at mealtimes.
4. Encourage the child to eat in the playroom.

780. A nursing instructor asks a student to describe the pathophysiology that occurs in Cushing's disease. Which statement by the student indicates an accurate understanding of this disorder?
1. "Cushing's disease is characterized by an oversecretion of insulin."
2. "Cushing's disease is characterized by an oversecretion of glucocorticoid hormones."
3. "Cushing's disease is characterized by an undersecretion of corticotropic hormones."
4. "Cushing's disease is characterized by an undersecretion of glucocorticoid hormones."

781. The nursing instructor asks the nursing student about the physiology related to the cessation of ovulation that occurs during pregnancy. Which response by the student indicates an understanding of this physiological process?
1. "Ovulation ceases during pregnancy because the circulating levels of estrogen and progesterone are high."
2. "Ovulation ceases during pregnancy because the circulating levels of estrogen and progesterone are low."
3. "The low levels of estrogen and progesterone increase the release of follicle-stimulating hormone and luteinizing hormone."
4. "The high levels of estrogen and progesterone promote the release of follicle-stimulating hormone and luteinizing hormone."

782. A nurse is assisting in collecting data on a child with seizures. The nurse is interviewing the child's parents to establish their adjustment to caring for their child with a chronic illness. Which statement by a parent would indicate a need for further teaching?
1. "Our child sleeps in our bedroom at night."
2. "We worry about injuries when our child has a seizure."
3. "Our child is involved in a swim program with neighbors and friends."
4. "Our babysitter just completed cardiopulmonary resuscitation (CPR) training."

783. A client is taking lansoprazole (Prevacid) for the chronic management of Zollinger-Ellison syndrome. The nurse advises the client to take which of the following products if needed for a headache?
1. Naprosyn (Aleve)
2. Ibuprofen (Advil)
3. Acetaminophen (Tylenol)
4. Acetylsalicylic acid (aspirin)

784. A depressed client verbalizes feelings of low self-esteem and self-worth typified by statements such as, "I'm such a failure. I can't do anything right!" The best nursing action would be to:
1. Tell the client that this is not true, and that we all have a purpose in life.
2. Remain with the client and sit in silence until the client verbalizes feelings.
3. Identify recent behaviors or accomplishments that demonstrate skill or ability.
4. Reassure the client that you know how the client is feeling and that things will get better.

785. A nurse is assigned to care for an infant with cryptorchidism. The nurse anticipates that diagnostic studies will be prescribed to evaluate:
1. DNA synthesis
2. Babinski reflex
3. Kidney function
4. Chromosomal analysis

786. A nurse is caring for a client with a diagnosis of pemphigus vulgaris. The nurse understands that a characteristic of this condition is:
1. Dry skin
2. Hard skin
3. Leathery skin
4. Blistering skin

787. A client asks the nurse about the causes of acne. The nurse most appropriately responds by telling the client:
1. "It is caused by oily skin."
2. "The exact cause of acne is not known."
3. "It is caused as a result of exposure to heat and humidity."
4. "Acne is caused by eating chocolate, nuts, and fatty foods."

❖ **788.** The nurse notes the appearance of skin breakdown on a client's hand at the site of an intravenous catheter that had medication infusing. The nurse determines that which adverse effect occurred? **Refer to figure.**

From Lewis, S.L., Dirksen, S.R., Heitkemper, M.M., et al. (2011). *Medical-surgical nursing: Assessment and management of clinical problems* (8th ed.). St. Louis: Mosby.

1. Phlebitis
2. Infiltration
3. Thrombosis
4. Extravasation

789. The nurse is reviewing the health record of a pregnant client at 16 weeks' gestation. The nurse should expect to note documentation that the fundus of the uterus is located at which of the following areas?
1. At the umbilicus
2. Just above the symphysis pubis
3. At the level of the xiphoid process
4. Midway between the symphysis pubis and the umbilicus

790. A nurse is assigned to care for a child with a compound (open) fracture of the arm that occurred as a result of a fall. The nurse plans care, knowing that this type of fracture involves:
1. The entire bone fractured straight across
2. A greater risk of infection than a simple fracture
3. One side of the bone being broken and the other side being bent
4. The bone being fractured but not producing a break in the skin

791. A nursing student is asked to discuss the topic of clubfoot at a clinical conference. The student plans to tell the group that clubfoot:
1. Is a congenital anomaly
2. Always occurs bilaterally
3. Affects girls more often than boys
4. Is a rare deformity of the skeletal system

792. A client with type 1 diabetes mellitus is to begin an exercise program, and the nurse is providing instructions to the client regarding the program. Which of the following should the nurse include in the teaching plan?
1. Try to exercise before mealtime.
2. Administer insulin after exercising.
3. Take a blood glucose test before exercising.
4. Exercise should be performed during peak times of insulin.

793. A nurse is caring for an older client who is terminally ill. Which of the following signs indicates to the nurse that death may be imminent?
1. Rubor and paresthesias
2. Eupnea and normal body temperature
3. Irregular, noisy breathing and cold, clammy skin
4. Presence of swallowing reflex and active bowel sounds

794. A nurse has given the client with tuberculosis instructions for proper handling and disposal of respiratory secretions. The nurse determines that the client understands the instructions if the client verbalizes which of the following?
1. Discard used tissues in a plastic bag.
2. Wash hands at least four times a day.
3. Brush teeth and rinse the mouth once a day.
4. Turn the head to the side if coughing or sneezing.

795. A client who has been taking isoniazid (INH) for 1½ months complains to the nurse about numbness, paresthesias, and tingling in the extremities. The nurse interprets that the client is experiencing:
1. Hypercalcemia
2. Peripheral neuritis
3. Small blood vessel spasm
4. Impaired peripheral circulation

796. A nurse is preparing a 2-year-old child with suspected nephrotic syndrome for a renal biopsy to confirm the diagnosis. The mother asks the nurse, "Will my child ever look thin again?" The nurse appropriately responds by saying:
1. "Do you feel guilty about your child's weight gain?"
2. "In most cases, medication and diet will control fluid retention."
3. "Wearing loose-fitting clothing should help conceal the extra weight."
4. "When children are little, it's expected that they'll look a little chubby."

❖ **797.** A nurse is caring for a client hospitalized with acute exacerbation of chronic obstructive pulmonary disease (COPD). Which of the following would the nurse expect to note in this client? **Select all that apply.**
  ❏ 1. Hypocapnia
  ❏ 2. Dyspnea on exertion
  ❏ 3. Presence of a productive cough
  ❏ 4. Difficulty breathing while talking
  ❏ 5. Increased oxygen saturation with exercise
  ❏ 6. A shortened expiratory phase of respiration

❖ **798.** A nurse is preparing to administer an enema to an adult client. Choose the interventions that the nurse would perform for this procedure. **Select all that apply.**
  ❏ 1. Apply disposable gloves.
  ❏ 2. Place the client in the right Sims' position.
  ❏ 3. Lubricate the enema tube and insert it approximately 4 inches.
  ❏ 4. Clamp the tubing if the client expresses discomfort during the procedure.
  ❏ 5. Hang the container containing the enema solution 24 inches above the client's anus.
  ❏ 6. Ensure that the temperature of the solution is between 100° F (37.8° C) and 105° F (40.5° C).

❖ **799.** A nurse is assigned to care for an adult client who had a brain attack (stroke) and is aphasic. Choose the appropriate interventions for communicating with the client. **Select all that apply.**
  ❏ 1. Face the client when talking.
  ❏ 2. Speak slowly and maintain eye contact.
  ❏ 3. Use gestures when talking to enhance words.
  ❏ 4. Avoid the use of body language when talking to the client.
  ❏ 5. Give the client directions using short phrases and simple terms.
  ❏ 6. Phrase what was said differently the second time, if there is a need to repeat it.

800. The nurse observes that a client with a nasogastric tube connected to continuous gastric suction is mouth breathing, has dry mucous membranes, and has a foul breath odor. In planning care, which nursing intervention would be best to maintain the integrity of this client's oral mucosa?
  1. Offer small sips of water frequently.
  2. Encourage the client to suck on sour, hard candy.
  3. Use lemon glycerin swabs to provide oral hygiene.
  4. Brush the client's teeth frequently. Use diluted mouthwash and water to rinse the mouth.

801. A client is admitted to the hospital with possible rheumatic endocarditis. The nurse would check the client for signs and symptoms of concurrent:
  1. Viral infection
  2. Yeast infection
  3. Streptococcal infection
  4. Staphylococcal infection

802. A client who is taking hydrochlorothiazide (HydroDIURIL, HCTZ) has been started on triamterene (Dyrenium) as well. The client asks the nurse why both medications are required. The nurse formulates a response, based on the understanding that:
  1. Both are weak potassium-losing diuretics.
  2. The combination of these medications prevents renal toxicity.
  3. Hydrochlorothiazide is an expensive medication, so using a combination of diuretics is cost-effective.
  4. Triamterene is a potassium-sparing diuretic, whereas hydrochlorothiazide is a potassium-losing diuretic.

803. A client who has begun taking fosinopril (Monopril) is very distressed, telling the nurse that he cannot taste food normally since beginning the medication 2 weeks ago. The nurse provides the best support to the client by:
  1. Telling the client not to take the medication with food
  2. Suggesting that the client taper the dose until taste returns to normal
  3. Informing the client that impaired taste is expected and generally disappears in 2 to 3 months
  4. Requesting that the health care provider (HCP) change the prescription to another brand of angiotensin-converting enzyme (ACE) inhibitor

804. A nurse is planning to administer amlodipine (Norvasc) to a client. The nurse plans to check which of the following before giving the medication?
  1. Respiratory rate
  2. Blood pressure and heart rate
  3. Heart rate and respiratory rate
  4. Level of consciousness and blood pressure

805. A client had an aortic valve replacement 2 days ago. This morning, the client says to the nurse, "I don't feel any better than I did before surgery." The appropriate response by the nurse is:
  1. "You will feel better in a week or two."
  2. "It's only the second day post-op. Cheer up."
  3. "This is a normal frustration. It'll get better."
  4. "You are concerned that you don't feel any better after surgery?"

❖ **806.** A nurse is preparing a list of home care instructions regarding stoma and laryngectomy care to a client. Choose the instructions that would be included in the list. **Select all that apply.**

- ❐ 1. Restrict fluid intake.
- ❐ 2. Obtain a Medic-Alert bracelet.
- ❐ 3. Keep the humidity in the home low.
- ❐ 4. Prevent debris from entering the stoma.
- ❐ 5. Avoid exposure to people with infections.
- ❐ 6. Avoid swimming and use care when showering.

807. A nurse administers an injection to a client with a diagnosis of acquired immunodeficiency syndrome (AIDS). After administering the medication, the nurse disposes of the used needle by:

1. Asking the client to recap the needle
2. Placing the needle and syringe in a puncture-resistant container
3. Recapping the needle before placing it in a puncture-resistant container
4. Laying the needle and syringe on the bedside table and carefully recapping the needle

808. A nurse is identifying clients in the community at risk for latex allergy. Which client population is most at risk for developing this type of allergy?

1. Children in day care centers
2. Individuals with spina bifida
3. Individuals with cardiac disease
4. Individuals living in a group home

809. A client has just had a cast removed and the underlying skin is yellow-brown and crusted. The nurse determines that further skin care instructions are required when the client states:

1. "I will soak the skin and then wash it gently."
2. "I need to scrub the skin vigorously with soap and water."
3. "I need to apply an emollient lotion to enhance softening."
4. "I need to use a sunscreen on the skin if it's exposed for a period of time."

810. A client has had skeletal traction applied to the right leg and has an overhead trapeze available for use. The nurse should monitor which of the following as a high-risk area for pressure and breakdown?

1. Scapulae
2. Left heel
3. Right heel
4. Back of the head

811. A client has been placed in Buck's extension traction. The nurse can provide for countertraction by:

1. Using a footboard

2. Providing an overhead trapeze
3. Slightly elevating the foot of the bed
4. Slightly elevating the head of the bed

812. A nurse would expect to note which interventions ❖ in the plan of care for a client with hypothyroidism? **Select all that apply.**

- ❐ 1. Provide a cool environment for the client.
- ❐ 2. Instruct the client to consume a high-fat diet.
- ❐ 3. Instruct the client about thyroid replacement therapy.
- ❐ 4. Encourage the client to consume fluids and high-fiber foods in the diet.
- ❐ 5. Instruct the client to contact the health care provider if episodes of chest pain occur.
- ❐ 6. Inform the client that iodine preparations will be prescribed to treat the disorder.

813. A nurse is admitting a client with Guillain-Barré syndrome to the nursing unit. The client has an ascending paralysis to the level of the waist. Knowing the complications of the disorder, the nurse brings which of the following items into the client's room?

1. Nebulizer and pulse oximeter
2. Blood pressure cuff and flashlight
3. Flashlight and incentive spirometer
4. Electrocardiographic monitoring electrodes and intubation tray

814. A client with chronic renal failure is receiving ferrous sulfate (Feosol). The nurse monitors the client for which common side effect associated with this medication?

1. Diarrhea
2. Weakness
3. Headache
4. Constipation

815. A nurse is attempting to communicate with a hearing-impaired client. Which of the following strategies by the nurse would be least helpful when talking to this client?

1. Reducing any background noise
2. Smiling continuously during conversation
3. Facing the client so that there is light on the nurse's face
4. Avoiding showing frustration through facial expression

816. A nurse is preparing to administer digoxin (Lanoxin), 0.125 mg orally, to a client with heart failure. Which vital sign is most **important for the nurse to check before administering the medication?**

1. Heart rate
2. Temperature
3. Respirations
4. Blood pressure

817. A postoperative client has a prescription to receive an intravenous (IV) infusion of 1000 mL normal saline solution over a period of 10 hours. The drop (gtt) factor for the IV infusion set is 15 gtt/mL. The nurse sets the flow rate at how many drops per minute? **Fill in the blank.**

_____ gtt/minute

818. A nurse is preparing to set up a sterile field using the principles of aseptic technique to perform a dressing change. Which of the following should the nurse include in the preparations? **Select all that apply.**
- ❏ 1. Use a dry table that is below waist level.
- ❏ 2. Open the distal flap of a sterile package first.
- ❏ 3. Prepare the sterile field just before the planned procedure.
- ❏ 4. Don clean gloves before touching items on the sterile field.
- ❏ 5. Place the sterile field 1 foot behind the working area and out of view of the client.
- ❏ 6. Avoid placing items within 1 inch of any area surrounding the outer edge of the sterile field.

819. A nurse is performing nasotracheal suctioning of a client. The nurse interprets that the client is adequately tolerating the procedure if which of the following observations are made?
1. Skin color becomes cyanotic.
2. Secretions are becoming bloody.
3. Coughing occurs with suctioning.
4. Heart rate decreases from 78 to 54 beats/minute.

820. A nurse inspects the oral cavity of a client with cancer and notes white patches on the mucous membranes. The nurse determines that this occurrence:
1. Is common
2. Suggests that the client is anemic
3. Is characteristic of a thrush infection
4. Is indicative that oral hygiene needs to be improved

821. A nurse is monitoring the laboratory results of a client preparing to receive chemotherapy. The nurse determines that the white blood cell count (WBC) is normal if which of the following results were present?

1. 2000 cells/mm^3
2. 3000 cells/mm^3
3. 5000 cells/mm^3
4. 15,000 cells/mm^3

822. A nurse instructs the client in breast self-examination (BSE). The nurse instructs the client to lie down and examine the left breast. The nurse instructs the client that while examining the left breast, to place a pillow:
1. Under the left shoulder
2. Under the right scapula
3. Under the right shoulder
4. Under the small of the back

823. A client suspected of having an abdominal tumor is scheduled for a computed tomography (CT) scan with dye injection. The nurse tells the client which of the following about the test?
1. The test may be painful.
2. The test takes approximately 2 to 3 hours.
3. Fluids will be restricted after the test.
4. The dye injected may cause a warm, flushing sensation.

824. A nurse is caring for a client dying of ovarian cancer. During care, the client states, "If I can just live long enough to attend my daughter's graduation, I'll be ready to die." Which phase of coping is this client experiencing?
1. Anger
2. Denial
3. Bargaining
4. Depression

825. A nurse is caring for a client who has been prescribed furosemide (Lasix) and is monitoring for adverse effects associated with this medication. Which of the following should the nurse recognize as a potential adverse effect? **Select all that apply.**
- ❏ 1. Nausea
- ❏ 2. Tinnitus
- ❏ 3. Hypotension
- ❏ 4. Hypokalemia
- ❏ 5. Photosensitivity
- ❏ 6. Increased urinary frequency

ANSWERS

741. 3

Rationale: Pertussis is transmitted by direct contact or respiratory droplets from coughing. The communicable period occurs primarily during the catarrhal stage. Respiratory precautions are not required during the convalescent phase. Options 1, 2, and 4 are components of home care instructions.

Test-Taking Strategy: Note the strategic words "convalescent" and "need for further instructions." These words indicate a negative event query and the need to select the incorrect statement. Options 1 and 4 can be easily eliminated because they are general interventions associated with convalescence. Knowing that coughing spells are associated with pertussis will assist in directing you to option 3 from the remaining options. In addition, a 2-week period of respiratory precautions is not required.

If you had difficulty with this question, review home care instructions for the child with pertussis.
Level of Cognitive Ability: Evaluating
Client Needs: Safe and Effective Care Environment
Integrated Process: Teaching and Learning
Content Area: Child Health: Integumentary/AIDS/Infectious Diseases
Reference: McKinney, James, Murray, Ashwill, pp. 1028–1029. 2009.

❖ **742. 1, 2, 3, 4, 5**
Rationale: Hypernatremia is described as having a serum sodium level that exceeds 145 mEq/L. Signs and symptoms would include dry mucous membranes, loss of skin turgor, thirst, flushed skin, elevated temperature, oliguria, muscle twitching, fatigue, confusion, and seizures. Interventions include monitoring fluid balance, monitoring vital signs, reducing dietary intake of sodium, monitoring electrolyte levels, and increasing oral intake of water. Sodium replacement therapy would not be prescribed for a client with hypernatremia.
Test-Taking Strategy: Focus on the data in the question. Noting that a sodium level of 172 mEq/L is elevated will direct you to the correct options. If you had difficulty with this question, review the care for the client experiencing hypernatremia.
Level of Cognitive Ability: Analyzing
Client Needs: Physiological Integrity
Integrated Process: Nursing Process/Planning
Content Area: Fundamental Skills: Fluids & Electrolytes/Acid-Base
Reference: Kunz, Steinmann, p. 495. 2010.

743. 4
Rationale: Glipizide (Glucotrol) is an oral hypoglycemic agent administered to decrease the serum glucose level and the signs and symptoms of hyperglycemia. Therefore, a decrease in both polyuria and polyphagia would indicate a therapeutic response. Laboratory values are also used to monitor a client's response to treatment. A fasting blood glucose level of 100 mg/dL is within normal limits. However, glycosylated hemoglobin of 12% indicates poor glycemic control.
Test-Taking Strategy: Note the strategic words "ineffective response." Recalling that glipizide is an oral hypoglycemic agent tells you to look for an option that would indicate hyperglycemia (lack of response to the medication). Options 1 and 2 are comparable or alike and are eliminated first. Next, eliminate option 3 because it is a normal blood glucose level. Review this medication if you had difficulty with this question.
Level of Cognitive Ability: Evaluating
Client Needs: Physiological Integrity
Integrated Process: Nursing Process/Evaluation
Content Area: Adult Health/Endocrine
References: Lehne, p. 687. 2010.
Pagana, Pagana, pp. 491–493. 2009.

744. 1
Rationale: Each dose of sulfisoxazole should be administered with a full glass of water, and the client should maintain a high fluid intake. The medication is more soluble in alkaline urine. The client should not be instructed to taper or discontinue the dose. Some forms of sulfisoxazole cause the urine to turn dark

brown or red. This does not indicate the need to notify the health care provider.
Test-Taking Strategy: Use the process of elimination. General principles related to medication administration will assist in eliminating options 2 and 4. From the remaining options, recalling that this medication is a sulfonamide will direct you to option 1. Review this medication if you had difficulty with this question.
Level of Cognitive Ability: Applying
Client Needs: Physiological Integrity
Integrated Process: Teaching and Learning
Content Area: Pharmacology
Reference: Lehne, p. 1030. 2010.

745. 3
Rationale: All the stomach contents are aspirated and measured before administering a tube feeding. This procedure measures the gastric residual volume. The gastric residual volume is checked to confirm whether undigested formula from a previous feeding remains, and thereby evaluates the absorption of the last feeding. It is important to check the gastric residual before administration of a tube feeding. A full stomach could result in overdistention, thus predisposing the client to regurgitation and possible aspiration. If residual feeding is obtained, the health care provider's prescription and agency policy are checked to determine the course of action (hold or reduce the volume of the intermittent tube feeding).
Test-Taking Strategy: Note that the subject of the question is the purpose of checking residual volume. Focusing on this subject should direct you to the correct option. Review the procedure for checking gastric residual volume if you had difficulty with this question.
Level of Cognitive Ability: Understanding
Client Needs: Physiological Integrity
Integrated Process: Nursing Process/Data Collection
Content Area: Adult Health/Gastrointestinal
Reference: Linton, pp. 779–781. 2012.

746. 2
Rationale: Simethicone is an antiflatulent used in the relief of pain caused by excessive gas in the gastrointestinal tract. Ondansetron is used to treat postoperative nausea and vomiting. Acetaminophen is a nonopioid analgesic. Magnesium hydroxide is an antacid and laxative.
Test-Taking Strategy: Use the process of elimination and note the strategic words "flatulence (gas pains)." Recalling the classifications of the medications in the options will direct you to the correct option. If this question was difficult, review this medication.
Level of Cognitive Ability: Applying
Client Needs: Physiological Integrity
Integrated Process: Nursing Process/Implementation
Content Area: Pharmacology
Reference: Hodgson, Kizior, pp. 1058–1059. 2012.

747. 4
Rationale: Change in appetite is one of the major symptoms of depression. Offering the client several small, frequent meals and the nurse's presence at that time to support, encourage,

or perhaps even feed the client is the most appropriate intervention. A client with depression experiences poor concentration and will not understand the importance of an adequate nutritional intake. Weighing the client does not address how to increase nutritional intake. Reporting the nutritional problems to the psychiatrist is correct to some degree, but does not address how one might increase food intake.
Test-Taking Strategy: Note the strategic word "initial" and focus on the subject, the poor nutritional intake. Option 4 is the only option that addresses the altered nutrition concretely and designs a method in which the client will feasibly increase the nutritional intake. Review care of the client with depression if you had difficulty with this question.
Level of Cognitive Ability: Applying
Client Needs: Physiological Integrity
Integrated Process: Nursing Process/Implementation
Content Area: Mental Health
Reference: Varcarolis, Halter, p. 229. 2009.

748. 1
Rationale: NPH is intermediate-acting insulin. Its onset of action is 1 to 2½ hours, it peaks in 4 to 12 hours, and its duration of action is 24 hours. Hypoglycemic reactions most likely occur during peak time.
Test-Taking Strategy: Focus on the subject, NPH insulin. Recalling that peak action is between 4 and 12 hours will direct you to the correct option. Review the characteristics of NPH insulin if you had difficulty with this question.
Level of Cognitive Ability: Applying
Client Needs: Physiological Integrity
Integrated Process: Nursing Process/Implementation
Content Area: Pharmacology
Reference: Lehne, pp. 665–666. 2010.

749. 3
Rationale: Hypercalcemia can occur in clients with hyperparathyroidism, and calcitonin is used to lower plasma calcium level. The highest priority outcome in this client situation would be a reduction in serum calcium level. Option 1 is unrelated to this medication. Although options 2 and 4 are expected outcomes, they are not the highest priority for administering this medication.
Test-Taking Strategy: Use the process of elimination. Noting the client diagnosis will assist in directing you to option 3. In addition, note the relation between the name of the medication and the word "calcium" in option 3. Review this medication if you had difficulty with this question.
Level of Cognitive Ability: Analyzing
Client Needs: Physiological Integrity
Integrated Process: Nursing Process/Planning
Content Area: Adult Health/Endocrine
Reference: Linton, p. 418. 2012.

750. 3
Rationale: The term "hemophilia" refers to a group of bleeding disorders. The identification of the specific factor deficiencies allows for definitive treatment with replacement agents. Hemophilia A results from a deficiency of factor VIII. Hemophilia B (Christmas disease) is a deficiency of factor IX. Hemophilia is inherited in a recessive manner via a genetic defect on the X chromosome, not the Y chromosome. Neither a bone marrow transplant nor splenectomy is used to treat this disorder.
Test-Taking Strategy: Knowledge regarding hemophilia and related causes and treatment is needed to answer the question. Remember, hemophilia A results from a deficiency of factor VIII. Review this disorder if you had difficulty with this question.
Level of Cognitive Ability: Understanding
Client Needs: Physiological Integrity
Integrated Process: Teaching and Learning
Content Area: Child Health: Hematological/Oncological
Reference: Leifer, pp. 632–633. 2011.

751. 3
Rationale: The confirmatory test for leukemia is microscopic examination of bone marrow obtained by bone marrow aspirate and biopsy. The WBC count may be high or low in leukemia. A lumbar puncture may be done to look for blast cells in the spinal fluid that are indicative of central nervous system disease. An altered platelet count occurs as a result of chemotherapy.
Test-Taking Strategy: Use the process of elimination and note the strategic word "confirm." Noting this strategic word and recalling that the bone marrow is affected in leukemia will direct you to the correct option. Review diagnostic studies related to leukemia if you had difficulty with this question.
Level of Cognitive Ability: Understanding
Client Needs: Physiological Integrity
Integrated Process: Nursing Process/Planning
Content Area: Child Health: Hematological/Oncological
Reference: McKinney, James, Murray, Ashwill, p. 1312. 2009.

752. 2
Rationale: When the child is nauseated, it is best to offer frequent intake of cool, clear liquids in small amounts because small portions are usually better tolerated. Cool, clear fluids are also soothing and better tolerated when a client is nauseated. It is best not to offer favorite foods when the child is nauseated because foods eaten during times of nausea will be associated with being sick. It is best to offer small, frequent meals of high-protein and high-calorie content once the nausea has been controlled with medication or has subsided.
Test-Taking Strategy: The subject of the question relates to nutritional status in a child with nausea. You should easily be able to eliminate options 1 and 3 because of the word "low" in these options. From the remaining options, recalling that the subject is related to nausea will assist in directing you to option 2. Review interventions related to relieving nausea if you had difficulty with this question.
Level of Cognitive Ability: Applying
Client Needs: Physiological Integrity
Integrated Process: Nursing Process/Implementation
Content Area: Child Health: Gastrointestinal/Renal
Reference: McKinney, James, Murray, Ashwill, p. 1317. 2009.

753. 1
Rationale: Safety of the child is the nursing priority. Seizure precautions should be implemented for any child with a brain tumor, both preoperatively and postoperatively. A thorough neurological assessment should be performed on the child,

and the child's safety should be assessed before allowing the child to get out of bed without help. Assessment of the child's gait should be assessed daily. However, options 2 and 3 are not required unless functional deficits exist. Isolating the child, option 4, is not necessary.

Test-Taking Strategy: Use the process of elimination and note the strategic words "safe environment." Eliminate options 2 and 3 first because they are comparable or alike. In addition, note the closed-ended word "all" in option 3. Eliminate option 4 because it is unnecessary. Review care of the child with a brain tumor if you had difficulty with this question.

Level of Cognitive Ability: Applying
Client Needs: Safe and Effective Care Environment
Integrated Process: Nursing Process/Planning
Content Area: Child Health: Neurological/Musculoskeletal
Reference: McKinney, James, Murray, Ashwill, p. 1323. 2009.

❖ **754. 1, 2, 5, 6**
Rationale: Intermittent suction is applied while rotating the catheter for 10 to 15 seconds. The nurse should hyperoxygenate the client with a resuscitator bag/Ambu-bag connected to an oxygen source before suctioning because suction depletes the client's oxygen supply (option 2). The catheter should be inserted quickly and gently until resistance is met or the client coughs; then pulled back 1 cm or ½ inch. Intermittent suction is applied while rotating and withdrawing the catheter. Option 3 is incorrect because wall suction should be set to 80 to 120 mm Hg. Pressure set at a higher level can cause trauma to respiratory tract tissues. Strict asepsis needs to be maintained, and the nurse would wear sterile gloves to perform this procedure. Suction is never applied when inserting the catheter because it will deplete oxygen and can traumatize tissues.

Test-Taking Strategy: Focus on the subject, suctioning procedure through a tracheostomy. The priority issues to think about when answering this question include maintaining oxygenation, maintaining asepsis, and preventing tissue trauma. This will assist in selecting the correct interventions. Review suctioning procedure if you had difficulty with this question.

Level of Cognitive Ability: Applying
Client Needs: Physiological Integrity
Integrated Process: Nursing Process/Implementation
Content Area: Adult Health/Respiratory
References: deWit, pp. 310–312. 2009.
Linton, pp. 1268–1269. 2012.

755. 2
Rationale: Because the placenta is implanted low in the uterus, cervical examination could cause the disruption of the placenta and initiate profound hemorrhage. The other options are also correct, but the profound hemorrhage is of the greatest concern in this case.

Test-Taking Strategy: Use the process of elimination and note the strategic word "primarily." Recalling that bleeding is a primary concern will direct you to the correct option. Review care of the client with placenta previa if you had difficulty with this question.

Level of Cognitive Ability: Understanding
Client Needs: Physiological Integrity
Integrated Process: Nursing Process/Implementation
Content Area: Maternity/Antepartum
Reference: McKinney, James, Murray, Ashwill, pp. 614–615. 2009.

756. 4
Rationale: Severe nipple soreness most often occurs as a result of poor positioning, incorrect latch-on, improper suck, or monilial infection. Comfort measures for nipple soreness include positioning the newborn with the ear, shoulder, and hip in straight alignment and with the baby's stomach against the mother's. Options 1, 2, and 3 do not identify measures that will alleviate the nipple soreness.

Test-Taking Strategy: Use the process of elimination to answer the question. Eliminate options 2 and 3 because they are comparable or alike. From the remaining options, careful reading of option 1 will assist in eliminating this option. Review these measures if you had difficulty with this question.

Level of Cognitive Ability: Applying
Client Needs: Health Promotion and Maintenance
Integrated Process: Teaching and Learning
Content Area: Maternity/Postpartum
Reference: McKinney, James, Murray, Ashwill, p. 571. 2009.

757. 1
Rationale: Agoraphobia is a fear of open spaces (i.e., leaving the house); panic attacks may occur when doing so. Option 2 describes a fear of closed spaces (claustrophobia). Option 3 describes a fear of public speaking (social phobia). Option 4 describes an obsessive-compulsive behavior.

Test-Taking Strategy: Use the process of elimination and focus on the strategic word "agoraphobia." Recalling the definition of agoraphobia will assist in directing you to the correct option. If you had difficulty with this question, review the various types of phobias.

Level of Cognitive Ability: Understanding
Client Needs: Psychosocial Integrity
Integrated Process: Nursing Process/Data Collection
Content Area: Mental Health
Reference: Morrison-Valfre, p. 197. 2009.

758. 3
Rationale: In the Orthodox Jewish tradition, members avoid meat from carnivores, pork products, and certain fish. The nurse would not deliver the food tray to the client and would ask the dietary department to deliver a different meal. Meat and dairy are served separately, thus the dairy-meat combination is not acceptable, making option 2 incorrect. Option 4 is incorrect because pork and pork products are also not allowed in the diet.

Test-Taking Strategy: Use the process of elimination. Recalling that the dairy-meat combination is not acceptable in the Orthodox Jewish tradition will direct you to the correct option. Review the dietary rules of this religious group if you had difficulty with this question.

Level of Cognitive Ability: Applying
Client Needs: Psychosocial Integrity
Integrated Process: Nursing Process/Implementation
Content Area: Fundamental Skills/Cultural Diversity
Reference: Nix, pp. 256, 522–523. 2009.

759. 3
Rationale: When a corneal donor dies, antibiotic eye drops, such as Neosporin or tobramycin may be prescribed and instilled. The eyes are closed and a small ice pack is placed on the closed eyes. The head of the bed is raised to 30 degrees.

Within 2 to 4 hours, the eyes are enucleated. The cornea is usually transplanted within 24 to 48 hours. Option 1 is incorrect because dry dressings are not applied. Some organ donation protocols indicate using normal saline-moistened gauze. Option 2 is not an immediate action. In addition, the client should have a signed donor card, living will, or an organ donor–identified driver's license stating his or her wishes. Additional legal documentation should not be required.

Test-Taking Strategy: Use the process of elimination. Note that the subject relates to preservation of the corneas and donation of the eyes. This should assist in eliminating options 2 and 4. From the remaining options, recalling that the head of the bed should be elevated will direct you to option 3. Review this procedure if you had difficulty with the question.

Level of Cognitive Ability: Applying
Client Needs: Safe and Effective Care Environment
Integrated Process: Nursing Process/Implementation
Content Area: Leadership/Management: Ethical/Legal
Reference: Ignatavicius, Workman, p. 1091. 2010.

760. 1

Rationale: Scopolamine is an anticholinergic medication that causes the frequent side effects of dry mouth, urinary retention, decreased sweating, and dilation of the pupils. The other options describe the opposite effects of cholinergic-blocking agents and therefore are incorrect.

Test-Taking Strategy: Use the process of elimination. Recalling that this medication is an anticholinergic will direct you to the correct option. If this medication is unfamiliar to you, review the side effects associated with anticholinergics.

Level of Cognitive Ability: Applying
Client Needs: Physiological Integrity
Integrated Process: Nursing Process/Implementation
Content Area: Pharmacology
Reference: Hodgson, Kizior, pp. 1048–1049. 2012.

761. 4

Rationale: Down syndrome is a form of mental retardation. It is a congenital condition that results in moderate to severe mental retardation. The syndrome has been linked to an extra group G chromosome, chromosome 21 (trisomy 21). Options 1, 2, and 3 are incorrect descriptions.

Test-Taking Strategy: Use the process of elimination. Eliminate options 1 and 2 first because average and above-average intelligence are not associated with this disorder. Eliminate option 3 because deficits in adaptive behavior do occur with Down syndrome. Also, recalling that Down syndrome is associated with an extra chromosome will help direct you to the correct option. Review the characteristics of this syndrome if you had difficulty with this question.

Level of Cognitive Ability: Understanding
Client Needs: Physiological Integrity
Integrated Process: Nursing Process/Implementation
Content Area: Child Health: Neurological/Musculoskeletal
Reference: Hockenberry, Wilson, pp. 619–620. 2009.

762. 1

Rationale: The behaviors identified in the question may be manifested by the client who is contemplating suicide. In clients who are depressed, anger may be self-directed in the form

of suicide. Many of these symptoms are those of the depressed client; however, with this client, these behaviors have increased. Hospitalization may actually lessen these symptoms in the depressed client, because a feeling of hope or relief may occur once treatment begins. Dealing with pertinent issues may be traumatic, but this is not the best interpretation of the behavior. Time off the unit for this client could put the client at risk for injury.

Test-Taking Strategy: Use the process of elimination and focus on the client behaviors addressed in the question. Noting the client's diagnosis and the words "becomes more anxious" will direct you to option 1. If you had difficulty with this question, review the characteristics and client behaviors related to suicide.

Level of Cognitive Ability: Analyzing
Client Needs: Psychosocial Integrity
Integrated Process: Nursing Process/Data Collection
Content Area: Mental Health
Reference: Morrison-Valfre, pp. 298–299, 301. 2009.

763. 1

Rationale: A serum potassium level less than 3.5 mEq/L is indicative of hypokalemia. Potassium deficit is the most common electrolyte imbalance and is potentially life threatening. Cardiac changes with hypokalemia may include peaked P waves, flattened T waves, depressed ST segment, and the presence of U waves.

Test-Taking Strategy: Use the process of elimination. From the information in the question, you need to determine that this client is experiencing hypokalemia. From this point, it is necessary to know the cardiac changes that are expected when hypokalemia exists. Options 2, 3, and 4 are all characteristic cardiac changes noted with hyperkalemia. Review these cardiac effects if you had difficulty with this question.

Level of Cognitive Ability: Analyzing
Client Needs: Physiological Integrity
Integrated Process: Nursing Process/Data Collection
Content Area: Fundamental Skills: Fluids & Electrolytes/Acid-Base
References: deWit, pp. 46, 48. 2009.
Linton, p. 188. 2012.

764. 3

Rationale: The normal serum ammonia level is 10 to 80 mcg/dL. In the client with hepatic encephalopathy, the serum level is not likely to drop below normal. The most optimal yet realistic change from the options provided would be to 70 mcg/dL, which falls in the normal range. A level of 100 mcg/dL represents an insufficient effect of the medication. Lactulose is administered for its hyperosmotic laxative effect, thus removing ammonia from the colon. The client should also be monitored for hypokalemia resulting from the severe purging lactulose causes.

Test-Taking Strategy: Familiarity with the normal serum ammonia level is needed to answer this question. It is also necessary to understand the association between hepatic encephalopathy and this laboratory value. Recalling that the normal level is 10 to 80 mcg/dL will direct you to the correct option. Review this test and the desirable effects of this medication if you had difficulty with this question.

Level of Cognitive Ability: Analyzing

Client Needs: Physiological Integrity
Integrated Process: Nursing Process/Data Collection
Content Area: Adult Health/Gastrointestinal
Reference: Pagana, Pagana, pp. 46–47. 2009.

765. 4

Rationale: Risk for ineffective cerebral tissue perfusion is the priority problem for the child with meningitis. Pain related to meningeal irritation may also be an appropriate problem, but is not the priority. There are no data in the question to indicate that options 2 and 3 are a problem.
Test-Taking Strategy: Use Maslow's Hierarchy of Needs theory to assist in eliminating options 2 and 3 because they are psychosocial problems. Next, use the ABCs—airway, breathing, and circulation—to direct you to option 4. Tissue perfusion relates to circulation. Review care of the child with meningitis if you had difficulty with this question.
Level of Cognitive Ability: Analyzing
Client Needs: Physiological Integrity
Integrated Process: Nursing Process/Planning
Content Area: Fundamental Skills: Fluids & Electrolytes/ Acid-Base
Reference: Hockenberry, Wilson, p. 1000. 2009.

766. 4

Rationale: In a postoperative client, a concern related to initiating a diet is aspiration. Initiating postoperative oral fluids may lead to distention and vomiting. Suction equipment must be available. A cardiac monitor and a code cart are unnecessary. A straw may help the client sip fluids, but is not necessary.
Test-Taking Strategy: Note the strategic words "postoperative" and "priority." Use the ABCs—airway, breathing, and circulation—to answer this question. Option 4 will maintain airway clearance. If you had difficulty with this question, review care to the postoperative client.
Level of Cognitive Ability: Applying
Client Needs: Safe and Effective Care Environment
Integrated Process: Nursing Process/Planning
Content Area: Fundamental Skills: Perioperative Care
References: deWit, pp. 94–95. 2009.
Potter, Perry, pp. 1401, 1405. 2009.

767. 4

Rationale: Ethambutol causes optic neuritis, which decreases visual acuity and the ability to discriminate between the colors red and green. This poses a potential safety hazard when driving a motor vehicle. The client is taught to report this symptom immediately. The client is also taught to take the medication with food if gastrointestinal upset occurs. Impaired hearing results from antitubercular therapy with streptomycin. Orange-red discoloration of secretions occurs with rifampin (Rifadin).
Test-Taking Strategy: Use the process of elimination. Option 2 is the least likely symptom to report; rather, it should be managed by taking the medication with food. Thus, this option can be eliminated first. From the remaining options, it is necessary to know that ethambutol may cause optic neuritis and difficulty with red-green discrimination. If this question was difficult, review the side effects of this medication.
Level of Cognitive Ability: Evaluating
Client Needs: Physiological Integrity
Integrated Process: Nursing Process/Evaluation
Content Area: Pharmacology

References: Hodgson, Kizior, p. 450. 2012.
Lehne, p. 1051. 2010.

768. 4

Rationale: The client with myasthenia gravis should be taught that timing of anticholinesterase medication is critical. It is important to instruct the client to administer the medication on time to maintain a chemical balance at the neuromuscular junction. If not given on time, the client may become too weak to swallow. Options 1, 2, and 3 include the necessary information that the client needs to understand to maintain health with this neurological degenerative disease.
Test-Taking Strategy: Use the process of elimination and note the strategic words "further teaching is necessary." These words indicate a negative event query and the need to select the incorrect client statement. Basic principles related to medication administration will direct you to the correct option. Remember, clients should not adjust dosage and medication times. If you had difficulty with this question, review the guidelines related to medication administration.
Level of Cognitive Ability: Evaluating
Client Needs: Physiological Integrity
Integrated Process: Teaching and Learning
Content Area: Pharmacology
References: Christensen, Kockrow, p. 693. 2011. *Adult health nursing.*
deWit, p. 607. 2009.

769. 1, 3, 6

Rationale: During a seizure, the child is placed on his or her side in a lateral position. Positioning on the side will prevent aspiration because saliva will drain out of the corner of the child's mouth. The child is not restrained because this could cause injury to the child. The nurse would loosen clothing around the child's neck and ensure a patent airway. Nothing is placed into the child's mouth during a seizure because this action may cause injury to the child's mouth, gums, or teeth. The nurse would stay with the child to reduce the risk of injury and allow for observation and timing of the seizure.
Test-Taking Strategy: Visualize this clinical situation. Recalling that airway patency and safety is the priority will assist in determining the appropriate interventions. Review care for the child experiencing a seizure if you had difficulty with this question.
Level of Cognitive Ability: Applying
Client Needs: Physiological Integrity
Integrated Process: Nursing Process/Implementation
Content Area: Child Health: Neurological/Musculoskeletal
Reference: Hockenberry, Wilson, pp. 1012–1013. 2009.

770. 0.7

Rationale: Use the medication calculation formula and note the prescribed (35 mg) and available doses (50 mg/mL).
Formula:

$$\frac{\text{Desired}}{\text{Available}} \times \text{Volume} = \text{mL per dose}$$

$$\frac{35 \text{ mg}}{50 \text{ mg}} \times 1 \text{ mL} = 0.7 \text{ mL}$$

Test-Taking Strategy: Follow the formula for the calculation of the correct dose, noting the prescribed dose and the available

dose. Note that the prescribed dose is a smaller amount than the dose available. This indicates that the amount to be given will be less than 1 mL. Once you have done the calculation, use a calculator to verify the answer. If you had difficulty with this question, review medication calculation problems.
Level of Cognitive Ability: Applying
Client Needs: Physiological Integrity
Integrated Process: Nursing Process/Implementation
Content Area: Fundamental Skills: Medications/Blood & IV Therapy
Reference: Potter, Perry, pp. 695–699. 2009.

❖ **771. 2520**
Rationale: The client consumed a total of 84 oz of fluid. Because 1 oz is equal to 30 mL, multiply 84 oz by 30 mL/oz. This yields 2520 mL.
Test-Taking Strategy: Focus on the subject, the total milliliters that the client consumed in a 24-hour period. Recalling that 1 oz equals 30 mL will assist in answering the question. Use a calculator to verify the amount. Review the procedure for changing ounces to milliliters if you had difficulty with this question.
Level of Cognitive Ability: Understanding
Client Needs: Physiological Integrity
Integrated Process: Nursing Process/Data Collection
Content Area: Fundamental Skills: Fluids & Electrolytes/ Acid-Base
References: Christensen, Kockrow, p. 689. 2011. *Foundations of nursing.*
Potter, Perry, pp. 695–698. 2009.

772. 4
Rationale: β-Adrenergic blocking agents, such as atenolol, inhibit the appearance of signs and symptoms of acute hypoglycemia, which would include nervousness, increased heart rate, and sweating. Therefore, the client receiving this medication should adhere to the therapeutic regimen and monitor blood glucose levels carefully. Option 4 is the most reliable indicator of hypoglycemia.
Test-Taking Strategy: Note the strategic words "most reliable" in the question. This indicates that more than one option could be partially or completely correct. Each option is, in fact, an indicator of hypoglycemia. Recalling the masking effects of β-adrenergic blocking agents helps you to choose the blood glucose level as the most reliable indicator. Review this medication if you had difficulty with this question.
Level of Cognitive Ability: Analyzing
Client Needs: Physiological Integrity
Integrated Process: Nursing Process/Data Collection
Content Area: Pharmacology
Reference: Skidmore-Roth, p. 169. 2012.

❖ **773. 17**
Rationale: The formula and calculation for this IV flow rate is:
Formula:

$$\frac{\text{Total volume} \times \text{drop factor}}{\text{Time (in minutes)}} = \text{drops per minute}$$

$$\frac{50\ \text{mL} \times 10\ \text{gtt/mL}}{30\ \text{minutes}} = 16.66,\ \text{or } 17\ \text{gtt/minute}$$

Test-Taking Strategy: To calculate the answer to this question correctly, you must be familiar with the standard formula for calculating IV flow rates. Use the formula and check your answer

with a calculator. Remember to round to the nearest whole number. Review this formula if you had difficulty with this question.
Level of Cognitive Ability: Applying
Client Needs: Physiological Integrity
Integrated Process: Nursing Process/Implementation
Content Area: Fundamental Skills: Medications/Blood & IV Therapy
Reference: Christensen, Kockrow, pp. 730–731. 2011. *Foundations of nursing.*

774. 2
Rationale: Sclerotic lesions occur as bone resorption increases and results in replacement of original bone with fibrous material. This condition occurs in Paget's disease, an age-related disorder. Options 1, 3, and 4 identify normal age-related changes in the musculoskeletal system.
Test-Taking Strategy: Use the process of elimination. Note the strategic words "potential complication." Recalling the normal age-related musculoskeletal findings will assist in directing you to the correct option. Review these normal findings and those that indicate a complication if you had difficulty with this question.
Level of Cognitive Ability: Understanding
Client Needs: Physiological Integrity
Integrated Process: Nursing Process/Data Collection
Content Area: Adult Health/Musculoskeletal
References: Christensen, Kockrow, pp. 1099–1100. 2011. *Foundations of nursing.*
Linton, p. 148. 2012.

775. 4
Rationale: The vomiting that occurs in Reye's syndrome is caused by cerebral edema and is a symptom of increased intracranial pressure. Small, frequent meals will not affect the amount of vomiting, and the health care provider is notified if vomiting occurs. Options 1, 2, and 3 are all correct statements. Decreasing stimuli and providing rest decrease stress on the brain tissue. Checking for jaundice will assist in identifying the presence of liver complications, which are characteristic of Reye's syndrome.
Test-Taking Strategy: Note the strategic words "need for further instruction." These words indicate a negative event query and the need to select the incorrect client statement. Recalling the causes of vomiting with Reye's syndrome will direct you to the correct option. Review the pathophysiology associated with Reye's syndrome if you had difficulty with this question.
Level of Cognitive Ability: Evaluating
Client Needs: Physiological Integrity
Integrated Process: Teaching and Learning
Content Area: Child Health: Neurological/Musculoskeletal
References: Hockenberry, Wilson, p. 1004. 2009.
Perry, Hockenberry, Lowdermilk, Wilson, pp. 1580–1581. 2010.

❖ **776. 10**
Rationale: Follow the formula for dosage calculation.
Formula: Desired

$$\frac{\text{Desired}}{\text{Available}} \times \text{Volume} = \text{mL per dose}$$

$$\frac{20\ \text{mEq}}{30\ \text{mEq}} \times 15\ \text{mL} = 10\ \text{mL}$$

Test-Taking Strategy: Follow the formula for the calculation of the correct dose and focus on the key information,

30 mEq/15 mL. Verify the answer with a calculator. Review medication calculations if you had difficulty with this question.
Level of Cognitive Ability: Applying
Client Needs: Physiological Integrity
Integrated Process: Nursing Process/Planning
Content Area: Fundamental Skills: Medications/Blood & IV Therapy
Reference: Potter, Perry, pp. 695–699. 2009.

777. 4
Rationale: Nizatidine, a histamine H_2-receptor blocker, is frequently used in the management of peptic ulcer disease. Histamine H_2-receptor blockers decrease the secretion of gastric acid (HCL). Antacids are used as adjunct therapy and neutralize acid in the stomach. Omeprazole is a proton pump inhibitor. Sucralfate (Carafate) promotes healing by covering the ulcer, thus protecting it from erosion caused by gastric acids.
Test-Taking Strategy: Focus on the pathophysiology associated with peptic ulcer disease. Next, recalling the actions of the medications in the options will direct you to the correct option. If you are unfamiliar with these medications or their actions, review this content.
Level of Cognitive Ability: Evaluating
Client Needs: Physiological Integrity
Integrated Process: Nursing Process/Evaluation
Content Area: Adult Health/Gastrointestinal
Reference: Linton, p. 807. 2012.

778. 2
Rationale: A depressed person suffers with depressed mood and is often withdrawn. Also, the person experiences difficulty concentrating, loss of interest or pleasure, low energy, fatigue, and feelings of worthlessness and poor self-esteem. The plan of care needs to provide successful experiences in a stimulating yet structured environment.
Test-Taking Strategy: Use the process of elimination. Options 1 and 4 are eliminated first because they are too restrictive and offer little or no structure and stimulation. Option 3 is eliminated next because of the word "insist" and the closed-ended word "all" in this option. Review care of the client with depression if you had difficulty with this question.
Level of Cognitive Ability: Applying
Client Needs: Psychosocial Integrity
Integrated Process: Nursing Process/Planning
Content Area: Mental Health
References: Morrison-Valfre, pp. 230–231. 2009.
Stuart, p. 307. 2009.

779. 4
Rationale: Mealtimes should center on pleasurable socialization. The child should be encouraged to eat meals with other children on the unit. A diet that is normal in protein with a sodium restriction is normally prescribed for a child with nephrotic syndrome. Parents or other family members should be encouraged to be present at mealtimes with a hospitalized child.
Test-Taking Strategy: Use the process of elimination. Eliminate options 1 and 2 first. A diet that is normal in protein with a sodium restriction is normally prescribed. Option 3 diminishes the importance of socialization at mealtime. This leaves option 4 as the correct option. Review dietary recommendations for the child with nephrotic syndrome if you had difficulty with this question.

Level of Cognitive Ability: Applying
Client Needs: Physiological Integrity
Integrated Process: Nursing Process/Planning
Content Area: Child Health: Gastrointestinal/Renal
References: Hockenberry, Wilson, pp. 960–961. 2009.
McKinney, James, Murray, Ashwill, p. 1159. 2009.

780. 2
Rationale: Cushing's syndrome is characterized by an oversecretion of glucocorticoid hormones. Addison's disease is characterized by the failure of the adrenal cortex to produce and secrete adrenocortical hormones. Options 1 and 4 are inaccurate regarding Cushing's syndrome.
Test-Taking Strategy: Use the process of elimination. Options 1 and 4 can be eliminated first because they are not associated with Cushing's syndrome. Remembering that in Cushing's ("u" as in "up") syndrome there is an oversecretion and in Addison's ("d" as in "down") there is an undersecretion will direct you to option 2. Review this disorder if you had difficulty with this question.
Level of Cognitive Ability: Understanding
Client Needs: Physiological Integrity
Integrated Process: Teaching and Learning
Content Area: Adult Health/Endocrine
Reference: Linton, p. 1019. 2012.

781. 1
Rationale: Ovulation ceases during pregnancy because the circulating levels of estrogen and progesterone are high, thus inhibiting the release of follicle-stimulating hormone and luteinizing hormone, which are necessary for ovulation. Options 2, 3, and 4 are incorrect.
Test-Taking Strategy: Knowledge regarding the hormonal changes that occur during the menstrual cycle and during pregnancy is required to answer this question. Remember, ovulation ceases during pregnancy because the circulating levels of estrogen and progesterone are high. Review these hormonal changes if you had difficulty with this question.
Level of Cognitive Ability: Understanding
Client Needs: Physiological Integrity
Integrated Process: Teaching and Learning
Content Area: Maternity/Antepartum
References: Leifer, p. 27. 2011.
Lowdermilk, Perry, Cashion, pp. 98–99, 101. 2010.

782. 1
Rationale: Parents are especially concerned about seizures that might go undetected at night. The nurse should suggest a baby monitor. Reassurance by the nurse should ensure parental confidence and decrease parental overprotection. Option 2 is a common concern. Options 3 and 4 demonstrate the parents' ability to choose respite care and activities appropriately. The parents need to be reminded that, as the child grows, they cannot always observe their child, but their knowledge of seizure activity and care are appropriate to minimize complications.
Test-Taking Strategy: Use the process of elimination and note the strategic words "need for further teaching." These words indicate a negative event query and the need to select the incorrect client statement. The correct option identifies a need to provide the parents with an alternative method to monitor for night seizures. Review parent teaching regarding seizures if you had difficulty with this question.
Level of Cognitive Ability: Evaluating

Client Needs: Psychosocial Integrity
Integrated Process: Teaching and Learning
Content Area: Child Health: Neurological/Musculoskeletal
Reference: Hockenberry, Wilson, p. 1014. 2009.

783. 3
Rationale: Zollinger-Ellison syndrome is a hypersecretory condition of the stomach. The client should avoid taking medications that are irritating to the stomach lining. Irritants would include aspirin and nonsteroidal antiinflammatory drugs (ibuprofen). The client should be advised to take acetaminophen for headache.
Test-Taking Strategy: Use the process of elimination. Remember that options that are comparable or alike are not likely to be correct. With this in mind, eliminate options 1 and 2 first. Choose acetaminophen over aspirin because it is least irritating to the stomach. Review this medication and this disorder if you had difficulty with this question.
Level of Cognitive Ability: Applying
Client Needs: Physiological Integrity
Integrated Process: Nursing Process/Implementation
Content Area: Pharmacology
References: Ignatavicius, Workman, p. 1279. 2010.
Skidmore-Roth, pp. 83–85. 2012.

784. 3
Rationale: Feelings of low self-esteem and worthlessness are common symptoms of the depressed client. An effective plan of care is to provide successful experiences for the client that are challenging but will not be met with failure to enhance the client's personal self-esteem. Reminders of the client's past accomplishments or personal successes are ways to interrupt the client's negative self-talk and distorted cognitive view of themselves. Options 1 and 4 offer false reassurance. Option 2 is not a therapeutic intervention with a depressed client.
Test-Taking Strategy: Use the process of elimination and therapeutic communication techniques. Eliminate options 1 and 4 because the nurse is offering an opinion and false reassurance. Eliminate option 2 because, in this situation, silence can be interpreted as agreeing with the client's feelings. Review care of the client with depression if you had difficulty with this question.
Level of Cognitive Ability: Applying
Client Needs: Psychosocial Integrity
Integrated Process: Nursing Process/Implementation
Content Area: Mental Health
References: Morrison-Valfre, p. 231. 2009.
Stuart, p. 289. 2009.

785. 3
Rationale: Cryptorchidism may be the result of hormone deficiency, intrinsic abnormality of a testis, or a structural problem. Diagnostic tests would assess kidney function, because the kidneys and testes arise from the same germ tissue. Babinski's reflex tests neurological function and is unrelated to this diagnosis. DNA synthesis and a chromosomal analysis are also unrelated to this diagnosis.
Test-Taking Strategy: Use the process of elimination and knowledge regarding the anatomical occurrence of cryptorchidism. Cryptorchidism, undescended or hidden testicles, relates

to the genitourinary system. Option 2 relates to neurological function. Options 1 and 4 relate to the structure of cells. Option 3 is the only option that relates to the genitourinary system. Review this disorder if you had difficulty with this question.
Level of Cognitive Ability: Understanding
Client Needs: Physiological Integrity
Integrated Process: Nursing Process/Planning
Content Area: Child Health: Gastrointestinal/Renal
Reference: McKinney, James, Murray, Ashwill, pp. 1151–1152. 2009.

786. 4
Rationale: Pemphigus vulgaris is a rare, chronic, blistering disease caused by an autoimmune disorder that occurs most often during middle and old age. The lesions occur on normal-appearing skin or mucous membrane surfaces as fragile, flaccid bullae. Breaking the bullae leaves partial-thickness wounds that bleed, weep, and eventually form crusts. The skin is not dry, hard, or leathery.
Test-Taking Strategy: Use the process of elimination. Eliminate options 2 and 3 first because they are comparable or alike. Next it is necessary to know that this condition results in blistering. If you had difficulty with this question, review the characteristics of pemphigus vulgaris.
Level of Cognitive Ability: Understanding
Client Needs: Physiological Integrity
Integrated Process: Nursing Process/Data Collection
Content Area: Adult Health/Integumentary
Reference: Ignatavicius, Workman, p. 516. 2010.

787. 2
Rationale: The exact cause of acne is unknown. Exacerbations that coincide with the menstrual cycle result from hormonal activity. Oily skin alone is not the cause of acne. Heat, humidity, and excessive perspiration also play a role in exacerbation of acne. There is no evidence that consumption of foods such as chocolate, nuts, or fatty foods affects acne.
Test-Taking Strategy: Use the process of elimination. Note the strategic words, "most appropriately" and focus on the subject, the causes of acne. Options 1, 3, and 4 are not causes of acne. Review this disorder and its causes if you had difficulty with this question.
Level of Cognitive Ability: Applying
Client Needs: Physiological Integrity
Integrated Process: Nursing Process/Implementation
Content Area: Adult Health/Integumentary
Reference: Christensen, Kockrow, p. 83. 2011. *Adult health nursing.*

788. 4
Rationale: Extravasation refers to the tissue injury that occurs from leakage of medication into surrounding skin and subcutaneous tissue; it can also cause tissue necrosis. Phlebitis is an inflammation of the vein that can occur from mechanical or chemical (medication) trauma or from a local infection. Phlebitis can cause the development of a clot (thrombophlebitis). Infiltration is seepage of the intravenous fluid out of the vein and into the surrounding interstitial spaces. It is a form of tissue injury but the injury is not to the extent that occurs with extravasation.
Test-Taking Strategy: Focus on the characteristics of the tissue injury in the figure. Eliminate options 1 and 3 first because they

are comparable or alike and relate to vein injury. Next noting that the injury in the figure illustrates an open wound will direct you to the correct option. Review the characteristics of extravasation if you had difficulty with this question.
Level of Cognitive Ability: Analyzing
Client Needs: Physiological Integrity
Integrated Process: Nursing Process/Data Collection
Content Area: Fundamental Skills: Medications/Blood & IV Therapy
Reference: Christensen, Kockrow, p. 323. 2011. *Adult health nursing.*

789. 4
Rationale: At 12 weeks' gestation, the uterus extends out of the maternal pelvis and can be palpated above the symphysis pubis. At 16 weeks, the fundus reaches midway between the symphysis pubis and the umbilicus. At 20 weeks, the fundus is located at the umbilicus. By 36 weeks, the fundus reaches its highest level at the xiphoid process.
Test-Taking Strategy: Knowledge regarding the patterns of uterine growth is required to answer this question. Focus on the weeks of gestation identified in the question to assist in directing you to the correct option. Review this uterine growth pattern if you had difficulty with this question.
Level of Cognitive Ability: Understanding
Client Needs: Physiological Integrity
Integrated Process: Nursing Process/Data Collection
Content Area: Maternity/Antepartum
Reference: McKinney, James, Murray, Ashwill, p. 259. 2009.

790. 2
Rationale: In a compound (open) fracture, a wound in the skin leads to the broken bone, and there is an added danger of infection. Option 1 describes a transverse fracture. Option 3 describes a greenstick fracture. Option 4 describes a closed or simple fracture.
Test-Taking Strategy: Use the process of elimination. Noting the strategic word "open" will assist in directing you to the correct option. Review the various types of fractures if you had difficulty with this question.
Level of Cognitive Ability: Understanding
Client Needs: Physiological Integrity
Integrated Process: Nursing Process/Planning
Content Area: Child Health: Neurological/Musculoskeletal
Reference: McKinney, James, Murray, Ashwill, pp. 1399–1401. 2009.

791. 1
Rationale: Clubfoot, one of the most common deformities of the skeletal system, is a congenital anomaly characterized by a foot that has been twisted inward or outward. The condition generally affects both feet, and boys are affected twice as often as girls.
Test-Taking Strategy: Use the process of elimination. Eliminate option 2 because of the closed-ended word "always" and option 4 because of the word "rare." From the remaining options, it is necessary to know that this disorder is a congenital anomaly. Review this disorder if you had difficulty with this question.
Level of Cognitive Ability: Understanding
Client Needs: Physiological Integrity

Integrated Process: Nursing Process/Planning
Content Area: Child Health: Neurological/Musculoskeletal
Reference: Perry, Hockenberry, Lowdermilk, Wilson, p. 775. 2010.

792. 3
Rationale: A blood glucose test performed before exercising provides information to the client regarding the need to eat a snack first. Exercising during the peak times of insulin effect or before mealtime places the client at risk for hypoglycemia. Insulin should be administered as prescribed.
Test-Taking Strategy: The subject of the question relates to the occurrence of a hypoglycemic reaction. Use the process of elimination, keeping in mind this subject and the effects of insulin and exercise on the blood glucose level. You should easily be able to eliminate the incorrect options. Review the effects of exercise on the blood glucose level if you had difficulty with this question.
Level of Cognitive Ability: Applying
Client Needs: Health Promotion and Maintenance
Integrated Process: Teaching and Learning
Content Area: Adult Health/Endocrine
Reference: Linton, pp. 1056–1058. 2012.

793. 3
Rationale: The clinical signs of impending or approaching death include inability to swallow; pitting edema; decreased gastrointestinal and urinary tract activity; bowel and bladder incontinence; loss of motion, sensation, and reflexes; cold or clammy skin; cyanosis; lowered blood pressure; noisy or irregular respiration; and Cheyne-Stokes respirations.
Test-Taking Strategy: Use the process of elimination and eliminate options 2 and 4 because these identify normal findings. Eliminate option 1 because it does not identify signs of approaching death. If you had difficulty with this question, review the signs associated with impending or approaching death.
Level of Cognitive Ability: Understanding
Client Needs: Physiological Integrity
Integrated Process: Nursing Process/Data Collection
Content Area: Fundamental Skills/End-of-Life Care
Reference: Linton, pp. 380–381. 2012.

794. 1
Rationale: Used tissues are discarded in a plastic bag, so contaminated respiratory secretions can be contained. The client with tuberculosis should wash hands carefully after each contact with respiratory secretions. Oral care should be performed more than once a day. The client should be instructed to cover the mouth and nose when laughing, sneezing, or coughing and to wear a mask when in contact with others until drug therapy suppresses the infection.
Test-Taking Strategy: Use the process of elimination. Note that the question specifically relates to information about handling and disposal of secretions. The only options that address this topic directly are options 1 and 4. Because turning the head to the side for coughing and sneezing does not specifically address the handling of secretions, eliminate option 4. Disposal of tissues in a plastic bag is correct. Review home care instructions related to tuberculosis if you had difficulty with this question.
Level of Cognitive Ability: Evaluating
Client Needs: Safe and Effective Care Environment

Integrated Process: Nursing Process/Evaluation
Content Area: Adult Health/Respiratory
References: Christensen, Kockrow, p. 403. 2011. *Adult health nursing.*
deWit, p. 327. 2009.

795. 2

Rationale: A common side effect of INH is peripheral neuritis. This is manifested by numbness, tingling, and paresthesias in the extremities. This side effect can be minimized with pyridoxine (vitamin B_6) intake.

Test-Taking Strategy: Use the process of elimination. Options 3 and 4 would not cause the signs and symptoms presented in the question, but instead would be manifested by pallor and coolness. Thus, options 3 and 4 can be eliminated first. From the remaining options, it is necessary to know either that peripheral neuritis is a side effect of the medication or that these signs and symptoms do not correlate with hypercalcemia. Review the side effects associated with isoniazid if you had difficulty with this question.
Level of Cognitive Ability: Analyzing
Client Needs: Physiological Integrity
Integrated Process: Nursing Process/Data Collection
Content Area: Adult Health/Respiratory
Reference: Christensen, Kockrow, p. 402. 2011. *Adult health nursing.*

796. 2

Rationale: It is important to give the mother information that addresses the issue that is the parent's concern. Most children experience remission with treatment. Options 1 and 3 are nontherapeutic and may add to the mother's guilt. Option 4 does not acknowledge the concern and is a stereotypical response.

Test-Taking Strategy: Use therapeutic communication techniques and focus on the mother's concern. Options 1, 3, and 4 do not address the mother's concern and are inappropriate and nontherapeutic responses. Remember to always address the mother's feelings and concerns. Review this disorder and therapeutic communication techniques if you had difficulty with this question.
Level of Cognitive Ability: Applying
Client Needs: Physiological Integrity
Integrated Process: Communication and Documentation
Content Area: Child Health: Gastrointestinal/Renal
References: Christensen, Kockrow, pp. 40–46. 2011. *Foundations of nursing.*
McKinney, James, Murray, Ashwill, pp. 1157–1159. 2009.
Perry, Hockenberry, Lowdermilk, Wilson, p. 1538. 2010.

❖ 797. 2, 3, 4

Rationale: Clinical manifestations of COPD include hypoxemia, hypercapnia, dyspnea on exertion and at rest, oxygen desaturation with exercise, use of accessory muscles of respiration, and a prolonged expiratory phase of respiration. The client may also exhibit difficulty breathing while talking, and may have to take breaths between every one or two words. Some clients with COPD, especially those with a history of smoking, often have a productive cough especially on arising in the morning. The chest x-ray will reveal a hyperinflated chest and a flattened diaphragm if the disease is advanced.

Test-Taking Strategy: Think about the pathophysiology associated with COPD. Eliminate option 5 because oxygen desaturation rather than saturation would occur. Next, eliminate option 6 because, in the client with COPD, a prolonged expiratory phase of respiration would be noted. From the remaining options, reading carefully will assist in eliminating option 1 because hypercapnia would occur. If you are unfamiliar with the manifestations associated with COPD, review this content.
Level of Cognitive Ability: Analyzing
Client Needs: Physiological Integrity
Integrated Process: Nursing Process/Data Collection
Content Area: Adult Health/Respiratory
References: Ignatavicius, Workman, pp. 596, 598, 624. 2010. Linton, pp. 588–589. 2012.

798. 1, 3, 4, 6 ❖

Rationale: The administration of an enema is a clean procedure, and standard precautions must be used. The nurse applies disposable gloves when administering an enema to prevent the transfer of microorganisms. To administer an enema, the nurse places the client in the left Sims' position because the enema solution will flow downward by gravity along the natural curve of the sigmoid colon and rectum, improving retention of the enema solution. The tube is lubricated for easy insertion and is inserted approximately 3 to 4 inches in an adult. If the client complains of cramping or discomfort during the procedure, the nurse clamps the tubing until the discomfort subsides. The container containing the enema solution is hung about 12 to 18 inches above the client's anus. A flow of solution that is too forceful can damage the bowel. The temperature of the solution should be between 100° F (37.8° C) and 105° F (40.5° C). Solution that is too hot will burn the client, and solution that is too cool will cause cramping.

Test-Taking Strategy: Visualize the procedure for administering an enema. Thinking about the anatomy of the bowel and the precautions that need to be taken to prevent trauma to rectal tissue will assist in identifying the correct interventions. Review the procedure for administering an enema if you had difficulty with this question.
Level of Cognitive Ability: Applying
Client Needs: Physiological Integrity
Integrated Process: Nursing Process/Implementation
Content Area: Adult Health/Gastrointestinal
Reference: Christensen , Kockrow, pp. 592–594. 2011. *Foundations of nursing.*

799. 1, 2, 3, 5 ❖

Rationale: A client who is aphasic has difficulty expressing or understanding language. The nurse would face the client when talking, establish and maintain eye contact, and speak slowly and distinctly. The nurse should use gestures and pantomime when talking to enhance words and use body language to enhance the message. The nurse would give the client directions using short phrases and simple terms, and phrase questions so that they can be answered with a yes or no. If there is a need to repeat something, the nurse should use the same words a second time.

Test-Taking Strategy: Recall that a client who is aphasic has difficulty expressing or understanding language. Using the principles related to communicating to a hearing-impaired client will assist in identifying the correct interventions. Review

the guidelines for communicating with an aphasic client if you had difficulty with this question.
Level of Cognitive Ability: Applying
Client Needs: Physiological Integrity
Integrated Process: Communication and Documentation
Content Area: Adult Health/Neurological
Reference: Linton, p. 508. 2012.

800. 4
Rationale: After the nasogastric tube is in place, mouth care is extremely important. With one naris occluded, the client tends to mouth breathe, drying the mucous membranes. Frequent oral hygiene may be required to prevent or care for dry, irritated mucous membranes. Frequent small sips of water would be contraindicated when the client is on gastric suction. The hard candy would increase the salivation but would not be useful in cleaning the oral cavity. Lemon glycerin swabs have a drying or irritating effect on the mucous membranes.
Test-Taking Strategy: Note the strategic word "best" and focus on the subject, maintaining the integrity of the oral mucosa. Recalling that a client on gastric suction will be NPO and swallowing water or other liquids would be prohibited will assist in eliminating options 1 and 2. From the remaining options, eliminate option 3 because lemon glycerin swabs are drying to the mucosa. Review care of the client with a nasogastric tube if you had difficulty with this question.
Level of Cognitive Ability: Applying
Client Needs: Physiological Integrity
Integrated Process: Nursing Process/Implementation
Content Area: Adult Health/Gastrointestinal
References: Linton, p. 791. 2012.
Lewis, Dirksen, Heitkemper, Bucher, Camera, p. 1034. 2011.

801. 3
Rationale: Rheumatic endocarditis, also called rheumatic carditis, is a major indicator of rheumatic fever, which is a complication of infection with group A β-hemolytic streptococcal infections. It is frequently triggered by streptococcal pharyngitis. Options 1, 2, and 4 are incorrect.
Test-Taking Strategy: Use the process of elimination. Recalling that streptococcal infections are largely responsible for rheumatic heart disease will direct you to option 3. Review the causes of endocarditis if you had difficulty with this question.
Level of Cognitive Ability: Applying
Client Needs: Physiological Integrity
Integrated Process: Nursing Process/Data Collection
Content Area: Adult Health/Cardiovascular
References: Christensen, Kockrow, pp. 345–346. 2011. *Adult health nursing.*
Ignatavicius, Workman, p. 787. 2010.

802. 4
Rationale: Potassium-sparing diuretics include amiloride (Midamor), spironolactone (Aldactone), and triamterene (Dyrenium). They are weak diuretics that are used in combination with potassium-losing diuretics. This combination is useful when medication and dietary supplement of potassium is not appropriate. The use of two different diuretics does not prevent renal toxicity. Hydrochlorothiazide is an effective and inexpensive generic form of the thiazide classification of diuretics.
Test-Taking Strategy: It is especially helpful to remember that hydrochlorothiazide is a potassium-losing diuretic and triamterene is a potassium-sparing diuretic; thus, option 1 can be eliminated. Toxicity from these medications is the result of fluid and electrolyte imbalances, so option 2 can be eliminated. Hydrochlorothiazide is a common and inexpensive diuretic, so option 3 can be eliminated. Review the action and uses of these medications if you had difficulty with this question.
Level of Cognitive Ability: Understanding
Client Needs: Physiological Integrity
Integrated Process: Nursing Process/Implementation
Content Area: Pharmacology
Reference: Lehne, pp. 453–454. 2010.

803. 3
Rationale: ACE inhibitors, such as fosinopril, cause temporary impairment of taste (dysgeusia). The nurse can tell the client that this effect usually disappears in 2 to 3 months, even with continued therapy, and provide nutritional counseling if appropriate to avoid weight loss. Options 1, 2, and 4 are inappropriate actions. Taking this medication with or without food does not affect absorption and action. The dosage should never be tapered without HCP approval and the medication should never be stopped abruptly.
Test-Taking Strategy: Use the process of elimination. Eliminate option 2 first because it is an inappropriate nursing action. The nurse does not advise the client to make dosage changes for any prescribed medication. Taking the medication with or without food is not going to change the taste of the food, so option 1 can be eliminated next. From the remaining options, you need to know that this effect occurs with medications in the ACE inhibitor group. Thus, you are left with the correct option, which is informing the client that impaired taste is expected. Review the effects of ACE inhibitors if you had difficulty with this question.
Level of Cognitive Ability: Applying
Client Needs: Physiological Integrity
Integrated Process: Nursing Process/Implementation
Content Area: Pharmacology
Reference: Kee, Hayes, McCuistion, p. 671. 2009.

804. 2
Rationale: Amlodipine is a calcium channel blocker. This medication decreases the rate and force of cardiac contraction. Before administering a calcium channel blocking agent, the nurse should check the blood pressure and heart rate, which could both decrease in response to the action of this medication. This action will help to prevent or identify early problems related to decreased cardiac contractility, heart rate, and conduction.
Test-Taking Strategy: To answer this question, you must know that amlodipine is a calcium channel blocker, and that this group of medications decreases the rate and force of cardiac contraction. This in turn lowers the pulse rate and blood pressure. Option 1 can be eliminated first because it is unrelated to the medication. With options 3 and 4, note that only half of the option is correct. When answering questions with two items per option, both of the items must be correct for that option to be correct. Review this medication if you had difficulty with this question.

Level of Cognitive Ability: Applying
Client Needs: Physiological Integrity
Integrated Process: Nursing Process/Data Collection
Content Area: Pharmacology
Reference: Hodgson, Kizior, pp. 56–57. 2012.

805. 4

Rationale: Paraphrasing is restating the client's message in the nurse's own words. Paraphrasing may be in the form of a question. Option 4 uses the therapeutic communication technique of paraphrasing. The client is frustrated and is searching for understanding. Options 1, 2, and 3 are inappropriate communication techniques. Option 1 belittles the client's concerns. Options 2 and 3 offer false reassurance by the nurse.
Test-Taking Strategy: Use therapeutic communication techniques to answer the question. Option 4 focuses on the client's feelings. Review therapeutic communication techniques if you had difficulty with this question.
Level of Cognitive Ability: Applying
Client Needs: Psychosocial Integrity
Integrated Process: Communication and Documentation
Content Area: Adult Health/Cardiovascular
References: Christensen, Kockrow, pp. 40–46. 2011. *Foundations of nursing.*
Lewis, Dirksen, Heitkemper, Bucher, Camera, pp. 853–854. 2011.

❖ 806. 2, 4, 5, 6

Rationale: The nurse would teach the client how to care for the stoma depending on the type of laryngectomy performed. Most interventions focus on protection of the stoma and the prevention of infection. Interventions include avoiding swimming and using caution when showering, avoiding exposure to people with infections, preventing debris from entering the stoma, and obtaining a Medic-Alert bracelet. Additional interventions include wearing a stoma guard or high-collar clothing to cover the stoma, increasing the humidity in the home, and increasing fluid intake to 3000 mL/day to keep the secretions thin.
Test-Taking Strategy: Recalling that most interventions focus on protection of the stoma and the prevention of infection will assist in identifying the client instructions for home care. Review these instructions if you had difficulty with this question.
Level of Cognitive Ability: Applying
Client Needs: Physiological Integrity
Integrated Process: Teaching and Learning
Content Area: Adult Health/Oncology
Reference: Christensen, Kockrow, p. 209. 2011. *Adult health nursing.*

807. 2

Rationale: The correct procedure for needle disposal is to discard uncapped needles and sharps in a hard-walled, puncture-resistant, leak-proof container immediately after use. Discarding the uncapped needle and attached syringe in a designated sharps container prevents injury to the client and health care personnel. Recapping needles increases the risk of needlestick injury. Options 1, 3, and 4 are unsafe actions.
Test-Taking Strategy: Use the process of elimination and principles related to the safe disposal of needles and syringes to answer the question. Note that options 1, 3, and 4 are comparable or alike in that they all address recapping the needle. Review these principles if you had difficulty with this question.
Level of Cognitive Ability: Applying
Client Needs: Safe and Effective Care Environment
Integrated Process: Nursing Process/Implementation
Content Area: Fundamental Skills: Safety/Infection Control
Reference: Christensen, Kockrow, p. 284. 2011. *Foundations of nursing.*

808. 2

Rationale: Individuals at risk for developing a latex allergy include health care workers; individuals who work with manufacturing latex products; individuals with spina bifida; individuals who wear gloves frequently such as food handlers, hairdressers, and auto mechanics; and individuals allergic to kiwis, bananas, pineapples, passion fruit, avocados, and chestnuts.
Test-Taking Strategy: Focus on the subject, a latex allergy. Recalling the cause and the source of the allergic reaction will easily direct you to the correct option. Review the cause of this type of allergy and the individuals at risk if you had difficulty with this question.
Level of Cognitive Ability: Analyzing
Client Needs: Health Promotion and Maintenance
Integrated Process: Nursing Process/Data Collection
Content Area: Adult Health/Immune
Reference: Perry, Potter, p. 197. 2010.

809. 2

Rationale: The skin under a casted area may be discolored and crusted with dead skin layers. The client should gently soak and wash the skin for the first few days. The skin should be patted dry, and a lubricating lotion should be applied. Clients often want to scrub the dead skin away, which irritates the skin. The client should avoid overexposing the skin to the sunlight.
Test-Taking Strategy: Note the strategic words "further skin care instructions are required." These words indicate a negative event query and the need to select the incorrect option. Option 3 is obviously helpful, and therefore cannot be the answer to the question as stated. Option 4 is good advice and is eliminated next. Options 1 and 2 seem to oppose each other, making it likely that one of them is correct. Because vigorous scrubbing is more likely to be irritating than providing a gentle wash, option 2 is the likely choice as the answer to the question. Review skin care measures after cast removal if you had difficulty with this question.
Level of Cognitive Ability: Evaluating
Client Needs: Physiological Integrity
Integrated Process: Teaching and Learning
Content Area: Adult Health/Musculoskeletal
Reference: Christensen, Kockrow, p. 156. 2011. *Adult health nursing.*

810. 2

Rationale: Common areas that are under pressure and are at risk for breakdown include the elbows (if they are used for repositioning instead of a trapeze) and the heel of the good leg (which is used as a brace when pushing up in bed). Other pressure points caused by the traction include the ischial tuberosity, popliteal space, and Achilles tendon.

Test-Taking Strategy: Note the strategic words "high-risk area." Thus, you would compare each of the options in terms of their relative risk, and choose the one that is highest. The right heel is eliminated first because it is off the bed in the traction setup. The overhead trapeze would diminish the likelihood that the scapulae and back of the head would be immobile. This leaves the left heel as the answer. This makes sense, given that the client would use the unaffected heel to push into the mattress during repositioning. With repeated use, this could cause the left heel to become reddened and break down. Review the complications of skeletal traction if you had difficulty with this question.
Level of Cognitive Ability: Applying
Client Needs: Physiological Integrity
Integrated Process: Nursing Process/Data Collection
Content Area: Adult Health/Musculoskeletal
Reference: Christensen, Kockrow, p. 157. 2011. *Adult health nursing.*

811. 3

Rationale: The part of the bed under an area in traction is usually elevated to aid in countertraction. For the client in Buck's extension traction (which is applied to a leg), the foot of the bed is elevated. Option 1 places undue pressure on the client's unaffected foot. Option 2 is not used for the purpose of countertraction. Buck's extension traction is applied to the leg therefore eliminate option 4.
Test-Taking Strategy: To answer this question correctly, you need to understand the principles of traction and countertraction and be familiar with Buck's extension traction. Option 2 is not used for the purpose of countertraction and is eliminated first. Knowing that Buck's extension traction is applied to the leg helps you eliminate option 4. Of the two remaining options, option 1 places undue pressure on the client's unaffected foot. Furthermore, a footboard is not used for the purpose of providing countertraction. Option 3 provides a force that opposes the traction force effectively without harming the client. Review care of the client in Buck's extension traction if you had difficulty with this question.
Level of Cognitive Ability: Applying
Client Needs: Physiological Integrity
Integrated Process: Nursing Process/Implementation
Content Area: Adult Health/Musculoskeletal
References: Christensen, Kockrow, p. 156. 2011. *Adult health nursing.*
deWit, p. 793. 2009.

❖ ## 812. 3, 4, 5

Rationale: The clinical manifestations of hypothyroidism are the result of decreased metabolism from low levels of thyroid hormone. Interventions are aimed at replacement of the hormones and providing measures to support the signs and symptoms related to a decreased metabolism. The nurse encourages the client to consume a well-balanced diet that is low in fat for weight reduction and high in fluids and high-fiber foods to prevent constipation. The client often has cold intolerance and requires a warm environment. The client would notify the health care provider if chest pain occurs since it could be an indication of overreplacement of thyroid hormone. Iodine preparations are used to treat hyperthyroidism. These medications decrease blood flow through the thyroid gland and reduce the production and release of thyroid hormone.
Test-Taking Strategy: Focus on the client's diagnosis—hypothyroidism. Recalling that the client has a decreased metabolic rate in this disorder will assist in determining the appropriate interventions. Review interventions for the client with hypothyroidism and hyperthyroidism if you had difficulty with this question.
Level of Cognitive Ability: Applying
Client Needs: Physiological Integrity
Integrated Process: Nursing Process/Implementation
Content Area: Adult Health/Endocrine
References: Christensen, Kockrow, pp. 498–500. 2011. *Adult health nursing.*
Linton, pp. 1036–1037. 2012.

813. 4

Rationale: The client with Guillain-Barré syndrome is at risk for respiratory failure because of ascending paralysis. An intubation tray should be available for use. Another complication of this syndrome is cardiac dysrhythmia, which necessitates the use of ECG monitoring. Because the client is immobilized, the nurse should routinely assess for deep vein thrombosis and pulmonary embolism.
Test-Taking Strategy: Use the process of elimination and the ABCs—airway, breathing, and circulation. With an ascending paralysis, the client is at risk for involvement of respiratory muscles and subsequent respiratory failure. This knowledge makes you look for an option that coincides with this line of thought. The correct option is the only one that includes an intubation tray, which would be needed if the client's status deteriorated to needing intubation and mechanical ventilation. It also addresses cardiac monitoring. This option most directly addresses the ABCs. Review care of the client with Guillain-Barré syndrome if you had difficulty with this question.
Level of Cognitive Ability: Applying
Client Needs: Physiological Integrity
Integrated Process: Nursing Process/Implementation
Content Area: Adult Health/Neurological
Reference: deWit, pp. 603–605. 2009.

814. 4

Rationale: Feosol is an iron supplement used to treat anemia. Constipation is a frequent and uncomfortable side effect associated with the administration of oral iron supplements. Stool softeners are often prescribed to prevent constipation. Options 1, 2, and 3 are not associated with this medication.
Test-Taking Strategy: Focus on the name of the medication. Recalling that oral iron can cause constipation will easily direct you to the correct option. If you had difficulty with this question, review the side effects of ferrous sulfate.
Level of Cognitive Ability: Understanding
Client Needs: Physiological Integrity
Integrated Process: Nursing Process/Data Collection
Content Area: Pharmacology
Reference: Hodgson, Kizior, p. 476. 2012.

815. 2

Rationale: Hearing-impaired clients rely on visual cues to help them comprehend the conversation of others. Smiling continuously is the least helpful strategy, because the smile distorts the appearance of the mouth if the client is trying to read lips. When beginning the conversation, it helps to reduce background noise such as turning off or lowering the volume of the television. Facing the client and standing so that there is light on the nurse's face are helpful strategies, because it assists the client to lip read. Taking care not to show frustration or annoyance with the client's impairment is also helpful to preserve the client's self-esteem.

Test-Taking Strategy: Note the strategic words "least helpful." Noting the words "smiling continuously" in option 2 will direct you to this option. If this question was difficult, review these communication strategies.

Level of Cognitive Ability: Applying
Client Needs: Psychosocial Integrity
Integrated Process: Communication and Documentation
Content Area: Adult Health/Ear
References: Christensen, Kockrow, p. 49. 2011. *Foundations of nursing.*
deWit, p. 630. 2009.

816. 1

Rationale: Digoxin is a cardiac glycoside that is used to treat heart failure and acts by increasing the force of myocardial contraction. Because bradycardia may be a clinical sign of toxicity, the nurse counts the apical heart rate for 1 full minute before administering the medication. If the pulse rate is less than 60 beats/minute in an adult client, the nurse would withhold the medication and report the pulse rate to the registered nurse, who would then contact the health care provider.

Test-Taking Strategy: Noting that the client has heart failure and recalling the action and nursing interventions related to administering this medication will assist in answering this question. Remember that bradycardia is a sign of toxicity. Review nursing interventions related to the administration of digoxin if you had difficulty with this question.

Level of Cognitive Ability: Applying
Client Needs: Physiological Integrity
Integrated Process: Nursing Process/Implementation
Content Area: Pharmacology
Reference: Hodgson, Kizior, p. 353. 2012.

❖ 817. 25

Rationale: Use the formula for calculating IV flow rates.
Formula:

$$\frac{\text{Total volume to infuse} \times \text{gtt factor}}{\text{Time in minutes}} = \text{gtt/minute}$$

$$\frac{1000 \text{ mL} \times 15 \text{ gtt/mL}}{600 \text{ minutes}} = 25 \text{ gtt/min}$$

Test-Taking Strategy: Follow the formula for calculating an IV flow rate and remember to change hours to minutes. Once you have done the calculation, recheck your work using a calculator and make sure that the answer makes sense. If you had difficulty with this question, review IV flow rates.

Level of Cognitive Ability: Applying
Client Needs: Physiological Integrity
Integrated Process: Nursing Process/Implementation
Content Area: Fundamental Skills: Medications/Blood & IV Therapy
Reference: Christensen, Kockrow, pp. 730–731. 2011. *Foundations of nursing.*

818. 2, 3, 6   ❖

Rationale: Sterile packages are opened away from the nurse's body, and the distal flap of a sterile package is opened first. This prevents contaminating the pack by reaching over the exposed sterile contents after the other flaps are opened (option 2). To avoid contamination, the sterile field should be prepared just before the planned procedure, and supplies should be used immediately (option 3). The outer 1-inch border of the sterile field must be considered unsterile, and sterile items are not placed within this 1-inch area (option 6). A dry table that is above waist level is used to set up a sterile field. Moisture will contaminate the sterile field and anything below waist level is considered contaminated, according to the principles of surgical asepsis. The sterile field must be kept in sight at all times, and the nurse should not turn away from it. If this happens, the nurse cannot be sure that it is still sterile. Sterile gloves, not clean gloves, are used. An unsterile item touching a sterile item contaminates the sterile item.

Test-Taking Strategy: Focus on the subject, the principles of aseptic technique. Thinking about these principles and visualizing each intervention will assist in identifying those that are appropriate. Review the principles of aseptic technique if you had difficulty with this question.

Level of Cognitive Ability: Applying
Client Needs: Safe and Effective Care Environment
Integrated Process: Nursing Process/Implementation
Content Area: Fundamental Skills: Safety/Infection Control
Reference: Christensen, Kockrow, pp. 295–296. 2011. *Foundations of nursing.*

819. 3

Rationale: Coughing is a normal response to suctioning for the client with an intact cough reflex, and it is not an indication that the client is not tolerating the procedure. The client should be encouraged to cough to help with removal of secretions from the lungs. The nurse should monitor for the adverse effects of suctioning, which include cyanosis (pulse oximetry falls below 90% or 5% from baseline), excessively rapid or slow heart rate (a 20 beat/minute change), or the sudden development of bloody secretions. If they occur, the nurse stops suctioning, administers oxygen as appropriate, and reports these signs to the health care provider immediately.

Test-Taking Strategy: Use the process of elimination and note the strategic words "adequately tolerating." Cyanosis and bradycardia are abnormal findings and are eliminated first. From the remaining options, the use of the word "becoming" in association with bloody secretions tells you that this has not been an ongoing problem, making this an incorrect option. Because the cough reflex is normally present, and suction triggers coughing, option 3 is preferable. Review this procedure if you had difficulty with this question.

Level of Cognitive Ability: Evaluating
Client Needs: Physiological Integrity
Integrated Process: Nursing Process/Evaluation
Content Area: Adult Health/Respiratory
References: Christensen, Kockrow, pp. 568–569. 2011. *Foundations of nursing.*
deWit, p. 312. 2009.

820. 3

Rationale: Candidiasis is a fungal infection caused by *Candida albicans.* When it occurs in the mouth, it is called thrush and

appears as white plaques. Although it can occur in an immuno-compromised client, it is not considered to be common. Options 2 and 4 are not accurate regarding this infection.
Test-Taking Strategy: Use the process of elimination. Options 1 and 4 can be eliminated first. Recalling that the anemic client is more likely to exhibit pallor will assist in eliminating option 2 and will direct you to option 3. If you are unfamiliar with the manifestations associated with thrush, review this content.
Level of Cognitive Ability: Understanding
Client Needs: Physiological Integrity
Integrated Process: Nursing Process/Data Collection
Content Area: Adult Health/Integumentary
Reference: Linton, p. 653. 2012.

821. 3
Rationale: The normal WBC count ranges from 4500 to 11,000 cells/mm³. Options 1 and 2 identify values lower than normal. Option 4 identifies a value higher than normal.
Test-Taking Strategy: Recalling the normal WBC count will direct you to the correct option. Remember the normal WBC count ranges from 4500 to 11,000 cells/mm³. Review the normal WBC count if you had difficulty with this question.
Level of Cognitive Ability: Understanding
Client Needs: Physiological Integrity
Integrated Process: Nursing Process/Data Collection
Content Area: Fundamental Skills: Laboratory Values
Reference: Christensen, Kockrow, p. 254. 2011. *Adult health nursing.*

822. 1
Rationale: The nurse would instruct the client to lie down and place a towel or pillow under the shoulder on the side of the breast to be examined. If the left breast is to be examined, the pillow would be placed under the left shoulder. Options 2 and 4 are incorrect.
Test-Taking Strategy: Visualize this procedure to select the correct option. Remember, to examine the left breast, the pillow is placed under the left shoulder; to examine the right breast, the pillow is placed under the right shoulder. If you are unfamiliar with the procedure for performing BSE, review this self-examination.
Level of Cognitive Ability: Applying
Client Needs: Health Promotion and Maintenance
Integrated Process: Teaching and Learning
Content Area: Adult Health/Oncology
Reference: Christensen, Kockrow, p. 573. 2011. *Adult health nursing.*

823. 4
Rationale: The CT scan causes no pain and takes about 15 to 60 minutes to perform. The dye may cause a warm flushing sensation when injected. Fluids are encouraged following the procedure. If an iodine dye is used, the client should be asked about allergies to seafood or iodine.

Test-Taking Strategy: Use the process of elimination and note the strategic words "dye injection." Noting the relationship between these strategic words and option 4 will assist in answering the question. Review this diagnostic test if you had difficulty with this question.
Level of Cognitive Ability: Understanding
Client Needs: Physiological Integrity
Integrated Process: Nursing Process/Implementation
Content Area: Adult Health/Oncology
References: Christensen, Kockrow, p. 116. 2011. *Adult health nursing.*
Pagana, Pagana, pp. 284–285. 2009.

824. 3
Rationale: Denial, bargaining, anger, depression, and acceptance are recognized stages that a person experiences when facing a life-threatening illness. The client's statement is indicative of bargaining. Denial is expressed as shock and disbelief and may be the first response to hearing bad news. Depression may be manifested by hopelessness, weeping openly, or remaining quiet or withdrawn. Anger may also be a first response to upsetting news, and the predominant theme is "Why me?" or the blaming of others.
Test-Taking Strategy: Focus on the client's statement as identified in the question to assist in selecting the correct option. From this point, you should be able to eliminate and the incorrect options. Review these stages if you had difficulty with this question.
Level of Cognitive Ability: Analyzing
Client Needs: Psychosocial Integrity
Integrated Process: Nursing Process/Data Collection
Content Area: Adult Health/Oncology
Reference: Christensen, Kockrow, p. 803. 2011. *Adult health nursing.*

825. 2, 3, 4
Rationale: Furosemide is a loop diuretic; therefore, an expected effect is increased urinary frequency. Nausea is a frequent side effect, not an adverse effect. Photosensitivity is an occasional side effect. Adverse effects include tinnitus (ototoxicity), hypotension, and hypokalemia and occur as a result of sudden volume depletion.
Test-Taking Strategy: Recalling that furosemide is a diuretic will assist in eliminating option 6. For the remaining options focus on the words "adverse effects" to assist in answering correctly. Review the side and adverse effects of furosemide if you had difficulty with this question.
Level of Cognitive Ability: Analyzing
Client Needs: Physiological Integrity
Integrated Process: Nursing Process/Data Collection
Content Area: Pharmacology
Reference: Hodgson, Kizior, pp. 526–528. 2012.

References

Alexander, M., Corrigan, A., Gorski, L., Hankins, J., & Perucca, R. (2010). *Infusion nursing: An evidence-based approach* (3rd ed.). St. Louis: Saunders.

Berg, R. A., Hemphill, R., Abella, B., et al. (2010). 2010 American Heart Association guidelines for cardiopulmonary resuscitation and emergency cardiovascular care. *Circulation, 122*, S685–S705. Available online at http://circ.ahajournals.org/cgi/reprint/122/18_suppl_3/S685.

Black, J. M., & Hawks, J. H. (2009). *Medical-surgical nursing: Clinical management for positive outcomes* (8th ed.). St. Louis: Saunders.

Christensen, B., & Kockrow, E. (2006). *Foundations of nursing* (5th ed). St. Louis: Mosby. Adapted from American Hospital Association (1992). A patient's bill of rights http://www.patienttalk.info/AHA-Patient_Bill_of_Rights.htm.

Christensen, B. L., & Kockrow, E. O. (2011). *Adult health nursing* (6th ed.). St. Louis: Mosby.

Christensen, B. L., & Kockrow, E. O. (2011). *Foundations and adult health nursing* (6th ed.). St. Louis: Mosby.

Clark, J., Queener, S., & Karb, V. (2000). *Pharmacologic basis of nursing practice* (6th ed.). St. Louis: Mosby.

deWit, S. C. (2009). *Fundamental concepts and skills for nursing* (3rd ed.). St. Louis: Saunders.

Edmunds, M. W. (2010). *Introduction to clinical pharmacology* (6th ed.). St. Louis: Mosby.

Fortinash, K., & Worret, P. (2012). *Psychiatric mental health nursing* (5th ed.). St. Louis: Mosby.

Gahart, B. L., & Nazareno, A. R. (2010). *2010 intravenous medications: A handbook for nurses and health professionals*. St. Louis: Mosby.

Gahart, B. L., & Nazareno, A. R. (2011). *2011 intravenous medications: A handbook for nurses and health professionals*. St. Louis: Mosby.

Hockenberry, M. J., & Wilson, D. (2009). *Wong's essentials of pediatric nursing* (8th ed.). St. Louis: Mosby.

Hodgson, B. B., & Kizior, R. J. (2011). *Saunders nursing drug handbook 2011*. St. Louis: Saunders.

Hodgson, B. B., & Kizior, R. J. (2012). *Saunders nursing drug handbook 2012*. St. Louis: Saunders.

Huszar, R. J. (2007). *Basic dysrhythmias: Interpretation and management* (3rd ed.). St. Louis: Mosby.

Ignatavicius, D. D., & Workman, M. L. (2010). *Medical-surgical nursing: Patient-centered collaborative care* (6th ed.). St. Louis: Saunders.

Jarvis, C. (2012). *Physical examination and health assessment* (6th ed.). St. Louis: Saunders.

The Joint Commission, National Patient Safety Goals Effective July 1, 2011, Hospital Accreditation Program. Available online at http://www.jointcommission.org/assets/1/6/NPSG_EPs_Scoring_HAP_20110706.pdf.

Kee, J. L., Hayes, E. R., & McCuistion, L. E. (2009). *Pharmacology: A nursing process approach* (6th ed.). St. Louis: Saunders.

Kee, J. L., Hayes, E. R., & McCuistion, L. E. (2012). *Pharmacology: A nursing process approach* (7th ed.). St. Louis: Saunders.

Kee, J. L., & Marshall, S. M. (2009). *Clinical calculations: With applications to general and specialty areas* (6th ed.). St. Louis: Saunders.

Keltner, N., Bostrom, C., & Mc Guinness, T. (2011). *Psychiatric nursing* (6th ed.). St. Louis: Mosby.

Kunz Howard, P., Steinmann, R. A., & Emergency Nurses Association. (2010). *Sheehy's emergency nursing: Principles and practice* (6th ed.). St. Louis: Mosby.

Lehne, R. L. (2010). *Pharmacology for nursing care* (7th ed.). St. Louis: Saunders.

Leifer, G. (2011). *Introduction to maternity & pediatric nursing* (6th ed.). St. Louis: Saunders.

Lewis, S. L., Dirksen, S. R., Heitkemper, M. M., et al. (2011). *Medical-surgical nursing: Assessment and management of clinical problems* (8th ed.). St. Louis: Mosby.

Linton, A. D. (2012). *Introduction to medical-surgical nursing* (5th ed.). St. Louis: Saunders.

Lowdermilk, D. L., Perry, S. E., & Cashion, M. C. (2010). *Maternity nursing* (8th ed.). St. Louis: Mosby.

Meiner, S. (2011). *Gerontologic nursing* (4th ed). St. Louis: Mosby.

McCance, K. L., & Huether, S. E. (2010). *Pathophysiology: The biologic basis for disease in adults and children* (6th ed.). St. Louis: Mosby.

McKinney, E. S., James, S. R., Murray, S. S., & Ashwill, J. (2009). *Maternal-child nursing* (3rd ed.). St. Louis: Saunders.

Monahan, F., Sands, J., Neighbors, M., Marek, J., & Green, C. (2007). *Phipps' medical-surgical nursing: Health and illness perspectives* (8th ed.). St. Louis: Mosby.

Morrison-Valfre, M. (2009). *Foundations of mental health care* (4th ed.). St. Louis: Mosby.

Mosby's dictionary of medicine nursing & health professions. (2009). St. Louis: Mosby.

National Council of State Boards of Nursing. (2011). *2011 NCLEX-PN® detailed test plan.* Chicago: National Council of State Boards of Nursing.

Newell, R., & Gournay, K. (2009). *Mental health nursing: An evidence-based approach* (2nd ed.). St. Louis: Churchill Livingstone.

Nix, S. (2009). *Williams' basic nutrition & diet therapy* (13th ed.). St. Louis: Mosby.

Ogden, S. J., & Fluharty, L. K. (2012). *Calculation of drug dosages: A work text* (9th ed.). St. Louis: Mosby.

Pagana, K. D., & Pagana, T. J. (2009). *Mosby's manual of diagnostic and laboratory tests* (4th ed.). St. Louis: Mosby.

Peckenpaugh, N. J. (2010). *Nutrition essentials and diet therapy* (11th ed.). St. Louis: Saunders.

Perry, S. E., Hockenberry, M. J., Lowdermilk, D. L., & Wilson, D. (2010). *Maternal child nursing care* (4th ed.). St. Louis: Mosby.

Perry, A. G., & Potter, P. A. (2010). *Clinical nursing skills and techniques* (7th ed.). St. Louis: Mosby.

Potter, P. A., & Perry, A. G. (2009). *Fundamentals of nursing* (7th ed.). St. Louis: Mosby.

Schlenker, E., & Roth, S. R. (2011). *Williams' essentials of nutrition and diet therapy* (10th ed.). St. Louis: Mosby.

Skidmore-Roth, L. (2009). *Mosby's 2009 nursing drug reference* (22nd ed.). St. Louis: Mosby.

Skidmore-Roth, L. (2010). *Mosby's 2010 nursing drug reference* (23rd ed.). St. Louis: Mosby.

Skidmore-Roth, L. (2012). *Mosby's 2012 nursing drug reference* (25th ed.). St. Louis: Mosby.

Stuart, G. W. (2009). *Principles and practice of psychiatric nursing* (9th ed.). St. Louis: Mosby.

Swearingen, P. L. (2012). *All-in-one care planning resource* (3rd ed.). St. Louis: Mosby.

Touhy, T. A., & Jett, K. (2010). *Ebersole and Hess' gerontological nursing & healthy aging* (3rd ed.). St. Louis: Mosby.

Varcarolis, E. M., & Halter, M. J. (2009). *Essentials of psychiatric mental health nursing: A communication approach to evidence-based care.* St. Louis: Mosby.

Varcarolis, E. M., & Halter, M. J. (2010). *Foundations of psychiatric mental health nursing.* St. Louis: Mosby.

Workman, M. L., LaCharity, L., & Kruchko, S. L. (2011). *Understanding pharmacology: Essentials for medication safety.* St. Louis: Saunders.

Index

A

Abacavir/Lamivudine (Epzicom), 882
Abacavir (Ziagen), 882, 883
Abandonment, fear of, in dying client, 939
ABCs, questions involving, 25, 26*b*
Abdomen
  examination of, 341
  in newborn exam, 283
  pain in, in peritoneal dialysis, 737
Abdominal aneurysm resection, positioning
  for, 192
Abdominal aortic aneurysm, 695
  resection of, 695
Abdominal binder, 179, 180*f*
Abdominal thrusts
  in adult, 169, 169*f*, 170*b*
    definition of, 165
  in child, 170
Abdominal wall defects, in child, 415
Abducens nerve, assessment of, 343*t*
Abduction
  child, 360, 945
  newborn, 287, 287*b*
ABGs. *See* Arterial blood gases (ABGs).
ABO
  compatibility and, 136
  definition of, 129
Abortion, 236, 236*b*
Abraxane (paclitaxel), 546
Abruptio placentae, 261, 261*f*
Absence seizures, 811
Absorption, definition of, 116
Abuse
  alcohol, 926, 928*b*
  of child, 361, 361*b*, 944. *See also* Child abuse.
  data collection questions for, 944*b*
  definition of, 310, 891
  as maternal risk factor, 224
  of older adult, 354, 945, 946*b*
  substance, 926, 926*b*, 928*b*
Abuser
  characteristics of, 944
  in cycle of violence, 943, 943*f*
Abusive behavior, 942
Accelerations, of fetal heart rate, 256
Acceptance, in pregnancy, 229
Accommodation, 335
  in cognitive development, 312
  in conflict resolution, 63
  definition of, 762
  in glaucoma, 768
Accountability
  definition of, 60
  of nurse, 62
Acculturation, definition of, 33
Acetabular dysplasia, 439

Acetaminophen (Tylenol), 830
  poisoning by, 419
  therapeutic levels of, 111*t*
Acetylcholine, in muscle contraction and
  relaxation, 839
Acetylsalicylic acid (aspirin), 830
  side effects of, 830
Acetylsalicylic acid (aspirin) poisoning, 420
Acid, 92
Acid base balance, 91–100
  kidneys in, 93
  lungs in, 92
  potassium in, 93, 93*f*
Acidity, homeostasis of, 722
Acidosis. *See also* Metabolic acidosis;
  Respiratory acidosis.
Acitretin (Soriatane), for psoriasis, 504
Acne vulgaris, 487
Acoustic nerve, assessment of, 343*t*
Acoustic neuroma, 778
Acquaintance rape, 946
Acquired immunity, 869
  definition of, 867
Acquired immunodeficiency syndrome
  (AIDS)
  in child, 466, 467*b*, 467*f*, 468*b*, 468*t*
  definition of, 867
  medications for, 882
  in newborn, 293
  in pregnancy, 240, 240*b*
  stages of, 240*b*
  testing for, 110
Acrocyanosis, in newborn, 283, 283*f*
Actinic keratoses, 486
  medications for, 503, 503*b*
Activated partial thromboplastin time (aPTT),
  103
Activity intolerance, in depression,
  interventions for, 940
Acute phase, of burn management, 494
Acute renal failure (ARF), 726
  continuous renal replacement therapy for,
    738
  definition of, 719, 726
  description and causes of, 726
  hemodialysis for, 731. *See also* Hemodialysis
  interventions for, 727
  peritoneal dialysis for, 735. *See also*
    Peritoneal dialysis (PD)
  phases of, 726, 726*b*
Acute respiratory distress syndrome, 635
Acute respiratory failure, 635
Adalat (nifedipine), for preterm labor, 301,
  301*t*
Adalimumab (Humira), 862
Adapalene (Differin), for acne, 506

Addiction(s), 924–935
  alcohol abuse as, 926
  codependency issues and, 931
  definition of, 891
  drug dependency as, 928
  dual diagnoses for, 931
  eating disorders as, 924. *See also* Eating
    disorders.
  in health care professionals, 931
  in newborn, 293
  substance abuse disorders as, 926, 926*b*
Addisonian crisis, 557, 557*b*
  definition of, 550
Addison's disease, 556, 556*t*
  definition of, 550
  mineralocorticoids for, 578, 578*b*
Adenectomy, pituitary, 555
Adenocarcinoma, definition of, 511
Adenoidectomy, 372
Adenoiditis, 372
Adenosine triphosphate, in muscle
  contraction and relaxation, 839
Administrative staff, in health care team, 65
Adolescent
  communication approaches to, 322
  development of, 327
  grief and, 937
  pregnancy in, 224
  psychosocial development of, 313*t*
Adrenal cortex, 552
Adrenal gland(s), 552
  anatomy and physiology of, 722
  disorders of, 556, 556*t*
Adrenal medulla, 552
Adrenalectomy, 558, 558*b*
  definition of, 550
Adrenergic agonists, nonselective, for
  glaucoma, 786
Adrenergic blockers, for hypertension, 709,
  709*b*
Adrenocortical insufficiency, glucocorticoids
  for, 578, 578*b*
Adult
  health and physical assessment of,
    332–350
    body systems data collection process in, 333
    documentation of, 346
    environment/setting for, 332, 333*b*
    health history in, 332
    mental status examination in, 332, 333*b*
    physical exam in, 332
    integumentary disorders in, 482. *See also*
      Integumentary disorders, in adult
      client.
  psychosocial development of, 313*t*
Advance directive, 55

Page numbers followed by *f*, *t*, and *b* indicate figures, tables, and boxes, respectively.

991